General Urology

10th edition

General Urology

DONALD R. SMITH, MD

Professor of Urology, Emeritus
University of California School of Medicine
San Francisco, California

Visiting Professor of Urology
University of Ain Shams
University of Cairo
Cairo, Egypt

Recent Consultant in Urology, Egypt,
under the auspices of People-to-People Health
Foundation, Inc. (PROJECT HOPE)
Washington, D.C.

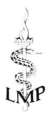

LANGE Medical Publications   **Los Altos, California 94022**

General Urology, 10th ed. $19.50

Copyright © 1957, 1959, 1961, 1963, 1966, 1969, 1972, 1975, 1978, 1981

A Concise Medical Library for Practitioner and Student

Current Medical Diagnosis & Treatment 1981 (annual revision). Edited by M.A. Krupp   1981
and M.J. Chatton. 1100 pp.

Current Pediatric Diagnosis & Treatment, 6th ed. Edited by C.H. Kempe, H.K. Silver,   1980
and D. O'Brien. 1122 pp, *illus.*

Current Surgical Diagnosis & Treatment, 5th ed. Edited by J.E. Dunphy and L.W. Way.   1981
1138 pp, *illus.*

Current Obstetric & Gynecologic Diagnosis & Treatment, 3rd ed. Edited by R.C. Benson.   1980
1001 pp, *illus.*

Harper's Review of Biochemistry, (formerly **Review of Physiological Chemistry**),   1981
18th ed. D.W. Martin, Jr., P.A. Mayes, and V.W. Rodwell. 614 pp, *illus.*

Review of Medical Physiology, 10th ed. W.F. Ganong. 628 pp, *illus.*   1981

Review of Medical Microbiology, 14th ed. E. Jawetz, J.L. Melnick, and E.A. Adelberg.   1980
593 pp, *illus.*

Review of Medical Pharmacology, 7th ed. F.H. Meyers, E. Jawetz, and A. Goldfien.   1980
747 pp, *illus.*

Basic & Clinical Immunology, 3rd ed. Edited by H.H. Fudenberg, D.P. Stites,   1980
J.L. Caldwell, and J.V. Wells. 782 pp, *illus.*

Basic Histology, 3rd ed. L.C. Junqueira and J. Carneiro. 504 pp, *illus.*   1980

Clinical Cardiology, 2nd ed. M. Sokolow and M.B. McIlroy. 718 pp, *illus.*   1979

General Ophthalmology, 9th ed. D. Vaughan and T. Asbury. 410 pp, *illus.*   1980

Correlative Neuroanatomy & Functional Neurology, 17th ed. J.G. Chusid. 464 pp, *illus.*   1979

Principles of Clinical Electrocardiography, 10th ed. M.J. Goldman. 415 pp, *illus.*   1979

Handbook of Obstetrics & Gynecology, 7th ed. R.C. Benson. 808 pp, *illus.*   1980

Physician's Handbook, 19th ed. M.A. Krupp, N.J. Sweet, E. Jawetz, E.G. Biglieri,   1979
R.L. Roe, and C.A. Camargo. 758 pp, *illus.*

Handbook of Pediatrics, 13th ed. H.K. Silver, C.H. Kempe, and H.B. Bruyn. 735 pp, *illus.*   1980

Handbook of Poisoning: Prevention, Diagnosis, & Treatment, 10th ed. R.H. Dreisbach.   1980
578 pp.

Lithographed in USA

Table of Contents

Preface

This edition of *General Urology* has been updated to keep the reader abreast of new developments in the field. We are pleased to note that past editions have been used not only by medical students but also by urologic residents, urologists, and physicians in other areas of practice.

Because many urologic disorders produce few or no symptoms, we have continued to stress the importance of careful history taking and physical examination in diagnosis. Perhaps most important is the personal study of urinary sediment and the PSP renal function test, from which the amount of residual urine can also be estimated. Voiding cystourethrograms and excretory urograms are being used to demonstrate vesicoureteral reflux (the most common cause of renal infection) and other lesions, including posterior urethral valves. The more sophisticated technics of angiography, venography, sonography, radioisotopic studies, and computed tomography are proving to be essential for diagnosis in many cases. Rapidly expanding knowledge of tumor immunology is contributing to diagnosis, treatment, and estimation of prognosis of genitourinary neoplasms.

As in past editions, I have called upon knowledgeable physicians to prepare definitive chapters in their fields of expertise. Dr. Emil A. Tanagho, a pioneer in the area of urodynamic study, has written a chapter on this essential diagnostic procedure. Dr. Jack W. McAninch, who has had wide experience in both civilian and military trauma practice, has rewritten the chapter on genitourinary tract injuries. Dr. Ira D. Sharlip has revised the section on sexual dysfunction.

It is a pleasure to note that this book is currently available in Spanish, Japanese, Polish, and Portuguese editions and that German and Italian translations are in preparation.

Donald R. Smith, MD

Cairo, Egypt
August, 1981

Authors

Mohamed M. Al-Ghorab, MB, ChB, DS, MCh
Professor and Chairman of Department of Urology, Faculty of Medicine, University of Alexandria (Alexandria, Egypt).

William J.C. Amend, Jr., MD
Associate Clinical Professor of Medicine, University of California School of Medicine (San Francisco).

Charles A. Barnett, MD
Assistant Clinical Professor of Radiology in Nuclear Medicine, University of California School of Medicine (Davis, California).

Granville C. Coggs, MD
Professor of Radiology, University of Texas Health Science Center; Chief of Radiology Service, Audie L. Murphy Memorial Veterans Administration Hospital (San Antonio, Texas).

Felix A. Conte, MD
Associate Professor of Pediatrics, University of California School of Medicine (San Francisco).

Nicholas J. Feduska, MD
Associate Professor of Surgery, Transplant Service, University of California School of Medicine (San Francisco).

Peter H. Forsham, MD
Professor of Medicine and Pediatrics and Director of Metabolic Research Unit, University of California School of Medicine (San Francisco).

H. Hugh Fudenberg, MD
Professor and Chairman of Basic and Clinical Immunology and Microbiology, Medical University of South Carolina (Charleston, South Carolina).

Melvin M. Grumbach, MD
Professor and Chairman of Department of Pediatrics, University of California School of Medicine (San Francisco); Director of Pediatric Services, University of California Hospitals (San Francisco).

Ernest Jawetz, MD, PhD
Professor of Microbiology and Medicine, University of California School of Medicine (San Francisco).

Felix O. Kolb, MD
Clinical Professor of Medicine and Research Physician, Metabolic Research Unit, University of California School of Medicine (San Francisco).

Melvyn T. Korobkin, MD
Professor of Radiology, Duke University School of Medicine, Durham, North Carolina.

Marcus A. Krupp, MD
Clinical Professor of Medicine Emeritus, Stanford University School of Medicine (Stanford); Director of Research, Palo Alto Medical Research Foundation (Palo Alto, California).

Jack W. McAninch, MD
Associate Professor and Vice Chairman of Department of Urology, University of California School of Medicine (San Francisco); Chief of Urology, San Francisco General Hospital (San Francisco).

Malcolm R. Powell, MD
Associate Clinical Professor of Medicine, University of California School of Medicine (San Francisco).

Rees B. Rees, Jr., MD, MS
Clinical Professor of Dermatology, University of California School of Medicine (San Francisco).

Oscar Salvatierra, Jr., MD
Professor of Surgery and Urology and Chairman of Transplant Service, University of California School of Medicine (San Francisco).

Ira D. Sharlip, MD, FACS
Assistant Clinical Professor of Urology, University of California School of Medicine (San Francisco).

Donald R. Smith, MD
Professor of Urology Emeritus, University of California School of Medicine (San Francisco).

Samuel D. Spivack, MD
Associate Clinical Professor of Medicine and Radiology, University of California School of Medicine (San Francisco).

Emil A. Tanagho, MD
Professor and Chairman of Department of Urology, University of California School of Medicine (San Francisco).

Flavio G. Vincenti, MD
Assistant Clinical Professor of Medicine, University of California School of Medicine (San Francisco).

J. Vivian Wells, MD, FRACP, FRCPA
Senior Staff Specialist in Clinical Immunology, Kolling Institute of Medical Research, Royal North Shore Hospital of Sydney (St. Leonards, New South Wales, Australia).

Anatomy of the Genitourinary Tract | 1

Emil A. Tanagho, MD

Urology deals with diseases and disorders of the genitourinary tract in the male and of the urinary tract in the female. Surgical diseases of the adrenal gland are also included. These systems are illustrated in Figs 1–1 and 1–2.

ADRENALS

Gross Appearance

A. Anatomy: Each kidney is capped by an adrenal gland, and both organs are enclosed within Gerota's (perirenal) fascia. Each adrenal weighs about 5 g. The right adrenal is triangular in shape; the left is more rounded and crescentic. Each gland is composed of a cortex, chiefly influenced by the pituitary gland, and a medulla derived from chromaffin tissue.

B. Relations: Fig 1–2 shows the relation of the adrenals to other organs. The right adrenal lies between the liver and the vena cava. The left gland lies close to the aorta and is covered on its lower surface by the pancreas; superiorly and laterally, it is related to the spleen.

Histology

The adrenal cortex is composed of 3 distinct layers: the outer zona glomerulosa, the middle zona fasciculata, and the inner zona reticularis. The medulla lies centrally and is made up of polyhedral cells containing eosinophilic granular cytoplasm. These chromaffin cells are accompanied by ganglion and small round cells.

Blood Supply

A. Arterial: Each adrenal receives 3 arteries: one from the inferior phrenic artery, one from the aorta, and one from the renal artery.

B. Venous: The right adrenal blood is drained by a very short vein which empties into the vena cava; the left adrenal vein terminates in the left renal vein.

Lymphatics

The lymphatic vessels accompany the suprarenal vein and drain into the lumbar lymph nodes.

KIDNEYS

Gross Appearance

A. Anatomy: The kidneys lie along the borders of the psoas muscles and are therefore obliquely placed. The position of the liver causes the right kidney to be lower than the left (Figs 1–2 and 1–3). The adult kidney weighs about 150 g.

The kidneys are supported by the perirenal fat (which is enclosed in the perirenal fascia), the renal vascular pedicle, abdominal muscle tone, and the general bulk of the abdominal viscera. Variations in these factors permit variations in the degree of renal mobility. The average descent on inspiration or on assuming the upright position is 4–5 cm. Lack of mobility suggests abnormal fixation (eg, perinephritis), but extreme mobility is not necessarily pathologic.

On longitudinal section (Fig 1–4), the kidney is seen to be made up of an outer cortex, a central medulla, and the internal calices and pelvis. The cortex is homogeneous in appearance. Portions of it project toward the pelvis between the papillae and fornices and are called the columns of Bertin. The medulla consists of numerous pyramids formed by the converging collecting renal tubules, which drain into the minor calices.

B. Relations: Fig 1–2 and 1–3 show the relations of the kidneys to adjacent organs and structures. Their intimacy with intraperitoneal organs explains, in part, some of the gastrointestinal symptoms which accompany genitourinary disease.

Histology

A. Nephron: The functioning unit of the kidney is the nephron, which is composed of a tubule which has both secretory and excretory functions (Fig 1–4). The secretory portion is contained largely within the cortex and consists of a renal corpuscle and the secretory part of the renal tubule. The excretory portion of this duct lies in the medulla. The renal corpuscle is composed of the vascular glomerulus, which projects into Bowman's capsule, which, in turn, is continuous with the epithelium of the proximal convoluted tubule. The secretory portion of the renal tubule is made up of the proximal

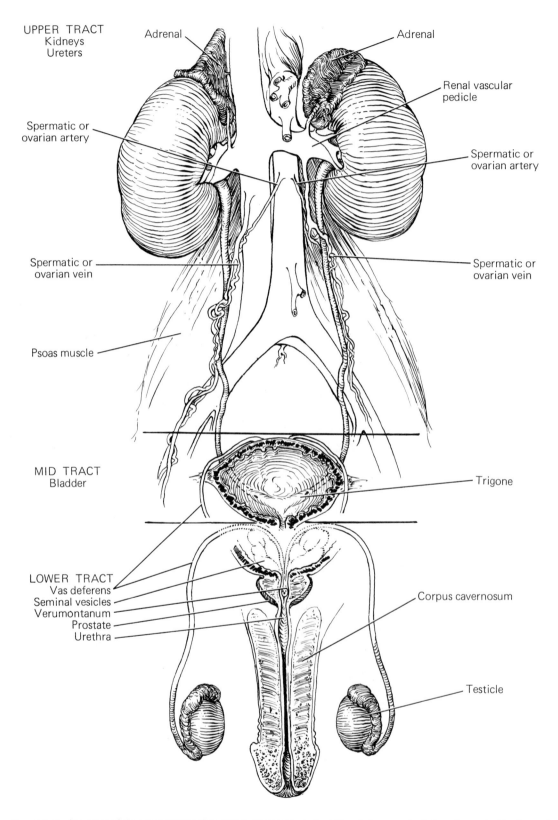

UPPER TRACT
Kidneys
Ureters

Adrenal

Adrenal

Renal vascular
pedicle

Spermatic or
ovarian artery

Spermatic or
ovarian artery

Spermatic or
ovarian vein

Spermatic or
ovarian vein

Psoas muscle

MID TRACT
Bladder

Trigone

LOWER TRACT
Vas deferens
Seminal vesicles
Verumontanum
Prostate
Urethra

Corpus cavernosum

Testicle

Figure 1–1. Anatomy of the male genitourinary tract. The upper and mid tracts have urologic function only. The lower tract has both genital and urinary functions.

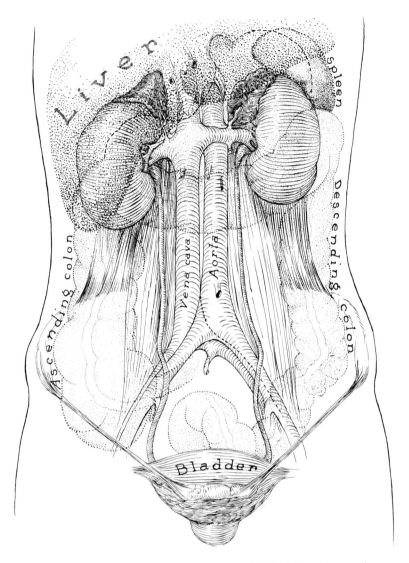

Figure 1–2. Relations of kidney, ureters, and bladder (anterior aspect).

convoluted tubule, the loop of Henle, and the distal convoluted tubule.

The excretory portion of the nephron is the collecting tubule, which is continuous with the distal end of the ascending limb of the convoluted tubule. It empties its contents through the tip (papilla) of a pyramid into a minor calix.

B. Supporting Tissue: The renal stroma is composed of loose connective tissue and contains blood vessels, capillaries, nerves, and lymphatics.

Blood Supply (Figs 1–2 and 1–4)

A. Arterial: Usually there is one renal artery, a branch of the aorta, which enters the hilum of the kidney between the pelvis, which normally lies posteriorly, and the renal vein. It may branch before it reaches the kidney, and 2 or more separate arteries

may be noted. In duplication of the pelvis and ureter, it is usual for each renal segment to have its own arterial supply.

This artery further divides into the interlobular arteries, which ascend in the columns of Bertin (between the pyramids) and then arch along the base of the pyramids (arcuate arteries). From these vessels, smaller (afferent) branches pass to the glomeruli. From the glomerular tuft, efferent arterioles pass to the tubules in the stroma.

B. Venous: The renal veins are paired with the arteries, but any of them will drain the entire kidney if the others are tied off.

Although the renal artery and vein are usually the sole blood vessels of the kidney, accessory renal vessels are common and may be of clinical importance if they are so placed as to compress the ureter, in which case hydronephrosis may result.

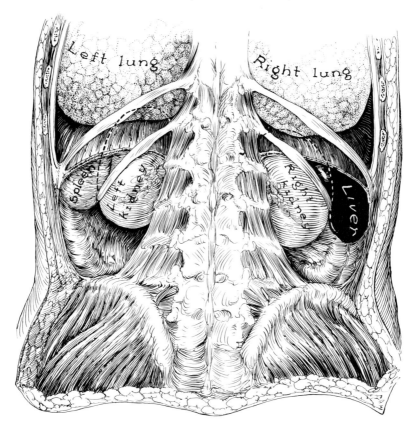

Figure 1–3. Relations of kidneys (posterior aspect).

Nerve Supply

The renal nerves derived from the renal plexus accompany the renal vessels throughout the renal parenchyma.

Lymphatics

The lymphatics of the kidney drain into the lumbar lymph nodes (Figs 18–1 and 18–2).

CALICES, RENAL PELVIS, & URETER

Gross Appearance

A. Anatomy:

1. Calices–The tips of the minor calices (8–12 in number) are indented by the projecting pyramids (Fig 1–4). These calices unite to form 2 or 3 major calices, which join the renal pelvis.

2. Renal pelvis–The pelvis may be entirely intrarenal or partly intrarenal and partly extrarenal. Inferomedially, it tapers to form the ureter.

3. Ureter–The adult ureter is about 30 cm long, varying in direct relation to the height of the individual. It follows a rather smooth S curve. Areas of relative narrowing are found (1) at the ureteropelvic junction, (2) where the ureter crosses over the iliac vessels, and (3) where it courses through the bladder wall.

B. Relations:

1. Calices–The calices are intrarenal and are intimately related to the renal parenchyma.

2. Renal pelvis–If the pelvis is partly extrarenal, it lies along the lateral border of the psoas muscle and on the quadratus lumborum muscle; the renal vascular pedicle is placed just anterior to it. The left renal pelvis lies at the level of the first or second lumbar vertebra; the right pelvis is a little lower.

3. Ureter–As followed from above downward, the ureters lie on the psoas muscles, pass medially to the sacroiliac joints, and then swing laterally near the ischial spines before passing medially to penetrate the base of the bladder (Fig 1–2). In the female, the uterine arteries are closely related to the juxtavesical portion of the ureters. The ureters are covered by the posterior peritoneum; their lowermost portions are closely attached to it, while the juxtavesical portions are embedded in vascular retroperitoneal fat.

The vasa, as they leave the internal inguinal rings, sweep over the lateral pelvic walls anteriorly to the ureters. They lie medial to the latter before penetrating the base of the prostate to become the ejaculatory ducts.

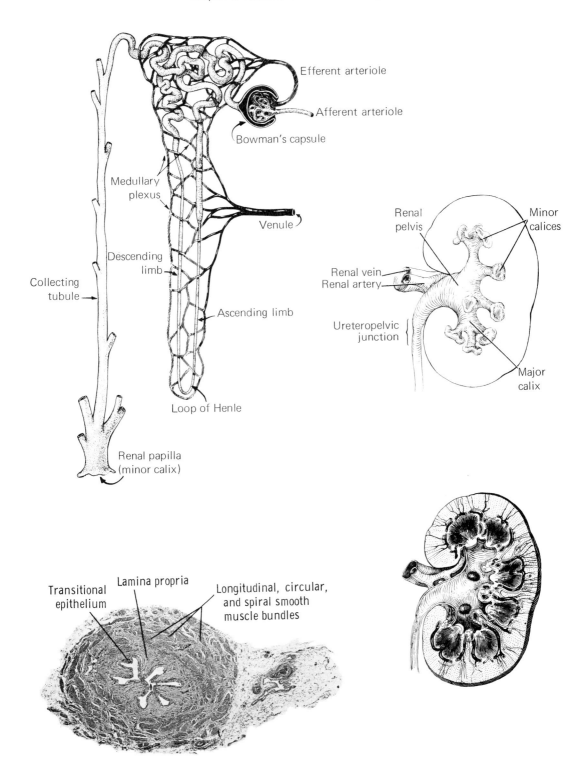

Figure 1–4. Anatomy and histology of the kidney and ureter. *Above left:* Diagram of the nephron and its blood supply. (Courtesy of Merck, Sharp, & Dohme: Seminar: 9[3], 1947.) *Above right:* Renal calices, pelvis, and ureter (posterior aspect). *Below left:* Histology of the ureter. The smooth muscle bundles are arranged in both a spiral and longitudinal manner. *Below right:* Longitudinal section of kidney showing calices, pelvis, ureter, and renal blood supply (posterior aspect).

Histology (Fig 1–4)

The walls of the calices, pelvis, and ureters are composed of transitional cell epithelium under which lies loose connective and elastic tissue (lamina propria). External to these are a mixture of spiral and longitudinal smooth muscle fibers. They are not arranged in definite layers. The outermost adventitial coat is composed of fibrous connective tissue.

Blood Supply

A. Arterial: The renal calices, pelvis, and upper ureters derive their blood supply from the renal arteries; the mid ureter is fed by the internal spermatic (or ovarian) arteries. The lowermost portion of the ureter is served by branches from the common iliac, hypogastric, and vesical arteries.

B. Venous: The veins of the renal calices, pelvis, and ureters are paired with the arteries.

Lymphatics

The lymphatics of the upper portions of the ureters as well as those from the pelvis and calices enter the lumbar lymph nodes. The lymphatics of the mid ureter pass to the hypogastric and common iliac lymph nodes; the lower ureteral lymphatics empty into the vesical and hypogastric lymph nodes (Figs 18–1 and 18–2).

BLADDER

Gross Appearance

The bladder is a hollow muscular organ which serves as a reservoir for urine. In women, its posterior wall and dome are invaginated by the uterus. The adult bladder has a capacity of 350–450 mL.

A. Anatomy: When empty, the adult bladder lies behind the pubic symphysis and is largely a pelvic organ. In infants and children, it is situated higher. When it is full, it rises well above the symphysis and can readily be palpated or percussed. When overdistended, as in acute or chronic urinary retention, it may cause the lower abdomen to bulge visibly.

Extending from the dome of the bladder to the umbilicus is a fibrous cord, the medial umbilical ligament, which represents the obliterated urachus. The ureters enter the bladder posteroinferiorly in an oblique manner and at these points are placed about 2.5 cm apart (Fig 1–5). The orifices are situated at the extremities of the crescent-shaped interureteric ridge which forms the proximal border of the trigone. The trigone occupies the area between the ridge and the bladder neck.

The internal sphincter, or bladder neck, is not a true circular sphincter but a thickening formed by interlaced and converging muscle fibers of the detrusor as they pass distally to become the smooth musculature of the urethra.

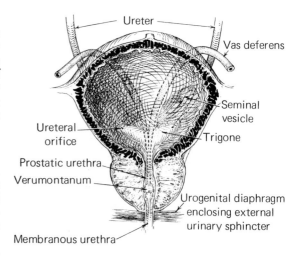

Figure 1–5. Anatomy and relations of the ureters, bladder, prostate, seminal vesicles, and vasa deferentia (anterior view).

B. Relations: In the male, the bladder is related posteriorly to the seminal vesicles, vasa deferentia, ureters, and rectum (Figs 1–7 and 1–8). In the female, the uterus and vagina are interposed between the bladder and rectum (Fig 1–9). The dome and posterior surfaces are covered by peritoneum; hence, in this area the bladder is closely related to the small intestine and sigmoid colon. In both male and female, the bladder is related to the posterior surface of the pubic symphysis, and, when distended, it is in contact with the lower abdominal wall.

Histology (Fig 1–6)

The mucosa of the bladder is composed of transitional epithelium. Beneath it is a well-developed submucosal layer formed largely of connective and elastic tissues. External to the submucosa is the detrusor muscle, made up of a mixture of smooth muscle fibers which are arranged at random in a longitudinal, circular, and spiral manner.

Blood Supply

A. Arterial: The arterial supply to the bladder comes from the superior, middle, and inferior vesical arteries, which arise from the anterior trunk of the hypogastric artery. Smaller branches from the obturator and inferior gluteal arteries also reach this organ. In the female, the uterine and vaginal arteries also send branches to the bladder.

B. Venous: Surrounding the bladder is a rich plexus of veins that ultimately empties into the hypogastric veins.

Lymphatics

The lymphatics of the bladder drain into the vesical, external iliac, hypogastric, and common iliac lymph nodes (Figs 18–1 and 18–2).

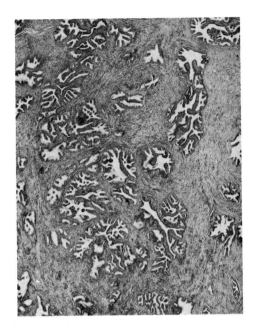 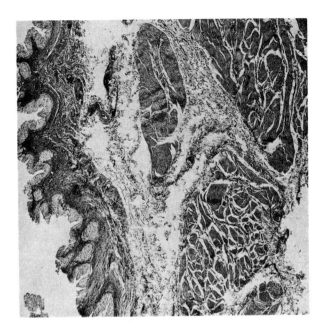

Figure 1–6. *Left:* Histology of the prostate. Epithelial glands embedded in a mixture of connective and elastic tissue and smooth muscle. *Right:* Histology of the bladder. The mucosa is transitional cell in type and lies upon a well-developed submucosal layer of connective tissue. The detrusor muscle is composed of interlacing longitudinal, circular, and spiral smooth muscle bundles.

PROSTATE GLAND

Gross Appearance

A. Anatomy: The prostate is a fibromuscular and glandular organ lying just inferior to the bladder (Figs 1–5 and 1–7). The normal prostate weighs about 20 g and contains the posterior urethra, which is about 2.5 cm in length. It is supported anteriorly by the puboprostatic ligaments and inferiorly by the urogenital diaphragm (Fig 1–5). The prostate is perforated posteriorly by the ejaculatory ducts, which pass obliquely to empty through the verumontanum on the floor of the prostatic urethra just proximal to the striated external urinary sphincter.

According to the classification of Lowsley, the prostate consists of 5 lobes: anterior, posterior, median, right lateral, and left lateral. The segment of urethra that traverses the prostate gland is the prostatic urethra. It is lined by an inner longitudinal layer of muscle (continuous with a similar layer of the vesical wall). Incorporated within the prostate gland is an abundant amount of smooth musculature derived primarily from the external longitudinal bladder musculature. This musculature represents the true smooth involuntary sphincter of the posterior urethra in the male.

Prostatic adenoma develops from the periurethral glands at the site of the median or lateral lobes. The posterior lobe, however, is prone to cancerous degeneration.

B. Relations: The prostate gland lies behind the pubic symphysis. Closely applied to the posterosuperior surface are the vasa deferentia and seminal vesicles (Fig 1–7). Posteriorly, it is separated from the rectum by the 2 layers of Denonvilliers' fascia, serosal rudiments of the pouch of Douglas, which once extended to the urogenital diaphragm (Fig 1–8).

Histology (Fig 1–6)

The prostate consists of a thin fibrous capsule under which are circularly oriented smooth muscle fibers and collagenous tissue that surrounds the urethra (involuntary sphincter). Deep to this layer lies the prostatic stroma, composed of connective and elastic tissues and smooth muscle fibers in which are embedded the epithelial glands. These glands drain into the major excretory ducts (about 25 in number) which open chiefly on the floor of the urethra between the verumontanum and the vesical neck. Just beneath the transitional epithelium of the prostatic urethra lie the periurethral glands.

Blood Supply

A. Arterial: The arterial supply to the prostate is derived from the inferior vesical, internal pudendal, and middle hemorrhoidal arteries.

B. Venous: The veins from the prostate drain into the periprostatic plexus, which has connections with the deep dorsal vein of the penis and the hypogastric veins.

Nerve Supply

The prostate gland receives a rich nerve supply

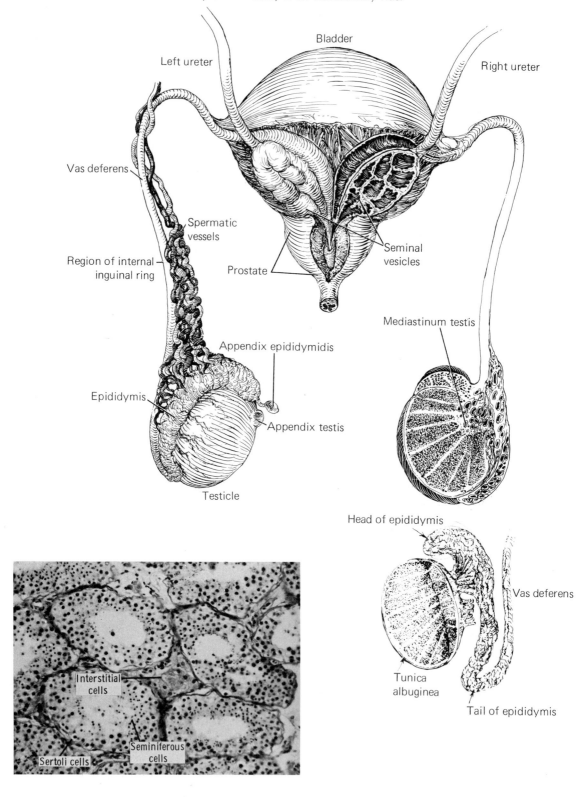

Figure 1–7. *Above:* Gross anatomy and relations of ureters, bladder, prostate, seminal vesicles, vasa deferentia, testes, and epididymides. *Below left:* Histology of the testis. Seminiferous tubules lined by supporting basement membrane for the Sertoli and spermatogenic cells. The latter are in various stages of development. *Below right:* Cross section of testis showing fibrous septa dividing organ into lobules.

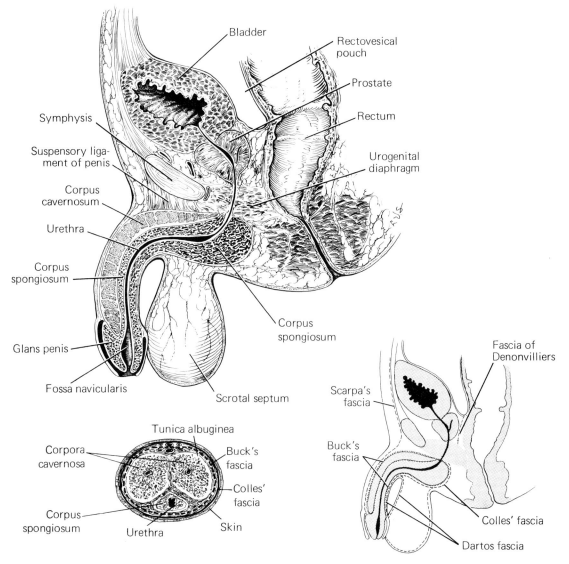

Figure 1–8. *Above:* Relations of the bladder, prostate, seminal vesicles, penis, urethra, and scrotal contents. *Below left:* Transverse section through the penis. The paired upper structures are the corpora cavernosa. The single lower body surrounding the urethra is the corpus spongiosum. *Below right:* Fascial planes of the lower genitourinary tract. (After Wesson.)

from the sympathetic and parasympathetic nerve plexuses.

Lymphatics

The lymphatics from the prostate drain into the hypogastric, sacral, vesical, and external iliac lymph nodes (Figs 18–1 and 18–2).

SEMINAL VESICLES

Gross Appearance

The seminal vesicles lie just cephalad to the prostate under the base of the bladder (Figs 1–5 and 1–7). They are about 6 cm long and quite soft. Each vesicle joins its corresponding vas deferens to form the ejaculatory duct. The ureters lie medial to each, and the rectum is contiguous with their posterior surfaces.

Histology

The mucous membrane is pseudostratified. The submucosa consists of dense connective tissue covered by a thin layer of muscle which in turn is encapsulated by connective tissue.

Blood Supply

The blood supply is similar to that of the prostate gland.

Nerve Supply

The nerve supply is mainly from the sympathetic nerve plexus.

Lymphatics

The lymphatics of the seminal vesicles are those that serve the prostate (Figs 18–1 and 18–2).

SPERMATIC CORD

Gross Appearance

The 2 spermatic cords extend from the internal inguinal rings through the inguinal canals to the testicles (Fig 1–7). Each cord contains the vas deferens, the internal and external spermatic arteries, the artery of the vas, the venous pampiniform plexus (which forms the spermatic vein superiorly), lymph vessels, and nerves. All of the above are enclosed in investing layers of thin fascia. A few fibers of the cremaster muscle insert on the cords in the inguinal canal.

Histology

The fascia covering the cord is formed of loose connective tissue which supports arteries, veins, and lymphatics. The vas deferens is a small, thick-walled tube consisting of an internal mucosa and submucosa surrounded by 3 well-defined layers of smooth muscle encased in a covering of fibrous tissue. Above the testes, this tube is straight. Its proximal 4 cm tend to be convoluted.

Blood Supply

A. Arterial: The external spermatic artery, a branch of the inferior epigastric, supplies the fascial coverings of the cord. The internal spermatic artery passes through the cord on its way to the testis. The deferential artery is close to the vas.

B. Venous: The veins from the testis and the coverings of the spermatic cord form the pampiniform plexus, which, at the internal inguinal ring, unites to form the spermatic vein.

Lymphatics

The lymphatics from the spermatic cord empty into the external iliac lymph nodes (Figs 18–1 and 18–2).

EPIDIDYMIS

Gross Appearance

A. Anatomy: The upper portion of the epididymis (globus major) is connected to the testis by numerous efferent ducts from the testis (Fig 1–7). The epididymis consists of a markedly coiled duct which, at its lower pole (globus minor), is continuous with the vas deferens. An appendix of the epididymis is often seen on its upper pole; this is a cystic body that in some cases is pedunculated but in others is sessile.

B. Relations: The epididymis lies posterolateral to the testis and is nearest to the testis at its upper pole. Its lower pole is connected to the testis by fibrous tissue. The vas lies posteromedial to the epididymis.

Histology

The epididymis is covered by serosa. The ductus epididymidis is lined by pseudostratified columnar epithelium throughout its length.

Blood Supply

A. Arterial: The arterial supply to the epididymis comes from the internal spermatic artery and the artery of the vas (deferential artery).

B. Venous: The venous blood drains into the pampiniform plexus, which becomes the spermatic vein.

Lymphatics

The lymphatics drain into the external iliac and hypogastric lymph nodes (Figs 18–1 and 18–2).

TESTIS

Gross Appearance

A. Anatomy: The average testicle measures about $4 \times 3 \times 2.5$ cm (Fig 1–7). It has a dense fascial covering called the tunica albuginea testis, which, posteriorly, is invaginated somewhat into the body of the testis to form the mediastinum testis. This fibrous mediastinum sends fibrous septa into the testis, thus separating it into about 250 lobules.

The testis is covered anteriorly and laterally by the visceral layer of the serous tunica vaginalis, which is continuous with the parietal layer that separates the testis from the scrotal wall.

At the upper pole of the testis is the appendix testis, a small pedunculated or sessile body which is similar in appearance to the appendix of the epididymis.

B. Relations: The testis is closely attached posterolaterally to the epididymis, particularly at its upper and lower poles.

Histology (Fig 1–7)

Each lobule contains 1–4 markedly convoluted seminiferous tubules, each of which is about 60 cm long. These ducts converge at the mediastinum testis, where they connect with the efferent ducts which drain into the epididymis.

The seminiferous tubule has a basement membrane containing connective and elastic tissue. This supports the seminiferous cells, which are of 2 types: (1) Sertoli (supporting) cells and (2) spermatogenic cells. The stroma between the seminiferous tubules contains connective tissue in which the interstitial Leydig cells are located.

Blood Supply

The blood supply to the testes is closely associated with that to the kidneys because of the common embryologic origin of the 2 organs.

A. Arterial: The arteries to the testes (internal spermatics) arise from the aorta just below the renal arteries and course through the spermatic cords to the testes, where they anastomose with the arteries of the vasa which branch off from the hypogastric artery.

B. Venous: The blood from the testis returns in the pampiniform plexus of the spermatic cord. At the internal inguinal ring, the pampiniform plexus forms the spermatic vein.

The right spermatic vein enters the vena cava just below the right renal vein; the left spermatic vein empties into the left renal vein.

Lymphatics

The lymphatic vessels from the testes pass to the lumbar lymph nodes, which, in turn, are connected to the mediastinal nodes (Figs 18–1 and 18–2).

SCROTUM

Gross Appearance

Beneath the corrugated skin of the scrotum lies the dartos muscle. Deep to this are the 3 fascial layers derived from the abdominal wall at the time of testicular descent. Beneath these is the parietal layer of the tunica vaginalis.

The scrotum is divided into 2 sacs by a septum of connective tissue. The scrotum not only supports the testes but, by relaxation or contraction of its muscular layer, helps to regulate their environmental temperature.

Histology

The dartos muscle, under the skin of the scrotum, is unstriated. The deeper layer is made up of connective tissue.

Blood Supply

A. Arterial: The arteries to the scrotum arise from the femoral, internal pudendal, and inferior epigastric arteries.

B. Venous: The veins are paired with the arteries.

Lymphatics

The lymphatics drain into the superficial inguinal and subinguinal lymph nodes (Figs 18–1 and 18–2).

PENIS & MALE URETHRA

Gross Appearance

The penis is composed of 2 corpora cavernosa and the corpus spongiosum, which contains the urethra, whose diameter is 8–9 mm. These corpora are capped distally by the glans. Each corpus is enclosed in a fascial sheath (tunica albuginea), and all are surrounded by a thick fibrous envelope known as Buck's fascia. A covering of skin, devoid of fat, is loosely applied about these bodies. The prepuce forms a hood over the glans.

Beneath the skin of the penis (and scrotum) and extending from the base of the glans to the urogenital diaphragm is Colles' fascia, which is continuous with Scarpa's fascia of the lower abdominal wall (Fig 1–8).

The proximal ends of the corpora cavernosa are attached to the pelvic bones just anterior to the ischial tuberosities. Occupying a depression on their ventral surface in the midline is the corpus spongiosum, which is connected proximally to the undersurface of the urogenital diaphragm, through which emerges the membranous urethra. This portion of the corpus spongiosum is surrounded by the bulbocavernosus muscle. Its distal end expands to form the glans penis.

The suspensory ligament of the penis arises from the linea alba and pubic symphysis and inserts into the fascial covering of the corpora cavernosa.

Histology

A. Corpora and Glans Penis: The corpora cavernosa, the corpus spongiosum, and the glans penis are composed of septa of smooth muscle and erectile tissue that enclose vascular cavities.

B. Urethra: The urethral mucosa that traverses the glans penis is formed of squamous epithelium. Proximal to this, the mucosa is transitional in type. Underneath the mucosa is the submucosa, which contains connective and elastic tissue and smooth muscle. In the submucosa are the numerous glands of Littre, whose ducts connect with the urethral lumen.

The urethra is surrounded by the vascular corpus spongiosum and the glans penis.

Blood Supply

A. Arterial: The penis and urethra are supplied by the internal pudendal arteries. Each artery divides into a profunda artery of the penis (which supplies the corpora cavernosa), a dorsal artery of the penis, and the bulbourethral artery. These branches supply the corpus spongiosum, the glans penis, and the urethra.

B. Venous: The superficial dorsal vein lies external to Buck's fascia. The deep dorsal vein is placed beneath Buck's fascia and lies between the dorsal arteries. These veins connect with the pudendal plexus, which drains into the internal pudendal vein.

Lymphatics

Lymphatic drainage from the skin of the penis is to the superficial inguinal and subinguinal lymph nodes. The lymphatics from the glans penis pass to

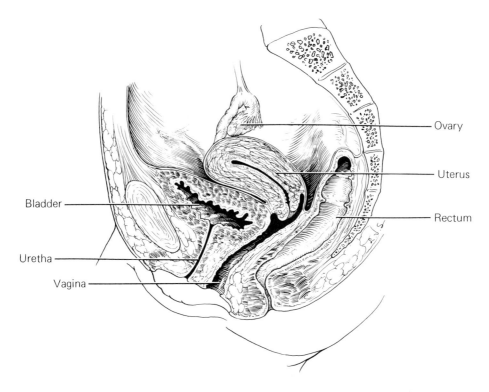

Ovary

Uterus

Rectum

Bladder

Uretha

Vagina

Figure 1–9. Anatomy and relations of the bladder, urethra, uterus and ovary, vagina, and rectum.

the subinguinal and external iliac nodes. The lymphatics from the deep urethra drain into the hypogastric and common iliac lymph nodes (Figs 18–1 and 18–2).

FEMALE URETHRA

The adult female urethra is about 4 cm long and 8 mm in diameter. It is slightly curved and lies beneath the pubic symphysis just anterior to the vagina.

The epithelial lining of the female urethra is squamous in its distal portion and pseudostratified or transitional in the remainder. The submucosa is made up of connective and elastic tissues and spongy venous spaces. Embedded in it are many periurethral glands, which are most numerous distally; the largest of these are the periurethral glands of Skene, which open on the floor of the urethra just inside the meatus.

External to the submucosa is a longitudinal layer of smooth muscle which is continuous with the inner longitudinal layer of the bladder wall. Surrounding this is a heavy layer of circular smooth muscle fibers which extend from the external vesical muscular layer. They constitute the true involuntary urethral sphincter. External to this is the circular striated (voluntary) sphincter surrounding the middle third of the urethra. It is part of the pelvic floor and levator muscles.

The arterial supply to the female urethra is derived from the inferior vesical, vaginal, and internal pudendal arteries. Blood from the urethra drains into the internal pudendal veins.

Lymphatic drainage from the external portion of the urethra is to the inguinal and subinguinal lymph nodes. Drainage from the deep urethra is into the hypogastric lymph nodes (Fig 18–1 and 18–2).

Nerve Supply to the Genitourinary Organs
See Figs 3–2, 3–3, and 19–1.

•   •   •

References

Adrenals

Ivemark B, Ekström T, Lagergren C: The vasculature of the developing and mature human adrenal gland. *Acta Paediatr Scand* 1967;**56**:601.

Johnstone FRC: The surgical anatomy of the adrenal glands with particular reference to the suprarenal vein. *Surg Clin North Am* 1964;**44**:1315.

Kidneys

Barger AC, Herd JA: The renal circulation. *N Engl J Med* 1971;**284**:482.

Cockett ATK: Lymphatic network of kidney. 1. Anatomic and physiologic considerations. *Urology* 1977;**9**:125.

Fetterman GH & others: The growth and maturation of human glomeruli and proximal convolutions from term to adulthood. *Pediatrics* 1965;**35**:601.

Fine H, Keen EN: Some observations on the medulla of the kidney. *Br J Urol* 1976;**48**:161.

Graves FT: The arterial anatomy of the congenitally abnormal kidney. *Br J Surg* 1969;**56**:533.

Hegedüs V: Arterial anatomy of the kidney: A three-dimensional angiographic investigation. *Acta Radiol [Diagn] (Stockh)* 1972;**12**:604.

Hodson J: The lobar structure of the kidney. *Br J Urol* 1972;**44**:246.

Layton JM: The structure of the kidney from the gross to the molecular. *J Urol* 1963;**90**:502.

Mayerson HS: The lymphatic system with particular reference to the kidney. *Surg Gynecol Obstet* 1963;**116**:259.

Meyers MA: The reno-alimentary relationships: Anatomic-roentgen study of their clinical significance. *Am J Roentgenol* 1975;**123**:386.

Potter EL: Development of the human glomerulus. *Arch Pathol* 1965;**80**:241.

Roddie IC: Modern views of physiology. 20. The kidney. *Practitioner* 1970;**205**:242.

Zamboni L, DeMartino C: Embryogenesis of the human renal glomerulus. 1. A histologic study. *Arch Pathol* 1968;**86**:279.

Calices, Renal Pelvis, & Ureters

Cussen LJ: The structure of the normal human ureter in infancy and childhood. *Invest Urol* 1967;**5**:179.

Elbadawi A, Amaku EO, Frank IN: Trilaminar musculature of submucosal ureter: Anatomy and functional implications. *Urology* 1973;**2**:409.

Hanna MK & others: Ureteral structure and ultrastructure. 1. Normal human ureter. *J Urol* 1976;**116**:718.

Osathanondh V, Potter EL: Development of human kidney shown by microdissection. 2. Renal pelvis, calyces, and papillae. 3. Formation and interrelationships of collecting tubules and nephrons. 4. Formation of tubular portions of nephrons. 5. Development of vascular pattern of glomerulus. *Arch Pathol* 1963;**76**:277, 290 and 1966;**82**:391, 403.

Sykes D: The morphology of renal lobulations and calyces, and their relationship to partial nephrectomy. *Br J Surg* 1964;**51**:294.

Weiss RM, Bassett AL, Hoffman BF: Adrenergic innervation of the ureter. *Invest Urol* 1978;**16**:123.

Bladder & Urethra

Elbadawi A, Schenk EA: A new theory of the innervation of bladder musculature. 2. Innervation of the vesicourethral junction and external urethral sphincter. *J Urol* 1974;**111**:613.

Fletcher TF, Bradley WE: Neuroanatomy of the bladder-urethra. *J Urol* 1978;**119**:153.

Gosling JA, Dixon DS: The structure and innervation of smooth muscle in the wall of the bladder neck and proximal urethra. *Br J Urol* 1975;**47**:549.

Hakky SI: Ultrastructure of the normal human urethra. *Br J Urol* 1979;**51**:394.

Hodges CV: Surgical anatomy of the urinary bladder and pelvic ureter. *Surg Clin North Am* 1964;**44**:1327.

Hutch JA: *Anatomy and Physiology of the Bladder, Trigone and Urethra.* Appleton-Century-Crofts, 1972.

Hutch JA: The internal urinary sphincter: A double loop system. *J Urol* 1971;**105**:375.

Olesen KP, Grau V: The suspensory apparatus of the female bladder neck. *Urol Int* 1976;**31**:33.

Tanagho EA, Miller ER: Functional considerations of urethral sphincteric dynamics. *J Urol* 1973;**109**:273.

Tanagho EA, Pugh RCB: The anatomy and function of the ureterovesical junction. *Br J Urol* 1963;**35**:151.

Tanagho EA, Smith DR: The anatomy and function of the bladder neck. *Br J Urol* 1966;**38**:54.

Tanagho EA & others: Observations in the dynamics of the bladder neck. *Br J Urol* 1966;**38**:72.

Prostate Gland

Bruschini H, Schmidt RA, Tanagho EA: The male genitourinary sphincter mechanism in the dog. *Invest Urol* 1978;**15**:284.

Hutch JA, Rambo ON Jr: A study of the anatomy of the prostate, prostatic urethra and the urinary sphincter system. *J Urol* 1970;**104**:443.

McNeal JE: The prostate and prostatic urethra: A morphologic study. *J Urol* 1972;**107**:1008.

Vaalsti A, Hervonen A: Autonomic innervation of the human prostate. *Invest Urol* 1980;**17**:293.

Wein AJ, Benson GS, Jacobowitz D: Lack of evidence for adrenergic innervation of external urethral sphincter. *J Urol* 1979;**121**:324.

Spermatic Cord

Ahlberg NE, Bartley O, Chidekel N: Right and left gonadal veins: An anatomical and statistical study. *Acta Radiol [Diagn] (Stockh)* 1966;**4**:593.

Bergman LL: The regional anatomy of the inguinal canal. *GP* (Oct) 1962;**26**:114.

Testis

Busch FM, Sayegh ES: Roentgenographic vidualization of human testicular lymphatics: A preliminary report. *J Urol* 1963;**89**:106.

Female Urethra

Lindner HH, Feldman SE: Surgical anatomy of the perineum. *Surg Clin North Am* 1962;**42**:877.

Zacharin RF: The anatomic supports of the female urethra. *Obstet Gynecol* 1968;**32**:754.

2 | Embryology of the Genitourinary System

Emil A. Tanagho, MD

At birth, the genital and urinary systems are related only in the sense that they share certain common passages. Embryologically, however, they are intimately related. Because of the complex interrelationships of the embryonic phases of the 2 systems, they will be discussed here as 5 subdivisions: the nephric system, the vesicourethral unit, the gonads, the genital duct system, and the external genitalia.

THE NEPHRIC SYSTEM

The nephric system develops progressively as 3 distinct entities: pronephros, mesonephros, and metanephros.

Pronephros

This is the earliest nephric stage in humans, and it corresponds to the mature structure of the most primitive vertebrate. It extends from the fourth to the fourteenth somites and consists of 6–10 pairs of tubules. These open into a pair of primary ducts that are also formed at that same level, extend caudally, and eventually reach and open into the cloaca. The pronephros is a vestigial structure that disappears completely by the fourth week of embryonic life (Fig 2–1).

Mesonephros

The mature excretory organ of the higher fish and amphibians corresponds to the embryonic mesonephros. It is the principal excretory organ during early embryonic life (4–8 weeks). It, too, gradually degenerates, although parts of its duct system become associated with the male reproductive organs. The mesonephric tubules develop from the intermediate mesoderm caudad to the pronephros shortly before pronephric degeneration. The mesonephric tubules differ from those of the pronephros in that they develop a cuplike outgrowth into which a knot of capillaries is pushed. This is called Bowman's capsule, and the tuft of capillaries is called a glomerulus. In their growth, the mesonephric tubules extend toward and estab-

lish a connection with the nearby primary nephric duct as it grows caudally to join the cloaca (Fig 2–1). This primary nephric duct is now called the mesonephric duct. After establishing their connection with the nephric duct, the primordial tubules elongate and become S-shaped. As the tubules elongate, a series of secondary branchings increases their surface exposure, thereby enhancing their capacity for interchanging material with the blood in adjacent capillaries. Leaving the glomerulus, the blood is carried by one or more efferent vessels that soon break up into a rich capillary plexus closely related to the mesonephric tubules. This is physiologically important. The mesonephros, which forms early in the fourth week, reaches its maximum size by the end of the second month.

Metanephros

The final phase of the development of the nephric system originates from both the intermediate mesoderm and the mesonephric duct. Development begins in the 5- to 6-mm embryo with a budlike outgrowth from the mesonephric duct as it bends to join the cloaca. This ureteral bud grows cephalad and collects mesoderm from the nephrogenic cord of the intermediate mesoderm around its tip. This mesoderm with the metanephric cap moves, with the growing ureteral bud, more and more cephalad from its point of origin. During this cephalad migration, the metanephric cap becomes progressively larger, and rapid internal differentiation takes place. Meanwhile, the cephalad end of the ureteral bud expands within the growing mass of metanephrogenic tissue to form the renal pelvis (Fig 2–1). Numerous outgrowths from the renal pelvic dilatation push radially into this growing mass and form hollow ducts that branch and rebranch as they push toward the periphery. These form the primary collecting ducts of the kidney. Mesodermal cells become arranged in small vesicular masses that lie close to the blind end of the collecting ducts. Each of these vesicular masses will form a uriniferous tubule draining into the duct nearest to its point of origin. As the kidney grows, increasing numbers of tubules are formed in its peripheral zone. These vesicular masses develop a central cavity and become S-shaped. One end of the

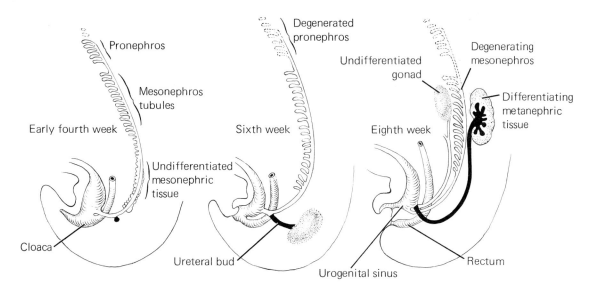

Figure 2–1. Schematic representation of the development of the nephric system. Only a few of the tubules of the pronephros are seen early in the fourth week, while the mesonephric tissue differentiates into mesonephric tubules that progressively join the mesonephric duct. The first sign of the ureteral bud from the mesonephric duct is seen. At 6 weeks, the pronephros has completely degenerated and the mesonephric tubules start to do so. The ureteral bud grows dorsocranially and has met the metanephrogenic cap. At the eighth week, there is cranial migration of the differentiating metanephros. The cranial end of the ureteric bud expands and starts to show multiple successive outgrowths. (Adapted from several sources.)

S coalesces with the terminal portion of the collecting tubules, resulting in a continuous canal. The proximal portion develops into the distal and proximal convoluted tubules and into Henle's loop; the distal end becomes the glomerulus and Bowman's capsule. At this stage, the undifferentiated mesoderm and the immature glomeruli are readily visible on microscopic examination (Fig 2–2). The glomeruli are fully developed by the thirty-sixth week or when the fetus weighs 2500 g (Potter). The metanephros arises opposite the 28th somite (fourth lumbar segment). At term, it has ascended to the level of the first lumbar or even the twelfth thoracic vertebra. This ascent of the kidney is due not only to actual cephalad migration but also to differential growth in the caudal part of the body. During the early period of ascent (seventh to ninth weeks), the kidney slides above the arterial bifurcation and rotates 90 degrees. Its convex border is now directed laterally, not dorsally. Further ascent proceeds more slowly until the kidney reaches its final position.

Certain features of these 3 phases of development must be emphasized: (1) The 3 successive units of the system develop from the intermediate mesoderm. (2) The tubules at all levels appear as independent primordia and only secondarily unite with the duct system. (3) The nephric duct is laid down as the duct of the pronephros and develops from the union of the ends of the anterior pronephric tubules. (4) This pronephric duct serves subsequently as the mesonephric duct and as such

gives rise to the ureter. (5) The nephric duct reaches the cloaca by independent caudal growth. (6) The embryonic ureter is an outgrowth of the nephric duct, yet the kidney tubules differentiate from adjacent metanephric blastema.

ANOMALIES OF THE NEPHRIC SYSTEM

Failure of the metanephros to ascend leads to **ectopic kidney.** An ectopic kidney may be on the proper side but low (simple ectopy) or on the opposite side (crossed ectopy) with or without fusion. Failure to rotate during ascent causes a **malrotated kidney.**

Fusion of the paired metanephric masses leads to various anomalies—most commonly **horseshoe kidney.**

The ureteral bud from the mesonephric duct may bifurcate, causing a **bifid ureter** at varying levels depending on the time of the bud's subdivision. An accessory ureteral bud may develop from the mesonephric duct, thereby forming a **duplicated ureter,** usually meeting the same metanephric mass. Rarely, each bud has a separate metanephric mass, resulting in **supernumerary kidneys.**

If the double ureteral buds are close together on the mesonephric duct, they will open near each other in the bladder. In this case, the main ureteral bud, which is the first to appear and the most caudal on the mesonephric ducts, will reach the bladder

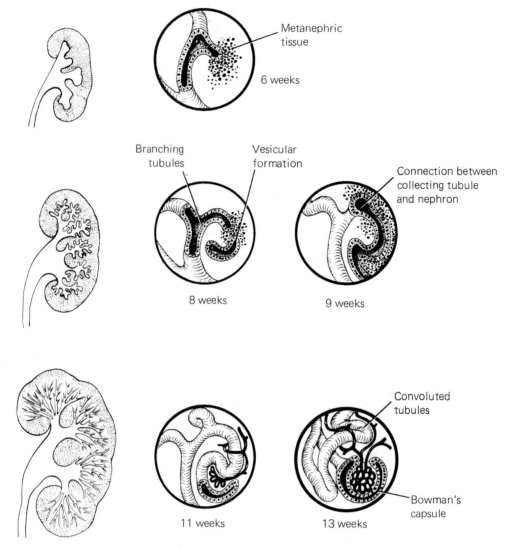

Figure 2–2. Progressive stages in the differentiation of the nephrons and their linkage with the branching collecting tubules. A small lump of metanephric tissue is associated with each terminal collecting tubule. These are then arranged in vesicular masses that later differentiate into a uriniferous tubule draining into the duct near which it arises. At one end, Bowman's capsule and the glomerulus differentiate; the other end establishes communication with the nearby collecting tubules.

first. It will then start to move upward and laterally and will be followed later by the second accessory bud as it reaches the urogenital sinus. The main ureteral bud (now more cranial on the urogenital sinus) will drain the lower portion of the kidney. The 2 ureteral buds have reversed their relationship as they moved from the mesonephric duct to the urogenital sinus. This is why double ureters always cross (Weigert-Meyer law). If the 2 ureteral buds are widely separated on the mesonephric duct, the accessory bud appears more proximal at the duct and will end in the bladder with an ectopic orifice lower than the normal one. This ectopic orifice could still be in the bladder close to its outlet, in the urethra, or even in the genital duct system (Fig 2–3). A single ureteral bud that arises higher

than normal on the mesonephric duct can also end in a similar ectopic location.

Lack of development of a ureteral bud will result in a **solitary kidney** and a hemitrigone.

THE VESICOURETHRAL UNIT

The blind end of the hindgut caudad to the point of origin of the allantois expands to form the cloaca, which is separated from the outside by an ectodermal depression under the root of the tail. This depression is called the proctodeum, and a thin plate of tissue closing the hindgut is the cloacal

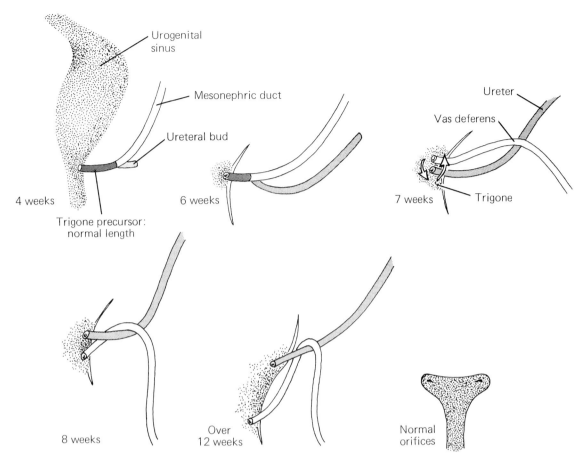

Figure 2–3. The development of the ureteral bud from the mesonephric duct and their relationship to the urogenital sinus. The ureteral bud appears at the fourth week. The mesonephric duct distal to this ureteral bud will be gradually absorbed into the urogenital sinus, resulting in separate endings for the ureter and the mesonephric duct. The mesonephric tissue that is incorporated into the urogenital sinus will expand and form the trigonal tissue.

membrane. At the 4-mm stage, starting at the cephalad portion of the cloaca where the allantois and gut meet, the cloaca progressively divides into 2 compartments by the caudad growth of a crescentic fold, the urorectal fold. The 2 limbs of the fold bulge into the lumen of the cloaca from either side, eventually meeting and fusing. The division of the cloaca into ventral (urogenital sinus) and dorsal (rectum) is completed during the seventh week. During the development of the urorectal septum, the cloacal membrane undergoes a reverse rotation so that the ectodermal surface is no longer directed toward the developing anterior abdominal wall but gradually faces caudally and slightly posteriorly. This growth change facilitates the subdivision of the cloaca and is brought about mainly by the development of the infraumbilical portion of the anterior abdominal wall and by regression of the tail. The mesoderm that passes around the cloacal membrane to the caudal attachment of the umbilical cord proliferates and grows, forming a surface elevation, the genital tubercle. The further growth of this part

of the abdominal wall progressively separates the umbilical cord from the genital tubercle. The division of the cloaca is completed before the cloacal membrane ruptures, and its 2 parts therefore open separately. The ventral part is the primitive urogenital sinus, which has the shape of an elongated cylinder and is continuous cranially with the allantois.

The urogenital sinus receives the mesonephric ducts. The caudad end of the mesonephric duct distal to the ureteral bud is progressively absorbed into the urogenital sinus. By the seventh week, both mesonephric duct and ureteral bud have independent opening sites. This will introduce an island of mesodermal tissue amid the surrounding endoderm of the urogenital sinus. As development progresses, the opening of the mesonephric duct (which will become the ejaculatory duct) migrates downward and medially. The opening of the ureteral bud (which will become the ureteral orifice) migrates upward and laterally. The absorbed mesoderm of the mesonephric duct expands with this migration to occupy the area limited by the final position of these tubes (Fig 2–3). This will later be differentiated as the trigonal structure, which is the only mesodermal inclusion in the endodermal vesicourethral unit.

The urogenital sinus can be divided into 2 main segments; the dividing line is the junction of the combined müllerian ducts with the urogenital sinus (Müller's tubercle), which is the most fixed reference point in the whole structure and which will be discussed below. The segments are as follows:

(1) The ventral and pelvic portion will form the bladder, part of the urethra in the male, and the whole urethra in the female. This portion receives the ureter.

(2) The urethral or phallic portion receives the mesonephric and the fused müllerian ducts. This will be part of the urethra in the male and forms the lower fifth of the vagina and the vaginal vestibule in the female.

During the third month, the ventral part of the urogenital sinus starts to expand and forms an epithelial sac whose apex tapers into an elongated, narrowed urachus. The pelvic portion remains narrow and tubular, and this will form the whole urethra in the female and the supramontanal portion of the prostatic urethra in the male. The splanchnic mesoderm surrounding the ventral and pelvic portion of the urogenital sinus begins to differentiate into interlacing bands of smooth muscle fibers and an outer fibrous connective tissue coat. By the twelfth week, the layers characteristic of the adult urethra and bladder are recognizable (Fig 2–4).

The part of the urogenital sinus caudad to the opening of the müllerian duct will form the vaginal vestibule and contribute to the lower fifth of the vagina in the female (Fig 2–5). In the male, it forms the inframontanal part of the prostatic urethra and the membranous urethra. The penile urethra is formed by the fusion of the urethral folds on the ventral surface of the genital tubercle. In the female, the urethral folds remain separate and form the labia minora. The glandular urethra in the male is formed by the canalization of the urethral plate.

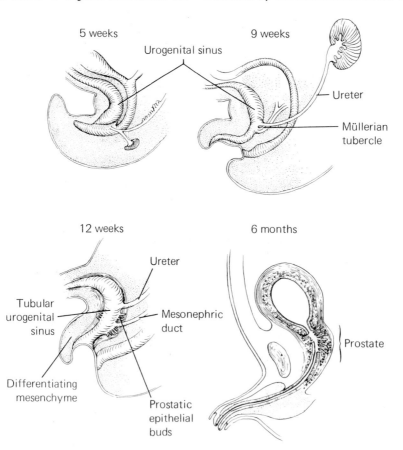

Figure 2–4. Differentiation of the urogenital sinus in the male. At the fifth week, the progressively growing urorectal septum is separating the urogenital sinus from the rectum. The former receives the mesonephric duct and the ureteral bud. It retains its tubular structure until the twelfth week, when the surrounding mesenchyme starts to differentiate into muscle fibers around the whole structure. The prostatic gland develops as multiple epithelial outgrowths just above and below the mesonephric duct. During the third month the ventral part expands to form the bladder proper while the pelvic part remains narrow and tubular, forming part of the urethra. (Reproduced, with permission, from Tanagho EA, Smith DR: Mechanisms of urinary continence. 1. Embryologic, anatomic, and pathologic considerations. *J Urol* 1969;**100**:640.)

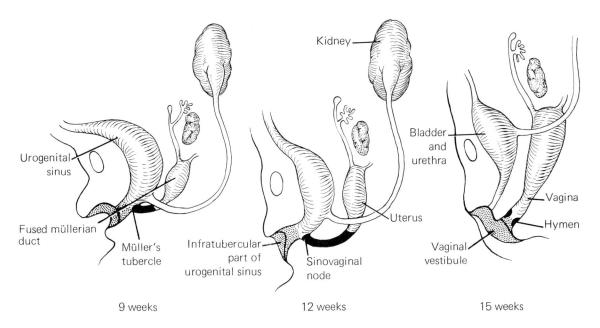

Figure 2–5. Differentiation of the urogenital sinus and the müllerian ducts in the female embryo. At 9 weeks, the urogenital sinus receives the fused müllerian ducts at Müller's tubercle (sinovaginal node), which is solidly packed with cells. As the urogenital sinus distal to Müller's tubercle becomes wider and shallower (15 weeks), the urethra and fused müllerian duct will have separate openings. The distal part of the urogenital sinus will form the vaginal vestibule and the lower fifth of the vagina (shaded area), and that part above Müller's tubercle will form the urinary bladder and the entire female urethra. The fused müllerian ducts will form the uterus and the upper four-fifths of the vagina. The hymen is formed at the junction of the sinovaginal node and the urogenital sinus.

The bladder originally extends up to the umbilicus, where it is connected to the allantois that extends into the umbilical cord. The allantois usually is obliterated at the level of the umbilicus by the fifteenth week. The bladder then starts to descend by the eighteenth week. As it descends, its apex becomes stretched and narrowed and it pulls on the already obliterated allantois, now called the urachus. By the twentieth week, the bladder is well separated from the umbilicus and the stretched urachus will become the middle umbilical ligament.

THE PROSTATE

The prostate develops as multiple solid outgrowths of the urethral epithelium both above and below the entrance of the mesonephric duct. These simple, tubular outgrowths begin to develop in 5 distinct groups at the end of the eleventh week and are complete by the sixteenth week (112 mm). They branch and rebranch, ending in a complex ductal system that encounters the differentiating mesenchymal cells around this segment of the urogenital sinus. These mesenchymal cells start to develop around the tubules by the sixteenth week and become denser at the periphery to form the prostatic capsule. By the twenty-second week, the muscular stroma is considerably developed and continues to progressively increase until birth.

From the 5 groups of epithelial buds, 5 lobes are eventually formed: anterior, posterior, median, and 2 lateral. Initially, these lobes are widely separated, but later they meet, with no definite septa dividing them. Tubules of each lobe do not intermingle with each other but simply lie side by side.

The anterior lobe tubules begin to develop simultaneously with those of the other lobes. Although in the early stages the anterior lobe tubules are large and show multiple branches, gradually they contract and lose most of these branches. They continue to shrink, so that at birth they show no lumen and appear as small, solid embryonic epithelial outgrowths. In contrast, the tubules of the posterior lobe are fewer in number yet relatively larger, with extensive branching. These tubules, as they grow, extend posterior to the developing median and lateral lobes and form the posterior aspect of the gland, which may be felt rectally.

ANOMALIES OF THE VESICOURETHRAL UNIT

Failure of the cloaca to subdivide is rare and results in a **persistent cloaca.** Incomplete subdivision is more frequent, ending with **rectovesical, rectourethral,** or **rectovestibular fistulas** (usually with **imperforate anus** or **anal atresia**).

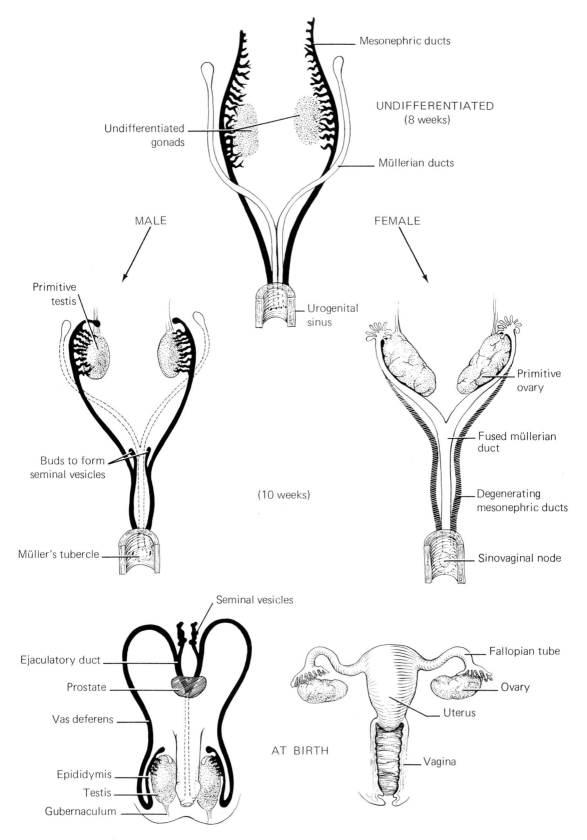

Figure 2–6. Transformation of the undifferentiated genital system into the definitive male and female systems.

Failure of descent or incomplete descent of the bladder leads to a **urinary umbilical fistula (urethral fistula), urachal cyst,** or **urachal diverticulum** depending on the stage and degree of maldescent.

Development of the genital primordia in an area more caudal than normal can result in formation of the corpora cavernosa just caudad to the urogenital sinus outlet, with the urethral groove on its dorsal surface. This defect results in complete or incomplete **epispadias** depending on its degree. A more extensive defect results in **vesical exstrophy.** Failure of fusion of urethral folds leads to various grades of **hypospadias.** This defect, because of its mechanism, never extends proximal to the bulbous urethra. This is in contrast to epispadias, which usually involves the entire urethra up to the internal meatus.

THE GONADS

Most of the structures which make up the embryonic genital system have been taken over from other systems, and their readaptation to genital function is a secondary and relatively late phase in their development. The early differentiation of such structures is therefore independent of sexuality. Furthermore, each embryo is at first morphologically bisexual, possessing all the necessary structures for either sex. The development of one set of sex primordia and the gradual involution of the other is determined by the sex type of the gonad.

The sexually undifferentiated gonad is a composite structure. Male and female potentials are represented by specific histologic elements (medulla and cortex) which have alternative roles in gonadogenesis. Normal differentiation involves the gradual predominance of one component.

The primitive sex glands make their appearance during the fifth and sixth weeks within a localized region of the thickening known as the urogenital ridge (this contains both the nephric and genital primordia). At the sixth week, the gonad consists of a superficial germinal epithelium and an internal blastema. The blastemal mass is derived mainly from proliferative ingrowth from the superficial epithelium that comes loose from its basement membrane.

During the seventh week, the gonad begins to assume the characteristics of a testis or ovary. Differentiation of the ovary usually occurs somewhat later than that of the testis.

If the gonad develops into a testis, the gland increases in size and shortens into a more compact organ while achieving a more caudal location. Its broad attachment to the mesonephros is converted into a gonadal mesentery known as the mesorchium. The cells of the germinal epithelium grow into the underlying mesenchyme and form cordlike masses. These are radially arranged and converge toward the mesorchium, where a dense portion of the blastemal mass is also emerging as the primordium of the rete testis. A network of strands soon forms which is continuous with the testis cords. The latter also split into 3–4 daughter cords. These eventually become differentiated into the seminiferous tubules by which the spermatozoa are produced. The rete testis unites with the mesonephric components that will form the male genital ducts, as discussed below (Fig 2–6).

If the gonad develops into an ovary, it (like the testis) gains a mesentery (mesovarium) and settles in a more caudal position. The internal blastema differentiates in the ninth week into a primary cortex beneath the germinal epithelium and a loose primary medulla. A compact cellular mass bulges from the medulla into the mesovarium and establishes the primitive rete ovarii. At 3–4 months of age, the internal cell mass becomes young ova. A new definitive cortex is formed from the germinal epithelium as well as from the blastema in the form of distinct cellular cords (Pflüger's tubes), and a permanent medulla is formed. The cortex differentiates into ovarian follicles containing ova.

Descent of the Gonads

A. The Testis: In addition to its early caudal migration, the testis later leaves the abdominal cavity and descends into the scrotum. By the third month of fetal life, the testis is located retroperitoneally in the false pelvis. A fibromuscular band (the gubernaculum) extends from the lower pole of the testis through the developing muscular layers of the anterior abdominal wall to terminate in the subcutaneous tissue of the scrotal swelling. The gubernaculum also has several other subsidiary strands that extend to adjacent regions. Just below the lower pole of the testis, the peritoneum herniates as a diverticulum along the anterior aspect of the gubernaculum, eventually reaching the scrotal sac through the anterior abdominal muscles (the processus vaginalis). The testis remains at the abdominal end of the inguinal canal until the seventh month. It then passes through the inguinal canal behind (but invaginating) the processus vaginalis. Normally, it reaches the scrotal sac by the end of the eighth month.

B. The Ovary: In addition to undergoing an early internal descent, the ovary becomes attached through the gubernaculum to the tissues of the genital fold and then attaches itself to the developing uterovaginal canal at its junction with the uterine tubes. This part of the gubernaculum between the ovary and uterus becomes the ovarian ligament; the part between the uterus and the labia majora becomes the round ligament of the uterus. This prevents extra-abdominal descent, and the ovary enters the true pelvis. It eventually lies posterior to the uterine tubes on the superior surface of the urogenital mesentery, which has descended with the ovary and now forms the broad ligament. A small processus vaginalis forms and passes toward the labial swelling, but it is usually obliterated at full term.

GONADAL ANOMALIES

Lack of development of the gonads leads to **gonadal agenesis.** Incomplete development with arrest at a certain phase leads to **hypogenesis. Supernumerary gonads** are rare. The commonest anomaly involves descent of the gonads, especially the testis. Retention of the testis in the abdomen or arrest of its descent at any point along its natural pathway leads to **cryptorchidism,** which may be either unilateral or bilateral. If the testis does not follow the main gubernaculum structure but follows one of its subsidiary strands, it will end in an abnormal position, resulting in **ectopic testis.**

Failure of union between the rete testis and mesonephros results in a testis separate from the male genital ducts (the epididymis).

THE GENITAL DUCT SYSTEM

Alongside the indifferent gonads, there are, early in embryonic life, 2 different yet closely related ducts. One is primarily a nephric duct (wolff-ian duct), yet it will also serve as a genital duct if the embryo develops into a male. The other (müllerian duct) is primarily a genital structure from the start.

Both ducts grow caudally to join the primitive urogenital sinus. The wolffian duct (known as the pronephric duct at the 4-mm stage) joins the ventral part of the cloaca, which will be the urogenital sinus. This duct gives rise to the ureteral bud close to its caudal end. The ureteral bud will grow cranially and meet metanephrogenic tissue. That part of each mesonephric duct caudad to the origin of the ureteric bud becomes absorbed into the wall of the primitive urogenital sinus so that the mesonephric duct and ureter open independently. This is achieved at the 15-mm stage (seventh week). During this period, starting at the 10-mm stage, the müllerian ducts start to develop. They reach the urogenital sinus relatively late—at the 30-mm embryonic stage (ninth week). This is the most constant and reliable point of reference in the whole system.

If the embryo develops into a male and the gonad starts to develop into a testis (17 mm, seventh week), the wolffian duct will start to differentiate into the male duct system, forming the epididymis, vas deferens, seminal vesicles, and ejaculatory ducts. At this time, the müllerian duct proceeds toward its junction with urogenital sinus and immediately starts to degenerate. It will only remain as a rudimentary structure.

If the embryo develops into a female and the gonad starts to differentiate into an ovary (22 mm,

Table 2–1. Male and female homologous structures.

Embryonic Structure	Male	Female
Mesonephric duct	Epididymis Vas deferens and seminal vesicles Ejaculatory ducts Appendix epididymidis Ureter, renal pelvis, etc Trigonal structure	Duct of epoophoron Gartner's duct Vesicular appendage Ureter, renal pelvis, etc Trigonal structure
Müllerian duct	Appendix testis Prostatic utricle	Fallopian tubes Uterus Vagina (upper four-fifths)
Müller's tubercle	Verumontanum	Hymen (site of)
Sinovaginal bulb from urogenital sinus	Part of prostatic utricle	Lower one-fifth of vagina
Junction of sinovaginal bulb and urogenital sinus	Disappears normally (remnants probably form posterior urethral valves)	Hymen
Urogenital sinus Ventral and pelvic part	Urinary bladder (except the trigone) Supramontanal part of prostatic urethra	Urinary bladder (except the trigone) Whole urethra
Phallic or urethral portion	Inframontanal part of prostatic urethra Membranous urethra	Vaginal vestibule
Genital tubercle	Penis	Clitoris
Urethral folds	Penile urethra	Labia minora
Genital swellings	Scrotum	Labia majora
Gubernaculum	Gubernaculum testis	Ligament of ovary Round ligament of uterus
Genital glands	Testis	Ovary
Germinal cords	Seminiferous tubules	Pflüger's tube

eighth week), the müllerian duct system forms the uterine (fallopian) tubes, uterus, and most of the vagina. The wolffian ducts, aside from their contribution to the urogenital sinus, remain rudimentary.

THE MALE DUCT SYSTEM

The Epididymis

Because of the proximity of the differentiating gonads and the nephric duct, some of the mesonephric tubules are retained as the efferent ductules, and their lumens become continuous with those of the rete testis. These tubules, together with that part of the mesonephric duct into which they empty, will form the epididymis. Each coiled ductule makes a conical mass known as the lobule of the epididymis. The cranial end of the mesonephric duct becomes highly convoluted, completing the formation of the epididymis. This is an example of direct inclusion of a nephric structure into the genital system. Additional mesonephric tubules, both cephalad and caudad to those that were included in the formation of the epididymis, will remain as rudimentary structures, ie, the appendix of the epididymis and the paradidymis.

Vas Deferens, Seminal Vesicles, & Ejaculatory Ducts

The mesonephric duct caudad to that portion forming the epididymis will form the vas deferens. Shortly before this duct joins the urethra (urogenital sinus), a localized dilatation (ampulla) develops and the saccular convoluted structure that will form the seminal vesicle is evaginated from its wall. The mesonephric duct between the origin of the seminal vesicle and the urethra will form the ejaculatory duct. The whole mesonephric duct now achieves its characteristic thick investment of smooth muscle, with a narrow lumen along most of its length.

Both above and below the point of entrance of the mesonephric duct into the urethra, multiple outgrowths of urethral epithelium mark the beginning of the development of the prostate. As these epithelial buds grow, they meet the developing muscular fibers around the urogenital sinus, and some of these fibers become entangled in the branching tubules of the growing prostate and become incorporated into it, forming its muscular stroma (Fig 2–4).

THE FEMALE DUCT SYSTEM

The müllerian ducts, which are a paired system, are seen alongside the mesonephric duct. It is not known whether they arise directly from the mesonephric ducts or separately as an invagination of the celomic epithelium into the parenchyma lateral to the cranial extremity of the mesonephric duct, but the latter theory is favored. The müllerian duct develops and runs lateral to the mesonephric duct. Its opening with the celomic cavity persists as the peritoneal ostium of the uterine tube (later it develops fimbriae). The other end grows caudally as a solid tip and then crosses in front of the mesonephric duct at the caudad extremity of the mesonephros. It continues its growth in a caudomedial direction until it meets and fuses with the müllerian duct of the opposite side. The fusion is partial at first, so there is a temporary septum between the 2 lumens. This later disappears, leaving one cavity that will form the uterovaginal canal. The potential lumen of the vaginal canal is completely packed with cells. The solid tip of this cord pushes the epithelium of the urogenital sinus outward, where it becomes Müller's tubercle (33-mm stage, ninth week). They actually fuse at the 63-mm stage (13th week), forming the sinovaginal node, which receives a limited contribution from the urogenital sinus. (This contribution will form the lower fifth of the vagina.)

The urogenital sinus distal to Müller's tubercle, originally narrow and deep, shortens, widens, and opens to form the floor of the pudendal or vulval cleft. This results in separate openings for the vagina and urethra and also brings the vaginal orifice to its final position nearer the surface. At the same time, the vaginal segment increases appreciably in length. The vaginal vestibule is derived from the infratubercular segment of the urogenital sinus (in the male, the same segment will form the inframontanal part of the prostatic urethra and the membranous urethra). The labia minora are formed from the urethral folds (in the male they will form the pendulous urethra). The hymen is the remnant of the müllerian tubercle. The lower fifth of the vagina is derived from the contribution of the urogenital sinus with the sinovaginal node. The remainder of the vagina and the uterus are formed from the lower fused third of the müllerian ducts. The fallopian tubes (oviducts) are the cephalad two-thirds of the müllerian ducts (Fig 2–6).

ANOMALIES OF THE GONADAL DUCT SYSTEM

Nonunion of the rete testis and the efferent ductules can occur and, if bilateral, lead to **azoospermia and sterility.** Failure of the müllerian ducts to approximate or incomplete fusion can lead to various degrees of **duplication** in the genital ducts. **Congenital absence** of one or both uterine tubes or of the uterus or vagina occurs rarely.

Arrested development of the infratubercular segment of the urogenital sinus leads to its persistence, with the urethra and vagina having a common duct to the outside (**urogenital sinus**).

THE EXTERNAL GENITALIA

During the eighth week, external sex differentiation begins to occur. Not until 3 months, however, do the progressively developing external genitalia attain characteristics that can be recognized as distinctively male or female. During the indifferent stage of sexual development, 3 small protuberances appear on the external aspect of the cloacal membrane. In front is the genital tubercle, and on either side of the membrane are the genital swellings.

By the breakdown of the urogenital membrane (17 mm, seventh week), the primitive urogenital sinus achieves a separate opening on the undersurface of the genital tubercle.

MALE EXTERNAL GENITALIA

The urogenital sinus opening extends on the ventral aspect of the genital tubercle as the urethral groove. The primitive urogenital orifice and the urethral groove are bounded on either side by the urethral folds. The genital tubercle becomes elongated to form the phallus. The corpora cavernosa are indicated in the seventh week as paired mesenchymal columns within the shaft of the penis. By the tenth week, the urethral folds start to fuse from the urogenital sinus orifice toward the tip of the phallus. At the fourteenth week, the fusion is complete and results in the formation of the penile urethra. The corpus spongiosum results from the differentiation of the mesenchymal masses around the formed penile urethra.

The glans penis becomes defined by the development of a circular coronary sulcus around the distal part of the phallus. The urethral groove and the fusing folds do not extend beyond the coronary sulcus. The glandular urethra develops as a result of canalization of an ectodermal epithelial cord that has grown through the glans. This canalization reaches and communicates with the distal end of the previously formed penile urethra. During the third month, a fold of skin at the base of the glans begins growing distally and, 2 months later, surrounds the glans. This forms the prepuce. Meanwhile, the genital swellings shift caudally and are recognizable as scrotal swellings. They meet and fuse, resulting in the formation of the scrotum, with 2 compartments partially separated by a median septum and a median raphe, indicating their line of fusion.

FEMALE EXTERNAL GENITALIA

Until the eighth week, the appearance of the female external genitalia closely resembles that of the male except that the urethral groove is shorter. The genital tubercle, which becomes bent caudally and lags in development, becomes the clitoris. As in the male (though on a minor scale), mesenchymal columns differentiate into corpora cavernosa and a coronary sulcus identifies the glans clitoridis. The most caudal part of the urogenital sinus shortens and widens, forming the vaginal vestibule. The urethral folds do not fuse but remain separate as the labia minora. The genital swellings meet in front of the anus, forming the posterior commissure, while the swellings as a whole enlarge and remain separated on either side of the vestibule and form the labia majora.

ANOMALIES OF THE EXTERNAL GENITALIA

Absence or duplication of the penis or clitoris is very rare. More commonly, the penis remains rudimentary or the clitoris may show hypertrophy. These may be seen alone or, more frequently, in association with **pseudohermaphroditism.** Concealed penis and transposition of penis and scrotum are relatively rare anomalies.

Failure or incomplete fusion of the urethral folds results in **hypospadias** (see above). Penile development is also anomalous in cases of **epispadias** and **exstrophy** (see above).

● ● ●

References

General

Allan FD: *Essentials of Human Embryology.* Oxford Univ Press, 1960.

Arey LB: *Developmental Anatomy: A Textbook and Laboratory Manual of Embryology,* 6th ed. Saunders, 1954.

Blechschmidt E: *The Stages of Human Development Before Birth: An Introduction to Human Embryology.* Saunders, 1961.

Frazer JES, Baxter JS: *Manual of Embryology: The Development of the Human Body,* 3rd ed. Williams & Wilkins, 1953.

Keith A: *Human Embryology and Morphology,* 6th ed. Williams & Wilkins, 1948.

Kjellberg SR, Ericsson NO, Rudhe U: *The Lower Urinary Tract in Childhood: Some Correlated Clinical and Roentgenologic Observations.* Year Book, 1957.

Patten BM: *Human Embryology,* 2nd ed. Blakiston, 1953.

Vaughan ED Jr, Middleton GW: Pertinent genitourinary embryology: Review for practicing urologist. *Urology* 1975;6:139.

Anomalies of the Nephric System

Akhtar M, Valencia M: Horseshoe kidney with unilateral renal dysplasia. *Urology* 1979;13:284.

Ayalon A & others: Ureterocele: A familial congenital anomaly. *Urology* 1979;13:551.

Brock WA, Kaplan GW: Ectopic ureteroceles in children. *J Urol* 1978;119:800.

Carrion H & others: Retrocaval ureter: Report of 8 cases and surgical management. *J Urol* 1979;121:514.

Correa RJ Jr, Paton RR: Polycystic horseshoe kidney. *J Urol* 1976;116:802.

Cowinn JL, Landry BW: Cystic diseases of the kidney in infants and children. *Radiol Clin North Am* 1968;6:191.

Douglas LL, Pott GA: Congenital ureteral diverticulum and solitary kidney. *J Urol* 1979;122:401.

Gribetz ME, Leiter E: Ectopic ureterocele, hydroureter, and renal dysplasia: An embryogenic triad. *Urology* 1978;11:131.

Heffernan JC, Lightwood RG, Snell ME: Horseshoe kidney with retrocaval ureter: Second reported case. *J Urol* 1978;120:358.

Hicks CC & others: Traumatic rupture of horseshoe kidney with partial ureteral duplication associated with supernumerary kidney. *Urology* 1976;8:149.

Johnson DK, Perlmutter AD: Single system ectopic ureteroceles with anomalies of heart, testis and vas deferens. *J Urol* 1980;123:81.

Koyanagi T & others: Everting ureteroceles: Radiographic and endoscopic observation, and surgical management. *J Urol* 1980;123:538.

Leiter E: Persistent fetal ureter. *J Urol* 1979;122:251.

Lockhard JL, Singer AM, Glenn JF: Congenital megaureter. *J Urol* 1979;122:310.

Magee MC: Ureteroceles and duplicated systems: Embryologic hypothesis. *J Urol* 1980;123:605.

Murphy WK, Palubinskas AJ, Smith DR: Sponge kidney: Report of 7 cases. *J Urol* 1961;85:866.

Osathanondh V, Potter EL: Pathogenesis of polycystic kidneys: Survey of results of microdissection. *Arch Pathol* 1964;77:510.

Osathanondh V, Potter EL: Pathogenesis of polycystic kidneys: Type 4 due to urethral obstruction. *Arch Pathol* 1964;77:502.

Romans DG, Jewett MAS, Robson CJ: Crossed renal ectopia with colic: A clinical clue to embryogenesis. *Br J Urol* 1976;48:171.

Soderdahl DW, Shiraki IW, Schamber DT: Bilateral ureteral quadruplication. *J Urol* 1976;116:255.

Traut HF: The structural unit of the human kidney. *Contribution to Embryology,* No. 76, Carnegie Inst Pub No. 332, 1923:15:103.

The Vesicourethral Unit

Begg RC: The urachus, its anatomy, histology and development. *J Anat* 1930;64:170.

Browne D: Some congenital deformities of the rectum, anus, vagina and urethra. (Hunterian Lecture.) *Ann R Coll Surg Engl* 1951;8:173.

Cullen TS: *Embryology, Anatomy and Diseases of the Umbilicus Together With Diseases of the Urachus.* Saunders, 1916.

Eagle JR Jr, Barrett GS: Congenital deficiency of abdominal musculature with associated genitourinary abnormalities: A syndrome. Report of nine cases. *Pediatrics* 1950;6:721.

Hinman F Jr: Surgical disorders of the bladder and umbilicus of urachal origin. *Surg Gynecol Obstet* 1961;113:605.

Lattimer JK: Congenital deficiency of the abdominal musculature and associated genitourinary anomalies: A report of 22 cases. *J Urol* 1958;79:343.

Lowsley OO: Persistent cloaca in the female: Report of two cases corrected by operation. *J Urol* 1948;59:692.

Stephens FD: *Congenital Malformations of the Rectum, Anus and Genitourinary Tracts.* Livingstone, 1963.

Stephens FD: The female anus, perineum and vestibule: Embryogenesis and deformities. *J Obstet Gynaecol Br Commonw* 1968;8:55.

Wainstein ML, Persky L: Superior vesical fistula: An unusual form of exstrophy of the urinary bladder. *Am J Surg* 1968;115:397.

Anomalies of the Vesicourethral Unit

Amar AD, Hutch JA: Anomalies of the ureter. Page 98 in: *Encyclopedia of Urology.* Vol 7: *Malformations.* Springer, 1968.

Ansell JS: Surgical treatment of exstrophy of bladder with emphasis on neonatal primary closure: Personal experience with 28 consecutive cases treated at University of Washington Hospitals from 1962 to 1977: Techniques and results. *J Urol* 1979;121:650.

Bauer SB & others: The bladder in boys with posterior urethral valves: A urodynamic assessment. *J Urol* 1979;121:769.

Chwalle R: The process of formation of cystic dilatations of the vesical end of the ureter and of diverticula at the ureteral ostium. *Urol Cutan Rev* 1927;31:499.

Das S, Brosman SA: Duplication of male urethra. *J Urol* 1977;117:452.

Ericsson NO: Ectopic ureterocele in infants and children: A clinical study. *Acta Chir Scand [Suppl]* 1954;197:1. [Entire issue.]

Escham W, Holt HA: Complete duplication of bladder and urethra. *J Urol* 1980;123:773.

Farkas A, Skinner DG: Posterior urethral valves in siblings. *Br J Urol* 1976;48:76.

Haralson IP: Double bladder and urethra with imperforate

anus and ureterorenal reflux: Case presentation with review of literature. *J Urol* 1980;**123**:776.

Landes RR, Melnick I, Klein R: Vesical exstrophy with epispadias: Twenty-year follow-up. *Urology* 1977;**9**:53.

Lattimer JK & others: Delayed development of scrotum in exstrophy. *J Urol* 1979;**121**:339.

Lattimer JK & others: Long-term follow-up after exstrophy closure: Late improvement and good quality of life. *J Urol* 1978;**119**:664.

Lenaghan D: Bifid ureters in children: An anatomical, physiological and clinical study. *J Urol* 1962;**87**:808.

Mackie GG: Abnormalities of the ureteral bud. *Urol Clin North Am* 1978;**5**:161.

Meyer R: Normal and abnormal development of the ureter in the human embryo: A mechanistic consideration. *Anat Rec* 1946;**96**:355.

Morgan RJ, Williams DI, Pryor JP: Müllerian duct remnants in the male. *Br J Urol* 1979;**51**:481.

Randall A, Campbell EW: Anomalous relationship of the right ureter to the vena cava. *J Urol* 1935;**34**:565.

Sellers BB & others: Congenital megalourethra associated with prune belly syndrome. *J Urol* 1976;**116**:814.

Shima H & others: Developmental anomalies associated with hypospadias. *J Urol* 1979;**122**:619.

Sohrabi A & others: Duplication of male urethra. *Urology* 1978;**12**:704.

Tanagho EA: Embryologic basis for lower ureteral anomalies: A hypothesis. *Urology* 1976;**7**:451.

Uehling DT: Posterior urethral valves: Functional classification. *Urology* 1980;**17**:27.

Gonadal Anomalies

Brosman SA: Mixed gonadal dysgenesis. *J Urol* 1979;**121**:344.

Grossman H, Ririe SDG: The incidence of urinary tract anomalies in cryptorchid boys. *Am J Roentgenol* 1968;**103**:210.

Honoré LH: Unilateral anorchism: Report of 11 cases with discussion of etiology and pathogenesis. *Urology* 1978;**11**:251.

Marshall FF, Shermeta DW: Epididymal abnormalities associated with undescended testis. *J Urol* 1979;**121**:341.

Pujol A & others: The value of bilateral biopsy in unilateral cryptorchidism. *Eur Urol* 1978;**4**:85.

Raiffer J, Walsh PC: Testicular descent: Normal and abnormal. *Urol Clin North Am* 1978;**5**:22.

Sugrue D: Male urogenital hypoplasia. *Am J Surg* 1968;**115**:390.

Walsh PC: The differential diagnosis of ambiguous genitalia in the newborn. *Urol Clin North Am* 1978;**5**:213.

Symptoms of Disorders of the Genitourinary Tract | 3

Donald R. Smith, MD

In the work-up of any patient, the history is of paramount importance; this is particularly true in urology. It will be necessary to discuss here only those urologic symptoms that are apt to be brought to the physician's attention by the patient. It is important to know not only whether the disease is acute or chronic but also whether it is recurrent, since recurring symptoms may represent acute exacerbations of chronic disease.

SYSTEMIC MANIFESTATIONS

Symptoms of fever, weight loss, and malaise should be sought. The presence of fever associated with other symptoms of urinary tract infection may be helpful in evaluating the site of the infection. Simple acute cystitis is essentially an afebrile disease. Acute pyelonephritis or prostatitis is apt to cause high temperatures (to 40 C [104 F]), often accompanied by violent chills. Infants and children suffering from acute pyelonephritis may have high temperatures without other localizing symptoms or signs. Such a clinical picture, therefore, *invariably* requires bacteriologic study of the urine.

A history of unexplained attacks of fever occurring even years before may have been due to an otherwise asymptomatic pyelonephritis. Renal carcinoma sometimes causes fever that may reach 39 C (102.2 F) or more. The absence of fever does not by any means rule out renal infection, for it is the rule that chronic pyelonephritis does not cause fever.

Weight loss is to be expected in the advanced stages of cancer, but it may also be noticed when renal insufficiency due to obstruction or infection supervenes.

General malaise may be noted with neoplasm, chronic pyelonephritis, or renal failure.

LOCAL & REFERRED PAIN

Two types of pain have their origins in the genitourinary organs: local and referred. The latter is especially common.

Local pain is felt in or near the involved organ. Thus, the pain from a diseased kidney (T10–12, L1)

is felt in the costovertebral angle and in the flank in the region of and below the 12th rib. Pain from an inflamed testicle is felt in the gonad itself.

Referred pain originates in a diseased organ but is felt at some distance from that organ. The ureteral colic (Fig 3–1) caused by a stone in the upper ureter may be associated with severe pain in the ipsilateral testicle; this is explained by the common innervation of these 2 structures (T11–12). A stone in the lower ureter may cause pain referred to the scrotal wall; in this instance, the testis itself is not hyperesthetic. The burning pain with voiding that accompanies acute cystitis is felt in the distal urethra in the female or in the glandular urethra in the male (S2–3).

Abnormalities of a urologic organ can also cause pain in any other organ (eg, gastrointestinal, gynecologic) that has a sensory nerve supply common to both (Figs 3–2 and 3–3).

Kidney Pain (Fig 3–1)

Typical renal pain is usually felt as a dull and constant ache in the costovertebral angle just lateral to the sacrospinalis muscle and just below the 12th rib. This pain often spreads along the subcostal area toward the umbilicus or lower abdominal quadrant. It may be expected in those renal diseases that cause sudden distention of the renal capsule. Acute pyelonephritis (with its sudden edema) and acute ureteral obstruction (with its sudden renal back pressure) both cause this typical pain. It should be pointed out, however, that many urologic renal diseases are painless because their progression is so slow that sudden capsular distention does not occur. Such diseases include cancer, chronic pyelonephritis, staghorn calculus, tuberculosis, and hydronephrosis due to mild ureteral obstruction.

Pseudorenal Pain (Radiculitis)

Mechanical derangements of the costovertebral or costotransverse joints can cause irritation or pressure on the costal nerves. Disorders of this sort are common in the cervical and thoracic areas, but the most common sites are T10–12 (Smith & Raney, 1976). Irritation of these nerves causes costovertebral pain, often with radiation into the ipsilateral lower abdominal quadrant. The pain is positional in

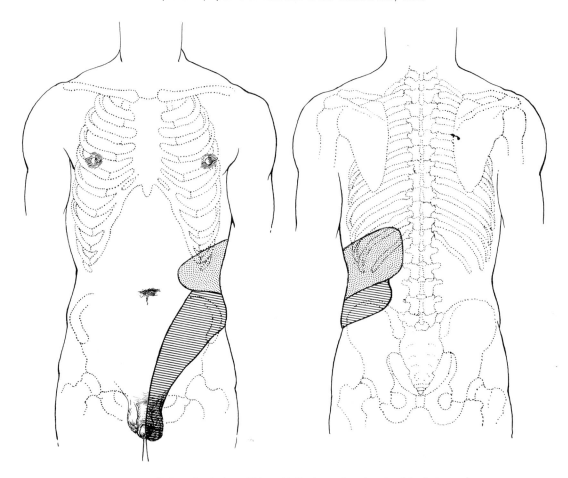

Figure 3–1. Referred pain from kidney (dotted areas) and ureter (shaded areas).

nature. Its first onset is usually quite acute, following the lifting of a heavy object, a blow to the costovertebral area, or a fall on the buttocks from a height. The pain is usually absent on arising from bed but is apt to increase as the day wears on. It is exacerbated by heavy physical work and is usually increased during an automobile trip over a rough road. It is apt to wake the patient up when a certain position is assumed (eg, lying on the right side) and is relieved by a change of position. Radiculitis may mimic ureteral colic or renal pain. True renal pain is seldom affected by movements of the spine.

Ureteral Pain (Fig 3–1)

Ureteral pain is typically stimulated by acute obstruction (passage of a stone or a blood clot). In this instance, there is back pain from capsular distention combined with severe colicky pain (due to renal pelvic and ureteral muscle spasm) that radiates from the costovertebral angle down toward the lower anterior abdominal quadrant, along the course of the ureter. In men it may also be felt in the bladder, scrotum, or testicle. In women it may radiate into the vulva. The severity and colicky nature of this pain are caused by the hy-

perperistalsis and spasm of this smooth muscle organ as it attempts to rid itself of a foreign body or to overcome obstruction. It should be remembered that radiculitis may mimic ureteral pain.

The physician may be able to judge the position of a ureteral stone by the history of pain and the site of referral. If the stone is lodged in the upper ureter, the pain radiates to the testicle, since the nerve supply of this organ is similar to that of the kidney and upper ureter (T11–12). With stones in the midportion of the ureter on the right side, the pain is referred to McBurney's point and may therefore simulate appendicitis; on the left side, it may resemble diverticulitis or other diseases of the descending or sigmoid colon (T12, L1). As the stone approaches the bladder, inflammation and edema of the ureteral orifice ensue, and symptoms of vesical irritability may occur. It is important to realize, however, that in mild ureteral obstruction, as seen in the congenital stenoses, there is usually no pain, either renal or ureteral.

Vesical Pain

The overdistended bladder of the patient in acute urinary retention will cause agonizing pain in the suprapubic area. Other than this, however, constant suprapubic pain not related to the act of urination is usually not of urologic origin. The relatively uncommon interstitial cystitis and vesical ulceration caused by tuberculosis or bilharziasis may cause suprapubic discomfort (usually relieved by urination) when the bladder becomes full.

The patient in chronic urinary retention due to bladder neck obstruction or to a neurogenic (neuropathic) bladder may experience little or no suprapubic discomfort even though the bladder reaches the umbilicus.

The most common cause of bladder pain is infection; the pain is usually not felt over the bladder but is referred to the distal urethra and is related to the act of urination. Terminal dysuria may be severe.

Prostatic Pain

Direct pain from the prostate gland is not common. Occasionally, when the prostate is inflamed, the patient may feel a vague discomfort or fullness in the perineal or rectal area (S2–4). Lumbosacral backache is occasionally experienced as referred pain from the prostate but is not a common symptom of prostatitis. Inflammation of the gland may cause symptoms of cystitis.

Testicular Pain

Testicular pain due to trauma, torsion of the spermatic cord, or infection is very severe and is felt locally, although there may be some radiation of the discomfort along the spermatic cord into the lower abdomen. It may involve the costovertebral area as well. Uninfected hydrocele and tumor of the testis do not commonly cause pain. A varicocele may cause a dull ache in the testicle that is increased after heavy exercise. At times, the first symptom of an early indirect inguinal hernia may be testicular pain (referred). Pain from a stone in the upper ureter may be referred to the testicle.

Epididymal Pain

Acute infection of the epididymis is the only painful disease of this organ and is quite common. Some degree of neighborhood inflammatory reaction involves the adjacent testis as well, further aggravating the discomfort. In the early stages of epididymitis, pain may first be felt in the groin or lower abdominal quadrant. (If on the right side, it may simulate appendicitis.) This may be a referred type of pain but can be secondary to associated inflammation of the vas deferens. The discomfort associated with epididymitis may reach the costal angle and mimic ureteral stone.

Back & Leg Pain

Pain low in the back and radiating down one or both legs, especially when associated with symptoms of vesical neck obstruction, suggests metastases to the pelvic bones from cancer of the prostate.

GASTROINTESTINAL SYMPTOMS OF UROLOGIC DISEASES

Whether renal or ureteral disease is painful or not, gastrointestinal symptoms are often present. The patient with acute pyelonephritis will suffer not only from localized back pain, symptoms of vesical irritability, chills, and fever but also from generalized abdominal pain and distention. The patient who is passing a stone down the ureter will have typical renal and ureteral colic and, usually, hematuria and may experience severe nausea and vomiting as well as abdominal distention. However, the urinary symptoms so far overshadow the gastrointestinal symptoms that the latter are usually ignored. Inadvertent overdistention of the renal pelvis (eg, with opaque material in order to obtain adequate retrograde urograms) may cause the patient to become nauseated, to vomit, and to complain of cramplike pain in the abdomen. This clinical experiment demonstrates the renointestinal reflex, which may lead to confusing symptomatology. In the very common "silent" urologic diseases, some degree of gastrointestinal symptomatology may be present that could mislead the clinician into seeking the diagnosis in the intraperitoneal zone.

Cause of the Mimicry

A. Renointestinal Reflexes: These account for most of the confusion. They arise because of the common autonomic and sensory innervations of the 2 systems (Figs 3–2 and 3–3). Afferent stimuli from the renal capsule or musculature of the pelvis may, by reflex action, cause pylorospasm (symptoms of peptic ulcer) or other changes in tone of the smooth muscles of the enteric tract and its adnexa.

B. Organ Relationships: The right kidney is closely related to the hepatic flexure of the colon, the duodenum, the head of the pancreas, the common bile duct, the liver, and the gallbladder (Fig 1–3). The left kidney lies just behind the splenic flexure of the colon and is closely related to the stomach, pancreas, and spleen. Inflammations or tumors in the retroperitoneum thus may extend into or displace intraperitoneal organs, causing them to produce symptoms.

C. Peritoneal Irritation: The anterior surfaces of the kidneys are covered by peritoneum. Renal inflammation, therefore, will cause peritoneal irritation, which leads to muscle rigidity and rebound tenderness.

The symptoms arising from chronic renal disease (eg, uninfected hydronephrosis, staghorn calculus, cancer, chronic pyelonephritis) may be entirely gastrointestinal and may simulate in every way the syndromes of peptic ulcer, gallbladder disease, appendicitis, or other less specific gastrointestinal complaints. If a thorough survey of the gastrointestinal tract fails to demonstrate suspected disease processes, the physician should give every consideration to study of the urinary tract.

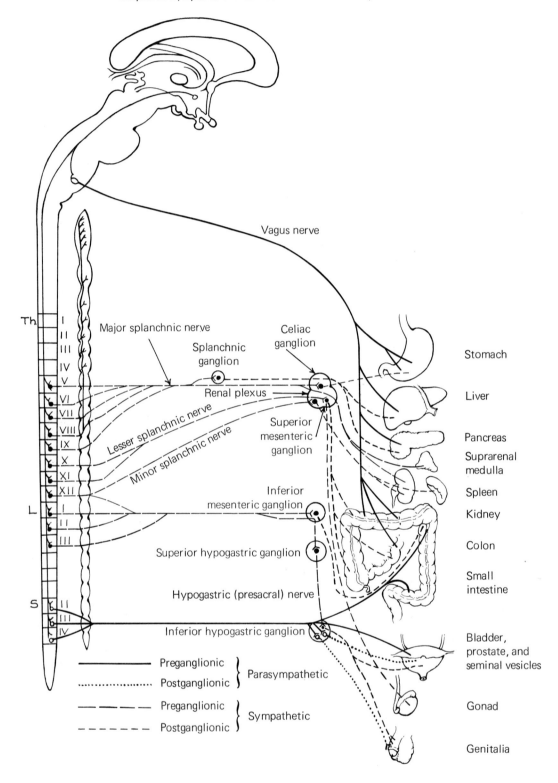

Figure 3–2. Diagrammatic representation of autonomic nerve supply to gastrointestinal and genitourinary tracts.

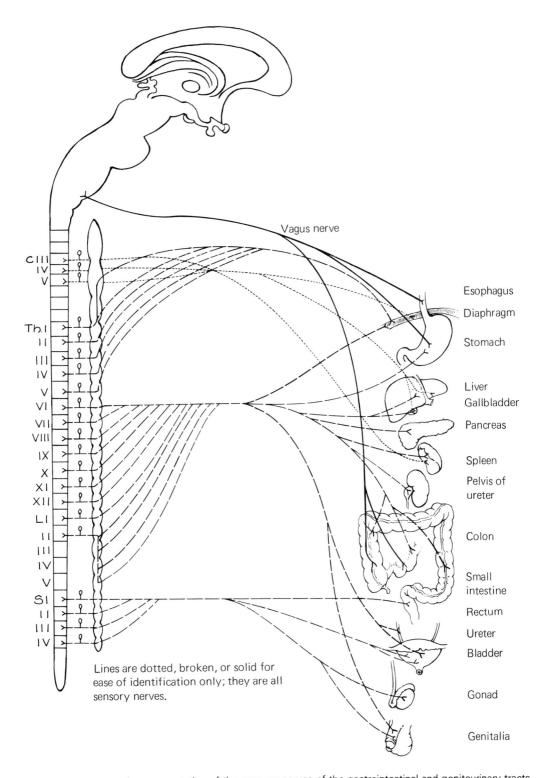

Figure 3–3. Diagrammatic representation of the sensory nerves of the gastrointestinal and genitourinary tracts.

SYMPTOMS RELATED TO THE ACT OF URINATION

Many conditions cause symptoms of "cystitis." These include infections of the bladder, vesical inflammation due to chemical or x-ray radiation reactions, interstitial cystitis, prostatitis, senile urethritis, psychoneurosis, torsion or rupture of an ovarian cyst, and foreign bodies in the bladder. Often, however, the patient with chronic cystitis notices no symptoms of vesical irritability. In children who have taken bubble baths, symptoms resembling cystitis may be noted secondary to the resulting urethritis.

Frequency, Nocturia, & Urgency

The normal capacity of the bladder is about 400 mL. Frequency may be caused by residual urine, which decreases the functional capacity of the organ. When the mucosa, submucosa, and even the muscularis become inflamed (eg, infection, foreign body, stones, tumor), the capacity of the bladder decreases sharply. This decrease is due to 2 factors: the pain resulting from even mild stretching of the bladder and the loss of bladder elasticity resulting from inflammatory edema. When the bladder is normal, urination can be delayed if circumstances require it, but this is not so in acute cystitis. Once the diminished bladder capacity is reached, any further distention may be agonizing, and the patient may actually urinate involuntarily if voiding does not occur immediately. During very severe acute infections, the desire to urinate may be constant, and each voiding may produce only a few milliliters of urine. Day frequency without nocturia and acute or chronic frequency lasting only a few hours suggest nervous tension (see Chapter 36).

Diseases that cause fibrosis of the bladder are accompanied by frequency of urination. Examples of such diseases are tuberculosis, interstitial cystitis, and bilharziasis. The presence of stones or foreign bodies causes vesical irritability, but secondary infection is almost always present.

Nocturia is often a symptom of renal disease related to a decrease in the functioning renal parenchyma with loss of concentrating power. Nocturia may occur in the absence of disease in persons who drink excessive amounts of fluids in the late evening. Coffee and alcoholic beverages, because of their specific diuretic effect, often produce nocturia if consumed just before bedtime. In older people who are ambulatory, some fluid retention may develop secondary to mild heart failure or varicose veins. With recumbency at night, this fluid is mobilized, leading to nocturia in these patients.

A very low or very high urine pH can irritate the bladder and cause frequency of urination. In chronic obstructive pulmonary disease, the Pa_{CO_2} is elevated. Compensation requires increased urinary excretion of chloride, leading to a low pH (Farcon & Morales, 1972). With hyperventilation, the urine becomes strongly alkaline.

Burning Upon Urination

This is common in acute cystitis and prostatitis. In men, it is usually felt in the distal urethra just proximal to or in the glans. In women, it is ordinarily referred to the urethra. It is important to remember that it is rarely felt in the suprapubic area. This burning sensation occurs in association with the act of urination, although it may be more marked at the beginning of, during, at the end of, or occasionally after urination. It may be very severe. Vague pain in the urethra not associated with the act of voiding is usually not caused by urinary system disease. In men, it is apt to be a psychosexual symptom; in women, however, it may occasionally be caused by chronic urethritis.

Enuresis

Strictly speaking, enuresis means bedwetting at night. It is physiologic during the first 2 or 3 years of life but becomes troublesome, particularly to parents, after that age. It may be functional or secondary to delayed neuromuscular maturation of the urethrovesical component, but it may present as a symptom of organic disease (eg, infection, distal urethral stenosis in girls, posterior urethral valves in boys, neurogenic or neuropathic bladder). If, however, wetting occurs also during the daytime or if there are other urinary symptoms—or if the enuresis persists beyond age 6 or 7—urologic investigation is essential. In adult life, enuresis may be replaced by nocturia for which no organic basis can be found.

Symptoms of Prostatic Obstruction

(See also Chapters 10 and 18.)

A. Hesitancy and Straining: Hesitancy in initiating the urinary stream is one of the early symptoms of enlarged prostate. As the degree of obstruction increases, hesitancy is prolonged; the patient may have to strain in order to initiate urination.

B. Loss of Force and Decrease of Caliber of the Stream: Progressive loss of force and caliber of the urinary stream is noted as urethral resistance increases despite the generation of increased intravesical pressure.

C. Terminal Dribbling: This becomes more and more noticeable as obstruction progresses and is a most distressing symptom.

D. Acute Urinary Retention: Sudden inability to urinate may supervene. The patient experiences increasingly agonizing suprapubic pain associated with severe urgency and may dribble only small amounts of urine.

E. Chronic Urinary Retention: This may cause little discomfort to the patient even though there is great hesitancy in starting the stream and marked reduction of its force and caliber. Constant dribbling of urine (paradoxic incontinence) may be experienced. It may be likened to water pouring over a dam.

F. Interruption of the Urinary Stream: Interruption may be abrupt and accompanied by severe pain radiating down the urethra. This type of reaction strongly suggests the complication of vesical calculus.

G. Sense of Residual Urine: The patient often feels that urine is still in the bladder even after urination has been completed.

H. Cystitis: Recurring episodes of acute cystitis suggest the presence of residual urine.

Symptoms of Urethral Obstruction

In the male, the combination of a slow and bifurcated stream suggests urethral stricture. A slow, weak stream in the male infant or little boy is compatible with posterior urethral valves or congenital urethral stricture.

Little girls with or without urinary infection may have a slow, hesitant, or interrupted stream. This should suggest involuntary spasm of the periurethral striated musculature secondary to distal urethral stenosis (see Chapter 30). Some women complain of constant impairment of urinary flow, in which case the possibility of urethral stricture should be investigated. Often, however, careful questioning will reveal that some voidings are slow, whereas others are quite free. This is compatible with periodic periurethral muscle spasm on a psychogenic basis, or with urethritis.

Incontinence

There are many reasons for incontinence. The history often gives a clue to its cause.

A. True Incontinence: The patient may lose urine without warning; this may be a constant or periodic symptom. The more obvious causes include exstrophy of the bladder, epispadias, vesicovaginal fistula, and ectopic ureteral orifice. Injury to the urethral smooth muscle sphincters may occur during prostatectomy or childbirth. Congenital or acquired neurogenic diseases may lead to dysfunction of the bladder and incontinence.

B. Stress Incontinence: When slight weakness of the sphincteric mechanisms is present, urine may be lost in association with physical strain (eg, coughing, laughing, rising from a chair). This is common with vesical neurogenic disease. The patient stays dry while lying in bed.

C. Urgency Incontinence: This type of urgency may be so precipitate and severe that there is involuntary loss of urine. Urgency incontinence not infrequently occurs with acute cystitis, particularly in women, since they seem to have relatively poor anatomic sphincters. Urgency incontinence is a common symptom of an upper motor neuron lesion. It is often seen also in tense, anxious women even in the absence of infection.

D. Paradoxic (Overflow or False) Incontinence: This is loss of urine due to chronic urinary retention or secondary to a flaccid bladder. The intravesical pressure finally equals the urethral resistance; urine then constantly dribbles forth.

Oliguria & Anuria

Oliguria and anuria may be caused by acute renal failure (due to shock or dehydration), fluid-ion imbalance, or bilateral ureteral obstruction.

Pneumaturia

The passage of gas in the urine almost always means that there is a fistula between the urinary tract and the bowel. This occurs most commonly in the bladder or urethra but may be seen also in the ureter or renal pelvis. Carcinoma of the sigmoid colon, diverticulitis with abscess formation, regional enteritis, and trauma cause most vesical fistulas. Congenital anomalies account for most ureteroenteric fistulas. Certain bacteria, by the process of fermentation, may rarely liberate gas.

Cloudy Urine

Patients often complain of cloudy urine, but it is most often cloudy merely because it is alkaline; this causes precipitation of phosphate. Chyluria is a rare cause of cloudy urine. A properly performed urinalysis will reveal the cause of cloudiness.

Bloody Urine

Hematuria is a danger signal that cannot be ignored. It is important to know whether urination is painful or not, whether the hematuria is associated with symptoms of vesical irritability, and whether blood is seen in all or only a portion of the urinary stream. Some individuals (particularly if they are anemic) will pass red urine after eating beets or taking laxatives containing phenolphthalein, in which case the urine is translucent rather than opaque and contains no red cells. Because of the wide use of rhodamine B as a coloring agent in cookies, cakes, cold drinks, and fruit juices, children commonly pass red urine after the ingestion of these foods. This is the so-called Monday morning disorder. The hemoglobinuria that occurs as a feature of the hemolytic syndromes may also cause the urine to be red.

A. Bloody Urine in Relation to Symptoms and Diseases: Hematuria associated with renal colic suggests ureteral stone, although a clot from a bleeding renal tumor can cause the same type of pain.

Hematuria is not uncommonly associated with nonspecific or tuberculous infection of the bladder. The bleeding is often terminal (bladder neck or prostate), although it may be present throughout urination (vesical or upper tract). Stone in the bladder often causes hematuria, but infection is usually present, and there are symptoms of bladder neck obstruction, neurogenic bladder, or cystocele. When a tumor of the bladder ulcerates, it is often complicated by infection and bleeding. Thus, symptoms of cystitis and hematuria are also compatible with neoplasm.

Dilated veins may develop at the bladder neck secondary to enlargement of the prostate. These may rupture when the patient strains to urinate.

Hematuria without other symptoms ("silent") must be regarded as a symptom of tumor of the bladder or kidney until proved otherwise. It is usually intermittent; bleeding may not recur for months. Complacency because the bleeding stops spontaneously must be condemned. Less common causes of silent hematuria are staghorn calculus, polycystic kidneys, solitary renal cyst, sickle cell disease, and hydronephrosis. Painless bleeding is common with acute glomerulonephritis. Recurrent bleeding is occasionally seen in children suffering from focal glomerulitis.

Richie & Kerr (1979) remind us that white patients can have sickle cell trait. Joggers frequently develop transient proteinuria and gross or microscopic hematuria (Boileau & others, 1980).

B. Time of Hematuria: Learning whether the hematuria is partial (initial, terminal) or total (present throughout urination) is often of help in identifying the site of bleeding. Initial hematuria suggests an anterior urethral lesion (eg, urethritis, stricture, meatal stenosis in young boys). Terminal hematuria usually arises from the posterior urethra, bladder neck, or trigone. Among the common causes are posterior urethritis and polyps and tumors of the vesical neck.

Total hematuria has its source at or above the level of the bladder (eg, stone, tumor, tuberculosis, nephritis).

Unusual Consequences of Micturition

Postmicturition syncope has been observed occasionally in men. Orthostatic hypotension and cardiac standstill have been observed in one patient. Psychomotor epilepsy and angina pectoris may be triggered by voiding.

MANIFESTATIONS RELATED TO SEXUAL ORGANS

Symptoms

Many people suffer from genitourinary complaints on a purely psychologic or emotional basis. In others, organic symptoms may be increased in severity because of tension states. It is therefore important to seek clues which might give evidence of emotional stress.

In women, the relationship of the menses to ureteral pain or vesical complaints should be determined, although menstruation may exacerbate both organic and functional vesical and renal difficulties.

Many patients, particularly women, recognize that the state of their "nerves" has a direct effect on their symptoms. They often realize that their "cystitis" develops following a tension-producing or anxiety-producing episode in their personal or occupational environment.

A. Sex Difficulties in the Male: Men may complain directly of sexual difficulty. However, they are often so ashamed of loss of sexual power that they cannot admit it even to a physician. In such cases they may ask for "prostate treatment" and hope that the physician will understand that they have sexual complaints and that they will be treated accordingly. The main sexual symptoms include impaired quality of erection, premature loss of erection, absence of ejaculate with orgasm, premature ejaculation, and even loss of desire. Since these symptoms are usually of psychologic origin, this area must therefore be explored.

B. Sex Difficulties in the Female: Women suffering from the psychosomatic cystitis syndrome almost always admit to an unhappy sex life. They notice that frequency or vaginal-urethral pain often occurs on the day following the incomplete sexual act. Many of them recognize the inadequacy of their sexual experiences as one of the underlying causes of urologic complaints; too frequently, however, the doctor either does not ask them pertinent questions or, if patients volunteer this information, ignores it.

In treating sex difficulties of suspected psychosomatic origin, the physician should explore pertinent facts concerning childhood, adolescence (sex education and experiences), marriage problems, and relationships with relatives, business associates, etc. Even if psychosomatic disease is strongly suspected before history-taking has been completed, a thorough examination and laboratory survey must be done. Both psyche and soma may be involved, and the patient must be assured that there is no serious organic disease. Although sexual interest and activity decline with advancing years, physically healthy men may continue to be sexually active into their eighth or ninth decades.

Objective Manifestations

(See also Infertility, Chapter 35).

On occasion, a patient may have objective signs. The most common include urethral discharge, lesions of the skin, and scrotal, perineal, or abdominal masses.

Another symptom referable to the sex organs is bloody ejaculation. This is usually caused by hypertrophy of the mucosa of the seminal vesicles.

•　•　•

References

Local & Referred Pain

DeWolf WC, Fraley EE: Renal pain. *Urology* 1975;6:403.

Dowd JB: Flank pain in nonurologic disease. *Med Clin North Am* 1963;47:437.

Smith DR, Raney FL Jr: Radiculitis distress as a mimic of renal pain. *J Urol* 1976;116:269.

Gastrointestinal Symptoms of Urologic Diseases

Takacs FJ: The interrelationships of gastrointestinal and renal diseases. *Med Clin North Am* 1966;50:507.

Symptoms Related to the Act of Urination

Bennett MA, Heslop RW, Meynell MJ: Massive haematuria associated with sickle-cell trait. *Br Med J* 1967;1:677.

Boileau M & others: Stress hematuria: Athletic pseudonephritis in marathoners. *Urology* 1980;15:471.

Davidson AIG, Matheson NA: Ovarian cysts and urinary symptoms. *Br J Surg* 1964;51:908.

Farcon EM, Morales PA: The association of chronic obstructive pulmonary disease (COPD) and lower urinary tract symptoms. *J Urol* 1972;108:619.

Fiala M & others: Role of adenovirus type II in hemorrhagic cystitis secondary to immunosuppression. *J Urol* 1974;112:595.

Glasgow EF, Moncrieff MW, White RHR: Symptomless haematuria in childhood. *Br Med J* 1970;2:687.

Hoffman RB, Zucker MO: A new technique in the treatment of renal bleeding: Epinephrine infusion in a patient with sickle cell trait. *Calif Med* (June) 1973;118:49.

Koehler PR, Kyaw MM: Hematuria. *Med Clin North Am* 1975;59:201.

Kounis NG, Kenmure AC: Micturition syncope, hypokalemia, and atrial fibrillation. *JAMA* 1976;236:954.

Levin S: Red urine: The Monday morning disorder of children. *Pediatrics* 1965;36:134.

Low AI, Matz LR: Haematuria and renal fornical lesions. *Br J Urol* 1972;44:681.

Marshall S: The effect of bubble bath on the urinary tract. *J Urol* 1965;93:112.

Morris JJ, McIntosh HD: Angina of micturition. *Circulation* 1963;27:85.

Richie JP, Kerr WS Jr: Sickle cell trait: Forgotten cause of hematuria in white patients. *J Urol* 1979;122:134.

Schoenberg BS, Kuglitsch JF, Varnes WE: Micturition syncope: Not a single entity. *JAMA* 1974;229:1631.

Spear GS & others: Idiopathic hematuria of childhood: Pathologic findings in the kidney in six patients. *Hum Pathol* 1973;4:349.

Tresidder GC: "Prostatism." *Practitioner* 1974;212:208.

Wiggelinkhuizen J, Landman C, Greenberg E: Chyluria. *Am J Dis Child* 1972;124:99.

Zivin I, Rowley W: Psychomotor epilepsy with micturition. *Arch Intern Med* 1964;113:8.

4 | Physical Examination of the Genitourinary Tract

Donald R. Smith, MD

The history will suggest whether a complete or partial examination is indicated. The symptom of urethral discharge probably does not require a thorough physical examination; on the other hand, painless hematuria would certainly require a careful examination of the genitourinary tract. In this chapter are discussed the urologic aspects of the physical examination of the patient.

EXAMINATION OF THE KIDNEYS

Inspection

On occasion, a mass may be visible in the upper abdominal area which, if soft (eg, as in hydronephrosis), may be difficult to palpate. Fullness in the costovertebral angle may be consistent with malignancy (eg, neuroblastoma in children) or perinephric infection. The presence and persistence of indentations in the skin from lying on wrinkled sheets suggest edema of the skin secondary to perinephric abscess. If this disease is suspected, have the patient lie on a rough towel and observe for indentations.

Palpation of the Kidneys

The kidneys lie rather high under the diaphragm and lower ribs and are therefore well protected from injury. Because of the position of the liver, the right kidney is lower than the left. The kidneys are difficult to palpate in men because of the resistance of abdominal muscle tone and because the kidneys in men are more fixed than those of women and move only slightly with change of posture or respiration. The lower part of the right kidney can sometimes be felt, but the left kidney cannot usually be felt unless it is grossly enlarged or displaced.

The most successful method of renal palpation is carried out with the patient lying supine on a hard surface (Fig 4–1). The kidney is lifted by one hand in the costovertebral angle. On deep inspiration, the kidney moves downward, and when it is lowest the other hand is pushed firmly and deeply beneath the costal margin in an effort to trap the kidney below that point. If this is successful, the anterior hand can palpate the size, shape, and consistency of the organ as it slips back into its normal position.

The kidney can sometimes best be palpated

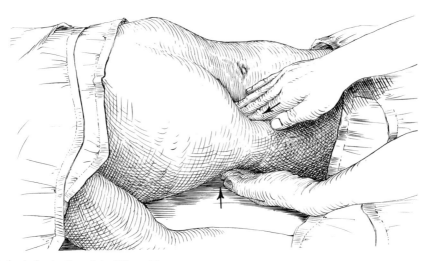

Figure 4–1. Method of palpation of the kidney. The posterior hand lifts the kidney upward. The anterior hand feels for the kidney. The patient then takes a deep breath; this causes the kidney to descend. As the patient inhales, the fingers of the anterior hand are plunged inward at the costal margin. If the kidney is mobile or enlarged, it can be felt between the 2 hands.

with the examiner standing behind the seated patient. At other times, if the patient is lying on one side, the uppermost kidney drops downward and medially, thereby making it more accessible to palpation.

Perlman & Williams (1976) have described a very effective method of identifying renal anomalies in the newborn. The fingers are placed in the costovertebral angle, with the thumb anterior. The thumb does the feeling. With this technic, the kidneys can be palpated 95% of the time. Anomalies were found in 0.5% of 11,000 neonates.

An enlarged renal mass suggests compensatory hypertrophy (if the other kidney is absent or atrophic), hydronephrosis, tumor, cyst, or polycystic disease. A mass in this area, however, may be a retroperitoneal tumor, the spleen, a lesion of the bowel (eg, tumor, abscess), a lesion of the gallbladder, or a pancreatic cyst. Tumors may have the consistency of normal tissue; they may also be nodular. Hydronephroses may be firm or soft. Polycystic kidneys are usually nodular.

An acutely infected kidney is tender, but this is difficult to elicit, since marked muscle spasm is usually present. Since normal kidneys are often tender also, this sign is not always helpful.

Although renal pain may be diffusely felt in the back, tenderness is usually well localized just lateral to the sacrospinalis muscle and just below the 12th rib. This may be brought out by palpation or, more sharply, by fist percussion over that area.

Percussion of the Kidneys

At times a greatly enlarged kidney cannot be felt on palpation, particularly if it is soft. This can be true of hydronephrosis. Such masses, however, may be readily outlined by percussion, both anteriorly and posteriorly; this part of the examination should never be omitted. Percussion is of particular value in outlining an enlarging mass in the flank following renal trauma (progressive hemorrhage), where tenderness and muscle spasm prevent proper palpation.

Transillumination

This maneuver may prove quite helpful in the child under age 1 year who presents with a suprapubic or flank mass. A 2- or 3-cell flashlight with an opaque flange protruding beyond the lens is an adequate instrument. The flashlight is applied at right angles to the abdomen. The fiberoptic light cord, used to illuminate various optical instruments, is an excellent source of cold light. A dark room is required. A distended bladder or cystic mass will transilluminate; a solid mass will not. Flank masses may also be tested by applying the light posteriorly.

Differentiation of Renal & Radicular Pain

Radicular pain (see p 27) is commonly felt in the costovertebral and subcostal areas. It may spread along the course of the ureter as well and is the most common cause of so-called "kidney" pain. Every patient who complains of flank pain should be examined for evidence of nerve root irritation. Frequent causes are poor posture, arthritic changes in the costovertebral or costotransverse joints, impingement of a rib spur on a subcostal nerve, hypertrophy of costovertebral ligaments pressing on a nerve, and intervertebral disk disease (Smith & Raney, 1976). Radicular pain may be noted as an aftermath of a flank incision wherein a rib may become dislocated, causing the costal nerve to impinge on the edge of a ligament (Krauss, Khonsari, & Lilien, 1977). Pain experienced during the preeruptive phase of herpes zoster involving any of the segments between T11 and L2 may also simulate pain of renal origin.

Radiculitis usually causes hyperesthesia of the area of skin served by the irritated peripheral nerve. This hypersensitivity can be elicited by means of the pinwheel or by grasping and pinching both skin and fat of the abdomen and flanks. Pressure exerted by the thumb over the costovertebral joints will reveal local tenderness at the point of emergence of the involved peripheral nerve.

Auscultation

Auscultation of the costovertebral areas and upper abdominal quadrants may reveal a systolic bruit which is often associated with stenosis or aneurysm of the renal artery. Bruits over the femoral arteries may be found in association with the Leriche syndrome, which may be a cause of impotence.

EXAMINATION OF THE BLADDER

The bladder cannot be felt unless it is moderately distended. In the adult, if it is percussible, it contains at least 150 mL of urine. In acute or (more commonly) in chronic urinary retention, the bladder may reach or even rise above the umbilicus, in which case its outline may be seen and usually felt. (In chronic retention, where the bladder wall is flabby, the bladder may be difficult to palpate. In this instance, percussion is of great value.)

In the male infant or little boy, palpation of a hard mass deep in the center of the pelvis is compatible with a thickened hypertrophied bladder secondary to obstruction caused by posterior urethral valves.

A sliding inguinal hernia containing some bladder wall can be diagnosed (when the bladder is full) by compressing the scrotal mass. The bladder will be found to further distend.

A few instances have been reported wherein marked edema of the legs has developed secondary to compression of the iliac vessels by a distended bladder. Bimanual (abdominorectal or abdominovaginal) palpation may reveal the extent of a vesical neoplasm. To be successful, it must be done under anesthesia.

EXAMINATION OF THE EXTERNAL MALE GENITALIA

PENIS

Inspection

If the patient has not been circumcised, the foreskin should be retracted. This may reveal tumor or balanitis as the cause of a foul discharge. If retraction is not possible (ie, phimosis), surgical correction (dorsal slit or circumcision) is indicated.

The observation of a poor urinary stream is significant. In the newborn, neurogenic (neuropathic) bladder or the presence of posterior urethral valves should be considered. In men, such a finding suggests urethral stricture or prostatic obstruction.

The scars of healed syphilis may be an important clue. An active ulcer requires bacteriologic or pathologic study (eg, syphilitic chancre, epithelioma). Superficial ulcers or vesicles are compatible with herpes simplex; they are often interpreted by the patient as a serious venereal disease, possibly syphilis. Venereal warts may be observed.

Meatal stenosis is a common cause of bloody spotting in the male infant. On rare occasions, it may be of such degree as to cause advanced bilateral hydronephrosis. It is easily corrected by meatotomy.

The position of the meatus should be noted. It may be located proximal to the tip of the glans on either the dorsum (epispadias) or the ventral surface (hypospadias). In either instance, there is apt to be abnormal curvature of the penis—dorsally with epispadias, ventrally with hypospadias. The urethral orifice is often stenotic in the latter.

Palpation

Palpation of the dorsal surface of the shaft may reveal a fibrous plaque involving the fascial covering of the corpora cavernosa. This is typical of Peyronie's disease. Tender areas of induration felt along the urethra may signify periurethritis secondary to urethral stricture.

Urethral Discharge

Urethral discharge is the most common complaint referable to the male sex organ. Gonococcal pus is usually profuse, thick, and yellow or gray-brown. Nonspecific discharges may be similar in appearance but are often thin, mucoid, and scanty. Although gonorrhea must be ruled out as the cause of a urethral discharge, a high percentage of such cases will be found to be nonspecific. Patients with urethral discharge should also be examined for other venereal diseases; double infection is not uncommon.

Bloody discharge should suggest the possibility of a foreign body in the urethra (male or female), urethral stricture, or neoplasm.

Urethral discharge must always be sought before the patient is asked to void.

SCROTUM

Infections and inflammations of the skin of the scrotum are not common. Small sebaceous cysts are occasionally seen. Malignant tumors are rare. The scrotum is bifid when midscrotal or perineal hypospadias is present.

Elephantiasis of the scrotum is caused by obstruction to lymphatic drainage. It is endemic in the tropics and is due to filariasis. Elephantiasis may result from radical resection of the lymph nodes of the inguinal and femoral areas, in which case the skin of the penis is also involved. Small hemangiomas of the skin are common and may bleed spontaneously.

TESTIS

The testes should be carefully palpated with the fingers of both hands. A hard area in the testis proper must be regarded as a malignant tumor until proved otherwise. Transillumination of all scrotal masses should be a routine procedure. With the patient in a dark room, a strong flashlight is placed against the scrotal sac posteriorly. A hydrocele will cause the intrascrotal mass to glow red. Light will not be transmitted through a solid tumor. Tumors are often smooth but may be nodular. They seem abnormally heavy. A testis replaced by tumor or damaged by gumma is insensitive to pressure, and the usual sickening sensation is absent. About 10% of tumors are associated with a secondary hydrocele that may have to be aspirated before definitive palpation can be done.

The testis may be absent from the scrotum. This may represent transient (physiologic retractile testis) or true cryptorchidism. Palpation of the groins may reveal the presence of the organ.

The atrophic testis (following postoperative orchiopexy, mumps orchitis, or torsion of the spermatic cord) is usually flabby and at times hypersensitive. Although spermatogenesis may be lost, androgen function is usually maintained.

EPIDIDYMIS

The epididymis is sometimes rather closely attached to the posterior surface of the testis, and at other times it is quite free of it. The epididymis should be carefully palpated for size and induration. Induration means infection (primary tumors are exceedingly rare).

In the acute stage of epididymitis, the testis and epididymis are indistinguishable by palpation; the testicle and epididymis may be adherent to the scrotum, which is usually quite red. Tenderness is exquisite.

Chronic painless induration should suggest tuberculosis, although nonspecific chronic epididymitis is also a possibility. Other signs of tuberculosis of the genitourinary tract usually present include "sterile" pyuria, a thickened seminal vesicle, a nodular prostate, and "beading" of the vas deferens.

SPERMATIC CORD & VAS DEFERENS

A swelling in the spermatic cord may be cystic (eg, hydrocele or hernia) or solid (eg, connective tissue tumor). The latter is rare. Lipoma in the investing fascia of the cord may simulate hernia. Diffuse swelling and induration of the cord are seen with filarial funiculitis.

Careful palpation of the vas deferens may reveal thickening (eg, chronic infection), fusiform enlargements (the "beading" caused by tuberculosis), or even its absence. The latter finding is of importance in the infertile male; it is rare.

TESTICULAR TUNICS & ADNEXA

Hydroceles are usually cystic but on occasion are so tense that they simulate solid tumors. Transillumination makes the differential diagnosis. They may develop secondary to nonspecific acute or tuberculous epididymitis, trauma, or tumor of the testis. The latter is a distinct possibility if hydrocele appears "spontaneously" between the ages of 18 and 35. It should be aspirated to permit careful palpation of underlying structures.

Hydrocele usually surrounds the testis completely. Cystic masses that are separate from but in the region of the upper pole of the testis are probably spermatoceles. Aspiration reveals the typical thin, milky fluid, which contains sperms.

VAGINAL EXAMINATION

Diseases of the female genital tract may secondarily involve the urinary organs, thereby making a thorough gynecologic examination essential. Commonly associated are urethrocystitis secondary to urethral diverticulitis or cervicitis, pyelonephritis during pregnancy, and ureteral obstruction from metastatic nodes or direct extension in cancer of the cervix.

Inspection

The urinary meatus may reveal a reddened, tender, friable lesion (urethral caruncle) or a reddened, everted posterior lip, which is often seen with senile urethritis and vaginitis. Biopsy is indicated if a malignant tumor cannot be ruled out. Smears of discharges should be made. The diagnosis of senile vaginitis (and urethritis) is established by staining a smear of the vaginal epithelium with Lugol's solution. It should be examined immediately after rinsing, because the brown dye in the cells fades quickly. Cells lacking glycogen (hypoestrogenism) do not take up the stain, whereas normal cells do.

Evidence of skenitis and bartholinitis may reveal the source of persistent urethritis or cystitis. The condition of the vaginal wall should be observed. Bacteriologic study of the secretions may be helpful. Urethrocele and cystocele may cause residual urine and lead to persistent infection of the bladder. They are often found in association with stress incontinence. A bulge in the anterior vaginal wall might represent a urethral diverticulum. The cervix should be inspected in order to note the presence of cancer or infection. Taking biopsy specimens or making Papanicolaou preparations may be indicated.

Palpation

At times the urethra, the base of the bladder, and the lower ureters may be tender on palpation, but little can be deduced from this. Induration of the urethra or trigonal area or a mass involving either may be a clue to an existing neoplasm. A soft mass found in this area could be a urethral diverticulum. Pressure on such a lesion may cause pus to extrude from the urethra. A stone in the lower ureter may be palpable. Evidence of enlargement of the uterus (eg, pregnancy, myomas) or diseases or inflammations of the colon or adnexa may afford a clue to the cause of urinary symptoms (eg, compression of a ureter by a malignant ovarian tumor, endometriosis, or diverticulitis of sigmoid colon adherent to the bladder).

Carcinoma of the cervix may invade the base of the bladder, causing vesical irritability or hematuria; or its metastases to iliac lymph nodes may compress the ureters.

Rectal examination may afford further information and is the obvious route of examination in children and virgins.

RECTAL EXAMINATION OF THE MALE

SPHINCTER & LOWER RECTUM

The estimation of sphincter tone is of great importance. Laxity of the muscle strongly suggests similar changes in the urinary sphincters and detrusor and may be a clue to the diagnosis of neurogenic disease. In addition to the digital prostatic examination, the examiner should palpate the entire lower rectum and rule out stenosis, internal hemorrhoids, cryptitis, rectal fistulas, mucosal polyps, and rectal malignancies.

PROSTATE

Before the rectal examination is made, a specimen of urine for routine analysis should be collected. This is of the utmost importance, since prostatic massage (or even palpation at times) will force prostatic secretion into the posterior urethra. If this secretion contains pus, a specimen of urine voided after the rectal examination will be contaminated by it.

Size

The average prostate is about 4 cm in length and width. It is widest superiorly at the bladder neck. As the gland enlarges, the lateral sulci become relatively deeper and the median furrow becomes obliterated. The prostate may also elongate. It is necessary to realize that the clinical importance of prostatic hyperplasia is measured by the severity of symptoms and the amount of residual urine and not by the size of the gland. On rectal examination,

the prostate may be of normal size and consistency in a patient with acute urinary retention.

Consistency

Normally, the consistency of the gland is similar to that of the contracted thenar eminence of the thumb (with the thumb completely opposed to the little finger). It is rather rubbery. It may be mushy if congested (due to lack of intercourse or to chronic infection with impaired drainage), indurated (due to chronic infection with or without calculi), or stony-hard (due to advanced carcinoma).

The difficulty lies in differentiating firm areas in the prostate: fibrosis from nonspecific infection, granulomatous prostatitis, nodulation from tuberculosis, or firm areas due to prostatic calculi or early cancer. Generally speaking, nodules caused by infection are raised above the surface of the gland. At their edges, the induration gradually fades to the normal softness of surrounding tissue. In cancer, conversely, the suspicious lesion is usually not raised; it is hard and has a sharp edge, ie, there is an abrupt change in consistency on the same plane. It tends to arise in the lateral sulcus (Fig 4–2).

Even the most experienced clinicians sometimes have trouble making this differentiation. In the absence of other signs of tuberculosis and in the absence of pus in the prostatic secretion, cancer is likely, particularly if an x-ray fails to show prostatic calculi (which are seen just behind or above the symphysis). Serum acid phosphatase determinations and radiographs of bones are of no help in diagnosing early carcinoma of the prostate.

Mobility

The mobility of the gland varies. Occasionally, it has great mobility; at other times, very little. With advanced carcinoma, it is fixed because of local extension through the capsule. The prostate

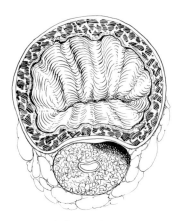

Inflammatory

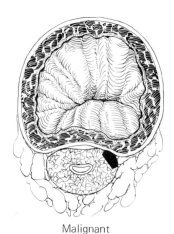

Malignant

Figure 4–2. Differential diagnosis of prostatic nodules. *Left:* Inflammatory area is raised above the surface of the gland; induration decreases gradually at its periphery. *Right:* Cancerous nodule is not raised; there is an abrupt change in consistency at its edges.

should be routinely massaged in the adult and its secretion examined microscopically. It should not be massaged, however, in the presence of an acute urethral discharge, acute prostatitis, or acute prostatocystitis; in men near the stage of complete urinary retention (because it may precipitate complete retention); or in men suffering from obvious cancer of the gland. Even without symptoms, massage is necessary, for prostatitis is commonly asymptomatic. Diagnosis and treatment of such silent disease is important in preventing cystitis and epididymitis.

Technic of Massage

The patient should lean over the examining table so that his body is horizontal. His legs should be straight and his feet somewhat apart.

Methods of massage vary, but the basic maneuver is to press the gland substance firmly with the pad of the index finger in order to express secretion into the prostatic urethra. Start laterally and superiorly and massage toward the midline. A rolling motion of the finger is less traumatic to the rectal mucosa and prostate gland and is better tolerated by the patient. Finally, the seminal vesicles should be stripped from above downward and medially (Fig 4–3).

Copious amounts of secretion may be obtained from some prostate glands and little or none from others. This of course depends to some extent upon the vigor with which the massage is carried out. If no secretion is obtained, have the patient void even a few drops of urine; this will contain adequate

secretion for examination. Microscopic examination of the secretion is done under low-power magnification. Normal secretion contains numerous lecithin bodies, which are refractile, like red cells, but much smaller than red cells. Only an occasional white cell is present. A few epithelial cells and, rarely, corpora amylacea are seen. Sperms may be present, but their absence is of no significance.

The presence of large numbers of pus cells is pathologic and suggests the diagnosis of prostatitis. Stained smears are usually impractical. It is difficult to fix this material on the slide, and even when this is successful, pyogenic bacteria are usually not found. Acid-fast organisms can often be found by appropriate staining methods.

On occasion it may be necessary to obtain cultures of prostatic secretion in order to demonstrate nonspecific organisms or *Mycobacterium tuberculosis*. After thorough cleansing of the glans and emptying of the bladder (to mechanically cleanse the urethra), massage is done. Drops of secretion are collected in a sterile tube of culture medium.

SEMINAL VESICLES

Palpation of the seminal vesicles should be attempted. The vesicles are situated under the base of the bladder and diverge from below upward (Figs 1–7 and 4–3). Normal seminal vesicles are usually not palpable, but when they are overdistended they may feel quite cystic. In the presence of chronic

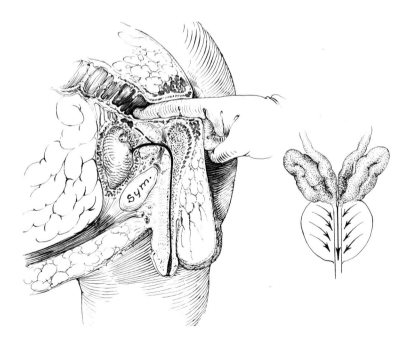

Figure 4–3. Technic of prostatic massage. The glandular substance is compressed from its lateral edges to the urethra, which lies in the center. (Drawing at right shows direction of pressure.) The seminal vesicles are then stripped from above downward.

infection (particularly tuberculosis) or in association with advanced carcinoma of the prostate, they may be markedly indurated. Stripping of the seminal vesicles should be done in association with prostatic massage, for the vesicles are usually infected when prostatitis is present. Primary tumors of the vesicles are very rare.

EXAMINATION OF LYMPH NODES
(Figs 18–1 and 18–2)

Inguinal & Subinguinal Lymph Nodes

With inflammatory lesions of the skin of the penis and scrotum or vulva, the inguinal and subinguinal lymph nodes may be involved. Such diseases include chancroid, syphilitic chancre, lymphogranuloma venereum, and, on occasion, gonorrhea.

Malignant neoplasms (squamous cell carcinoma) involving the penis, glans, scrotal skin, or distal urethra in women metastasize to the inguinal and subinguinal nodes. Testicular tumors do not spread to these nodes unless they have invaded the scrotal skin or the patient has been subjected to previous orchiopexy.

Other Lymph Nodes

Tumors of the testis and prostate may involve the left supraclavicular nodes. Tumors of the bladder and prostate typically metastasize to the hypogastric, external iliac, and preaortic nodes, although only occasionally are they so large as to be palpable. Masses near the midline in the upper abdomen in a young man should suggest metastases from cancer of the testis; the primary growth may be minute and completely hidden in the substance of what appears to be a normal testicle.

NEUROLOGIC EXAMINATION

A careful neurologic survey may uncover sensory or motor impairment that will account for residual urine (neuropathic bladder) or incontinence. Since the bladder and its sphincter are innervated by the second to fourth sacral segments, much information can be gained by testing anal sphincter tone and the sensation of the perianal skin and by eliciting the Achilles tendon and bulbocavernosus reflexes. The bulbocavernosus reflex is normal if, with a finger in the rectum, the external anal sphincter and bulbocavernosus muscle can be felt to contract when the glans penis or clitoris is squeezed or an indwelling Foley catheter is jerked. If no contraction occurs, interruption of the sacral reflex arc (lower motor neuron lesion) is present.

It is wise, particularly in children, to seek a dimple over the lumbosacral area. Palpate the sacrum to be sure it is present and normally formed. Sacral agenesis or partial development is compatible with deficits of S2–4. If findings seem abnormal, x-ray examination is indicated.

•   •   •

References

Examination of the Kidneys

Hodges CV, Barry JM: Non-urologic flank pain: A diagnostic approach. *J Urol* 1975;113:644.

Koop CE: Abdominal mass in the newborn infant. *N Engl J Med* 1973;289:569.

Krauss DJ, Khonsari F, Lilien OM: Incapacitating flank pain of questionable origin. *Urology* 1977;9:51.

Marshall S, Lapp M, Schulte JW: Lesions of the pancreas mimicking renal disease. *J Urol* 1965;93:41.

Mofenson HC, Greensher J: Transillumination of the abdomen in infants. *Am J Dis Child* 1968;115:428.

Perlman M, Williams J: Detection of renal anomalies by abdominal palpation in newborn infants. *Br Med J* 1976;3:347.

Smith DR, Raney FL Jr: Radiculitis distress as a mimic of renal pain. *J Urol* 1976;116:269.

Examination of the Bladder

Boyarsky S, Goldenberg J: Detection of bladder distention by suprapubic percussion. *NY State J Med* 1962;62:1804.

Carlsson E, Garsten P: Compression of the common iliac vessels by dilatation of the bladder. *Acta Radiol* 1960;53:449.

Patil UB: Estimation of residual urine in bladder: Use of vesical "thrill" test. *Urology* 1974;4:737.

External Genitalia in the Female

Redman JF, Bissada NK: How to make a good examination of the genitalia of young girls. *Clin Pediatr (Phila)* 1976;15:907.

Neurologic Examination

Bors E, Blenn KA: Bulbocavernosus reflex. *J Urol* 1959;82:128.

Urologic Laboratory Examination | 5

Donald R. Smith, MD

BLOOD COUNT

Hypochromic anemia may occur in association with chronic pyelonephritis, uremia, and carcinoma. Most infections will be accompanied by an increased white cell count with a shift to the left.

Erythrocytosis has been noted in association with 3–4% of urologic renal diseases, including carcinoma, hydronephrosis, and simple cyst. A number of instances have also been seen in association with uterine myomas and hepatoma. The erythropoietin level in the plasma is increased. Following definitive surgery, the erythropoietin level and the increased red cell count return to normal. If metastases develop later, erythrocytosis returns. (**Note:** Platelets, leukocytes, and other blood elements are usually not increased; the term polycythemia as applied to red blood cell count elevation in these disorders is a misnomer.)

EXAMINATION OF URETHRAL DISCHARGE IN THE MALE

A specimen of the discharge should be obtained before the patient voids. If discharge is absent at the time of examination, the urethra should be "milked," or the first portion of the voided urine can be collected and centrifuged. This sediment is similar to gross discharge. Since many men harbor gonococci in the absence of discharge, the first portion of the urine should be cultured if gonorrhea is suspected. The combination of stained smear of discharge and urine culture has yielded a positive diagnosis in 99% of subjects (Feng, Medeiros, & Murray, 1977).

The sediment or the actual discharge should be examined while wet. Trichomonads are seen as motile round bodies that are a little larger than pus cells. They may be cultured in a liquid liver or other suitable medium. The presence of lecithin bodies suggests that the discharge may be of prostatic origin. Pus and epithelial cells should be noted. If many epithelial cells are seen, chronic infection is probably present.

These secretions should also be stained. Methylene blue preparations permit clear observation of bacterial morphology. If cocci are present, Gram's stain (for gonococci) must be done.

EXAMINATION OF THE URINE

Urinalysis is without doubt the most important and most fruitful of all laboratory screening tests, yet it is the most poorly performed laboratory test in all medicine. There are 3 reasons for the inadequacy of so many urinalyses: (1) the urine is too often improperly collected, (2) it is not examined when fresh, and (3) examination of the sediment is frequently incomplete.

It is essential that the urine specimen be collected before the rectal examination is made. This guarantees that the urine will not be contaminated by infected prostatic secretion that may drain into the posterior urethra following this manipulation.

Proper Collection of Urine

In both men and women, the urethra harbors bacteria and a few pus cells. Any urine specimen voided into a single container will for this reason be contaminated by the normal urethral flora. This immediately clouds the interpretation of microscopic findings or urine cultures and often leads to the diagnosis of cystitis when the bladder urine actually contains no pus cells or bacteria. This applies particularly to women, in whom voiding causes urine to flow over the vulva and, at times, into the vagina.

A. Collecting Specimens From Men: The simplest method of collecting urine from a man is to give him a clean glass and instruct him to start his stream into the toilet bowl or urinal. He should be instructed to retract a redundant foreskin. After the stream has thoroughly cleansed the urethra, it should be directed into the glass (without interrupting the act of urination); before voiding has been completed, the glass should be removed. This affords a "midstream" (second glass) specimen that is as clean as that obtained by catheter.

A "2-glass" test affords the most information. The patient is instructed to begin voiding in one glass. After 10–15 mL have been passed, the stream should be directed into the second glass. If the patient complains of a scant discharge but none can be expressed at the time of examination, the first glass will contain the elements of the discharge. It should be centrifuged and examined as discharge. Pus in the first glass without white cells in the second suggests urethritis.

B. Collecting Specimens From Women: Women should be placed in the lithotomy position. The labia are held apart. After the vulva has been cleansed—and with the labia still separated—the patient is instructed to start voiding into a bowl held close to the vulva. The midportion of the stream should be collected in a sterile container. It is almost impossible for a woman to accomplish this without help.

Catheterization is also satisfactory and should not be avoided because of the fear of introducing infection with the catheter; the advantages of obtaining a "sterile" specimen far overshadow this slight risk, which may be further diminished by thorough irrigation of the bladder and the instillation of 30–60 mL of 1:5000 aqueous chlorhexidine solution or 0.5% neomycin. The passage of a catheter of moderate size (22F) in women also permits exploration of the urethra and may reveal stenosis, which may be the predisposing cause of the urinary infection.

C. Collecting Specimens From Children: If the boy or girl is old enough to cooperate, a midstream specimen can be collected as described above for men and women. The use of a plastic bag (after thorough antiseptic cleansing) for collection of urine in the neonate and infant is unsatisfactory from the bacteriologic standpoint (Hardy, Furnell, & Brumfitt, 1976). Kelalis & others (1973) have shown that when little girls void in the supine position, more than half of them reflux urine into the vagina. Boehm & Haynes (1966), utilizing a technic they call "midstream catch," report minimal bacterial contamination. After feeding, and before the infant voids, the genital area is thoroughly cleansed with hexachlorophene detergent. The child is then held in the prone position (Fig 5–1). The spinal reflex of Perez is then elicited by stroking the back along the paravertebral muscles. Spontaneous voiding usually occurs within 5 minutes. The stream is directed into a sterile container.

One should not hesitate to catheterize little girls if other methods of urine collection fail (Redman & Bissada, 1976). If an immediate specimen is needed, suprapubic aspiration should be considered. Complications are rare (Pass & Waldo, 1979).

Examination While Fresh

The "morning urine" is not an adequate urine specimen for routine examination of the urinary sediment. Even though the specific gravity of such a specimen is acceptable as a fairly dependable renal function test, the urinary sediment is abnormally altered after standing a few hours. Red cells break up and casts disintegrate as the urine becomes al-

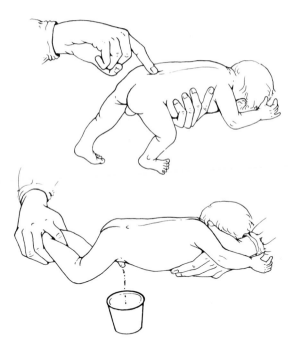

Figure 5–1. "Midstream catch" urine by the method of Boehm and Haynes. (Redrawn from Boehm JJ, Haynes JL: Bacteriology of "midstream catch" urines: Studies in newborn infants. *Am J Dis Child* 1966;111:366.)

kaline; bacteria, if not present in the fresh urine, enter the container and multiply rapidly. This can lead to the erroneous diagnosis of "urinary tract infection." Whether the physician is interested in the presence of red cells, casts, pus cells, or bacteria, a specimen that is not fresh is of little value. If urinalysis is to be a dependable technic, the specimen must be collected properly and examined immediately.

Schumann, Harris, & Henry (1978) have found that the study of urinary casts is enhanced by utilizing the Papanicolaou stain.

Microscopic Examination of Sediment After Centrifuging

The stained smear of urinary sediment, examined personally by the physician caring for the patient, is of the greatest importance as a screening test for the presence of bacteriuria. On occasion, although bacteria are seen on a stained smear, the cultures are reported as "negative." Since finding bacteria on a stained smear means that there are at least 10,000 organisms per milliliter, such a finding is pathognomonic of infection, and a negative culture report in this instance should be ignored. A stained smear gives quick information so that immediate treatment can be instituted; a culture takes many hours to complete, with loss of valuable time. Studies show that the correlation of stained smears with cultures is good (Littlewood, Jacobs, & Ramsden, 1977). If the patient has symptoms compatible with cystitis but pyuria and bacteriuria are absent, a culture should be obtained. This may negate the few errors encountered with the stained smear.

A. Wet Smear: This should be examined under low and medium power. White cells, red cells, crystals, and casts should be searched for, and the types of casts present should be noted (Fig 5–2). Squamous epithelial cells from the urethra and bladder neck are to be expected in the urine of the female; they are absent in men except in patients who are receiving estrogen therapy for cancer of the prostate. Trichomonads and yeast cells may also be seen.

B. Staining of the Sediment: Whether the wet smear reveals abnormalities or not, a stained smear must be examined. If pus cells appear to be present in a wet smear, staining of the sediment will aid in differentiating leukocytes and epithelial cells. The finding of transitional (mononuclear) epithelial cells, singly or in clumps, strongly suggests vesical neoplasm (Fig 5–3). The stained smear will also tentatively identify the bacteria. This will allow the physician to select an antibiotic or chemotherapeutic agent immediately and on the basis of objective clinical information. Staining the urine when pus is present may also reveal that no bacteria can be seen. Such a "sterile" pyuria strongly suggests tuberculosis of the urinary tract. Death from renal

tuberculosis may occur if the diagnosis is delayed, and late diagnosis is usually due to improperly performed urinalyses.

If no pus is found in the wet preparation, the sediment must still be stained, since about 30% of patients with chronic urinary tract infection or urinary stasis have apyuric bacteriuria. One should not wait for the presence of pyuria or symptoms suggesting urinary tract diseases before considering such a possibility. This means that routine urinalysis in all patients, no matter what their symptoms, requires staining of the urinary sediment; until this has been done, urinary tract infection has not been ruled out.

1. For pyogenic organisms–

a. Triple-strength methylene blue is the stain of choice:

Methylene blue	1.5
Alcohol	30.0
0.1 N potassium hydroxide	2.0
Distilled water, qs ad	120.0

An ampule of methylene blue prepared for intravenous use is also satisfactory.

Fix the sediment on the slide with heat. Take care to only *warm* the slide, since too much heat will distort the stained cells. Flood the slide with the dye for 10–20 seconds, then rinse and dry with mild heat. Do not blot, since this is apt to remove the sediment. It is helpful to mark the slide through

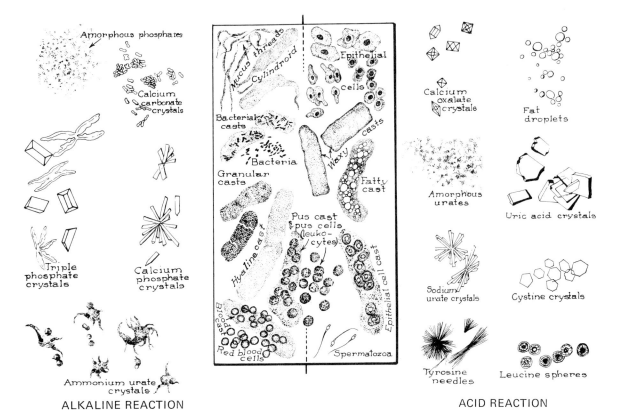

ALKALINE REACTION   ACID REACTION

Figure 5–2. Microscopic examination of urine sediment. (Redrawn after Todd & Sanford.)

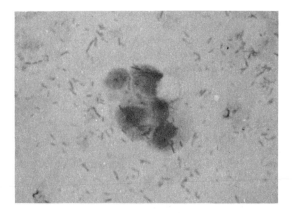

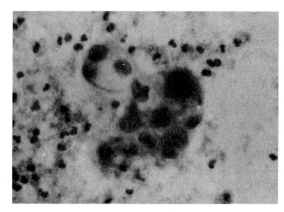

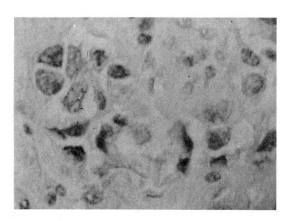

Figure 5–3. Urinary cytology. *Above left:* Triple-strength methylene blue stain of urinary sediment showing clumps of transitional cells with irregular and relatively large nuclei. Note presence of bacteria. *Above right:* Papanicolaou stain from same urinary sediment. Note similarity to methylene blue stain. *Left:* Biopsy of papillary vesical neoplasm from same patient. Clump of transitional cells in upper left hand corner is similar to those seen in urinary sediment.

the area containing the stained sediment with a red wax pencil before the immersion oil is applied. This allows the microscopist to find the plane of the sediment with ease when the oil immersion lens is used. A cover slip is not necessary.

b. Gram's stain is of limited value in the study of urinary sediment. If rods are found, they are usually gram-negative; if cocci are found, they are usually gram-positive. Gram's stain has the disadvantage of repeated staining and washing, which may cause the sediment to be washed from the slide. It is useful in the identification of the gonococcus.

(1) Fix smear by heat.

(2) Cover with crystal violet for 1 minute.

(3) Wash with water. Do not blot.

(4) Cover with Gram's iodine for 1 minute.

(5) Wash with water. Do not blot.

(6) Decolorize for 10–30 seconds with gentle agitation in acetone (30 mL) and alcohol (70 mL).

(7) Wash with water. Do not blot.

(8) Cover for 10–30 seconds with safranin (2.5% solution in 95% alcohol).

(9) Wash with water and let dry.

2. Acid-fast (Ziehl-Neelsen) stains–Acid-fast staining should be done if a "sterile pyuria" is found or if urinary tuberculosis is suspected. The centrifuged sediment from 15 mL of urine discloses

tubercle bacilli in half of such cases. If a 24-hour urine specimen is centrifuged, it will reveal tubercle bacilli in about 70–80%. The technic for Ziehl-Neelsen staining is as follows:

a. Stain heat-fixed smear with steaming Ziehl's carbolfuchsin for 5 minutes, or leave in cold stain for 24 hours. Cold Kinyoun carbolfuchsin acid-fast stain may be applied for 5 minutes.

b. Wash in tap water.

c. Decolorize with acid-alcohol until only a slight pink tinge remains.

d. Wash in tap water.

e. Counterstain with triple-strength methylene blue for 10–20 seconds.

f. Wash in tap water and dry with heat.

Cultures for Bacteria

A. Quantitative Cultures: Some type of quantitative estimation of the number of bacteria must be made. It is essential that the colony count be judged in the light of the specific gravity of the specimen (Friedman & Gladstone, 1971). A count of 1000 organisms per milliliter in urine with a specific gravity of 1.002 is significant. A similar count in 1.030 urine might be compatible with urethral contamination. If urine which is not too dilute has been collected properly and plated immediately, a count of fewer than 1000 organisms per milliliter is compatible with urethral contamination. Only counts above 1000 organisms per milliliter are significant. The acceptance of the popular concept that 100,000 organisms per milliliter is the "breaking point" between contamination and true infection causes many urinary tract infections to be missed. This high count was chosen to allow for errors in collection of urine and delays in transport to the laboratory. Quantitative cultures are also useful in antibiotic sensitivity tests, which are helpful in the definitive treatment of infections.

Kunin & others (1976) have evaluated the usefulness of a nitrite indicator strip in the detection of infection in little girls. False-positive results were rare. It would appear to be a good simple screening test.

Many authors* have described and evaluated simplified methods of quantitative urine culture applicable to office practice. The advantages of such office procedures are absolute control of the method of collection of urine by the physician and the opportunity for immediate plating. Few hospitals can compete with these technics, which make available a quantitative culture within hours. With such a method, a colony count of 1000 per milliliter is significant. Drug sensitivity disks can be placed on another plate, thus affording quick guidance in the choice of antibiotic.

B. Cultures for Tubercle Bacilli: If stained smears are negative for tubercle bacilli, cultures should be made. Even if the smears reveal acid-fast organisms, cultures should be done, since the finding of the bacteria in the stained sediment, although it is strong presumptive evidence, is not definitive proof of the presence of tuberculosis.

Antibody-Coated Bacteria

It is assumed by many investigators that the finding of antibody-coated bacteria establishes the diagnosis of infection of renal origin. Gleckman (1979), however, finds the test quite inaccurate. Lorentz and Resnick (1979) found that elevation of urinary LDH was a much more accurate test. Gleckman & Crowley (1979) found antibody-coated bacteria associated with epididymitis, prostatitis, and cystitis complicating bladder tumor or stone.

Summary

The stained smear of the sediment from a properly collected urine is all that is needed to diagnose most cases of urinary tract infection. Bacteriologic cultures and sensitivity tests are required in patients who are acutely ill or in those who suffer from chronic or recurrent disease.

Other Tests of the Urine

A. Urinary pH: Normal kidneys contribute to the control of body pH by excreting urine in the pH range of 4.5 to about 7.5. The former figure is

*McLin & Tavel, 1971; Kunin & DeGroot, 1975; and Gillenwater & others, 1976.

typical of diabetic acidosis. Readings above 7.5 mean that urea-splitting organisms are present. Despite a low blood pH, the urinary pH in renal tubular acidosis is fixed between 6.0 and 7.0.

Cytologic Examination: (Fig 5–3.) Transitional cells shed from tumors of the urinary tract may be demonstrated either by the Papanicolaou technic (Tannenbaum, 1975) or by methylene blue stain (Schulte & others, 1963). The latter is as efficient as the former and therefore lends itself to office practice. Men do not shed epithelial cells unless they are taking estrogens, in which case squamous cells are seen. Women commonly shed squamous cells from the bladder neck and urethra. Both may pass small round transitional cells, however, if acute cystitis is present.

These stains correlate well with the presence of transitional cell neoplasms of the renal pelvis, ureter, or bladder but have not been too helpful in suggesting the presence of adenocarcinoma of the kidney.

C. Hormone Tests: In the presence of a testicular tumor, estimates of the amount of chorionic gonadotropin are of great importance in calculating the prognosis and may help to evaluate the presence or absence of metastases after the primary tumor has been removed. Determination of the amounts of plasma testosterone, pituitary gonadotropins, corticosteroids, and estrogens in the urine may be helpful in certain endocrine disorders, including infertility in the male. (See Chapters 20, 32, and 34.)

D. Sulkowitch Test: The Sulkowitch test affords a rough estimate of the amount of calcium excreted in the urine. The patient should be instructed to refrain from drinking milk or eating cheese for 3–4 days before the test is done. The Sulkowitch test is useful in uncovering hyperparathyroidism or idiopathic hypercalciuria as a cause of urinary calculus formation. Sulkowitch reagent is made up according to the following formula:

Oxalic acid	2.5
Ammonium oxalate	2.5
Glacial acetic acid	5.0
Distilled water, qs ad	150.0

To 5 mL of urine add 2 mL of Sulkowitch reagent. The amount of calcium is estimated by the speed of precipitation and the intensity of the cloud; it is graded from 0 to 4+.

Lack of reaction is compatible with hypoparathyroidism (it may be negative in acute pancreatitis), whereas a strongly positive test means hypercalciuria and suggests the possibility of hypercalcemia. This test is indispensable in the study and management of patients suffering from urinary stone; it must, however, be correlated with the specific gravity of the urine.

E. Lactate Dehydrogenase (LDH): This enzyme has been found to be significantly elevated in most potentially fatal medical renal diseases and chronic pyelonephritis. Increased levels are also observed in patients with cancer of the kidney, bladder, and prostate.

Amador, Dorfman, & Wacker (1965) have studied the urinary levels of LDH and alkaline phosphatase activities in the differential diagnosis of renal and other diseases. The levels of both enzymes are normal in renal cyst, adrenocortical hyperplasia, benign prostatic hyperplasia, benign essential hypertension, and acute cystitis and pyelonephritis. Since the LDH test is rather nonspecific and since 75% of patients with an elevated level of the enzyme prove to have urinary infection, the simple test of urinalysis is usually definitive. Gault & Geggie (1969) have found LDH estimation to be a poor diagnostic step.

F. Vanilmandelic Acid (VMA): Vanilmandelic acid is the urinary metabolite of the catecholamines, including dopa, dopamine, norepinephrine, normetanephrine, and metanephrine. VMA levels are elevated in patients with pheochromocytoma, neuroblastoma, and ganglioneuroma. VMA determination is, therefore, a simple yet efficient screening test for these conditions. Estimation of the various catecholamines probably affords somewhat greater diagnostic accuracy.

RENAL FUNCTION TESTS

The kidneys have 3 primary functions: (1) regulation of sodium chloride, potassium, and water (fluid and ion) balance; (2) regulation of body pH; and (3) excretion of the end products of metabolism.

Proteinuria

The presence of proteinuria as measured by sulfosalicylic acid or indicator papers must be explained, although random tests may be misleading. Proteinuria must be correlated with the specific gravity of the specimen. A mere trace of protein in urine with a specific gravity of 1.004–1.010 is compatible with a significant 24-hour loss of protein in a patient with marked impairment of renal function, even uremia. Amounts of protein up to 100 mg per 24 hours are normal.

Sulfosalicylic acid (but not Albustix) gives a positive test for proteinuria in the presence of some radiopaque chemicals used in excretory urography.

Heavy proteinuria is seen in nephrosis and, at times, glomerulonephritis; but the clinical picture and other findings in the urinary sediment usually lead to the proper diagnosis. The heaviest proteinuria may be noted in children with high fever and severe dehydration and in orthostatic proteinuria. Proteinuria is not, therefore, necessarily pathognomonic of intrinsic renal disease.

Urine Specific Gravity

The specific gravity of the urine is a simple and significant test of renal function, although determination of osmolality may be more accurate. Normal kidneys in young persons can concentrate to 1.040; at age 40, to 1.036; at age 50, to 1.030. Thus, a specific gravity of 1.030 in a man age 70 implies not only excellent renal function but also intense dehydration. With marked hydration, the specific gravity may fall to 1.000. Urine densities above 1.040 suggest that the specimen contains radiopaque fluid.

In the presence of diminishing renal function, there is progressive loss of concentrating power until 1.006–1.010 is reached. The power of dilution, however, tends to be maintained until renal damage is extreme. Even in uremia, although the concentrating power is limited to 1.010, dilution in the range of 1.002–1.004 may still be found. Therefore, a specific gravity of 1.004 in a random urine specimen does not guarantee adequate renal function. Oddly, the fixation point of specific gravity with advanced hydronephrosis is closer to 1.006, and even in this circumstance dilution may reach 1.002.

Estimation of urine osmolality is undoubtedly more meaningful, but determination of the specific gravity lends itself to office diagnosis.

Urinary specific gravity rises as the radiopaque medium used in excretory urography is excreted. Total renal function may be estimated by subtracting the specific gravity of the preinjection specimen from the specific gravity of the urine voided any time up to 2 hours after the infusion. An increase of 0.025 units or more indicates good total renal function. Less than this implies impaired function. In the uremic patient, little change is observed (Marshall, 1964).

The PSP (Phenol Red) Test

(Also a measure of residual urine.)

The patient is instructed to void. Exactly 1 mL of phenolsulfonphthalein (containing 6 mg of the dye) is then given intravenously with a tuberculin syringe (the ampule contains 1.2 mL). The patient should drink no more than 200 mL of water during each of the 2 subsequent half-hour periods. (Do not force fluids before or during the test, since excretion of PSP is not dependent upon urine flow. Furthermore, rapid vesical filling causes an obstructed bladder to lose tone, and the amount of residual urine is thereby increased.) Collect urine specimens one-half hour and, if excretion is less than 50%, 1 hour after the injection. Alkalinize with 5–10 mL of 10% NaOH to bring out the red color. Dilute the specimen with water to a volume of 1000 mL if the dye appears in good concentration. If the specimen is pale, dilute with only 250 mL or 500 mL, in which case the resulting percentage should be divided by 4 or 2, respectively. The percentage of dye recovered is measured by means of colorimetry. Collections beyond the first hour are of no value.

At times the urine may have a brownish hue; this usually occurs in "stagnant" (residual) urine. The azo dyes (eg, Azo Gantrisin, Pyridium) and Bromsulphalein interfere with accurate estimation of PSP excretion. Probenecid (Benemid) depresses PSP excretion by 67% because it interferes with the transport of the dye.

If a catheter is in the bladder, it is necessary to irrigate it at the time of collection of each specimen, because an indwelling catheter does not completely empty the bladder. The PSP excretion may be low if the test is done shortly after excretory urography, for both the radiopaque fluid and PSP compete for transport on protein molecules.

The average amount of dye normally recovered in the first half-hour specimen is 50–60%; the second specimen contains 10–15%. The normal total, then, for 1 hour is 60–75%. The normal PSP in children (infants excepted) is 5–10% higher than in the adult. An unusually high PSP in an adult is compatible with surgical or congenital absence of one kidney, with compensatory hypertrophy of its mate.

A "diaper" PSP test can be done on infants, even the newborn. The dye is given intramuscularly, and the diaper is removed after 3 hours. It is placed in a graduate which is filled to the 1000 mL mark. The normal PSP in infants is 50% or more in 3 hours. Even at the age of 3 days, at least 30% will be excreted in 3 hours. In the presence of vesical outlet obstruction, bilateral renal damage, or vesicoureteral reflux, little of the dye may be recovered. Such a finding requires explanation.

The PSP test is a test of renal blood flow and tubular function. Since urologic renal diseases primarily affect the tubules, the test has obvious value as an index of the presence and extent of urologic renal damage. The test has the advantage of being simple, and in most cases it also affords a fairly accurate estimate of residual urine. If the urine specimen collected half an hour after the intravenous injection contains 50% or more of the dye, renal function is good, and if the urine volume is small (eg, 25–50 mL), there can be no significant residual urine. The test can therefore be stopped at that point, for nothing further can be learned from a second specimen. If the first specimen does not contain the normal amount of dye, a second specimen should be collected at the end of the second half-hour.

The presence of residual urine (vesical or bilateral ureterorenal) is suggested if a "flat" or "uphill" curve is obtained in association with (1) a fairly good total PSP in 1 hour, (2) a morning specific gravity of 1.024 or better, or (3) a normal serum creatinine. With increasing degrees of renal damage and in the absence of residual urine, the following PSP curves are to be expected in 1 hour: 40%–15%, 30%–10%, and 20%–10%. Even poorly functioning kidneys do

Table 5–1. Examples of PSP excretion.

	I		II		III	
½ hour	25 mL	15%	30 mL	35%	25 mL	25%
1 hour	55 mL	25%	40 mL	25%	50 mL	25%
Totals	80 mL	40%	70 mL	60%	75 mL	50%

From such excretion curves the approximate amounts of residual urine can be estimated:

$$\frac{\text{Vol}^1\ (50\ \text{or}\ 60\ -\ \text{PSP}^1)}{\text{PSP}^1} = \frac{\text{Approximate amount of}}{\text{residual urine (in mL)}}$$

Vol^1 = the volume of the first specimen.
PSP^1 = the percentage of PSP recovered in the first specimen.
"50 or = the expected normal PSP excretion after ½ hour.
 60"
(The second half-hour does not enter into this calculation.)

The amount of residual urine in each of the above examples can therefore be calculated as follows:

$$\text{I} \quad \frac{25\ (60\ -\ 15)}{15} = \frac{1125}{15} = \text{About 75 mL residual urine}$$

$$\text{II} \quad \frac{30\ (60\ -\ 35)}{35} = \frac{750}{35} = \text{About 21 mL residual urine}$$

$$\text{III} \quad \frac{25\ (60\ -\ 25)}{25} = \frac{875}{25} = \text{About 35 mL residual urine}$$

not produce an "uphill" curve, since 70% of the dye is cleared the first time around. When damage is severe, the total PSP is low and the curve "flat" (10%–10%, 5%–5%, Trace–Trace).

The examples of PSP excretion in Table 5–1 therefore imply the presence of residual urine, for the curves are "flat" or nearly so, or "uphill."

When PSP curves are flat and their totals are low (eg, 20%–15%, 10%–10%, or 5%–5%), a serum creatinine should be obtained. If normal, a PSP of 50%–60% in the first half-hour can be assumed and the calculation of the amount of residual urine made. The same would be true if the specific gravity of the urine were 1.024 or higher. If there is doubt in the physician's mind, immediate catheterization should be performed and the PSP content of the retained urine added to that obtained during the test. This maneuver will show total PSP excretion and give an estimation of residual urine.

The use of the PSP test for estimation of total renal function and of residual urine, if present, makes it one of the most valuable routine office diagnostic procedures. It is a more useful test of renal function than measurement of nitrogen retention. It is inexpensive and affords real information in one-half hour, and it estimates degrees of renal damage before the uremic stage is reached. This test should be a routine laboratory procedure like the complete blood count and urinalysis. Since so many serious renal diseases are silent, the PSP test may occasionally pick up such a case. Many patients in uremia both feel and look well. A PSP of better than 30% in the first half-hour rules out uremia due to renal failure; only when it is 30% or less should tests for nitrogen retention be done.

In unilateral renal disease (eg, hydronephrosis), the specific gravity or concentration tests may show impairment because of the mixing of the urine from the good kidney with that from the diseased. The PSP, however, will usually be normal, because of the compensatory hypertrophy of the good kidney. In this instance, then, the PSP is a more dependable test of total renal function than concentrating power.

Gault & Fox (1969) have described the 60-minute plasma PSP concentration as a test of renal function. One milligram of PSP per kilogram body weight is given intravenously. The residual plasma level at 1 hour is estimated by colorimetry. The normal value is in the range of 110 μg. A high level implies impaired renal function. This method is of value if the urine is bloody, but in other circumstances the routine PSP test or determination of the blood urea nitrogen and creatinine levels seems simpler.

Endogenous Creatinine Clearance

Although creatinine is filtered through the glomerulus and PSP is excreted by the tubules, these tests tend to parallel each other because most renal diseases involve both renal elements (Table 5–2). Thus, the creatinine clearance is roughly equal to twice the excretion of PSP in the first half-hour. The clearance of endogenous creatinine approximates the glomerular filtration rate (GFR) as measured by inulin. The normal values vary between 72 and 140 mL/min.

The same is true when residual urine is present in the bladder. A dilute urine retained in the bladder will lower the specific gravity of the concentrated fluid produced by dehydration, and the inference of renal impairment may be made. The PSP, however, will give a "flat" curve with a fairly normal total (eg, 25%–20%: total, 45%), which suggests the presence of residual urine.

For these reasons, concentration tests should be performed in conjunction with the PSP. This will help to prevent errors that might occur in the interpretation of the concentration test in certain disorders.

Blood Nitrogen Levels

In the face of bilateral ureteral or bladder neck obstruction, bilateral vesicoureteral reflux, shock, or heart failure, the flow of urine down the tubules is slowed. This allows overreabsorption of urea nitrogen; creatinine is not so affected. Such a phenomenon is compatible with the countercurrent theory of renal function. When the urinary tract is normal and unobstructed, the plasma urea:creatinine ratio is 10:1. When there is significant bilateral urinary stasis or diminished renal blood flow, the urea:creatinine ratio rises to 20–30:1. A similar pattern is seen when there is extravasation of urine into the peritoneal cavity. Thus, the combination of both blood urea nitrogen and creatinine determinations is of considerable diagnostic importance as a screening test (Baum, Dichoso, & Carlton, 1975).

In the adult, the upper limits of normal are creatinine, 1.4 mg/dL, and blood urea nitrogen, 20 mg/dL. Up to age 5, the normal creatinine is 0.6 mg/dL and the blood urea nitrogen 8 mg/dL.

Young children with advanced bilateral hydronephrosis may have a fixed specific gravity of 1.006 with a trace of protein and yet have a serum creatinine level within the normal range. A "diaper" PSP test will reveal the renal damage or suggest residual urine.

Serum Electrolytes

(See Appendix.)

The estimation of the concentration of serum electrolytes is important in patients with suspected fluid-ion imbalance or oliguria, hyperparathyroidism, hyperaldosteronism, and chronic renal failure.

Urine Chloride Concentration
(Bedside Test of Scribner)

One of the prime functions of the kidneys is the regulation of body sodium chloride in relation to body water. In the face of sodium chloride excess, the kidneys can excrete up to 375 mEq/L of salt. With sodium chloride deprivation, normal kidneys can so efficiently withhold salt that its concentration in the urine falls to zero. As renal function fails, the specific gravity becomes fixed at 1.006–1.010 (stage of uremia); with further damage, the PSP excretion finally falls to a trace. The last measurable function the kidneys lose is sodium chloride regulation. In lower nephron nephrosis (acute tubular necrosis), the chloride concentration becomes fixed at 30–40 mEq/L. The only exception to this rule is the relatively rare incomplete tubular lesion in which the chloride concentration may be fixed at a point between 20 and 100 mEq/L.

It is obvious, then, that estimation of the urine

Table 5–2. Correlation of PSP test, serum creatinine, and creatine clearance (no residual urine).

Half-Hour PSP	Specific Gravity	Serum Creatinine (mg/dL)	Creatinine Clearance (mL/min)
50 and higher	1.015–1.040	to 1.4 (normal)	100 and higher
30	1.010	1.7	60
20	1.010	2.0	40
10	1.010	2.4	20
5	1.010	3.4	10
0	1.010	4.0 and higher	5 or less

chloride is helpful in the treatment of fluid and electrolyte derangements and in the estimation of renal function. A urine chloride of 250 mEq/L implies good renal tubular function and sodium chloride excess. Similarly, a chloride concentration of 1–2 mEq/L also implies adequate tubular function but sodium chloride depletion or retention (eg, heart failure).

When specific gravity becomes fixed, those mechanisms having to do with ammonia and bicarbonate substitution are sharply limited. Under these circumstances, the urine sodium concentration tends to equal the level of chloride in the urine unless the patient is receiving excess base (sodium lactate or bicarbonate).

●　●　●

References

Examination of the Urine

Amador E, Dorfman LE, Wacker WEC: Urinary alkaline phosphatase and LDH activities in the differential diagnosis of renal disease. *Ann Intern Med* 1965;**62**:30.

Brody LH, Salladay JR, Armbruster K: Urinalysis and the urinary sediment. *Med Clin North Am* 1971;**55**:243.

Emanuel B, Aronson N: Neonatal hematuria. *Am J Dis Child* 1974;**128**:204.

Feng WC, Medeiros AA, Murray ES: Diagnosis of gonorrhea in male patients by culture of uncentrifuged first-voided urine. *JAMA* 1977;**237**:896.

Friedman SA, Gladstone JL: The effects of hydration and bladder incubation time on urine colony counts. *J Urol* 1971;**105**:428.

Gault MH, Geggie PHS: Clinical significance of urinary LDH, alkaline phosphatase and other enzymes. *Can Med Assoc J* 1969;**101**:208.

Gavan TL: In vitro antimicrobial susceptibility testing: Clinical implications and limitations. *Med Clin North Am* 1974;**58**:493.

Gillenwater JY & others: Home urine cultures by the dip-strip method: Results in 289 cultures. *Pediatrics* 1976;**58**:508.

Gleckman R: A critical review of the antibody-coated bacteria test. *J Urol* 1979;**122**:770.

Gleckman R, Crowley M: Epididymitis as cause of antibody-coated bacteria in urine. *Urology* 1979;**14**:241.

Hakulinen A: Urinary excretion of vanilmandelic acid of children in normal and certain pathological conditions. *Acta Paediatr Scand [Suppl]* 1971;**212**:1. [Entire issue.]

Hardy JD, Furnell PM, Brumfitt W: Comparison of sterile bag, clean catch and suprapubic aspiration in the diagnosis of urinary infection in early childhood. *Br J Urol* 1976;**48**:279.

Hendler ED, Kashgarian M, Hayslett JP: Clinicopathological correlations of primary haematuria. *Lancet* 1972;**1**:458.

Jonsson K: Renal angiography in patients with hematuria. *Am J Roentgenol* 1972;**116**:758.

Kelalis PP & others: Urinary vaginal reflux in children. *Pediatrics* 1973;**51**:941.

Kunin CM, DeGroot JE: Self-screening for significant bacteriuria: Evaluation of dip-strip combination nitrite/culture test. *JAMA* 1975;**231**:1349.

Kunin CM, DeGroot JE: Sensitivity of a nitrite indicator strip method in detecting bacteriuria in preschool girls. *Pediatrics* 1977;**60**:244.

Kunin CM & others: Detection of urinary tract infections in 3- to 5-year-old girls by mothers using a nitrite indicator strip. *Pediatrics* 1976;**57**:829.

Labovits ED & others: "Benign" hematuria with focal glomerulitis in adults. *Ann Intern Med* 1972;**77**:723.

Lindberg U & others: Asymptomatic bacteriuria in schoolgirls: Clinical and laboratory findings. *Acta Paediatr Scand* 1975;**64**:425.

Littlewood JM, Jacobs SI, Ramsden CH: Comparison between microscopical examination of unstained deposits of urine and quantitative culture. *Arch Dis Child* 1977;**52**:894.

Lorentz WB, Resnick MI: Comparison of urinary lactic dehydrogenase with antibody-coated bacteria in the urine sediment as means of localizing the site of urinary tract infection. *Pediatrics* 1979;**64**:672.

McLin P, Tavel FR: Urine culture and direct sensitivity testing: A rapid simple method for use in the office. *Clin Med* 1971;**78**:16.

Pass RF, Waldo FB: Anaerobic bacteremia following suprapubic bladder aspiration. *J Pediatr* 1979;**94**:748.

Redman JF, Bissada NK: Direct bladder catheterization in infant females and young girls. *Clin Pediatr (Phila)* 1976;**15**:1060.

Ritter S, Spencer H, Smachson J: The Sulkowitch and quantitative urine calcium excretion. *J Lab Clin Med* 1960;**56**:314.

Rubin MI, Baliah T: Urinalysis and its clinical interpretation. *Pediatr Clin North Am* 1971;**18**:245.

Schulte JW & others: A simple technic for recognizing abnormal epithelial cells in the urine. *J Urol* 1963;**89**:615.

Schumann GB, Harris S, Henry JB: An improved technic for examining urinary casts and a review of their significance. *Am J Clin Pathol* 1978;**69**:18.

Tannenbaum M: Urinary cytology: The microscopic cystoscope. *Urology* 1975;**6**:750.

Tunnessen WW, Smith C, Oski FA: Beeturia: A sign of iron deficiency. *Am J Dis Child* 1969;**117**:424.

Wyatt RJ, McRoberts JW, Holland NH: Hematuria in childhood: Significance and management. *J Urol* 1977;**117**:366.

Renal Function Tests

Albert MS: Acid-base disorders in pediatrics. *Pediatr Clin North Am* 1976;**23**:639.

Barsocchini LM, Smith DR: Diaper phenolsulfonphthalein test in the newborn infant. *J Urol* 1964;**91**:195.

Baum N, Dichoso CC, Carlton CE Jr: Blood urea nitrogen and serum creatinine: Physiology and interpretations. *Urology* 1975;**5**:583.

Berliner RW, Bennett CM: Concentration of urine in the mammalian kidney. *Am J Med* 1967;**42**:777.

Galambos JT, Herndon EG Jr, Reynolds GH: Specific-gravity determination: Fact or fancy. *N Engl J Med* 1964;**270**:506.

Gault MH, Fox I: The sixty-minute plasma phenolsulfon-phthalein concentration as a test of renal function. *Am J Clin Pathol* 1969;**52**:345.

Greenhill A, Gruskin AB: Laboratory evaluation of renal function. *Pediatr Clin North Am* 1976;**23**:661.

Griner PF, Liptzin B: Use of the laboratory in a teaching hospital: Implications for patient care, education and hospital costs. *Ann Intern Med* 1971;**75**:157.

Jensen H, Henriksen K: Proteinuria in non-renal infectious disease. *Acta Med Scand* 1974;**196**:75.

Kampmann J & others: Rapid evaluation of creatinine clearance. *Acta Med Scand* 1974;**196**:517.

Laboratory tests: Misuse and abuse. (Editorial.) *JAMA* 1971;**218**:90.

Lindeman RD, Van Buren HC, Raisz LG: Osmolar renal concentrating ability in healthy young men and hospitalized patients without renal disease. *N Engl J Med* 1960;**262**:1306.

Lyon RP: Measurement of urine chloride as a test of renal function. *J Urol* 1961;**85**:884.

Marshall S: A test of renal function: Excretion of contrast medium as measured by urinary specific gravity. *Br J Urol* 1964;**36**:519.

Newcombe DS, Cohen AS: Uricosuric agents and phenol-sulfonphthalein excretion. *Arch Intern Med* 1963;**112**:738.

Richardson JA, Philbin PE: The one-hour creatinine clearance rate in healthy men. *JAMA* 1971;**216**:987.

Scribner BH: Bedside determination of chloride. *Proc Staff Meet Mayo Clin* 1950;**25**:209.

Smith DR: Estimation of the amount of residual urine by means of the phenolsulfonphthalein test. *J Urol* 1960;**83**:188.

Young JD Jr, de Mendonca PP, Bendhack D: A comparison of phenolsulfonphthalein excretion with the renal clearance of creatinine and PAH. *Am Surg* 1969;**169**:724.

Roentgenographic Examination of the Urinary Tract | 6

Donald R. Smith, MD, & Melvyn T. Korobkin, MD

PLAIN FILM OF ABDOMEN

A plain film of the abdomen, also called a KUB (kidney, ureter, and bladder), is a helpful step in the presumptive diagnosis of genitourinary disease (Figs 6–1 and 6–2). Since gastrointestinal and urologic diseases tend to mimic each other, it may be helpful in differential diagnosis as well.

Renal Shadows
A. Kidney Size: A plain film of the abdomen will usually show the renal outlines. They may be obscured, however, by bowel content, lack of perinephric fat, or a perinephric hematoma or abscess, which typically obliterates the renal shadow. This difficulty, however, may be overcome by tomography. Congenital absence or possible ectopy of a kidney may be suggested. If both kidneys are unusually large, polycystic kidney disease, multiple myeloma, lymphoma, amyloid disease, or hydronephrosis may be present. If both are small, the end stage of glomerulonephritis or bilateral atrophic pyelonephritis must be considered. Unilateral enlargement should suggest renal tumor, cyst, or hydronephrosis, whereas a small kidney on one side is compatible with congenital hypoplasia, atrophic pyelonephritis, or an ischemic kidney. Normally, the left kidney is 0.5 cm longer than its mate. Discrepancy in the relative size of one kidney may imply renal ischemia.

The normal kidney extends from the top of the first to the bottom of the third to fourth lumbar vertebra (Hunter, Howey, & Hocken, 1975).

B. Position: In 90% of cases, the right kidney is lower than the left, because of displacement by the liver. If a kidney appears to be abnormally displaced, a retroperitoneal tumor should be suspected (eg, adrenal tumor, pancreatic pseudocyst).

The axes of the kidneys are oblique to the spine; their lower poles are farther apart than their upper poles because they lie along the borders of the psoas muscles. If their axes are parallel to the spine (which means that the lower ends of the kidneys are lying on the psoas muscles), the possibility of "horseshoe" kidney should be considered.

C. Shape: The shape of the kidney should be studied. A lobulated edge might suggest polycystic

kidney disease. An expansion of one pole of a kidney is compatible with tumor, cyst, or carbuncle. Indentations on the lateral border of a small kidney suggest scarring from previous attacks of pyelonephritis.

Calcification
Because a plain film of the abdomen is 2-dimensional, it is practically impossible to make a positive diagnosis of stone in the urinary tract except in the instance of a staghorn calculus, which forms a perfect cast of the pelvis and calices, thereby simulating a urogram. All one can usually say from study of a plain film is that there are opaque bodies in the region of the adrenal, kidney, ureter, bladder, or prostate. Oblique and lateral films, as well as visualization of the urinary tract with radiopaque fluids, are necessary in order to actually determine the position of the calcification in the respective organs.

Punctate calcification in the adrenals suggests tuberculous involvement (Fig 13–2) or neuroblastoma (Fig 21–16). Adrenal calcification follows spontaneous hemorrhage into the gland (Fig 6–12) (Brill, Krasna, & Aaron, 1976). Numerous small calcific bodies in the parenchyma of a kidney may suggest tuberculosis (Fig 6–2) or medullary sponge kidney (Fig 22–10), although nephrocalcinosis (Fig 15–5) caused by primary or secondary hyperparathyroidism or hypercalciuria should be considered. About 7% of malignant renal tumors contain some calcification. Calcifications in the veins in the perivesical area (phleboliths) may simulate stone in the ureter, but as a rule they are perfectly round, often laminated, and contain radiolucent centers. Calcified mesenteric lymph nodes may also resemble stone. Linear calcification lying to the left of the lumbar spine is compatible with aneurysm of the abdominal aorta. An aneurysm of the right renal artery (Fig 22–12) may be confused with a gallstone. Calcifications at the junction of the hypogastric and iliac arteries are often seen just below the sacroiliac joints and may therefore be confused with ureteral stones. A stone in the appendix may occasionally be confused with stone in the ureter. Radiopaque gallstones may overlie the kidney, but an oblique or lateral film will demonstrate that the opacity is an-

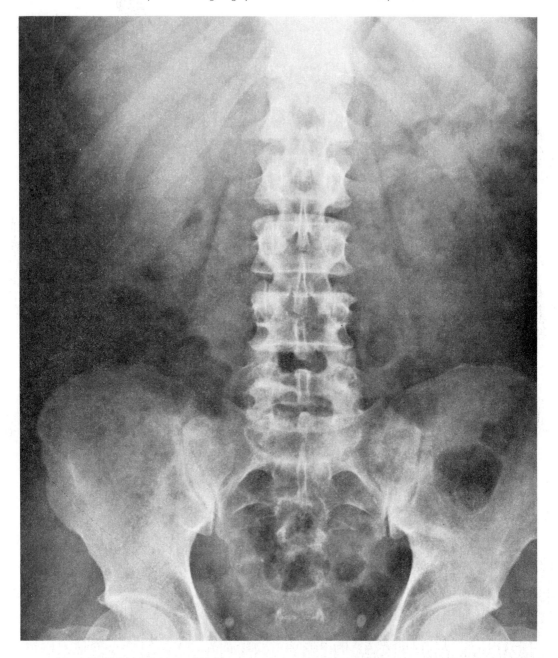

Figure 6–1. Normal plain film of abdomen. Bones are normal, psoas shadows well demarcated, renal shadows normal. The bladder contains some urine. Two phleboliths are seen in the region of the lower ureters and bladder.

terior to the kidney. Uterine fibroids and, occasionally, diseased ovaries may undergo pathologic calcification. Moles on the skin and swallowed pills or foreign bodies may be radiopaque. The wall of an adrenal or renal cyst may contain calcium.

The use of tomography will show indistinct calcifications often missed on a plain film.

Psoas Shadows

The psoas muscles usually stand out sharply. If one is obliterated and the kidney shadow on that

side is absent, and if there is scoliosis of the spine with its concavity on the side of the defect, perinephric or paranephric abscess or hematoma is a possibility.

Bone Shadows

Survey of the bones may reveal arthritic change, which may suggest that what was thought to be kidney pain is really caused by radiculitis. Gross spina bifida may be noted; such findings would suggest the presence of neurogenic bladder

(Fig 19–10). Metastases should also be sought. If osteoblastic, they almost certainly arise from the prostate; if osteolytic, the common primary sites are in the breast, thyroid, lung, and kidney (Fornasier & Horne, 1975).

Complete absence or partial agenesis of the sacrum is compatible with neurogenic (neuropathic) bladder (Braren & Jones, 1979). Price & Loveday (1975), utilizing "soft tissue radiography" (similar to mammography), observed that testicular tumors were opaque; benign lesions were more radiolucent.

Gastrointestinal Shadows

A plain film, by demonstrating gas in the small bowel, may lead to the diagnosis of bowel obstruction, although the initial impression may have been disease of the urinary tract. Gas under the diaphragm with the patient in an upright posture makes the diagnosis of a ruptured viscus (eg, perforated peptic ulcer). A large renal mass may displace all intestinal gas from that area (Fig 6–2).

Plain Film of Abdomen With Tomography

Tomography enhances the renal and psoas outlines, thus clarifying renal size, shape, and position. It may also reveal extrarenal (eg, suprarenal) masses and zones of calcification invisible on the plain film. Should the excretory urograms reveal a space-occupying lesion of the renal pelvis, a tomogram may show a faint opaque body compatible with stone but not tumor.

EXCRETORY UROGRAMS

During the past 30 years, improvements in intravenous radiographic media have been such that they now rival retrograde urograms in quality, and their efficiency has impaired the usefulness of the latter as a test of renal function. Although nausea, vomiting, and pain in the arm are occasionally experienced after intravenous injection of radiopaque material, these reactions are usually less disturbing to the patient than the sequelae of retrograde urography (nausea and vomiting, abdominal and renal pain). Rare allergic reactions, (eg, urticaria, asthma, shock) following intravenous infusion of these iodized substances are apparently usually aborted by adding an antihistamine to the radiopaque fluid.

Excretory urograms illustrate the urinary excretory tract in the most physiologic manner. The renal pelves and calices are not distorted by the overdistention which may be produced with retrograde filling.

The cystogram which is obtained on the later films may reveal trabeculation, diverticula, or a space-occupying lesion (Fig 18–12). A postvoiding film may demonstrate residual urine in the bladder. *Note:* For 1–2 hours after injection of the radiopaque medium, the normal specific gravity of the urine is 1.040–1.060. Under these circumstances, a specific gravity of 1.020 or less indicates that renal function is severely impaired.

Indications

Excretory urograms are indicated when disease of the urinary tract is suspected. Diseases which should be investigated by this means include cysts and tumors of the kidney (space-occupying lesions), tuberculosis of the kidney (ulceration of calices), pyelonephritis, hydronephrosis, vesicoureteral reflux, hypertension, and stone in the urinary tract.

Excretory urograms may also be of value in patients suffering from gastrointestinal complaints in whom no organic disease of the gastrointestinal tract can be demonstrated. A urologic cause for the symptoms may be shown.

Because the radiographic fluid increases the density of the kidneys to x-rays, the size of the kidneys and their outlines become clearer. This is an advantage when evidence of expansion of the renal parenchyma (eg, tumor) or change in size of the kidney is sought. Tomography more clearly delineates renal morphology.

If renal injury is suspected, excretory urograms should be obtained as soon as practicable (primarily to make certain that the uninjured contralateral kidney is normal). This is invaluable information if emergency removal of the injured kidney becomes imperative as a lifesaving measure.

Excretory urograms are indispensable in infants, particularly male infants, where cystoscopy may be unduly traumatic. During the first month of life, delayed concentration and prolonged excretion of urographic contrast medium are observed. In this age group, the usual early films should be deleted and late films (1–2 hours) taken. A few months later, however, the best film may be noted 6 minutes after injection in the nondehydrated child.

Untoward Reactions & Contraindications

Excretory urograms are contraindicated if there is evidence of hypersensitivity: history of allergic reactions to previous intravenous urography, iodine sensitivity, or other allergic manifestations such as hives or asthma. Although the routine addition of an antihistamine to the contrast medium may reduce the incidence of allergic reactions, it would be unwise to depend upon this precaution if the patient has manifested hypersensitivity in the past. Excretory radiopaque material may be lethal in patients with multiple myeloma, congenital adrenal hyperplasia (Silverman & Nyham, 1976), diabetes, or primary hyperparathyroidism (Carvallo, Rakowski, & Argy, 1978). Fluids in these cases should be forced beforehand. In fact, Dure-Smith (1976) claims that restriction of fluids before administration of radiopaque fluid does not enhance concentration of the medium. Lalli (1975) has adduced

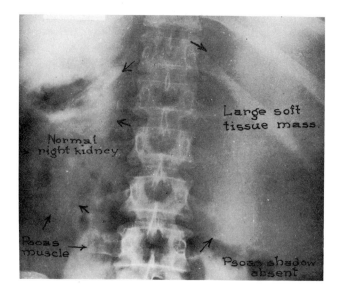

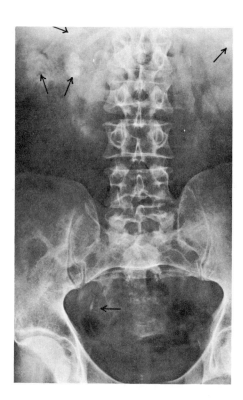

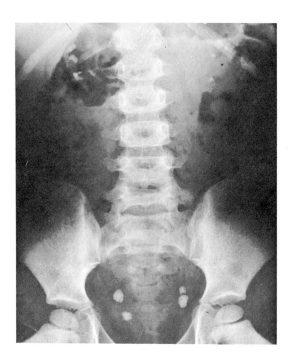

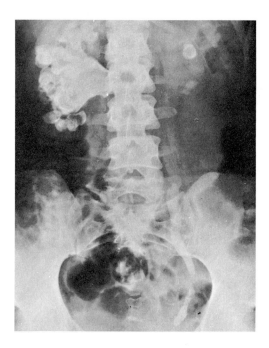

Figure 6–2. Abnormal plain films of the abdomen. *Above left:* Large soft tissue mass in left upper abdomen (simple cyst of kidney). Absence of intestinal gas (displacement of bowel) over mass (see Fig 6–32, below left and right, same patient). *Above right:* Calcification in small functionless right kidney and lower right ureter typical of advanced tuberculosis. There is a stone in the left kidney. *Below left:* Multiple renal and ureteral calcium oxalate stones in 12-year-old boy suffering from hyperoxaluria. *Below right:* Large staghorn calculus in right kidney and multiple stones in left kidney and lower half of ureter.

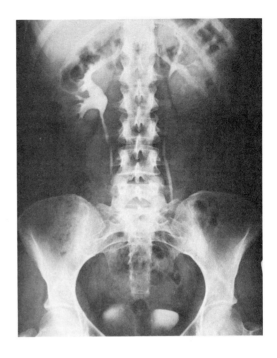
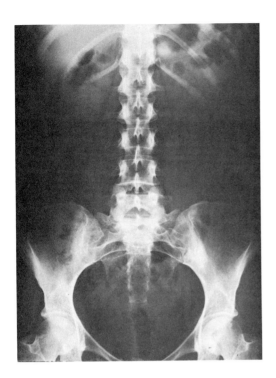
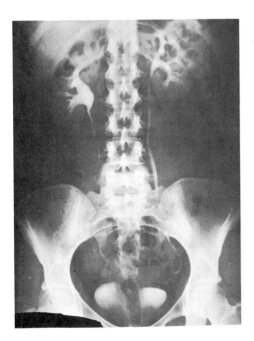
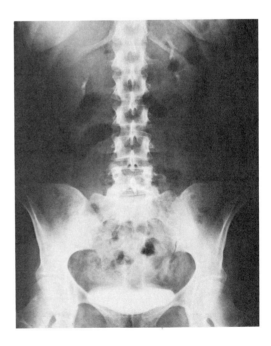

Figure 6–3. Normal excretory urogram. *Above left:* Plain abdominal film. Bones normal, renal shadows fairly well seen, psoas margins distinct. Black oblong shadow below coccyx is a vaginal menstrual tampon. *Above right:* Five minutes after injection of radiopaque material. Prompt excretion in good concentration. Lower calices of left kidney indistinct, upper ureters well outlined. Note area of systole in both upper ureters. Some radiopaque material in bladder. *Below left:* Fifteen-minute film. Calices of left kidney now well filled. All calices are well cupped. Differences in ureteral diameter are caused by systolic contractions. *Below right:* Twenty-five-minute film, prone. Excellent drainage of opaque material. Each kidney drops a distance equal to height of one-half vertebra.

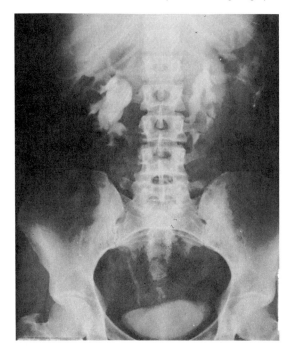
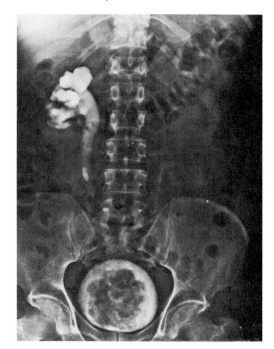
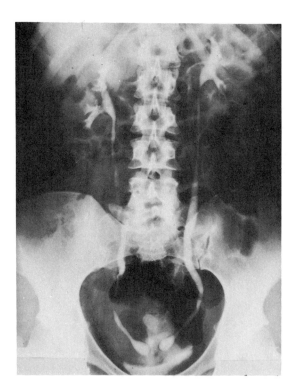
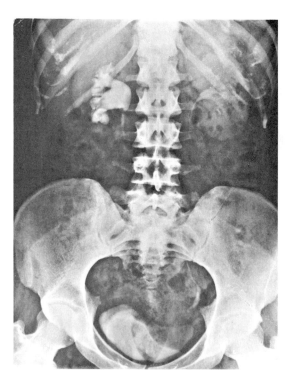

Figure 6–4. Abnormal excretory urograms. *Above left:* Horseshoe kidney. Axes of renal masses vertical, lower calices on psoas muscles. *Above right:* Right ureteral stone causing hydronephrosis. Large irregular filling defect from unsuspected vesical neoplasm. *Below left:* Bilateral ureteroceles causing a minimum of obstruction. *Below right:* Moderate right hydronephrosis with obstruction at ureteropelvic junction due to aberrant vessel. Compression of left side of bladder from enlarged uterus.

evidence to the effect that many adverse reactions are caused by fear. Lalli (1980) also believes that most reactions are due to a specific effect on the central nervous system.

A few deaths due to pulmonary injury have been reported in infants. This is thought to be caused by the hypertonicity of the contrast medium. Preliminary dehydration should therefore be condemned.

If the PSP test is less than 30% in 1 hour or if blood nitrogen retention is demonstrated, it will be necessary to administer a larger dose of radiopaque fluid (eg, double the usual dose or use a 90% concentration of the medium) or to perform infusion urography. Adequate films may thus be obtained when the blood urea nitrogen is as high as 100 mg/dL.

In women, urography is most safely performed during the 10 days following the onset of menses. It presents a genetic hazard during pregnancy.

Technic

A. Preparation of the Patient: No food or fluids should be taken for at least 6 hours before the procedure is scheduled, although in infants dehydration should not be practiced. A cathartic (eg, castor oil) taken the night before will decrease the amount of gas and fecal material in the bowel, thus ensuring clearer delineation of the urinary tract. An enema is less effective. If urograms are urgently desired and the patient is hydrated, satisfactory films are still obtainable. A 3-minute film should be added to the series, since the radiopaque material under these circumstances is excreted more promptly. A double dose of the iodide will further enhance the quality of the films.

B. Procedure:

1. Preliminary plain film–This must be taken not only to check on the quality of the radiographic technic and the position of the patient but also to demonstrate urinary stones that might be obscured by the radiopaque medium.

2. Injection of the radiopaque fluid–The amount of fluid that should be injected varies with the type of fluid and the age of the patient. (Follow the manufacturer's directions.) One of the antihistamines should be added to the infusion material.

a. Intravenous injection–This is the method of choice if venipuncture is feasible. Since allergic reactions may occur and death may ensue (rarely), preliminary tests for hypersensitivity should be performed. If one or more tests are positive, this examination should not be done. Unfortunately, none of these tests guarantees complete safety, although the intravenous test is more reliable than the ocular or subcutaneous test.

(1) Tests for sensitivity–

(a) Ocular test–One drop of the contrast medium is instilled into the eye. If erythema is produced, the test is positive.

(b) Subcutaneous test–Inject 0.1 mL sub-cutaneously. If induration and erythema develop promptly, the test is positive.

(c) Intravenous test–Inject 1 mL of the medium intravenously. If no signs of hypersensitivity (eg, urticaria, asthma) are observed, the test is negative.

(2) Manifestations of sensitivity–If symptoms and signs of hypersensitivity are manifested by the patient during the injection, it should be stopped immediately. Warning signs of allergic reaction include respiratory difficulty; sneezing, itching, or urticaria; nausea and vomiting; and fainting. Treatment consists of oxygen for anoxia, hypertensive drugs and intravenous dextrose solutions for shock, intravenous barbiturates for convulsions, and the intravenous injection of an antihistamine if allergic reactions are observed (Siegle & Lieberman, 1978).

b. Extravascular infusion–This procedure is indicated if venipuncture is impossible (eg, in the infant). (See manufacturer's directions for dosage.) The ocular and intradermal tests should be performed first. If sensitivity is demonstrated by these tests, the infusion should be withheld. The ampule of radiopaque medium (to which an antihistamine has been added) is diluted to 100 mL with normal saline solution. Equal parts of the solution are given subcutaneously over the scapular areas. Excretion is maximal on the 30- to 60-minute films.

3. Routine urograms–The infusion should be given rapidly. Radiograms are taken at 10 seconds for the nephrogram effect, and at 5, 10, and 15 minutes with the patient in the supine position. Films taken 2 and 3 minutes after the beginning of the injection (minute sequence) should be routine in all patients who are hypertensive, for these radiograms, by revealing delayed concentration of the dye in one kidney, may suggest decreased renal function and blood flow. At 25 minutes, a film is also taken with the patient erect in order to demonstrate the mobility of the kidneys, to obtain ureterograms, and to observe the efficiency with which the renal pelves and ureters drain. All films should include the kidney, ureter, and bladder areas, since subtle changes in the ureters that imply the presence of vesicoureteral reflux may otherwise be missed.

In infants and children, the films should be taken at 3, 5, 8, and 12 minutes, for their kidneys excrete the fluid more rapidly than do those of the adult. If the renal areas are obscured by bowel content, the child should be offered 150–240 mL of a carbonated beverage (Geraghty, 1966). The resulting gas-filled stomach displaces the bowel and thus improves visualization of the kidneys.

Ureteral compression may be helpful if the first urogram shows poor concentration of the medium. The urine is thus held in the upper urinary tracts, affording enhanced filling. Compression, however, may cause spontaneous extravasation of urine in the region of the pelvis. This is not pathologic.

4. Supplementary urograms–As soon as the routine exposures are taken and developed, they should be viewed. Oblique, lateral, or supine films may then be indicated in order to localize calcific bodies more accurately and to gain a third dimension of the urogram; this may be helpful if caliceal distortion is suspected. Taking films in the prone position, particularly in children, may lead to improved filling of some calices and the ureter. Troublesome gas shadows may also be displaced.

If excretion of the urographic fluid is delayed, films should be taken periodically for as long as 4 hours or even 24 hours after the injection. Advanced hydronephrosis and dilated ureters may become apparent only then. It is feasible to inject additional radiopaque medium if there is impaired concentration on the initial films.

5. X-ray of the bladder region after voiding– This should be routine in all urologic patients, no matter what age or sex. At the conclusion of the urographic study, the patient should be instructed to void; a film of the bladder area should be taken immediately. This will demonstrate the presence or absence of residual urine. Partial urinary retention is common but is often not suspected. Normal and abnormal urograms are shown in Figs 6–3 and 6–4.

6. Urethrography–Boltuch & Lalli (1975) recommend that in conjunction with excretory urography, satisfactory urethrograms can be obtained in the male by placing a zipper clamp on the distal penile shaft. The patient is instructed to void; films are then exposed.

Janson, Roberts, & Evans (1977) have noted displacement of the left kidney in infants, suggesting adrenal enlargement. Deflation of the stomach by gastric tube caused the kidney to ascend to a normal position. Renal tomography may reveal the renal fascia (Marx & Patel, 1979). Barbaric (1976) believes that this implies an abnormality caused by renal scarring, acute renal infection, calculi, or intra- and perirenal masses.

Kabakian & others (1976) report that medial deviation of the right lower ureter is the rule in females. Saldino & Palubinskas (1972) find a similar medial deviation of the upper and mid ureters that simulates the change compatible with retroperitoneal fibrosis.

Lateral displacement of the bladder usually implies pathologic change (Korobkin, Minagi, & Palubinskas, 1975). Such causes include vesical diverticulum, fecal impaction, inguinal hernia, and prostatic carcinoma.

INFUSION UROGRAPHY

This technic of excretory urography is indicated in patients suffering from renal insufficiency (blood urea nitrogen up to 100 mg/dL) and when maximum detail is required. Preliminary dehydration is unnecessary. Give 25% sodium diatrizoate (Hypaque) or similar radiopaque fluid, 2–4 mL/kg

in a similar volume of normal saline. This is infused through an 18-gauge needle over a period of 5–10 minutes. Films are exposed at 10, 20, and 30 minutes, though additional films and views may be indicated. This technic lends itself well to tomography, which can be executed at the completion of the infusion (Greene, Fraser, & Hartman, 1976).

In the presence of ureteral obstruction, eg, stone, perirenal extravasation of the radiopaque solution will be observed in 25% of patients (Bernardino & McClennan, 1976).

The routine use of this type of urography, particularly in children, should be condemned. Preliminary hydration plus the marked osmotic diuresis stimulated by the larger dose of the radiopaque fluid causes the ureters to be completely full and somewhat dilated, thus simulating the changes compatible with vesicoureteral reflux.

If the patient is being studied for hypertension, exposure should be made at 2, 3, 4, and 5 minutes as well. This procedure also lends itself to the urea washout test, which can be done as the final step.

In a few instances, opacification of the uterus and even myomas may be noted (Golimbu & others, 1975). Cystic and mixed ovarian tumors may be detected (Imray, 1975).

UREA WASHOUT TEST

Since the basic phenomenon in renal ischemia is the overreabsorption of water by the renal tubules, a hyperconcentration of the radiopaque medium in this kidney should be seen on urography. This change can be accentuated by osmotic diuresis produced by urea.

After preliminary dehydration, (1) infuse 50 mL of 50% sodium diatrizoate (Hypaque)—or other opaque medium—rapidly through a 16-gauge needle; (2) expose films at 30 seconds and at 2, 3, 5, 8, 15, and 20 minutes; (3) give 40 g urea and 30 mL of sodium diatrizoate in 500 mL of normal saline in a 15-minute period; and (4) take a film every 3 minutes until one or both kidneys have "washed out" the radiopaque medium. Normally, both are washed out in 15 minutes. If one kidney retains the "dye" 6–9 minutes longer than the other kidney, the test is considered positive for renal ischemia.

ANGIONEPHROTOMOGRAMS
(Intravenous Renal Angiograms)

Nephrotomography has its greatest usefulness in the differentiation of renal cyst and tumor. Briefly, this technic involves the rapid intravenous injection of a bolus of radiopaque material that opacifies vascularized tissues in the kidney. The space occupied by a cyst or abscess fails to opacify (Fig 6–5); a malignant tumor shows normal or increased opacification because of its increased blood

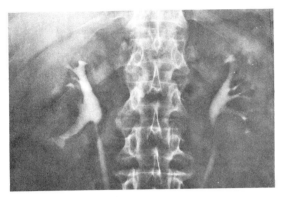

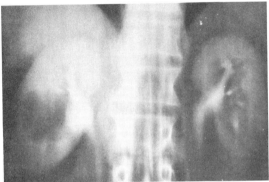

Figure 6–5. Angionephrotomogram. *Above:* Excretory urogram showing space-occupying lesion in the center of the right kidney; calices distorted and displaced. *Below:* Nephrotomogram showing lack of opacification of the lesion, which, therefore, is a simple cyst. Note the similarity of this urogram to that in Fig 18–3 (bottom right), which proved to be cancer.

supply (Fig 18–4). Renal angiography is, however, more efficient in this differential diagnosis.

Technic

(1) Preparation of the patient and tests for sensitivity to the radiographic fluid are carried out as described for excretory urograms.

(2) Take a plain film of the renal areas, and then take test tomograms to demonstrate the kidneys (usually 8–11 cm from the tabletop). Insert a No. 12 needle into one antecubital vein or one No. 16 needle into each antecubital vein. Establish the circulation time by injecting 2.5 mL of 20% sodium dehydrocholate (Decholin) in 10 mL of normal saline solution. Inject 30–50 mL of 50% sodium diatrizoate (Hypaque) or other opaque medium to enhance the nephrogram. Rapidly inject 50 mL of 90% sodium diatrizoate, take a plain film at the predetermined circulation time, and follow immediately with 4–6 tomograms. The immediate film may reveal opacification of the renal arteries (Lee & Henderson, 1977).

RETROGRADE UROGRAMS

Only this type of radiography requires special training in urologic instrumentation. The indications, contraindications, and technic of the preliminary cystoscopy and ureteral catheterization are discussed in Chapter 9.

After catheters have been passed to the renal pelves, a "split" renal function test (PSP) should be performed (see Chapter 5) and urine specimens obtained for microscopic examination and culture. Undiluted radiopaque material is then allowed to flow up the catheters. The average normal renal pelvis has a capacity of 3–4 mL. Overdistention causes painful renal pelvic and ureteral spasms (colic) and capsular (costovertebral) pain. Overfilling may also distort the urogram; if the pelvis is extrarenal, a normal pelvis and calices may appear hydronephrotic (Figs 6–6 and 6–7).

Indications

A. Infection: When upper tract abnormality is suspected and pyuria is present, catheterization of the ureters affords separate urine specimens from the kidneys for bacteriologic study, thus establishing the site of the infection. Retrograde urograms can then be done.

B. Inadequate Excretory Urograms: If excretory urograms (even the infusion type) do not adequately demonstrate ureteropelvic detail, retrograde urograms may be needed.

C. Impaired Total Renal Function: If renal function is decreased to the point where excretory urograms will prove inadequate, retrograde filling of the renal pelves will be necessary.

D. Assessment of Degree of Ureteral Obstruction: If excretory urograms portray ureteropelvic junction or ureteral obstruction, its degree may be best judged by instilling radiopaque fluid into the renal pelvis. The catheter is then removed. In the absence of significant obstruction, most of the medium will have drained out in 15 minutes, whereas marked stenosis may cause retention of the iodide for hours.

E. Sensitivity to Intravenous Radiopaque Fluid: If excretory urograms are contraindicated because of allergy, retrograde urograms must be substituted.

F. Need for Oblique and Lateral Radiograms: Since the radiopaque medium given intravenously is diluted by urine, the density of the excreted fluid is less than that obtained with retrograde filling. If oblique and lateral films are desired, the density of the tissues through which the x-rays must pass is increased; retrograde instillation may prove more satisfactory in some instances.

Contraindications

Although there are contraindications to cystoscopy and ureteral catheterization, there are none to retrograde urography itself.

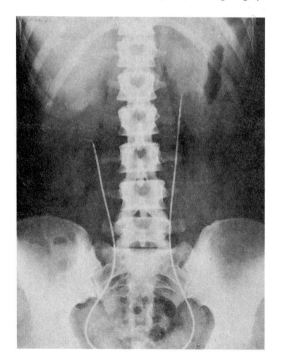 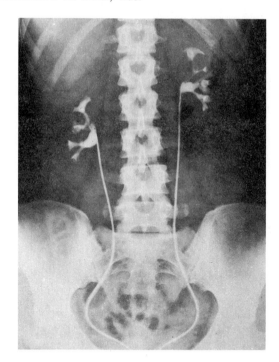

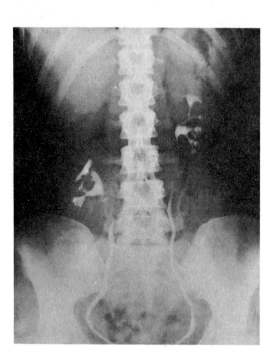 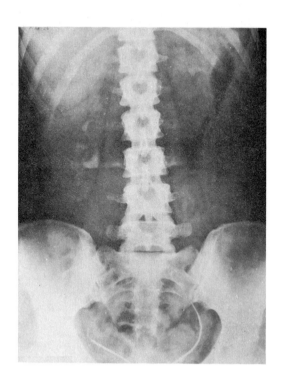

Figure 6–6. Normal retrograde urogram. *Above left:* Plain abdominal film showing radiopaque ureteral catheters in the renal pelves. *Above right:* Film taken in the supine position. Calices are well cupped and there is no dilatation of the pelves. *Below left:* Urogram taken in the upright position with catheters drawn down into the lower ureters. The right kidney drops the height of one and one-half vertebrae, causing some redundancy of the upper ureter. The left kidney drops the height of one vertebra. *Below right:* Film taken 15 minutes later, showing almost complete drainage of both kidneys.

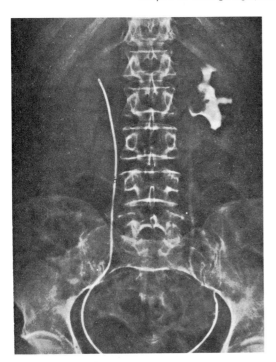
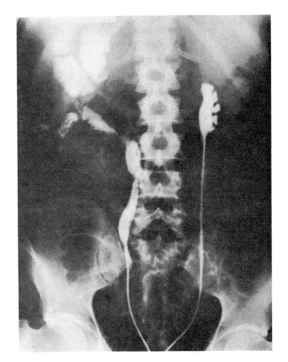
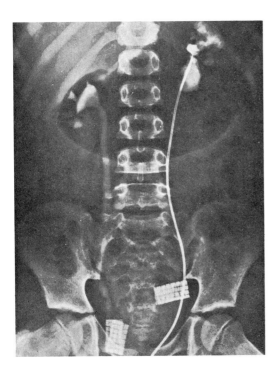
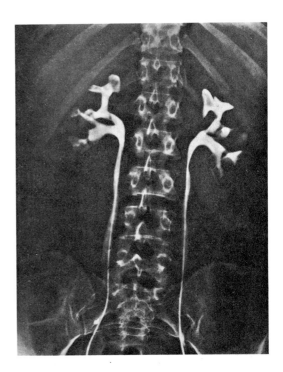

Figure 6–7. Abnormal retrograde urograms. *Above left:* Space-occupying lesion of left renal pelvis. Transitional cell carcinoma. *Above right:* Stones in right renal pelvis and upper ureter; calculus pyonephrosis. Atrophic kidney, left. *Below left:* Bilateral renal tuberculosis. Moth-eaten appearance of calices of left kidney, obliteration of upper calix, and dilated and foreshortened ureter on right. *Below right:* Bilateral papillary necrosis. All papillae have sloughed. Upper medial and lowest calices on left show "negative" shadows representing retained papillae.

Technic

A. Preparation of the Patient: Fluids can be taken as tolerated unless general anesthesia is to be employed for the procedure. The bowel should first be cleansed by catharsis (eg, castor oil).

B. Procedure:

1. Cystoscopy and ureteral catheterization– These are done first.

2. Preliminary plain film of abdomen (supine)–This checks on the position of the patient and the catheters and on the radiographic technic, and demonstrates calcific densities in the urinary tract which might be obscured by the radiopaque medium.

3. Instillation of the radiopaque fluid–

a. Supine urogram–If the capacity of the renal pelvis is not known, 3–4 mL of undiluted urographic medium should be instilled by gravity under low pressure (20 cm of water). A radiogram is then taken, developed, and viewed. If filling is incomplete, another x-ray film can be exposed after more fluid is introduced.

b. Oblique or lateral radiograms–These should then be taken as indicated.

c. Upright ureteropyelogram–The patient is then placed in the semierect position, and, while the urographic fluid is still being introduced, the catheters are slowly withdrawn into the lower ureters and a film taken. This affords good ureterograms and shows the degree of mobility of the kidneys.

If ureteral filling is inadequate, the patient should be placed in the Trendelenburg position and more of the contrast medium instilled; an x-ray exposure is again made.

d. "Emptying" or delayed films–If the ureteropyelograms reveal evidence of obstruction, an x-ray should be taken 15 minutes after the previous one, without further introduction of radiopaque medium. If some of the medium is still retained, later films should be made in order to assess the degree of obstruction.

4. Pneumopyelography–In differentiating between a nonopaque stone and a papillary tumor of the renal pelvis, 4–6 mL of air may be instilled into the catheter. A stone may show some opacification; a tumor will not, though both may cause a filling defect in the pelvis or calices that shows up on excretory urograms.

BULB URETEROPYELOGRAM

If optimum ureteral detail is essential, a bulb ureteropyelogram should be obtained. This is accomplished by forcing a bulbous tipped catheter tightly into the ureteral orifice. Radiopaque fluid is then instilled with a syringe.

OPACIFICATION OF RENAL CYSTS

One of the most difficult problems in diagnosis is the differentiation of renal cyst and tumor. Some urologists, fearing the complications of cancer on the wall of a cyst, tend to explore all kidneys showing evidence of a space-occupying lesion as revealed by urography. Others will not resort to surgery if the diagnosis of cyst can be established. Renal angiography (particularly of the selective type) establishes the diagnosis of vascular adenocarcinomas, but what appears to be a nonvascular mass, although almost always a cyst, could be a necrotic tumor or an abscess. In this instance, renal cystography can be performed.

Under fluoroscopic or ultrasonic control and after administration of a radiopaque fluid intravenously (although some clinicians needle blindly, using previous urograms as a guide), a 7-inch, 18-gauge needle is introduced into the presumed cyst. In most instances, clear fluid will be obtained; this should be subjected to cytologic study. Radiopaque fluid is then instilled into the cystic cavity and a film taken. If the radiopaque fluid is homogeneous, the edges of the cavity smooth, and cytology negative, the diagnosis of simple cyst is warranted, thus negating the need for surgery (Fig 22–5). The return of bloody fluid or just a little blood implies the presence of carcinoma; surgery is indicated. The needle may also be introduced under guidance with ultrasound (see Chapter 7).

ANTEGRADE UROGRAMS

If excretory or infusion urograms reveal the presence of advanced hydronephrosis or a large nonfunctioning renal mass and radiopaque fluid introduced into the lower ureter fails to reach the renal pelvis because of ureteral stenosis, antegrade urograms can be procured. A high-dose infusion urogram should first be obtained. Under fluoroscopic or ultrasonic (Weinstein & Skolnick, 1978) control, an 18-gauge needle, 15 cm long, should be passed into a dilated calix or pelvis. Radiopaque material can then be instilled and appropriate films taken.

In order to afford temporary drainage, a small plastic catheter can be passed through the needle as a nephrostomy tube. The needle can then be removed.

CYSTOGRAMS

Cystograms are made by instilling radiopaque fluid into the bladder through a catheter. Roentgenograms then show an outline of the bladder wall, including diverticula. In addition,

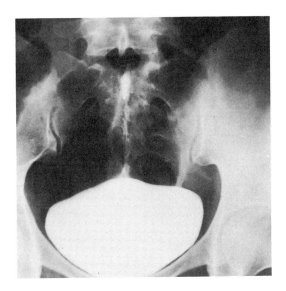
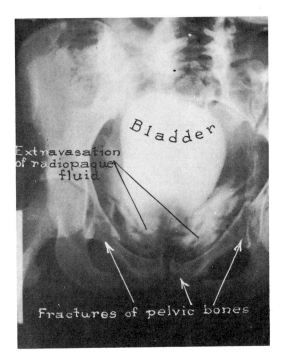
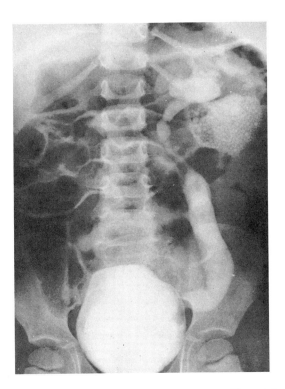
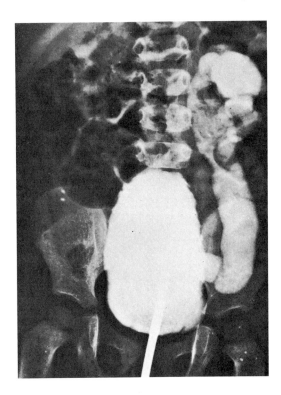

Figure 6–8. Normal and abnormal cystograms. *Above left:* Normal cystogram. *Above right:* Avulsion of prostatic urethra secondary to pelvic fracture. Extraperitoneal extravasation. *Below left:* Light iodized oil (Lipiodol) instilled into bladder to seek evidence of residual urine. Lipiodol refluxed up second left ureter to fill hydronephrotic lower pole (same patient as below right). *Below right:* Trabeculated bladder and left ureteral reflux demonstrating marked hydroureteronephrosis.

ureteropyelograms may be obtained if the ureterovesical "valves" are incompetent (see Chapter 11).

RETROGRADE CYSTOGRAMS

Indications

A. When Cystoscopy Is Not Feasible: In male infants, the small caliber of the urethra may preclude passage of the smallest cystoscope or panendoscope. If mechanical difficulties prevent passage of an optical instrument to the bladder but a catheter can be successfully passed, a cystogram may reveal a vesical tumor, vesicoureteral reflux, or protrusion of an enlarged prostate into the vesical cavity.

If a catheter cannot be introduced through the urethra, a small plastic tube can be placed in the bladder through the barrel of a needle passed suprapubically.

B. Study of the Neurogenic (Neuropathic) Bladder: Particularly in the spastic type of neurogenic bladder, ureterovesical reflux is common. Cystograms will reveal this reflux as well as the degree of damage from hydronephrosis or pyelonephritis.

C. Rupture of the Bladder: Cystography is the best method of testing for extravasation of urine.

D. Recurrent Infection: Cystography should be routine in the study of any patient suffering from recurrent infection, particularly children. Vesicoureteral reflux is one of the common causes of perpetuation of infection. This procedure may also delineate vesical fistulous communications and is of great help in the study of urinary incontinence in both males and females.

E. Lateral Cystogram: This is an important step in the evaluation of the woman with stress incontinence. (See Chapter 28.)

Contraindications

During acute attacks or exacerbations of chronic urinary infection, the instillation of radiopaque medium under pressure may increase the seriousness of the infection (eg, bacteremia), particularly if reflux exists.

Technic

Maskell, Pead, & Vinnicombe (1978) noted that 22% of their patients undergoing this procedure developed bacteriuria. They recommend prophylactic antibiotics.

(1) If vesicoureteral reflux is suspected, a KUB should be made. If vesical disease only is to be studied (eg, rupture), a film of the bladder area alone is sufficient.

(2) A catheter is passed to the bladder. The urine it contains should be drained off.

(3) Introduction of radiopaque fluid: In the adult, 250–350 mL are sufficient. In a child 1 year old, the normal vesical capacity is 75–100 mL. Any fluid used for excretory or retrograde urography diluted with 3 parts of water or normal saline solution can be used.

(4) The catheter is then clamped off and an x-ray taken with the patient supine. This may reveal trabeculation and diverticula, intravesical protrusion of an enlarged prostate, vesical tumors, or vesicoureteral reflux.

(5) Left and right oblique radiograms will visualize diverticula that lie behind the bladder or a fistulous tract into the vagina.

(6) Cystograms taken in the true lateral position are helpful in delineating the cause of urinary

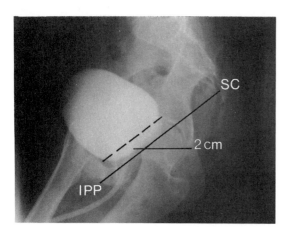
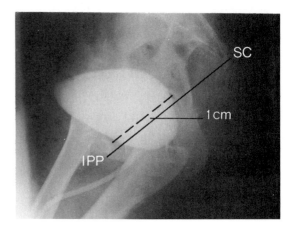

Figure 6–9. Lateral cystogram in stress incontinence. The dashed line shows the normal position of the base of the normal bladder. Line SCIPP is a reference line drawn from the sacrococcygeal (SC) joint to the inferior point of the pubic bone (IPP). *Left:* Resting cystogram in stress incontinence. The bladder base lies 2 cm below the normal position. *Right:* Cystogram taken with straining in a patient with stress incontinence. Normally, the base of the bladder should lie on the dashed line. The base of the bladder descends about 4 cm, revealing poor support of the urethrovesical junction.

incontinence, particularly in women (Figs 6–9 and 28–2).

(7) The vesical fluid is then allowed to drain out and another x-ray film exposed. Diverticula or a fistulous tract into the vagina will still contain the radiopaque fluid and will be clearly defined. Intraperitoneal or extraperitoneal extravasation of the contrast medium behind the bladder will be shown. Fig 6–8 demonstrates the normal and some abnormal cystograms.

DELAYED CYSTOGRAMS

Simple cystography often fails to demonstrate ureterovesical reflux, although incompetency of the vesicoureteral valves exists. Stewart (1955) has shown that "delayed" cystograms reveal this reflux more efficiently. If voiding cystourethrography is attempted but the patient cannot void, delayed cystograms should be resorted to.

Technic

(1) Preliminary film of abdomen should be made.

(2) A small catheter is passed to the bladder and the urine drained off.

(3) Radiopaque fluid is then introduced into the bladder. The amount varies from 30 mL in an infant to 120 mL for a child age 8 years and 20–300 mL for adults. The least noxious fluid is urographic medium diluted with 3 parts of water or normal saline solution.

(4) The catheter is then removed.

(5) Serial x-ray films are then exposed every 15–30 minutes during the next 1–3 hours. Ureteral reflux may appear on one "delayed" film only to be absent on the next. One kidney may reveal reflux, whereas on the next exposure only the opposite kidney may contain the radiopaque fluid.

VOIDING CYSTOURETHROGRAMS

Because of the increased intravesical pressure generated at the time of voiding, this technic often shows ureteral reflux when both the simple and delayed cystograms fail to do so. The voiding cystourethrogram may also reveal the presence of posterior urethral valves (Fig 29–1) or urethral strictures (Fig 29–4). If catheterization is impossible or thought to be contraindicated, radiopaque fluid can be instilled by suprapubic vesical puncture.

Immediately following the conclusion of the series of delayed cystograms or after filling the bladder with the radiopaque medium, the patient is instructed to void. During the act of urination, one or more x-rays are taken.

CYSTOURETHROGRAMS

Cystourethrograms combine simple cystography with urethrography. Vesical and urethral abnormalities are thereby visualized.

A catheter is passed to the bladder and a plain film of the bladder area is taken. About 200–300 mL of radiopaque fluid or air are then introduced into the bladder, a plain x-ray film exposed, and oblique views made. With the patient lying at a 45-degree angle, 20 mL of radiopaque water-soluble lubricant are injected into the urethra and a radiogram made (Fig 6–10).

• • •

RETROGRADE URETHROGRAMS

Stenoses of the urethra and enlargements of the prostate and even some posterior urethral valves (Fig 29–1) can be shown on films by introducing into the urethra 20–30 mL of a water-soluble lubricant in which there is an equal amount of radiopaque fluid. Oily media (eg, iodized oil [Lipiodol] are contraindicated, since they may cause pulmonary emboli. The radiogram should be taken while the fluid is being injected. Oblique films of the area of the urethra and prostate will demonstrate narrowings, diverticula, fistulas, and other diseases of these organs (Fig 6–10).

ESTIMATION OF RESIDUAL URINE IN CHILDREN

Instill 5 mL of ascendant iodized oil (Lipiodol) into the bladder. If the child does not retain urine, a film taken 24 hours later will show no retention of the opaque material. If some urinary retention does exist, the fluid may remain in the bladder for many days. If vesicoureteral reflux is present, the iodized oil may be visualized in the kidney (Fig 6–8).

CINERADIOGRAPHY

Cineradiography, formerly only a research tool, is now of practical value in clinical diagnosis. It reveals a higher incidence and degree of reflux than cystography and the voiding cystourethrogram and affords a dynamic picture of this abnormality.

The bladder is gradually filled with radiopaque fluid. The ureters are studied for transient or persistent reflux. The efficiency of peristalsis may also be studied. Reflux may only be demonstrated during the act of voiding, when intravesical pressure is high. About half of children suffering from urinary tract infection will show vesicoureteral reflux. This phenomenon is also revealed in a significant number of adults with chronic pyelonephritis.

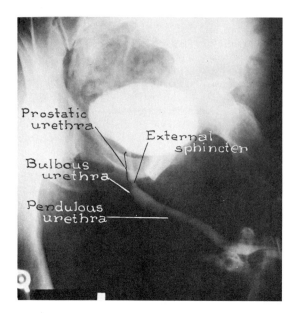

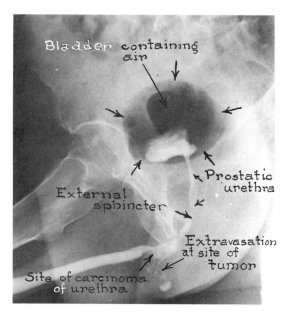

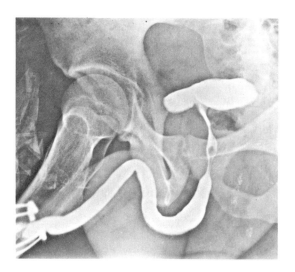

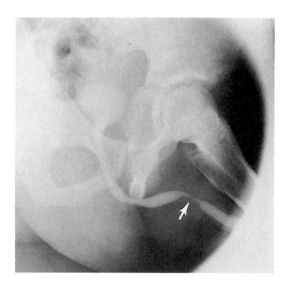

Figure 6–10. Normal and abnormal cystourethrograms and retrograde urethrograms. *Above left:* Normal cystourethrogram. *Above right:* Cystourethrogram showing carcinoma of urethra. *Below left:* Normal urethrogram. Note "negative" shadow over pubic bone representing the verumontanum. *Below right:* Oblique retrograde urethrogram showing stricture of pendulous urethra.

RENAL ANGIOGRAPHY

Although renal angiograms can be procured by direct lumbar needle puncture of the aorta, this technic has been superseded by percutaneous femoral angiography, wherein a catheter is passed to the level of the renal arteries under fluoroscopic control. Percutaneous catheterization of the brachial or axillary artery is also feasible. Twelve to 24 mL of radiopaque fluid suitable for intravenous urography (eg, meglumine diatrizoate, 66%, and sodium diatrizoate, 10%, [Renografin-76]) are rapidly introduced into the aorta, and serial films are immediately taken (midstream technic). About 10 exposures are made over a period of 10 seconds, but 2 per second are exposed for the first 3 seconds. A second or even a third injection may be indicated for oblique views. Besides demonstrating the caliber of the great vessels, this procedure shows the renal arterial circulation (Fig 6–11). Fig 34–3 reveals stenosis of the renal artery as the cause of hypertension. A pheochromocytoma is shown in Fig 21–15.

Selective renal angiography is accomplished by passing a femoral catheter into one of the renal arteries under fluoroscopic control. About 8 mL of contrast medium are injected, and approximately 16 exposures are made during the first few seconds (Fig 6–11). The intrarenal vascular detail demonstrated by this technic is superior to the midstream method and is therefore of particular value in the differential diagnosis of renal cyst (Fig 22–6) and tumor (Fig 18–3). The space occupied by a cyst fails to opacify. Neovascularity followed by increased density on late films is typical of tumor.

In cases where the lesion is small or obscured by overlying arteries, epinephrine can first be injected into the catheter, followed by instillation of radiopaque medium. This technic causes spasm of normal vessels but has no effect on arteries in tumors.

Though renal angiography is reported to be complicated by acute renal failure in 12% of cases (Swartz & others, 1978), Eisenberg, Bank, & Hedgcock (1980) failed to see this in well-hydrated patients.

VESICAL ANGIOGRAPHY

In order to judge the size and depth of penetration of vesical neoplasms, the following technic can be employed. A Seldinger catheter is passed to the bifurcation of the aorta, and the vessels are "flooded" with 30 mL of 90% contrast material. As an alternative, each hypogastric artery is selectively catheterized and into each of them are instilled 10 mL of radiopaque fluid. Films are rapidly exposed over a period of 8 seconds. The series is repeated in the oblique position, affording a tangential view of the tumor. These roentgenograms reveal the typical pattern or "stain" of an invasive tumor (Fig 18–12), thus improving accuracy of staging of the lesion. The study may be enhanced if 60 mL of CO_2 are first instilled into the bladder.

LYMPHANGIOGRAPHY

Cannulation of a lymphatic vessel in the foot and injection of an oily contrast medium leads to x-ray opacification of the inguinal, pelvic, ret-

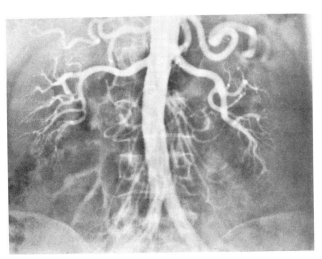 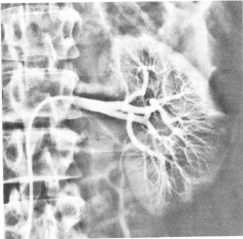

Figure 6–11. Normal percutaneous femoral renal angiograms. *Left:* Midstream technic. Renal arteries and their branches are of normal caliber and distribution. The celiac axis, splenic artery, and branches of the superior mesenteric arteries are well outlined. *Right:* Selective renal angiogram. Detail of smaller arterial branches is enhanced. They are evenly distributed throughout the kidney.

roperitoneal, and supraclavicular lymphatic systems (Fig 6–12). The main value of this procedure is the demonstration of metastatic infiltration in regional lymph nodes (Fig 6–13). It therefore lends itself to the study of patients with cancers of the testes (Fig 18–20), penis, bladder, or prostate. It can demonstrate the lymphatic connections to the kidney in patients with chyluria.

VENACAVOGRAPHY

Retrograde catheterization of the femoral veins affords a route for the injection of radiopaque material into the vena cava (Fig 27–5). Evidence of masses in the right retroperitoneal areas is demonstrated by encroachment on the vessel. Thus, this technic is one of particular value in outlining enlarged retroperitoneal lymph nodes (eg, testicular tumor; Fig 6–14). This technic may also reveal tumor thrombus in the adrenal vein or vena cava.

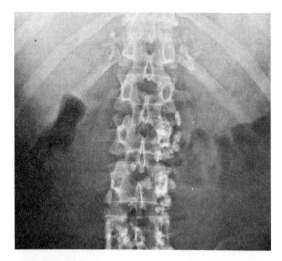

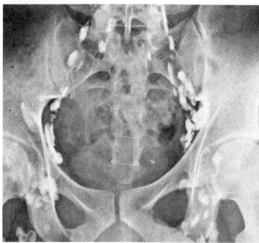

Figure 6–12. Normal lymphangiogram. (Composite of 2 films.) Note calcifications of both adrenal glands, probably secondary to spontaneous hemorrhage. Compare with Fig 6–13.

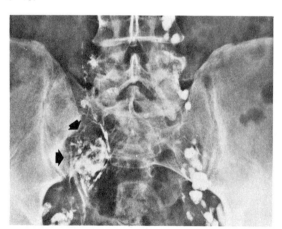

Figure 6–13. Abnormal lymphangiogram. Carcinoma of the penis with metastases to right common iliac nodes, overlying sacroiliac joint, which have blocked ascent of contrast medium.

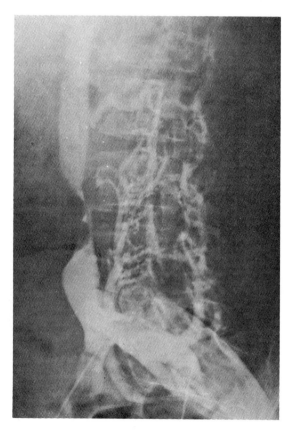

Figure 6–14. Venacavogram. Right posterior oblique exposure revealing defect caused by metastases to lumbar lymph nodes from seminoma of right testis. (See Fig 18–20 for retrograde ureterogram on same patient.)

SELECTIVE RENAL VENOGRAPHY

While venacavography may reveal gross extension of renal carcinoma into the vena cava, it may miss minor defects in the renal veins themselves because of the "washout" of the veins by a large volume of blood. Selective renal venography overcomes this deficiency. It is an excellent method of demonstrating renal vein thrombosis (Fig 22–13).

The washout effect can be decreased by injection of epinephrine into the renal artery 10 seconds before the venous infusion of 35–60 mL of radiopaque material. If indicated, a blood sample from the renal vein can be subjected to analysis for renin.

Renal phlebography can differentiate between an absent and a nonfunctioning kidney (Braedel & others, 1976). Oleaga & others (1978), using this technic, found it helpful in diagnosing obscure cancers and chronic pyelonephritis.

SELECTIVE ADRENAL VENOGRAPHY

Transfemoral catheterization of one or both adrenal veins can be accomplished. This allows estimation of the concentration of hormones (eg, aldosterone, cortisol, 11-deoxycortisol) in the venous blood and phlebography. It is particularly useful in the endocrinologic and radiographic diagnosis of Cushing's disease, hyperaldosteronism, carcinoma, and bilateral adrenal hyperplasia.

COMPUTED TOMOGRAPHY (CT SCAN) OF THE URINARY TRACT

Computed tomography (CT) differs from conventional radiography in several ways. Although x-rays pass through the patient during CT examination, the detector system is usually a scintillation phototube or gas-filled ionization chamber rather than the usual x-ray film. The x-ray tube and detector system are on opposite sides of the patient, and during a scan they rotate around the patient while recording information about the internal structure of the thin transverse cross section through which the x-ray beam is passing. Through a complex series of mathematical manipulations, the computer "reconstructs" the cross-sectional image as an array or grid of individual picture elements and displays it as an integrated picture on a television monitor. The image on the screen bears a remarkable resemblance to photographs from standard textbooks of cross-sectional anatomy. The approximate density of any tissue within the image being displayed can be determined by simple manipulation of the control dials.

Several important advances in CT technology during the past 4 years have significantly improved the image quality and clinical utility of body scanning. The major advance has been the development of more rapid scanning cycles. Most CT scanners now generate the data needed to reconstruct an image in approximately 2–5 seconds, so that most patients can be examined during suspended respiration. This and other technologic improvements are providing images of remarkable clarity and accuracy.

Most CT scanners function in the same way. The patient lies supine on an adjustable tabletop that extends through a circular opening of the scanning gantry. The patient is asked to suspend respiration for the required scanning time. Usually, multiple scans are performed at various levels of the body, depending on the clinical question being pursued, the type of collimation available, and the time available for examination. For most areas of the abdomen, a slice thickness of 5–10 mm is chosen. A typical examination of the kidneys consists of a series of 10-mm contiguous transverse slices through both kidneys. When small lesions are discovered, or when the region to be examined is especially small, collimation down to a slice thickness of 4 or 5 mm is often selected when this option is available.

Because collapsed or fluid-filled loops of bowel can simulate a pathologic mass on CT images, it is often desirable to have the patient ingest dilute oral contrast material prior to examination of the abdomen. Intravenous injection of standard urographic contrast material is also frequently given. The indications for intravenous contrast material and the necessity for precontrast scans are matters of current debate. Because most renal masses "enhance" less than normal parenchyma, they are easier to detect after injection of contrast material. This is particularly true for small masses that do not produce a recognizable alteration in the external contour of the kidney.

Renal Masses

Several reports (McClennan & others, 1979; Magilner & Ostrum, 1978; Sagel & others, 1977) document a very high accuracy for CT in differentiating simple renal cyst from a more complicated mass. A renal mass that does not conform to the criteria for a simple renal cyst usually turns out to be a renal carcinoma, though other lesions such as abscess or hemorrhagic renal cyst are occasionally diagnosed. In general, CT assessment of a renal mass is obtained either as part of the evaluation of a mass detected by urography and incompletely characterized by ultrasound examination, or as part of the evaluation of a mass discovered during CT examination ordered for other reasons.

In CT examination, a renal mass is considered to be a simple benign cyst if it has a homogeneous attenuation value (density) similar to that of water and has a wall thickness that is virtually unmeasurable (Fig 6–15). A typical renal cancer has a density

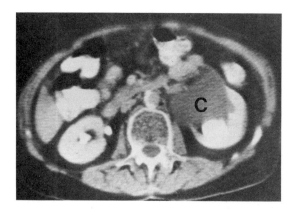

Figure 6–15. Simple renal cyst. CT shows a homogeneous, thin-walled mass (C) that had an attenuation value near that of water.

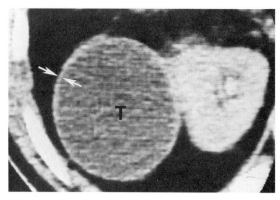

Figure 6–17. Necrotic renal cancer. Although CT showed a homogeneous mass (T) with water density, the measurable wall thickness (arrows) correctly suggested that this was not a simple renal cyst. (Courtesy of W Foster.)

similar to that of normal renal parenchyma, although occasionally its density is slightly higher or lower than that of normal tissue (Fig 6–16). Necrosis of a renal cancer renders the lesion of nonhomogeneous density; some completely necrotic tumors may be mostly of homogeneous water density but typically have a thick wall that indicates they are not simple benign cysts (Fig 6–17).

The above density criteria apply to scans obtained without the injection of intravenous contrast material. Because the material is excreted and concentrated by normal renal parenchyma, nonfunctioning renal masses are more easily visible following its use. Noncystic renal masses increase in density following contrast injection, though not to the same degree as the surrounding normal parenchyma. Renal cysts maintain a density close to that of water. Nonenhanced imaging may not detect a small intrarenal mass that does not alter the ex-

pected renal contour. Therefore, intravenous contrast medium should almost always be used unless a specific contraindication exists. A precontrast scan of the kidneys is not usually necessary, since the enhanced scan alone provides adequate diagnostic information (Engelstad & others, 1980).

In most radiology departments, demonstration of a solitary renal mass during urography leads to evaluation by diagnostic ultrasound. If the ultrasound examination demonstrates all of the findings characteristic of a simple benign cyst, there is probably no reason to perform any other diagnostic imaging examination. If the ultrasound examination is technically unsatisfactory or fails to demonstrate the classic criteria of a simple benign cyst, CT offers an accurate and noninvasive method of evaluating the lesion. The most frequent causes of an indeterminate ultrasound examination are (1) a mass in the upper pole of the left kidney, (2) a mass in the region

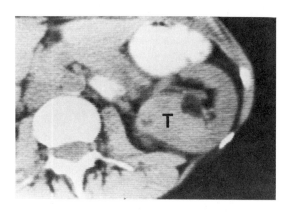

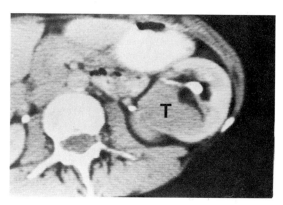

Figure 6–16. Renal carcinoma. *Left:* CT shows a renal mass (T) with an attenuation value slightly higher (more opaque) than adjacent renal parenchyma. *Right:* After intravenous injection of contrast material, the mass appears less dense than opacified normal parenchyma, although its attenuation value had increased and was much higher than that of water.

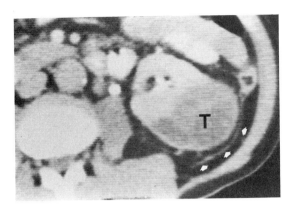

Figure 6–18. Intracapsular renal carcinoma. CT shows a well-demarcated renal mass (T) with preservation of perirenal fat between it and Gerota's fascia (arrows).

of the renal pelvis, (3) the presence of multiple renal masses, and (4) a markedly obese patient.

CT is accurate for preoperative staging of renal cancer (Levin, Lee, & Weigel, 1979; Love & others, 1979). Weyman & others (1980) have demonstrated that CT is as accurate as angiography in determining the local extent of the cancer (Fig 6–18), the presence of enlarged regional lymph nodes, and the presence of tumor thrombus within the main renal vein and the inferior vena cava (Fig 6–19) (Marks & others, 1978).

CT is also uniquely valuable in assessing a suspected recurrence of renal cancer (Bernardino & others, 1979; Alter, Uehling, & Zwiebel, 1979). Following a left nephrectomy, the tail of the pancreas and loops of small bowel tend to occupy the site of the resected kidney. Following a right nephrectomy, the duodenum and head of the pancreas migrate to the right renal bed in a similar manner. CT will detect even a small mass in these cases (Fig 6–20).

Adrenal Mass

In the brief interval since this book was last revised, it has become widely accepted that CT is the method of choice for evaluation of a known or suspected adrenal mass. The basis for this widespread acceptance is the accurate CT visualization of normal adrenal glands in most patients (Montagne & others, 1978; Karstaedt & others, 1978). When both glands are adequately visualized, as is true in over 90% of cases, the absence of a demonstrable adrenal mass essentially excludes a lesion larger than 1 cm in diameter.

The adrenal glands have a characteristic appearance in CT images (Fig 6–21). Either 2 or 3 thin limbs are visualized on images of normal glands, usually in the overall shape of an inverted letter V or Y. It is important to try to identify each of the limbs, because some masses arise from only one limb, with the rest of the gland appearing to be normal.

In patients with functioning adrenal disorders such as pheochromocytoma, Cushing's syndrome, and primary aldosteronism, CT can detect and localize an adrenal mass (Fig 6–22). CT accuracy in these patients is remarkably high (Karstaedt & others, 1978; Korobkin & others, 1979; Dunnick & others, 1979; Laursen & Damgaard-Pedersen, 1980). Virtually no false-positive examinations have been reported. If CT reveals normal adrenal glands in patients with pheochromocytoma, it is essential to continue with the examination to evaluate the para-aortic region and the bladder. Approximately half of patients with Cushing's syndrome due to a pituitary lesion rather than an adrenal mass (so-called "adrenal hyperplasia"), have glands of normal size by CT (Korobkin & others, 1979). The rest have diffuse thickening of the limbs of the adrenal glands corresponding to macroscopic enlargement. It is obvious, then, that demonstration of bilateral normal adrenal glands can never exclude a diagnosis of Cushing's syndrome: Normal adrenal CT excludes

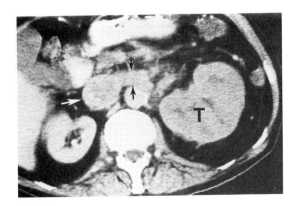

Figure 6–19. Vascular extension of renal carcinoma. CT shows marked enlargement of the left renal vein (black arrows) and inferior vena cava (white arrow) due to tumor thrombus from a carcinoma (T) in the left kidney.

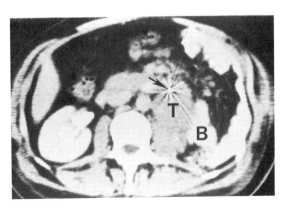

Figure 6–20. Recurrent renal carcinoma. CT shows a small soft tissue mass (T) in the bed of the resected kidney. A surgical clip (arrow), and contrast-filled small bowel (B) are adjacent to the locally recurrent tumor.

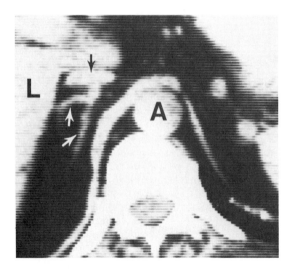

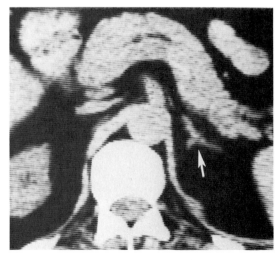

Figure 6–21. Normal adrenal glands. *Left:* CT shows both major limbs (white arrows) of the right adrenal gland. (A, aorta; L, liver; black arrow, vena cava.) *Right:* CT section caudal to (A) shows all 3 limbs of the left adrenal (arrow).

only a unilateral adrenal tumor as the cause of the syndrome.

CT detects most lesions of primary aldosteronism, in which tumors are typically less than 2 cm in diameter (White & others, 1980). However, if the scan shows normal adrenal glands or fails to clearly demonstrate both glands, radionuclide scanning or adrenal vein sampling should be performed if the clinical and biochemical evidence for a unilateral tumor is compelling.

Adrenal carcinoma is almost always quite large when it first comes to clinical presentation and is always detectable by CT. It is sometimes difficult to differentiate such a large mass from other lesions in contiguous structures. Adrenal metastases (Fig 6–23), either unilateral or bilateral, are commonly identified in patients with current primary tumors of the lung or breast, with melanoma, and occasion-

ally with other lesions. The CT characteristics of metastases are almost identical to those of primary functioning adrenal masses, and therefore it may be impossible to differentiate primary from metastatic neoplasm in a patient with known metastatic disease and a unilateral adrenal mass lesion.

CT is also useful in evaluating suspected adrenal mass lesions detected on a urogram. In addition to confirming the presence of an adrenal mass, CT occasionally shows a normal adrenal gland surrounded by abundant retroperitoneal fat (Fig 6–24), thereby obviating any further diagnostic evaluation.

Retroperitoneum

Because of the large amount of fat normally present in the retroperitoneum, CT is the most accurate imaging method available for detection of

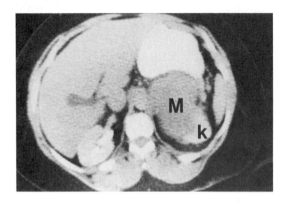

Figure 6–22. Unilateral adrenal mass. CT shows a large mass (M) replacing the left adrenal gland. (k, upper pole of left kidney.)

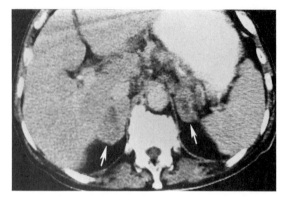

Figure 6–23. Adrenal metastases. CT section cephalad to both kidneys shows bilateral solid adrenal masses (arrows).

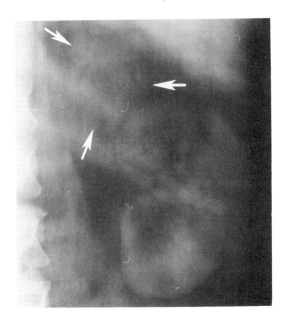

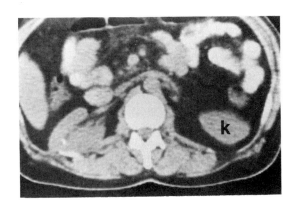

Figure 6–24. Normal fat simulating adrenal mass during urography. *Left:* Urogram shows lateral displacement of upper pole of left kidney and a suspected adrenal mass (arrows). *Right:* CT shows that only retroperitoneal fat is present medial to upper pole of left kidney (k). CT section more cephalad showed a normal left adrenal gland.

mass lesions in that anatomic compartment.

A. Fluid Collections: The presence of a hematoma, abscess, benign fluid collection, or benign or metastatic tumor can be accurately assessed with CT. Although large mass lesions are frequently detected by other imaging technics, only CT can almost routinely display the entire retroperitoneal space, thus warranting a high degree of confidence in a report indicating the absence of a mass lesion. However, the precise nature of a mass is often not apparent by CT criteria alone. (Two prominent exceptions are the high density of an acute hematoma [Fig 6–25] and the extraluminal gas often present within an abscess.)

B. Lymphadenopathy: The most frequent use of CT for the retroperitoneal space is in the evaluation of suspected lymph node disease. Retroperitoneal lymph nodes that are enlarged due to malignant disease are easily demonstrated. Para-aortic lymph node enlargement is most easily identified (Fig 6–26), whereas pelvic nodes are more difficult to assess because they are usually accompanied by contiguous blood vessels of variable caliber. The abdominal aorta and inferior vena cava

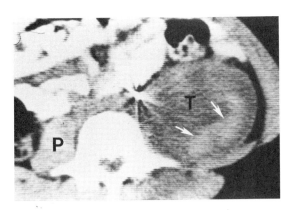

Figure 6–25. Subacute psoas hematoma. CT shows a huge mass (T) involving the left psoas muscle. The clumps of higher density tissue (arrows) within the mass indicate the presence of fresh blood. Note the normal right psoas muscle (P).

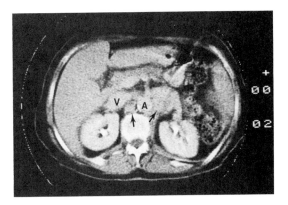

Figure 6–26. Enlarged para-aortic lymph nodes. CT shows enlarged nodes (arrows) adjacent to the aorta (A) and vena cava (V).

are normally surrounded only by fat, making enlarged lymph nodes in these areas easy to visualize. It must be recognized that CT cannot identify filling defects within normal-sized lymph nodes; therefore, a negative CT examination for lymph node enlargement should never be considered definitive for exclusion of metastatic disease to these nodes. Although CT accuracy in assessment of retroperitoneal lymph node disease is well documented for lymphoma, its accuracy for nodal metastases from pelvic cancer has not been fully defined.

CT has certain advantages over lymphography in evaluation of lymph node metastases. Nodes between the renal hilum and the diaphragm are usually not adequately visualized on lymphography, but enlarged nodes in that region are usually well delineated by CT. This has particular relevance in testicular cancer because of the well-known preferential drainage of metastases to lymph nodes in and around the hilum of the kidneys with this disease. Also of significance for urologic cancer is CT demonstration of the internal iliac lymph node chain, which is not normally opacified during lymphography. It is prudent to obtain a CT scan first when evaluating pelvic and retroperitoneal lymph nodes in patients with pelvic cancer. Lymphangiography can be reserved for patients with a normal CT examination, some of whom will have metastatic disease in normal-sized nodes. Percutaneous aspiration biopsy for confirmation of malignant cells can then be performed for histologic evaluation of enlarged lymph nodes detected by CT or abnormal nodes identified on a lymphogram.

Bladder & Prostate

The bladder, prostate gland, and seminal vesicles are clearly delineated on all CT scans through the pelvis. Only in exceptional cases is contrast material needed to assess the bladder. Normally, the urine-filled bladder is easily identifiable. Because the perivesical fat and the intravesical urine

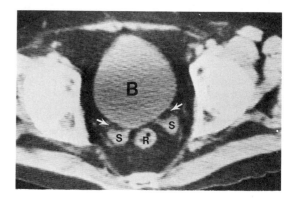

Figure 6–28. Normal seminal vesicles. The seminal vesicles (S) are normally well demonstrated by CT, between the bladder (B) anteriorly and the rectum (R) posteriorly. The arrows point to the normally preserved fat plane between the seminal vesicles and the bladder.

have densities different from that of the bladder wall, wall thickness is usually easy to evaluate. Focal thickening of the bladder wall may be the only CT evidence of a bladder cancer (Fig 6–27). The seminal vesicles are remarkably well delineated by CT (Fig 6–28); visualization of normal fat planes between the vesicles and the bladder is considered important evidence against direct involvement by cancer of the bladder or the prostate gland (Seidelmann & others, 1977).

Preliminary evidence indicates that CT is accurate for staging of the local extent of bladder cancer (Hodson, Husband, & MacDonald, 1979; Seidelmann & others, 1978). Its accuracy appears to be greatest in assessing the extent of large tumors, precisely where clinical assessment may be most problematic. Detection of direct spread to the pelvic wall by a large bladder cancer is also easily and accurately obtained (Fig 6–29), as is differentiation

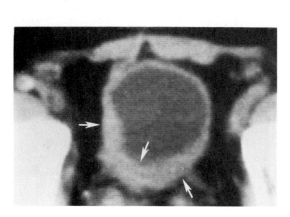

Figure 6–27. Bladder carcinoma. Thickening of the posterior wall (arrows) of the bladder was due to infiltrating carcinoma.

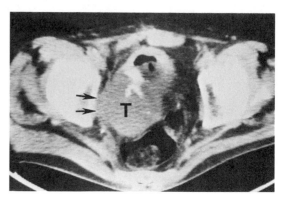

Figure 6–29. Extension of bladder carcinoma. CT shows that a known bladder cancer (T) has extended to involve the lateral side walls of the pelvis (arrows).

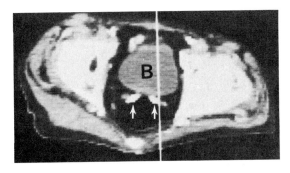
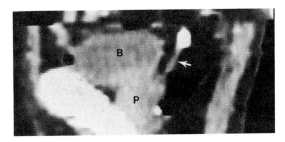

Figure 6–30. *Left:* Conventional transaxial CT images of pelvis from which parasagittal image was reconstructed. The vertical line represents the parasagittal plane chosen. (B, bladder; arrows, calcified seminal vesicles.) *Right:* Parasagittal reconstructed image shows the bladder (B), prostate (P), and junction of vas deferens and seminal vesicle (arrow).

of tumors confined to the deep muscles of the bladder wall from those extending into the perivesical fat, although this distinction often does not affect therapeutic management.

The value of CT in the staging of prostatic cancer has not been adequately evaluated. It is known that most of these cancers do not have a density different from normal or hypertrophic prostatic tissue. CT may be helpful in detecting seminal vesicle involvement by prostatic cancer, especially with the newly emerging computer technics for reconstruction of images in coronal and sagittal planes of section (Fig 6–30).

CT availability should make diagnosis of pelvic lipomatosis certain in all cases (Fig 6–31). Compression or displacement of the bladder or pelvic ureters due to the presence of pelvic fat can be accurately visualized. Abnormalities such as bilateral iliac lymph node enlargement sometimes deform the bladder in a manner similar to pelvic lipomatosis; CT permits a definitive diagnosis in all problematic cases.

OTHER X–RAY STUDIES

Roentgenograms of the gastrointestinal tract, chest, and bones may contribute to urologic diagnosis.

Gastrointestinal Series (Fig 6–32)

A barium enema may show displacement of the colon—a cardinal sign of retroperitoneal tumor. The stomach may also be displaced by large retroperitoneal masses (eg, kidney, spleen, pancreas).

Cholecystograms

Films of the gallbladder may show evidence of gallbladder disease. Extensive renal carcinoma may invade the common duct. Cholecystitis or cholelithiasis may be the cause of pseudorenal pain.

Chest Film

An x-ray of the chest may reveal the source of a tuberculous infection of the kidney or may show

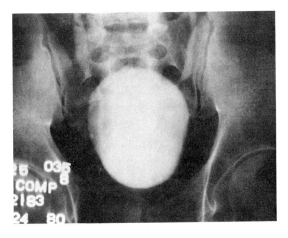
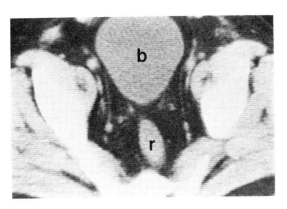

Figure 6–31. *Left:* Urogram shows findings suggestive of pelvic lipomatosis. *Right:* CT confirms the presence of abundant pelvic fat. No mass lesions are present. The bladder (b) and rectum (r) are characteristically elongated in the anteroposterior dimension.

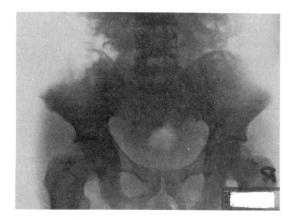

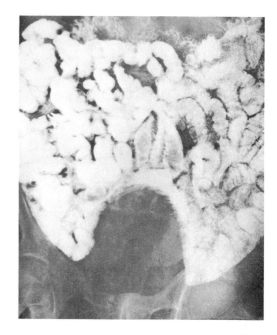

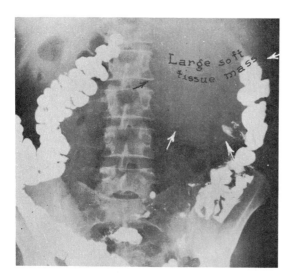

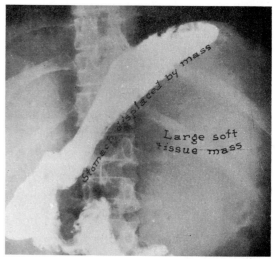

Figure 6–32. Miscellaneous x-ray studies. *Above left:* Study of bones reveals hemisacrum, which is often associated with findings of neuropathic bladder. *Above right:* Patient with low midline mass and cramping abdominal pain. Gastrointestinal series showing the cause of the symptoms—a distended bladder. *Below left:* Barium enema showing displacement of transverse colon by large cyst of left kidney. *Below right:* Gastrointestinal series (same patient) showing displacement of stomach by cyst of left kidney.

metastasis from renal, testicular, or other tumors (Fig 18–4).

Osteograms

Films of bones may reveal evidence of metas-

tases (Figs 18–4 and 18–17), spina bifida (Fig 19–10), or changes compatible with hyperparathyroidism (Fig 15–4), or osteitis fibrosa generalisata as often seen in patients with renal tubular acidosis.

•   •   •

References

General

Friedland GW: Pediatric urography. *Urol Clin North Am* 1979;6:375.

Lowman RM: Retroperitoneal tumors: A survey and assessment of Roentgen techniques. *Radiol Clin North Am* 1965;3:543.

Pfister RC, Newhouse JH: Radiology of ureter. *Urology* 1978;12:15.

Symposium on urinary tract (radiologic aspects). *Radiol Clin North Am* 1965;3:3.

Plain Film of Abdomen

Ambos MA, Bosniak MA: Tomography of the kidney bed as an aid in differentiating renal pelvic tumor and stone. *Am J Roentgenol* 1975;125:331.

Babaian RJ, Lucey DT, Fried FA: Significance and evaluation of calcifications associated with renal masses. *Urology* 1978;12:109.

Braren V, Jones WB: Sacral agenesis: Diagnosis, treatment and follow-up of urological complications. *J Urol* 1979;121:543.

Brill PW, Krasna IH, Aaron H: An early rim sign in neonatal adrenal hemorrhage. *Am J Roentgenol* 1976;127:289.

Elkin M, Cohen G: Diagnostic value of the psoas shadow. *Clin Radiol* 1962;13: 210.

Fornasier VL, Horne JG: Metastases to the vertebral column. *Cancer* 1975;36:590.

Hunter AM, Howey S, Hocken AG: Normal radiological renal size: Simple estimation from single urogram series. *NZ Med J* 1975;81:409.

Madsen EH: The value of tomography for the demonstration of small intrarenal calcifications. *Br J Radiol* 1972;45:203.

Olurin EO, Olurin O: Pancreatic calcification: A report of 45 cases. *Br Med J* 1969;4:534.

Price JL, Loveday BJ: Soft tissue radiography of the testicles. *Br J Radiol* 1975;48:179.

Shemilt P: The origin of phleboliths. *Br J Surg* 1972;59:695.

Stevenson J, MacGregor AM, Connelly P: Calcification of the adrenal glands in young children. *Arch Dis Child* 1961;36:316.

Excretory Urograms

Allen TD: Extensive displacement of the kidney by intraperitoneal disease. *J Urol* 1967;97:823.

Barbaric Z: Renal fascia in urinary tract disease. *Radiology* 1976;118:561.

Boltuch RL, Lalli AF: A new technique for urethrography. *Radiology* 1975;115:736.

Carvallo A, Rakowski TA, Argy WP Jr: Acute renal failure following drip infusion pyelography. *Am J Med* 1978;65:38.

Cerny JC, Kendall AR, Nesbit RM: Subcutaneous pyelography in infants: A reappraisal. *J Urol* 1967;98:405.

Chait A & others: Vascular impressions on the ureter. *Am J Roentgenol* 1971;111:729.

Cohen MD: Intravenous urography in neonates and infants: What dose of contrast should be used? *Br J Radiol* 1979;52:942.

Cunningham JJ: Radiologic features of the interureteric ridge. *Am J Roentgenol* 1975;125:688.

Daughtridge TG: Mucosal folds in the upper urinary tract. *Am J Roentgenol* 1969;107:743.

Dunbar JS, Nogrady B: Excretory urography in the first year of life. *Radiol Clin North Am* 1972;10:365.

Dure-Smith P: Fluid restriction before excretory urography. *Radiology* 1976;118:487.

Filly RA & others: Urinary tract infections in children. 2. Roentgenologic aspects. *West J Med* 1974;121:374.

Fischer HW, Doust VL: An evaluation of pretesting in the problem of serious and fatal reactions to excretory urography. *Radiology* 1972;103:497.

Fletcher EWL, Lecky JW: The normal position of the upper ureter in lateral intravenous pyelography. *Br J Urol* 1969;41:554.

Ford WH Jr, Palubinskas AJ: Renal extravasation during excretory urography using abdominal compression. *J Urol* 1967;97:983.

Gates DF, Ceccarelli FE: Benadryl and the IVP reaction. *J Urol* 1972;108:627.

Geraghty JA: An approach to the problem of intestinal gas in diagnostic radiology. *Br J Radiol* 1966;39:42.

Gilbert EF & others: Hemorrhagic renal necrosis in infancy: Relationship to radiopaque compounds. *J Pediatr* 1970;76:49.

Grainger RG: Renal toxicity of radiological contrast media. *Br Med Bull* 1972;28:191.

Janson KL, Roberts JA, Evans BB: Displacement of left kidney suggesting adrenal tumor. *Urology* 1977;9:91.

Kabakian HA & others: Asymmetry of the pelvic ureters in normal females. *Am J Roentgenol* 1976;137:723.

Kassner EG, Elguezabal A, Pochaczevsky R: Death during intravenous urography: Overdose syndrome in young infants. *NY State J Med* 1973;73:1958.

Korobkin M, Minagi H, Palubinskas AJ: Lateral displacement of the bladder. *Am J Roentgenol* 1975;125:337.

Kumar D, Cigtay OS, Klein LH: Aberrant renal papilla. *Br J Radiol* 1977;50:141.

Lalli AF: Contrast media reactions: Data analysis and hypothesis. *Radiology* 1980;134:1.

Lalli AF: Urography, shock reaction and repeated urography. (Editorial.) *Am J Roentgenol* 1975;125: 264.

Lopez FA & others: The nephrogram: A valuable indication of renal abnormalities. *Am J Roentgenol* 1969;106:614.

Martin DJ, Gilday DL, Reilly BJ: Evaluation of the urinary tract in the neonatal period. *Radiol Clin North Am* 1975;13:359.

Marx WJ, Patel SK: Renal fascia: Its radiographic importance. *Urology* 1979;13:1.

Nogrady MB, Dunbar JS: Delayed concentration and prolonged excretion of urographic contrast medium in the first month of life. *Am J Roentgenol* 1968;104:289.

Olsson O: Excretion of sodium metrizoate through the liver during urography. *Acta Radiol [Diagn] (Stockh)* 1971;11:85.

Peck AG, Yoder IC, Pfister RC: Tomography of pelvic-abdominal masses during intravenous urography. *Am J Roentgenol* 1975;125:322.

Pollack HM: Some limitations and pitfalls of excretory urography. *J Urol* 1976;116:537.

Riggs W Jr, Hagood JH, Andrews AE: Anatomic changes in the normal urinary tract between supine and prone urograms. *Radiology* 1970;94:107.

Saldino RM, Palubinskas AJ: Medial placement of the ureter: A normal variant which may simulate retroperitoneal fibrosis. *J Urol* 1972;**107**:582.

Siegle RL, Lieberman P: A review of untoward reactions to iodinated contrast material. *J Urol* 1978;**119**:581.

Silverman SH, Nylan WL: Shock following intravenous pyelography in patients with congenital adrenal hyperplasia. *J Pediatr* 1976;**88**:269.

Swick M: Uroradiographic media. *Urology* 1974;**4**:750.

Wilkiemeyer RM, Boyce WH, Malek RS: Validity of the intravenous pyelogram in assessment of renal function. *Surg Gynecol Obstet* 1972;**135**:897.

Infusion Urography

Bernardino ME, McClennan BL: High dose urography: Incidence and relationship to spontaneous peripelvic extravasation. *Am J Roentgenol* 1976;**127**:373.

Bosniak MA: Nephrotomography: A relatively unappreciated but extremely valuable diagnostic tool. *Radiology* 1974;**113**:313.

Golimbu M & others: Adventitious hysterogram during intravenous pyelography. *Urology* 1975;**6**:394.

Greene LF, Fraser RA, Hartman GW: Bolus nephrotomography in diagnosis of lesions of kidney. *Urology* 1976;**7**:221.

Imray TJ: Evaluation of pelvic masses during infusion excretory urography. *Am J Roentgenol* 1975;**125**:60.

Urea Washout Test

Harwood-Nash DCF, Lansdown EL: Evaluation of the urea washout pyelogram and urography in the assessment of renovascular hypertension. *Can Med Assoc J* 1967;**96**:245.

Angionephrotomograms

Athanasoulis CA & others: Angionephrotomography and subtraction: Relative value in renal mass lesions. *Am J Roentgenol* 1973;**117**:108.

Lee TG, Henderson DC: Intravenous renal angiography revisited. *J Urol* 1977;**117**:267.

Pfister RC, Shea TE: Nephrotomography: Performance and interpretation. *Radiol Clin North Am* 1971;**9**:41.

Retrograde Urograms

Khan AU, Leary FJ, Greene LF: Pneumopyelography. *Urology* 1976;**8**:921.

Taylor RJ & others: Use and abuse of retrograde pyelography. *Urology* 1979;**14**:536.

Opacification of Renal Cysts

Buttarazzi PJ & others: Aspiration of renal cyst. *J Urol* 1968;**100**:591.

Lalli AF: Percutaneous aspiration of renal masses. *Am J Roentgenol* 1967;**101**:700.

Antegrade Urograms

Fletcher EWL, Gough MH: Antegrade pyelography in children. *Br J Radiol* 1973;**46**:191.

Sherwood T, Stevenson JJ: Antegrade pyelography: A further look at an old technique. *Br J Radiol* 1972;**45**:812.

Weinstein BJ, Skolnick ML: Ultrasonically guided antegrade pyelography. *J Urol* 1978;**120**:323.

Cystourethrograms

Colapinto V, McCallum RW: The role of urethrography in urethral disease. 2. Indications for transphincter urethroplasty in patients with primary bulbous strictures. *J Urol* 1979;**122**:612.

Currarino G: Narrowings of the male urethra caused by contractions or spasm of the bulbocavernosus muscle: Cystourethrographic observations. *Am J Roentgenol* 1970;**108**:641.

Hutch JA, Shopfner CE: The lateral cystogram as an aid to urologic diagnosis. *J Urol* 1968;**99**:202.

McAlister WH, Cacciarelli A, Shackelford GD: Complications associated with cystography in children. *Radiology* 1974;**111**:167.

McCallum RW, Colapinto V: The role of urethrography in urethral disease. 1. Accurate radiological localization of the membranous urethra and distal sphincters in normal male subjects. *J Urol* 1979;**122**:607.

Maskell R, Pead L, Vinnicombe J: Urinary infection after micturating cystography. *Lancet* 1978;**2**:1191.

Simon G, Berdon WE: Suprapubic bladder puncture for voiding cystourethrography. *J Pediatr* 1972;**81**:555.

Stewart CM: Delayed cystography and voiding cystourethrography. *J Urol* 1955;**74**:749.

Theander G: Roentgen appearance of prostatic channels in infancy and childhood. *Acta Radiol [Diagn] (Stockh)* 1971;**11**:467.

Retrograde Urethrograms

McClennan BL, Becker JA, Robinson T: Venous extravasation at retrograde urethrography: Precautions. *J Urol* 1971;**106**:412.

Mukerjee MG & others: Urethrovascular reflux and its significance in urology. *J Urol* 1974;**112**:608.

Mullin EM, Peterson LJ, Paulson DF: Retrograde urethrogram: Diagnostic aid and hazard. *J Urol* 1973;**110**:464.

Estimation of Residual Urine in Children

Young BW, Anderson WG, King GG: Radiographic estimation of residual urine in children. *J Urol* 1956;**75**:263.

Cineradiography

Tanagho EA, Hutch JA, Miller ER: Diagnostic procedures and cinefluoroscopy in vesico-ureteral reflux. *Br J Urol* 1966;**38**:435.

Renal Angiography

Alfidi RJ, Gill WM, Klein HJ: Arteriography of adrenal neoplasms. *Am J Roentgenol* 1969;**106**:635.

Ambos MA & others: Replacement lipomatosis of the kidney. *AJR* 1978;**130**:1087.

Casarella WJ: Magnification renal arteriography. *Urology* 1973;**1**:501.

Eisenberg RL, Bank WO, Hedgcock MW: Renal failure after major angiography. *Am J Med* 1980;**68**:43.

Elkin M: Radiology of the urinary tract: Some physiological considerations. *Radiology* 1975;**116**:259.

Feldman AE & others: Renal pseudotumors: An anatomic-radiologic classification. *J Urol* 1978;**120**:133.

Goldstein HM, Reuter SR, Wallace S: Pseudotumor of the renal pelvis caused by arterial impression. *J Urol* 1974;**111**:735.

Hegeöus V: Three-dimensional selective angiography in the diagnosis of renal masses. *Acta Radiol [Diagn] (Stockh)* 1974;**15**:401.

Jander HP & others: Selective angiography in renal and perirenal inflammatory lesions: Correlation with histopathology. *Br J Radiol* 1979;**52**:536.

Kahn PC, Wise HM Jr: The use of epinephrine in selective angiography of renal masses. *J Urol* 1968;**99**:133.

Killen DA, Foster JH: Spinal cord injury as a complication of contrast angiography. *Surgery* 1966;**59**:969.

Lang EK: Roentgenographic assessment of asymptomatic renal lesions: An analysis of the confidence level of diagnoses established by sequential roentgenographic investigation. *Radiology* 1973;**109**:257.

Meyers MA, Whalen JP, Evans JA: Diagnosis of perirenal and subcapsular masses: Anatomic-radiologic correlation. *Am J Roentgenol* 1974;**121**:523.

Moes CAF, Burrington JD: The use of aortography in the diagnosis of abdominal masses in children. *Radiology* 1971;**98**:59.

Pearson JC, Tanagho EA, Palubinskas AJ: Nonoperative diagnosis of pyelocalyceal deformity due to venous impressions. *Urology* 1979;**13**:207.

Roy P: Percutaneous catheterization via the axillary artery. *Am J Roentgenol* 1965;**94**:1.

Swartz RD & others: Renal failure following major angiography. *Am J Med* 1978;**65**:31.

Vesical Angiography

Wise HW Jr, Fainsinger MH: Angiography in the evaluation of carcinoma of the bladder. *JAMA* 1965;**192**:1027.

Lymphangiography

Fraley EE, Clouse M, Litwin SB: The uses of lymphography, lymphadenography and color lymphadenography in urology. *J Urol* 1965;**93**:319.

Kolbenstvedt A: Normal lymphographic variations of lumbar, iliac and inguinal lymph vessels. *Acta Radiol* [*Diagn*] (*Stockh*) 1974;**15**:662.

Oritz F, Walzak MP, Marshall VF: Chyluria: Lymphatic-urinary fistula demonstrated by lymphangiography. *J Urol* 1964;**91**:608.

Wallace S & others: Lymphangiographic interpretation. *Radiol Clin North Am* 1965;**3**:467.

Venacavography

Berdon WE, Baker DH, Santulli TV: Factors producing spurious obstruction of the inferior vena cava in infants and children with abdominal tumor. *Radiology* 1967;**88**:111.

Hayt DB: Upright inferior vena cavography. *Radiology* 1966;**86**:865.

Hipona FA, Crummy AB: The roentgen diagnosis of renal vein thrombosis. *Am J Roentgenol* 1966;**98**:122.

Wendel RG, Evans AT, Wiot JF: A new technique for inferior venacavography. *J Urol* 1968;**100**:705.

Selective Renal Venography

Braedel HU & others: Renal phlebography: An aid in the diagnosis of the absent or non-functioning kidney. *J Urol* 1976;**116**:703.

Oleaga JA & others: Renal venography: New applications in pathologic conditions. *Urology* 1978;**12**:609.

Selective Adrenal Venography

Nicolis GL & others: Percutaneous adrenal venography: A clinical study of 50 patients. *Ann Intern Med* 1972;**76**:899.

Computed Tomography of Urinary Tract

Alter AJ, Uehling DT, Zwiebel WJ: Computed tomography of the retroperitoneum following nephrectomy. *Radiology* 1979;**133**:663.

Bernardino ME & others: Computed tomography in the evaluation of post-nephrectomy patients. *Radiology* 1979;**130**:183.

Brownlie K, Kreel L: Computer assisted tomography of normal suprarenal glands. *J Comput Assist Tomogr* 1978;**2**:1.

Dunnick NR & others: Computed tomography in adrenal tumors. *AJR* 1979;**132**:43.

Engelstad BL & others: The role of pre-contrast images in computed tomography of the kidney. *Radiology* 1980;**136**:153.

Hodson NJ, Husband JE, MacDonald JS: The role of computed tomography in the staging of bladder cancer. *Clin Radiol* 1979;**30**:389.

Karstaedt N & others: Computed tomography of the adrenal gland. *Radiology* 1978;**129**:723.

Korobkin M & others: Computed tomography in the diagnosis of adrenal disease. *AJR* 1979;**132**:231.

Laursen K, Damgaard-Pedersen K: CT for pheochromocytoma diagnosis. *AJR* 1980;**134**:277.

Levin E, Lee KR, Weigel J: Preoperative determination of abdominal extent of renal cell carcinoma by computed tomography. *Radiology* 1979;**132**:395.

Love L & others: Computed tomography staging of renal carcinoma. *Urologic Radiology* 1979;**1**:3.

McClennan BL & others: CT of the renal cyst: Is cyst aspiration necessary? *AJR* 1979;**133**:671.

Magilner AD, Ostrum BJ: Computed tomography in the diagnosis of renal masses. *Radiology* 1978;**126**:715.

Marks WM & others: CT diagnosis of tumor thrombosis of the renal vein and inferior vena cava. *AJR* 1978;**131**:843.

Montagne JP & others: Computed tomography of the normal adrenal glands. *AJR* 1978;**130**:963.

Sagel SS & others: Computed tomography of the kidney. *Radiology* 1977;**124**:359.

Seidelmann FE & others: Accuracy of CT staging of bladder neoplasms using the gas-filled method: Report of 21 patients with surgical confirmation. *AJR* 1978;**130**:735.

Seidelmann FE & others: Computed tomography of the seminal vesicles and seminal vesicle angle. *Computed Axial Tomography* 1977;**1**:281.

Weyman PJ & others: Comparison of computed tomography and angiography in the evaluation of renal cell cardinoma. *Radiology* 1980;**137**:417.

White EA & others: Use of computed tomography in diagnosing the cause of primary aldosteronism. *N Engl J Med* 1980;**303**:1503.

7 | Ultrasonic Examination of the Urinary Tract

Granville C. Coggs, MD

EXAMINATION TECHNICS & NORMAL ANATOMY

During the past few years, progress in ultrasound has led to the production of machines capable of producing images of greater resolution and superior diagnostic quality. Renal parenchymal detail is now shown with great clarity.

High-resolution images are now produced by static B scanners and also by high-resolution real time instruments. The clearest images are produced during suspended respiration.

With the static B scanner, the transducer is moved at a constant speed in a single sweep along the skin overlying the organ to be imaged. The kidneys are usually first demonstrated with the patient prone (Fig 7–1). Beginning at the iliac crest, transverse scans (Fig 7–2) are made at 1-cm intervals until the upper poles of the kidneys are completely visualized. The lateral and medial borders of the kidneys are marked on the skin with grease pencil. The midpoints of these marks indicate the longest longitudinal axis of the kidneys. Longitudinal, somewhat oblique scans (Fig 7–3) are then made at 1-cm intervals until the entire kidney (Fig 7–4) has been visualized. In order for the sound beam to intercept the kidney surfaces perpendicularly, the transducer is often angled somewhat cephalad and medially.

The supine position also usually allows good visualization of the right kidney (Fig 7–5), because a good sound pathway is provided by the overlying liver (Fig 7–6). However, gas in the stomach and in the splenic flexure of the colon often interferes with imaging of the left kidney when the patient is supine. The left kidney is best imaged with the patient in the right lateral decubitus position, where the spleen serves as a sound pathway for both longitudinal and transverse scans. Conventional static B scan and real time instruments also visualize the bladder and prostate with the patient supine (Fig 7–5).

The greatest progress in higher resolution and diagnostic quality has been in the development of real time ultrasound instruments. The most recent real time instruments produce a high-resolution live image with a single placement of the transducer. Fig 7–7 shows a real time instrument being used to produce a longitudinal scan of the right kidney with the patient supine; Fig 7–8 shows a longitudinal scan of the left kidney with the patient prone. Real time instruments are particularly useful with children, who are less likely to cooperate in suspending respiration. A longitudinal scan of the right kidney of a supine child, produced with a high-resolution real time instrument, is shown in Fig 7–9. The pelvocaliceal structures are seen in the central portion of the kidney as strong echoes, with the more sonolucent renal pyramids radiating toward the periphery of the kidney. The renal cortex, containing echoes of intermediate intensity, surround the renal pyramids. In general, the echo intensity of the renal cortex is slightly less than that of liver parenchyma. Real time sector scanners with small fields of view are particularly useful for viewing images between the ribs of the thorax and behind the symphysis pubica.

DIFFERENTIAL DIAGNOSIS OF RENAL CYSTS & TUMORS

With the continuing refinement of urographic technics, unsuspected renal masses—most of them benign—are being found more frequently. The increased use of ultrasound in evaluating right upper quadrant pain has made this a primary technic in detecting and characterizing renal masses. It may be useful in cases of hematuria even if the intravenous urogram is normal, because a urogram will not detect a peripheral renal lesion that does not deform the caliceal system or renal outline.

Most authors now feel that renal sonography should follow urography in evaluation of a renal mass. If necessary, renal sonography should be followed by percutaneous puncture or arteriography for definitive diagnosis, which can be made with nearly 100% accuracy if symptoms or other findings suggest tumor. Many authors now feel that in an asymptomatic patient over 60 years of age, if a renal mass is incidentally discovered with the ultrasonic appearance characteristic of a benign cyst, no further work-up is needed.

In general, patients younger than 60 years of

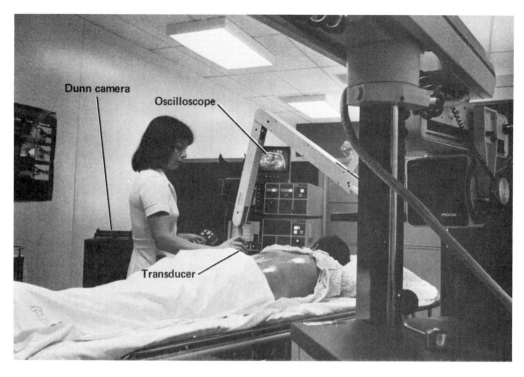

Figure 7–1. Production of a transverse B scan of the renal areas. An example of a transverse cross section of the kidneys is shown in detail in Fig 7–2.

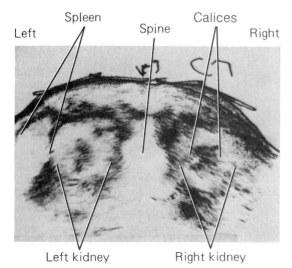

Figure 7–2. Prone transverse section through the mid portion of normal kidneys.

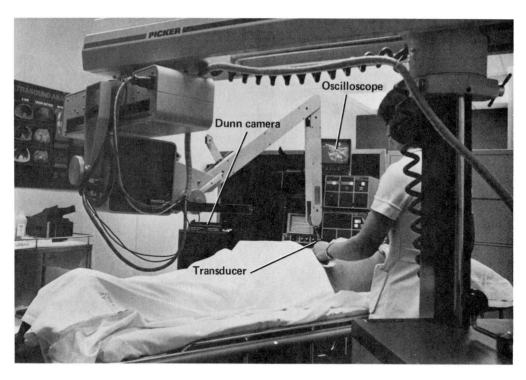

Figure 7–3. Production of a longitudinal B scan through the renal area. An example of a longitudinal section of the left kidney usually obtained is shown in Fig 7–4.

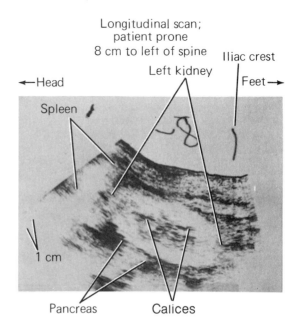

Figure 7–4. Longitudinal B scan through the left renal area outlining the kidney, the spleen, and the tail of the pancreas.

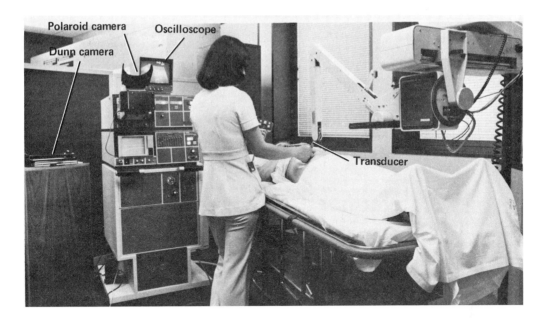

Figure 7–5. Production of a longitudinal B scan through the liver and right kidney with the patient supine.

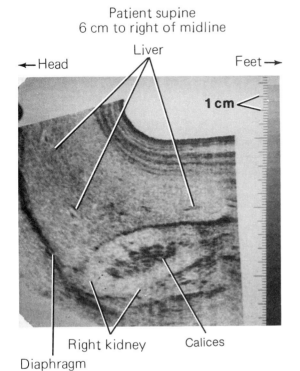

Figure 7–6. Longitudinal section through the liver and right kidney with the patient supine.

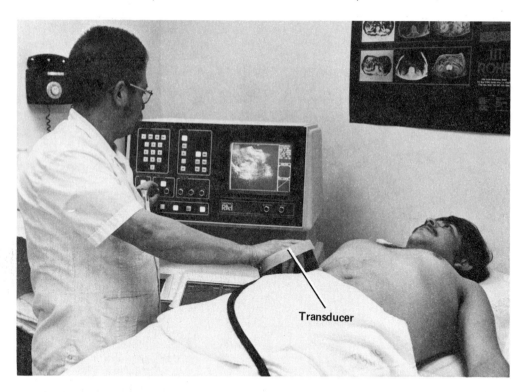

Figure 7–7. Production of a longitudinal scan of the right kidney with the patient supine, using a high-resolution real time sector scanner. (Patient's head to the left of the screen and feet to the right.)

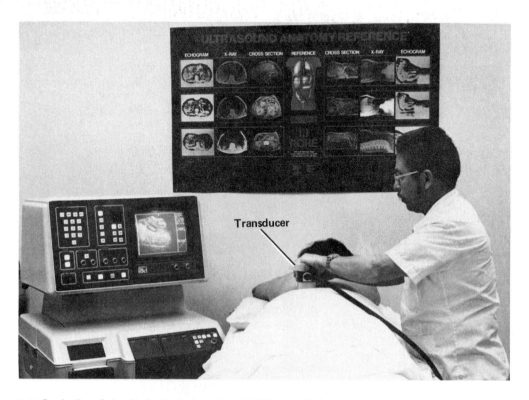

Figure 7–8. Production of a longitudinal scan through the left kidney with the patient prone. (Patient's head to the left of the screen and feet to the right.)

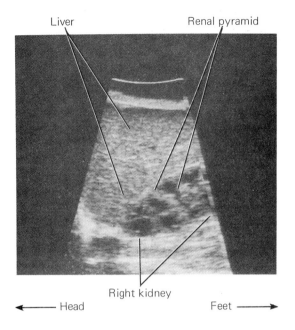

Liver　　　　　　Renal pyramid

Right kidney

◄──── Head　　　　　　Feet ────►

Figure 7–9. Longitudinal scan of the liver and right kidney of a supine pediatric patient by a high-resolution real time sector scanner.

age whose renal sonograms show a cystic pattern should undergo cyst puncture, whereas patients whose sonograms show a pattern of solid mass should be examined by arteriography.

Most authorities believe that a mass requires no further investigation if it yields clear fluid on aspiration and is shown to be a smooth-walled area on an x-ray film made following injection of contrast medium. However, Ambrose & others (1977) have reported 4 cases of 55 presumed cysts in which clear aspirated fluid and negative cytologic findings were found to be associated with renal neoplasm.

The typical findings with cyst are displacement of the caliceal echoes, an anechoic area with a sharply defined border, and increased sound transmission from the far wall of the mass. The center of the mass remains quite anechoic despite increasing intensity of the sound beam (Fig 7–10).

A renal tumor also generally shows displacement of the caliceal echoes. Increasing gain produces an increased number of echoes within the mass. The outline of the mass is usually irregular and does not allow increased sound transmission of the far wall (Fig 7–10).

Sonography is about 95% accurate in distinguishing between solid and cystic renal masses. Angiomyolipoma is a benign tumor that seems to have a characteristic sonographic appearance which permits accurate diagnosis. These tumors have very strong echoes because they contain large amounts of fat. If complementary plain films show increased radiolucency or if CT scans

show densities consistent with fat content, the diagnosis can be made with more confidence. Open biopsy or segmental resection should then be done, or—depending upon the clinical circumstances— the need for surgery can be ruled out.

Kumari & others (1981) have recently described the appearance of leukemic infiltration of the kidneys. Characteristic features are enlargement of the kidneys, diffuse coarse echoes within the renal cortex, and loss of definition and distortion of the renal sinus echo complex, which shows central anechoic rounded or oblong defects simulating hydronephrosis. Acute nephritis or an abscess may resemble cysts or tumors with sonography. The echo pattern in focal bacterial nephritis usually resembles that of a solid mass, but it has an echo pattern of slightly less intensity than that of normal parenchyma. If clinical signs suggest infection, changes in focal masses of the kidney can be monitored with ultrasound to evaluate response to therapy. Ultrasound and CT scans of the kidneys of a diabetic patient with the clinical diagnosis of renal abscess are shown in Fig 7–11.

EVALUATION OF POLYCYSTIC KIDNEYS

The sonographic picture of adult-onset polycystic kidney disease shows cysts that are usually of different sizes with sonolucent patterns similar to those of isolated cysts (Fig 7–12). In late stages of the disease, the kidneys are usually markedly enlarged and have irregular borders. Gray scale technics now permit earlier detection of the disease during childhood and facilitate genetic counseling.

When comparing the effectiveness of ultrasonography, CT scanning, and nephrotomography in polycystic kidney and liver disease, Rosenfield & others (1977) found ultrasound to be most consistent in identifying these lesions. Adult-onset polycystic kidney disease is often associated with polycystic liver disease, where cysts sometimes involve the pancreas, spleen, or ovary.

In infantile polycystic kidney disease, cysts are small but are visualized by urography. Sonography demonstrates enlargement of both kidneys and distorted renal architecture, but cysts as such may not be recognized.

ASSISTANCE IN PERCUTANEOUS ASPIRATION OF RENAL CYSTS & PERCUTANEOUS RENAL BIOPSY

Kristensen & Holm in Copenhagen (1972) and Goldberg & Pollack in Philadelphia (1972) were leaders in the use of transducers with central holes to accommodate percutaneous puncture of renal cysts (Fig 7–13). Since these reports were published, real time transducers containing holes for percutaneous needle puncture have become avail-

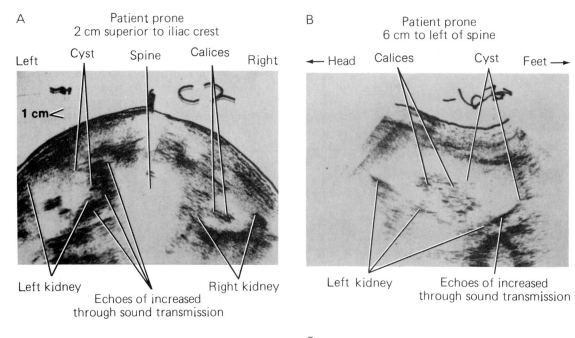

A Patient prone
2 cm superior to iliac crest

Left   Cyst   Spine   Calices   Right

1 cm<

Left kidney   Right kidney
Echoes of increased
through sound transmission

B Patient prone
6 cm to left of spine

← Head   Calices   Cyst   Feet →

Left kidney   Echoes of increased
through sound transmission

C Patient prone
5 cm to right of spine

←Head   Feet →

1 cm <

Right kidney   Spherical tumor mass of
lower pole, containing
echoes, no increased
through sound transmission

Figure 7–10. Transverse *(A)* and longitudinal *(B)* sections through the left kidney showing a cyst of the medial aspect of the lower pole of the kidney. Note increased back wall echoes showing good through sound transmission. *C:* Longitudinal section through the right kidney showing a tumor of the lower pole. Note bulge in contour of lower pole with echoes within the mass and no increased through sound transmission.

able. Linear array or sector real time scanners, which do not contain holes, can also be used to facilitate puncture of these cysts or other masses that can be sonographically visualized. During these procedures, the cyst or mass is visualized by placing the real time scanner over the appropriate area, and a needle is then passed percutaneously using the scanner to direct its introduction. With a cyst, the bright echoes of the needle tip can usually be observed as the tip enters the mass. The tip can also be seen by introducing a small amount of air through the needle and observing the bright echoes of air bubbles as they float upward within the cyst.

Visualization of the needle tip within a solid mass is not so easily accomplished, but with real time observation, movements of the mass may be seen as it is encountered by the tip.

Fluid aspirated from a benign cyst is usually clear. Clear fluid is the most characteristic indication of nonmalignancy. If aspirated fluid is not clear, arteriography or surgical exploration is usually indicated.

Some authors feel that percutaneous aspiration of cysts is not always appropriate, because it will not reveal the tumor that occasionally occurs within a cyst. However, Von Schreeb (1967) studied 150

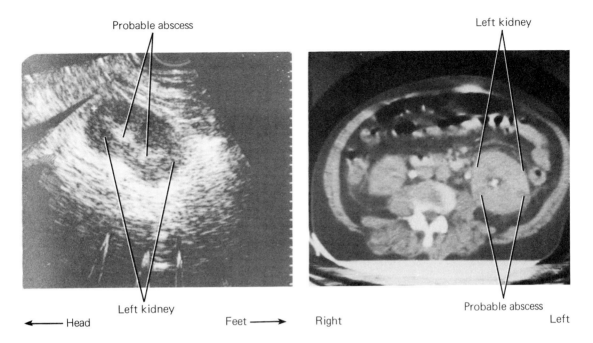

Probable abscess   Left kidney

Left kidney

Probable abscess

◄——— Head   Feet ———►   Right   Left

Figure 7–11. *Left:* Longitudinal scan of the left kidney with the patient prone. Sonolucent area of the posterior aspect of the kidney probably represents a renal abscess. *Right:* Renal CT scan of the same patient made 1 day following the sonogram examination.

renal tumors treated with nephrectomy and found that 5-year survival rates were not significantly different for 77 patients who had percutaneous puncture and instillation of contrast medium prior to nephrectomy and for 73 patients who underwent nephrectomy without prior percutaneous puncture.

Prior to biopsy, the B scan can be used to locate and outline the position of the kidney on the patient's skin while the patient breathes quietly or suspends inspiration. B scan will also show the depth to which the biopsy needle should penetrate. Percutaneous puncture should be performed during suspended inspiration in the same position in which sonographic localization was performed.

Gerzof (1979) has been a leader in percutaneous aspiration and drainage of pararenal fluid collections and other fluid collections and abscesses within the abdomen.

EVALUATION OF UNILATERAL NONVISUALIZING KIDNEY

In the pediatric age group, the most common reasons for nonvisualization of one kidney by urography are renal agenesis, renal hypoplasia, polycystic kidney, hydronephrosis, and renal vein thrombosis. Polycystic kidney is the most common cause of an abnormal abdominal mass in the first few days of life, and hydronephrosis is the most common

cause of such a mass shortly after the first few days. These conditions have characteristic sonographic appearances, and sonography is better than 90% accurate in identifying them.

In adults, hydronephrosis, polycystic kidney, hypoplastic or chronically infected kidney, renal vein thrombosis, renal artery occlusion, and tumor invading an entire kidney are causes of unilateral nonvisualization that may be identified by sonography.

Renal vein thrombosis usually causes enlargement of a kidney, whereas with arterial embolism, the kidney is usually normal in size and shape. Late stage hydronephrosis produces a sonolucent renal pelvis (Fig 7–14). If the cause of obstruction is in the lower urinary tract, a dilated ureter may be seen. A distended urinary bladder may produce dilatation of the ureter and renal pelvis; therefore, before an ultrasonic diagnosis of hydronephrosis is made, the urinary bladder should be scanned.

EVALUATION OF BILATERAL NONVISUALIZING KIDNEYS

Ultrasound can distinguish hydronephrosis, polycystic kidneys, and small end-stage kidneys. Sanders & Jeck (1976) report on 23 patients with blood urea nitrogen levels above 70 mg/dL who were thought to be in renal failure. With ultrasound, kidney size was determined and hy-

7 cm superior to iliac crest

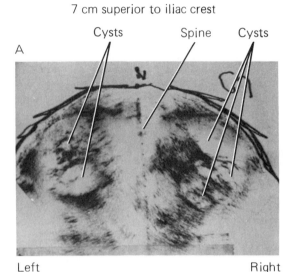

A

Left   Right

8 cm to left of midline

B

←Head   Feet→

9 cm to right of midline

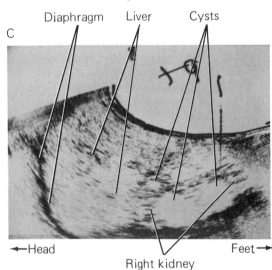

C

←Head   Feet→
           Right kidney

Figure 7–12. *A:* Prone section showing cysts of various sizes in both kidneys. *B:* Longitudinal section of cysts of various sizes in kidneys. *C:* Supine view showing overlying liver and multiple cysts in the right kidney.

dronephrosis or polycystic kidney was diagnosed, if present, in all but one instance. In 10 patients, urography (in 4 cases with tomography) failed to adequately demonstrate the kidney. Hydronephrosis and polycystic kidneys differ in appearance. Kidneys in end stage renal disease are never more than 9 cm long. Fig 7–15 shows an instance of inadequate visualization by urogram of hydronephrosis of the left kidney and very poor visualization of the right kidney. The sonogram demonstrated marked hydronephrosis of the right kidney and right hydroureter.

DIAGNOSIS OF PERIRENAL ABSCESS & RETROPERITONEAL LESIONS

McCullough & Leopold (1976) reported on 18 patients who had retroperitoneal fluid collections that had been demonstrated at surgery. When infection is present, this condition has a mortality rate of about 45%. Ultrasound was the most valuable technic in diagnosing these lesions, which included urinoma, perinephric abscess, lymphocele, infected perinephric hematoma, and psoas abscess. The diagnosis can be easily made when these fluid collections or a tumor mass causes displacement of a kidney. Visualization of progressive kidney displacement can help in determining the rate of tumor growth or the presence of continued bleeding. Greene & Steinbach (1975) visualized several cases of hypernephroma in which sonography revealed extension to the inferior vena cava. Conrad & others (1976) have reported sonographic identification of 3 perinephric fluid collections that were causing hypertension as a consequence of the Page kidney phenomenon. Figs 7–16 and 7–17 show perinephric abscesses. Fig 7–18 illustrates a large retroperitoneal hematoma secondary to adrenal carcinoma.

INTRAOPERATIVE LOCALIZATION & CLINICAL RECOGNITION OF RENAL CALCULI

Cook & Lytton (1977) used a small 10-MHz frequency probe during lithotomy to localize renal calculi. The presence of calculi can be confirmed by intraoperative x-rays using mammography film. The ultrasound probe will then display the stone in 3 dimensions to facilitate passage of the small needle through a slot guide of the probe into the stone. Stones 2–3 mm in diameter are readily detected. Small stones or residual fragments were completely removed in 7 of 11 patients treated by this technic.

In clinical examinations, calcific renal stones sometimes cast acoustic shadows similar to the shadow of cholelithiasis. Nonradiopaque renal stones that contain uric acid may also cast acoustic shadows. Fig 7–19 shows a calcific renal stone with characteristic acoustic shadowing that had not been detected by an excretory urogram using plain films and tomography. Intestinal gas obscured the stone on plain films, and the density of the iodinated

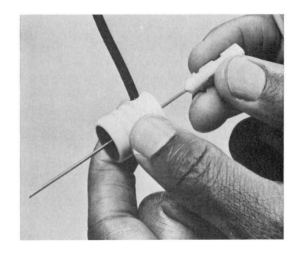

Figure 7–13. Needle aspiration transducer.

contrast medium obscured the stone during tomography.

PEDIATRIC UROLOGIC EVALUATION

Ultrasonic technics in children are similar to those used with adults. However, when the static B scanner is used, children under age 3 usually require sedation. High-resolution real time instruments have greatly facilitated pediatric examinations. A high-resolution real time sector scanner was used to image the liver and right kidney of a pediatric patient shown in Fig 7–9.

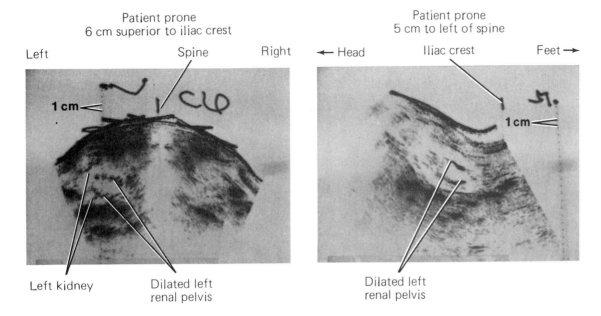

Patient prone
6 cm superior to iliac crest

Left — Spine — Right

1 cm

Left kidney — Dilated left renal pelvis

Patient prone
5 cm to left of spine

← Head — Iliac crest — Feet →

1 cm

Dilated left renal pelvis

Figure 7–14. Transverse and longitudinal pictures showing markedly advanced hydronephrosis with oval-shaped echo-free area of the left renal pelvis.

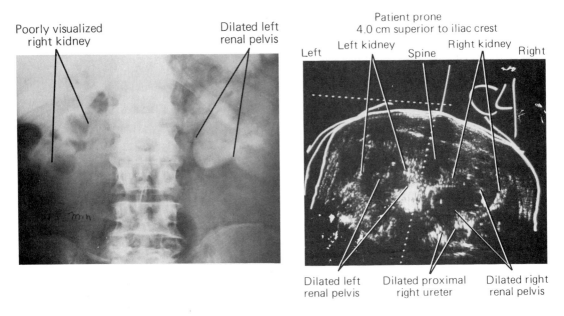

Figure 7–15. *Left:* Radiograph showing moderately dilated left renal pelvis but very poor visualization of the right kidney and ureter. *Right:* Transverse B scan through the renal areas showing moderate dilation of the left renal pelvis and marked dilation of the right renal pelvis and ureter.

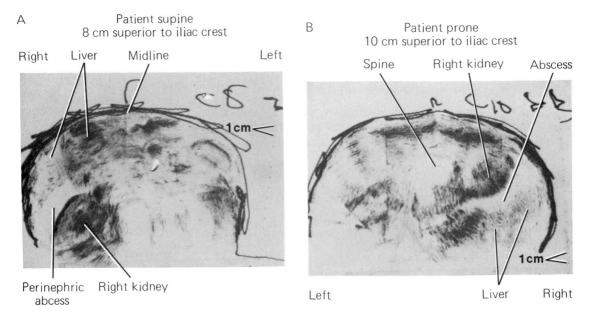

Figure 7–16. *A:* Supine transverse section showing echo-free perinephric abscess between the right kidney and liver. *B:* Prone view showing the perinephric abscess of the lateral aspect of the right kidney.

Paranephric abcess

Left kidney

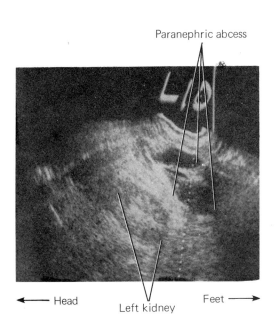
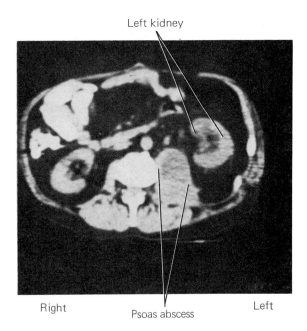

⟵ Head   Left kidney   Feet ⟶   Right   Psoas abscess   Left

Figure 7–17. *Left:* Longitudinal sonogram of the left renal area, showing a large abscess posterior to the left kidney resulting in forward displacement of the kidney. *Right:* Transverse CT scan through the renal areas produced 1 day later. A large abscess involving the left psoas muscle is shown displacing the left kidney anteriorly and laterally.

In 28 pediatric cases, Shkolnik (1977) used B mode scanning to delineate one or both kidneys that had not been visualized by intravenous urography. B scan imaging was also successful in 10 cases of renal failure in which intravenous urography was not attempted. Following demonstration of poor function on intravenous urogram, Sample, Gyepes, & Ehrlich (1977) used ultrasonography to clearly

8 cm superior to iliac crest
Liver   Hematoma
Midline
Right   Left

Figure 7–18. Supine transverse section showing large echo-free space representing hematoma secondary to a carcinoma of the left adrenal gland.

delineate hypoplasia, polycystic kidney, hydronephrosis, and vascular accidents, usually renal vein thrombosis. Sonography has clearly elucidated cases of infantile polycystic disease, bilateral hydronephrosis, and transient renal failure that demonstrated bilateral poor function on the intravenous urogram.

Using a high-resolution real time scanner in infants under 6 months of age, Leopold (1980) has clearly imaged the spinal canal, the fluid surrounding the spinal cord, the cord itself, and even the central canal of the cord.

Large abdominal masses representing Wilms's tumor and pheochromocytoma have been characterized. A diverticulum of the bladder or a ureterocele may appear as a cystic mass in the pelvis. Rhabdomyosarcomas of the prostate appear as echolucent pelvic masses. Testicular neoplasms are characterized by asymmetric echoes within the testis.

Garrett, Kossoff, & Osborn (1975) have reported 2 cases of intrauterine diagnosis of fetal hydronephrosis and megaureter secondary to urethral obstruction.

EVALUATION OF RENAL TRANSPLANTS

The relatively superficial position of renal transplants in the body and the accuracy of current gray scale technics make transplant evaluation by

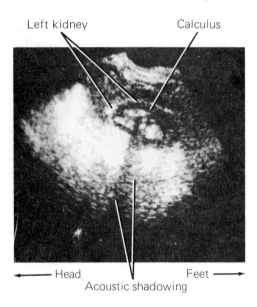

Left kidney   Calculus

←———— Head   Feet ————→
Acoustic shadowing

Figure 7–19. Longitudinal scan of the left kidney made with the patient prone. The strong echo with dependent acoustic shadowing is characteristic of renal calculus.

diagnostic ultrasound relatively easy. Baseline measurements should be made about 7–10 days after transplantation. The kidney usually enlarges slowly during the first 6 months after transplant. A sudden enlargement to 20% more than the initial donor size occurring soon after transplant usually indicates acute rejection.

In 70% of cases studied, Hillman, Birnholz, & Busch (1979) found that echographic and histologic assessments of chronic rejection were the same. Early rejection is characterized by indistinctness of the cortical medullary boundary; in chronic rejection, decreased cortical thickness is a prominent feature. Frick & others (1981) report an overall accuracy rate of 85% for sonographic diagnosis of rejection when correlated with biopsy findings. In addition to increased size of the transplant, they noted decreased echogenicity of renal pyramids, focal zones of sonolucency in the renal cortex, and patchy sonolucent areas indicating coalescence of both cortex and medulla.

Rosenfield & Taylor (1976) have observed both the development and resolution of pyelocaliectasis in transplants. Ultrasound clearly shows the various fluid collections—abscesses, lymphoceles, urinomas, or hematomas (Fig 7–20)—that commonly occur following transplant. Spigos (1977) has used ultrasound to monitor the percutaneous biopsy of transplants; the biopsy needle should be guided into the upper pole of the transplant.

ESTIMATION OF RESIDUAL URINE

The urine-filled bladder is readily outlined by sonography. Holmes (1974) has used a planimeter to calculate the volume of urine in the bladder to an accuracy of ± 10%. Harrison, Parks, & Sherwood (1975) described the usefulness of ultrasound in children with neuropathic bladders. This simple, noninvasive method requires no preparation of the patient, can be performed repeatedly, and is well accepted by children. These authors and Teele (1977) advocate sagittal scanning of the bladder for useful semiquantitative information. McLean & Edell (1978) and Pedersen, Bartrum, & Grytter (1975) have also described methods for determination of residual urine volume. Sonography is useful in older patients for determining the amount of residual urine after voiding, dispensing with the need for catheterization. Bladder contour in a normal woman before and after voiding is shown in Fig 7–21.

EVALUATION OF BLADDER & PROSTATE

B scanning of the bladder has been used to evaluate the intravesical extent of tumors, identify seminal vesicle cysts, characterize congenital urachal anomalies, and identify overdistended bladders in some patients with pelvic symptoms. The development of gray scale technic and computerized digital image processing has greatly enhanced the transrectal approach to evaluation of the bladder and prostate.

Boyce & others (1976) found the transrectal approach useful in detecting early asymptomatic tumors of the prostate, in accurately staging local disease of the prostate, and in evaluating treatment. Although this approach is not used to detect bladder tumors, it will reliably evaluate the degree of tumor invasion so that proper therapy can be chosen. Boyce found that when prostatic hyperplasia was diagnosed by gray scale technics, no other disease was later noted.

Henneberry, Carter, & Neiman (1979), utilizing static gray scale B scanners and the suprapubic approach, have accurately estimated prostate size. A prostate of normal size delineated by the suprapubic approach is shown in Fig 7–22.

Sonography cannot differentiate between prostatic calculi, severe inflammation, and prostatic carcinoma.

DIAGNOSIS OF SCROTAL LESIONS

Recent improvements in gray scale technics have led to increased use of sonography in evaluating scrotal lesions. Jellins (1977) used specialized sonographic equipment for preoperative assess-

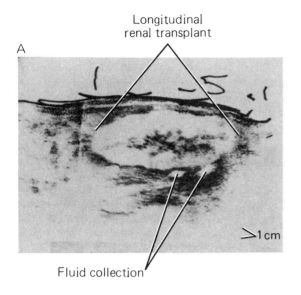

A: Longitudinal renal transplant

Fluid collection

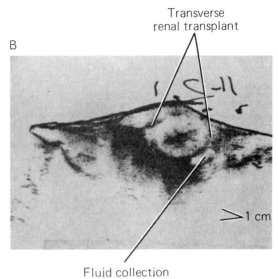

B: Transverse renal transplant

Fluid collection

Right inguinal fossa, postvoiding

C

Symphysis

1 cm

Renal transplant

Lymphocele

Figure 7–20. *A:* Longitudinal section through transplant in left iliac fossa with a small amount of fluid located posterior to renal transplant. *B:* Transverse section of transplant showing small pocket of fluid posterior to renal transplant. *C:* Longitudinal section through a renal transplant, showing nearby fluid collection (lymphocele). The picture was taken after voiding, thus differentiating this collection of fluid from the urinary bladder.

ment when the diagnosis was unclear on clinical examination. Hydroceles were readily differentiated, and other testicular abnormalities measuring a few millimeters in cross section were recognized. Sample, Gyepes, & Ehrlich (1977) reported on the evaluation of 55 patients with scrotal diseases. Sonography was accurate in detecting abnormalities in the contents of normal-sized scrotums that were painful and was highly reliable in detecting occult neoplasms in patients with mediastinal or retroperitoneal metastases when there was no clinical evidence of disease within the scrotum. Hydrocele, spermatocele, and epididymitis were readily distinguished from testicular masses. However, chronic torsions could not be distinguished from testicular tumors. A correct distinction between testicular and extratesticular abnormalities was made in 80% of their patients. A normal sonogram proved to be highly reliable.

Leopold (1980) used a high-resolution real time scanner to delineate in exquisite detail the tissues within the scrotum. He even noted the frequent occurrence of a small amount of fluid surrounding normal testes. Most testicular tumors were more sonolucent than normal parenchyma; however, the type of tumor could not be distinguished. The smallest tumor found was 8 mm in diameter and was not palpable. A high-resolution real time sector scanner produced the sonogram of the normal testis and hydrocele shown in Fig 7–23. A static gray scale B scanner produced the images of hemorrhagic infarction of the testis shown in Fig

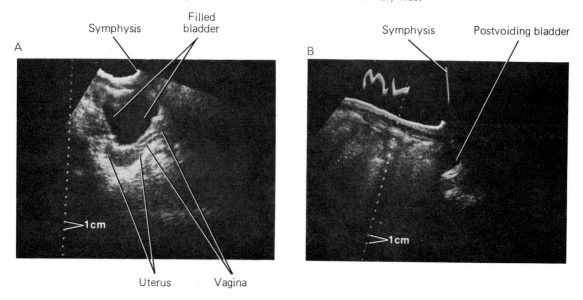

Figure 7–21. *A:* Sagittal section through filled urinary bladder. *B:* Postvoiding film showing little residual urine. ML = midline.

7–24 and anaplastic seminoma of the testes shown in Fig 7–25.

DIAGNOSIS OF TORSION OF THE TESTIS USING DOPPLER ULTRASOUND

The distinguishing feature of torsion of the testis is loss of blood flow. Hahn & others (1975) have used isotope scans to demonstrate this, but the procedure is cumbersome. Levy (1975) and Pedersen, Holm, & Hald (1975) have used the

Doppler ultrasonic stethoscope to distinguish acute testicular torsion from epididymitis in 8 patients.

Pocket-sized ultrasonic stethoscopes or table models with speakers may be used. These machines function according to the Doppler shift principle. Two transducers are incorporated into the head of

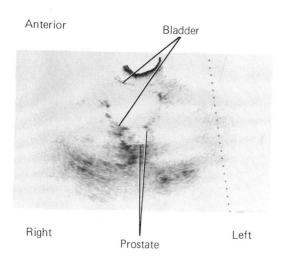

Figure 7–22. Transverse scan of the bladder and prostate produced by scanning from the suprapubic approach. Normal size and shape of the prostate is shown.

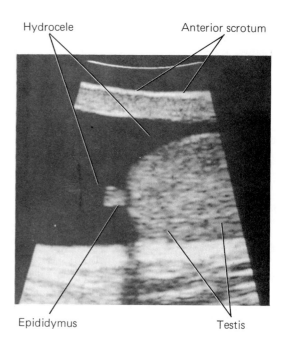

Figure 7–23. Longitudinal section through the scrotum made with a high-resolution sector scanner. The testis and epididymis appear normal; a small hydrocele is present.

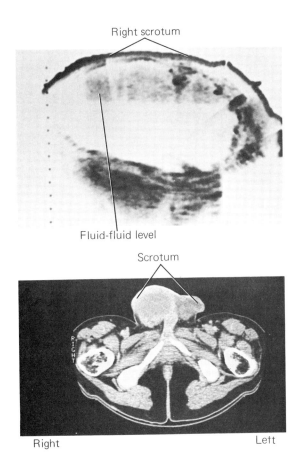

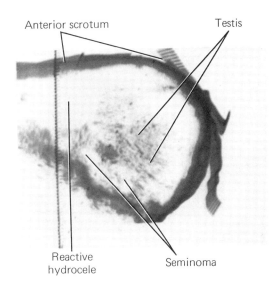

Figure 7–25. Longitudinal sonogram of the left testis demonstrating a somewhat sonolucent anaplastic seminoma posterior to the testis. (Courtesy of T Collins.)

Figure 7–24. *Top:* Longitudinal sonogram through the scrotum demonstrating a fluid-fluid level produced by hemorrhagic infarction of the testes. *Bottom:* Transverse CT scan through the scrotum showing enlargement of the right scrotum. The fluid-fluid level detected sonographically is not demonstrated. (Courtesy of M Slaysman.)

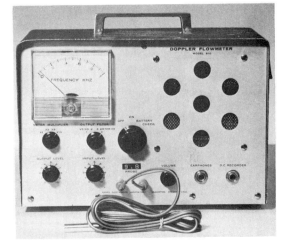

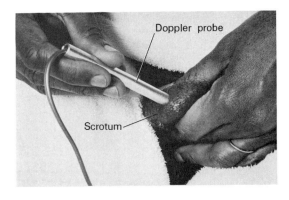

the stethoscope. One transducer continuously sends high-frequency sound waves into the tissues; the other continuously receives high-frequency sound waves reflected back from the tissues. If the tissue is stationary, no sound will be heard. The periodic intermittent blood flow in vessels is received and heard as pulsatile sound.

The testis to be examined is supported against the scrotal skin with one hand, and the instrument is guided over the surface with the other (Fig 7–26). The testis is systematically auscultated, beginning posteriorly directly over the testicular artery as it enters the gonad. The instrument is then guided anteriorly over the ventral surface, and the change in sound intensity is recorded. The examination takes about 5 minutes.

Absence of pulsatile sound from the painful testis is diagnostic of testicular torsion. Examination of the noninvolved testis serves as a control. Nasrallah, Manzone, & King (1977) caution against re-

Figure 7–26. Doppler probe *(top)* and its application in the diagnosis of testicular torsion *(bottom)*.

liance on a single test and recommend clinical assessment. They report 4 cases of surgically confirmed testicular torsion in which false-negative results had been obtained with Doppler ultrasound.

• • •

References

General References

Arger PH, Zarembok I: Source of diagnostic pitfalls in renal sonography. *Urology* 1977;**9**:353.

Ferrucci JT: Body ultrasonography. *N Engl J Med* 1979;**300**:538.

Rosenfield AT, Taylor KJW: Gray scale nephrosonography: Current status. *J Urol* 1977;**117**:2.

Rosenfield AT & others: Anatomy and pathology of the kidney by gray scale ultrasound. *Radiology* 1978;**128**:737.

Rosenfield AT & others: Gray scale ultrasonography in medullary cystic disease of the kidney and congenital hepatic fibrosis with tubular ectasia: New observations. *AJR* 1977;**129**:297.

Russell JM, Resnick MI: Ultrasound in urology. *Urol Clin North Am* 1979;**6**:445.

Sanders RC: The complimentary uses of nuclear medicine and ultrasound in the kidney. *J Urol* 1978;**120**:521.

Sanders RC: Renal ultrasound. *Radiol Clin North Am* 1975;**13**:417.

Scheible W: Gray scale ultrasound and the genitourinary tract: A review of clinical applications. *Radiol Clin North Am* 1979;**17**:281.

Physical Background & Examination Technics

Buddemeyer EU: Physics of diagnostic ultrasound. *Radiol Clin North Am* 1975;**13**:391.

Differential Diagnosis of Renal Cysts & Tumors

Ambrose SS & others: Unsuspected renal tumors associated with renal cysts. *J Urol* 1977;**117**:704.

Asher WM, Leopold GR: A streamlined diagnostic approach to renal mass lesions with renal echogram. *J Urol* 1972;**108**:205.

Bush WH: Angiomyolipoma: Characteristic images by ultrasound and computed tomography. *Urology* 1979;**14**:531.

Edell SL, Bonavita JA: The sonographic appearance of acute pyelonephritis. *Radiology* 1979;**132**:683.

Goldberg BB, Capitanio MA, Kirkpatrick JA: Ultrasonic evaluation of masses in pediatric patients. *Am J Roentgenol* 1972;**116**:677.

Goldstein HM: Ultrasonic detection of renal tumor extension into the inferior vena cava. *AJR* 1978;**130**:1083.

Kay CJ & others: Ultrasonic characteristics of chronic atrophic pyelonephritis. *AJR* 1979;**132**:47.

Kumari SS & others: Sonographic findings in leukemic infiltration of the kidneys. Scientific Exhibit at the Annual Meeting of the American Roentgen Ray Society, San Francisco, 1981.

Lee TG & others: Ultrasound findings of renal angiomyolipoma. *J Clin Ultrasound* 1978;**6**:150.

McDonald DG: The complete echographic evaluation of solid renal masses. *J Clin Ultrasound* 1978;**6**:402.

Munechika H & others: Gray scale ultrasound in identifica-tion of lymphoma complicating lymphomatoid granulomatosis. *Urology* 1979;**13**:443.

Ralls PW & others: Severe hydronephrosis and severe renal cystic disease: Ultrasonic differentiation. *AJR* 1980;**134**:473.

Shawker TH & others: Renal angiomyolipoma: Diagnosis by combined ultrasound and computerized tomography. *J Urol* 1979;**121**:675.

Silverman JF, Kilhenny C: Tumor in the wall of a simple renal cyst. *Radiology* 1969;**93**:95.

Walzer A, Weiner SN, Koenigsberg M: The ultrasound appearance of tumor extension into the left renal vein and inferior vena cava. *J Urol* 1980;**123**:945.

Evaluation of Polycystic Kidneys

Kelsey JA, Bowie JD: Gray-scale ultrasonography in the diagnosis of polycystic kidney disease. *Radiology* 1977;**122**(Suppl 2):791.

Lawson TL, McClennan BL, Shirkhoda A: Adult polycystic kidney disease: Ultrasonographic and computed tomographic appearance. *J Clin Ultrasound* 1978;**6**:297.

Rosenfield AT & others: Gray scale ultrasonography, computerized tomography and nephrotomography in evaluation of polycystic kidney and liver disease. *Urology* 1977;**9**:436.

Rosenfield AT & others: Ultrasonography and nephrotomography in the presymptomatic diagnosis of dominantly inherited (adult-onset) polycystic kidney disease. *Radiology* 1980;**135**:423.

Assistance in Percutaneous Aspiration of Renal Cysts and Percutaneous Renal Biopsy

Gerzof S & others: Percutaneous catheter drainage of abdominal abscesses guided by ultrasound and computed tomography. *AJR* 1979;**133**:1.

Goldberg BB, Pollack HM: Ultrasonic aspiration transducer. *Radiology* 1972;**102**:187.

Kristensen JK & others: Ultrasonically guided percutaneous puncture of renal masses. *Scand J Urol Nephrol* 1972;**6**(Suppl 15):49.

Lalli AF: Percutaneous aspiration of renal masses. *Am J Roentgenol* 1967;**101**:700.

Leopold GR & others: Renal ultrasound: An updated approach to the diagnosis of renal cysts. *Radiology* 1973;**109**:671.

Smith EH, Bartrum RJ: Ultrasonically guided percutaneous aspiration of abscesses. *Am J Roentgenol* 1974;**122**:308.

Von Schreeb T: Is there a risk of spreading tumor in diagnostic puncture? *Scand J Urol Nephrol* 1967;**1**:270.

Evaluation of Unilateral Nonvisualizing Kidneys

Ellenbogen PH & others: Sensitivity of gray scale ultrasound in detecting urinary tract obstruction. *AJR* 1978;**130**:731.

Marangola JP, Bryan PJ, Azimi F: Ultrasonic evaluation of the unilateral nonvisualized kidney. *Am J Roentgenol* 1976;**126**:853.

Taylor KJW, Kraus V: Gray-scale ultrasound imaging: Assessment of acute hydronephrosis. *Br J Urol* 1975;**47**:593.

Evaluation of Bilateral Nonvisualizing Kidneys

Behan M, Wixson D, Kazam E: Sonographic evaluation of the nonfunctioning kidney. *J Clin Ultrasound* 1979;**7**:449.

Morin ME, Baker DA: The influence of hydration and bladder distension on the sonographic diagnosis of hydronephrosis. *J Clin Ultrasound* 1979;**7**:192.

Sanders RC, Jeck DL: B-scan ultrasound in the evaluation of renal failure. *Radiology* 1976;**119**:199.

Winston M, Pritchard J, Paulin P: Ultrasonography in the management of unexplained renal failure. *J Clin Ultrasound* 1978;**6**:23.

Diagnosis of Perirenal Abscess & Retroperitoneal Lesions

Asher WM & others: Echographic evaluation of splenic injury after blunt trauma. *Radiology* 1976;**118**:411.

Conrad MB & others: Sonography of the Page kidney. *J Urol* 1976;**116**:293.

Greene D, Steinbach HL: Ultrasonic diagnosis of hypernephroma extending into the inferior vena cava. *Radiology* 1975;**115**:679.

McCullough DL, Leopold GR: Diagnosis of retroperitoneal fluid collections by ultrasonography: A series of surgically proved cases. *J Urol* 1976;**115**:656.

Intraoperative Localization and Clinical Recognition of Renal Calculi

Cook JH, Lytton B: Intraoperative localization of renal calculi during nephrolithotomy by ultrasound scanning. *J Urol* 1977;**117**:543.

Edell S, Zegel H: Ultrasonic evaluation of renal calculi. *AJR* 1978;**130**:261.

Mulholland SG & others: Ultrasonic differentiation of renal pelvic filling defects. *J Urol* 1979;**122**:14.

Pediatric Urologic Evaluation

Boineau FG, Rothman J, Lewy JE: Nephrosonography in the evaluation of renal failure and masses in infants. *J Pediatr* 1975;**87**:195.

Friedberg JE, Mitnick JS, Davis DA: Antepartum ultrasonic detection of multicystic kidney. *Radiology* 1979;**131**:198.

Garrett WJ, Kossoff G, Osborn RA: The diagnosis of fetal hydronephrosis, megaureter and urethral obstruction by ultrasonic echography. *Br J Obstet Gynaecol* 1975;**82**:115.

Kay R, Lee TG, Tank ES: Ultrasonographic diagnosis of fetal hydronephrosis in utero. *Urology* 1979;**13**:286.

Leopold G: Ultrasonography of superficially located structures. *Radiol Clin North Am* 1980;**18**:161.

Rosenberg ER & others: Ultrasonic diagnosis of renal vein thrombosis in neonates. *AJR* 1980;**134**:35.

Sample WF, Gyepes MT, Ehrlich RM: Gray scale ultrasound in pediatric urology. *J Urol* 1977;**117**:518.

Shkolnik A: B-mode ultrasound and the nonvisualizing kidney in pediatrics. *AJR* 1977;**128**:121.

Slovis TL, Perlmutter AD: Recent advances in pediatric urological ultrasound. *J Urol* 1980;**123**:613.

Teele RL: Ultrasonography of the genitourinary tract in children. *Radiol Clin North Am* 1977;**15**:109.

Evaluation of Renal Transplants

Bartrum RJ Jr & others: Evaluation of renal transplants with ultrasound. *Radiology* 1976;**118**:405.

Frick MP & others: Ultrasound in acute renal transplant rejection. *Radiology* 1981;**138**:657.

Hillman BJ, Birnholz JC, Busch GJ: Correlation of echographic and histologic findings in suspected renal allograft rejection. *Radiology* 1979;**132**:673.

Leopold GR: Renal transplant size measured by reflected ultrasound. *Radiology* 1970;**95**:687.

Phillips JF, Neiman HL, Brown TL: Ultrasound diagnosis of posttransplant renal lymphocele. *Am J Roentgenol* 1976;**126**:1194.

Rosenfield AT, Taylor KJW: Obstructive uropathy in the transplant kidney: Evaluation by gray scale sonography. *J Urol* 1976;**116**:101.

Spigos D, Capek V, Jonasson O: Percutaneous biopsy of renal transplants using ultrasonographic guidance. *J Urol* 1977;**117**:699.

Estimation of Residual Urine

Barrett E, Morley P: Ultrasound in the investigation of space-occupying lesions of the urinary tract. *Br J Radiol* 1971;**44**:733.

Goldberg BB, Meyer H: Ultrasonically guided suprapubic urinary bladder aspiration. *Pediatrics* 1973;**51**:70.

Harrison NW, Parks C, Sherwood T: Ultrasound assessment of residual urine in children. *Br J Urol* 1975;**47**:805.

Holmes JH: Urologic ultrasonography. Pages 242–259 in: *Diagnostic Ultrasound.* King DL (editor). Mosby, 1974.

McLean GK, Edell SL: Determination of bladder volumes by gray scale ultrasonography. *Radiology* 1978;**128**:181.

Pedersen JF, Bartrum RJ, Grytter C: Residual urine determination by ultrasonic scanning. *Am J Roentgenol* 1975;**125**:474.

Teele RL: Ultrasonography of the genitourinary tract in children. *Radiol Clin North Am* 1977;**15**:109.

Evaluation of Bladder & Prostate

Boyce WH & others: Ultrasonography as an aid in the diagnosis and management of surgical diseases of the pelvis: Special emphasis on the genitourinary system. *Ann Surg* 1976;**184**:477.

Henneberry M, Carter MF, Neiman HL: Estimation of prostatic size by suprapubic ultrasonography. *J Urol* 1979;**121**:615.

Holm HH, Northeved A: A transurethral ultrasonic scanner. *J Urol* 1974;**111**:238.

Lee TG, Reed TA: Ultrasonic diagnosis of the bladder as a symptomatic pelvic mass. *J Urol* 1977;**117**:283.

Resnick MI, Willard JW, Boyce WH: Recent progress in ultrasonography of bladder and prostate. *J Urol* 1977;**117**:444.

Walls WJ, Lin F: Ultrasonic diagnosis of seminal vesicle cyst. *Radiology* 1975;**114**:693.

Watanabe H & others: Development and application of new equipment for transrectal ultrasonography. *J Clin Ultrasound* 1974;**2**:91.

Watanabe H & others: Mass screening program for prostatic diseases with transrectal ultrasonotomography. *J Urol* 1977;**117**:746.

Watanabe H & others: Transrectal ultrasonotomography of the prostate. *J Urol* 1975;**114**:734.

Diagnosis of Scrotal Lesions

Gottesman JE & others: Diagnostic ultrasound in the evaluation of scrotal masses. *J Urol* 1977;**118**:601.

Jellins J: Ultrasonic imaging of the scrotum. Presentation at the 22nd Annual Meeting of the American Institute of Ultrasound in Medicine, 1977.

Leopold G: Ultrasonography of superficially located structures. *Radiol Clin North Am* 1980;**18**:1.

Leopold G & others: High-resolution ultrasonography of scrotal pathology. *Radiology* 1979;**131**:719.

Sample WF, Gyepes MT, Ehrlich RM: Gray scale ultrasound in pediatric urology. *J Urol* 1977;**117**:518.

Shawker TH: B-mode ultrasonic evaluation of scrotal swellings. *Radiology* 1976;**118**:417.

Diagnosis of Torsion of the Testis Using Doppler Ultrasound

Hahn LC & others: Testicular scanning: A new modality for the preoperative diagnosis of testicular torsion. *J Urol* 1975;**113**:60.

Levy BJ: The diagnosis of torsion of the testicle using the Doppler ultrasonic stethoscope. *J Urol* 1975;**113**:63.

Milleret R: Doppler ultrasound diagnosis of testicular cord torsion. *J Clin Ultrasound* 1976;**4**:643.

Miskin M, Bain J: B-mode ultrasonic examination of the testes. *J Clin Ultrasound* 1974;**2**:307.

Nasrallah PF, Manzone D, King LR: Falsely negative Doppler examinations in testicular torsion. *J Urol* 1977;**118**:194.

Pedersen JF, Holm HH, Hald T: Torsion of the testis diagnosed by ultrasound. *J Urol* 1975;**113**:66.

Perri AJ & others: Necrotic testicle with increased blood flow on Doppler ultrasonic examination. *Urology* 1976;**8**:265.

Radioisotopic Kidney Studies | 8

Malcolm R. Powell, MD, & Charles A. Barnett, MD

Radioisotopic technics provide a means of investigating the structure and function of internal organs without disturbing normal physiologic processes. The radiopharmaceuticals used in evaluation of kidney function do not impose the hypertonic and chemical stress associated with intravenous contrast media, and the low iodide content in the iodinated radiopharmaceuticals does not pose a sensitivity risk. Radiopharmaceuticals in the kidney are detected by an external instrument after peripheral intravenous injection, so that the instrumentation common to other methods of urologic evaluation is avoided. The level of radiation is acceptable for all age groups, although some methods are modified with children. The distribution of radiotracers in tissue can be quantitated and analyzed by computer. Unlike the images obtained by sonography or CT scan, radionuclide images show the entire organ that concentrates the tracer.

The role of radioisotopic imaging in genitourinary diagnosis is not yet well defined. However, radiotracers provide information concerning kidney and bladder function that may not be easily obtained in other ways. Current nuclear imaging for urologic diagnosis includes renal blood flow imaging, static imaging of the kidney and urinary tract, renal function quantitation and imaging, bladder reflux and emptying studies, testicular imaging, and detection of abscesses by gallium- or indium-labeled leukocytes.

TECHNICS OF RENAL EVALUATION WITH RADIOPHARMACEUTICALS

Radiopharmaceuticals

Four general types of renal radioisotopic labels are in current use. Classified according to the mechanisms of labeling, they are as follows: (1) renal cortex labels, which are retained in the renal tubular cells; (2) intravascular compartment labels; (3) renal tubular function labels, which briefly label the renal cortex as they are accumulated by renal tubular cells and then are passed into the urine and cleared from the kidney; and (4) substances cleared solely by glomerular filtration, allowing for determination of glomerular filtration rate. Tables 8–1A and B list the characteristics of the more useful radiopharmaceuticals in these categories, and Fig

Table 8–1A. Radiopharmaceuticals for urologic diagnosis: Characteristics of the commonly used radionuclide labels.

Radionuclide	Physical Half-Life	Gamma Ray Energies (keV) and Abundance	Gamma Camera Sensitivity (dots/min/μCi for Various Collimators)	Advantages and Disadvantages
Technetium-99m (^{99m}Tc)	6.0 hours	140 (90%)	336–1080*	Very large numbers of gamma rays (photons) for radiation absorbed doses (no beta particles). Photon energy ideal. Readily available.
Iodine-131 (^{131}I)	8.1 days	364 (82%) 637 (6.8%) 284 (5.4%) etc	101*	Easy to bind to complex molecules without significant denaturation. Radiation absorbed dose per available photon high.
Iodine-125 (^{125}I)	60.2 days	27 (K x-ray) 35 (7%)	Not useful (energy too low for resolution)	Long shelf life when used to tag complex molecules. Low energy most suitable for in vitro measurements.
Gallium-67 citrate (^{67}Ga)	3.24 days	93 (68%) 184 (23%) 296 (21%) 388 (8%)	Low sensitivity (improved by dual spectrometer)	Specially ordered for each test. Cost relatively high. Best currently available tracer to detect neoplasms and abscesses.

*Data from Anger HO: Radioisotope cameras. Chapter 10 in: *Instrumentation in Nuclear Medicine.* Hine GJ (editor). Academic Press, 1967.

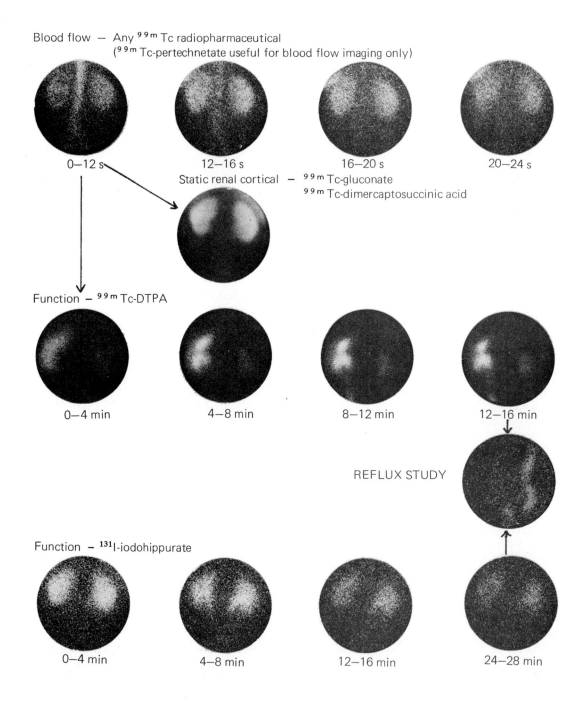

Blood flow — Any ^{99m}Tc radiopharmaceutical
(^{99m}Tc-pertechnetate useful for blood flow imaging only)

0–12 s   12–16 s   16–20 s   20–24 s

Static renal cortical — ^{99m}Tc-gluconate
^{99m}Tc-dimercaptosuccinic acid

Function — ^{99m}Tc-DTPA

0–4 min   4–8 min   8–12 min   12–16 min

REFLUX STUDY

Function — ^{131}I-iodohippurate

0–4 min   4–8 min   12–16 min   24–28 min

Figure 8–1. Sequence required for nuclear medicine imaging procedures for the kidneys and urinary tract. As diagrammed by this illustration, a single radiopharmaceutical can be used for more than one purpose. Any ^{99m}Tc-labeled agent can be used to obtain a blood flow study, since each photograph requires only a large number of radioactive disintegrations per brief time interval. Some of these agents localize in the renal cortex and allow for excellent static images of the kidney 20 minutes to an hour or more after injection. Typical agents used are ^{99m}Tc gluconate and ^{99m}Tc dimercaptosuccinic acid. A function evaluation can be performed either with ^{99m}Tc-DTPA, as it is excreted by glomerular filtration, or with sodium iodohippurate ^{131}I, which is excreted by tubular filtration. Once bladder filling occurs, these agents can be used for a reflux study, either during micturition or with compression of a filled bladder. Thus, the "triple isotope study" is currently used for scintiphotographic evaluation of kidney structure, blood flow, and function using usually 2 agents or sometimes only one agent. s = seconds; min = minutes.

Table 8—1B. Radiopharmaceuticals for urologic diagnosis.

Radiopharma-ceutical	Usual Dose (μCi)	Radiation-Absorbed Dose (Rads) From Usual Doses		Usual Scintiphoto Exposure Time and Imaging Time Postdose	Use
		Renal	Whole Body		
Urologic Radiopharmaceuticals					
^{99m}Tc-Fe ascorbate DTPA ^{99m}Tc glucohep-tonate ^{99m}Tc methyl-succinate	20,000	1.0	0.008	Serial: 4-second photos at 0—30 seconds; static: 2- to 4-minute photos at 30 minutes.	Localized in renal cortex by deposition and retention in renal tubular cells. Uptake is proportionate to regional renal blood flow. Rapid serial photos show renal blood flow distribution.
^{99m}Tc (Sn)-DTPA	20,000	0.10	0.030	Serial: 1- or 2-minute photos at 0—20 minutes or longer. Also useful to image blood flow.	Excreted solely by glomerular filtration. Useful for function imaging, but cortical definition vs background less than with other ^{99m}Tc agents.
Sodium iothala-mate ^{125}I	50	Negligible	0.00015	Not useful for imaging.	Glomerular filtration rate measurement.
^{99m}Tc (Sn)-DTPA	1000	0.03 (bladder)	0.001	Static views during filling of bladder; 6-second images during voiding.	Direct radionuclide cystography to detect and measure reflux.
^{99m}Tc pertech-netate	20,000	0.1 (testis)	0.020	Serial: Photos every 3—4 seconds to image blood flow. Static: Photos every 10—15 minutes.	Evaluation of testicular masses and differentiation of torsion from epididymitis.
Sodium iodohip-purate ^{131}I	200	0.080	0.0042 (assumes normal clearance)	2- to 10-minute photos (depending on renal function): 0—30 minutes for normal function to 1—2 hours for poor function.	Excreted by tubular function (like para-aminohippurate). 70—80% extraction causes rapid clearance in normal tissue. Prolonged cortical transit time occurs in ischemic or other forms of tubular damage with increased water reabsorption.
Sodium iodohip-purate ^{123}I	2000	0.01	0.0005	Serial images for 30 minutes or longer for poor function.	Excreted by tubular function. Same uses as for ^{131}I hippurate.
Other Nonrenal Radiopharmaceuticals Useful in Urology					
^{99m}Tc-diphos-phonate	15,000	1.05	0.15	2—4 minutes per view at 2—4 hours (30 minutes for whole body scan).	Bone imaging to detect reactive bone formation at sites of metastases before x-rays show abnormalities (prostatic, renal cell, and testicular cancer). Excreted by kidney yields genitourinary tract information.
^{67}Ga citrate	4000	6.0	1.0	5 minutes per view at 4—6 hours for abscesses and 48 hours for tumors (1 hour for whole body scan).	Detects occult neoplasms and abscesses. Used to stage testicular neoplasms by detecting lymph node involvement. Requires bowel preparation before scanning.

8–1 illustrates their use in evaluation of the kidneys and urinary tract.

A. Renal Cortex Labels: Until about 1973, the most commonly used renal cortical labels were the radioactive mercury–labeled chlormerodrins. More recently, renal cortical labels employing ^{99m}Tc in various compounds have been introduced. These compounds deliver a smaller radiation absorbed dose to the kidneys than do the radioactive mercury agents and provide more radioactive emissions for static imaging. Following peripheral intravenous injection, these tracers are accumulated in renal tubular epithelium, thereby labeling the renal cortex, while a portion of the injected dose passes into the urine. These substances are dependent upon renal blood flow for cortical labeling and, once fixed in the renal tubular cells, provide for imaging of the renal cortex.

B. Intravascular Compartment Labels: The intravascular compartment of the kidney can be imaged immediately after peripheral intravenous injection of 5 or preferably 10 mCi of any ^{99m}Tc-labeled radiopharmaceutical. A series of 3- to 5-second posterior view photographs of the kidneys is obtained during the first pass filling of the kidneys before the tracer is lost by active uptake or by dilution in the blood and exchange with other spaces. Since ^{99m}Tc agents can be used in amounts that provide large numbers of disintegrations per minute at quite acceptable radiation exposures, good definition of renal blood flow is recorded. These photographs are different from arteriograms in that they depict transit times of the tracer through various portions of the kidney rather than momentary intravascular distributions. In a normal renal vascular flow study, film exposure in renal cortical areas should be similar to that used during maximal aortic filling in the same series of pictures. A renal vascular flow study can also be performed with nonrenal agents such as ^{99m}Tc pertechnetate or ^{99m}Tc-labeled human serum albumin, since with this procedure, imaging is not dependent upon renal uptake of the tracer but only upon renal blood flow, which constitutes over 20% of the cardiac output. Following the blood flow study, static renal imaging can be performed with the same radiopharmaceutical if one of the renal cortical labeling agents such as ^{99m}Tc glucoheptonate was used.

C. Renal Tubular Function Labels: Sodium iodohippurate ^{131}I is used for renal tubular function studies and renograms. It is excreted into the urine by the renal tubular epithelium. A radioisotope renogram is a recording of the amount of radioactivity detected over each kidney from the time of peripheral intravenous injection of the labeled iodohippurate. Following injection, the count rate increases in a few seconds as 20% of the injected tracer is delivered to the kidneys by renal blood flow. The kidney with normal plasma flow rapidly accumulates iodohippurate, so that an increasing amount of radioactivity is detected over the kidney until the amount of radioactivity lost by urine drainage exceeds the amount accumulated by the renal cortex. Thereafter, if renal drainage is normal, the amount of radioactivity in the kidney continues to decrease, because the radiopharmaceutical was given as a single injection and the amount available in the blood for clearance has decreased throughout the period of observation. In uremia there is slower accumulation and prolonged cortical retention of iodohippurate, so that late scintiphotographs usually show an image similar to the image produced with renal cortical agents. Iodohippurate evaluations can be done in patients with severe uremia when neither intravenous urograms nor ^{99m}Tc glucoheptonate images can be obtained. Iodohippurate is also useful for detection of poorly functioning renal tissue in conditions other than uremia.

D. Glomerular Filtration Labels: Several other radiopharmaceuticals are useful in special circumstances. Agents that are excreted solely by glomerular function can be used to determine the glomerular filtration rate. The 2 that are most commonly available are ^{99m}Tc (Sn)-DTPA, a pure chelate of technetium, and radioiodinated iothalamate. It should be noted that ^{99m}Tc-DTPA must be prepared with tin reduction of the technetium as indicated by the designation ^{99m}Tc (Sn)-DTPA or it will not be a true glomerular agent because of incomplete reduction. Several commercial agents have been available which were referred to as ^{99m}Tc-DTPA but which actually are complex mixtures of ^{99m}Tc pertechnetate, ^{99m}Tc (Sn)-DTPA, and other complexing agents such as iron ascorbate. The ^{99m}Tc (Sn)-DTPA can also be used for renal imaging, although the renal cortex is not defined as

clearly as with agents that localize within the cortex and remain there. The ^{99m}Tc (Sn)-DTPA excretion study is useful for constructing a radioisotope urogram and can be used for studies of ureteral reflux in the same way as sodium iodohippurate ^{131}I. Both of these agents can be imaged during reflux from the bladder following initial peripheral intravenous administration.

E. Other Radiopharmaceuticals: Other radiopharmaceuticals of urologic interest are those used for detection of primary malignancies and their metastases and for the detection of abscesses. Since most genitourinary tumors tend to metastasize to bone, radionuclide bone imaging is an important evaluation when these malignancies are suspected. Bone metastases may be detected much earlier by a radionuclide study than by conventional radiographic screening methods. The most commonly used bone imaging agent is ^{99m}Tc methylene diphosphonate (see Table 8–1B).

Occult malignant tumors and abscesses can be detected by the so-called "tumor scan." For this technic, gallium-67 citrate seems to be as useful an agent as any presently available. It is injected intravenously, and the scans are performed after a variable delay as described in Table 8–1B. Bowel preparation is necessary before scanning. Since uptake in purulent abscesses is usually much greater than in neoplasms or normal tissue, an abscess will usually be seen quite clearly against surrounding structures.

Instrumentation

All of the radiopharmaceuticals discussed above are labeled with gamma radiation–emitting isotopes, which is necessary for external detection of radiation during in vivo studies. Gamma rays penetrate tissue as do x-rays; beta particles have charge and mass, which cause rapid absorption during passage through tissue.

A. Probe Counter: In the past, probe counters were used extensively in renal function studies. The probe counter has 2 or more detectors that record the amount of radioactivity in each kidney and, with additional detectors, in one or 2 other areas such as the bladder or cardiac blood pool. Each detector has a scintillation crystal with a cylindric collimator that limits the field of view to a cone-shaped area. Radioactive disintegrations detected in each field of view are continuously converted to average count rates by rate meters and are then plotted as functions of time by a recorder. The probe counter therefore provides a graphic and numerical recording of radiopharmaceutical content versus time in each kidney, and the other areas viewed. The averaging of functional activity of an entire kidney that is provided by this method may be misleading, since abnormalities are not localized and regional events may be obscured.

Probe counters have been used less frequently in renal studies since scintillation cameras have become generally available that can obtain both radioactive counts versus time and kidney images. Computers interfaced with the scintillation camera also provide analysis of function in specific portions of the kidney; for example, cortical areas can be analyzed while pelvocaliceal areas are excluded. Regional function can be evaluated as well. Neither is possible with the probe counter. However, the probe counter does have one virtue that assures its continued use in some instances: its sensitivity in detecting radiation. A cylindric collimator is much more sensitive than a scintillation camera detector and requires very small amounts of tracer, so that tests can be repeated frequently at less cost.

B. Anger Scintillation Camera (Gamma Camera): Radionuclide imaging instrumentation is designed to portray both the distribution of radioactivity in an organ or a tissue and the count rate of radioactivity emitted. In the past, 2 general types of radionuclide imaging equipment were used: radionuclide scanners and stationary detector radionuclide imaging devices. Only the Anger scintillation camera, a stationary detector gamma-imaging instrument, is now in general use. The camera's detector consists of a disk of sodium iodide 12 inches or more in diameter and one-half inch or less in thickness. The field of view is limited to a diameter approximately 2 inches less than the crystal diameter by a lead collimator with parallel holes perpendicular to the crystal surface. These holes allow only vertically oriented gamma rays to enter the detector. The scintillations produced in the crystal are detected by photomultiplier tubes connected to a computer in the instrument that determines the location of an event. This information is relayed to an oscilloscope that displays the location by a point of light. The oscilloscope display is photographed continuously, so that photographs are composed of large numbers of dots. Each dot recorded represents a gamma ray traveling vertically from its point of origin in the subject; therefore, the dots accumulate in a pattern representative of the in vivo distribution of radioactivity. The result is referred to as a "scintiphoto."

Because the scintillation camera detector is stationary, continuous photographs can be made showing all the scintillations detected from both kidneys over an interval of time. The scintiphotograph may record an interval as brief as a few seconds or as long as many minutes. Thus, this camera will photograph either static or rapidly changing distributions of radionuclide labels. Radioactivity concentrations are imaged both in rapid dynamic studies such as those showing blood flow or in slower dynamic studies such as those showing urine concentration and excretion. In addition, the information collected can be electronically processed to provide numerical information from small defined areas within the field of view. This numerical information can be analyzed by computer to provide quantification of regional renal function.

SCINTIPHOTOGRAPHY

Since evaluation of kidney structure and function by means of the scintillation camera combines aspects of most of the other nuclear medicine methods—and since the image sequences are an effective device for explaining the clinical uses of nuclear medicine tests—scintiphotography will be discussed most extensively.

The scintillation camera can visualize up to 3 distributions of a single radiopharmaceutical, or 2 or 3 different radiopharmaceuticals can be used to image the structure, function, and blood flow distributions of the kidney. Sequential studies performed in the same position can provide more information than a single evaluation. The studies are performed rapidly and without patient discomfort. Each radioactive label can be seen without distortion from previously injected labels.

The original multiple radiopharmaceutical study was the "triple isotope study," which used chlormerodrin ^{203}Hg for positioning and static imaging of renal structure, sodium iodohippurate ^{131}I for evaluation of renal function and imaging of poorly functioning renal tissue, and ^{99m}Tc pertechnetate for imaging renal blood flow distribution. Although it was not necessary to use all 3 radiopharmaceuticals in every patient, triple studies were generally performed for mass lesions, renal ischemia, and trauma. In a uremic patient, sodium iodohippurate ^{131}I alone was usually used, and a blood flow study was performed if indicated. Iodohippurate alone was also used for sequential evaluation of renal function following acute tubular necrosis, transplantation, or other forms of renal damage.

The newer ^{99m}Tc-labeled radiopharmaceuticals, which are cortical labeling agents, will evaluate both renal structure and blood flow. Iodohippurate remains an important agent for evaluation of renal function.

Kidney scintiphotography is best performed with the patient prone and the abdomen compressed. This prevents renal rotation and positions the kidneys closer to the detector and to the midline of the patient, with the long axes of the kidneys parallel to the plane of the detector. Scintiphotographs can be obtained in other positions to evaluate the dynamic effects of patient position on renal function or blood flow, and, when necessary, adequate images can be obtained with the patient supine and the detector viewing the kidneys through the table.

It is now customary to first inject a small portion of the ^{99m}Tc cortical agent for renal localization and positioning and then the remainder of the dose for blood flow studies. The rapid sequence scintiphotographs of blood flow will show the agent appearing first in the abdominal aorta, then in the kidneys and the spleen at about the same time, and, much later, in the liver. Renal blood flow is sufficient to show the kidneys as well-defined structures; much less tracer will be seen in surrounding structures. Normal renal blood flow distribution will cause the kidney to appear about as bright as the aorta at the level of the kidney. This study will determine vascularity in any renal mass lesion. A corresponding cold area on the ^{99m}Tc blood flow study suggests a lack of vascularity and, if spherical, a cyst. A mass lesion that is densely labeled by ^{99m}Tc in the blood flow study suggests a vascular tumor, usually a renal cell carcinoma. Vascular tumors often fill at a time differing from the time of renal cortical filling. A renal cell carcinoma is often better visualized during the blood flow study than is the remainder of the renal cortex, particularly in the frequent instance where the tumor mass causes relative ischemia in surrounding tissue. This may be due to a direct pressure effect from the neoplasm or to the invasion of vascular structures, particularly the renal vein. On the other hand, simple cysts tend to cause discrete spherical defects without other disturbance of renal cortical blood flow. Therefore, in static studies, the cortex around a cyst is generally better labeled than the cortex around a neoplasm. An apparent cyst surrounded by poorly labeled cortex suggests necrosis of a renal cell carcinoma and formation of a cyst—a frequent occurrence.

After the blood flow information is obtained, some renal cortical agents can be used immediately to obtain a urogram, if sufficient tracer is filtered and not reabsorbed. Avascular spaces adjacent to or within the kidney can be visualized when scintiphotographs are taken immediately after injection of the technetium-labeled agents, before they are diffused into extravascular spaces. This may be particularly important in identifying exophytic renal cysts that do not disrupt the cortex enough to cause a defect in the image. After an hour or more, the ^{99m}Tc cortical agents are cleared from the calices and renal pelvis, leaving tracer in the cortex only. Excellent high-resolution images of the cortex can then be obtained, showing small details such as scars, masses, or other lesions that displace normal tissue. The amount of agent in the cortex is related to renal blood flow; areas retaining little of the agent may thus be ischemic. When there are focal lesions in the kidney, it often becomes important to obtain special views using oblique orientation or even a different collimator such as a single pinhole collimator, which allows for a larger field of view.

Static renal images are particularly effective for evaluation of suspected renal mass lesions. Glucoheptonate imaging is more sensitive than intravenous urography for detection of renal masses, especially in cortical and medullary areas where peripheral parenchymal bulges and central "masses" distorting calices could represent either true masses or columns of Bertin on intravenous urography. Peripelvic lesions are more difficult to evaluate by radionuclide imaging because defects in this area are also produced by normal pelvic fat and other pelvic structures. Questionable pelvic masses on urography are probably best studied by computed tomography, which can identify fat density and better distinguish normal from abnormal structures in this area. Neoplasm must be suspected when a renal defect is detected by static radionuclide imaging. Perfusion of the defect region, which can be determined by comparing the defect study with the blood flow study, suggests neoplasm or arteriovenous malformation. Vascular cortical lesions are usually renal cell carcinomas. Renal carcinomas often cause decreased blood flow in the affected kidney due to mass effect within the kidney capsule or to direct invasion of the renal vein, so a mass lesion with general reduction of tracer uptake in the rest of the kidney suggests neoplasm.

Iodohippurate imaging studies continue to be extremely useful even though the images contain fewer data points than those of the newer renal cortical labeling agents. With the patient remaining in exactly the same position as in the static scintiphotographs, a series of photographs is obtained beginning immediately after peripheral intravenous injection of the iodohippurate dose. For comparison, the photographic parameters—including exposure time—should be kept constant throughout the series. A simultaneous recording of count rate over each kidney provides radioisotope renograms. If renal function is normal, serial iodohippurate scintiphotographs are usually obtained with a 2- to 4-minute exposure time, but with decreased function it may be best to obtain exposures of as long as 10 minutes each to record significant numbers of counts in each photograph. With extreme reduction of renal function, there is usually insufficient uptake of renal cortical agents to allow for visualization, whereas iodohippurate will be accumulated slowly and allow for imaging. In iodohippurate studies of uremic patients, renal cortical labeling eventually will reveal considerable information about kidney structure and function. Delayed views may even show enough detail of the renal pelvis and ureters to rule out obstruction in the severely uremic patient.

Iodohippurate appearance in the kidneys is dependent initially upon renal blood flow. When blood levels of tracer fall as a result of renal accumulation and other extravascular loss, the rate of renal accumulation of iodohippurate slows. As the rate of accumulation is exceeded by iodohippurate loss through urine drainage from the kidney, the radioactivity count rate over the kidney peaks and then falls. Iodohippurate scintiphotographs show the location of radioactivity in the kidney during the different phases of iodohippurate excretion. The simultaneously recorded renogram tracing is obtained by computer analysis. Interpretation of iodohippurate scintiphotographs is performed both by observing whether the rate of iodohippurate accumulation and excretion is within normal limits and by comparing the function of the 2 kidneys or of part of one kidney with other tissue in the same kidney. Generally, if there is no dilatation of intra-renal drainage structures or obstruction of urine drainage, the most frequent cause of regional or unilateral decrease of renal function is renal isch-emia. Most other causes of decreased renal function will result in generalized changes affecting both kidneys equally—as is usually seen in glomerular nephritis, pyelonephritis, acute tubular necrosis, and vasculitis. When ischemia is present, not only is the accumulation of iodohippurate in the kidneys slowed but there is increased reabsorption of water by the ischemic tubules, causing decreased urine volume from the area of the ischemic renal cortex and a prolongation of the transit time of iodohippu-rate through the cortex. The scintiphotographs will therefore show late labeling of the ischemic kidney when normal renal cortex in the same patient has completely cleared the iodohippurate. During the drainage phase of an iodohippurate study, various obstructive problems are easily demonstrated. Even with abdominal compression in the prone position, the normal kidney is rapidly emptied of labeled urine by ureteral peristalsis. Fifteen min-utes after injection, the kidney usually contains less than half the number of counts detected at the maximum count rate. Postvoiding residual urine volume in the bladder can be readily estimated by scintiphotographs, and cine studies will detect and evaluate vesicoureteral reflux. Urine reflux from the bladder can be easily differentiated from the trace amounts of radiopharmaceutical remaining in the ureter.

This extensive renal evaluation can be per-formed in about 40 minutes if there are no signifi-cant abnormalities but may take an hour or more if there are major abnormalities. Depending upon patient tolerance for a complicated procedure, this evaluation can be considerably shortened and tai-lored to the clinical situation.

EXAMPLES OF CLINICAL UTILIZATION OF RADIONUCLIDE IMAGING STUDIES

The value of nuclear medicine methods in the investigation of renal structure and function can be best appreciated by a review of common clinical findings.

Most renal imaging studies with radionuclides are obtained with the patient prone and the kidneys viewed posteriorly. In this position, with the appli-cation of mid and lower abdominal compression, the kidneys assume a somewhat different position than that seen on the common supine intravenous urograms. In the prone position, the liver shape also changes, creating a space above the right kid-ney that permits this kidney to move cephalad.

Figs 8–2 and 8–3 demonstrate renal scin-tiphoto studies in which vascular tumors are dif-ferentiated from nonvascular tumors. A tumor of the renal cortex will produce a static image defect either by displacing normal cortex from the tumor site, or by interfering with the mechanism of tissue labeling, or both (Fig 8–2). In order for normal tissue labeling to occur, blood flow to the area must be normal and the tissue must have appropriate metabolic activity. Thus, renal masses will appear in a scan or scintiphoto as "cold areas," with absent or reduced labeling surrounded by labeled cortex. Typically, a cyst (Fig 8–3) will be seen as a discrete spherical defect that is not associated with de-creased localization of tracer in the adjacent cortex. Carcinomas tend to cause much more extensive changes, with large, irregular areas of decreased perfusion in the region of the neoplasm. An irregu-larly shaped renal cortex due to fetal lobulations will be labeled in its entirety, since it is composed of normal parenchyma.

To evaluate vascularity of a focal defect, the patient is given a rapid peripheral intravenous in-jection of a ^{99m}Tc-labeled radiopharmaceutical, and a series of 4-second scintiphotographs is ob-tained. If the lesion is seen to be vascular, it is presumed to be a neoplasm or arteriovenous mal-formation. After the rapid sequence of blood flow pictures is obtained, an immediate 1-minute expo-sure using greatly diminished dot intensity on the scintillation camera oscilloscope will produce an image of high quality (high data density) showing the renal vascular pool prior to localization of the label in extravascular spaces. This method can be particularly valuable in differentiating neoplasms that are less well vascularized, particularly the transitional cell carcinomas.

It is essential that the relative positions of the patient and the camera detector be kept constant for each radiopharmaceutical used, so that regional findings with one agent can be precisely compared with findings of others. For this reason, it is best to avoid changing collimators by using a medium energy collimator for the entire study when sodium iodohippurate ^{131}I is used.

The camera study is limited by the spatial reso-lution of the instrument for the number of counts detected. This is a function of the density of radioac-tivity in the area studied, intrinsic resolution of the detector system, and lack of renal motion during the study. In practice, it may not be possible to vis-ualize renal lesions much less than 1 inch in diame-ter, although much smaller lesions can theoretically be identified. The effects of a neoplasm on sur-rounding tissues often cause the lesion to appear larger than its true dimensions.

The scintiphoto renogram can detect regional renal ischemia causing renal vascular hypertension. Fig 8–4 shows the sequential use of 2 radiophar-maceuticals for this purpose. A renal blood flow study is performed first. A ^{99m}Tc-labeled agent such as glucoheptonate is used most commonly. Ischemic areas are directly identified in this study. Next, immediate static images of the kidneys are

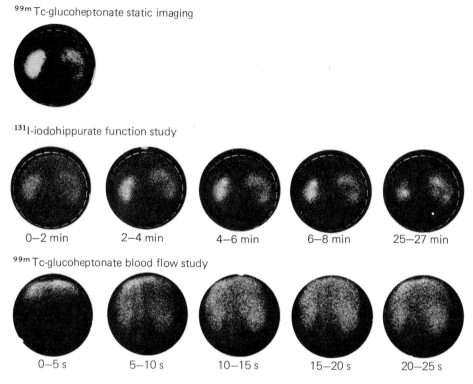

Figure 8–2. Renal cell carcinoma. A "triple" renal evaluation showing alterations in kidney structure, function, and blood flow typical of renal cell carcinoma. The tumor has invaded the renal vein, causing abnormal renal hemodynamics; a distinct defect in the cortex of the right kidney (gluconate image) shows normal or increased blood flow. Kidney cortex affected by the tumor shows decreased gluconate localization, a reduced rate of iodohippurate accumulation, and prolongation of iodohippurate transit time owing to increased free water reabsorption. s = seconds; min = minutes.

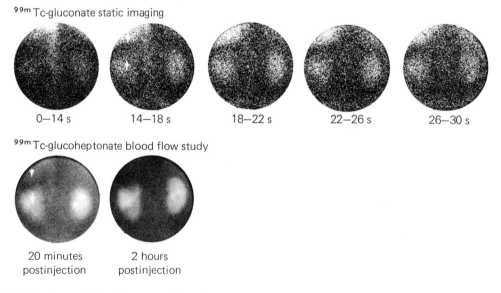

Figure 8–3. Renal cyst. Evaluation was performed using a single radiopharmaceutical to obtain both blood flow and structure studies. The area above the left kidney and below the spleen image remains relatively free of radioactive blood content during a blood flow study; it is clearly defined as a defect of the upper pole of the kidney after localization of the gluconate in the kidney cortex. Typically, a renal cyst does not interfere with blood flow to the remainder of the cortex of the affected kidney. Renal cysts are often exophytic, protruding from the kidney and showing as a cold defect in background radioactivity surrounding the kidney. s = seconds.

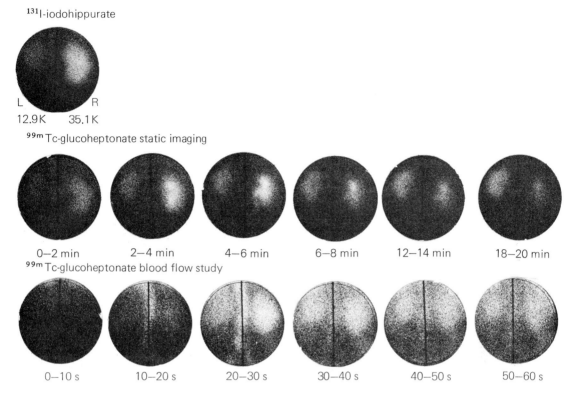

131I-iodohippurate

L   R
12.9K   35.1K

99mTc-glucoheptonate static imaging

0–2 min   2–4 min   4–6 min   6–8 min   12–14 min   18–20 min

99mTc-glucoheptonate blood flow study

0–10 s   10–20 s   20–30 s   30–40 s   40–50 s   50–60 s

Figure 8–4. Renovascular hypertension secondary to arteriosclerotic disease. Typical of renovascular hypertension, the left kidney has diminished uptake of glucoheptonate as a result of reduced renal blood flow, which is confirmed in the blood flow study. There is a slowed rate of iodohippurate accumulation in this small kidney and a prolongation of iodohippurate transit time through the cortex secondary to increased water reabsorption, so that the latter part of this study shows cortical retention of iodohippurate at a time when the normal kidney shows only a slight degree of retention in a superior caliceal system and normal clearance from other areas. s = seconds; min = minutes; K = thousands of counts.

obtained using the same agent. A sodium iodohippurate 131I series study is then done to show accumulation and drainage of labeled urine from the kidneys. If available, a computer can be used to produce a renogram curve of cortical area counts as a function of time. Iodohippurate will accumulate less rapidly in an ischemic kidney or in an ischemic area of a kidney; however, ischemia is not defined by this slow labeling, since it also occurs in other disorders of renal function. Renal ischemia causing hypertension is strongly suggested by a prolonged iodohippurate transit time through cortical tissue when other parts of the same kidney or the other kidney show normal transit times. The prolonged transit time results from increased water reabsorption by the ischemic area and consequent delayed washout of label from the kidney. Such labeling may be differentiated from that of obstruction, since it occurs in the cortex and not in drainage structures. The iodohippurate study therefore defines a characteristic physiologic abnormality as accurately as the Howard, Stamey, or Rappaport tests, and may locate the region of the abnormality within the kidney.

The renogram curve is produced by computer analysis of cortical areas as a function of time. In

essence, there are 3 parts to the curve—a vascular phase, a function phase, and a drainage phase. The vascular phase is the period during which the rate of accumulation rapidly rises in each kidney, as the iodohippurate enters the intravascular spaces. During the function phase, the increase of count rate in the kidneys is nearly linear. The iodohippurate blood level is almost constant for the first few minutes after postinjection mixing, and the cortex extracts tracer from the blood at a constant rate for 3–8 minutes after injection until drainage of urine from the kidney begins to occur. The rate of drainage eventually exceeds the rate of accumulation of iodohippurate, and the count rate begins to decrease. A normally hydrated prone patient with normal urine drainage will show peaking of count rate at 3–8 minutes and then a fall of count rate to no less than half of the maximum within 15 minutes. In the sitting position, the peak occurs somewhat earlier and the fall is more rapid. Fig 8–5 summarizes the various abnormalities that may be detected by the iodohippurate function study.

The study of kidney transplant illustrated in Fig 8–6 shows several uses of iodohippurate renography by the scintillation camera. First, this study evaluates the success of the vascular and ureteral anastomoses in the period immediately following transplantation. Good early labeling of the entire renal cortex attests to normal perfusion. If urine is seen to drain normally, patency of the ureteral anastomosis is confirmed. Second, the transplant renogram often demonstrates general reduction of function that may occur with a rejection reaction, acute tubular necrosis, or other similar processes. Focal areas of decreased iodohippurate labeling may be observed if there is regional ischemia, partial infarction, or other local change. The rate at which iodohippurate is accumulated and drained charac-

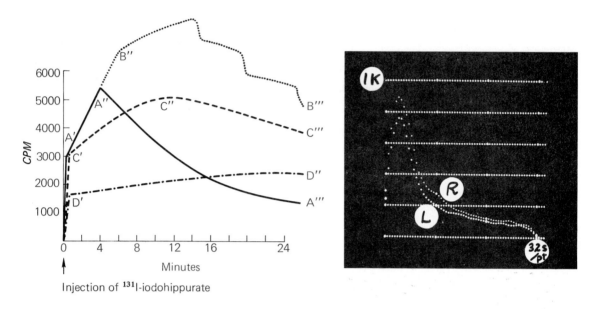

Figure 8–5. Summary of several abnormalities detected by radioisotope renography using sodium iodohippurate 131I. CPM = counts per minute. *Solid line:* Normal renogram idealized as O–A'–A''–A'''. O–A' = vascular phase. Initial vascular labeling detected. A'–A'' = function phase. Iodohippurate accumulation by renal cortical cells recorded. A''–A''' = drainage phase. Drainage exceeds accumulation; count rate decreases. *Dotted line:* Renogram of mild obstruction. O–A' = no change from normal. A'–B'' = accumulation of counts prolonged in function phase. B''–B''' = poorly defined broad peak and slowed drainage phase. Steps down in count rate suggest intermittent flow. *Dashed line:* Renogram of renovascular ischemia, normal renovascular volume. O–C' = vascular labeling delayed but similar in amount to normal. C'–C'' = decreased function; decreased rate of accumulation. C''–C''' = increased water reabsorption; decreased urine volume; slowing of iodohippurate drainage. *Dash-dotted line:* Renogram typical of severe ischemia or nephritis and reduced function. O–D' = delayed and reduced vascular labeling. D'–D'' = extreme slowing of iodohippurate accumulation; little drainage. The finding of normal function in one kidney and abnormal function in the other kidney indicates that renograms O–C''' and O–D'' are related to unilateral disease typical of renovascular ischemia that may be functionally significant in causing hypertension. The finding of bilateral and symmetric renogram abnormalities would indicate a generalized renal disease that, in terms of the renogram, could be glomerulonephritis, pyelonephritis, acute tubular necrosis, or the result of renal vascular disease. The diagram of possible abnormalities can be compared with the normal renogram at right.

¹³¹I-iodohippurate

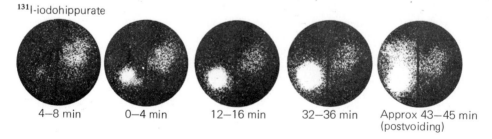

| 4–8 min | 0–4 min | 12–16 min | 32–36 min | Approx 43–45 min (postvoiding) |

Figure 8–6. Cadaver transplant; urine extravasation with voiding. After intravenous administration of sodium iodohippurate 131I, accumulation occurs in a transplanted kidney, with generalized and localized reduction of accumulation related to rejection reaction or acute tubular necrosis. In this example the kidney is functioning, with considerable excretion of urine into the bladder, but obvious extravasation of urine occurs when the patient attempts to void. The iodohippurate study is particularly sensitive in the detection of minor amounts of urine extravasation that would ordinarily be seen only on retrograde studies and even then with difficulty. min = minutes.

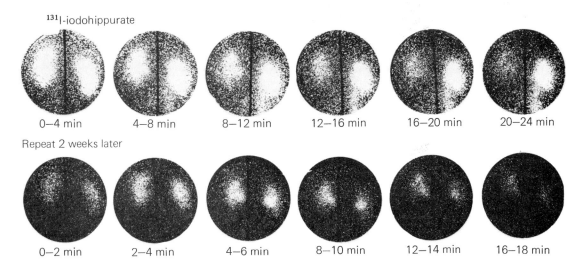

Figure 8–7. Renal trauma. This patient, who was allergic to contrast media, was evaluated with serial sodium iodohippurate ^{131}I studies. The iodohippurate study is in any case a most sensitive way to serially evaluate kidney function and is very helpful following trauma. Here the right kidney and ureter show delay of iodohippurate drainage and retention of iodohippurate within the ureter immediately after flank injury but complete clearing of abnormality 2 weeks after the initial study. There was never any evidence of extravasation of urine. min = minutes.

terizes progressive changes in renal function that occur in rejection activity or other processes. Last, the slow iodohippurate transit through a kidney allows for high data density scintiphotos or even scans of the renal cortex. In uremia, this often allows better renal visualization than the static images obtained with other agents.

In evaluation of renal trauma, radioisotopic studies are useful in the diagnosis of extrarenal hematoma, renal lacerations, reduction of renal function secondary to contusion, or urine extravasation. Fig 8–7 demonstrates a case of simple renal contusion and the clearing of abnormalities 2 weeks later. The iodohippurate study is particularly useful in demonstrating extravasation of urine either due to trauma or after surgery (Fig 8–6). Small concentrations of extravasated dye that are completely inapparent on simultaneous intravenous urograms are readily visualized by tracer technics.

The iodohippurate gamma-imaged urogram is also useful in studying the renal pelvis, ureters, and bladder. In renal obstructive disease, the renogram often defines structures well enough to provide a general idea of the severity of the obstruction without retrograde urography or other involved procedures. Gamma-imaged urograms can be used in patients hypersensitive to contrast media, since the amount of iodide in radioiodinated hippurate is insufficient to cause iodide sensitivity. Other uses include the screening of uremic patients for obstructive uropathy, evaluation of male infants, follow-up of surgically corrected obstruction for patency and functional status, and evaluation of ureteral reflux. Fig 8–8 demonstrates a study for ureteral reflux where the reflux occurred only during micturition. This study did not require catheterization, since it used tracer excreted after peripheral intravenous injection. The study was performed approximately one-half hour after injection of ^{99m}Tc-DTPA, when most of the tracer had been

Left ureteral reflux with voiding (anterior view of bladder after ^{99m}Tc-DTPA excretion)

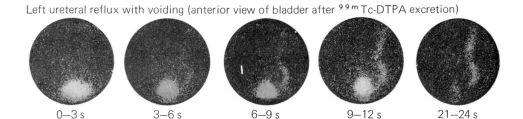

Figure 8–8. Left ureteral reflux with voiding. After the bladder is filled from renal excretion of an intravenously administered radionuclide, ureteral reflux studies may be obtained without catheterization. The patient was asked to void in a sitting position while the anterior aspect of the bladder and ureteral area were viewed. Ureteral reflux can be seen beginning at 3–6 seconds as the bladder contracts, and it becomes maximal after voiding is completed. s = seconds.

excreted and the ureters were relatively free of radioactivity.

While definition of individual caliceal structure and other fine detail is not within even an order of magnitude of the resolution available on a conventional radiographic study, a radionuclide imaging study is sufficient for many clinical purposes. It presents enough detail so that more complicated studies may not be required. An important advantage of these radiopharmaceuticals is the generally low radiation absorbed doses even in serial studies.

OTHER RADIONUCLIDE IMAGING PROCEDURES USEFUL IN UROLOGY

Bladder Scanning

Radioisotopes have been used since 1959 to demonstrate vesicoureteral reflux. The nuclear cystogram is accurate in diagnosing reflux, and, because of its quantification capabilities, has several advantages over conventional roentgenographic cystography. These advantages include greater sensitivity for detecting reflux, much less radiation exposure, and provision of quantitative data on bladder function. These data include precise calculations of the total bladder volume, the bladder volume at which reflux occurs, the volume of reflux into the upper tracts, and the postvoiding residual bladder volume. The procedure of the nuclear cystogram is more consistent than that of roentgenographic cystography, so that patients can be more easily quantitated over a period of time. For example, the technic has shown that prior to becoming clinically stable, children with improving reflux have a progressively increased bladder volume at which reflux occurs.

The test can be performed by either the direct or indirect method. The indirect method does not require catheterization (Fig 8–8). It relies on rapid and relatively complete renal clearance of sodium iodohippurate ^{131}I or ^{99m}Tc-DTPA. Standard renal flow and static images can be obtained before the cystogram. When most of the radioactivity has been concentrated in the bladder, the patient is placed before the camera in a sitting or standing position and monitored during voiding. A sudden increase in radioactivity over the ureters or kidneys indicates reflux. Normal voiding mechanics are present, because catheterization is not necessary. Quantitative evaluation of improvement in the volume at which reflux occurs does require the direct method and catheterization.

This technic has certain disadvantages, however: The patient must be cooperative and able to retain urine and must void on command. Indirect cystography is thus not suitable for infants and most young children. The study is dependent upon renal function; bladder volume cannot be varied; and the amount of bladder volume necessary to produce reflux may not be achieved.

For these reasons (especially in children), direct radionuclide cystography is the technic of choice. The patient is placed supine on the scanning table with the gamma camera underneath the table. The urethra is catheterized and connected to a bottle of sterile normal saline. The bottle is placed 100 cm above the tabletop. After flow is started, 1 mCi of ^{99m}Tc tracer is injected into the stream of saline. Bladder filling and possible reflux can be monitored during the course of the study by a persistence oscilloscope. The camera and computer can be set up to allow for acquisition of data during the entire course of bladder filling. If reflux occurs, the bladder filling volume at which it occurs is noted. After filling, scintigrams are obtained in the anterior view and both posterior oblique views. The patient may then sit on a bedpan in front of the gamma camera. The catheter is removed, and the patient is encouraged to void. A voiding scintigram of the bladder and upper abdomen is obtained. The volume of urine voided is measured. From this volume and from counts of the bladder before and after voiding, total bladder volume and residual volume can be calculated. The amount of urine reflux is also calculated from data obtained from the involved ureter.

Testicular Scanning

The blood-brain barrier concept developed from the observation that some injected dyes stained most tissues but not the brain. It was noted that the seminiferous tubules were also not stained. Scrotal imaging, based on the relative lack of vascular permeability in normal testicular tissue, was first performed in 1973. It was believed that the loss of blood supply to a testis in torsion would show as an area of decreased perfusion on imaging. Conversely, increased uptake would be noted in areas of increased capillary permeability resulting from inflammation, as in epididymitis.

The study is performed with the patient supine and the legs abducted. The penis is taped back over the pubis. The scrotum is placed parallel to the face of the low energy collimator by a tape sling. Lead shielding can be used if scrotal separation from the thighs cannot be obtained by abduction. The tracer dose is 15 or 20 mCi of ^{99m}Tc pertechnetate for adults. A series of 10-second exposures should be made to show blood flow characteristics, and then higher resolution static images should be made immediately postinjection to better define perfusion volume distribution.

Scrotal scans are most helpful when the angiographic phase and the delayed tissue phase are interpreted together. The findings can then be compared to other clinical signs associated with painful scrotal swelling. The dynamic phase demonstrates the iliac arteries, the spermatic cords, and the testicular tissue itself. Relative blood flow into the testicular area is low. With imaging, flow to the affected testis is compared with that of the normal testis. Small testes in children or adults are not as easily diagnosed by the scan. Lead or cobalt markers placed over each testis may help define the affected organ on static images.

The testicular scan is most valuable in differentiating torsion from epididymitis when other clinical signs are not clear. In epididymitis, perfusion is seen to be markedly increased on the flow study in the affected side lateral to the testis. Static images show a "hot" epididymis. In acute testicular torsion, perfusion on the flow study is decreased or normal—never increased. On static images, the testis shows as a rounded cold area. Unfortunately, many of these cases are not evaluated immediately.

Delayed evaluation will show normal perfusion with a rounded cold area surrounded by hyperemic tissue. Later, the testes and hemiscrotum are smaller. Areas of low isotope localization must be correlated with the distribution of scrotal contents and clinical symptoms. Areas of decreased uptake may represent torsion, a hematoma of the scrotal wall or testicular capsule, an abscess, a hydrocele, or a poorly perfused area of necrotic tumor.

An abscess shows markedly increased perfusion with intense radionuclide angiographic definition of the vessels. The static image will show areas of hyperemia, but the most prominent finding is a

Metastatic renal cell carcinoma

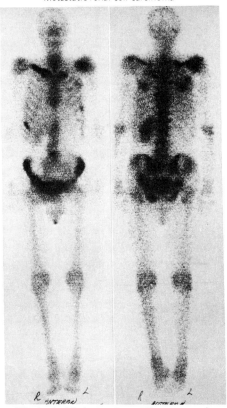

(Obtained with dual-probe rectilinear scanner)

Metastatic prostatic carcinoma

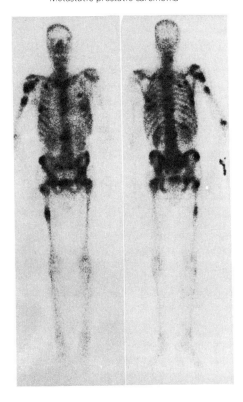

(Obtained with whole body imaging modification of scintillation camera)

Figure 8–9. Whole body bone scanning. Whole body bone scanning can be accomplished using either conventional rectilinear scanners, usually with dual probes and image minification to show the entire body on a single x-ray film; or with a whole body imaging adaptation of the scintillation camera, also with image minification. Illustrated here are bone scans using both methods with ^{99m}Tc phosphate bone scanning agent. The metastatic renal cell carcinoma scan shows extensive pelvic metastases as well as right clavicular, left shoulder, and several rib metastases. It should be noted that the scans obtained with a dual probe whole body scanner are usually shown with the right side to the viewer's left in both the anterior and posterior views. This is done so that they can be readily superimposed. With whole body imaging adaptations of the scintillation camera, it is conventional to show a "fluoroscopic view" with the patient's left on the viewer's left in a posterior view. In the illustration of metastatic prostatic carcinoma, there are numerous pelvic, spine, rib, and long bone metastases. Bone scans will image the kidneys and bladder (the left kidney in the renal cell carcinoma patient has been surgically removed), so that urologic diagnoses are frequently obtained from bone scans.

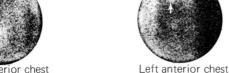

Right anterior chest   Left anterior chest

Gallium-67 tumor imaging study

Figure 8–10. Testicular carcinoma metastatic to the lungs, evaluated with gallium-67 citrate tumor imaging. Several agents have a propensity to accumulate in tumors and abscesses. After intravenous administration, whole body scans at 48–72 hours postinjection will show gallium-67 citrate localization in the liver, to a lesser extent in bone, and to a slight extent in soft tissues, as well as in any site of neoplasm or abscess that has the characteristic of accumulating this tracer. The method is useful for preoperative staging of metastases of testicular and other urologic neoplasms. The areas of gallium uptake shown in the lungs and mediastinum are consistent with metastasis.

cool or even cold area within the scrotum that may be separated by palpation from the testis. Torsion of the testicular appendages may produce slightly increased perfusion, but the scrotal structures frequently appear to be normal on both sides on static images. Testicular tumors demonstrate slightly increased perfusion on the flow study. Static images show normal homogeneous or irregular activity that is slightly warmer and of larger dimensions than in the normal testis. Hydroceles and spermatoceles show normal perfusion with lucencies either surrounding the testis in hydrocele or adjacent to the superior lateral aspect of the testis in spermatocele.

Testicular scanning, then, is a technic that can provide early evaluation of acute scrotal problems. The high rate of clinical misdiagnosis in the emergency room could perhaps be lowered with immediate scrotal scanning, and testicular survival rates improved. The demonstration of a normal and well-perfused testis could help prevent unnecessary exploration of the scrotum in clinically uncertain cases.

Bone & Tumor Scanning

Bone scanning and tumor scanning are 2 other radionuclide imaging procedures that have relatively frequent applications in urology. Both tests are best performed by a combination of whole body imaging technics and spot views of suspicious areas. These procedures are performed after intravenous administration of tracer, allowing time for tracer localization. In bone scanning with the technetium-labeled agents described in Table 8–1, the postinjection interval before scanning is generally 2 hours. Patients are asked to empty their bladders prior to scanning, since a significant portion of the tracer is excreted in the urine. The bone-seeking tracer localizes in areas of bone mineral turnover in normal bone, but especially in areas of bone formation stimulated by the presence of neoplasm, inflammation, or bone repair. The bone scan is usually much more efficient in detecting early metastatic neoplastic involvement of bone than are conventional x-ray studies. Since both prostatic and

renal cell carcinoma have a marked tendency toward early bone metastasis, bone scans are frequently advisable in the work-up of these patients prior to planning definitive treatment. Fig 8–9 compares 2 imaging technics: an evaluation for metastatic renal cell carcinoma recorded by a conventional dual probe whole body scanner and an evaluation for metastatic prostatic carcinoma recorded by a whole body imaging modification of the scintillation camera. The spatial resolution of small lesions is obviously better with the adapted scintillation camera study. These bone scans can be used both for detection of lesions that do not appear on x-rays and for evaluation of response of lesions to therapy. If a bony lesion heals, it will show on scan as a lessened accumulation of tracer compared to control scans.

Fig 8–10 demonstrates tumor scanning with gallium-67 citrate. This is administered intravenously and the scan is done 48–72 hours later, when blood levels of tracer have decreased to very low concentrations. Bowel preparation is required prior to scanning, because bowel secretion of the tracer will interfere with evaluation of the abdominal and pelvic areas. Radiogallium localizes in a wide variety of neoplastic lesions, in abscesses, and even in kidneys involved with active pyelonephritis. The technic may therefore be used to detect both occult neoplasms and occult abscesses or infection. Concentrations of the tracer tend to be greater in abscesses than in neoplastic lesions, and with abscesses, there is less interference by normal uptake of tracer in structures such as the liver, spleen, bones, and gut, which always show some gallium accumulation. Tumor localization may be somewhat more difficult in the abdomen, but the gallium-67 citrate scan has been used in staging testicular tumors, where it reportedly has been more efficient than lymphography. Because of the greater uptake in abscesses, these scans can be performed as early as 4 hours after tracer injection, compared to the 48–72 hours required for differentiation of neoplastic lesions.

•   •   •

References

Hine GJ (editor): *Instrumentation in Nuclear Medicine.* Academic Press, 1967.

Holder LE & others: Testicular radionuclide angiography and static imaging: Anatomy, scintigraphic interpretation and clinical indications. *Radiology* 1977;**125**:739.

Leonard JC & others: Renal cortical imaging and the detection of renal mass lesions. *J Nucl Med* 1979;**20**:1018.

Maxwell MH & others: Radioisotope renogram in renal arterial hypertension. *J Urol* 1968;**100**:376.

Morris JG & others: The diagnosis of renal tumors by radioisotope scanning. *J Urol* 1967;**97**:40.

Nadel NS & others: Preoperative diagnosis of testicular torsion. *Urology* 1973;**1**:478.

Nasrallah PF & others: Quantitative nuclear cystogram aid in determining spontaneous resolution of vesicoureteral reflux. *Urology* 1978;**6**:654.

Older RA & others: Accuracy of radionuclide imaging in distinguishing renal masses from normal variants. *Radiology* 1980;**136**:443.

Pistemia DD, McDougall R, Kriss JP: Screening for bone metastases. *JAMA* 1975;**231**:46.

Powell MR: Evaluation of kidney structure and function by radioisotope imaging. Page 447 in: *Clinical Uses of Radionuclides: Critical Comparison with Other Techniques.* AEC Symposium Series No. 27. US Atomic Energy Commission, 1972.

Radionuclide studies of the genitourinary system. (2 parts.) *Semin Nucl Med* 1974;**4**:3, 97. [Entire issues.]

Rosenthal J: Ortho-iodohippurate-I-131 kidney scanning in renal failure. *Radiology* 1966;**78**:298.

Shuler SE: The scintillation camera in pediatric renal disease. *Am J Dis Child* 1970;**120**:115.

Symposium on advances in imaging techniques. *Urol Clin North Am* 1979;**6**:307. [Entire issue.]

9 | Instrumental Examination of the Urinary Tract

Donald R. Smith, MD

PRELIMINARY PROCEDURES

Aseptic Technic

Instruments must be prepared and used in an aseptic manner. Metal sounds and rubber or plastic catheters can be autoclaved. Optical instruments are gas sterilized. Soaking instruments in antiseptic solutions is inadequate.

The glans penis should be washed thoroughly with soap and water or an antiseptic solution. The vulva must be cleansed and the labia held apart as the instrument is introduced.

It should be pointed out that because of the presence of bacteria in the distal urethra, it is impossible to pass an instrument in a completely sterile manner. Secondary cystitis rarely occurs, however, unless there is residual urine in the bladder.

Lubrication of Urethra

Catheters and other instruments must not be passed into the urinary tract without proper lubrication. In women, it is sufficient to dip the instrument in the lubricant. In men, however, such a procedure is inadequate because the meatus removes the lubricant and the instrument then passes over a relatively dry mucous membrane. The male urethra can be lubricated only by instilling at least 15 mL of a sterile water-soluble lubricant. This is best accomplished with a syringe with a rubber bulb on one end. It should have a blunt tip so that it does not have to be passed down the urethra. Oils (eg, mineral oil or olive oil) must not be used, since fatal oil emboli have resulted from their use. The syringe serves not only to introduce the column of lubricant into the canal but also, by virtue of the constant, steady pressure required, to overcome the normal tone of the external sphincter muscle. This resistance may be increased if the patient is apprehensive. Inexperienced instrumentalists frequently have difficulty introducing catheters against the force of this spasm, and this has resulted in many false diagnoses of "urethral stricture."

Anesthesia

A barbiturate administered 30–45 minutes before instrumentation allays apprehension. As an alternative measure, morphine, 8 mg, or a similar narcotic can be given intravenously 5–10 minutes before the instrument is inserted. Intravenous injection of a tranquilizing drug such as diazepam (Valium Injectable) is also effective. Inject it slowly, and stop when the patient exhibits drowsiness.

Local anesthesia is indicated before instrumentation, although this is less effective in men than in women. The female urethra is best anesthetized by introducing a solution of 10% cocaine on a cotton applicator and leaving it in the canal for 5 minutes. With this technic, instrumentation is almost without discomfort. In men, really effective anesthetic agents (ie, cocaine) cannot be instilled, for they are easily absorbed through the posterior urethra and prostate into the circulatory system and may cause sudden collapse and even death. Less toxic drugs must therefore be used, and these are usually less effective. They may be incorporated into the lubricating jelly. These solutions or jellies are retained in the urethra by placing a clamp on the glans for 5 minutes. Useful anesthetic agents include 2% lidocaine (Xylocaine) and 0.5% dyclonine (Dyclone).

General anesthesia should be used if the patient is apprehensive or if biopsy or other painful manipulations are necessary. Thiopental is ideal for short cystoscopic procedures, but spinal anesthesia may prove more useful if x-rays are to be taken, since patients can be asked to cooperate by holding their breath at the proper time. Explosive agents (eg, ether) are contraindicated if electrocoagulation is to be employed.

Warning to Patient

Instrumentation is always uncomfortable and may be painful. It is essential to warn all patients that this discomfort will occur and to warn men that the discomfort will be greater as the instrument passes through the prostatic urethra. No movement should be rough or abrupt; pick up the instrument slowly, introduce it gently, and advance it gradually. Failure to do these things will cause distrust and apprehension on the part of the patient. Spasm of the external sphincter may develop, in which case instrumentation is made more difficult or even impossible.

Calibration & Size of Instruments

Instruments are most commonly calibrated in the USA according to the French (F) scale. Each number on the scale equals 0.33 mm. Therefore, a 30F sound has a diameter of 10 mm.

Each number on the American (A) and English (E) scales equals 0.5 mm; the English scale is 2 numbers less than the American. Hence, 10 mm = 30F = 20A = 18E; and 6 mm = 18F = 12A = 10E.

THE CATHETER

Catheters are used for diagnostic purposes to explore the urethra for stenoses or injury, to discover residual urine in the bladder after voiding, and to introduce contrast medium into the bladder. They are used therapeutically to relieve urinary retention.

Types & Sizes of Catheters (Fig 9–1)

Soft rubber catheters should be used in most instances since they cause less trauma and are easier to manipulate past enlarged prostatic lobes than less flexible instruments. If for any reason a soft rubber catheter fails to pass (eg, it may impinge on the base of a lobe which occupies most of the posterior part of the bladder neck), a stiffer silk-woven coudé (elbow) catheter (which has a bent tip) should be tried. If the catheter is to be left in place (indwelling), a self-retaining (balloon) catheter should be utilized. It may be necessary or advantageous to leave a plain catheter (Robinson) in the bladder; it must then be taped in place (Fig 9–3).

In general, it is a mistake to try to pass small catheters in men (12–14F); they lack body and are apt to coil up at the external sphincter. Catheterization is really less traumatic and more successful if instruments of adequate size (20–22F) are used. The larger catheters are also better suited for exploring the urethra for stricture. The urethra of a girl age 6 will easily accept a 14F catheter. The urethra of a boy of the same age will take a 12F catheter.

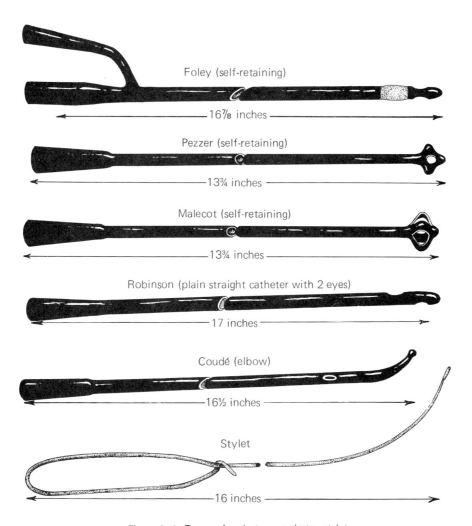

Foley (self-retaining)

16⅞ inches

Pezzer (self-retaining)

13¾ inches

Malecot (self-retaining)

13¾ inches

Robinson (plain straight catheter with 2 eyes)

17 inches

Coudé (elbow)

16½ inches

Stylet

16 inches

Figure 9–1. Types of catheters; catheter stylet.

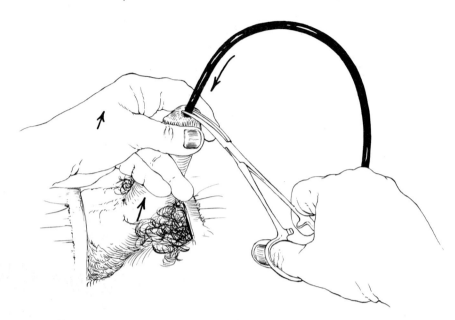

Figure 9–2. Technic of catheterization. A sterile water-soluble lubricant is first instilled into the urethra by means of a bulb syringe. The penis is drawn taut with one hand. The catheter, held near its tip with a sterile clamp, is introduced into the urethra; the other end of the catheter is held between the fourth and fifth fingers of the hand holding the clamp. The clamp is then moved up on the catheter and the catheter introduced farther into the urethra.

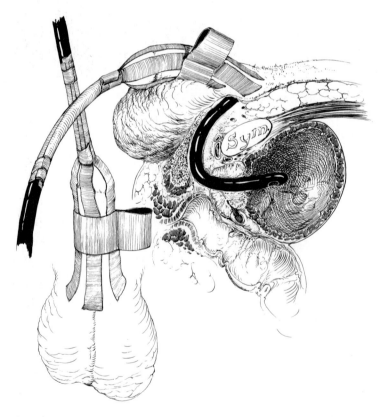

Figure 9–3. Taping the plain catheter in place in the male. Four strips of half-inch adhesive tape are placed on the penis and catheter. They are bound to the catheter by 2 pieces of half-inch tape just distal to the glans and at the point where they terminate on the catheter. A piece of 1-inch tape is placed about the mid penis in such a manner that a loop is formed which will separate if erection occurs.

Technic of Catheterization

A. In Men: After proper cleansing and anesthesia, the catheter can be manipulated with a sterile-gloved hand. It is simpler, however, to grasp the catheter near its tip with a sterile clamp and to hold the other end of the catheter between the fourth and fifth fingers of the same hand. The catheter can then be advanced with the clamp without being touched by the unsterile hand (Fig 9–2). The penis must be stretched taut with the other hand to eliminate urethral redundancy.

If an impassable stricture is encountered, it will be necessary to dilate the urethra with sounds (Fig 9–4) or with filiforms and followers (Figs 9–5 and 9–6).

If a stylet is used (Fig 9–1), the lumen of the catheter should be lubricated before the stylet is inserted; otherwise the stylet will be difficult to remove after passage of the instrument. The technic of passing a catheter with a stylet is similar to that for passing sounds. The catheter should be drawn taut over the stylet so that its tip cannot become dislodged, pass out through the "eye" of the catheter, and traumatize the urethra.

Do not partially withdraw the styleted catheter and then readvance it. The resulting drag on the catheter may allow the tip of the stylet to protrude through the distal opening of the catheter and cause urethral injury. At times it is helpful to guide stiff instruments with a finger in the rectum. When the catheter has been successfully passed, the stylet is removed.

B. In Women: A short metal catheter is more satisfactory than other types, since it can be manipulated with one hand while the other holds the labia apart. Rubber catheters can also be used. Those made of glass are contraindicated; small cracks or chips may abrade the mucosa. A self-retaining (Foley) catheter can be used if constant drainage is indicated. A Pezzer or Malecot catheter introduced on a catheter stylet is also satisfactory. A plain catheter can be used for this purpose by taping it to the labial area (after shaving).

METAL SOUNDS

Metal (stainless steel or nickel-plated steel) sounds may be used instead of catheters to explore the urethra for stenoses. Their major use, however, is in the treatment of stricture.

Technic of Passing a Sound

A. In Men: With the penis stretched taut and the instrument held almost horizontally (over the groin), the tip of the sound is introduced into the urethra. When the tip reaches the bulb (at the external sphincter), the handle is brought to the vertical position, which usually enables the tip to pass through the sphincter. Moving the handle to the horizontal position (parallel to the thighs) causes the sound to advance into the bladder (Fig 9–4).

The first sound passed should be a 24F, even though the patient says he has a narrow stricture. This size has a broad tip that will not perforate a friable urethral wall and is therefore ideal for urethral exploration. If a 24F sound cannot be passed, smaller sounds can be tried. If a 20F will not pass, do not use the smaller sizes, for their tips are relatively sharp and may pierce the urethral wall. In this instance, use filiforms and followers, which are much safer (Figs 9–5 and 9–6).

B. In Women: Because of the short and relatively straight canal of the female urethra, the passage of sounds is quite simple in women. Significant stricture is rare, although moderate stenoses are commonly found and are often the cause of chronic or recurrent cystitis, particularly in little girls.

FILIFORMS & FOLLOWERS

Filiforms and followers are the instruments of choice for dilating narrow strictures. Catheterizing followers may be used to catheterize men with narrow strictures.

Types & Sizes

Filiforms are made of woven silk or plastic material and must be quite pliable. Useful sizes are 3–6F. Numerous filiform tips are available, but the coudé and corkscrew types are most useful. The free end of the filiform is equipped with a female thread.

The follower may be made of metal or of woven pliable silk. Useful sizes are 8–30F. It may be solid or it may be hollow to allow simultaneous catheterization. Its end has a male thread that may be easily screwed into the filiform.

Technic of Passing Filiforms

After lubricant jelly has been instilled into the urethra, the filiform is introduced. If it is arrested, it must be partially withdrawn, rotated, and readvanced. If this fails, one or more filiforms should be added and all manipulated in turn. When one finally passes down to its hilt without resistance, its tip has entered the bladder. The appropriate follower is then screwed into the filiform in a clockwise direction and advanced down the urethra (Figs 9–5 and 9–6).

BOUGIES A BOULE

These olive-tipped bougies (Fig 9–7) are useful in calibrating the urethra, particularly in little girls (see Chapter 30). Bougies of increasing size should be used until one passes with some resistance. On withdrawal, there will be a snap as the bougie's broad shoulders pass through the stenotic area.

Example of a sound

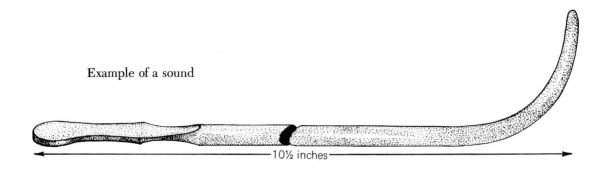

10½ inches

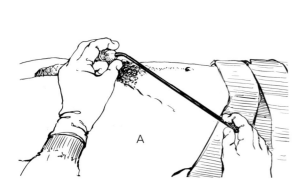

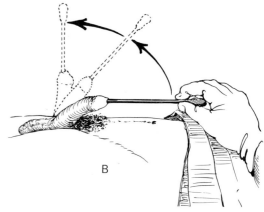

After proper urethral lubrication, the tip of the sound enters the urethra. The sound is in the horizontal position over the groin.

The penis is pulled taut on the sound, which is advanced down the urethra and moved simultaneously to the midline; its handle is gradually moved to the vertical position.

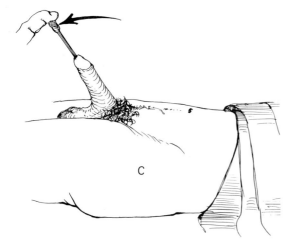

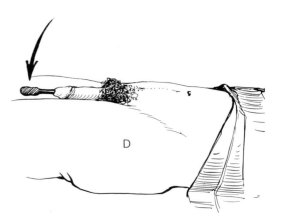

The sound will usually pass through the external urinary sphincter if pressure is exerted on the handle at right angles to its shaft with one finger.

When the sound has passed all the way into the bladder it should be possible to rotate it freely. (The curved part of the sound is lying free in the vesical cavity.)

Figure 9–4. Passing a sound through the male urethra.

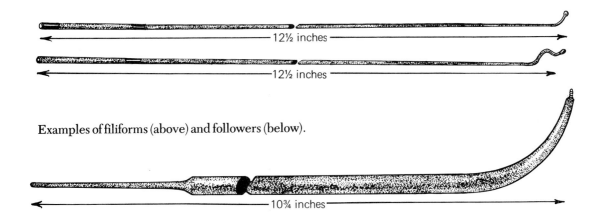

Examples of filiforms (above) and followers (below).

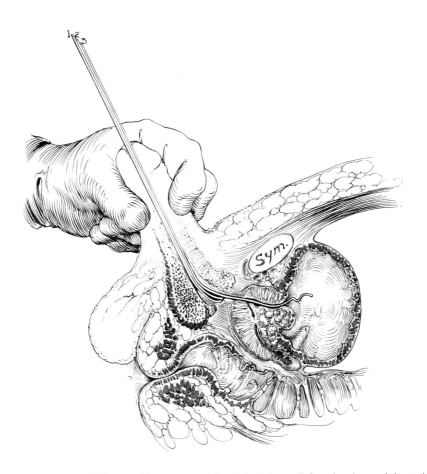

Figure 9–5. Technic of passage of filiforms. After proper urethral lubrication, a filiform is advanced down the urethra; the penis is held taut. If the filiform is arrested at any point, it is partially withdrawn, rotated, and advanced again. If it still fails to pass, 2 or more filiforms are inserted into the urethra. Each filiform in turn is advanced, withdrawn, rotated, and readvanced. One of them will usually pass to the bladder. (Passing of follower is shown in Fig 9–6.)

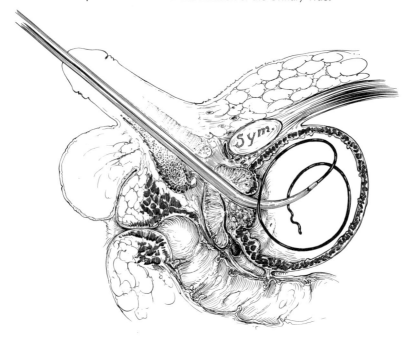

Figure 9–6. Passing the follower. When a filiform passes into the bladder, a small follower is screwed into the filiform and advanced to the bladder, using the same technic as for passage of a sound (Fig 9–5).

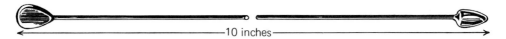

←——————————————10 inches——————————————→

Figure 9–7. Bougie à boule.

CYSTOMETER

The cystometer is a diagnostic instrument that measures the tone of the detrusor in relation to the volume of fluid in the bladder. It evaluates both normal and pathologic physiology of bladder function and contributes much to the management of the patient suffering from vesical dysfunction secondary to disease or trauma of the nervous system. A simple cystometer is illustrated in Fig 9–8.

Technic

The apparatus is so arranged that the zero mark on the manometer is level with the pubic symphysis. Care should be taken that all air is removed from the tubing. As sterile water or normal saline solution is slowly introduced (60–120 drops/min) into the indwelling catheter, the intravesical pressure is measured on the manometer. As each 50 mL is added, the pressure on the manometer is recorded in relation to the total volume of fluid introduced. The patient is asked to describe all sensations experienced, including the desire to void. These remarks are recorded at the appropriate points on the cystometrogram. When a strong involuntary urge to void occurs, this pressure should be noted.

CYSTOSCOPY & PANENDOSCOPY

Useful Instruments

Many instruments have been devised for the visual inspection of the bladder and urethra, but the 2 most useful are the cystoscope and the panendoscope. They come in sizes varying between 12 and 26F; therefore, even very young patients may be examined.

A. Cystoscope: The cystoscopic view is largely at right angles to the shaft of the instrument. It has a wide-angle lens and is therefore best for inspection of the bladder. It visualizes the prostatic urethra only fairly well and the distal (and female) urethra not at all.

B. Panendoscope: The panendoscope has a smaller field of vision; its view is almost in line with the shaft of the instrument. Therefore, the portion of the bladder near the bladder neck cannot be seen unless a "retrograde" lens is used with it. This instrument, however, is excellent for visualization of the urethra distal to the neck of the bladder. These instruments, then, complement each other.

Uses

A. Diagnostic Uses: Complete endoscopic studies are among the most precise diagnostic tests in all medicine.

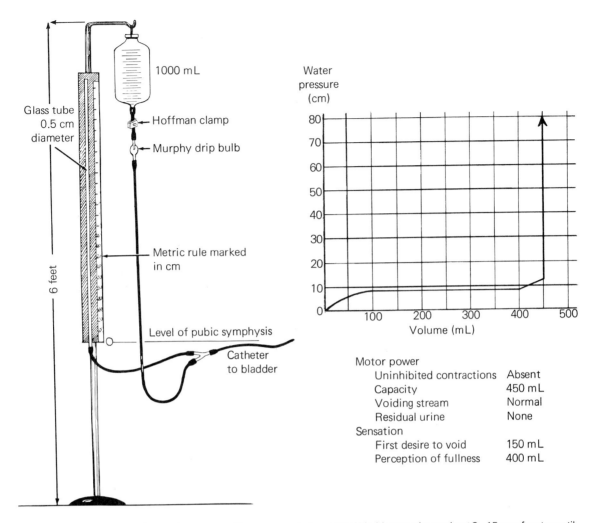

Figure 9–8. Cystometer and normal cystogram. The pressure in the normal bladder remains at about 8–15 cm of water until capacity (350–550 mL) is reached, at which time the intravesical pressure rises sharply to or above 100 cm of water. Involuntary voiding then occurs around the catheter. No uninhibited contractions occur, and there is no residual urine. A spastic neurogenic (neuropathic) bladder (Fig 19–3) exhibits uninhibited contractions, as demonstrated by transient increases in intravesical pressure as fluid is introduced into the bladder. In either case, involuntary voiding around the catheter occurs at relatively low volumes (50–300 mL). The tone of the flaccid neurogenic bladder (Fig 19–7) is impaired. Thus, intravesical pressure remains low (6–10 mL), there are no uninhibited contractions, and no final involuntary voiding pressure develops even when the bladder is filled with 500 or even 1000 mL of water; vesical capacity is increased.

1. Direct inspection–The cystoscope and panendoscope make possible visualization of the bladder wall for such diseases as tumor, stone, and ulcer. The configuration and position of the ureteral orifices are of paramount importance when vesicoureteral reflux is suspected. The degree of obstruction from an enlarged prostate and urethral stricture, polyp, or tumor may be seen. Biopsy of neoplasms can be made.

2. "Sterile" urine specimen, relative renal function–Through these instruments clean specimens of urine can be taken from the bladder for bacteriologic study. Catheters can be passed to the renal pelves for the collection of urine specimens and the separate measurement of renal function (PSP test).

3. Radiography–Through these ureteral catheters, radiopaque material can be introduced so that perfect "casts" of the calices, pelves, and ureters can be observed on x-ray films.

4. Reflux–The presence of vesicoureteral reflux can be ascertained by filling the bladder with sterile water to which indigo carmine or methylene blue dye has been added. After the patient voids, cystoscopy is performed. If blue fluid is seen emanating from a ureteral orifice, reflux has been demonstrated.

B. Therapeutic Uses: Many diseases of the

bladder and urethra lend themselves to transure-. thral treatment. Tumors can be biopsied and resected. Ureteral stones can be manipulated.

Major Indications for Cystoscopy or Panendoscopy & Ureteral Catheterization

These technics are indicated for the evaluation of hematuria, chronic or recurrent urinary infection, unexplained urologic symptoms (eg, enuresis, frequency), and evaluation of congenital anomalies, which are very commonly found in the genitourinary tract. They are useful also in any clinical situation in which excretory urograms have suggested pathologic change but have not furnished all the information necessary for definitive diagnosis and treatment.

Contraindications to Cystoscopy or Panendoscopy

Cystoscopy and panendoscopy are contraindicated in acute urinary tract infection (trauma may exacerbate the infection) and in the presence of severe symptoms of prostatic obstruction, since trauma may produce just enough edema of the bladder neck to cause complete urinary retention. Of course, if cystoscopy must be done, this risk must be taken.

RESECTOSCOPE & LITHOTRITE

Resectoscope

The resectoscope is a commonly used visual instrument with which transurethral resection of the prostate or of vesical carcinoma is performed.

Lithotrite

The lithotrite allows the urologist to crush smaller vesical calculi transurethrally.

REACTIONS TO INSTRUMENTATION

Urethra & Bladder (Sounds, Cystoscopy)

Some bleeding is to be expected in men. Burning on urination and frequency may be noted because of trauma to the mucous membrane. Acute urinary retention may develop in men suffering from moderate prostatism. This may be due to edema from the instrumentation. Exacerbation of lower tract infection may occur. Epididymitis may develop if prostatocystitis is present. "Urethral chill" (which is really due to bacteremia from an infected prostate traumatized by instrumentation or vesicoureteral reflux) may occur.

Ureters & Kidney (Ureteral Catheterization, Urography)

Nausea, vomiting, and abdominal cramps are often experienced from overdistention of the renal pelves with radiopaque material. Renal and ureteral pain and colic (from overdistention) or ureteral edema (from trauma) may ensue. Bleeding may occur if the tip of a catheter pierces the renal parenchyma. Exacerbation of kidney infection may develop, or new infection may be introduced. Temporary anuria is rare; it may be caused by excessive ureteral edema from instrumentation or sensitivity to the urographic medium.

●   ●   ●

References

Preliminary Procedures

Bodner H & others: Sodium methohexol amnesia for urethral instrumentation. *J Urol* 1973;**110**:208.

Getzoff PL: A safe and effective topical anesthetic for office cystoscopy. *J Urol* 1968;**99**:118.

Ulm AH, Wagshul EC: Pulmonary embolization with an oily medium. *N Engl J Med* 1960;**263**:137.

The Catheter

Desautels RE: The causes of catheter-induced urinary infections and their prevention. *J Urol* 1969;**101**:757.

Desautels RE: Managing the urinary catheter. *Geriatrics* (Sept) 1974;**29**:67.

Cystometer

Marshall S: A disposable cystometer. *J Urol* 1964;**91**:458.

Cystoscopy & Panendoscopy

Amar AD, Chabra K: Reduction of radiation exposure of children during urologic diagnosis including a nonradiographic method of demonstrating vesicoureteral reflux. *Pediatrics* 1965;**35**:960.

Urinary Obstruction & Stasis | 10

Emil A. Tanagho, MD

Because of their damaging effect on renal function, obstruction and stasis of urinary flow are among the most important of urologic disorders. Either leads eventually to hydronephrosis, a peculiar type of atrophy of the kidney that may terminate in renal insufficiency or, if unilateral, complete destruction of the organ. Furthermore, obstruction leads to infection, which causes additional damage to the organs involved.

Classification

Obstruction may be classified according to etiology (congenital or acquired), duration (acute or chronic), degree (partial or complete), and level (upper or lower urinary tract).

Etiology

Congenital anomalies, more common in the urinary tract than in any other organ system, are generally obstructive. In adult life, many types of acquired obstruction can occur.

A. Congenital: The common sites of congenital narrowing are the meatus in boys (meatal stenosis) or just inside the external urinary meatus in little girls; the posterior urethral valves; and the ureterovesical and ureteropelvic junctions. Another congenital cause of urinary stasis is damage to sacral roots 2–4 as seen in spina bifida and myelomeningocele (Fig 19–10). Vesicoureteral reflux causes both vesical and renal stasis (see Chapter 11).

B. Acquired: Acquired obstructions are numerous and may be primary in the urinary tract or secondary to retroperitoneal lesions that invade or compress the urinary passages. Among the common causes are (1) urethral stricture secondary to infection or injury; (2) benign prostatic hyperplasia or cancer of the prostate; (3) vesical tumor involving the bladder neck or one or both ureterovesical orifices; (4) local extension of cancer of the prostate or cervix into the base of the bladder, occluding the ureters; (5) compression of the ureters at the pelvic brim by metastatic nodes from malignancy of the prostate or cervix; (6) ureteral stone; (7) retroperitoneal fibrosis or malignancy; and (8) pregnancy.

Neurogenic dysfunction affects principally the bladder. The upper tracts are damaged secondarily by ureterovesical obstruction or reflux and, often, complicating infection. Severe constipation, especially in children, can cause bilateral hydroureteronephrosis from compression of the lower ureters.

Elongation and kinking of the ureter secondary to vesicoureteral reflux commonly lead to ureteropelvic obstruction and hydronephrosis. Unless a voiding cystourethrogram is obtained in all children having this lesion, the primary cause may be missed and improper treatment applied.

Pathogenesis & Pathology

Obstruction and neurovesical dysfunction have the same effects upon the urinary tract. These changes can best be understood by considering (1) the effects upon the lower tract (distal to the bladder neck) of severe external urinary meatal stricture and (2) the effects upon the mid tract (bladder) and upper tract (ureter and kidney) of benign prostatic hyperplasia.

A. Lower Tract: Hydrostatic pressure proximal to the obstruction causes dilatation of the urethra. The wall of the urethra may become thin, and a diverticulum may form. If the urine becomes infected, spontaneous urethral rupture with urinary extravasation may occur. The prostatic ducts may become widely dilated (Fig 29–4).

B. Mid Tract: In the earlier stages (compensatory phase), the muscle wall of the bladder becomes thickened. With decompensation, it may be thinned and, therefore, weakened.

1. Stage of compensation–In order to balance the increasing urethral resistance, the bladder musculature hypertrophies. Its thickness may double. Complete emptying of the bladder is thus made possible.

Little more than hypertrophied muscle may be seen microscopically, although the effects of infection are often superimposed. In case of secondary infection, there may be edema of the submucosa, which may be infiltrated with plasma cells, lymphocytes, and polymorphonuclear cells.

At cystoscopy, surgery, or autopsy, visual evidence of this compensation is demonstrated in the following ways (Fig 10–1).

a. Trabeculation of the bladder wall–The wall of the distended bladder is normally quite smooth. With hypertrophy, individual muscle bundles stand out taut and give a coarsely interwoven appearance to the mucosal surface. The trigonal muscle and the interureteric ridge, which normally are only slightly raised above the surrounding tissues, respond to obstruction by hypertrophy of their smooth musculature. The ridge then becomes a prominent structure. This trigonal hypertrophy causes increased resistance to urine flow in the intravesical ureteral segments owing to accentuated downward pull upon them. It is this mechanism that causes relative functional obstruction of the ureterovesical junctions, leading to back pressure on the kidney and hydroureteronephrosis. In the presence of significant residual urine, which further stretches the ureterotrigonal complex, this obstruction increases. (A urethral catheter will relieve it somewhat by eliminating the trigonal stretch. Definitive prostatectomy leads to permanent release of stretch and gradual softening of trigonal hypertrophy with relief of the obstruction.)

b. Cellules–Normal intravesical pressure is about 30 cm of water at the beginning of micturition. Pressures 2–4 times as great may be reached by the trabeculated (hypertrophied) bladder in its attempt to force urine past the obstruction. This pressure tends to push mucosa between the superficial muscle bundles, causing the formation of small pockets, or cellules (Fig 10–1).

c. Diverticula–If cellules force their way en-

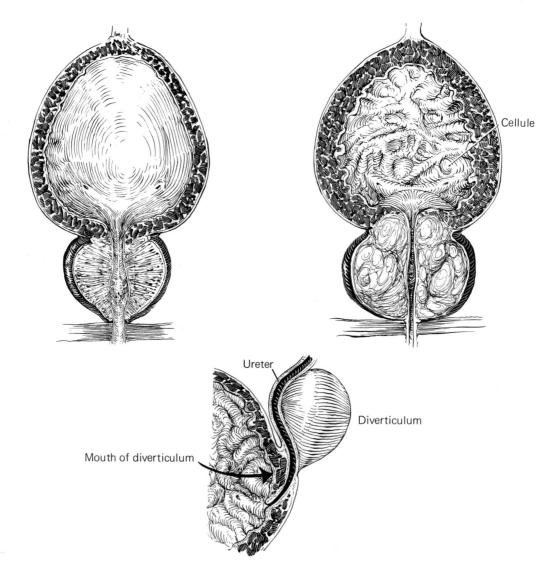

Figure 10–1. Changes in the bladder developing from obstruction. *Above left:* Normal bladder and prostate. *Above right:* Obstructing prostate causing trabeculation, cellule formation, and hypertrophy of the interureteric ridge. *Below:* Marked trabeculation (hypertrophy) of the vesical musculature; diverticulum displacing left ureter.

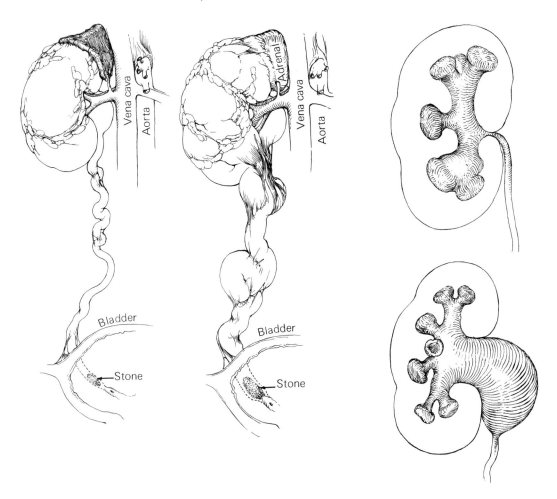

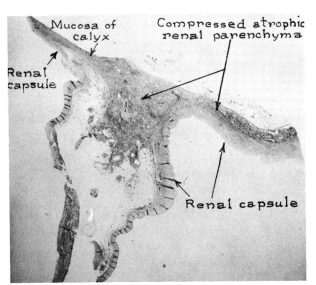

Figure 10–2. Mechanisms and results of obstruction. *Above left:* Early stage. Elongation and dilatation of ureter due to mild obstruction. *Above center:* Later stage. Further dilatation and elongation with kinking of the ureter; fibrous bands cause further kinking. *Below left:* Photomicrograph of advanced hydronephrosis. Thin layer of renal parenchyma covered by fibrous capsule. *Above right:* Intrarenal pelvis. Obstruction transmits all back pressure to parenchyma. *Below right:* Extrarenal pelvis, when obstructed, allows some of the increased pressure to be dissipated by the pelvis.

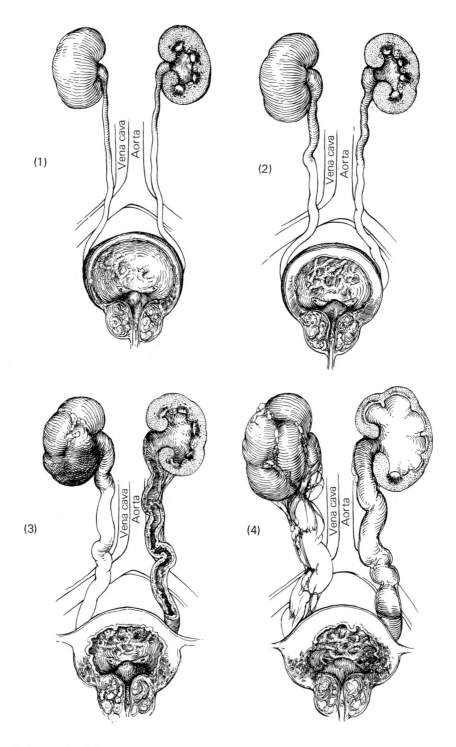

Figure 10–3. Pathogenesis of bilateral hydronephrosis. Progressive changes in bladder, ureters, and kidneys from obstruction of an enlarged prostate: thickening of bladder wall, dilatation and elongation of ureters, and hydronephrosis.

tirely through the musculature of the bladder wall, they become saccules, then actual diverticula, which may be embedded in perivesical fat or covered by peritoneum, depending upon their location. They have no muscle wall and are therefore unable to expel their contents into the bladder efficiently even after the primary obstruction has been removed. When this occurs, secondary infection is difficult to eradicate, and surgical removal of the diverticula may be required. If a diverticulum pushes through the bladder wall on the anterior surface of the ureter, the ureterovesical junction will become incompetent. (See Chapter 11.)

d. Mucosa–In the presence of acute infection, the mucosa may be reddened and edematous. This may lead to temporary vesicoureteral reflux in the presence of a "borderline" junction. The chronically inflamed membrane may be thinned and pale. In the absence of infection, the mucosa appears normal.

2. Stage of decompensation–The compensatory power of the bladder musculature varies greatly. One patient with prostatic enlargement may have only mild symptoms of prostatism but a large obstructing gland that can be palpated rectally and observed cystoscopically; another may suffer acute retention and yet have a gland of normal size on rectal palpation and what appears to be only a mild obstruction cystoscopically.

In the face of progressive urethral obstruction, possibly aggravated by prostatic infection with edema or by congestion from lack of intercourse, decompensation of the detrusor may occur, resulting in the presence of residual urine after voiding. The amount may range up to 500 mL or more.

C. Upper Tract:

1. Ureter–In the early stages of obstruction, intravesical pressure during the filling phase of the bladder is normal. It is only during the act of voiding that this pressure is increased. It is not transmitted to the ureters and renal pelves because of the competence of the ureterovesical "valves." (A true valve is not present; the ureterotrigonal unit, by virtue of its intrinsic structure, resists the retrograde flow of urine.) However, owing to the trigonal hypertrophy discussed earlier and to the resultant increase in resistance to urine flow across the terminal ureter, there is progressive back pressure on the kidney, resulting in ureteral dilatation and hydronephrosis. Later, with the phase of decompensation accompanied by residual urine, there is an added stretch effect on the already hypertrophied trigone that increases appreciably the resistance to flow at the lower end of the ureter and induces further hydroureteronephrosis. With decompensation of the ureterotrigonal complex, the valvelike action may be lost, vesicoureteral reflux occurs, and the increased intravesical pressure is then transmitted to the renal pelves.

Secondary to the back pressure from reflux or obstruction from the hypertrophied and stretched

trigone or a ureteral stone, the ureteral musculature thickens in its attempt to push the urine downward by increased peristaltic activity (stage of compensation). This causes elongation and some tortuosity of the ureter (Fig 10–2). At times this change becomes marked; bands of fibrous tissue develop that on contraction further angulate the ureter so that secondary ureteral stenosis develops. Under these circumstances, removal of the obstruction below may not prevent the kidney from undergoing complete destruction from the acquired ureteral obstruction.

Finally, because of increasing pressure, the ureteral wall becomes attenuated and therefore loses all of its contractile power (stage of decompensation). Dilatation may be so extreme that the ureter resembles a loop of bowel (Figs 10–3 and 11–8, top right).

2. Kidney–The pressure within the renal pelvis is normally close to zero. When this pressure increases because of obstruction or reflux, the pelvis and calices dilate. The degree of hydronephrosis that develops depends upon the duration, degree, and site of the obstruction (Fig 10–4). The higher the obstruction, the greater the effect upon the kidney. If the renal pelvis is entirely intrarenal and the obstruction is at the ureteropelvic junction, all the pressure will be exerted upon the parenchyma. If the renal pelvis is extrarenal, a ureteropelvic stenosis will exert only part of the resulting pressure on the parenchyma. The pelvis, being embedded in fat, dilates more readily, thus "decompressing" the calices (Fig 10–2).

In the earlier stages, the pelvic musculature undergoes compensatory hypertrophy in its effort to force urine past the obstruction. Later, however, the muscle becomes stretched and atonic (and decompensated).

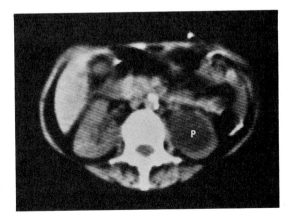

Figure 10–4. Hydronephrotic left renal pelvis. Low density mass (P) in left renal sinus had attenuation value similar to that of water, suggesting the correct diagnosis. Unless intravenous contrast material is used, differentiation from peripelvic cyst may be difficult.

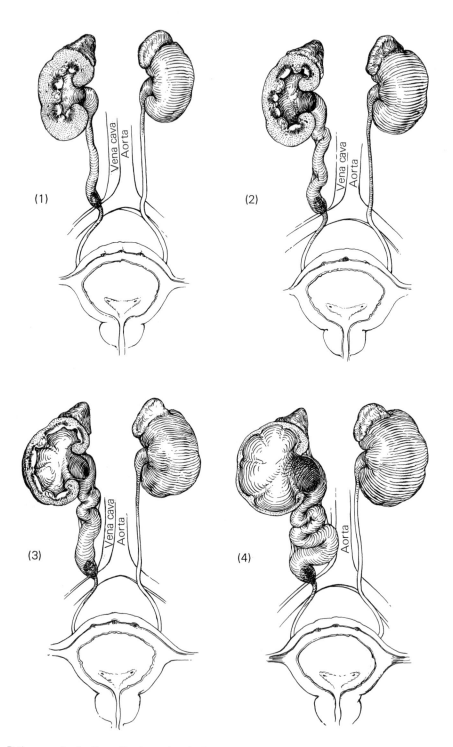

Figure 10–5. Pathogenesis of unilateral hydronephrosis. Progressive changes in ureter and kidney secondary to obstructing calculus. As the right kidney undergoes gradual destruction, the left kidney gradually enlarges (compensatory hypertrophy).

The progression of hydronephrotic atrophy is as follows:

(1) The earliest changes in the development of hydronephrosis are seen in the calices. The end of a normal calix (as seen on a urogram, Fig 6–6) is concave because of the calix that projects into it; with increase in intrapelvic pressure, the fornices become blunt and rounded. With persistence of increased intrapelvic pressure, the papilla becomes flattened, then convex (clubbed) as a result of compression, enhanced by ischemic obstruction. The parenchyma between the calices is affected to a lesser extent. The changes in the renal parenchyma are due to (1) compression atrophy from increase in intrapelvic pressure (more accentuated with intrarenal pelves) and (2) ischemic atrophy from hemodynamic changes, mainly manifested in arcuate vessels running at the base of the pyramids parallel to the kidney outline which become more vulnerable to compression between the renal capsule and the centrally increasing intrapelvic pressure.

This spotty atrophy is caused by the nature of the blood supply of the kidney. The arterioles are "end arteries"; therefore, ischemia is most marked in the areas farthest from the interlobular arteries. As the back pressure increases, hydronephrosis progresses, with the cells nearest the main arteries exhibiting the greatest resistance.

This increased pressure is transmitted up the tubules. The tubules become dilated, and their cells atrophy from ischemia.

(2) Only in unilateral hydronephrosis are the advanced stages of hydronephrotic atrophy seen. Eventually the kidney is completely destroyed and appears as a thin-walled sac filled with clear fluid (water and electrolytes) or pus (Fig 10–5).

If obstruction is unilateral, the increased intrarenal pressure will cause some suppression of renal function on that side. The closer the intrapelvic pressure approaches the glomerular filtration pressure (6–12 mm Hg), the less urine can be secreted. Glomerular filtration rate and renal plasma flow are reduced. Concentrating power is gradually lost. The urine urea:creatinine concentration ratio is low when compared to that of the normal kidney.

Hydronephrotic atrophy is an unusual type of pathologic change. Other secretory organs (eg, the submaxillary gland) cease secreting when their ducts are obstructed. This causes primary (disuse) atrophy. The completely obstructed kidney, however, continues to secrete urine. (If this were not so, hydronephrosis could not occur, since it depends upon increased intrarenal pressure.) As urine is excreted into the renal pelvis, fluid and, particularly, soluble substances are reabsorbed, through either the tubules or the lymphatics. This has been demonstrated by injecting PSP into the obstructed renal pelvis. It disappears (is reabsorbed) in a few hours and is excreted by the other kidney. With an increase in intrapelvic pressure that rapidly approaches filtration pressure, there is a safety mechanism that permits a break in the surface lining of the collecting structure at the weakest point—the fornices. This leads to escape and extravasation of urine from the pelvis into the parenchymal interstitium (pyelointerstitial backflow). This extravasated fluid will be absorbed by the renal lymphatics but will allow a drop in pressure in the renal pelvis, with further concomitant filtration of urine. This is why the fluid in the renal pelvis is constantly changing by reabsorption followed by secretion. Other evidence is the fact that the markedly hydronephrotic kidney does not contain urine in the true sense; only water and a few salts are present.

Functional impairment in unilateral hydronephrosis, as measured by PSP or excretory urograms, will be greater and will increase faster than that seen in bilateral hydronephrotic kidneys showing comparable damage on urography. As unilateral hydronephrosis progresses, the normal kidney undergoes compensatory hypertrophy of its nephrons (renal counterbalance), thereby assuming the function of the diseased kidney in order to maintain normal total renal function. For this reason, successful anatomic repair of the ureteral obstruction of such a kidney may fail to improve its powers of waste elimination.

If both kidneys are equally hydronephrotic, a strong stimulus is continually being exerted on both to maintain maximum function. This is also true of a solitary hydronephrotic kidney. Consequently, the return of function in these kidneys after repair of their obstructions is at times remarkable.

Physiologic Explanation of Symptoms of Bladder Neck Obstruction

The following hypothesis has been brought forward to explain the syndrome known as "prostatism," which occurs with progressive vesical obstruction.

The bladder, like the heart, is a hollow muscular organ that receives fluid and forcefully expels it. And, like the heart, it reacts to an increasing work load by going through the successive phases of compensation and finally decompensation.

Normally, contraction of the detrusor muscle and the trigone pulls the bladder neck open and forms a funnel through which the urine is expelled. The intravesical pressure generated in this instance varies between 20 and 40 cm of water; this force further widens the bladder neck.

With bladder neck obstruction, hypertrophy of the vesical musculature develops, allowing intravesical pressure to rise to 50–100 cm or more of water in order to overcome the increased outlet resistance. Despite this, the encroaching prostate appears to interfere with the mechanisms that ordinarily open the internal orifice. Also, the contraction phase may not last long enough for all of the urine to be expelled; "exhaustion" of the muscle occurs prematurely. The refractory phase then sets in, and the detrusor is temporarily unable to respond to further stimuli. A few minutes later, voiding may be initiated again and completed.

A. Compensation Phase:

1. Stage of irritability–In the earliest stages of obstruction of the bladder neck, the vesical musculature begins to hypertrophy. The force and size of the urinary stream remain normal because the balance is maintained between the expelling power of the bladder and urethral resistance. During this phase, however, the bladder appears to be hypersensitive. As the bladder is distended, the need to void is felt. In the individual with a normal bladder these early urges can be inhibited, and the bladder relaxes and distends to receive more urine. However, in the patient with hypertrophied detrusor, the contraction of the detrusor is so strong that it virtually goes into spasm, producing the symptoms of an irritable bladder. The earliest symptoms of bladder neck obstruction, therefore, are urgency (even to the point of incontinence) and frequency, both day and night.

2. Stage of compensation–As the obstruction increases, further hypertrophy of the muscle fibers of the bladder occurs, and the power to empty the bladder completely is thereby maintained. During this period, in addition to urgency and frequency, the patient notices hesitancy in initiating urination while the bladder develops contractions strong enough to overcome resistance at the bladder neck. The obstruction causes some loss in the force and size of the urinary stream, and the stream becomes slower as vesical emptying nears completion (exhaustion of the detrusor as it nears the end of the contraction phase).

B. Decompensation Phase: If vesical tone becomes impaired or if urethral resistance exceeds detrusor power, some degree of decompensation (imbalance) occurs. The contraction phase of the vesical muscle becomes too short to completely expel the contents of the bladder, and residual urine is the result.

1. Acute decompensation–The tone of the compensated vesical muscle can be temporarily embarrassed by rapid filling of the bladder (high fluid intake) or by overstretching of the detrusor (postponement of urination though the urge is felt). This may cause increased difficulty of urination, with marked hesitancy and the need for straining to initiate urination; a very weak and small stream; and termination of the stream before the bladder completely empties (residual urine). Acute and sudden complete urinary retention may also occur.

2. Chronic decompensation–As the degree of obstruction increases, a progressive imbalance between the power of the bladder musculature and urethral resistance develops. Therefore, it becomes increasingly more difficult to expel all the urine during the contraction phase of the detrusor. The symptoms of obstruction become more marked. This residuum gradually increases, thus diminish-

ing the functional capacity of the bladder. Progressive frequency of urination is noted. On occasion, as the bladder decompensates, it becomes overstretched and attenuated. It may contain 1000–3000 mL of urine. It loses its power of contraction, and overflow (paradoxic) incontinence results.

Clinical Findings

A. Symptoms:

1. Lower and mid tract (urethra and bladder)–Symptoms of obstruction of the lower and mid tract are typified by the symptoms of urethral stricture, benign prostatic hyperplasia, neurogenic bladder, and tumor of the bladder involving the vesical neck. The principal symptoms are hesitancy in starting urination, lessened force and size of the stream, and terminal dribbling; hematuria, which may be initial with stricture and total with prostatic obstruction or vesical tumor; and burning on urination, cloudy urine (complicating infection), and acute urinary retention.

2. Upper tract (ureter and kidney)–Symptoms of obstruction of the upper tract are typified by the symptoms of congenital ureteral stenosis or ureteral or renal stone. The principal complaints are pain in the flank radiating along the course of the ureter, gross total hematuria (from stone), gastrointestinal symptoms, chills, fever, burning on urination, and cloudy urine with onset of infection, which is the common sequel to obstruction or vesicoureteral reflux. Nausea, vomiting, loss of weight and strength, and pallor are due to uremia secondary to bilateral hydronephrosis.

Obstruction of the upper tract may be silent even when uremia supervenes.

B. Signs:

1. Lower and mid tract–Palpation of the urethra may reveal induration about a stricture. Rectal examination may show atony of the anal sphincter (damage to the sacral nerve roots) or benign or malignant enlargement of the prostate. Vesical distention may be found.

Although observation of the force and caliber of the urinary stream affords a rough estimate of maximum flow rate, the rate can be measured accurately with a urine flowmeter or, even more simply, by the following technic: Have the patient begin to void. When observed maximum flow has been reached, interpose a container to collect the urine, and simultaneously start a stopwatch. After exactly 5 seconds, remove the container. The flow rate in milliliters per second can easily be calculated. The normal urine flow rate is 20–25 mL/s in males and 25–30 mL/s in females. Any flow rate under 15 mL/s is to be regarded with suspicion. A flow rate under 10 mL/s is indicative of obstruction or of weak detrusor function. Flow rates associated with an atonic neurogenic (neuropathic) bladder (diminished detrusor power), urethral stricture, or prostatic obstruction (increased urethral resistance) may be as low as 3–5 mL/s. A cystometrogram will differentiate between these 2 causes of impaired flow rate. After definitive treatment of the cause, flow rate should return to normal.

In the presence of a vesical diverticulum or vesicoureteral reflux, although detrusor power is normal, the urinary stream may be impaired because of the diffusion of intravesical pressure into the diverticulum and vesicoureteral junctions as well as the urethra. Excision of the diverticulum or repair of the vesicoureteral junctions leads to efficient expulsion of urine via the urethra.

2. Upper tract–An enlarged kidney may be discovered by palpation or percussion. Renal tenderness may be elicited if infection has supervened. Cancer of the cervix may be noted; it may invade the base of the bladder and occlude one or both ureteral orifices, or its metastases to the iliac lymph nodes may compress the ureters. A large pelvic mass (tumor, pregnancy) can displace and compress the ureters. Children with advanced urinary tract obstruction (usually due to posterior urethral valves) may develop ascites. Rupture of the renal fornices allows leakage of urine, which passes into the peritoneal cavity through a tear in the peritoneum.

C. Laboratory Findings: Anemia may be found secondary to chronic infection or in advanced bilateral hydronephrosis (stage of uremia). Leukocytosis is to be expected in the acute stage of infection. Little if any elevation of the white blood count accompanies the chronic stage.

Large amounts of protein are usually not found in the obstructive uropathies. Casts are not common from hydronephrotic kidneys. Microscopic hematuria may indicate renal or vesical infection, tumor, or stone. Pus cells and bacteria may or may not be present.

In the presence of unilateral hydronephrosis, the PSP test will be normal because of the contralateral renal hypertrophy. Suppression of the PSP indicates bilateral renal damage, residual urine (vesical or bilateral ureterorenal), or vesicoureteral reflux.

In the presence of significant bilateral hydronephrosis, urine flow through the renal tubules is slowed. Thus, urea is significantly reabsorbed but creatinine is not. Blood chemistry therefore reveals a urea:creatinine ratio well above the normal 10:1 relationship.

D. X-Ray Findings: (Fig 10–6.) A plain film of the abdomen may show enlargement of renal shadows, calcific bodies suggesting ureteral or renal stone, or metastases to the bones of the spine or pelvis. If metastases are present in the spine, they may be the cause of spinal cord damage (neuropathic bladder); if osteoblastic, cancer of the prostate is almost certainly the cause.

Excretory urograms will reveal almost the entire story unless renal function is severely impaired. They are more informative when obstruction is present because the opaque material is retained.

These urograms will demonstrate the degree of dilatation of the pelves, calices, and ureters. The point of ureteral stenosis will be revealed. Segmental dilatation of the lower end of a ureter implies the possibility of vesicoureteral reflux (Fig 11–7), which can be revealed by cystography. The accompanying cystogram may show trabeculation as an irregularity of the vesical outline and may show diverticula. Vesical tumors, nonopaque stones, and large intravesical prostatic lobes may cause radiolucent shadows. A film taken immediately after voiding will show residual urine. Few tests that are as simple and inexpensive give the physician so much information.

Retrograde cystography shows changes of the bladder wall caused by distal obstruction (trabeculation, diverticula) or demonstrates the obstructive lesion itself (enlarged prostate, posterior urethral valves, vesical neoplasm). If the ureterovesical valves are incompetent, ureteropyelograms will be obtained by reflux (Fig 6–8).

Retrograde urograms may show better detail than the excretory type, but care must be taken not to overdistend the passages with too much opaque fluid; small hydronephroses can be made to look quite large. The degree of ureteral or ureterovesical obstruction can be judged by the degree of delay of drainage of the radiopaque fluid instilled.

Computerized tomography scanning and sonography can also help determine the extent of dilatation and of parenchymal atrophy.

E. Isotope Scanning: In the presence of obstruction, the radioisotope renogram may show depression of both the vascular and secretory phases and a rising rather than a falling excretory phase due to retention of the radiopaque urine in the renal pelvis.

The ^{131}I activity recorded on the gamma camera will reveal poor uptake of the isotope, slow transport of the isotope through the parenchyma, and accumulation of scintillations in the renal pelvis. (See Chapter 8.)

F. Instrumental Examination: Exploration of the urethra with a catheter or other instrument is a valuable diagnostic measure. Passage may be blocked by a stricture or tumor. External sphincter spasm may make passage difficult. Passage of the catheter immediately after voiding allows estimation of the amount of residual urine in the bladder. Residual urine is common in bladder neck obstruction (enlarged prostate), cystocele, and neurogenic (neuropathic) bladder. Even though the urinary stream may be markedly impaired with urethral stricture, residual urine is usually absent.

Measurement of vesical tone by means of cystometry is helpful in diagnosing the neurogenic bladder and in differentiating between bladder neck obstruction and vesical atony.

Inspection of the urethra and bladder by means of cystoscopy and panendoscopy may reveal the primary obstructive agent. Catheters may be

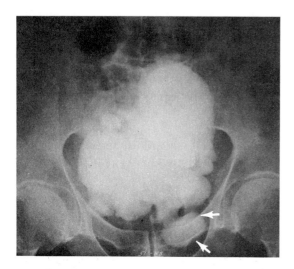

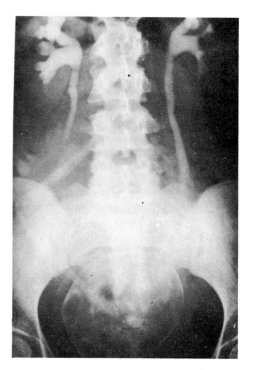

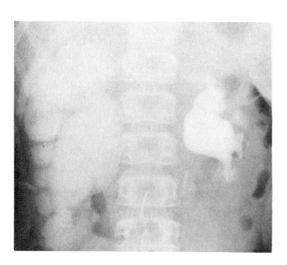

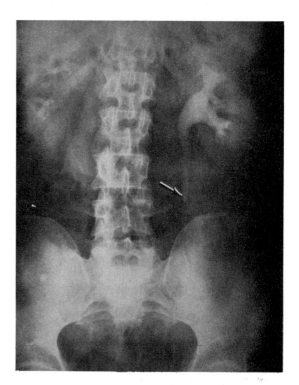

Figure 10–6. Changes in bladder, ureters, and kidneys caused by obstruction. *Above left:* Cystogram showing benign prostatic enlargement and multiple diverticula. Arrows point to femoral hernia that probably developed as a result of straining to urinate. *Above right:* Pregnancy. Significant dilatation and elongation of upper right ureter due to compression at the pelvic line. Left side normal. *Below left:* Excretory urogram, 70 minutes after injection. Advanced right hydronephrosis secondary to ureteropelvic obstruction. Mild ureteropelvic obstruction on left. *Below right:* Stone in right ureter (see arrow) with mild hydronephrosis.

passed to the renal pelves and urine specimens obtained. Measurement of the function of each kidney may be done (PSP test), and retrograde ureteropyelograms can be made.

Differential Diagnosis

A thorough examination usually leaves no doubt about the diagnosis. The differential diagnosis under these circumstances is rarely difficult. If seemingly simple infection does not respond to medical therapy, or if infection recurs, obstruction or vesicoureteral reflux is the probable cause, and complete study of the urinary tract is indicated.

Complications

Stagnation of urine leads to infection, which then may spread throughout the entire urinary system. Once established, infection is difficult and at times impossible to eradicate even after the obstruction has been relieved.

Often the invading organisms are ureasplitting (proteus, staphylococci). This causes the urine to become alkaline, in which case calcium salts precipitate and form bladder or kidney stones more easily.

If both kidneys are affected, the result may be renal insufficiency. Secondary infection increases renal damage.

Pyonephrosis is the end stage of a severely infected and obstructed kidney. The kidney is functionless and is filled with thick pus. At times, a plain film of the abdomen may show an air urogram caused by gas liberated by infecting organisms.

Treatment

A. Relief of Obstruction: Treatment of the main causes of obstruction and stasis is described in detail elsewhere: benign prostatic hyperplasia, cancer of the prostate, neurogenic bladder, ureteral stone, posterior urethral valves, and ureteral stenosis.

1. Lower tract obstruction (distal to the bladder)–With patients in whom secondary renal or ureterovesical damage (reflux in the latter) is minimal or nonexistent, correction of the obstruction is sufficient. If significant reflux is demonstrated and does not subside spontaneously after relief of obstruction, surgical repair might be needed. Repair becomes imperative if there is considerable hydronephrosis in addition to reflux. Preliminary drainage of the bladder by indwelling catheter or other means of diversion (eg, loop ureterostomy) is indicated in order to preserve and improve renal function. If, after a few months of drainage, reflux persists, surgical repair of the incompetent intravesical portion of the ureter should be done.

2. Upper tract obstruction (above the bladder)–If tortuous, kinked, dilated, or atonic ureters have developed secondary to lower tract obstruction (so that they are themselves obstructive), vesical drainage will not protect the kidneys from further damage; the urine proximal to the obstruction must be diverted by nephrostomy or ureterostomy. The kidneys then may regain some function. Over a period of many months, the ureter may become less tortuous and less dilated; its obstructive areas may open up. If radiopaque material instilled into the nephrostomy tube passes readily to the bladder, it may be possible to remove the nephrostomy tube. If obstruction or reflux persists, surgical repair is indicated. Permanent urinary diversion (eg, ureteroileal conduit) may be necessary.

If one kidney has been badly damaged, as measured by tests of function and urography, nephrectomy may be necessary.

B. Eradication of Infection: Once the obstruction is removed, every effort should be made to eradicate infection. If it has been severe and prolonged, antibiotics may fail to sterilize the urinary tract.

Prognosis

No simple statement can be made about the prognosis in this group of patients. The outcome depends upon the cause, site, degree, and duration of the obstruction. The prognosis is also definitely influenced by complicating infection, particularly if it has been present for a long time.

If renal function is fair to good, if the obstruction or other causes for stasis can be corrected, and if complicating infection can then be eradicated, the prognosis is generally excellent.

•   •   •

References

Aaronsen IA: Compensated obstruction of the renal pelvis. *Br J Urol* 1980;**52**:79.

Almgård LE, Fernström I: Percutaneous nephropyelostomy. *Acta Radiol [Diagn] (Stockh)* 1974;**15**:288.

Alton DJ, McDonald P: Urinary obstruction in the neonatal infant. *Radiol Clin North Am* 1975;**13**:343.

Aron B, Tessler A, Morales P: Angiography in hydronephrosis. *Urology* 1973;**2**:231.

Barbaric ZL & others: Percutaneous nephropyelostomy in the management of acute pyohydronephrosis. *Radiology* 1976;**118**:567.

Belman AB, King LR: Vesicostomy: Useful means of reversible urinary diversion in selected infants. *Urology* 1973;**1**:208.

Berdon WE & others: Hydronephrosis in infants and children: Value of high dosage excretory urography in predicting renal salvageability. *Am J Roentgenol* 1970;**109**:380.

Bergstrom H: The diagnostic value of renography in suspected obstruction of the urinary tract during pregnancy. *Acta Obstet Gynecol Scand* 1975;**54**:65.

Borden TA, Gill WB, Lyon ES: Further experience with circle tube nephroureterostomy urinary diversion. *Surg Gynecol Obstet* 1975;**140**:547.

Bourne RB: Intermittent hydronephrosis as a cause of abdominal pain. *JAMA* 1966;**198**:1218.

Bredin HC & others: The surgical correction of congenital ureteropelvic junction obstructions in normally rotated kidneys. *J Urol* 1974;**111**:460.

Bryan PJ, Azimi F: Ultrasound in diagnosis of congenital hydronephrosis due to obstruction of pelviureteric junction. *Urology* 1975;**5**:17.

Cohen B & others: Ureteropelvic junction obstruction: Its occurrence in 3 members of a single family. *J Urol* 1980;**120**:361.

Cremin BJ: Urinary ascites and obstructive uropathy. *Br J Urol* 1975;**48**:113.

Devine CJ Jr, Devine PC: Urethral strictures. (Editorial.) *J Urol* 1980;**123**:506.

Edelmann CM Jr, Spitzer A: The maturing kidney: A modern view of well-balanced infants with imbalanced nephrons. *J Pediatr* 1969;**75**:509.

Emmott RC, Tanagho EA: Ureteral obstruction due to fecal impaction in patient with colonic loop urinary diversion. *Urology* 1980;**15**:496.

Engel RME: Permanent urinary diversion in childhood: Indications and types. *Urology* 1974;**3**:178.

Fanestil DD, Blackard CE: Etiology of postobstructive diuresis: Ouabain-sensitive adenosine triphosphate deficit and elevated solute excretion in the postobstructed dog kidney. *Invest Urol* 1976;**14**:148.

Fayad MM & others: The ureterocalyceal system in normal pregnancy: A study using isotope renography and intravenous pyelography. *Acta Obstet Gynecol Scand* 1973;**53**:69.

Fourcroy JL, Azoury B, Miller HC: Bilateral ureteral obstruction as a complication of vascular graft surgery. *Urology* 1980;**15**:556.

Fowler JE Jr, Meares EM Jr, Goldin AR: Percutaneous nephrostomy: Techniques, indications, and results. *Urology* 1975;**6**:428.

Fowler R, Jensen F: Percutaneous antegrade pyelography in small infants and neonates. *Br J Radiol* 1975;**48**:987.

Gill WB, Curtis GA: The influence of bladder fullness on upper urinary tract dimensions and renal excretory function. *J Urol* 1977;**117**:573.

Gillenwater JY & others: Renal function after release of chronic unilateral hydronephrosis in man. *Kidney Int* 1975;**7**:179.

Guyer PB, Delany D: Urinary tract dilatation and oral contraceptives. *Br Med J* 1970;**4**:588.

Halpern GN, King LR, Belman AB: Transureteroureterostomy in children. *J Urol* 1973;**109**:504.

Hanna MK, Jeffs RD: Primary obstructive megaureter in children. *Urology* 1975;**6**:419.

Hawtrey CE & others: Clinical experience with loop nephrostomy for urinary diversion. *J Urol* 1974;**112**:36.

Hull JC, Kumar S, Pletka PG: Reflex anuria from unilateral ureteral obstruction. *J Urol* 1980;**123**:265.

Hutch JA, Tanagho EA: Etiology of non-occlusive ureteral dilatation. *J Urol* 1965;**93**:177.

Ibrahim A, Asha HA: Prediction of renal recovery in hydronephrotic kidneys. *Br J Urol* 1978;**50**:222.

Johnston JH: The presentation of management of neonatal obstructive uropathies. *Postgrad Med J* 1972;**48**:486.

Johnston JH & others: Pelvic hydronephrosis in children: A review of 219 personal cases. *J Urol* 1977;**117**:97.

Kelalis PP: Urinary diversion in children by the sigmoid conduit: Its advantages and limitations. *J Urol* 1974;**112**:666.

Kelalis PP & others: Ureteropelvic obstruction in children: Experiences with 109 cases. *J Urol* 1971;**106**:418.

Kendall AR, Karafin L: Intermittent hydronephrosis: Hydration pyelography. *J Urol* 1967;**98**:653.

Krohn AG & others: Compensatory renal hypertrophy: The role of immediate vascular changes in its production. *J Urol* 1970;**103**:564.

Leff LO, Smith JP: Achalasia in children and adults. *Urology* 1973;**2**:139.

Lupton EW & others: Diuresis renography and morphology in upper urinary tract obstruction. *Br J Urol* 1979;**51**:10.

Maizels M, Stephens FD: Valves of ureter as cause of primary obstruction of ureter: Anatomic, embryologic and clinical aspects. *J Urol* 1980;**123**:742.

Marshall S: Urea-creatinine ratio in obstructive uropathy and renal hypertension. *JAMA* 1964;**190**:719.

Mattsson T: Frequency and management of urological and some other complications following radical surgery for carcinoma of the cervix uteri, stages I and II: A five-year analysis of 202 cases. *Acta Obstet Gynecol Scand* 1975;**54**:271.

Mayor G & others: Renal function in obstructive nephropathy: Long-term effects of reconstructive surgery. *Pediatrics* 1975;**56**:740.

Michaelson G: Percutaneous puncture of the renal pelvis, intrapelvic pressure and the concentrating capacity of the kidney in hydronephrosis. *Acta Med Scand [Suppl]* 1974;**559**:1. [Entire issue.]

Milewski PJ: Radiograph measurements and contralateral renal size in primary pelvic hydronephrosis. *Br J Urol* 1978;**50**:289.

Perlmutter AD, Kroovand RL, Lai Y-W: Management of ureteropelvic obstruction in first year of life. *J Urol* 1980;**123**:535.

Perlmutter AD, Patil J: Loop cutaneous ureterostomy in infants and young children: Late results in 32 cases. *J Urol* 1972;**107**:655.

Peterson JC & others: Severe hypernatremia complicating urinary tract obstruction. *Urology* 1980;**15**:505.

Remigailo RV & others: Ileal conduit urinary diversion: Ten-year review. *Urology* 1976;**7**:343.

Roberts JA: Hydronephrosis of pregnancy. *Urology* 1976;8:1.

Rose JS & others: B-mode sonographic evaluation of abdominal masses in the pediatric patient. *Am J Roentgenol* 1974;120:691.

Schmidt JD & others: Complications, results and problems of ileal conduit diversions. *J Urol* 1973;109:210.

Schulman A, Herlinger H: Urinary tract dilatation in pregnancy. *Br J Radiol* 1975;48:638.

Shapiro SR, Bennett AH: Recovery of renal function after prolonged unilateral ureteral obstruction. *J Urol* 1976;115:136.

Sharma D: Scrotal flap urethroplasty in the primary management of the "watering-can perineum." *Br J Urol* 1979;51:400.

Sholem SL, Lattimer JK, Uson AC: Further experience with loop cutaneous ureterostomy to save badly damaged kidneys. *J Urol* 1974;111:827.

Smart WR: Chapter 55 in: *Urology*, 3rd ed. Campbell MF, Harrison JH (editors). Saunders, 1970.

Stephens FD: Idiopathic dilatations of the urinary tract. *J Urol* 1974;112:819.

Tanagho EA, Meyers FH: Trigonal hypertrophy: A cause of ureteral obstruction. *J Urol* 1965;93:678.

Tanagho EA, Smith DR, Guthrie TH: Pathophysiology of functional ureteral obstruction. *J Urol* 1970;104:73.

Thompson IA, Bruns TNC: Neonatal ascites: A reflection of obstructive disease. *J Urol* 1972;107:509.

Walsh PC & others: Percutaneous antegrade pyelography in hydronephrosis: Preoperative assessment. *Urology* 1973;1:537.

Walther PC, Parsons CL, Schmidt JD: Direct vision internal urethrotomy in management of urethral strictures. *J Urol* 1980;123:497.

Waterhouse K, Laungani G, Patil U: Surgical repair of membranous urethral strictures: Experience with 105 consecutive cases. *J Urol* 1980;123:500.

Wedge JJ, Grosfeld JL, Smith JP: Abdominal masses in the newborn: 63 cases. *J Urol* 1971;106:770.

Weiss RM, Schiff M Jr, Lytton B: Reflux and trapping. *Radiology* 1976;118:129.

Whalley PJ, Cunningham FG, Martin FG: Transient renal dysfunction associated with acute pyelonephritis of pregnancy. *Obstet Gynecol* 1975;46:174.

Whitfield HN & others: Frusemide intravenous urography in the diagnosis of pelviureteric junction obstruction. *Br J Urol* 1979;51:445.

Youssef AMR, Cockett ATK, Mee AD: Internal urethrotomy using Sachse knife for managing urethral strictures. *Urology* 1980;15:562.

Zincke H, Malek RS: Experience with cutaneous and transureteroureterostomy. *J Urol* 1974;111:760.

11 | Vesicoureteral Reflux

Emil A. Tanagho, MD

Under normal circumstances, the ureterovesical junction allows urine to enter the bladder but prevents urine from regurgitating into the ureter, particularly at the time of voiding. In this way, the kidney is protected from high pressure in the bladder and from contamination by infected vesical urine. When this valve is incompetent, the chance for development of urinary infection is significantly enhanced, and pyelonephritis is then inevitable. With few exceptions, pyelonephritis—acute, chronic, or healed—is secondary to vesicoureteral reflux.

ANATOMY OF THE URETEROVESICAL JUNCTION

An understanding of the causes of vesicoureteral reflux requires a knowledge of the anatomy of the ureterovesical valve. Anatomic studies performed by Hutch (1972) and by Tanagho & Pugh (1963) are incorporated into the following discussion (Fig 11–1).

Mesodermal Component

This structure, which arises from the wolffian duct, is made up of 2 parts that are innervated by the sympathetic nervous system:

A. The Ureter and the Superficial Trigone: The smooth musculature of the renal calices, pelvis, and extravesical ureter is composed of helically oriented fibers that allow for peristaltic activity. As these fibers approach the vesical wall, they are reoriented into the longitudinal plane. The ureter passes obliquely through the vesical wall; the intravesical ureteral segment is thus composed of longitudinal muscle fibers only and therefore cannot undergo peristalsis. As these smooth muscle fibers approach the ureteral orifice, those that form the roof of the ureter swing dorsally to join the fibers that form its floor. They then spread out and join equivalent muscle bundles from the other ureter and also continue caudally, thus forming the superficial trigone. The trigone passes over the neck of the bladder, ending at the verumontanum in the male and just inside the external urethral orifice in the female. Thus, the ureterotrigonal complex is

one structure. Above the ureteral orifice, it is tubular; below that point, it is flat.

B. Waldeyer's Sheath and the Deep Trigone: Beginning at a point about 2–3 cm above the bladder, an external layer of longitudinal smooth muscle surrounds the ureter. This muscular sheath passes through the vesical wall, to which it is connected by a few detrusor fibers. As it enters the vesical lumen, its roof fibers diverge to join its floor fibers, which then spread out, joining muscle bundles from the contralateral ureter and forming the deep trigone, which ends at the bladder neck.

Endodermal Component

The vesical detrusor muscle bundles are intertwined and run in various directions. However, as they converge upon the internal orifice of the bladder, they tend to become oriented into 3 layers:

A. Internal Longitudinal Layer: This layer continues into the urethra submucosally and ends just inside the external meatus in the female and at the caudal end of the prostate in the male.

B. Middle Circular Layer: This layer is thickest anteriorly and stops at the vesical neck.

C. Outer Longitudinal Layer: These muscle bundles take a circular and spiral course about the external surface of the female urethra and are incorporated within the peripheral prostatic tissue in the male. They constitute the true vesicourethral sphincter.

The vesical detrusor muscle is innervated by the parasympathetic nerves (S2–4).

PHYSIOLOGY OF THE URETEROVESICAL JUNCTION

Although many investigators had suspected that normal trigonal tone tended to occlude the intravesical ureter, it remained for Tanagho & others (1965) to prove it. Using nonrefluxing dogs, they demonstrated the following:

(1) Interruption of the continuity of the trigone resulted in reflux. An incision was made in the trigone 3 mm below the ureteral orifice, resulting in an upward and lateral migration of the ureteral orifice with shortening of the intravesical ureter.

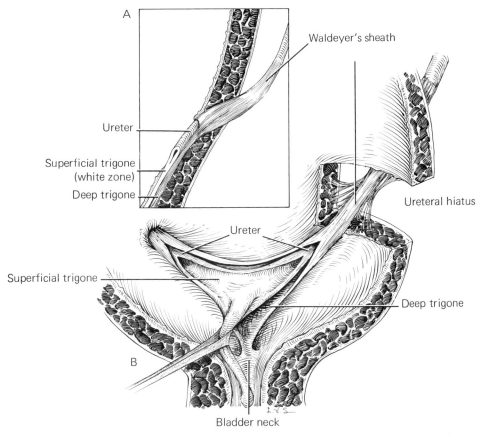

A

Waldeyer's sheath

Ureter

Superficial trigone
(white zone)

Deep trigone

Ureter

Ureteral hiatus

Superficial trigone

Deep trigone

B

Bladder neck

The ureteral muscle extends downward
and becomes the superficial trigone.

Waldeyer's sheath extends downward
and becomes the deep trigone.

Figure 11–1. Normal ureterotrigonal complex. **A:** Side view of ureterovesical junction. Waldeyer's muscular sheath invests the juxtavesical ureter and continues downward as the deep trigone, which extends to the bladder neck. The ureteral musculature becomes the superficial trigone, which extends to the verumontanum in the male and stops just short of the external meatus in the female. **B:** Waldeyer's sheath is connected by a few fibers to the detrusor muscle in the ureteral hiatus. This muscular sheath, inferior to the ureteral orifices, becomes the deep trigone. The musculature of the ureters continues downward as the superficial trigone. (Redrawn and modified, with permission, from Tanagho EA, Pugh RCB: The anatomy and function of the ureterovesical junction. *Br J Urol* 1963;**35**:151.)

Reflux was demonstrable. After the incision healed, reflux ceased.

(2) Unilateral lumbar sympathectomy resulted in paralysis of the ipsilateral trigone. This led to lateral and superior migration of the ureteral orifice and reflux.

(3) Electrical stimulation of the trigone caused the ureteral orifice to move caudally, thus lengthening the intravesical ureter. This maneuver caused a marked rise in resistance to flow through the ureterovesical junction. Ureteral efflux of urine ceased. The intravenous injection of epinephrine caused the same reaction. On the other hand, isoproterenol caused the degree of occlusion to drop below normal. If, however, the trigone was incised, electrical stimulation of the trigone or the administration of epinephrine failed to increase ureteral occlusive pressure.

(4) During gradual filling of the bladder, intravesical pressure increased only slightly, whereas pressure within the intravesical ureter rose progressively—due, apparently, to increasing trigonal stretch. A few seconds before the expected sharp rise in intravesical pressure generated for voiding, the closure pressure in the intravesical ureter rose sharply and was maintained for 20 seconds after detrusor contracture had ceased. This experiment demonstrated that ureterovesical competence is independent of detrusor action and is governed by the tone of the trigone, which contracts vigorously just before voiding, thus helping to open and funnel the vesical neck. At the same time, significant pull is placed upon the intravesical ureter, so that it is occluded during the period when intravesical pressure is high. During the voiding phase, there is naturally no efflux of ureteral urine.

One may liken this function to the phenomenon of the Chinese thimble: The harder the finger (trigone) pulls, the tighter the thimble (intravesical ureter) becomes. Conversely, a deficient pull may lead to incomplete closure of the ureterovesical junction.

It was concluded from these experiments that normal ureterotrigonal tone prevents vesicoureteral reflux. Electrical or pharmacologic stimulation of the trigone caused increased occlusive pressure in the intravesical ureter and increased resistance to flow down the ureter, whereas incision or paralysis of the trigone led to reflux. The theory that ureterovesical competence was maintained by intravesical pressure crushing the intravesical ureter against its backing of detrusor muscle was thereby disproved.

Biopsy of the trigone (and the intravesical ureter) in patients with primary reflux revealed marked deficiency in the development of its smooth muscle (Fig 11–2). Electrical stimulation of such a trigone caused only a minor contraction of the ureterotrigonal complex. This work led to the conclusion that the common cause of reflux, particularly in children, is congenital attenuation of the ureterotrigonal musculature.

THE CAUSES OF REFLUX

The major cause of vesicoureteral reflux is attenuation of the trigone and its contiguous intravesical ureteral musculature. Any condition that shortens the intravesical ureter may also lead to reflux, but this is less common. Familial vesicoureteral reflux has been observed by a number of authors. It appears to be a genetic trait.

Congenital Causes
A. Trigonal Weakness ("Primary Reflux"): This is by far the most common cause of ureteral regurgitation. It is most often seen in little girls,

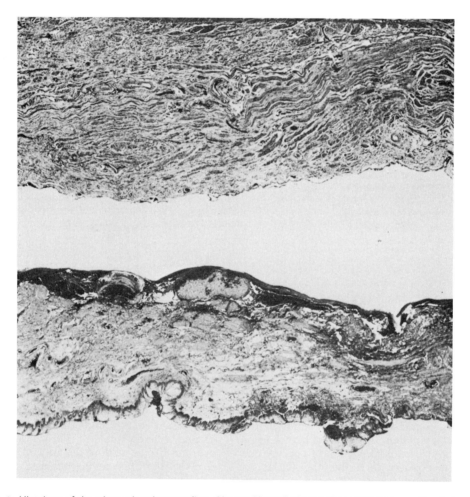

Figure 11–2. Histology of the trigone in primary reflux. *Above:* Normal trigone demonstrating wealth of closely packed smooth muscle fibers. *Below:* The congenitally attenuated trigonal muscle that accompanies vesicoureteral reflux. Note absence of inflammatory cells. (Reproduced, with permission, from Tanagho EA & others: Primary vesicoureteral reflux: Experimental studies of its etiology. *J Urol* 1965;**93:**165.)

though occasionally also in boys. Reflux in adults—usually women—probably represents the same congenital defect. Weakness of one side of the trigone leads to decrease in the occlusive pressure in the ipsilateral intravesical ureter. Diffuse ureterotrigonal weakness causes bilateral reflux.

It is postulated that ureteral trigonal weakness is related to the development of the ureteral bud on the mesonephric duct. It is known that the ureter acquires its musculature from its cranial end caudally, so that if a segment is muscularly deficient, it is deficient in its most caudad part. It is also postulated that if the ureter is too close to the urogenital sinus on the mesonephric duct, it will join the latter relatively early in embryonic life, before acquiring adequate mesenchymal tissue around itself to be differentiated later into proper trigonal musculature as well as lower ureter. This embryologic hypothesis explains all the known features of refluxing ureters—their muscular weakness, their lateral placement on the bladder base with a very short submucosal segment, and their usual association with weak ureteral musculature and gaping ureteral orifices (which, in severe cases, will assume a golf-hole endoscopic appearance at their junction with the bladder wall). It also explains why, in duplicated systems, if there is only one refluxing unit, it is the upper orifice (originally closer to the urogenital sinus on the mesonephric duct, thus the one with the least muscular development).

In the normal state, the intravesical ureterotrigonal muscle tone exerts a downward pull, whereas the extravesical ureter tends to pull cephalad (Fig 11–3). If trigonal development is deficient, not only is its occlusive power diminished but the ureteral orifice tends to migrate upward toward the ureteral hiatus. The degree of this retraction relates to the degree of incompetence of the junction (Fig 11–4). If the ureteral orifice lies over the ureteral hiatus in the bladder wall (so-called golf-hole orifice), it is completely incompetent. The degree of incompetency is judged by the findings on excretory urography and cystography and the cystoscopic appearance of the ureteral orifices.

B. Ureteral Abnormalities:

1. Complete ureteral duplication–(Fig 11–5.) The intravesical portion of the ureter to the upper renal segment is usually of normal length, whereas that of the ureter to the lower pole is abnormally short; this orifice is commonly incompetent. However, Stephens (1964) has demonstrated that the musculature of the superiorly placed orifice is attenuated, which further contributes to its weakness.

2. Ectopic ureteral orifice–A single ureter or one of a pair may open well down on the trigone, at the vesical neck, or in the urethra. In this instance, vesicoureteral reflux is the rule. This observation makes it clear that the length of the intravesical ureter is not the sole factor in reflux. Stephens (1964) has observed that such intravesical ureteral

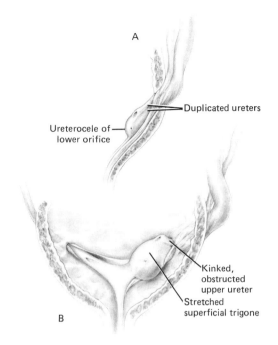

Figure 11–3. *A:* Small ureterocele developing in a duplicated system (where it always involves a lower ureteral orifice). *B:* Expansion of submucosal segment leads to lifting and angulation of ipsilateral lower pole ureteral orifice. Duplicated system ureteroceles are rarely so small. (Diagrammatic representation.) (Reproduced, with permission, from Tanagho EA: Ureteroceles: Embryogenesis, pathogenesis and management. *J Cont Educ Urol* (Feb) 1979;**18**:13.)

segments are usually devoid of smooth muscle. Thus, they have no occlusive force.

3. Ureterocele–A ureterocele involving a single ureter rarely allows reflux, but this lesion usually involves the ureter that drains the upper pole of a duplicated kidney. Because the ureteral orifice is obstructed, the intramural ureter becomes dilated. This increases the diameter of the ureteral hiatus, thus further shortening the intravesical segment of the other ureter, which therefore may become incompetent. Resection of the ureterocele usually causes its ureter to reflux freely as well.

Vesical Trabeculation

Occasionally, a heavily trabeculated bladder may be associated with reflux. The causes include the spastic neurogenic bladder and severe obstruction distal to the bladder. These lesions, however, are associated with trigonal hypertrophy as well; the resultant extra pull on the ureterotrigonal muscle tends to protect the junction from incompetency. In a few such cases, however, the vesical mucosa may protrude through the ureteral hiatus just above the ureter, thus forming a diverticulum, or saccule (Fig 11–6). The resulting dilatation of the hiatus shortens the intravesical segment; reflux may then occur.

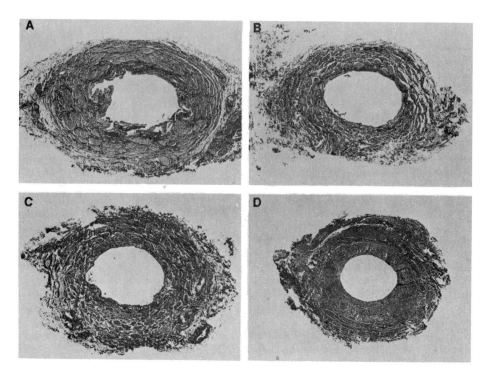

Figure 11–4. Histology of the various grades of submucosal muscular weakness of the ureteral orifice. (See also Fig 11 –9.) *A:* Normal. Minimal deficiency. (Cone orifice.) *B:* More marked muscular weakness. (Stadium orifice.) *C:* Marked muscular deficiency. (Horseshoe orifice.) *D:* Extreme muscular deficiency. Only a few muscle fibers can be seen; the rest is collagen tissue.

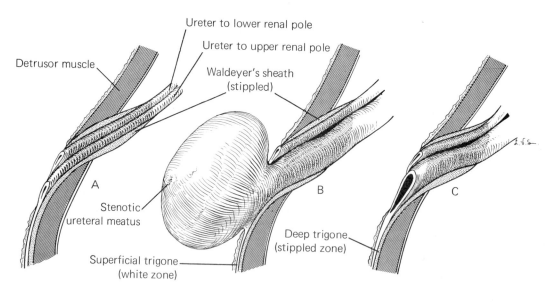

Figure 11–5. Ureteral duplication and ureterocele as causes of vesicoureteral reflux. *A:* Ureteral duplication showing juxtavesical and intravesical ureters encased in common sheath (Waldeyer's). The superior ureter, which always drains the lower renal pole, has a shorter intravesical segment; in addition, it is somewhat devoid of muscle. It therefore tends to allow reflux. *B:* Duplication with ureterocele that always involves caudal ureter, which drains upper renal pole. Pinpoint orifice is obstructive, causing hydroureteronephrosis. Resulting wide dilatation of ureter and ureteral hiatus shortens the intravesical segment of the other ureter, often causing it to reflux. *C:* Resection of ureterocele allows reflux into that ureter.

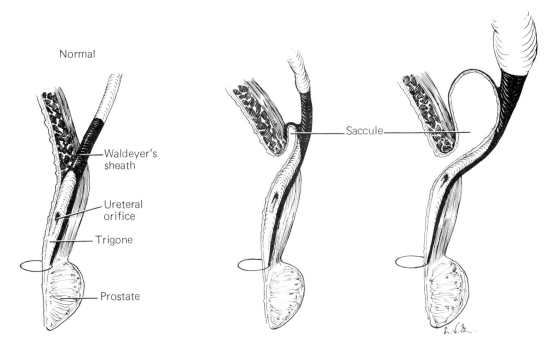

Figure 11–6. Development of ureteral saccule, seen occasionally in cases of primary reflux but more commonly in obstructed or neurogenic bladders with marked trabeculation. Note that the vesical mucosa herniates through the ureteral hiatus, pulling the ureteral orifice upward with it. The latter may ultimately open inside the saccule rather than inside the bladder.

Edema of the Vesical Wall Secondary to Cystitis

As noted above, valves vary in their degrees of incompetency. A "borderline" junction may not allow reflux when the urine is sterile, but the edema involving the trigone and intravesical ureter associated with cystitis may impair valvular function. In addition, the abnormally high voiding pressure may lead to reflux, in which case secondary pyelonephritis may ensue. After cure of the infection, cystography again reveals no reflux. It is believed that a completely normal junction will not decompensate even under these circumstances.

It has been shown that pyelonephritis of pregnancy is associated with vesicoureteral reflux. Many patients give a history of urinary tract infections during childhood. The implication is that they "outgrew" reflux at puberty but that if bacteriuria becomes established during pregnancy their "borderline" valves may become incompetent. This condition may be aggravated by the hormones of pregnancy, which may contribute to a further loss of tone of the ureterotrigonal complex. After delivery, the reflux is usually no longer demonstrable (Hutch & Amar, 1972).

Eagle-Barrett (Prune Belly) Syndrome

This is a relatively rare condition in which there is failure of normal development of the abdominal muscles and the smooth muscle of the ureters and bladder. Bilateral cryptorchidism is the rule. At times, talipes equinovarus and hip disloca-

tion are also noted. Because of deficiency of the smooth muscle of the ureterotrigonal complex, reflux is to be expected; advanced hydroureteronephrosis is therefore found.

Iatrogenic Causes

Certain operative procedures may lead to either temporary or permanent ureteral regurgitation.

A. Prostatectomy: With any type of prostatectomy, the continuity of the superficial trigone is interrupted at the vesical neck. If the proximal trigone moves upward, temporary reflux may occur. This mechanism may account for the high fever (even bacteremia) that is sometimes observed when the catheter is finally removed. Fortunately, in 2–3 weeks the trigone again becomes anchored and reflux ceases.

Preexisting trigonal hypertrophy (due to prostatic obstruction) helps to compensate for the effect of trigonal interruption; thus, reflux may never occur.

B. Wedge Resection of the Posterior Vesical Neck: This procedure, often performed in conjunction with plastic revision of the vesical neck for supposed vesical neck stenosis or dysfunction, may also upset trigonal continuity and allow reflux.

C. Ureteral Meatotomy: Extensive ureteral meatotomy may be followed by reflux. Fortunately, however, limited incision of the roof of the intravesical ureter divides few muscle fibers, since they have left the roof to join muscle fibers on the floor. Wide resection in the treatment of vesical neoplasm is often followed by ureteral regurgitation.

D. Resection of Ureterocele: If the ureteral hiatus is widely dilated, this procedure is often followed by reflux.

Contracted Bladder

A bladder that is contracted secondary to interstitial cystitis, tuberculosis, radiotherapy, carcinoma, or schistosomiasis may be associated with ureteral reflux.

COMPLICATIONS OF VESICOURETERAL REFLUX

Vesicoureteral reflux damages the kidney through one or both of 2 mechanisms: (1) pyelonephritis and (2) hydroureteronephrosis (Fig 11–7).

Pyelonephritis

Vesicoureteral reflux is one of the common contributing factors leading to the development of cystitis, particularly in females. When reflux is present, bacteria reach the kidney and the urinary tract cannot empty itself completely, so that infection is perpetuated. (See Pathogenesis, p 157, for a discussion of this phenomenon.)

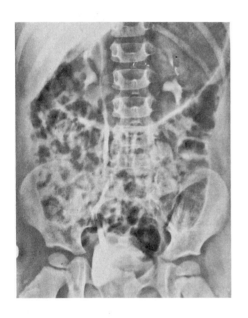
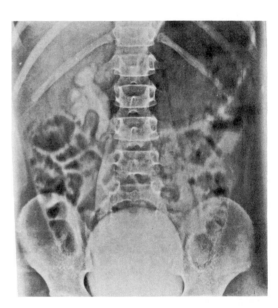
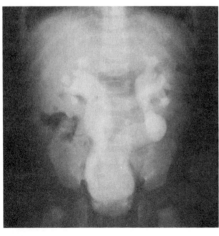
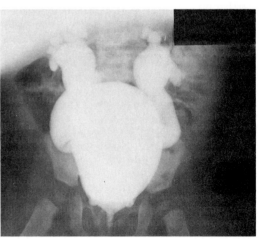

Figure 11–7. Excretory urogram with changes that imply right vesicoureteral reflux. *Top left:* Excretory urogram showing normal right urogram and a ureter that is mildly dilated and remains full through its entire length. The ureteral change implies reflux. *Top right:* Cystogram demonstrates the reflux. Note, now, the degree of dilatation of the ureter, pelvis, and calices. *Bottom left:* Excretory urogram shows bilateral hydroureteronephrosis with pyelonephritic scarring. These findings imply the presence of reflux. *Bottom right:* Voiding cystourethrogram. Free reflux bilaterally.

Hydroureteronephrosis

Dilatation of the ureter, renal pelvis, and calices is usually observed in association with reflux, sometimes to an extreme degree (Fig 11–8). Such changes are often seen in the absence of infection in the male because of the relatively long segment of sterile urethra in that sex. Sterile reflux is less damaging than infected reflux.

There are 3 reasons for the dilatation: (1) **Increased workload:** The ureter is meant to transport the volume of urine secreted by the kidney toward the bladder only once. In the presence of reflux, there are variable volumes going back and forth, and the workload may be doubled, quadrupled, or increased 10 times or even more. Eventually, the ureter is not able to transport the increased volume, and stasis of dilatation results. (2) **High hydrostatic pressure:** The ureter is protected from the high pressures of the urinary bladder by the competent ureterovesical junction. If there is free reflux, the high intravesical pressure will be directly transmitted to the ureteral and pelvic walls, which results in marked stretching and dilatation. (3) **Weak ureteral musculature:** In reflux, the ureteral wall is invariably deficient in musculature to some degree. The more severe the reflux, the more apparent this phenomenon. Some cases show more massive dilatation than others. The properly muscularized ureter is better able to resist and compensate for overwork and hydrostatic pressure than the muscularly deficient ureter. The latter tends to undergo further dilatation once it is subjected to any increased intraluminal pressure.

Whether sterile reflux is harmful or not is the subject of controversy. We feel there is conclusive evidence that even in the absence of infection, severe sterile reflux can lead to parenchymal damage. Pyelointerstitial backflow or pyelorenal backflow under the high pressures of reflux (not infrequently seen during cystographic studies) leads to extravasation of urine in the interstitium of the kidney. The presence of urine in any interstitium will result in marked inflammatory response with cellular infiltration, resulting finally in fibrosis and scarring. On a long-term basis, this can lead to parenchymal changes indistinguishable from bacterial inflammatory pyelonephritic scarring. This damage may be termed reflux nephropathy. If severe, it will produce parenchymal damage serious enough to lead to end stage kidneys.

Intravesical pressure is transmitted through the incompetent ureteral orifice. This back pressure is quite high at the time of voiding. Furthermore, the ureteropelvic and ureterovesical junctions are less distensible than the rest of the ureter. Either junction may have trouble passing the volume of normal urinary secretion plus the refluxed urine; functional obstruction may result. The common cause of ureteropelvic and ureterovesical "obstruction" is vesicoureteral reflux. Such changes indicate the need for cystography.

THE INCIDENCE OF REFLUX

Incompetency of the ureterovesical junction is an abnormal condition. Peters and others found no reflux in 66 premature infants; Lich and co-workers found none in 26 infants studied during the first 2 days of life. Leadbetter and others noted normal cystograms in 50 adult males. (See Smith, 1978, reference.)

The incidence of vesicoureteral reflux is 50% in children with urinary tract infection but only 8% in adults with bacteriuria. This discrepancy is explained by the fact that the female child usually has pyelonephritis whereas the adult female usually has cystitis only. The concept that bacteriuria implies the presence of pyelonephritis must be condemned.

The fairly competent ("borderline") valve refluxes only during an acute attack of cystitis. Since cystography is performed in such cases only after the infection has been eradicated, the incidence of reflux is abnormally low. On the other hand, reflux is demonstrable in 85% of patients whose excretory urograms reveal significant changes typical of healed pyelonephritis.

When infection associated with reflux occurs during the first few weeks of life, many patients are septic and uremic. Most are boys who have posterior urethral valves. After age 6 months, the female:male ratio of infection with reflux is 10:1.

CLINICAL FINDINGS

A history compatible with acute pyelonephritis implies the presence of vesicoureteral reflux. This is most commonly seen in females, particularly little girls. Persistence of recurrent "cystitis" should suggest the possibility of reflux. Often, in these instances, the patient has an asymptomatic low-grade pyelonephritis.

Symptoms Related to Reflux

A. Symptomatic Pyelonephritis: The usual symptoms in the adult are chills and high fever, renal pain, nausea and vomiting, and symptoms of cystitis. In children, only fever and vague abdominal pains and sometimes diarrhea are apt to occur.

B. Asymptomatic Pyelonephritis: The patient may have no symptoms whatsoever. The incidental findings of pyuria and bacteriuria may be the only clues. This points up the need for a proper urinalysis in all children.

C. Symptoms of Cystitis Only: In these cases, bacteriuria is resistant to antimicrobials or infection quickly recurs following treatment. These patients may have reflux with asymptomatic chronic pyelonephritis.

D. Renal Pain on Voiding: Surprisingly, this is a rare complaint in the refluxing patient.

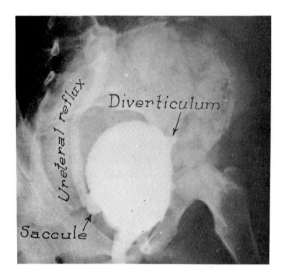

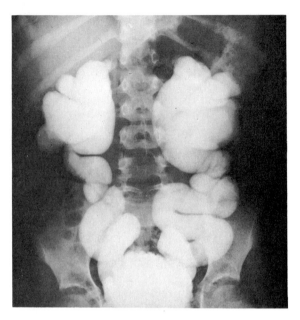

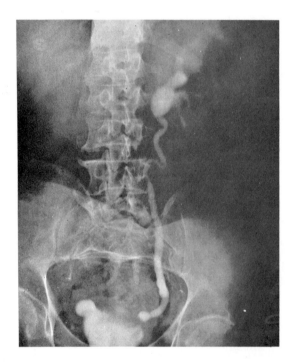

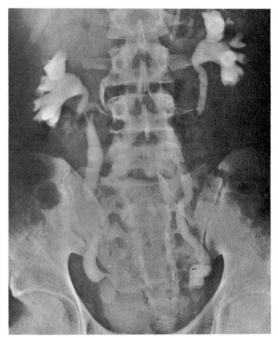

Figure 11–8. Cystograms revealing vesicoureteral reflux. ***Above left:*** Saccule at right ureterovesical junction. ***Above right:*** Meningomyelocele. Reflux with severe bilateral hydroureteronephrosis; serum creatinine, 0.6 mg/dL; PSP excretion, 5% in 1 hour. ***Below left:*** Postprostatectomy patient with reflux on left and bilateral saccules. ***Below right:*** Ten-year-old boy with meningomyelocele. Bladder has been emptied. Impairment of drainage at ureterovesical junctions is demonstrated. (Courtesy of JA Hutch.)

E. Uremia: The last stage of bilateral reflux is uremia due to destruction of the renal parenchyma by hydronephrosis or pyelonephritis (or both). The patient often adjusts to renal insufficiency and may appear quite healthy. Many renal transplants are performed in patients whose kidneys have deteriorated secondarily to reflux and accompanying infection. Early diagnosis, based upon careful urinalysis, would have led to the proper diagnosis in childhood. Progressive pyelonephritis is, with few exceptions, a preventable disease.

F. Hypertension: In the later stages of atrophic pyelonephritis, a significant incidence of hypertension is observed.

Symptoms Related to the Underlying Disease

The clinical picture is often dominated by the signs and symptoms of the primary disease.

A. Urinary Tract Obstruction: The little girl may have hesitancy in initiating the urinary stream and an impaired or intermittent stream secondary to spasm of the periurethral striated muscle (see Distal Urethral Stenosis, Chapter 30). In males, the urinary stream may be slow as a result of posterior urethral valves (infants) or prostatic enlargement (men over 50).

B. Spinal Cord Disease: The patient may have a serious neurogenic disease such as paraplegia, quadriplegia, multiple sclerosis, or meningomyelocele. Symptoms may be limited to those of neurogenic bladder: incontinence of urine, urinary retention, and vesical urgency.

Physical Findings

During an attack of acute pyelonephritis, renal tenderness may be noted. Its absence, however, does not rule out chronic renal infection.

Palpation and percussion of the suprapubic area may reveal a distended bladder secondary to obstruction or neurogenic disease.

The finding of a hard midline mass deep in the pelvis in a male infant is apt to represent a markedly thickened bladder caused by posterior urethral valves.

Examination may reveal a neurologic deficit compatible with a paretic bladder.

Laboratory Findings

The most common complication, particularly in the female, is infection. Bacteriuria without pyuria is not uncommon. In the male, urine may be normal because of the long, sterile urethra.

PSP excretion will be diminished in uremia. The curve, even when renal function is normal, may be "flat" because some of the first half-hour excretion may be refluxed back up to the kidneys; with gross bilateral reflux, the total PSP may be alarmingly low. The serum creatinine may be elevated in the advanced stage of renal damage, but it may be normal even when the degree of reflux and hydronephrosis is marked (Fig 11–8, above right).

The PSP test is the superior screening test in this instance.

X-Ray Findings

The plain film may reveal evidence of spina bifida, meningomyelocele, or absence of the sacrum, thus pointing to a neurologic deficit. Even in vesicoureteral reflux, excretory urograms may be normal, but usually one or more of the following clues to the presence of reflux is noted (Fig 11–7): (1) A persistently dilated lower ureter. (2) Areas of dilatation in the ureter. (3) Ureter visualized throughout its entire length. (4) Presence of hydroureteronephrosis with a narrow juxtavesical ureteral segment. (5) Changes of healed pyelonephritis: caliceal clubbing with narrowed infundibula or cortical thinning.

A normal intravenous urogram does not rule out reflux.

The presence of ureteral duplication suggests the possibility of reflux into the lower pole of the kidney. In this case, hydronephrosis or changes compatible with pyelonephritic scarring may be seen. Abnormality of the upper segment of a duplicated system can be caused by the presence of an ectopic ureteral orifice with reflux or by obstruction secondary to a ureterocele.

Reflux is diagnosed by demonstrating its existence with one of the following technics: simple or delayed cystography, voiding cystourethrography, or voiding cinefluoroscopy. A radionuclide technic can be used. One mCi of ^{99m}Tc is instilled into the bladder along with sterile saline solution. The gamma camera will reveal ureteral reflux.

Amar (1966) has shown that reflux can be demonstrated by filling the bladder with sterile water containing 5 mL of indigo carmine per 100 mL. The patient then voids and the bladder is thoroughly flushed out with sterile water. The ureteral orifices are viewed cystoscopically for blue-tinged efflux. This technic protects the patient from radiation exposure, and its efficiency is equal to that of voiding cystourethrography. In general, reflux that is demonstrated only with voiding implies a more competent valve than that which allows low-pressure regurgitation. As has been pointed out, failure to demonstrate reflux on one study does not rule out intermittent reflux.

The voiding phase of the cystogram may reveal changes compatible with distal urethral stenosis with secondary spasm of the voluntary periurethral muscles in the female child (Fig 30–1) or changes in the small boy that are diagnostic of posterior urethral valves.

Instrumental Examination

A. Urethral Calibration: In females, urethral calibration using bougies à boule should be done. Distal urethral stenosis is almost routinely found in little girls suffering from urinary infection. Destruction of the ring is an important step in improving the hydrodynamics of voiding: lowered intravesical voiding pressure and the abolition of residual vesical urine (see Chapter 29). Less commonly, urethral stenosis is discovered in the adult female and should be treated.

B. Cystoscopy: Most little girls with reflux have smooth-walled or only slightly trabeculated bladders. Chronic cystitis, ureteral duplication, or ureterocele may be evident. An orifice may be found to be ectopic at the bladder neck or even in the urethra. As the bladder is filled, a small diverticulum may form on the roof of the ureteral orifice (Fig 11–6). These findings imply the possibility of reflux. The major contribution of cystoscopy is to allow study of the morphology of the ureteral orifice and its position in relation to the vesical neck (Fig 11–9).

1. Morphology–The orifice of a normal ureter has the appearance of a volcanic cone. That of a slightly weaker valve looks like a football stadium; an even weaker one has the appearance of a horseshoe with its open end pointing toward the vesical neck. The completely incompetent junction has a "golf-hole" orifice that lies over the ureteral hiatus.

2. Position–By and large, the more defective the appearance of the ureteral orifice, the farther from the vesical neck it lies. The degree of retraction of the orifice reflects the degree of ureterotrigonal deficiency.

DIFFERENTIAL DIAGNOSIS

Functional (nonocclusive) vesicoureteral obstruction may cause changes similar to those suggesting the presence of reflux on excretory urography. Multiple cystograms fail to show reflux. Tanagho, Smith, & Guthrie (1970) have shown that this congenital obstruction is due to a heavy layer of circularly oriented smooth muscle fibers surrounding the ureter at this point. Its action is sphincteric.

Significant obstruction distal to the vesical neck leads to hypertrophy of both the detrusor and trigonal muscles. The latter exert an exaggerated pull upon the intravesical ureter, thus causing functional obstruction (see Tanagho & Meyers, 1965). Hydroureteronephrosis is therefore to be expected; vesicoureteral reflux is uncommon.

Other lesions that may cause hydroureteronephrosis without reflux include low ureteral stone, ureteral occlusion by cervical or prostatic cancer, urinary tract tuberculosis, and schistosomiasis.

TREATMENT

It is impossible to give a concise and definitive discourse on the treatment of vesicoureteral reflux because of the many factors involved and because there is no unanimity of opinion among urologists

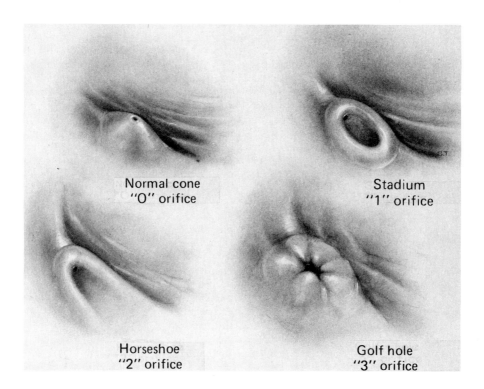

Figure 11–9. Cystoscopic appearance of the normal ureteral orifice and 3 degrees of incompetency of the ureterovesical junction. (Reproduced, with permission, from Lyon RP, Marshall SK, Tanagho EA: The ureteral orifice: Its configuration and competency. *J Urol* 1969;**102**:504.)

on this subject. In general, probably more than half of children with primary reflux can be controlled by nonsurgical means and the rest will require some form of operative procedure. Adults exhibiting reflux will usually require vesicoureteroplasty.

Medical Treatment

A. Indications: The child with primary reflux (attenuated trigone) who has fairly normal upper tracts on urographic study and whose ureterovesical valves on cystoscopy appear fair to good has an excellent chance of "outgrowing" the defect, particularly if cystograms show only transient or "high-pressure" reflux.

The male child with posterior urethral valves may cease to reflux once these valves are destroyed.

The adult female who occasionally develops acute pyelonephritis following intercourse but whose urine quickly clears on antimicrobial therapy will probably be controlled if she takes steps to prevent vesical infections (see Treatment, p 176). This is particularly true if, when her urine is sterile, reflux cannot be demonstrated on cystography. The maintenance of sterile urine will allow her "borderline" valve to remain competent.

B. Methods of Treatment: Destruction of the ring of distal urethral stenosis in little girls or of posterior urethral valves in boys usually gives excellent results, reducing voiding intravesical pressure and abolishing vesical residual urine and reflux.

Definitive treatment of the urinary infection with bactericidal drugs should be given, followed by chronic suppressive therapy for 6 months or more.

Triple voiding is the least effective method. Since vesicoureteral reflux prevents the urinary tract from emptying itself completely, thus destroying the vesical defense mechanism, triple voiding once a day is helpful if the child is old enough to be trained. When reflux is present, the bladder empties itself on voiding, but some urine ascends to the kidneys and then returns to the bladder. Voiding again a few minutes later will push less urine into the ureters. A third voiding will usually completely empty the urinary tract. Thus, the patient's own natural resistance can operate to a maximum degree.

Children with reflux often have thin-walled bladders and do not perceive the normal urge to void when the bladder is full. Further detrusor tone is lost with overfilling, thus contributing to residual urine. Such children should "void by the clock" every 3–4 hours whether they have the urge or not. Vesical residual urine may then be minimized.

The infant female with markedly dilated upper urinary tracts may be tided over by means of an indwelling urethral catheter. Over a period of months, ureteral dilatation and elongation may regress; renal function is protected. At a convenient and strategic time, more definitive therapy can be accomplished.

C. Evaluation of Success of Medical Treatment: Urinalysis should be done at least once a month for a year or more. Maintenance of sterile urine is an encouraging sign. Cystograms should be repeated every 4–6 months. Excretory urography should be ordered at 6 and 12 months to be sure that renal deterioration does not occur.

About half of children with reflux are cured by medical treatment.

Surgical Treatment

A. Indications: Reflux caused by the following abnormalities will not disappear spontaneously: (1) ectopic ureteral orifice, (2) ureteral duplication, (3) ureterocele associated with ureteral duplication and reflux into the uninvolved ureter, (4) "golf-hole" ureteral orifice, and (5) low-pressure reflux with significant hydroureteronephrosis.

Surgery is indicated (1) if it is not possible to keep the urine sterile and reflux persists; (2) if acute pyelonephritis recurs despite a strict medical regimen and chronic suppressive antimicrobial therapy; (3) if there is increased renal damage as portrayed by serial excretory urograms; or (4) if reflux persists for 1 year after institution of therapy.

B. Types of Surgical Therapy: In cases of markedly impaired kidney function and massively dilated ureters, surgical treatment may require preliminary urinary diversion to improve renal function and to allow dilated ureters to regain tone. Later, definitive relief of obstruction (eg, posterior urethral valves) and ureterovesicoplasty can be performed at the optimum time. Some patients with irreversible lesions causing reflux (eg, meningomyelocele) or badly damaged and atonic ureters may require permanent diversion of the urine (ie, ureteroileocutaneous anastomosis).

1. Temporary urinary diversion–If drainage of refluxed urine into the bladder is free, cystostomy (or an indwelling urethral catheter in girls) may prove helpful. If the ureters are dilated and kinked, a redundant loop can be brought to the skin. The ureter is opened at this point and urine collected into an ileostomy bag. Later, the loop can be resected and its ends anastomosed, and ureteral reimplantation can then be done. Nephrostomy may be necessary if ureteral redundancy is absent.

2. Permanent urinary diversion–If it is felt that successful ureterovesicoplasty cannot be accomplished, a Bricker type of diversion is indicated. If renal function is poor and the ureters are widely dilated and atonic, ureterocutaneous diversion may be the procedure of choice.

3. Other surgical procedures–

a. If reflux is unilateral, with the affected kidney badly damaged and the other kidney normal, nephrectomy is indicated.

b. If one renal pole of a duplicated system is essentially functionless, heminephrectomy with removal of its entire ureter should be done. If there is moderate hydronephrosis of one renal pole with duplication, an alternative is anastomosis of the dilated ureter or pelvis to the normal ureter or pelvis. The remainder of the dilated refluxing ureter should be removed.

c. In unilateral reflux, anastomosis of the lower end of the refluxing ureter into the side of its normal mate (transureteroureterostomy) has a few proponents.

4. Definitive repair.

Definitive Repair of Ureterovesical Junction (Ureterovesicoplasty)

A. Principles of Repair: (Tanagho, 1970.)

1. Resect the lower 2–3 cm of the ureter whose muscle is underdeveloped.

2. Free up enough extravesical ureter so that an intravesical segment 2.5 cm long can be formed.

3. Place the intravesical ureter in a submucosal position.

4. Suture the wall of the new ureteral orifice to the cut edge of the trigonal muscle.

B. Types of Operation: The following procedures satisfy the above principles and have been successful in a high percentage of cases: the advancement operation (Hutch, 1963; Glenn & Anderson, 1967), and the Politano-Leadbetter (1958), the Paquin (1959), and the Cohen (1975) transtrigonal operations.

If the ureters are unduly tortuous, the redundant portions must be resected. If widely dilated, the lower ends must be tailored to a more normal size.

C. Results of Ureterovesicoplasty: About 93% of patients no longer show reflux after ureterovesicoplasty. About 3% develop ureterovesical stenosis that requires reoperation. At least 75% have and maintain sterile urine without antimicrobials 3–6 months after surgery. Many patients in whom bacteriuria persists have cystitis only. Febrile attacks cease. This has been demonstrated by finding that the renal urines collected by ureteral catheters are sterile. Considering that only the most severe and advanced cases are submitted to surgical repair, these are impressive results, and they exceed by far the cure rates reported when only antimicrobials are used (10–15%). This operation is rightly considered one of the most significant accomplishments of modern urology.

PROGNOSIS

In patients with reflux who are judged to have fairly competent valves, conservative therapy as outlined above is highly successful in the cure of the reflux and therefore infection.

Patients with very incompetent ureterovesical valves subjected to surgical repair also have an excellent prognosis. A few children, however, have such badly damaged urinary tracts when finally submitted to diagnostic procedures that little help other than permanent urinary diversion can be offered.

●   ●   ●

References

Ahmed S, Smith AJ: Results of ureteral reimplantation in patients with intrarenal reflux. *J Urol* 1978;**120**:332.

Amar AD: Cystoscopic demonstration of vesicoureteral reflux: Evaluation in 250 patients. *J Urol* 1966;**95**:776.

Amar AD: Eradication of reflux in adults by excision of chronic infection reservoirs without antireflux operation. *J Urol* 1975;**113**:175.

Amar AD: Vesicoureteral reflux in adults: A 12-year study of 122 patients. *Urology* 1974;**3**:184.

Amar AD, Singer B, Chabra K: The practical management of vesicoureteral reflux in children: A review of 12 years' experience with 236 patients. *Clin Pediatr* 1976;**15**:562.

Ambrose SS & others: Observations on small kidney associated with vesicoureteral reflux. *J Urol* 1980;**123**:349.

Angel JR, Smith TW Jr, Roberts JA: Hydrodynamics of pyelorenal renal reflux. *J Urol* 1979;**122**:20.

Arap S & others: The extra-vesical antireflux plasty: Statistical analysis. *Urol Int* 1971;**26**:241.

Atwell JD, Allen NH: The interrelationship between paraureteric diverticula, vesicoureteric reflux and duplication of the pelvicaliceal collecting system: A family study. *Br J Urol* 1980;**52**:269.

Babcock JR, Keats GK, King LR: Renal changes after uncomplicated antireflux operation. *J Urol* 1976;**115**:720.

Baker R, Barbaris HJ: Comparative results of urological evaluation of children with initial and recurrent urinary tract infection. *J Urol* 1976;**116**:503.

Bakshandeh K, Lynne C, Carrion H: Vesicoureteral reflux and end stage renal disease. *J Urol* 1976;**116**:557.

Bourne HH & others: Intrarenal reflux and renal damage. *J Urol* 1976;**115**:304.

Burkholder GV, Harper RC, Beach PD: Congenital absence of the abdominal muscles. *Am J Clin Pathol* 1970;**53**:602.

Burko H, Rhamy RK: Lower urinary tract problems related to infection: Diagnosis and treatment. *Pediatr Clin North Am* 1970;**17**:233.

Carter TC, Tomskey GC, Ozog LS: Prune-belly syndrome: Review of 10 cases. *Urology* 1974;**3**:279.

Cattolica EV: Renal scarring and primary reflux in adults. *Urology* 1974;**4**:397.

Cohen SJ: Ureterozystoneostomie: Eine neue antireflux Technik. (Ureterocystoneostomy: A new technique for reflux prevention.) *Aktuelle Urologie* 1975;**6**:1.

Coleman JW, McGovern JH: Ureterovesical reimplantation in children: Surgical results in 491 children. *Urology* 1978;**12**:514.

Cremin BJ: The urinary tract anomalies associated with agenesis of the abdominal walls. *Br J Radiol* 1971;**44**:767.

DeKlerk DP, Reiner WG, Jeffs RD: Vesicoureteral reflux and ureteropelvic junction obstruction: Late occurrence of ureteropelvic obstruction after successful ureteroneocystostomy. *J Urol* 1979;**121**:816.

Devine PC & others: Vesicoureteral reflux in children: Indications for surgical and nonsurgical treatment. *Urology* 1974;**3**:315.

Fair WR & others: Urinary tract infections in children. 1. Young girls with non-refluxing ureters. *West J Med* 1974;**121**:366.

Fehrenbaker LG, Kelalis PP, Stickler GB: Vesicoureteral reflux and ureteral duplication in children. *J Urol* 1972;**107**:862.

Garrett RA, Schlueter DP: Complications of antireflux operations: Causes and management. *J Urol* 1973;**109**:1002.

Geist RW, Antolak SJ Jr: The clinical problems of children with sterile ureteral reflux. *J Urol* 1972;**108**:343.

Glenn JF, Anderson EE: Distal tunnel ureteral reimplantation. *J Urol* 1967;**97**:623.

Gonzales ET, Leitner WA, Glenn JF: An analysis of various modes of therapy for vesicoureteral reflux. *Int Urol Nephrol* 1972;**4**:235.

Govan DE & others: Urinary tract infections in children. 3. Treatment of ureterovesical reflux. *West J Med* 1974;**121**:382.

Helin I: Clinical and experimental studies on vesico-ureteric reflux. *Scand J Urol Nephrol* 1975;**28** (**Suppl**):1.

Hendren WH: Complications of megaureter repair in children. *J Urol* 1975;**113**:228.

Hendren WH: Reoperation for the failed ureteral reimplantation. *J Urol* 1974;**111**:403.

Hodson CJ: The radiological contribution toward the diagnosis of chronic pyelonephritis. *Radiology* 1967;**88**:857.

Huland H & others: Vesicoureteral reflux in end stage renal disease. *J Urol* 1979;**121**:10.

Hutch JA: The mesodermal component: Its embryology, anatomy, physiology and role in prevention of vesicoureteral reflux. *J Urol* 1972;**108**:406.

Hutch JA: Ureteric advancement operation: Anatomy, technique, and early results. *J Urol* 1963;**89**:180.

Hutch JA, Amar AD: *Vesicoureteral Reflux and Pyelonephritis.* Appleton-Century-Crofts, 1972.

Johnston JH: Vesicoureteric reflux with urethral valves. *Br J Urol* 1979;**51**:100.

Johnston JH, Farkas A: The congenital refluxing megaureter: Experiences with surgical reconstruction. *Br J Urol* 1976;**48**:153.

Kiesavan P, Fowler R: Vesicoureteric reflux and ureterovesical obstruction. *Urology* 1977;**10**:105.

Kogan SJ, Freed SZ: Postoperative course of vesicoureteral reflux associated with benign obstructive prostatic disease. *J Urol* 1974;**112**:322.

Leadbetter GW Jr: Skin ureterostomy with subsequent ureteral reconstruction. *J Urol* 1972;**107**:462.

Lenaghan D & others: The natural history of reflux and long-term effects of reflux on the kidney. *J Urol* 1976;**115**:728.

Lewy PR, Belman AB: Familial occurrence of nonobstructive, noninfectious vesicoureteral reflux with renal scarring. *J Pediatr* 1975;**86**:851.

Lome LG, Williams DI: Urinary reconstruction following temporary cutaneous ureterostomy diversion in children. *J Urol* 1972;**108**:162.

Lyon RP: Renal arrest. *J Urol* 1973;**109**:707.

Lyon RP, Marshall SK, Scott MP: Treatment of vesicoureteral reflux: Point system based on twenty years of experience. *Urology* 1980;**16**:38.

Lyon RP, Marshall SK, Tanagho EA: The ureteral orifice: Its configuration and competency. *J Urol* 1969;**102**:504.

MacGregor M: Pyelonephritis lenta: Consideration of childhood urinary infection as the forerunner of renal insufficiency in later life. *Arch Dis Child* 1970;**45**:159.

Majd M, Belman AB: Nuclear cystography in infants and children. *Urol Clin North Am* 1979;**6**:395.

Marshall S & others: Ureterovesicoplasty: Selection of patients, incidence and avoidance of complications: A review of 3527 cases. *J Urol* 1977;**118**:829.

Middleton AW Jr, Nixon GW: Lack of correlation between upper tract changes on excretory urography and significant vesicoureteral reflux. *J Urol* 1980;**123**:227.

Miller HC, Caspari EW: Ureteral reflux as genetic trait. *JAMA* 1972;**220**:842.

Mulcahy JJ, Kelalis PP: Non-operative treatment of vesicoureteral reflux. *J Urol* 1978;**120**:336.

Nasrallah PF & others: Quantitative nuclear cystogram: Aid in determining spontaneous resolution of vesicoureteral reflux. *Urology* 1978;**12**:654.

Orikasa S & others: Effect of vesicoureteral reflux on renal growth. *J Urol* 1978;**119**:25.

Paquin AJ Jr: Ureterovesical anastomosis: The description and evaluation of a technique. *J Urol* 1959;**82**:573.

Parrott TS, Woodard JR: Reflux in opposite ureter after successful correction of unilateral vesicoureteral reflux. *Urology* 1976;**7**:276.

Politano VA, Leadbetter WF: An operative technique for correction of vesicoureteral reflux. *J Urol* 1958;**79**:932.

Rabinowitz R & others: Primary massive reflux in children. *Urology* 1979;**13**:248.

Rabinowitz R & others: Surgical treatment of the massively dilated ureter in children. 1. Management by cutaneous ureterostomy. *J Urol* 1977;**117**:658.

Randel DE: Surgical judgment in the management of vesicoureteral reflux. *J Urol* 1978;**119**:113.

Ransley PG: The renal papilla and intrarenal reflux. In: *Scientific Foundations of Urology.* Williams PI, Chisholm GD (editors). Year Book, 1976.

Ransley PG: Vesicoureteral reflux: Continuous surgical dilemma. *Urology* 1978;**12**:246.

Rees RWM: The effect of transurethral resection of the intravesical ureter during the removal of bladder tumours. *Br J Urol* 1969;**41**:2.

Roberts JA: Experimental pyelonephritis in the monkey. 4. Vesicoureteral reflux and bacteria. *Invest Urol* 1976;**14**:198.

Rolleston GL, Maling TMJ, Hodson CJ: Intrarenal reflux and the scarred kidney. *Arch Dis Child* 1974;**49**:531.

Rose JS, Glassberg KI, Waterhouse K: Intrarenal reflux and its relationship to renal scarring. *J Urol* 1975;**113**:400.

Sala NL, Rubi RA: Ureteral function in pregnant women. 5. Incidence of vesicoureteral reflux and its effect upon ureteral contractility. *Am J Obstet Gynecol* 1972;**112**:871.

Salvatierra O Jr, Kountz SL, Belzer FO: Primary vesicoureteral reflux and end-stage renal disease. *JAMA* 1973;**226**:1454.

Salvatierra O Jr, Tanagho EA: Reflux as a cause of end stage kidney disease: Report of 32 cases. *J Urol* 1977;**117**:441.

Savage DCL & others: Covert bacteriuria of childhood: A clinical and epidemiological study. *Arch Dis Child* 1973;**43**:8.

Schmidt JD & others: Vesicoureteral reflux: An inherited lesion. *JAMA* 1972;**220**:821.

Scott JES: The management of ureteric reflux in children. *Br J Urol* 1977;**49**:109.

Servadio C, Nissenkorn I, Baron J: Radioisotope cystography using ^{99m}Tc sulfur colloid for the detection and study of vesicoureteral reflux. *J Urol* 1974;**111**:750.

Siegel SR, Sokoloff B, Siegel B: Asymptomatic and symptomatic urinary tract infection in infancy. *Am J Dis Child* 1973;**125**:45.

Smith DR: Vesicoureteral reflux and other abnormalities of the ureterovesical junction. Chapter 10 in: *Urology*, 4th ed. Campbell MF, Harrison JH (editors). Saunders, 1978.

Snyder HM & others: Urodynamics in the prune belly syndrome. *Br J Urol* 1976;**48**:663.

Stephens FD: Intramural ureter and ureterocele. *Postgrad Med J* 1964;**40**:179.

Stephens FD: Treatment of megaloureters by multiple micturition. *Aust NZ J Surg* 1957;**27**:130.

Stickler GB & others: Primary interstitial nephritis with reflux: A cause of hypertension. *Am J Dis Child* 1971;**122**:144.

Tanagho EA: The pathogenesis and management of megaureter. Pages 85–116 in: *Reviews in Paediatric Urology*. Johnston JH, Goodwin WE (editors). North-Holland Publishing Co., 1974.

Tanagho EA: Surgical revision of the incompetent ureterovesical junction: A critical analysis of techniques and requirements. *Br J Urol* 1970;**42**:410.

Tanagho EA: Ureteral tailoring. *J Urol* 1971;**106**:194.

Tanagho EA, Guthrie TH, Lyon RP: The intravesical ureter in primary reflux. *J Urol* 1969;**101**:824.

Tanagho EA, Jonas U: Reduced bladder capacity: Cause of ureterovesical reflux. *Urology* 1974;**4**:421.

Tanagho EA, Meyers FH: Trigonal hypertrophy: A cause of ureteral obstruction. *J Urol* 1965;**93**:678.

Tanagho EA, Pugh RCB: The anatomy and function of the ureterovesical junction. *Br J Urol* 1963;**35**:151.

Tanagho EA, Smith DR, Guthrie TH: Pathophysiology of functional ureteral obstruction. *J Urol* 1970;**104**:73.

Tanagho EA & others: Primary vesicoureteral reflux: Experimental studies of its etiology. *J Urol* 1965;**93**:165.

Timothy RP, Decter A, Perlmutter AD: Ureteral duplication: Clinical findings and therapy in 46 children. *J Urol* 1971;**105**:445.

Tremewan RN & others: Diagnosis of gross vesico-ureteral reflux using ultrasonography. *Br J Urol* 1976;**48**:431.

Udall DA & others: Transureteroureterostomy. *Urology* 1973;**2**:401.

Uehling DT, Wear JB Jr: Concentrating ability after antireflux operation. *J Urol* 1976;**116**:1.

Vesicoureteral reflux and its familial distribution. (Editorial.) *Br Med J* 1975;**4**:726.

Wacksman J, Anderson EE, Glenn JF: Management of vesicoureteral reflux. *J Urol* 1978;**119**:814.

Waldbaum RS, Marshall VF: The prune belly syndrome: A diagnostic therapeutic plan. *J Urol* 1970;**103**:668.

Warren MM, Kelalis PP, Stickler GB: Unilateral ureteroneocystostomy: The fate of the contralateral ureter. *J Urol* 1972;**107**:466.

Welch KJ, Kearney GP: Abdominal muscular deficiency syndrome: Prune belly. *J Urol* 1974;**111**:693.

Whitaker RH: Reflux induced pelvi-ureteric obstruction. *Br J Urol* 1976;**48**:555.

Whitaker RH, Flower CDR: Ureters that show both reflux and obstruction. *Br J Urol* 1979;**51**:471.

Williams DI: The natural history of reflux. *Urol Int* 1971;**26**:350.

Williams GL & others: Vesicoureteric reflux in patients with bacteriuria in pregnancy. *Lancet* 1968;**2**:1202.

Willscher MK & others: Infection of the urinary tract after antireflux surgery. *J Pediatr* 1967;**89**:743.

Woodard JR, Holden S: The prognostic significance of fever in childhood urinary infections: Observations in 350 consecutive patients. *Clin Pediatr (Phila)* 1976;**15**:1051.

Zel G, Retik AB: Familial vesicoureteral reflux. *Urology* 1973;**2**:249.

Nonspecific Infections of the Urinary Tract | 12

Emil A. Tanagho, MD

The "nonspecific" infections of the genitourinary tract are a group of diseases having similar manifestations and caused by the gram-negative rods (eg, *Escherichia coli, Proteus vulgaris*) and gram-positive cocci (staphylococci and streptococci). They are to be distinguished from infections caused by "specific" organisms, each of which causes a clinically unique disease (eg, tuberculosis, gonorrhea, actinomycosis). In acute infections, a single organism is usually found; mixed infections are often seen in chronic stages.

By far the most common invaders are the gram-negative bacteria, particularly *E coli*. Others in this group are *Enterobacter aerogenes, P vulgaris* and *Proteus mirabilis*, and *Pseudomonas aeruginosa*. *Streptococcus faecalis* and *Staphylococcus aureus* are found on occasion. A pure coccal infection may suggest renal stone.

These infections can involve any of the urinary organs (or genital organs in the male) and can spread from a given locus to any or all of the others. Renal infections are of the greatest importance because of the parenchymal destruction they cause.

Identification of the type of bacteria (ie, rods or cocci) may be important in the empiric selection of medication.

PATHOGENESIS

Four Main Pathways of Entry Into the Urinary Tract

It is not always possible to trace the mode of entry of bacteria into the genitourinary tract. There are 4 major possibilities.

A. Ascending Infection: There is increasing evidence that ascending infection is the most common cause of urinary tract infection. The incidence of urinary infection—judged by age group and sex—permits certain inferences. Urosepsis is common from birth to age 10. At least 80% of cases are in females, and the incidence of pyelonephritis is relatively high. However, during the first 6 months of life, infection predominates in the male because of the presence of posterior urethral valves (Cohen, 1976; Bahna & Torp, 1975; Winberg & others, 1974). New infections are seldom seen from this age until age 20, at which time urinary infection again becomes common. Again, the great majority are in women, and the incidence parallels the years of sexual activity. This high incidence appears to be related to the short urethra of the female, which often harbors urinary pathogens that migrate from the perineum to the vaginal vestibule. Most of these infections involve the bladder only. At age 60 and beyond, the incidence of infection again increases; and because bladder neck obstruction and the inevitable vesical residual urine commonly affect males of this age, most of these patients are men. Secondary pyelonephritis in this latter group is uncommon.

These data strongly support the inference that the most common route of infection is up the urethra, particularly in the female. Pyelonephritis is quite common in very young people and is usually associated with demonstrable vesicoureteral reflux. Infection in older men is usually secondary to prostatitis or obstruction with or without reflux.

B. Hematogenous Spread: This is an uncommon pathway of bacterial invasion of the kidneys, prostate, and testes. During the course of many infections elsewhere in the body, bacteria are apt to enter the bloodstream; in fact, this may occur in a healthy person. These invaders are usually destroyed by normal body processes; however, if the number of bacteria is great, if they are virulent, and particularly if the field is receptive (eg, renal stone), infection of the genitourinary tract may occur. In experimental animals, intravenous injection of urinary pathogens leads to pyelonephritis only if the ureter is temporarily obstructed or the kidney traumatized. It seems conceivable that ureteral or ureteropelvic obstruction or vesicoureteral reflux could prepare the ground for hematogenous pyelonephritis by this mechanism.

The most obvious examples of renal infection via hematogenous invasion are tuberculosis (metastatic from the lungs) and renal carbuncle (metastatic from skin infection). Conversely, in the course of acute infections of the kidney or prostate, bacteria often enter the bloodstream.

C. Lymphatogenous Spread: There is firm evidence that infection can spread to the urinary tract through the lymphatic channels, but this

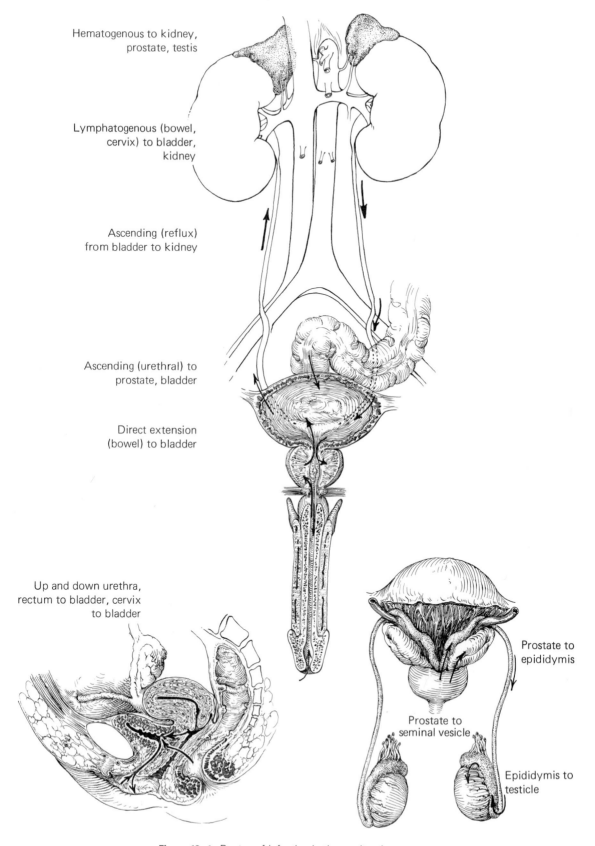

Hematogenous to kidney, prostate, testis

Lymphatogenous (bowel, cervix) to bladder, kidney

Ascending (reflux) from bladder to kidney

Ascending (urethral) to prostate, bladder

Direct extension (bowel) to bladder

Up and down urethra, rectum to bladder, cervix to bladder

Prostate to epididymis

Prostate to seminal vesicle

Epididymis to testicle

Figure 12–1. Routes of infection in the genitourinary tract.

probably occurs rarely. A few investigators believe that infections spread from the large bowel to the urinary tract through the lymphatics. Others think that cervicitis may cause vesical or renal infection by the spread of bacteria via the periureteral lymph vessels. Bloodstream infections of lymphatic origin are also a theoretic possibility.

D. Direct Extension From Another Organ: Intraperitoneal abscesses (appendiceal abscess, diverticulitis of the sigmoid) may involve and infect the urinary organs (bladder).

Factors Predisposing to Infection

Other factors that contribute to the establishment of bacteria in the genitourinary organs include the following:

A. Stasis and Obstruction: Bacteria are better able to gain a foothold if there is stasis or obstruction, as seen with distal urethral stenosis in little girls, enlarged prostate, and vesicoureteral reflux. Under these circumstances, pathogenic urethral bacteria ascending to the bladder become established in the bladder because the vesical defense mechanism is made inoperative by the presence of vesical residual urine.

Constipation in children has been related to urinary tract infection of both sexes (Neumann, de Domenico, & Nogrady, 1973). Many have great difficulty voiding. When the constipation is relieved, most of the children cease having infections.

B. Presence of a Foreign Body: A kidney containing a stone is apt to become infected even in the absence of obstruction. A foreign body introduced into the bladder (eg, indwelling catheter) will lead to infection. Such objects seem to lower the normal resistance to successful invasion by bacteria.

C. Continuous Source of Infection: This can occur from fistulas communicating between skin or bowel and urinary channels.

D. General Body Resistance: Resistance may be lowered in the course of debilitating illnesses and during periods of chronic or excessive fatigue, in which case infection gains a foothold more easily. Diabetes predisposes to urinary infection.

Organs & Pathways of Infection Within the Urinary Tract (Fig 12–1)

A. Kidney: It is becoming increasingly clear that the most common cause of renal infection is vesicoureteral reflux. Reflux is found in association with most instances of atrophic pyelonephritis. Hematogenous invasion is a rare route of infection.

B. Bladder: The bladder may become involved by bacteria descending from the kidney or, more commonly, ascending from the urethra or prostate. Direct bloodstream invasion of the bladder is undoubtedly rare. Lymphatogenous spread from cervical or uterine infection seems possible. Infections of the bowel may spread to the bladder by contiguity (diverticulitis of the sigmoid colon).

C. Prostate: The prostate is most commonly

infected by ascent of the urethral flora, whose numbers are increased in urethritis. Hematogenous invasion is a possibility.

D. Urethra: The urethra in both sexes usually becomes infected by ascending bacteria. These infections are usually nonvenereal. Deep ascent of these bacteria may cause cystitis and, if there is ureteral reflux, pyelonephritis. Infection may also descend to the urethra from prostate or bladder.

E. Epididymis: Infection usually reaches the epididymis by descent (reflux of urine) along the vas or the perivasal lymphatics from an infected prostate.

F. Testis: The testis is commonly invaded hematogenously by bacteria (pneumococci, brucellae, etc) or viruses (mumps, etc). Occasionally it becomes infected by direct extension from epididymal inflammation (both tuberculous and nonspecific).

Relation of Symptoms to Onset of Infection

If lower tract symptoms precede the onset of chills, fever, and renal pain, a primary (ascending) urologic infection is probably present. In this instance, vesicoureteral reflux should be suspected. If, however, the systemic symptoms precede the complaints referable to the lower urinary tract, metastatic infection or spread from some other area of infection may have occurred. In the latter instance, the extraurologic focus must be identified if possible.

Correlation of Factors That Cause & Perpetuate Urinary Tract Infections

The cause of urinary tract infections and their perpetuation can now be explained on a scientific basis. With few exceptions, the offending organism ascends the urethra and gains a foothold in the presence of vesical residual urine. The complication of pyelonephritis implies incompetency of the ureterovesical junction.

A. Source of Bacteria: Years ago, Helmholz showed that, with few exceptions, bacteria are found in significant numbers only in the distal 3–4 cm of the male urethra. Furthermore, it is unusual to find urinary pathogens in the male urethra. It is for these reasons that bladder or kidney infection develops late or not at all in males even in the presence of significant vesical residual urine (posterior urethral valves, enlarged prostate). It may be that anything that slows the voiding flow rate might allow further ascent of bacteria in males, so that the organisms finally reach the bladder.

In the female, however, the short urethra presents an entirely different problem. Cox, Lacy, & Hinman (1968) studied the urethral flora in women. In those without a history of urinary tract infections, 50% had bacteria in the proximal one-fourth of the urethra; of these bacteria, 27% were urinary pathogens. These organisms have their source in the perineum. In a group of women suffering from recurrent infections, 77% had bacteria in the proximal 1 cm of the urethra and 55% of the organisms were pathogenic to the urinary tract. Unfortunately, successful eradication of the urinary infection is not accompanied by sterilization of the urethra. The same organism may remain, in which case the next infection is caused by that bacterium; or a new pathogen may become established and cause a new infection.

These findings readily explain the common but mistaken observation that urinary infections are "difficult to cure." Infection usually is eradicated, but new infections develop in a high percentage of cases (Turck, Ronald, & Petersdorf, 1968). Certainly, a new organism represents a new infection, but the reappearance of the same bacterium does not necessarily imply relapse. The nature of the urethral flora governs the bacteriologic findings in the urine (Stamey & Mihara, 1980). Measures to correct vesical outlet obstruction (posterior urethral valves, distal urethral stenosis in little girls) usually stop recurrent urinary infection, but the pathogenic urethral bacteria are still present.

We may say, then, that with few exceptions the bacteria infecting the bladder ascend from the urethra.

B. The Vesical Defense Mechanism: Clinical experience demonstrates that the bladder has an intrinsic defense against bacteria. It is impossible to pass a catheter to the bladder without carrying bacteria into the bladder, but cystitis secondary to this procedure is rare unless there is vesical residual urine. Hinman (1968) showed that though significant numbers of bacteria were introduced into the bladders of normal young men by catheter, all had sterile urine within 72 hours without the use of antimicrobials. A similar observation was made in a group of women who required indwelling catheters for some days following certain gynecologic operations. Without the use of antimicrobials, their urine became sterile spontaneously. These workers were able to show experimentally that a bladder that completely empties itself seldom becomes infected. Complete voiding washes out most of the bacteria. Those few left in a film of urine on the vesical mucosa are killed. The implication is that the mucosa represents the intrinsic vesical defense mechanism against bacteria. Shom, Parsons, & Mulholland (1977) believe that mucoprotein on the mucosal surface of the bladder contributes to the defense mechanism.

C. Factors Causing Perpetuation of Urinary Infection: The urinary tract that completely empties itself at the time of voiding tends to remain sterile even though bacteria ascend to the bladder. If, however, there is some urologic abnormality that defeats this normal mechanism, the bacteria not only gain a foothold but the infection is perpetuated.

1. Vesical residual urine–Any defect that causes residual urine contributes to persistence of infection. Such diseases include neurogenic bladder, urethral obstruction, enlarged prostate, and cystocele. Although drugs may fail to keep the urine sterile, correcting the urologic disease will often cause the urine to clear spontaneously. If it does not, antimicrobials will then usually bring about cure.

2. Foreign bodies in the bladder–Even though meticulous hygiene and antibiotic coverage are practiced when an indwelling catheter is in place, after 10–21 days bacteriuria is almost always found. It cannot be eradicated until the catheter is removed. Following certain gynecologic operations, it has been customary to leave a urethral catheter in place for 3–10 days, and infection in such cases was almost inevitable. Recently, enthusiasm has developed for draining the bladder suprapubically with a small (8–10F) plastic catheter. The majority do not become infected, and spontaneous sterilization of the urine occurs on removal of the catheter. The remaining 10% respond promptly to antimicrobials. The presence of a stone in the bladder will cause infection to persist.

3. Vesicoureteral reflux–At the time of voiding, in the presence of vesicoureteral reflux, the bladder usually empties itself completely but some urine is forced into the ureter and kidney. Within a few minutes after voiding, this urine drains back to the bladder; in essence, the patient has not emptied the bladder. This defeats the vesical defense mechanism.

4. Urethrovesical reflux–In a child who suffers from spasm of the external periurethral sphincter caused by distal urethral stenosis (Tanagho & Miller, 1972), the proximal urethra becomes distended with voiding. The turbulent flow of urine in this segment washes urinary pathogens back into the bladder, which never quite empties itself (Hinman, 1966). Cystitis supervenes. In some adult women, periodic spasm of the external sphincter occurs as a result of anxiety or tension. This, too, may cause urethral bacteria to ascend to the bladder.

5. Residual urine in the upper urinary tract–Any disease causing retention of urine in the renal pelvis (ureteral stone, ureteropelvic junction obstruction) will perpetuate infection once it gains a foothold.

6. Foreign bodies in the kidney–Once renal infection ensues, the presence of a stone will tend to defeat efforts to sterilize the urine.

NONSPECIFIC INFECTIONS OF THE KIDNEYS

ACUTE PYELONEPHRITIS

The term "pyelonephritis" is used because infections of the renal pelvis alone ("pyelitis") do not occur; however, it is the "nephritis" that is important.

Bacteria can reach the kidney through the bloodstream, or they may travel up a ureter that has an incompetent ureterovesical valve. The latter mechanism is by far the most common. It has been shown that vesicoureteral reflux may occur during acute cystitis but ceases when the infection has been cured. This explains the onset of secondary pyelonephritis. If obstruction, reflux, or stasis is present, the chances for the bacteria to gain a foothold are increased. These factors also tend to perpetuate the infection.

One-third of pregnant women with pyelonephritis will exhibit reflux. After termination of the pregnancy, reflux disappears. It is for this reason that the not uncommon bacteriuria seen in pregnancy (6% incidence) is potentially dangerous.

Pathology

A. Gross: The kidney may be greatly enlarged as a result of edema. The surface may be dull. On cut section, the sharp demarcation between cortex and medulla is lost; multiple small abscesses may be visible. The pelvic mucosa is often injected and roughened.

B. Microscopic: There is diffuse or spotty inflammation characterized by leukocytic infiltration, edema, and small hemorrhagic areas. The tubular epithelium may desquamate if the infection is severe. The glomeruli are much less involved; in fact, they are peculiarly immune to inflammatory change except in the most severe cases.

Pathogenesis (Fig 12–2)

With few exceptions, acute pyelonephritis develops from infection in the bladder through the mechanism of vesicoureteral reflux. If the ureterovesical junction, anatomically and physiologically, is of "borderline" quality, cure of the infection will cause the "valve" to revert to competency; a cystogram taken at this time will fail to reveal reflux. When the junction is grossly abnormal, response to antimicrobial therapy may be slow; sterilization of the urine may not be possible. Even in the presence of sterile urine, reflux persists. This inability to completely empty the urinary tract makes the vesical defense mechanism inoperative; recurring infections are therefore common.

If the urine becomes sterile, the renal lesion has been healed, although new infections may occur. Some of these patients may become afebrile, although bacteriuria persists. This represents the asymptomatic stage of chronic pyelonephritis.

Each acute infection leads to healing by scar. The kidney becomes smaller and its edge irregular. In the past, these radiographic findings have been called "chronic pyelonephritis." This is not correct, since these scars represent evidence of previous infections, and such a patient may have had sterile urine for many years. The x-ray, then, is of no help in judging whether active infection exists, although the findings of bacteriuria and reflux imply the presence of chronic pyelonephritis.

Clinical Findings

A. Symptoms: At the onset, there is a severe

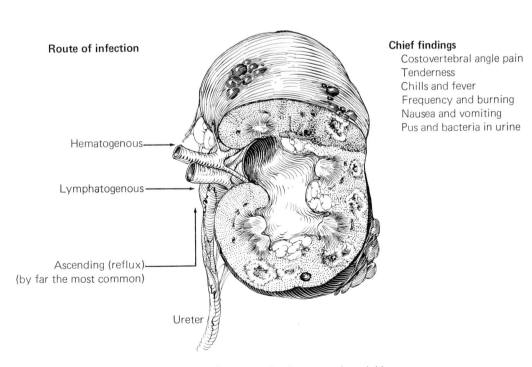

Route of infection

Hematogenous

Lymphatogenous

Ascending (reflux)
(by far the most common)

Ureter

Chief findings
Costovertebral angle pain
Tenderness
Chills and fever
Frequency and burning
Nausea and vomiting
Pus and bacteria in urine

Figure 12–2. Pathogenesis of acute pyelonephritis.

constant ache over one or both kidneys (flank and back) due to distention of the renal capsule caused by edema. The pain may radiate to the lower abdominal quadrant. Young children seldom complain of localized renal pain, which is apt to be referred as poorly localized abdominal discomfort. Symptoms of cystitis develop: frequency, nocturia, urgency, and burning on urination. The patient is quite prostrated, and nausea and vomiting are usually present.

B. Signs: The patient appears to be quite sick. Intermittent high fever with chills is to be expected. The pulse rate is, however, the best index of the severity of the infection. If the infection is due to *E coli*, the pulse rate may be only 90/min; with staphylococci, it may reach 140. Tenderness is present over the affected kidney, which is usually not palpable because of muscle spasm. Fist percussion over the costovertebral angle will be quite painful. Abdominal distention may be marked and rebound tenderness may be present, suggesting an intraperitoneal lesion. Auscultation usually reveals a quiet intestine.

C. Laboratory Findings: The white blood count may reach 40,000/μL, and the neutrophil count is elevated. The sedimentation rate is increased. The urine is usually cloudy, shows a little protein, and contains large amounts of pus and bacteria. A few red cells may also be noted. Quantitative cultures will be positive and may be helpful in treatment of refractory infections, in which case sensitivity studies should be done. Renal function as measured by specific gravity of urine or PSP will be only slightly affected unless there is overwhelming sepsis, with bilateral multiple cortical abscesses or necrotizing papillitis. Serial blood cultures should be done on any patient with urinary tract infection who has chills and fever, since bacteremia is not uncommon in such cases.

D. X-Ray Findings: A plain film of the abdomen may show some obliteration of the renal shadow owing to edema of the kidney and perinephric fat. Suspicious calcifications (stones) should be sought. Excretory urograms during the acute stage usually show little diminution in function, although the pelvis and calices on the affected side may be small because of secretion of a small volume of urine as compared to the uninvolved kidney. These films are most valuable in surveying the tract for the presence of obstruction or possible vesicoureteral reflux. When the infection is severe, the involved kidney may be enlarged, show a decreased nephrogram effect on the immediate film, and reveal little or no caliceal radiopaque material. After appropriate therapy, the urograms return to normal (Davidson & Talner, 1973).

Although cystography might reveal vesicoureteral reflux during the acute stage of infection, such an examination is contraindicated at this time. Excretory urography and cystography should be done later, after the infection is controlled.

E. Radionuclide Imaging: Imaging the kidneys with gallium-67 can be used to localize the site of infection. Hurwitz & others (1976) claim 86% accuracy, although some false positives and false negatives were encountered.

Differential Diagnosis

Pancreatitis causes pain, which may be posterior, and the position and degree of pain may cause confusion with pyelonephritis. Serum amylase, however, will be elevated and pyuria will not be found.

Basal pneumonia may cause pain in the subcostal area, but it is usually pleuritic in type. Examination of the chest should make that diagnosis.

Acute appendicitis or acute disease of the gallbladder may be suspected if the patient's pain is largely anterior and if there is muscle spasm and rebound tenderness in the right upper or lower quadrant. Careful palpation over the kidney should reveal some tenderness, and proper urinalysis should be definitive.

Acute diverticulitis of the descending colon may cause pain in the left flank. Usually, however, a history of change in bowel habits may be elicited. The urine is normal. A barium enema will reveal evidence of changes in the bowel.

Herpes zoster affecting the somatic segments of the renal area (T12, L1) can simulate pain arising from the kidney. However, the pain is superficial, and skin hypersensitivity can be demonstrated. The onset of the typical skin changes of shingles will settle the problem.

Complications

If diagnosis is delayed and treatment inadequate, the infection may become chronic. This is particularly true if vesicoureteral reflux is present. The chronic form is seldom recognized because it is usually silent and because few or no pus cells are found in the urine. The bacteria can be found, however, if they are diligently sought. The chronic infection may lead to (1) renal insufficiency; (2) secondary arteriolar sclerosis, which may cause renal ischemia and, in turn, hypertension; or (3) stone formation and further renal damage.

Bacteremia or septicemia of renal origin may develop in the acute stage of fulminating pyelonephritis and may cause infection or even multiple cortical abscesses of the other kidney. Metastatic abscesses may develop in other organs. Bacteremic shock is occasionally seen, especially when gram-negative rods invade the bloodstream.

In the late stage of infected hydronephrosis or pyonephrosis, particularly in diabetic patients, gas may be liberated in the kidney, leading to an air urogram on the plain film. The mortality rate from this type of sepsis is significant.

Prevention

Pyelonephritis in the male infant implies the

presence of significant urinary obstruction (eg, posterior urethral valves). Excretory urography and, when indicated, retrograde cystography—or even endoscopy—should be done once the first infection is controlled.

Renal infection in a little girl suggests the presence of vesicoureteral reflux. Intravenous urograms and a voiding cystourethrogram are therefore essential. Treatment of the accompanying distal urethral stenosis will improve vesical hydrodynamics and lessen the chance for the development of cystitis. If there is no cystitis, there can be no pyelonephritis.

Pyelonephritis in a woman suggests incompetency of the ureterovesical segment. Radiologic study is indicated. Steps should be taken to prevent the onset of cystitis (see section on prevention of acute cystitis).

Infection of the kidney in the male is usually secondary to obstruction, eg, by ureteral stone or an enlarged prostate. Such lesions should be sought and treated.

Treatment

A. Specific Measures: Urine should first be obtained for microscopy, cultures, and sensitivity tests. Based upon the findings gained from the stained smear of the sediment, a relatively nontoxic drug, chosen empirically, should be started. Preferably it should afford both a high urine and tissue concentration (eg, one of the tetracyclines, ampicillin). Ureteral obstruction may have to be relieved by cystoscopic means. This may mean extraction of a ureteral stone or temporary drainage with an indwelling ureteral catheter, as in acute ureteral obstruction due to pregnancy or to extrinsic pressure on the ureter from cancer.

If other methods fail, surgical treatment of obstruction may be necessary (eg, removal of a ureteral stone).

B. General Measures: Pain must be relieved by appropriate drugs. Vesical irritability can be minimized by alkalinizing the urine (which may require 12–20 g/d of sodium bicarbonate) or by giving an antispasmodic such as belladonna or atropine with phenobarbital. Bed rest is definitely indicated during the acute phase of the infection. Adequate urinary output (1000 mL/d) should be maintained, but indiscriminate forcing of fluids only leads to urinary dilution of the antimicrobial drug being administered. Nausea and vomiting may necessitate the administration of parenteral fluids.

C. Failure of Response: If no clinical improvement occurs in 48–72 hours, either the wrong drug is being used or obstruction or stasis is present. Obtain excretory urograms, and look for changes suggesting vesicoureteral reflux or obstruction. Obtain a report on the culture and sensitivity tests and switch to an appropriate bactericidal drug, observing the usual precautions against toxicity.

D. Follow-Up Care: Even when a satisfactory clinical response is achieved, the urinary sediment must be examined for pathogens periodically for 2 months. Absence of symptoms is not proof of cure, nor is absence of pus cells in the urine.

Prognosis

The prognosis is good if the response to antibiotics is complete, ie, if all infecting organisms are eliminated. If obstruction or reflux is present but is not discovered, recurrences are to be expected. Persistence of bacteriuria requires explanation. Estimation of vesical residual urine, excretory urograms, and cystograms must then be done.

CHRONIC PYELONEPHRITIS

Etiology & Pathogenesis

The term chronic pyelonephritis implies the persistent presence of bacteria in the kidney. An outdated medical tenet states that once a kidney becomes infected it is difficult to cure by medical means. The implication is that renal infection is not often curable by the administration of appropriate drugs, as are infections of the lungs, meninges, and other organs and structures. It has become increasingly clear that if the urine of such a patient can be made sterile, another attack represents a new infection. The failure of medical treatment is readily explained by the omission of a proper urologic work-up seeking evidence of stasis of urine and, particularly, vesicoureteral reflux. The cure rate of recurrent or chronic pyelonephritis is at least 80% if refluxing ureterovesical valves are corrected by medical means or by surgery, whereas medical treatment alone permanently cures only 40–50% of a similar group of patients. The cure of a disease requires understanding of its cause.

The source of the bacteria is, with few exceptions, the urethra; they ascend to the bladder with ease, particularly in women after sexual intercourse. If the ureterovesical valves are entirely normal, the infection is confined to the bladder. In the presence of a "borderline" valve, acute cystitis may cause such a valve to become temporarily incompetent, thus causing pyelonephritis. Cure by antibiotics again leads to competency of the ureterovesical junction. If the vesical urine can be kept sterile, pyelonephritis is prevented. If, however, the ureterovesical junction is grossly abnormal, bacteria in the bladder reach the kidney and, since the infection is then perpetuated, true chronic pyelonephritis persists. Recent observations have made it clear that healed or atrophic pyelonephritis, portrayed on x-rays, is usually associated with vesicoureteral reflux.

In the absence of reflux, hematogenous pyelonephritis may occur secondary to ureteral obstruction or the presence of a renal stone. Again, treatment of the cause must be considered if infection is to be permanently relieved.

It should be pointed out that "chronic pyelo-nephritis" cannot be diagnosed on urograms. Evidence of scarring may be noted, but this represents healing from previous infections and tells us nothing about the presence or absence of renal bacteriuria. These changes should be read as "healed pyelonephritis."

Pathology

Grossly, the kidney is of normal size or small, depending upon the stage and duration of the disease. The capsule is pale and strips poorly. The surface of the kidney is often pitted and depressed, with scarred areas. The cut surface may show fairly well defined cortical and medullary zones, but in a more advanced stage the tissues may be pale and fibrotic. The pelvic mucosa is pale and fibrotic also (Fig 12–3).

Microscopically, the parenchyma is diffusely infiltrated with plasma cells and lymphocytes. The tubules show varying stages of degeneration; some may show considerable dilatation and may contain proteinaceous casts. The glomeruli may be fibrotic, even hyalinized. Considerable thickening of arteries and arterioles is obvious. Not infrequently, the kidney shows areas of acute infection as well as varying degrees of healed disease.

It is often stated that evidence of pyelonephritis is found in 10–15% of autopsies. As diagnostic criteria for this entity are tightened, the incidence is now considered to be in the range of 1–2% (Freedman, 1967).

Many instances of xanthogranulomatous pyelonephritis have been reported. The kidney is usually functionless. It is enlarged, often nodular, and may suggest carcinoma. Sheets of lipid-filled histiocytes, plasma cells, and lymphocytes in a fibrous stroma are microscopically visible; these signs may be confused with those of renal cancer even after radiographic study.

Clinical Findings

A. Symptoms: Except during acute exacerbations, there are apt to be few symptoms. There may be mild discomfort over the kidney and some degree of vesical irritability. These, however, may be entirely absent. Vague gastrointestinal complaints may be noted, particularly in children. Unexplained low-grade fever or anemia may be the only clue to the presence of disease. Hypertension is common, particularly in children (Still & Cotton, 1967).

When acute exacerbations occur, localized renal pain may be present and the patient may complain of vesical symptoms. This clinical picture may be misinterpreted as a recurrent acute infection rather than an acute stage of chronic infection.

If the disease is advanced and bilateral (atrophic pyelonephritis), the presenting symptoms may be those of uremia.

B. Signs: There are usually no physical findings unless exacerbation is present, in which case some degree of localized renal tenderness may be elicited. Hypertension may be discovered.

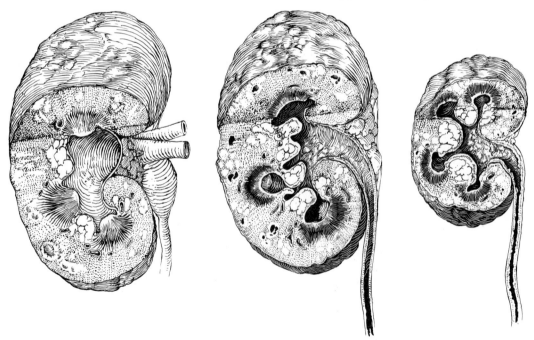

Figure 12–3. Progressive pathologic changes in kidney resulting from repeated attacks of acute pyelonephritis with progressive scarring. **Left:** Early stage of focal parenchymal scarring. **Center:** Progressive scarring with narrowing of the necks of the calices, which therefore become dilated (Fig 12–4). **Right:** End stage of recurrent pyelonephritis (stage of atrophy).

C. Laboratory Findings: Anemia may be found, especially if the patient is uremic. The white blood count may be elevated during an acute stage but otherwise is usually normal.

The urinary sediment may or may not contain white cells, but some bacteria can almost always be demonstrated in the stained smear or culture. The degree of seriousness of an infection cannot be gauged by numbers of pus cells or organisms.

Quantitative cultures should be obtained and sensitivity tests performed.

Some type of renal function test should be done. If the PSP is low, bilateral renal damage, residual urine, or reflux should be suspected.

D. X-Ray Findings: A plain film of the abdomen may show that one or both kidneys are small (atrophic). Evidence of stone may be noted. Excretory urograms may be normal, but changes are usually seen that suggest scarring from repeated attacks of renal infection (small kidney; indentations of the lateral borders, representing scars; narrowing of the infundibula where they join the pelvis; dilatation and roughening of the calices; and delayed excretion and poor concentration of the medium; see Figs 12–3 and 12–4). Dilatation or fullness of the ureter may signify vesicoureteral reflux (Fig 11–7).

Retrograde urograms will show similar changes. Voiding cystourethrography demon-strates vesicoureteral reflux in at least half of patients with scarred kidneys.

E. Instrumental Examination: On cystoscopy, the bladder wall may show evidence of chronic infection. Abnormal configuration and position of a ureteral orifice may be compatible with a refluxing ureterovesical junction. Stained smears and cultures of vesical and renal urine specimens will place the site of infection accurately. Only in this way can the presence of active renal infection be established. Renal function tests (PSP) will measure the functioning of each kidney separately. Diminution may be noted in cases of advanced disease.

Differential Diagnosis

Recurrent acute cystitis may cause symptoms identical to those of a mild attack of pyelonephritis. A history of recurrent attacks of vesical irritability associated with bacteriuria indicates the need for excretory urograms and possibly cystograms. These should allow differentiation.

Chronic cystitis can only be differentiated from chronic pyelonephritis by the absence of renal infection as demonstrated by ureteral catheterization. Urograms are normal in cystitis but show evidence of scarring in pyelonephritis.

Tuberculosis may mimic chronic pyelonephritis perfectly. The absence of bacteria on the methylene blue stain or culture of sediment con-

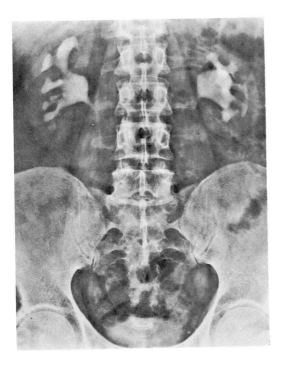
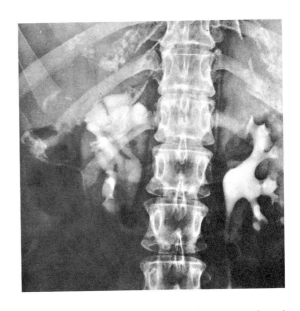

Figure 12–4. Healed pyelonephritis. *Left:* Excretory urogram showing flattening and clubbing of the calices; edge of renal shadow close to ends of the calices. These changes reflect numerous past episodes of acute pyelonephritis. *Right:* Excretory urogram showing marked atrophy of parenchyma of right kidney, with calices of upper pole extending to renal capsule. Left kidney normal.

taining pus cells should suggest tuberculosis. Further bacteriologic studies will confirm this. Urography may reveal parenchymal calcifications and moth-eaten (ulcerated) caliceal changes typical of tuberculosis.

Xanthogranulomatous pyelonephritis and cancer of the kidney may be confused on urography. In the former, the kidney is usually functionless, whereas with cancer the kidney can almost always be visualized by means of excretory urography. Angiography or an isotope scan (see Chapter 8) should differentiate the two.

Complications

A. Unilateral Infection: In the atrophic stage, hypertension may develop owing to renal ischemia from severe arteriolar sclerosis. During the stage of exacerbation, bacteremia may occur, with involvement of the other kidney.

B. Bilateral Infection: In the late stage of bilateral renal infection, the incidence of hypertension is high. The end stage is often uremia.

C. General: Stone formation is enhanced in the presence of urea-splitting organisms, which produce an alkaline urine, since calcium salts are less soluble in an alkaline medium.

Prevention

Recurrent or chronic renal infection is usually secondary to vesicoureteral reflux or obstruction. (See section on prevention of acute pyelonephritis.)

Treatment

The finding of pus and bacteria in the urine does not establish the diagnosis of pyelonephritis. The most common cause of these abnormal elements is acute or chronic cystitis, particularly in adults.

A. Specific Measures:

1. Medical–Intensive chemotherapeutic and antibiotic therapy is needed. The choice of drug depends upon antimicrobial sensitivity tests prepared from cultures of the urine. The drug should be given for 2–3 weeks. This should be followed by suppressive therapy for months or years. Suitable drugs include the sulfonamides, methenamine plus a urinary acidifier, or nitrofurantoin. Palmer (1974) has shown that a severely infected kidney fails to concentrate many drugs because of tubular damage, thus lessening their effectiveness.

In pyelonephritis of pregnancy, an acute attack should be treated with a relatively nontoxic drug. Even if this is successful, chronic suppressive therapy should be continued until a few weeks after delivery.

2. Local–Eradication of chronic prostatic infection or treatment of urethral stricture may contribute to the ultimate control of the renal infection.

3. Surgical–Correction of obstructive lesions may be indicated. If vesicoureteral reflux has been demonstrated and sterilization of the urine cannot

be achieved or maintained, repair of the ureterovesical junction must be considered. If one kidney is badly damaged, nephrectomy may be the procedure of choice.

B. Treatment of Complications: If the disease is bilateral and function is impaired (loss of concentrating power), a urine output of 1000–1500 mL is necessary to facilitate the removal of metabolic waste products. If hypertension is present in association with a unilateral atrophic kidney (and provided the other kidney functions perfectly), nephrectomy should be considered.

Prognosis

If the diagnosis is delayed until both kidneys are badly scarred, only medical therapy is indicated in the hope of conserving what functioning tissue is left. Dialysis or even renal transplantation may become necessary (see Chapters 25 and 26). Fortunately, repair of the incompetent ureterovesical junction leads to permanent sterilization of the urine in a high percentage of patients with chronic pyelonephritis.

BACTEREMIC SHOCK

Etiology

The genitourinary tract is one of the common sources of bacteremia. Bacteremia may develop spontaneously following obstruction (eg, an infected kidney suddenly occluded by a calculus) or instrumentation of an infected prostatic urethra, or vesical bacteria may be forced up through incompetent ureterovesical valves under the hydrostatic pressure of an irrigating solution.

There is an increased incidence of bacteremia wherever antibiotics are used indiscriminately. Patients receiving immunosuppressive drugs (eg, renal transplantation) and those with diabetes, cirrhosis, cancer, burns, and peritonitis are at greater risk.

Most cases of septic shock are seen in patients over age 40, although it is not uncommon following septic abortion. Rowe, Buckner, & Newmark (1975) have observed this complication in many surgical pediatric patients. An increasing incidence of shock caused by *Serratia* and *Candida* infections has been observed.

Shock is caused by cardiac decompensation or inadequate circulating blood volume. It reflects a failure of blood flow to the cells; the hypotension is secondary. Perhaps 30% of patients with gram-negative bacteriuria will go into shock. The immediate cause is liberation of endotoxin from the walls of dead bacteria. Septic shock is relatively rare in gram-positive infections, since these organisms liberate an exotoxin.

Pathogenesis & Pathology

Shock due to trauma or heart failure causes

constriction of the precapillary sphincters (increased peripheral resistance) and is associated with decreased cardiac output. Shock caused by gram-negative bacteremia initially reflects increased peripheral resistance, but in most cases this rapidly progresses to decreased peripheral resistance and increased cardiac output. It seems that—though capillary resistance persists—this resistance is overcome by the opening of arteriovenous shunts that deprive cells of both oxygen and nutrition. The postcapillary sphincters remain closed. Plasma and, to a lesser extent, red cells leak into the interstitial tissues because of increased hydrostatic pressure, leading to diminished circulating blood volume. Patients with bacteremic shock who have a low cardiac output probably have suffered prior myocardial damage; this group, therefore, has a poorer prognosis.

The heart and brain suffer relatively less anoxia than other tissues and organs, for vasoconstriction does not occur in these vital organs. Cerebral anoxia is manifested by apathy or even stupor. The anoxic myocardium may fail.

The liver normally converts lactate to pyruvate. In shock, this process is impaired and serum lactic acid rises. This implies diminution of hepatic blood flow. Diminished renal blood flow results in oliguria with retention of water and salt. If treatment is delayed, acute tubular necrosis may supervene.

Disseminated intravascular coagulation is always present in shock. This diffuse coagulation consumes large numbers of platelets, fibrinogen, and other clotting factors, thus depleting the blood of normal coagulating power. Hemorrhages are common, particularly from the gastrointestinal tract. Ischemia of gastric mucosa may also lead to bleeding. Damage to the reticuloendothelial system will lower the host's resistance to bacteria.

The most serious lesions occur in the lungs. There is a decrease in surfactant; edema or even hemorrhage into the intra-alveolar septa occurs, leading to increased pulmonary compliance. Fibrin thrombi and even hyaline membranes may be noted. Loss of plasma from congested capillaries contributes to interstitial edema. Because of sludging, disseminated intravascular coagulation may develop throughout the body, but particularly in the lungs. When peripheral and visceral capillaries open up as a consequence of definitive treatment, this sludged material is filtered by the lungs, which may be overwhelmed.

Perhaps 20–40% of the alveoli become nonfunctioning because of the development of these lesions. Their blood receives no oxygen, and venous admixture occurs. For this reason, Pa_{O_2} is low (50–60 mm Hg) despite the addition of O_2 to the inspired air. Because of shunting across the capillary beds throughout the body, the partial pressure of O_2 in the veins approaches that in the arterial tree, reflecting serious tissue anoxia.

Anoxia leads to an increase in respiratory rate. CO_2 is blown off, leading to respiratory alkalosis. As anoxia persists, anaerobic metabolism develops, leading to the accumulation of lactic acid and metabolic acidosis. Cellular damage and even death of cells ensues.

The most common cause of death in septic shock is pulmonary failure (shock lung). The problem, then, is to immediately attack the cause of the shock (ie, bacteremia) and the shock itself.

Clinical Findings

A. Symptoms: The patient develops fever ranging from 38.5 to 40 C (101–104 F) and associated chills. Anxiety may be present early, followed by apathy as the process continues. There is evidence of bacterial infection (eg, urinary tract, peritoneum) and often a history of urethral instrumentation a few hours previously.

B. Signs: Cloudy mentation is usual when hypotension supervenes. Peripheral cyanosis with a moist, pale skin is present. Respirations are shallow and rapid. The pulse is rapid and thready. The blood pressure is about 70/40 mm Hg, or 25 mm Hg below the hypertensive patient's normal systolic pressure. Capillary refill of the nail beds is prolonged. Oliguria is to be expected. Hours may pass, however, before hypotension develops.

C. Laboratory Findings: Leukopenia is usually observed in infants. The white count is elevated, with a shift to the left. The number of platelets is diminished because of consumption coagulopathy. The PCV is usually increased as a result of loss of plasma into the interstitial tissues. Blood volume studies may be misleading. Because of diminished renal blood flow, urine specific gravity is increased, and the ratio of serum blood urea nitrogen to creatinine may exceed the normal 10:1 ratio. In most instances, the ECG will suggest myocardial infarction, but these changes merely reflect diminished coronary artery blood flow. There is an increase in the blood levels of fatty acids and glucose.

Since the source of the bacteremia is often the urinary tract, pyuria and bacteriuria may be found. Urine cultures and serial blood cultures with sensitivity testing are mandatory. *E coli* is the most common offender.

Since pulmonary insufficiency is the rule, frequent estimates of arterial pH and Pa_{O_2} as well as serum electrolytes are necessary. Serum lactate levels (normal, 0.44–1.8 mmol/L) are important in estimating prognosis. Values of 5 mmol/L or more are associated with a high mortality rate and reflect the degree of tissue anoxia. On the other hand, a progressive decrease in the serum lactate level following therapy is a most encouraging sign.

If possible, the cardiac index should be measured. A high output improves prognosis. Estimation of peripheral resistance is helpful. Progressive increase from an initial low level after therapy has been instituted implies increased tissue oxygenation via opening capillaries.

D. X-Ray Findings: A chest film may show diffuse alveolar infiltrates that may progress to complete consolidation as part of "shock lung."

Differential Diagnosis

Simple bacteremia is accompanied by chills and fever, but hypotension and oliguria do not occur. This is particularly true of coccal infections. Secondary heart failure may lead to hypotension, thus obscuring the diagnosis. Estimation of central venous pressure will facilitate differentiation (see below).

Acute cardiac failure, especially when secondary to myocardial infarction, may cause sudden hypotension. Evidence of overwhelming infection is absent.

Hypovolemic shock may be caused by marked dehydration (eg, vomiting, diarrhea) or hemorrhage. Symptoms and signs of infection are absent. Basically, treatment of this condition is as for bacteremic shock, ie, restoration of circulating blood volume.

Complications

The primary infection may not respond to antibiotic therapy. Prolonged hypoxia and hypotension may lead to acute renal tubular necrosis or myocardial infarction. Heart failure may ensue. Hemorrhages from bowel ulceration or disseminated intravascular coagulation (consumptive coagulopathy) may develop. The most serious complication is, however, acute respiratory failure. Even though infection is conquered and the microcirculatory lesion is improved, irreversible and progressive pulmonary damage may lead to death.

Prevention

If urologic instrumentation is necessary, the urine should first be sterilized. There is no convincing evidence that prophylactic antibiotic therapy reduces the incidence of bacteremia.

If an indwelling catheter is necessary, aseptic technic must be used in its passage. A closed drainage system should be used to decrease the chances of ascent of bacteria to the bladder, but the development of bacteriuria is inevitable. Careful intermittent catheterization markedly decreases the incidence of infection but creates a problem of availability of personnel to perform the procedure.

Treatment

Since early diagnosis and immediate treatment significantly influence prognosis, the clinician must be on the alert for this impending catastrophe. If a patient at risk—eg, one undergoing urethral instrumentation—is observed to develop anxiety or lethargy, fever, rapid and shallow respiration, and an accelerated, thready pulse, the possibility of bacteremia with impending shock should be considered and preventive measures instituted. Begin appropriate antibiotic therapy immediately and give 1 L of crystalloid or (preferably) colloid solution intravenously. An intravenous bolus of a corticosteroid should be administered (see below).

If the patient is in shock, the aim of treatment is to combat the infection, restore circulating blood volume, and improve the perfusion of vital organs (heart, brain, and lungs). Abscesses must be drained. With septic abortion, hysterectomy must be considered. An obstructing ureteral stone should be removed or bypassed by catheter.

A. Specific Measures:

1. Initial step–

a. Insert a urethral catheter to monitor urine flow.

b. Introduce a small plastic catheter into the superior vena cava or right atrium so that central venous pressure can be estimated. Its position should be checked by x-ray. Pressures of 0–4 cm of water imply poor filling of the heart due to diminished circulating blood volume; levels of 6–12 cm of water are compatible with adequate filling of the right heart but can occur if both cardiac failure and diminished blood volume are present. A pressure above 15 cm of water is diagnostic of heart failure. The central venous pressure affords a rough estimate of blood volume.

2. Antibiotics–If the organism from the primary site has been identified and sensitivity tests have been obtained, the best drug or combination of drugs should be administered. If the offending organism has not yet been identified, gram-negative bacillary infection should be assumed. Empiric therapy should be begun immediately. Gentamicin is the drug of choice. Give 1.5 mg/kg intramuscularly every 8 hours. Kanamycin plus cephalothin or chloramphenicol is also efficacious. Subsequent bacteriologic reports may suggest the use of other antimicrobial drugs. If oliguria or renal failure is present, less frequent administration will be necessary. (See Table 12–1.)

3. Steps to improve circulating blood volume and perfusion of vital organs–

a. Parenteral fluids–If the central venous pressure is low, immediately begin infusion of a crystalloid solution (eg, normal saline or Ringer's injection). The hematocrit will probably be elevated because of selective loss of plasma from the engorged capillaries. Colloid solutions should be administered as soon as possible, because more than 75% of crystalloids and water enter the extravascular space. The colloids include low-molecular-weight dextran, pooled plasma (risk of hepatitis), blood, or albumin (5% solution). Their oncotic pressure tends to draw plasma back into the capillaries, thus lessening tissue and cellular edema and helping to wash sludged red and white cells and platelets into the general circulation. Low-molecular-weight dextran decreases blood viscosity and combats platelet adhesiveness. These fluids can be pushed until the central venous pressure approaches 12–14 cm of water, care being taken to seek signs of cardiac overload.

Even though the central venous pressure is within the normal range, a test loading dose of 500 mL of a crystalloid or colloid solution should be rapidly infused. An immediate rise in pressure of 5 cm of water suggests that more fluid may lead to heart failure. If the patient tolerates this amount, additional fluid should be given. Increased urine secretion as determined by hourly measurements of output and clearing mentation are favorable signs even though the peripheral blood pressure rises only moderately or not at all. Evidence of improving tissue perfusion is far more important than an increase in peripheral blood pressure.

In most instances, antibiotic therapy plus correction of the diminished circulating blood volume is all that is needed for complete recovery.

b. Glucocorticoids–If the above steps do not result in significant improvement within 3–4 hours, corticosteroids should be administered in pharmacologic doses (20–50 times physiologic doses). These agents appear to protect the cellular mitochondrial membrane from rupturing and releasing lysosomal enzymes that would destroy the cell. They may also preserve the integrity of small vessels and decrease adhesiveness of platelets. In addition, they may also have an inotropic effect. Since the antibiotics continually kill the bacteria, there is a constant liberation of endotoxin. Evidence suggests that corticosteroids protect the capillaries from the action of endotoxin. Give one of the following as a bolus intravenously: dexamethasone, 3–6 mg/kg; methylprednisolone succinate, 15–30 mg/kg; or hydrocortisone sodium succinate, 50–150 mg/kg. Repeat this dose every 4–6 hours. These drugs can be given for as long as 3 or even 4 days and then stopped abruptly without apparent harm. In a controlled study, Schumer (1976) noted a significant reduction in the mortality rate when steroids were used instead of saline only.

c. Vasodilators–If, after restoration of circulating blood volume and the administration of corticosteroids, significant improvement has not occurred, the use of vasodilators should be considered.

(1) Alpha-adrenergic blocking agent–Phenoxybenzamine (Dibenzyline) blocks the vasoconstricting action of the catecholamines, which are circulating in large amounts during shock. The usual dose is 1 mg/kg in 100 mL of saline given over a period of 2 hours. Since it is a long-acting drug, titration cannot be done.

(2) Beta-adrenergic stimulating agent–Isoproterenol decreases venous pooling and arterial tone and increases venous return. In addition, this drug has both inotropic and chronotropic effects. Overdose may lead to tachycardia and arrhythmias. Add 2.5–5 mg of the drug to 500 mL of 5% dextrose in water and run the infusion at a rate of about 1 mL/min. If there is no change in central venous

pressure, pulse pressure, or urine output, the rate of drip should be increased.

Infused desipramine hydrochloride (200 mg in 500 mL normal saline) increases cardiac output, blood pressure and renal blood flow, and urinary output. Infusion should be rapid initially, and then should be slowed to the minimum needed to maintain adequate organ perfusion.

Before adrenergic drugs are used, blood volume must be corrected (central venous pressure at 12–15 cm of water). Even then central venous pressure may drop, necessitating immediate further infusion of colloids or crystalloid solutions.

d. Vasopressors–Vasopressors are rarely indicated except to support coronary artery flow in the late stages of shock. The patient who is already in shock has vasospasm from excessive amounts of circulating catecholamines. Such a drug merely treats the blood pressure cuff and has no clinical effect other than to cause further tissue anoxia.

4. Support of vital organs–

a. Lungs–The pulmonary complications of shock are the most serious, since they interfere with normal oxygenation of the blood. Oxygen (5–8 L/min) should be administered by mask and a nasal tube, though significant increase in Pa_{O_2} is seldom seen, because of blood admixture. Intubation or tracheostomy may be necessary so that assisted or controlled ventilation can be accomplished if the Pa_{O_2} remains at 60 mm Hg or below. An attempt should be made to raise the Pa_{O_2} to 70–90 mm Hg and hold the Pa_{CO_2} between 32 and 40 mm Hg. The treatment of heart failure may reduce pulmonary edema and improve aeration.

b. Heart–Steps taken to raise the central venous pressure will improve cardiac output. Immediate digitalization is necessary in the face of heart failure. Vasodilators seem to have an inotropic effect, as do the corticosteroids also. Acidosis has a deleterious effect upon the myocardium. Give $NaHCO_3$ intravenously.

c. Kidneys–In the early stage of shock, oliguria usually develops. Aggressive infusion of fluids usually corrects this defect. It may be further improved by corticosteroids and vasodilating drugs. If these measures fail, give a diuretic, eg, furosemide (Lasix), 20–40 mg intravenously. Should this fail to increase urine flow, assume the presence of acute tubular necrosis and limit fluids thereafter.

B. Other Measures:

1. Problems in fluid and electrolyte balance–Difficulties are to be expected—particularly hyperkalemia due to leakage of K^+ from the anoxic cell as Na^+ enters it. Cell death further liberates K^+, and lactic acidosis, which develops in shock, causes further loss of potassium from the cell. (Banked whole blood contains 10–30 mEq of K^+ per liter.) Treat the acidosis with intravenous $NaHCO_3$ and give 200 mL of 50% glucose containing 20 units of insulin. Sodium polystyrene sulfonate (Kayexalate) enemas (50 g in 200 mL of glucose) every 4 hours

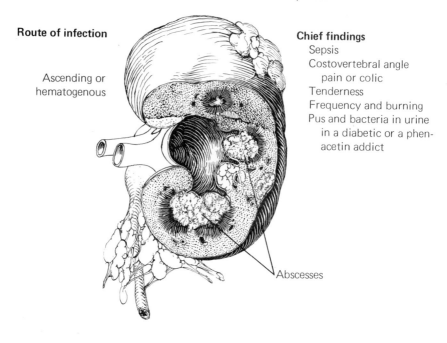

Route of infection

Ascending or
hematogenous

Chief findings
Sepsis
Costovertebral angle
  pain or colic
Tenderness
Frequency and burning
Pus and bacteria in urine
  in a diabetic or a phen-
  acetin addict

Abscesses

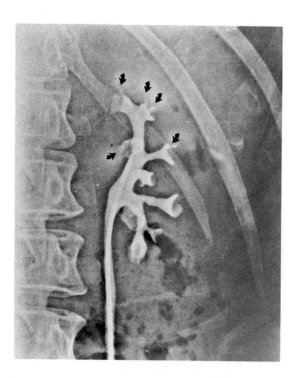

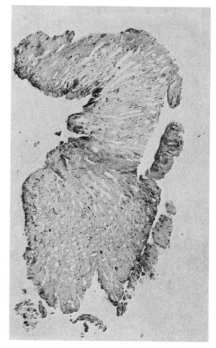

Figure 12–5. Papillary necrosis. *Above:* Pathogenesis. *Left:* Arrows point to "cracks" into parenchyma in a patient in the earliest stage of papillitis (medullary type). *Right:* Papilla passed spontaneously in urine, recovered by patient. (Reduced 30% from × 10.)

may prove efficacious. Dialysis may be necessary. Constant electrocardiographic monitoring is essential.

2. Disseminated intravascular coagulation (DIC)—This condition contributes to circulatory and respiratory failure, especially the latter. The infusion of low-molecular-weight dextran, in addition to expanding circulating blood volume, decreases the viscosity of blood. One to 2 units should be given the first day and 1 unit per day thereafter. If blood studies show evidence of consumption coagulopathy or if hemorrhagic phenomena develop, give heparin, 1000–2000 units intravenously every 4–6 hours. Periodic measurements of blood clotting are necessary. Improvement in pulmonary function may supervene.

Prognosis

Prompt diagnosis and the immediate institution of treatment afford a fairly good prognosis. Encouraging signs include clearing mentation, establishment of good urine flow, control of fever, and increasing P_{aO_2}. The most serious sign is progressive pulmonary failure. High levels of serum lactate are also of great concern. If, however, there is underlying lethal disease (eg, leukemia), the mortality rate approaches 85%. In favorable cases, particularly those of urologic origin, the survival rate approaches 85%.

NECROTIZING PAPILLITIS
(Papillary Necrosis)

Etiology

This is an uncommon type of renal inflammation, though Harrow believes that the necrosis is primary and the infection secondary. Formerly, it was usually a complication of pyelonephritis in diabetes or in patients suffering from urinary obstruction. Today, most patients with papillitis give a history of excessive and prolonged ingestion of analgesics containing phenacetin and aspirin for the relief of migraine or arthritic pain. Patients with sickle cell trait may develop papillary necrosis (Pandya & others, 1976). The combination of infection and vesicoureteral reflux may also cause this lesion. The association of papillary necrosis and cirrhosis has been cited. Papillary necrosis appears to be caused by ischemic necrosis of the papilla or the entire pyramid, leading to the diagnostic urographic changes. A few cases have been reported in infancy, though most are seen in women with migraine.

Pathogenesis & Pathology (Figs 12–5 and 12–6)

The disease is usually bilateral; a few or all of the calices may become progressively more severely involved. Although most patients have pyelonephritis as well, a few are found to have sterile urine. This latter group has associated chronic in-

terstitial nephritis, which is seen in association with analgesic abuse.

Some degree of renal atrophy secondary to infection may be noted. In fact, in adults, only 2 renal lesions will cause shrinking of the kidney in a period of a few weeks: an acute vascular lesion and acute papillary necrosis. Simple pyelonephritis in the adult will not cause this phenomenon. One or more papillae are absent. The line of demarcation is vague. Retained or calcified papillae may be found free in the pelvis. Infiltration of neutrophils, small round cells, and plasma cells is microscopically visible at the site of papillary slough. Changes typical of chronic pyelonephritis are usually evident. Heptinstall (1976) believes that many patients suspected of having healed pyelonephritis really represent examples of interstitial nephritis and papillary necrosis due to analgesic abuse. In the case of analgesic abuse, the interstitial tissues are infiltrated by fibrous tissue and round cells (chronic interstitial nephritis). Severe ischemia of the pyramids may be noted.

Clinical Findings

A. Symptoms: In the rare fulminating type of papillitis, severe sepsis may come on abruptly. Renal pain may be noted. Oliguria with uremic coma may develop rapidly, culminating in death. More commonly, the patient complains of symptoms of chronic cystitis, often with exacerbations of pyelonephritis. Attempts at sterilization of the urine usually fail. Recurrent renal colic may be experienced as sloughed papillae are passed. Known sickle cell trait, vesicoureteral reflux, diabetes, cirrhosis, or a history of prolonged use of analgesics (6–60 pills a day for years) may be significant.

B. Signs: In acute papillitis, fever is high and prostration marked. Renal tenderness may be noted. In the chronic form, no abnormal signs are usually elicited. At the time of febrile flare-up, renal tenderness may be found.

C. Laboratory Findings: In the fulminating form, the white blood count is significantly elevated. Urinalysis reveals pyuria and bacteriuria. Blood cultures may be positive. Shock may ensue. Glycosuria and acidosis will be noted in the uncontrolled diabetic. Progressive azotemia is to be expected.

Most of the patients in the chronic phase have infected urine. Anemia may be found in association with renal insufficiency. PSP excretion is usually depressed, often below 30% in one-half hour. At this level, nitrogen retention will be increased.

D. X-Ray Findings: Satisfactory excretory urograms in the uremic patient may only be obtained by infusing increased amounts of radiopaque material. In the earliest stages, before papillary slough, the urograms may show no anatomic abnormality. Later, ulceration of the central portion of a papilla (medullary necrosis; Fig 12–5) or delinea-

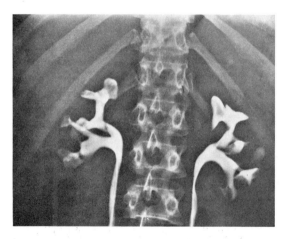 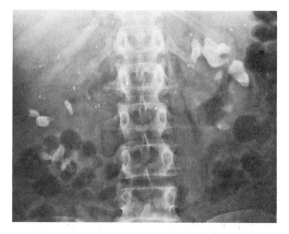

Figure 12–6. Papillary necrosis. *Left:* Retrograde urogram showing papillary necrosis. Calices seem enlarged because of sloughed papillae. "Negative" shadows in upper medial calices and in lowest calices on left represent sloughed papillae. *Right:* (Same patient 5 years later.) Multiple renal stones caused by calcification of retained sloughed papillae. The papillae are represented by the relatively translucent centers in peculiarly shaped stones.

tion of cavities caused by sloughed papillae may be seen (Fig 12–6). "Negative" shadows representing retained papillae may be noted. During the later phase, irregular calcified bodies containing radiolucent centers (the papillae) are diagnostic.

If uremia is of such severity as to preclude excretory urography, retrograde urography must be performed. Retrograde urography either will establish the diagnosis or will reveal a urologic lesion that may be amenable to therapy.

Differential Diagnosis

Uncomplicated diabetic coma can be diagnosed on the basis of blood glucose and serum electrolytes. Treatment of the coma should cause prompt response. If bilateral necrotizing papillitis is present as a complication, the diabetic patient will not improve under insulin therapy; progressive renal impairment will be observed, and death from renal failure and sepsis may ensue. In contrast, patients with acute pyelonephritis are not so prostrated, nor does acute renal failure develop.

Bilateral renal cortical abscesses secondary to bacteremia may simulate acute papillitis clinically. Both may show progressive loss of renal function. Urograms made early in the course of either disease may be normal or may show evidence of chronic infection. After 2 or 3 weeks, when the necrotic papillae have sloughed, the urographic demonstration of necrotizing papillitis is diagnostic.

Complications

If the patient with bilateral papillary necrosis recovers, persistent chronic pyelonephritis is usually seen; bacteriuria resists antimicrobial therapy.

The passage of a sloughed papilla may cause ureteral colic and obstruction. If the sloughed papil-

lae are not passed down the ureter, they may undergo peripheral calcification. The clinical picture is then compatible with nephrolithiasis.

Prevention

Because of the relatively high incidence of papillitis in diabetics and cirrhotics, careful urinalyses and periodic urine cultures should be obtained whether symptoms of urologic infection are present or not. Infection, once discovered, should be treated vigorously. Pharmaceutical compounds containing aspirin and particularly phenacetin should be considered nephrotoxic; their long-term and persistent use must be condemned. If the patient stops taking these drugs, renal function may improve to some extent.

Treatment

A. Specific Therapy: Intensive treatment with an appropriate antibiotic is indicated, although the results have been disappointing insofar as sterilization of the urine is concerned. The choice of drug depends upon the type of bacteria found in the urine and the results of antibiotic sensitivity studies.

B. General Measures: Diabetes must be carefully controlled. The aspirin or phenacetin addict must stop taking the drug.

C. Surgical Therapy: If the disease is unilateral and fulminating (as demonstrated by physical examination, urography, and renal function tests) and if drug therapy does not result in prompt improvement, nephrectomy must be considered. This procedure must be undertaken with caution, however, since the other kidney may later become involved. If a sloughed papilla should obstruct a ureter, it can usually be removed by cystoscopic manipulation.

Prognosis

The rare fulminating form is rapidly fatal. Patients with the chronic type usually do fairly well. Although renal function may be depressed, progressive uremia is unusual if chronic suppression with antimicrobial drugs is instituted.

RENAL ABSCESS
(Renal Carbuncle)

Etiology

Until 3 decades ago, renal abscesses caused by *Staphylococcus aureus* and arising as metastases from skin lesions far outnumbered those that were a consequence of primary suppurative renal disease. Today, however, two-thirds of such abscesses fall into the latter category. It is thought that with the advent of antibiotic therapy, immediate administration of such drugs has cured many lesions before they could be accurately diagnosed as having a staphylococcal origin. A few such cases in drug addicts have been reported.

Pathogenesis & Pathology (Fig 12–7)

An abscess (carbuncle) caused by *S aureus* develops from hematogenous spread of the organisms from a primary skin lesion. Multiple cortical abscesses develop that are usually focal. They coalesce to form a multilocular abscess. If the diagnosis is not made until late in the course of infection, the ab-

scess may rupture into the pelvicaliceal system or into the perinephric space (perinephric abscess). In the first instance, pus and cocci are found in the urine only after rupture into the renal pelvis has occurred. With a perinephric abscess, pyuria and organisms on stained smear of the sediment may be absent, although urine cultures may be positive.

The more common type of renal abscess, however, is secondary to long-standing renal infection caused by chronic ureteral obstruction or, more commonly, calculus disease (calculous pyonephrosis) (Malgieri, Kursh, & Persky, 1977). Timmons & Perlmutter (1976) feel that renal abscesses in children may be a complication of vesicoureteral reflux, with invasion of the renal collecting tubules by gram-negative organisms. In adults, the kidney is usually damaged by chronic suppurative pyelonephritis that may culminate in one or more abscesses. These, too, may rupture into the perinephric space. One-third of patients in this category are diabetics (Thorley, Jones, & Sanford, 1974).

Clinical Findings

A. Symptoms: Staphylococcal renal abscess usually has an abrupt onset, with fever, chills, and localized costovertebral pain. There are no symptoms of vesical irritability, because in the early stages, the urinalysis is normal. The patient is often quite septic. The picture is that of acute pyelonephritis.

In most patients, however, there is a long his-

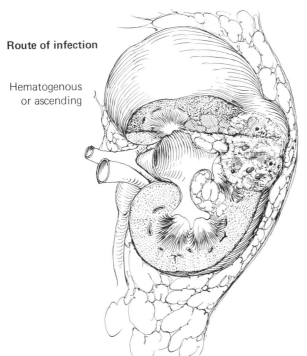

Route of infection

Hematogenous or ascending

Chief findings

Fever (high- or low-grade)
Costovertebral angle pain
Tenderness or no localizing
signs or bladder symptoms

Figure 12–7. Pathogenesis of renal carbuncle.

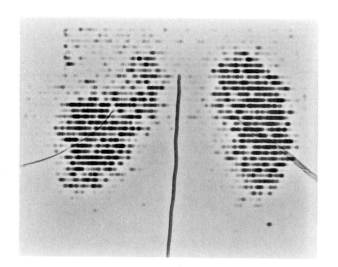

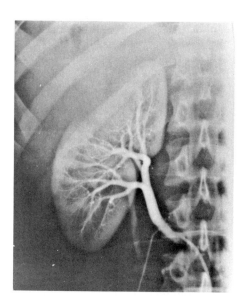

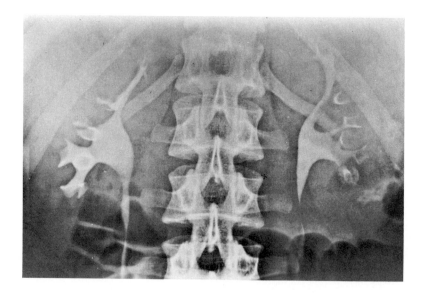

Figure 12–8. Renal carbuncle. *Above left:* Renal scan revealing absence of functional renal tissue in superolateral portion, right kidney. *Above right:* Selective renal angiogram, same patient, showing avascular mass in superolateral portion, right kidney. Surgical diagnosis: renal carbuncle. *Below:* Excretory urogram. Elongation of upper calix, right kidney. Carbuncle was a complication of measles.

tory of recurrent urinary tract infections with exacerbations. Previous passage of stones may be noted. There is usually a past diagnosis of chronic renal infection with or without stones. Corrective renal surgery may have been done.

B. Signs: In acute cases, the localizing signs are flank tenderness and possibly a palpable mass, as well as edema of the skin of the costovertebral area. The latter is best revealed by having the patient lie on a rough towel. Quite often in the patient with chronic renal infection, the development of an abscess causes few findings.

C. Laboratory Findings: In the early stages of staphylococcal infection, urinalysis is negative, although urine culture may reveal the organism. The urinalysis is abnormal only if the abscess ruptures into the renal pelvis. In patients with a history of long-standing infection, the urine always contains pus and bacteria, usually gram-negative rods. The white count is elevated, with an absolute increase in polymorphonuclear neutrophils.

A diagnosis of diabetes mellitus is often made. Patients with an acute staphylococcal infection usually have a normal blood urea nitrogen and serum creatinine; those with long-standing infection are apt to exhibit some degree of nitrogen retention.

Blood cultures in both groups are apt to be positive (Thorley, Jones, & Sanford, 1974).

D. X-Ray Findings: The plain film usually shows an enlarged kidney or a bulge of the external contour of the kidney if its outline is visible. However, perinephric edema often obliterates the outline. The psoas shadow is usually indistinct or absent. Scoliosis of the spine is usually not observed unless the abscess has ruptured into the perinephric space. Renal stones may be delineated.

Excretory urograms usually demonstrate a space-occupying lesion representing the abscess (Fig 12–8). In patients with chronic infection, hydronephrosis, pyelonephritic changes, and often stones are to be expected. Such kidneys often reveal delayed opacification. A few will be functionless.

Angiography usually makes the diagnosis (Koehler & Nelson, 1976). The abscess fails to opacify; its walls are irregular. Surrounding vessels are displaced, and hypervascularity is common. The most important sign is the presence of an increased number of capsular vessels over the area of the abscess.

E. CT Scans: Very few patients with renal abscesses have been examined by means of computed tomography (CT). Depending on the relative amount of pus or solid debris present, the attenuation value or density of an abscess can overlap that of a cyst or neoplasm. The appearance of an abscess on CT scans is probably indistinguishable from that of a necrotic neoplasm.

F. Isotope Scanning: The rectilinear scan will depict a space-occupying lesion (Fig 12–8). With the use of technetium and iodine compounds, the Anger camera will show an avascular space-

occupying lesion. These findings are also compatible with simple cyst. However, gallium-67 localizes in inflammatory tissue; an abscess will therefore "light up" on dynamic scanning. It may reveal an abscess even though excretory urograms are normal (Hopkins, Hall, & Mende, 1976).

Differential Diagnosis

In acute pyelonephritis, symptoms and signs may be similar to those of abscess, but no space-occupying lesion is shown on urography, and a ^{67}Ga scan will be negative for abscess.

Acute cholecystitis may resemble a staphylococcal renal abscess when the urine is normal. The presence of a palpable and tender gallbladder may make the diagnosis. Radiographic visualization of the gallbladder and kidneys should be definitive.

Acute appendicitis may be confused with renal abscess, since renal pain often radiates to the lower abdominal quadrant. However, the finding of infected urine plus signs and symptoms referred to the flank should suggest renal disease. Excretory urograms should differentiate between the 2 disorders.

Complications

Complications include both bacteremia with general sepsis and rupture of the abscess into the perinephrium.

Treatment

When the diagnosis of staphylococcal abscess is made, the patient should be treated with a penicillin resistant to β-lactamase. In the early stages, cure is often possible, but if not, surgical operation will be required. This may consist of drainage of the abscess, heminephrectomy, or even nephrectomy if the kidney is diffusely involved.

In the case of abscess secondary to long-standing renal infection, appropriate antimicrobial therapy should be employed, although failure is to be expected. Drainage must be instituted. Primary nephrectomy or nephrectomy at a later date is usually necessary.

Prognosis

Administration of the appropriate drug early in the course of infection due to *S aureus* may effect a cure. If the diagnosis is not made until late in the disease or if medical treatment fails, surgery will be necessary.

Abscess that is secondary to chronic pyelonephritis and is often complicated by stone will require surgical treatment.

PERINEPHRIC ABSCESS

Etiology

Perinephric abscess can be secondary to a staphylococcal infection of the kidney but is usually

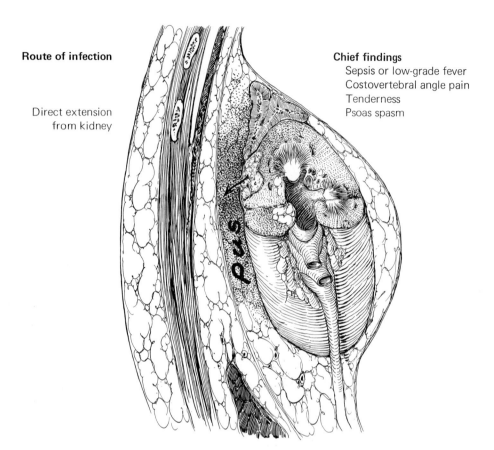

Route of infection

Direct extension
from kidney

Chief findings
   Sepsis or low-grade fever
   Costovertebral angle pain
   Tenderness
   Psoas spasm

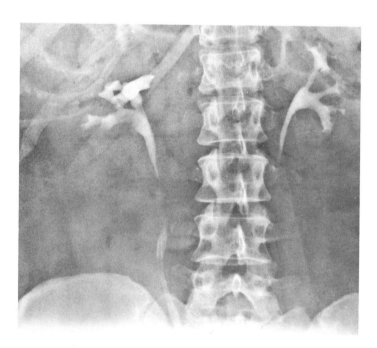

Figure 12–9. Perinephric abscess. *Above:* Pathogenesis. *Below:* Excretory urogram showing lateral displacement of lower pole of right kidney, scoliosis of spine, and absence of right psoas shadow. Note compression of upper right ureter by abscess.

a complication of an advanced chronic nonspecific renal infection.

Pathogenesis & Pathology (Fig 12–9)

Perinephric abscess lies between the renal capsule and the perirenal (Gerota's) fascia. The staphylococcal type probably originates from rupture of a small renal cortical abscess or, less commonly, from a renal carbuncle. The primary renal lesion may heal although the perinephric abscess progresses.

Perinephric cellulitis and abscess, however, usually complicate severe chronic renal infection such as calculous pyonephrosis or infected hydronephrosis. The presumption is that spontaneous extravasation of infected material occurs. In this instance, pus and bacteria (usually gram-negative rods) are found in the urine.

Perirenal abscesses may become quite large. When advanced, they tend to point over the iliac crest (Petit's triangle) posterolaterally.

Clinical Findings

A. Symptoms: In the more common type (secondary to advanced chronic renal infection), a history of prolonged or recurrent urinary infection may be elicited. In the staphylococcal type, there is often a history of a skin infection a few weeks before the onset of symptoms. Malaise may be mild or severe, depending upon the virulence of the invading organism. Pain in the flank varies in degree. The patient may note a tender mass in the renal area.

B. Signs: Fever may be low-grade or septic. Marked tenderness over the kidney and in the costovertebral angle is usually found. A large mass may be felt or percussed in the flank. Some rebound tenderness may be elicited. The diaphragm on the affected side may be high and fixed. Ipsilateral pleural effusion is common. Scoliosis of the spine, with its concavity to the affected side, is usually seen. This is due to spasm of the psoas muscle, which also causes the patient to lie with the ipsilateral leg flexed on the abdomen. Edema of the skin over the abscess may be evident. Minimal edema is best demonstrated by having the patient lie on a rough towel for a few minutes.

C. Laboratory Findings: Anemia may be found. The white count may be markedly or only slightly elevated. The sedimentation rate is usually accelerated. The urine may be free of pus and bacteria if the renal organism is a *Staphylococcus*. If the abscess is secondary to other chronic renal disease, pus and bacteria (usually rods) are found. Renal function tests are usually normal except in chronic bilateral renal disease.

D. X-Ray Findings: A plain film of the abdomen typically shows evidence of a mass in the flank. The renal and psoas shadows are obliterated because of neighboring edema. Scoliosis of the spine, with its concavity to the affected side, is usually seen. The presence of a calcific body in this area

should suggest an abscess secondary to calculous pyonephrosis. Occasionally, a localized collection of gas caused by gas-forming (coliform) organisms may be observed in the perirenal area.

Excretory urograms may show delayed visualization due to parenchymal disease. Changes suggesting a space-occupying lesion (eg, carbuncle) may be noted, but evidence of advanced hydronephrosis or calculous pyonephrosis is most commonly seen. Lack of mobility of the kidney with change in position of the patient or with respiration strongly suggests acute or chronic perinephritis. The entire kidney or only one pole may be displaced laterally by the abscess (Fig 12–9).

A barium enema may show displacement of the bowel anteriorly, laterally, or medially.

A chest film may demonstrate an elevated diaphragm on the ipsilateral side, and fluoroscopy often shows fixation on respiration. Some free pleural fluid and disk atelectasis may be seen.

Retrograde urograms may be necessary if the excretory films are equivocal.

Gallium-67 localizes in inflammatory tissue, and the diagnosis may often be made using the scintillation camera.

Differential Diagnosis

Chronic renal infection may cause many of the symptoms that accompany perinephric abscess: fever, localized pain, and tenderness. The urine shows evidence of infection. The plain abdominal x-ray and excretory urograms should reveal a clearly defined renal shadow; the psoas shadow should be present and the spine straight. Urographic evidence of chronic pyelonephritis may be seen.

Infected hydronephrosis may cause fever and localized pain and tenderness and may account for the presence of a mass in the flank. The urine is infected. Excretory urograms should make the differentiation.

Paranephric abscess is a collection of pus external to the perirenal fascia and is often secondary to inflammatory disease of the spine (eg, tuberculosis). Many of the signs of perinephric abscess may be seen on a plain x-ray film, but the finding of a bone lesion in the low thoracic area should suggest the proper diagnosis. Urograms are normal.

Complications

Rarely, the perinephric abscess may point just above the iliac crest posterolaterally or extend downward into the iliac fossa and inguinal region. It can cross the spine within the perirenal fascia and involve the other side, but this, too, is rare.

Considerable ureteral compression from the abscess may develop, giving rise to hydronephrosis. Even after drainage of the abscess, ureteral stenosis may develop during the healing process.

Prevention

Since most instances of perinephric abscess

complicate a pyelonephrotic kidney, its removal might be indicated.

Treatment

A. Specific Measures: In the stage of perinephritis, resolution of the infection, when due to staphylococci, may be expected when proper antibiotics are used. When a frank abscess is present, surgical drainage through the flank is indicated. If the cause is primary renal disease (eg, calculous pyonephrosis, infected hydronephrosis), nephrectomy may be necessary. Whether this should be done at the time of drainage of the abscess or later depends upon the judgment of the surgeon.

Pederson, Hancke, & Kristensen (1973) suggest aspiration of the collection of pus so that sensitivity tests can be performed and optimal chemotherapy instituted. This would appear to be useful if urine cultures are negative.

B. General Measures: In the early stages, local heat may be helpful in relieving pain and muscle spasm.

C. Follow-Up Care: Even though the kidney itself is normal, excretory urograms must be obtained 2 or 3 months after drainage of the abscess to be sure ureteral stenosis has not developed.

Prognosis

If the abscess is uncomplicated by primary renal disease and if proper treatment is used, the prognosis is good. Removal of the kidney may be necessary if the organ is badly damaged.

NONSPECIFIC INFECTIONS OF THE URETER

Isolated infection of the ureter does not occur. Although ureteritis accompanies pyelonephritis, the former contributes few symptoms and is clinically of little importance. In the presence of chronic renal and ureteral infection, the ureteral wall may become fibrotic. This may lead to stricture formation or interfere with normal peristalsis. Except in these unusual circumstances, cure of the renal infection leads to resolution of ureteral inflammation.

NONSPECIFIC INFECTIONS OF THE BLADDER

ACUTE CYSTITIS

Etiology

Cystitis is far more common in women than in men. In women, cystitis is caused by ascent of bacteria from the urethra. Symptoms usually develop 36–48 hours after intercourse, which is why the patient seldom recognizes the association. Many women state that they have difficulty in urinating (eg, hesitancy and slow stream), but careful questioning usually reveals that voiding is free most of the time. These obstructive symptoms are therefore not suggestive of urethral stenosis; they must arise from periodic spasm of the striated periurethral sphincter, ordinarily caused by anxiety and tension. Under these circumstances, there is wide dilatation of the proximal urethra, leading to turbulent urinary flow that washes the flora of the deep urethra into the bladder. Cystitis also accompanies the rare hematogenous renal infection. Lymphatogenous spread from an infected cervix seems possible but must be rare.

In men, cystitis is always secondary to some other factor: infection in the prostate or kidney or residual urine associated with the enlarged prostate. The presence of a vesical calculus or an ulcerated vesical neoplasm is often complicated by cystitis.

Bowel infections (eg, diverticulitis, appendiceal abscess) may involve the bladder by contiguity.

Pathogenesis & Pathology

The infected bladder, unless it is constantly insulted by an infected prostate or kidney or contains residual urine, tends to heal spontaneously. With antibiotic therapy, acute infection usually resolves without residual structural or functional injury.

In acute cystitis, the bladder either is diffusely reddened or contains multiple foci of submucosal hemorrhage. The mucosa is edematous; its surface may be covered by a purulent membrane. Superficial ulcers are occasionally seen. The muscularis is usually not involved. Microscopically, in addition to the edema, some desquamation of the mucosa occurs. Dilatation of capillaries is striking. Leukocytic infiltration may extend into the muscle. Temporary ureteral reflux through a "borderline" ureterovesical junction may occur, thus leading to secondary acute pyelonephritis.

Clinical Findings

A. Symptoms: Symptoms include burning on urination, urgency to the point of incontinence, frequency and nocturia, and often hematuria, which is usually terminal (on the toilet tissue). Fever is low-grade or absent unless prostatic or renal infection is present. Urinary complaints predominate; little malaise occurs. There may be mild low backache or suprapubic discomfort.

In women, the attack usually follows intercourse ("honeymoon cystitis"). In men, quiescent prostatitis may be activated by sexual excitement or alcoholic indulgence and thus cause secondary cystitis. A preceding urethral discharge (either nonspecific or gonorrheal) may imply prostatitis.

With nonspecific urethritis in men, it is possible that these microorganisms may ascend to the prostate or bladder.

In children, most instances of cystitis really represent chronic pyelonephritis, because of the high incidence of reflux at this age. There is a group of children who develop symptoms of acute hemorrhagic cystitis that has been shown to be caused by adenovirus type 11 or 21. It is a self-limiting disease.

A history of recurrent attacks of cystitis suggests the presence of unrecognized prostatitis or residual urine, exacerbations of chronic cystitis or pyelonephritis, or, most commonly in women, ascent of bacteria in association with sexual intercourse.

Cyclophosphamide (Cytoxan) not infrequently causes acute cystitis with hemorrhage. Although stopping the drug may be followed by resolution, in a few instances cystectomy has been necessary as a lifesaving procedure. In association with this vesical inflammation, vesicoureteral reflux may develop.

B. Signs: Examination of the abdomen is usually normal. Tenderness is occasionally found over the bladder. The presence of a tender epididymis points to prostatitis as an obvious cause for the cystitis. Rectal examination may reveal a relaxed anal sphincter, suggesting neurogenic dysfunction and the presence of residual urine. In men, the prostate may be enlarged, firm, and tender—even hot. (These findings are compatible with acute prostatitis.) Not until the acute phase has abated should the gland be massaged to prove the presence of infection, since bacteremia with pyelonephritis, acute epididymitis, and prostatic abscess can occur.

Pelvic examination may reveal acute urethritis (nonspecific or gonorrheal), urethral diverticulum, vaginitis (including trichomonal vaginitis), or cystocele (with residual urine) as causes of cystitis. The urethra may be markedly tender. Infection in Skene's glands should be sought. Vaginal discharge should be examined bacteriologically. A partially imperforate hymen or urethrohymenal fusion may be noted.

C. Laboratory Findings: The white blood count is usually elevated. Urinalysis shows pus cells and bacteria; red blood cells may be present. In acute infection, great amounts of pus are common. (In chronic disease, little or no pus is found.) Renal function is not affected.

D. X-Ray Findings: X-rays are not indicated unless stasis or renal infection is suspected. They may be needed, however, if the patient fails to respond to adequate therapy for the cystitis or if infection is recurrent; obstruction, vesicoureteral reflux, tuberculosis, or calculus may be the cause.

E. Instrumental Examination: Cystoscopy is contraindicated during the acute phase. It should be done 7–10 days later, however, if hematuria has been noticed; an ulcerating vesical neoplasm, stone, or foreign body may be found.

Differential Diagnosis

Chronic prostatitis may cause similar symptoms, yet the urine may be normal. Prostatic massage will reveal pus in the secretion.

Allergic cystitis may have an abrupt onset. A few pus cells, eosinophils, and monocytes are found. No bacteria are seen on the stained smear. A history of ingestion of food that has caused a similar reaction in the past may be elicited. Allergy to certain spermatocidal jellies may cause vesical irritability. A history of other allergies may be helpful.

Acute exacerbation of a chronic bladder infection may simulate a new infection, for chronic cystitis often causes no symptoms. Such exacerbation usually resists routine treatment, thereby suggesting chronic disease. Cystoscopy will be of help in differentiation.

Psychosomatic cystitis syndrome may cause symptoms similar to those of acute cystitis. However, urinalysis shows no evidence of infection. A history of recurrent attacks precipitated by anxiety or emotional upset can usually be obtained (see Chapter 35).

Tuberculous cystitis may be differentiated by the finding of "sterile" pyuria on the stained smear or on culture. Tubercle bacilli usually are demonstrable on an acid-fast stain or on culture. There is no response to adequate therapy for a nonspecific infection. This should cause the physician to be suspicious.

Neoplasm involving the bladder may be primary or due to direct extension from the colon or cervix. With invasion and ulceration, infection is inevitable and will not respond to antibiotics. Since this calls for cystoscopy, the diagnosis will become obvious.

Many children, reacting to the detergents in bubble bath, may complain of symptoms suggesting cystitis. Urinalysis shows no infection.

Complications

Acute pyelonephritis is a common complication of ascending acute cystitis in little girls because of the relatively high incidence of vesicoureteral reflux in this age group. It is relatively rare in the adult.

Prevention

In women who are suspected of suffering recurrent attacks of cystitis following intercourse, postcoital voiding with vigor followed by a similar effort the next morning will abolish infections in 80% of cases. If this is ineffective, give 1 g of a sulfonamide or 100 mg of nitrofurantoin orally at the time of vigorous voiding. Landes, Melnick, & Hoffman (1970) have observed a marked decrease in incidence of recurrent cystitis in women following application of povidone-iodine (Betadine) ointment to the periurethral area following the last voiding in the evening and the first voiding in the morning.

Treatment

A. Specific Measures: Nitrofurantoin, ampicillin, penicillin G, nalidixic acid, and the tetracyclines are the most useful drugs for the treatment of acute cystitis. The sulfonamides are also efficacious and the least expensive. If they fail to sterilize the urine within 2 weeks, thorough urologic investigation is indicated.

B. General Measures: The irritable bladder may be sedated by one of the following measures:

1. Alkalinization of the urine–It may be necessary to give 16–20 g of sodium bicarbonate. Fruit juices are also helpful.

2. Antispasmodics–Many of the antispasmodics used in the treatment of gastrointestinal disorders are useful. Tincture of belladonna or atropine combined with phenobarbital may afford relief.

3. Local heat–Hot sitz baths may ease severe pain and spasm. An adequate fluid intake is desirable, but forcing fluids is not helpful, increases urinary frequency, and decreases the urinary concentration of antimicrobial drugs.

4. Hymenotomy–Urethrohymenal fusion or incomplete hymenal perforation should be treated appropriately.

Prognosis

In the absence of stasis, acute cystitis resolves promptly with proper medical therapy. No vesical injury should result. If the infection recurs, the underlying cause must be determined.

CHRONIC CYSTITIS

Etiology & Pathogenesis

Chronic infection of the bladder is often secondary to chronic infection of the upper tract. It may also be due to residual urine, ureteral reflux, or urethral stenosis. Too frequently it is the result of incomplete treatment of simple acute cystitis. The most common cause of pyuria and bacteriuria is cystitis. The presence of these abnormal urinary constituents is not pathognomonic of pyelonephritis, which must be proved by thorough urologic examination.

Pathology

In the chronic stage, the mucosa is often pale and appears thinned. Ulceration is rare. The surface may be studded with cysts (cystitis cystica). Capacity is diminished if fibrosis of the detrusor is extensive. Pericystic fibrosis is a rare complication. Microscopic section usually shows thinning of the epithelium. The submucosa and muscle layers are infiltrated with fibroblasts, small round cells, and plasma cells.

Clinical Findings

A. Symptoms: Complaints may be those of constant or recurrent mild vesical irritability, or there may be none at all. In men, chronic cystitis may be secondary to chronic prostatitis but is more often due to obstruction distal to the bladder with residual urine. In women, it may persist because of chronic urethritis or residual urine (eg, urethral diverticulum, cystocele, urethral stenosis). In both sexes, chronic kidney infection is often the cause. Symptoms suggesting such disease should be sought.

B. Signs: Renal tenderness (infection) or enlargement (hydronephrosis) may be noted. A distended bladder may be found. Examination of the external genitalia in the male is usually noncontributory. Rectal examination may demonstrate impaired tone of the anal sphincter, which suggests detrusor weakness related to neurogenic bladder. Prostatic enlargement, cancer, or infection may be discovered. Pelvic examination may show cervicitis, vaginitis, or inflammation of Skene's or Bartholin's glands. Palpation of the urethra may reveal a mass that, when pressure is applied to it, causes pus to exude from the meatus. This finding is typical of urethral diverticulum.

C. Laboratory Findings: The blood count is usually not remarkable. If anemia is present, something other than bladder infection is the cause. In many instances, few or no pus cells are found; nevertheless, the stained smear or culture reveals bacteria.

Renal function tests in simple chronic cystitis are normal. If the excretion of PSP is depressed, it means either bilateral renal damage (obstruction or infection), reflux, or vesical residual urine. In either case, such a finding is an important clue suggesting further search for the cause of chronicity.

D. X-Ray Findings: A plain film of the abdomen may reveal a large kidney (hydronephrosis) or a small one (atrophic pyelonephritis). An excretory urogram shows no abnormality in uncomplicated cystitis. However, since a significant number of cases of chronic cystitis are secondary to upper urinary tract infection or vesical residual urine, this examination should always be performed. Renal calcification suggesting stone or tuberculosis may be seen.

This examination may reveal hydronephrosis due to ureteral obstruction or changes compatible with healed pyelonephritis. The cystogram may demonstrate trabeculation of the bladder wall, suggesting obstruction distal to the bladder. Ureteral reflux may be observed. The film taken after voiding may reveal residual urine. Retrograde urograms may be required.

E. Instrumental Examination: The passage of a large catheter (22F) may reveal a urethral stricture or residual urine. Either can perpetuate chronic infection.

Cystoscopy will demonstrate the degree of a cystocele or prostatic obstruction. Ulceration of the vesical wall may be seen (tuberculosis); foreign bodies may be found. Panendoscopy may reveal the orifice of a urethral diverticulum.

Ureteral catheterization for relative renal function studies and separate urine specimens for bacteriologic survey may be needed to determine the source of the infection and the presence of ureteral obstruction.

Differential Diagnosis

Chronic prostatitis may cause symptoms of cystitis, but the finding of pus in the prostatic secretion makes the diagnosis.

Since chronic pyelonephritis is often without symptoms referable to the kidneys, thorough urologic investigation (including a voiding cystourethrogram) is needed to establish the cause of the infection in all cases of chronic cystitis.

Tuberculosis of the kidney and bladder is a chronic disease that may mimic chronic cystitis in every way. Certain findings should suggest the presence of tuberculosis: (1) "sterile" pyuria on a stained smear or culture of urinary sediment, (2) lack of response to the usual antibiotics, (3) evidence of a renal lesion by urography, (4) the finding of acid-fast organisms by smear or culture, and (5) ulceration of the bladder wall, with biopsy positive for tuberculosis.

Emotional tension as a cause of chronic bladder symptoms should be suspected if urinalysis is normal and emotional instability is noted. (See Chapter 36.)

Senile urethritis in women past the menopause commonly causes symptoms suggesting chronic cystitis. Urinalysis is normal, and the appearance of the vaginal mucosa is typical of senile change.

Interstitial cystitis causes frequency, nocturia, and suprapubic pain when the contracted bladder becomes full. The urine is free of pus cells and bacteria. Cystoscopy reveals the typical vesical contracture, and when the bladder is overdistended the mucosa on the dome may split and bleed.

Irradiation cystitis may occur following radiotherapy of tumors in the region of the bladder (eg, cancer of the cervix). The urine may become infected if vesical ulceration develops. The history of previous x-ray or radium therapy as well as the cystoscopic finding of a pale, edematous, or telangiectatic vesical mucosa and, at times, ulceration make the differentiation. Biopsy may be indicated to rule out neoplasm.

Chronic urethritis in women may also cause long-standing symptoms suggestive of chronic cystitis. The urine, however, is negative. Panendoscopy will reveal inflammation of the urethral mucosa. Some urethral stenosis is usually found as well.

Complications

Renal infection may occur either because of an incompetent ureterovesical valve or, rarely, by the hematogenous route. Occasionally, fibrosis of the bladder wall may cause contracture with loss of capacity. Stenosis of the intramural portion of the ureters or vesicoureteral reflux may develop, whereupon hydronephrosis follows.

Prevention

Most cases are secondary to vesical residual urine (eg, cystocele, enlarged prostate). Treatment designed to improve vesical emptying is indicated.

Treatment

A. Specific Measures: One of the less expensive, less toxic drugs should be tried first (eg, a sulfonamide or nitrofurantoin; or trimethoprim alone or in combination with sulfamethoxazole); if it fails to cure the infection, further drug therapy should be based on the results of sensitivity tests. Antibiotic treatment must be intensive and prolonged (3–4 weeks). Even under these conditions, therapy is often unsuccessful. Chronic antimicrobial suppression treatment (eg, sulfonamides, methenamine with an acidifier) should then be instituted.

Thorough studies are essential in order to identify the underlying cause of the infection (eg, urethral stenosis, prostatitis). Unless these conditions are corrected, treatment will be unsatisfactory.

B. General Measures: Since symptoms of vesical irritability are usually not as severe as those accompanying acute infection, they can usually be relieved by the measures listed on p 176.

Prognosis

Simple drug therapy often fails to eradicate the infection unless steps are taken to treat the cause (eg, enlarged prostate, chronic prostatitis, chronic urethritis in the female).

NONSPECIFIC INFECTIONS OF THE PROSTATE GLAND

ACUTE PROSTATITIS & PROSTATIC ABSCESS

Etiology

Acute prostatic infection may be hematogenous or may occur as a result of ascent of bacteria up the urethra. It is seen occasionally in childhood and has been observed in the neonatal period. A chronic quiescent prostatic infection can become acute following too vigorous prostatic massage or urethral instrumentation.

Pathogenesis & Pathology

Acute bacterial prostatic infection is usually complicated by acute cystitis and even by acute urinary retention. It may resolve (especially with proper medication), or, rarely, it may progress to abscess formation. Microscopic examination of the acutely infected gland reveals diffuse leukocytic infiltration; abscesses may be noted. Edema is marked. Similar changes are found also in the seminal vesicles, for these are usually involved when the prostate is infected.

Granulomatous prostatitis is a second form of acute prostatitis. It, too, is usually a febrile disease at onset and is usually associated with pyuria. Resolution is slow, and the gland becomes hard. It can, therefore, suggest carcinoma. Microscopically, a granulomatous reaction is noted. The stroma is infiltrated with polymorphonuclear leukocytes, lymphocytes, plasma cells, and multinucleated giant cells. The stroma shows increased fibrosis. Many of the acini have ruptured, releasing prostatic secretion into the connective tissue. It is thought that this is the cause of the severe inflammatory reaction.

Towfighi & others (1972) find many eosinophils in the tissues as well as a frequent history of allergic phenomena.

Clinical Findings

A. Symptoms: Vesical irritability (burning, frequency, urgency, nocturia) may be extreme. Hematuria may be present; it is usually initial or terminal but may be total. Purulent urethral discharge may be noted. There may be perineal aching or low back pain. Moderate to high fever is usual. Cloudy urine is to be expected. Symptoms may have developed during an acute upper respiratory infection, following the extraction of infected teeth, or after urethral instrumentation. Swelling of the gland may cause urinary retention.

B. Signs: The patient ordinarily is not prostrated, but fever may be high. Urethral discharge may be present. Rectal examination reveals an exquisitely tender, enlarged, "hot" prostate. It may be quite firm. Fluctuation means abscess formation. The prostate should not be massaged while acutely inflamed. After the acute phase is over, however, massage is indicated for both diagnosis and treatment.

In the granulomatous form, the prostate may persist in its enlargement and become quite indurated, thus simulating carcinoma. Three to 6 months may be required for resolution.

C. Laboratory Findings: The white blood count is usually elevated in the range of $20,000/\mu L$. Urinalysis shows pus and bacteria on stain and culture. Sensitivity tests should be done. Prostatic secretion should be subjected to culture and sensitivity tests, though the cultures are usually negative.

D. Instrumental Examination: Instrumentation is contraindicated during the acute stage. The only exception to this rule is to relieve acute urinary retention due to prostatic edema or abscess. If an abscess is suspected, the diagnosis may be established by perineal needle puncture.

Differential Diagnosis

Acute pyelonephritis may also be marked by severe vesical irritability. The backache with prostatitis is usually sacral, whereas in pyelonephritis it is in the lumbar area. Rectal examination should establish the diagnosis of acute prostatitis.

Amicrobic pyuria may cause exactly the same symptoms as acute prostatitis. Urinalysis or culture, however, reveals no demonstrable organisms in amicrobic pyuria. Rectal findings also help in differentiation.

Acute congestive prostatitis (prostatosis), often due to lack of sexual activity, may cause perineal, back, and testicular pain as well as urethral discharge. The prostate may be swollen and moderately tender. There are, however, no symptoms of vesical irritability and no fever. Massage of the prostate will produce copious secretion, often containing pus cells, with prompt cessation of symptoms.

Carcinoma of the prostate may be confused with subsiding granulomatous prostatitis. Perineal or transrectal needle biopsy may be indicated in order to arrive at the correct diagnosis.

Complications

Acute urinary retention may occur from swelling of the gland. If an abscess forms, it may rupture spontaneously into the urethra, rectum, or perineum. Acute pyelonephritis may occur by the hematogenous route. This is particularly apt to happen if the prostate is massaged or if instrumentation is done during the acute stage. Acute epididymitis is not uncommon. It, too, is apt to occur from prostatic manipulation or instrumentation during the acute stage.

Prevention

Prostatic massage should be part of the physical examination of all men. The discovery and treatment of asymptomatic prostatitis may prevent the later development of an acute process. Too vigorous prostatic massage may exacerbate a chronic infection.

In the presence of bacteriuria, the urine should be sterilized before catheterization or endoscopy is done.

Treatment

A. Specific Measures: Only 5 antimicrobials are active in prostatic tissue: erythromycin, oleandomycin, cefazolin and cephalexin, and trimethoprim. Since the bacteria are usually gram-negative rods, a combination of sulfamethoxazole, 160 mg, and trimethoprim, 800 mg, should be administered. Give one tablet ("double-strength") containing these amounts orally twice daily for 10–14 days. The urine (and the acute symptoms) should respond in a few days. After subsidence of the acute symptoms and the development of sterile urine, the prostate should be massaged to note the pus content and to obtain material for culture.

Instrumentation is contraindicated at first unless urinary retention occurs. If a frank abscess develops, drainage by perineal needle in addition to antimicrobial medication may lead to resolution. Surgical perineal drainage or transurethral unroofing of the abscess may be necessary.

Granulomatous prostatitis may respond to corticosteroids.

B. General Measures: Perineal pain may require analgesics; sitz baths may afford some relief and may hasten resolution of the inflammation. Vesical irritability can be relieved by antispasmodics. Bed rest is essential. An adequate fluid intake is needed.

Prognosis

The prognosis is good if antibiotic therapy is instituted. If treatment is inadequate, the infection may become chronic and more difficult to eradicate.

CHRONIC PROSTATITIS

Etiology

Chronic prostatitis usually develops as a result of invasion of bacteria from the urethra. It may also have a hematogenous source. Inadequate treatment of acute prostatitis may lead to the chronic form. It may develop secondary to cystitis or pyelonephritis. A few cases of coccidioidal granuloma of the prostate have been reported.

The cause of chronic prostatitis remains unclear. Positive bacterial cultures of prostatic secretions are rarely obtainable. In most cases, there are pus cells in the urine, yet the results of culture are negative. Currently, chlamydial infection is highly suspect as a cause of nonbacterial prostatitis and epididymitis, but chlamydial cultures are very difficult to obtain except in specialized laboratories. If chlamydial causation of chronic prostatitis is verified, the impact on therapy will be significant.

Pathogenesis & Pathology

An acute or subacute prostatic infection may become chronic. Chronic infection may rarely lead to contracture of the bladder neck. Function (eg, potency, fertility) is not impaired.

Chronic prostatic infection usually causes the gland to be firmer than normal as a result of fibrosis. The ducts may contain pus; their lining cells may degenerate. Similar changes are found in the seminal vesicles, for these are usually involved when the prostate is infected.

Clinical Findings

A. Symptoms: There are usually no symptoms. Most men with chronic prostatitis have no reason to suspect it. A few men may note an aching or "fullness" in the perineum, low back pain, or an unexpected low-grade fever. Urethral discomfort with ejaculation may be felt.

Symptoms accompanying a mild exacerbation may include urethral discharge (which may be the only symptom) and symptoms of cystitis. If the patient has symptoms of prostatic obstruction, these may suddenly increase as a result of swelling of the gland. Acute epididymitis may occur; this usually signifies that prostatitis exists.

Other symptoms often incorrectly attributed to prostatitis include infertility (uncomplicated chronic prostatitis rarely causes sterility), impotence (exceedingly rare if it occurs at all), and such psychosomatic complaints—usually associated with sexual difficulties—as nervousness, insomnia, and emotional tension.

B. Signs: Epididymitis is usually caused by prostatitis, though reflux of sterile urine down the vas may cause a type of chemical epididymitis. Rectal examination may reveal a normal, boggy, or indurated prostate. There may be areas of fibrosis. Crepitation may sometimes be felt if stones are present. Massage of the prostate will produce secretion that contains pus. A few pathogens may be found on culture, but sensitivity tests have not proved helpful. The degree of tenderness is of little help in diagnosis, since tenderness is generally determined by the pain threshold of the patient and the degree of apprehension from which he suffers.

C. Laboratory Findings: Urethral discharge should be examined both unstained (trichomonads, lecithin bodies from the prostate) and stained. The white blood count is generally normal unless an exacerbation or complication (epididymitis) is present. The urine may contain pus and bacteria. The PSP test is normal unless there is a silent bilateral renal disease (infection) or residual urine (bladder neck obstruction).

D. X-Ray Findings: Plain films or excretory urograms will be normal unless there are complications (eg, prostatic enlargement, urethral stricture, chronic pyelonephritis).

E. Instrumental Examination: Instrumentation is not indicated unless there is evidence of complications (eg, prostatic enlargement, urethral stricture, upper tract infection).

Differential Diagnosis

Symptoms of acute or chronic urethritis may suggest prostatitis, but the prostatic secretions in those instances will be clear.

Cystitis may be confused with prostatitis, but one must remember that cystitis in men is always secondary to renal or prostatic infection or residual urine. Again, examination of the prostatic secretion will make the differentiation.

Diseases of the anus (eg, fissure, thrombosed hemorrhoid) may cause perineal pain and, at times, urinary urgency, but proper examination of this area should make the correct diagnosis.

Complications

Acute or chronic cystitis may occur secondary to prostatic infection. Pyelonephritis by the hematogenous route may develop from exacerbation of the prostatic infection. Acute epididymitis may follow physical strain, prostatic massage, or urethral instrumentation. An exacerbation of the infection may occur spontaneously or after prostatic massage or urethral instrumentation. Contracture of the bladder neck caused by fibrosis of the prostatic parenchyma is occasionally seen. In such cases, there are symptoms of prostatism and, at times, residual urine.

Prevention

Vigorous treatment of acute prostatitis may prevent the development of chronic disease. Since prostatitis is often secondary to urethral infection, appropriate treatment of both nonspecific and gonorrheal urethritis is indicated.

Treatment

A. Specific Measures: Bacterial prostatitis is resistant to medical treatment. A complicating cystitis will often respond rapidly to the commonly used antimicrobials (eg, sulfonamides, nitrofurantoin), but Stamey, Mears, & Winningham (1970) and Madsen & others (1968) find that the usual chemotherapeutic drugs do not reach the prostate even when adequate serum and urine levels are achieved. However, 2 drugs would seem to be active in the prostate: trimethoprim and minocycline. Trimethoprim-sulfamethoxazole, one "double-strength" tablet twice a day as described on p 178 should be administered for 10–14 days. Drach (1974) suggests a course of 28 days, but even then some relapses occur and it may be necessary to continue to give suppressive antimicrobial drugs to prevent recurrent cystitis. Minocycline has been shown by Hensle, Prout, & Griffin (1977) to diffuse readily into prostatic tissue. Full doses should be given for 2 weeks. A prostatic massage every 2 weeks may promote drainage. Intercourse should therefore be encouraged. Transurethral prostatic resection may be indicated in recalcitrant cases to remove the infected tissue.

If chlamydial infection is suspected, treatment should be with erythromycin, 500 mg 4 times daily for 3–4 weeks.

B. General Measures: Daily sitz baths may hasten resolution of the infection.

Prognosis

Although chronic prostatic infection causes little harm in itself, the complications arising from it are important. This points up the need for routine prostatic massage with microscopic examination of the secretion in all men so that silent chronic prostatitis may be discovered and treated.

NONSPECIFIC INFECTIONS OF THE SEMINAL VESICLES

Almost all infections of the prostate involve the seminal vesicles as well, but it is doubtful if seminal vesiculitis causes any specific symptoms. Infection of the seminal vesicles without prostatitis probably does not occur. For these reasons, seminal vesiculitis is covered in the discussion of prostatic infections.

NONSPECIFIC INFECTIONS OF THE MALE URETHRA*

ACUTE URETHRITIS

Etiology

Acute urethritis is usually an ascending infection, but it can be caused by an infection descending from an infected prostate. Both gram-negative rods and gram-positive cocci are occasionally found. In most cases, however, stained smears or cultures of the secretion are usually negative for bacteria. No specific microorganism has yet been incriminated. In normal controls, 27% of young men harbor *Ureaplasma urealyticum* (T mycoplasmas). In those with urethral discharge, 76% have this organism. After treatment of the nonspecific urethritis, only 28% have positive cultures for *U urealyticum* organism (McChesney & others, 1973). *Mycoplasma hominis* is also often found. It should be pointed out that the mycoplasmas are normal inhabitants of both the vagina and the urethra in both sexes. Whether they are truly the etiologic agents is moot. *Chlamydia* is also suspect. Trichomonads occasionally cause urethritis.

Pathogenesis & Pathology

Urethritis may ascend to the prostate and bladder. If urethritis is severe enough, a periurethral abscess may form, and urethral stricture may then develop; but this is rare. In the acute stage of infection, the mucosa is red, edematous, and covered with a purulent exudate. It may be ulcerated. Microscopic examination shows marked edema and infiltration by leukocytes, plasma cells, and lymphocytes. Capillaries are markedly dilated. The glands of Littre may be engorged or plugged by masses of pus cells.

Acute urethritis in the female is seldom seen except in association with gonorrhea.

Clinical Findings

A. Symptoms: Urethral discharge is the lead-

---

*See Chapters 14 and 30 for nonspecific infection of the female urethra and for gonorrheal urethritis.

ing symptom; it may be as profuse as in gonorrhea. There may be a constant itching or burning sensation in the urethra and on urination.

The onset of symptoms often seems to be related to intercourse. Symptoms may develop a few days thereafter, or the interval may be longer. A history of intercourse during menstruation, when the vaginal bacterial flora is increased, may be obtained. Usually, however, no obvious cause can be discovered.

B. Signs: The discharge may be profuse or scanty and either thick and purulent or thin or mucoid. The lips of the meatus are often red, edematous, and everted.

C. Laboratory Findings: The discharge must be examined unstained and stained. Wet preparations may show trichomonads or may reveal lecithin bodies (typical of prostatic secretion). Rods and cocci may be found on the stained slide, but in most instances no bacteria are seen; this raises the question of possible infection with *U urealyticum* or chlamydiae. This step is the important one in differentiating nonspecific from gonorrheal urethritis. Cultures may be necessary in doubtful cases. Sensitivity tests are of little help in treatment.

If no discharge is available at the time of examination, the first portion of the voided urine will contain "subclinical" discharge. This should be centrifuged and the sediment examined as discharge.

The midstream specimen of urine will be free of pus and bacteria unless complications (prostatitis, cystitis) are present.

D. Instrumental Examination: Instrumentation is contraindicated during the acute stage. Later, however, the passage of a sound will rule out urethral stricture as a cause of the urethritis.

Differential Diagnosis

Gonorrheal urethritis often causes the same symptoms. The stained smear makes the differentiation.

Amicrobic pyuria may start with acute urethritis but is also associated with severe symptoms of acute cystitis. Sterile pyuria and discharge are the rule.

Trichomonal urethritis is differentiated by microscopic identification of the motile organisms, though cultures of prostatic secretion or the ejaculate are much more rewarding.

Nonspecific prostatitis is often accompanied by urethral discharge. The absence of pus in the prostatic secretion differentiates the 2 conditions.

Complications

Prostatitis or cystitis may occur by direct extension. These complications are usually caused, however, by the passage of instruments or the use of forceful urethral irrigations.

Periurethral abscess may develop, but this also is usually a complication of injudicious urologic treatment. The abscess may rupture into the ure-

thra or may drain through the skin. The complications of periurethral abscess are urinary fistula and urethral stricture caused by the fibrosis in the healing process.

Prevention

Acute urethritis may develop from an indwelling urethral catheter made of latex. Use the smallest catheter that is practical, preferably coated with (or made of) silicon. Since nonspecific urethritis due to chlamydiae is usually transmitted by intercourse, empiric treatment of the partner should be considered if that group of organisms is the suspected offender.

Treatment

A. Specific Measures: Although antimicrobial therapy is not often spectacular, the combination of a sulfonamide and either tetracycline or erythromycin seems to give the best result. These drugs are efficacious for both chlamydial and *U urealyticum* infections.

Prostatitis is often the cause of urethral discharge. Prostatic massage is contraindicated in the early stages of acute urethritis; if prostatitis is present, massage may exacerbate its symptoms. However, massage is indicated after a few days for differential diagnostic purposes (silent chronic prostatitis). A course of massage is indicated if prostatitis is found.

B. General Measures: Experience has shown that intercourse should be temporarily discontinued, since it prolongs the acute phase of the disease.

Prognosis

Acute nonspecific urethritis is at times difficult to eradicate (see Chronic Urethritis, below). Underlying causes (eg, prostatitis, urethral stricture) must be sought. Fortunately, little harm is done organically by this disease, although it does cause the patient considerable anxiety.

CHRONIC URETHRITIS

Etiology

Chronic urethral infection may represent the end stage of an incompletely healed acute urethritis or may be an infection that has spread from a chronic prostatitis or has developed at the point of urethral stricture. One or more types of pyogenic organisms are usually found.

The urethral discharge may develop in men who have had no intercourse for months. Others, after a period of abstinence followed by sexual activity (frequently accompanied by moderate alcoholic intake), may develop discharge even though a condom has been used. Recurrent discharge is often a symptom of psychosexual trouble and is probably caused by psychic overstimulation of the glands of Littre. In this instance, pus cells are absent from the secretion.

Pathogenesis & Pathology

In chronic urethritis, the mucosa is usually granular and often appears dull but may be reddened. Microscopically, one sees lymphocytes, plasma cells, and a few leukocytes; fibroblasts are increased.

Clinical Findings

A. Symptoms: Urethral discharge is the primary symptom. It varies in amount and consistency and may appear and disappear spontaneously. The discharge may only be noticed before the first urination after waking. Some urethral irritation may be noted that is not usually related to urination. If there are symptoms of vesical irritability, prostatitis or cystitis is probably present. Psychosexual problems may be uncovered.

B. Signs: The discharge may or may not be present at the time of examination. Prostatic examination may reveal a gland that is boggy and congested or, conversely, firm, even containing fibrotic nodules. It may be normal on palpation. Many cases of chronic urethritis are secondary to chronic prostatitis.

C. Laboratory Findings: The unstained discharge should be examined for lecithin bodies and in saline for trichomonads. Culture (if available) should be done if trichomoniasis is suspected. The former suggests a prostatic source for the urethral secretions. The discharge should be stained with methylene blue and with Gram's stain. Nonspecific organisms (rods and cocci) and gonococci should be sought. Quite often, no bacteria are seen at all; this suggests infection with *U urealyticum* or *Chlamydia* or a psychosomatic reaction. Cultures may be needed in equivocal cases.

If no discharge is present at the time of examination, the first part of the voided urine can be centrifuged, since it contains the pus cells, microorganisms, and mucus that make up the discharge. It is then examined in the same manner as the discharge itself. A less satisfactory technic is to give the patient slides on which he can place any discharge for later examination.

The midstream specimen of urine should be free of pus and bacteria unless complications are present (eg, cystitis).

D. Instrumental Examination: The passage of a sound may be arrested by a urethral stricture, which may prove to be an important factor in producing the discharge. Panendoscopy will visualize the inflamed urethral wall. It may demonstrate a urethral tumor or a diverticulum containing pus.

Differential Diagnosis

Gonorrheal urethritis develops 2–5 days following exposure. The discharge is usually profuse and purulent. The stained smear tells the story. If any doubt exists, cultures can be made.

Reiter's syndrome is characterized by iritis and arthritis as well as urethritis. The discharge is usually free of bacteria. The infective agent is not established but is thought to be one of the chlamydiae.

Trichomonal urethritis is difficult to diagnose because the organism is often hard to demonstrate in a wet preparation. Culture of prostatic secretion or the ejaculate is necessary.

Complications

The urethral infection can ascend to the prostate or bladder, but this is not usual unless instrumentation is done injudiciously.

Prevention

See under Acute Urethritis.

Treatment

The usual chemotherapeutic and antibiotic drugs do not usually cure the disease, but they should be tried. A combination of a sulfonamide and an antibiotic such as one of the tetracyclines or erythromycin may prove helpful.

A congested or infected prostate requires periodic massage. A urethral stricture must be dilated. Sexual problems should be resolved if possible. This may require psychiatric referral.

Prognosis

The disease itself is not harmful, although urinary tract complications occasionally develop from it. The psychologic effect is usually the most serious result of the infection.

NONSPECIFIC INFECTIONS OF THE EPIDIDYMIS

ACUTE EPIDIDYMITIS

Etiology

There are 3 common causes of epididymitis: (1) Preexisting prostatitis, or prostatic infection introduced by an interval or indwelling urethral catheter. (2) Prostatectomy, particularly the transurethral type, where the ejaculatory ducts are laid open in the prostatic fossa. The hydrostatic pressure with voiding or with physical strain may force urine (which may contain bacteria for 8–12 weeks after the operation) down the vas. The infection may also reach the epididymis through the perivasal lymphatics. (3) Reflux of sterile urine down the vas deferens will lead to a chemical epididymitis. Recurrent epididymitis in a young boy suggests the possibility of ureteral drainage into a seminal vesicle. Recurrent epididymitis has been described in a few patients with sarcoidosis.

Pathogenesis & Pathology

In its early stages, epididymitis is a cellular inflammation (cellulitis). It starts in the vas deferens and descends to the lower pole of the epididymis. The initial symptoms may be pain in the groin and even in the flank secondary to the vasitis.

In the acute stage, the epididymis is swollen and indurated. The infection spreads from the lower to the upper pole. On section, small abscesses may be seen. The tunica vaginalis often secretes serous fluid (inflammatory hydrocele), and this fluid may contain pus. The spermatic cord becomes thickened. The testis becomes swollen secondarily from passive congestion but rarely becomes involved in the inflammation.

Microscopically, changes range from edema and infiltration with leukocytes, plasma cells, and lymphocytes to actual abscess formation. The tubular epithelium may show necrosis. Resolution may be complete without residual injury, but peritubular fibrosis often develops, occluding the ducts. If bilateral, it may result in sterility.

Clinical Findings

A. Symptoms: Epididymitis often follows severe physical strain such as lifting a heavy object. It may develop after considerable sexual excitement. The trauma of urethral instrumentation may initiate the complication. It is not uncommon after prostatectomy. Prostatitis is usually the underlying cause.

Pain develops rather suddenly in the scrotum. It may radiate along the spermatic cord and even reach the flank. The pain is generally quite severe and the epididymis exquisitely sensitive. Swelling is rapid and may cause the organ to become twice the normal size in the course of 3 or 4 hours. The temperature may reach 40 C (104 F). Urethral discharge may be noted. Symptoms of cystitis, with cloudy urine, may accompany the painful swelling.

B. Signs: There may be tenderness over the groin (spermatic cord) or in the lower abdominal quadrant on the affected side. The scrotum is enlarged. The overlying skin may be reddened. If abscess is present, the skin may appear dry, flaky, and thinned; it may rupture spontaneously. If seen early, the enlarged, indurated, tender epididymis may be distinguished from the testis. After a few hours, however, the testis and epididymis become one mass.

The spermatic cord is thickened by edema. Hydrocele secondary to the inflammation may develop within a few days. Urethral discharge may be seen.

Palpation of the prostate may reveal changes suggesting acute or chronic prostatitis. The gland should not be massaged during the acute phase, since the epididymitis may be made worse.

C. Laboratory Findings: The white blood count often reaches 20,000–30,000/μL. Urethral discharge, if present, should be examined both unstained and stained. Urinalysis may or may not reveal evidence of infection.

Differential Diagnosis

Tuberculous epididymitis is usually not painful. The epididymis is usually distinguishable from the testis on palpation. "Beading" of the vas may be noted. Induration of the prostate and a thickened ipsilateral seminal vesicle are compatible with tuberculosis. The finding of a "sterile" pyuria by smear and of tubercle bacilli on culture will establish the diagnosis.

Testicular tumor is almost always painless; on occasion, however, because of internal hemorrhage, there may be sudden distention of the tunica albuginea that will cause pain. The mass may be found to be separate from a normal epididymis. Prostatic examination and urinalysis will be normal. If doubt exists, urinary chorionic gonadotropins should be measured, although only 15% of testicular tumors elaborate this substance. If testicular tumor cannot be ruled out, orchiectomy should be done.

Torsion of the spermatic cord is usually an affliction of children just before puberty, although it is occasionally seen in men. Epididymitis occurs in an older age group. In the early phase of torsion, the examiner may palpate the epididymis anterior to the testis. The testis is apt to be retracted. Later, however, the testis and epididymis become one enlarged, tender mass. Prehn's sign may be helpful in differentiation: If pain is relieved when the scrotum is gently lifted onto the symphysis, the pain is due to epididymitis; if pain is increased, torsion is the more probable diagnosis. If torsion cannot be ruled out, the testis should be explored.

Torsion of the appendages of the testis or epididymis is a rare disease of prepuberal boys. These pedunculated bodies may become twisted, causing localized pain and swelling. In the early stages, palpation discloses a tender nodule at the upper pole of the testicle; the epididymis is normal. Later, the entire testis becomes swollen, making the differential diagnosis between epididymitis and torsion of the cord or rudimentary appendages difficult. Early surgery is necessary in this instance, since torsion of the cord must receive prompt treatment.

Testicular trauma may simulate acute epididymitis in every way, but the history of the injury and the absence of pyuria will help in differentiation.

Mumps orchitis is usually accompanied by parotitis. There are no urinary symptoms, and the urinary sediment is free of pus cells and bacteria.

Complications

Abscess formation may occur but is rare unless urethral instrumentation or prostatic massage has been done. The abscess may drain spontaneously through the scrotum or may require surgical drainage.

Epididymal abscess may extend into and destroy the testis (epididymo-orchitis), but this is rare.

Prevention

Once the process has subsided, the presence of prostatitis should be sought and, if present, treated. Recurrent acute attacks may indicate the need for ipsilateral vasoligation.

Treatment

A. Specific Measures: If the patient is seen within 24 hours after onset, the disease may be almost completely aborted by infiltrating the spermatic cord just above the testicle with 20 mL of 1% procaine hydrochloride or other local anesthetic agent, thereby obtaining complete anesthesia. Fever usually falls abruptly. Pain may disappear almost completely. The inflammatory mass may resolve in a few days rather than the usual 2 or 3 weeks. If one injection does not afford relief, it should be repeated the next day.

Antibiotics are helpful but not curative. Secondary cystitis will usually clear quickly.

After the epididymitis has subsided (usually 2 or 3 weeks), treatment of the prostatitis is indicated.

B. General Measures: Bed rest is necessary during the acute phase (3–4 days). Support for the enlarged heavy testicle partially relieves the discomfort. Scrotal supporters are too small; the more roomy athletic supporter, lined with cotton, is best.

Analgesics should be used as necessary to combat pain. Local heat usually affords comfort and probably hastens resolution of the inflammatory process. The sitz bath is a useful means of applying heat to the infected prostate and epididymis. If heat increases the pain, an ice bag should be used instead.

Sexual excitement or physical strain (eg, with defecation) may exacerbate the infection and must therefore be controlled.

Prognosis

Almost all acutely inflamed epididymides resolve spontaneously, although it may take 1 or 2 weeks before all pain is gone and 4 weeks or longer for the epididymis to approach normal size and consistency. Complications are not common, although sterility is always a threat if the disease is bilateral.

CHRONIC EPIDIDYMITIS

Chronic epididymitis is the irreversible end stage of a severe acute epididymitis that has been followed by frequent mild attacks.

In chronic epididymitis, fibroplasia has caused induration of the organ. Microscopically, the scarring is so marked that tubular occlusion is usually seen. The tissues are infiltrated with lymphocytes and plasma cells.

There are usually no symptoms except during a mild exacerbation, at which time there may be some degree of local discomfort. The patient may notice a lump in the scrotum.

The epididymis is thickened and somewhat enlarged. It may or may not be tender. It is easily distinguished from the testis on palpation. Often the spermatic cord is thickened, and at times the diameter of the vas is increased. The prostate may be firm or may contain areas of fibrosis. Its secretion will usually contain pus.

Urinalysis may show infection secondary to prostatitis.

Tuberculous epididymitis mimics nonspecific chronic epididymitis in every way. Beading of the vas, thickening of the ipsilateral seminal vesicle, and the finding of "sterile" pyuria and tubercle bacilli in the urine will make the diagnosis of tuberculous epididymitis. Cystoscopy may reveal vesical ulcers; urograms are of further help.

Testicular tumor may present with a "lump in the testicle." Palpation will show either a thickened epididymis or a hard, insensitive testis (tumor).

Tumors of the epididymis are very rare. Differentiation from chronic epididymitis may ultimately be made only by the pathologist.

If chronic epididymitis is bilateral, sterility is to be expected.

Little benefit can be derived from the administration of antibiotics alone. The prostatitis that is often present must be treated. If prostatic massages cause exacerbation of the epididymal infection, vasoligation should be done during a quiescent interval. The prostatitis can then be treated. Epididymectomy may at times be necessary.

Except for recurring pain and the threat of infertility in bilateral involvement, chronic epididymitis is of little consequence. Once the stage of fibrosis is reached, nothing can be done to resolve it.

NONSPECIFIC INFECTIONS OF THE TESTIS

ACUTE ORCHITIS

Etiology

The testis may become inflamed from a hematogenous source. Orchitis may occur with any infectious disease (eg, coxsackievirus infection, dengue). Patients with mumps parotitis excrete the virus in the urine. Therefore, it would appear that a complicating mumps epididymo-orchitis may also be a descending infection. The edema that develops probably leads to death of the spermatogenic cells from ischemia. Primary infection of an epididymis may involve its testis by direct extension.

Pathogenesis & Pathology

Grossly, in nonspecific orchitis, the testis is much enlarged, congested, and tense. On section, small abscesses may be noted. Microscopically, there is edema of the connective tissue, with diffuse neutrophilic infiltration. The seminiferous tubules also show involvement; necrosis is present. In the healed stage, the seminiferous tubules are embedded in fibrous tissue. On histologic study they may show considerable atrophy. The interstitial cells are usually preserved.

Mumps is the most common cause of inflammation of the testis, which occurs only after puberty. It is usually unilateral but may be bilateral. Grossly, the testis is much enlarged and bluish in color. On section, because of the interstitial reaction and edema, the tubules do not extrude. Microscopically, edema and dilatation of blood vessels are noted. Neutrophils, lymphocytes, and macrophages are abundant. Tubular cells show varying degrees of degeneration. In the healed stage, the testis is small and flabby. Microscopic study in this instance shows marked tubular atrophy, although the Leydig cells are usually normal in appearance. The epididymis usually shows similar changes.

Clinical Findings

A. Symptoms: Onset is sudden, with pain and swelling of the testicle. The scrotum becomes reddened and edematous. There are no urinary symptoms, as are often seen with epididymitis. Fever may reach 40 C (104 F), and prostration may be marked.

B. Signs: The parotitis of mumps may be present, or evidence of other infectious disease may be found. One or both testes may be enlarged and very tender. The epididymis cannot be distinguished from the testis on palpation. The scrotal skin may be reddened. An acute transilluminating hydrocele may develop.

C. Laboratory Findings: The white blood count is usually elevated. Urinalysis is usually normal, although some protein may be found. Abnormal renal function is found in all patients with mumps. Microhematuria and proteinuria are common. The specific virus can be found in the urine. Later, renal function and urine return to normal.

Differential Diagnosis

Acute epididymitis, when seen early, will be obvious because the involvement is solely epididymal. Later, this sign will become obscure. Urethral discharge, pyuria, and absence of a generalized infectious disease should point to epididymitis.

Torsion of the spermatic cord may present difficulties in differentiation. In torsion, the epididymis may be felt anterior to the testis during the early stages. Absence of infection tends to rule out orchitis.

Complications

In one-third to one-fourth of patients, the involved testis becomes infertile due to irreversible damage to spermatogenic cells. Androgenic function, however, is usually maintained.

Prevention

The incidence of mumps orchitis may possibly be lessened by administering mumps convalescent serum, 20 mL, during the incubation period or very early in the disease. Mumps attenuated virus vaccine is highly effective and safe and is recommended for all susceptible persons over age 1. Routine administration of estrogens or corticosteroids to all postpuberal males who develop mumps has been suggested as a prophylactic against orchitis. However, there seems to be little evidence that this practice is effective.

Treatment

A. Specific Measures: Appropriate antibiotics are helpful in controlling some infections but are of no value in the treatment of mumps orchitis. Infiltration of the spermatic cord just above the involved testis with 20 mL of 1% procaine sometimes causes rapid resolution of the swelling and thereby relieves pain. There is evidence that this may protect spermatogenic activity as well by improving blood supply.

B. General Measures: Bed rest is necessary. Local heat is helpful and may relieve the pain. Support to the organ affords some comfort. An athletic supporter containing cotton padding is useful even when the patient is in bed.

Prognosis

Destruction of spermatogenic cells is to be feared, particularly if the disease is bilateral. This is one of the causes of infertility. The acute phase lasts about 1 week. Noticeable atrophy may be observed in 1 or 2 months.

ANTIMICROBIAL TREATMENT OF URINARY TRACT INFECTIONS
Ernest Jawetz, MD, PhD

Choice of Drug

A. Type of Infecting Organism and Confirmation of Diagnosis: A clinical impression of urinary tract infection (UTI) should be confirmed by microscopic examination of uncentrifuged urine under coverslip or of stained sediment of centrifuged urine and by quantitative screening culture (more than 10^5 bacteria of one kind confirms the diagnosis). Detailed identification of the organism and its antimicrobial sensitivity is not usually necessary in the first attack of urinary tract infection but is important in recurrent or chronic infection or in a patient with severe systemic symptoms. In women, dysuria is often caused by vaginitis or urethral syndrome. Urethral syndrome consists of dysuria and frequency as in urinary tract infection but with few or no bacteria in the urine.

B. Identification of Site of Infection: Infections of the lower urinary tract (urethra and bladder) tend to respond more quickly to drug treatment than infections of the upper urinary tract (kidneys) and are less likely to recur after treatment. Initially, symptoms and signs are most important in determining the site of infection; later, immunofluorescence staining of bacteria in urine (to detect coating immunoglobulin, which suggests tissue infection) or bladder washout is useful.

Lower tract infection tends to respond to antibacterial drug concentrations in urine, without the need for high systemic drug levels. Urinary antiseptics and low doses of systemic drugs that are excreted into the urine in high concentration produce effective drug levels in urine. In upper tract infection, particularly when there are symptoms of possible bacteremia and tissue involvement, initial high systemic drug levels are preferable.

C. Acute Versus Chronic and Initial Versus Recurrent Infection: Acute initial infections have a tendency to subside and heal spontaneously. Low-dose treatment with a soluble sulfonamide (eg, sulfisoxazole, 0.5 g 4–8 times daily) for 7–10 days generally results in remission or cure. Even a single large dose of an effective drug—eg, amoxicillin, 3 g orally—can be curative. By contrast, recurrent infection is often caused by organisms resistant to previously used drugs, and selection of a suitable drug must rely on laboratory results. Treatment with higher doses for 4–6 weeks may be required to cure a long-standing infection, especially if it involves the upper tract. In low-grade chronic infections, low-dose trimethoprim-sulfamethoxazole or a urinary antiseptic may suppress bacterial growth for months and permit healing. It is clear that the concentration of an effective antibacterial drug in urine is of primary importance in successful treatment. However, full systemic doses of antibacterial drugs should be considered for management of pyelonephritis patients who show signs of systemic toxicity or sepsis.

D. Adverse Reaction to Drug: A history of hypersensitivity reaction to a particular drug usually requires the use of a substitute drug. Patients who have a history of a reaction to penicillin should receive no penicillin and probably no cephalosporin for urinary tract infections—although they might well tolerate either. Similarly, patients who have reacted adversely to nitrofurantoin or sulfonamides should not be given these drugs. However, a history of reactions probably caused by changes in

microbial flora following the use of tetracyclines or ampicillin is not a definite contraindication to use of these drugs.

E. Antimicrobial Drug Susceptibility Tests: In urologic office practice, microscopic examination of the urine suffices to guide drug selection in many acute infections. Screening cultures are inexpensive ($3 in 1980), provide an approximate quantification of bacterial numbers, and may provide a culture for subsequent susceptibility testing if this is required. Precise quantitative culture and identification of the organism is usually reserved for recurrent or chronic urinary tract infection. In such cases, disk sensitivity tests are often done. However, results of disk tests commonly indicate susceptibility of the organism to the **blood** concentration of drug, which is many times lower than the **urine** concentration, and the latter is the most important therapeutic concern in urinary tract infection. Results of disk tests for nitrofurantoin, nalidixic acid, and sometimes sulfonamides do indicate bacterial susceptibility to urine concentrations. However, the disk test results for many systemically employed antimicrobial drugs have limited relevance to the selection of drugs for urinary tract infection.

Since 1979–1980, the commercial availability of microtiter plates with measured drug concentrations and simple inoculation methods has made possible a return to sensitivity testing of drugs in broth dilution. Results are stated as minimal **inhibitory** concentration (MIC) of a given drug. This permits interpretation in terms of usual urine concentrations and is helpful in treatment of urinary infections that did not respond to or relapsed following initial treatment. Microtiter broth dilution assays can also reveal the minimal **bactericidal** concentration (MBC) of a drug for the infecting organism.

Drug Dosage & Renal Function

Most antimicrobial drugs are excreted by the kidneys and appear in the urine in much higher concentration than in blood or tissues. So-called "urinary doses" are a fraction of the usual systemic dose and result in urinary drug levels inhibitory for many bacteria in the urine. However, such "urinary doses" should not be used in acute urinary infections—at least until a clinical response is evident. To maintain adequate drug levels, the urine cannot be too dilute. Fluid intake should be between 1500 and 2000 mL/d for an adult.

The excretion of many drugs is greatly reduced with renal insufficiency. This results in drug retention and added nephrotoxicity. To avoid accumulation of the drug in the bloodstream and tissues, either the dose must be reduced or the interval between doses increased. In Table 12–1, the half-life of drugs in serum of normal subjects is compared with that in patients with creatinine clearance of 10 mL/min, and possible dosage adjustments are suggested. The kidneys of uremic individuals do not

Table 12–1. Use of antibiotics in patients with renal failure.

	Principal Mode of Excretion or Detoxification	Approximate Half-Life in Serum		Proposed Dosage Regimen In Renal Failure		Significant Removal of Drug by Dialysis (H = Hemodialysis; P = Peritoneal Dialysis)
		Normal	Renal Failure*	Initial Dose†	Give Half of Initial Dose at Interval of	
Penicillin G	Tubular secretion	0.5 h	6 h	6 g IV	8–12 h	H, P no
Ampicillin	Tubular secretion	1 h	8 h	6 g IV	8–12 h	H yes, P no
Carbenicillin	Tubular secretion	1.5 h	16 h	4 g IV	12–18 h	H, P yes
Ticarcillin	Tubular secretion	1.5 h	16 h	3 g IV	12–18 h	H, P yes
Nafcillin	Kidney 20%, liver 80%	0.5 h	2 h	2 g IV	4–6 h	H, P no
Cephalothin	Tubular secretion	0.8 h	8 h	4 g IV	18 h	H, P yes
Cephalexin Cephradine	Tubular secretion and glomerular filtration	2 h	15 h	2 g orally	8–12 h	H yes, P no
Cefazolin	Tubular secretion and glomerular filtration	2 h	30 h	2 g IM	24 h	H yes, P no
Cefoxitin, cefamandole	Tubular secretion and liver	1 h	16–20 h	2 g IV	12–18 h	H, P yes
Amikacin	Glomerular filtration	2.5 h	3 d	15 mg/kg IM	3 d	H, P yes
Gentamicin	Glomerular filtration	2.5 h	2–4 d	3 mg/kg IM	2–3 d	H, P yes‡
Tobramycin	Glomerular filtration	2.5 h	3 d	3 mg/kg IM	2 d	H, P yes
Vancomycin	Glomerular filtration	6 h	6–9 d	1 g IV	5–8 d	H, P no
Polymyxin B	Glomerular filtration	6 h	2–3 d	2.5 mg/kg IV	3–4 d	P yes, H no
Tetracycline	Glomerular filtration	8 h	3 d	1 g orally or 0.5 g IV	3 d	H, P no
Chloramphenicol	Mainly liver	3 h	4 h	1 g orally or IV	8 h	H, P no
Erythromycin	Mainly liver	2.5 h	5 h	1 g orally or IV	8 h	H, P no
Clindamycin	Glomerular filtration and liver	2.5 h	4 h	600 mg IV or IM	8 h	H, P no

*Considered here to be marked by creatinine clearance of 10 mL/min or less.
†For a 60-kg adult with a serious systemic infection. The "initial dose" listed is administered as an intravenous infusion over a period of 1–8 hours, or as 2 intramuscular injections during an 8-hour period, or as 2–3 oral doses during the same period.
‡Aminoglycosides are removed irregularly in peritoneal dialysis. Gentamicin is removed 60% in hemodialysis.

excrete some drugs in sufficient quantities to reach antibacterial concentrations in the urine. Nitrofurantoin, methenamine salts, polymyxin B, colistimethate, nalidixic acid, tetracyclines, and trimethoprim-sulfamethoxazole should *not* be given in renal failure.

Duration of Treatment & Follow-Up

For the first attack of symptomatic urinary tract infection, a 7- to 10-day course of a suitable drug is planned. On day 3, the urine should be examined by smear or culture to ascertain that bacteria are suppressed. If they are not, a different drug must be used. Two weeks after treatment ends, the urine is again examined. If the patient is asymptomatic and the urine free of bacteria, the infection is assumed to be cured.

If symptoms return or if the urine contains significant numbers of bacteria, either a relapse (same organism) or reinfection (different organism) has occurred. Culture and susceptibility tests are advisable, and a second course of an appropriate drug is begun. Treatment should be continued for 3 weeks or longer if tolerated. Two weeks after the second course of therapy has ended, follow-up examination is performed. If the urine is free of bac-

teria and the patient is asymptomatic, subsequent follow-up examinations are planned. If relapse is ascertained, complete urologic examination, including intravenous urography, is carried out to exclude an organic cause that may be surgically remediable. If there is reinfection, 7-day courses of an appropriate drug, selected by culture and sensitivity tests, usually suffice to suppress each episode. However, long-term prophylaxis with either daily or alternate-day nitrofurantoin, 100 mg, or trimethoprim-sulfamethoxazole, 1–2 tablets, can be given to sexually active women who are prone to develop frequently recurring urinary infections. Other patients with frequent recurrences of symptomatic urinary infection or with evidence of chronic urinary tract infection should receive urinary antiseptics for many months, in the hope that chronic suppression of infection will permit healing.

Use of Antimicrobial Drugs During Pregnancy

Oral tetracyclines should not be given after the fourth month of pregnancy because they produce hypoplasia and staining of bones and teeth in the fetus. Parenteral tetracyclines may be severely toxic to the liver of a pregnant woman. Sulfonamides and trimethoprim-sulfamethoxazole should be avoided during the third trimester, because they may contribute to kernicterus in the newborn.

Women who have significant bacteriuria in early pregnancy are at risk of developing symptomatic pyelonephritis in later pregnancy. Screening for bacteriuria in the third or fourth month is widely practiced. If results are positive, a 3- to 4-week course of treatment is often recommended to avoid later complications.

SYSTEMIC ANTIMICROBIAL DRUGS

Sulfonamides

This large group of drugs inhibits the growth of many bacteria by blocking the uptake of extracellular p-aminobenzoic acid required for synthesis of folate. The most soluble sulfonamides, sulfisoxazole and trisulfapyrimidines, rarely (if ever) precipitate in urine to cause crystalluria. However, they may cause other side-effects of sulfonamides (rash, fever, hematologic disturbances, vasculitis, etc). Soluble sulfonamides are drugs of choice for the initial treatment of a first urinary tract infection, which is commonly caused by coliform bacteria. Many coliform bacteria are still susceptible to sulfonamides, although many common bacteria (eg, streptococci, staphylococci) have become resistant. Sulfisoxazole or trisulfapyrimidines, 2–4 g/d (150 mg/kg/d for children), are given orally for 7–10 days. Long-acting sulfonamides should never be given for urinary tract infections. Sulfonamides (0.5 g 2–4 times daily) may be effective in suppressing asymptomatic bacteriuria (eg, in early pregnancy) and preventing later pyelonephritis. Whenever sulfonamides are administered, the urine should be kept alkaline and the daily urine volume kept above 1500 mL/d. A complete blood count should be done once a week.

Trimethoprim

This substituted pyrimidine inhibits bacterial dihydrofolate reductase thousands of times more efficiently than the same enzyme of mammalian cells and thus blocks synthesis of purines in bacteria. It inhibits many gram-negative enteric bacteria that commonly cause urinary tract infection (eg, *Escherichia coli*, *Proteus*, *Klebsiella*, *Enterobacter*). About 2–8% of organisms carry plasmids that make them resistant to trimethoprim. The usual dose of trimethoprim is 100 mg by mouth every 8–12 hours, which gives urine levels of 50–180 μg/mL. This is sufficient for the treatment of urinary tract infections due to susceptible bacteria. Trimethoprim also concentrates by nonionic diffusion in prostatic and vaginal fluids and thus may be effective in bacterial prostatitis. Side-effects include fever, rashes, gastrointestinal symptoms, and

hematologic abnormalities attributable to folate deficiency. Trimethoprim alone or in combination (see below) should not be given to patients with a creatinine clearance below 15 mL/min.

Trimethoprim-Sulfamethoxazole (Co-Trimoxazole)

Fixed-dose combinations of sulfamethoxazole, 400 mg, and trimethoprim, 80 mg, are available for urinary tract and other infections. The 2 drugs interrupt sequential steps leading to the synthesis of purines and may be synergistic.

The usual oral dose is 2 tablets 2–3 times daily, particularly in relapsing, chronic urinary tract infections. In children, pregnant women, or patients with renal failure, the dose must be reduced. An investigational intravenous formulation of trimethoprim-sulfamethoxazole can be used in serious illness due to bacteria not susceptible to other drugs (eg, *Serratia*). The side-effects may include all of those mentioned for each component of the mixture, and others. A dose of 1 tablet daily or 3 times weekly has a prophylactic effect in sexually active women and others prone to develop recurrent urinary tract infections.

Penicillins

All penicillins share the same chemical nucleus, which contains the β-lactam ring necessary for biologic activity, and act on bacteria by inhibiting the final step (transpeptidation) in the synthesis of cell wall mucopeptide. Part of the bactericidal action of penicillins is due to activation of lytic enzymes in the cell wall. The commonest cause of resistance to some penicillins is bacterial production of enzymes (β-lactamases) that break the lactam ring and inactivate the drug. Penicillin resistance on this basis is common among staphylococci and gram-negative rods.

All penicillins taken by mouth must be given 1 hour before or after a meal. Penicillin G remains a drug of choice for streptococci, non-β-lactamase-producing staphylococci and gonococci, treponemes, clostridia, and other anaerobes. Oral penicillin G, 800,000 units 4 times daily; or ampicillin, 500 mg 4 times daily; or amoxicillin, 250 mg 4 times daily, each can be effective in acute cystitis caused by E coli or Proteus mirabilis. Each of these drugs, until and unless (before being) inactivated by β-lactamase, appears in the urine in sufficiently high concentration to suppress the causative bacteria. Carbenicillin indanyl sodium, in a dosage of 1–2 tablets orally every 6 hours, can be effective in urinary tract infections caused by Proteus or Pseudomonas.

For severe systemic infection, these lactamase-susceptible penicillins are injected intravenously in doses 5–50 times larger than those given above (see Table 12–2). Carbenicillin or ticarcillin is often combined with gentamicin to treat major infections caused by *Pseudomonas*. Ampicil-

Table 12–2. Antimicrobials often used in urology.

Drug	Route	Daily Adult Dose	Daily Pediatric Dose	Untoward Effects
Soluble sulfonamide (sulfisoxazole, trisulfapyrimidines)	Oral	1 g 4 times	100–150 mg/kg	Rashes, fever, nausea, vomiting, diarrhea, arthritis, stomatitis, thrombocytopenia, hemolytic or aplastic anemia, granulocytopenia, hepatitis, vasculitis, Stevens-Johnson syndrome, psychosis, etc. Crystalluria and hematuria rare.
Trimethoprim	Oral	100 mg twice	15–30 mg/kg	
Trimethoprim-sulfamethoxazole (co-trimoxazole)	Oral	4 tablets	Trimethoprim, 15 mg/kg, and sulfamethoxazole, 150 mg/kg	
Ampicillin	Oral	2–4 g	50–100 mg/kg	Hypersensitivity: rashes, fever, anaphylaxis, dermatitis, serum sickness, nephritis, eosinophilia, vasculitis, hemolytic anemia, granulocytopenia. Nausea, vomiting, diarrhea especially with oral penicillins. CNS toxicity with very high doses and renal insufficiency.
	IV	2–10 g	100–300 mg/kg	
Amoxicillin	Oral	0.75–1.5 g	20–40 mg/kg	
Carbenicillin	Oral	1.5–3 g	50–70 mg/kg	
	IV	30 g	100–600 mg/kg	
Ticarcillin	IV	200–300 mg/kg	200–300 mg/kg	
Nafcillin	Oral	2–4 g	50–100 mg/kg	
	IV	3–12 g	100–200 mg/kg	
Dicloxacillin	Oral	1–2 g	25–50 mg/kg	
Penicillin V or G	Oral	1.6–3.2 million units	0.05–0.1 million units/kg	
Penicillin G	IV	1.2–20 million units	0.05–0.3 million units/kg	
Cefazolin	IV	3–6 g	25–100 mg/kg	Same as with penicillins.
Cephalothin	IV	3–12 g	60–100 mg/kg	
Cefoxitin	IV	3–12 g	?	
Cefamandole	IV	2–10 g	50–150 mg/kg	
Cephalexin	Oral	1–4 g	25–50 mg/kg	
Cephradine	Oral	1–4 g	25–50 mg/kg	
Tetracycline	Oral	1–2 g	20–40 mg/kg	Fever, rashes, anorexia, nausea, diarrhea, yellow mottling of teeth and bones, liver damage, vestibular reactions, renal tubular damage.
Oxytetracycline	Oral	1–2 g	20–40 mg/kg	
Doxycycline	Oral	200 mg	2.5–4 mg/kg	
Minocycline	Oral	200 mg	2.5–4 mg/kg	
Chloramphenicol	Oral	1–3 g	50 mg/kg	Anorexia, nausea, diarrhea, aplastic anemia (rare), gray syndrome in neonates.
	IV	2–4 g	50–100 mg/kg	
Erythromycin	Oral	1–2 g	30–50 mg/kg	Anorexia, nausea, diarrhea; cholestatic hepatitis as a hypersensitivity reaction.
Gentamicin	IM or IV	3–5 mg/kg	3–5 mg/kg	Nephrotoxicity and ototoxicity.
Tobramycin	IM or IV	3–5 mg/kg	3–5 mg/kg	
Amikacin	IM or IV	15 mg/kg	15 mg/kg	
Kanamycin	IM or IV	15 mg/kg	15 mg/kg	
Polymyxin B	IV	2.5 mg/kg	1.5–2.5 mg/kg	Paresthesias, dizziness, nephrotoxicity.
Colistimethate	IM	2.5–5 mg/kg	2.5 mg/kg	
Nitrofurantoin	Oral	200–400 mg	5–7 mg/kg	Nausea, vomiting, rashes, pulmonary infiltrates, rare neurotoxicity.
Methenamine hippurate	Oral	2 g	75 mg/kg	Vesical irritation.
Methenamine mandelate	Oral	4 g	75 mg/kg	
Nalidixic acid	Oral	4 g	30–60 mg/kg	Rashes, gastrointestinal disturbances, visual and CNS disturbances, photosensitization (rare).
Oxolinic acid	Oral	4 g	—	

lin combined with gentamicin or tobramycin is the drug of choice for systemic infections caused by enterococci.

The β-lactamase-resistant penicillins are principally used against lactamase-producing staphylococci. For minor infections, nafcillin or dicloxacillin can be given by mouth; for major infections, nafcillin, 3–12 g, is injected intravenously (see Table 12–2).

All penicillins cross-react in hypersensitive patients, and persons with a history of penicillin reactions are also about 4 times more likely to have hypersensitivity reactions to a cephalosporin than persons without such a history. However, a history of penicillin reaction is far from reliable in predicting a patient's response. Penicillin excretion is reduced in renal failure, and the dose should be adjusted downward (Table 12–1).

Cephalosporins

These drugs are chemically similar to penicillins, cross-react to a certain extent with them, and have an identical mode of action. Cephalosporins are relatively resistant to β-lactamases and can be effective against bacteria producing these enzymes. The number of available cephalosporins (and related cephamycins) grows every month, with special claims being made for the efficacy and safety of each drug.

Oral cephalosporins, including cephalexin, cephradine, and cefaclor, are sufficiently well absorbed so that 0.25–1 g taken every 6 hours results in high urine levels, suitable for treatment of acute urinary tract infection due to coliform organisms. Parenteral cephalosporins, including cefazolin or cephradine in dosages of 4 g/d and cefamandole or cephalothin in dosages of 4–12 g/d, must be given intravenously for major systemic infections or severe pyelonephritis caused by gram-negative enteric bacteria. Cefoxitin, 3–12 g/d intravenously, has activity against anaerobes as well. Cefazolin, 1 g every 6 hours pre- and postoperatively for 24 hours, has found favor in surgical prophylaxis. Cephalosporins should never be used for infections of the central nervous system. All cephalosporins can induce hypersensitivity reactions, but hematologic or renal disorders are rare. Their toxic potential may be enhanced by diuretics or aminoglycosides.

Tetracyclines

This large group of bacteriostatic drugs is active against many different organisms. Tetracycline hydrochloride and oxytetracycline are most commonly used in oral doses of 0.5 g 4 times daily. Because of a high frequency of resistance among coliform bacteria and enterococci, these drugs are not at present preferred in urinary tract infections. However, many gonococcal infections are cured by treatment for 5 days, and nongonococcal urethritis and other chlamydial infections are cured by treatment for 10–14 days.

The absorption of tetracyclines is impaired by divalent cations (milk, antacids, ferrous sulfate), and a large proportion of the oral drug is excreted in feces and modifies normal flora in the gut. Because they are deposited in bone and teeth, tetracyclines should not be given to pregnant women or children under age 7. Tetracyclines, except doxycycline, accumulate in renal insufficiency.

Chloramphenicol

This bacteriostatic drug is effective against many bacteria, but because of its potential serious toxicity (aplastic anemia, gray syndrome in infants) it is only used for very specific indications. Oral doses of 0.5 g 4 times daily are sometimes used for serious anaerobic infections or gram-negative sepsis. However, chloramphenicol has little place in general urologic practice.

Aminoglycosides

Drugs in this large group share antimicrobial, pharmacologic, and toxic features. They act as potent inhibitors of protein synthesis in bacteria and are often bactericidal. All aminoglycosides are ototoxic and nephrotoxic, and all are more effective at alkaline pH. All can accumulate in renal failure; to avoid serious toxicity, adjustments must be made in dosage or the time interval between injections when the serum creatinine is elevated. No aminoglycosides are absorbed from the gut; they must be injected intramuscularly or intravenously to yield systemic or urinary levels. The usefulness of a given aminoglycoside varies with time and place, since susceptible bacterial populations are replaced by resistant ones owing to overuse of the drug. Susceptibility testing is essential.

A. Neomycin and Kanamycin: These 2 aminoglycosides are too ototoxic and nephrotoxic to be used systemically. When taken orally, they remain principally in the gut lumen and affect the gut flora. These drugs, 1 g every 6 hours, sometimes combined with erythromycin base, 0.5 g 4 times daily, are used preoperatively for 1–2 days to prepare for intestinal surgery. Occasionally, solutions of these drugs are used for irrigation of contaminated or infected spaces, but the total daily dose must not exceed 10 mg/kg. Placement of 2–4 g of these drugs into the peritoneal cavity may result in respiratory arrest.

B. Gentamicin and Tobramycin: These drugs are active against many gram-negative bacteria in concentrations of 1–5 μg/mL, but streptococci and *Bacteroides* are unaffected. There is significant cross resistance between the drugs, and strains of *Pseudomonas*, *Serratia*, *Proteus*, and *Enterobacter* must be tested for individual susceptibility. After injection of 5–7 mg/kg/d in divided doses, serum levels reach 3–8 μg/mL—sufficient to treat gram-negative systemic and bacteremic infections. With injected doses of 2–3 mg/kg/d, urine drug levels are ample to control most of the common infecting organisms in urinary tract infection.

Upon prolonged use, these drugs may affect both the auditory and vestibular portions of the eighth nerve. The loss of high-frequency sound perception is often a premonitory sign on audiograms. These drugs are nephrotoxic, particularly in renal failure, and dose adjustment is required. This can be done best by laboratory monitoring of drug levels (to be kept below peak levels of 10 μg/mL) or by adjustments suggested in Table 12–1. The initial dose of tobramycin for a patient with renal insufficiency can be estimated as follows: 1 mg/kg intramuscularly every (6 × serum creatinine level [in mg/dL]) hours. Tobramycin is believed to be less nephrotoxic than gentamicin, but this is not established.

Both drugs sometimes act synergistically with carbenicillin or ticarcillin against gram-negative rods, especially *Pseudomonas*, but laboratory confirmation is required in individual cases.

C. Amikacin: Give 15 mg/kg/d intramuscularly of this derivative of kanamycin to achieve peak serum levels of 10–30 μg/mL. In systemic infections, some gram-negative bacteria that are resis-

Table 12–3. Choices of drugs for microorganisms commonly encountered in infections of the urinary and genital tracts.

	Drug(s) of Choice	Alternative Drug(s)
Gram-positive cocci		
Staphylococcus aureus (β-lactamase – producing)	Nafcillin or cephradine*	Vancomycin
Staphylococcus (non – β-lactamase – producing)	Penicillin G	Erythromycin
Streptococcus, group D		
Streptococcus faecalis (also *Streptococcus faecium,* enterococci)	Ampicillin plus gentamicin†	Penicillin G plus amikacin
Streptococcus bovis	Penicillin G	Vancomycin
Streptococcus, group B	Ampicillin	Cephalexin*
Gram-negative cocci		
Gonococcus	Penicillin G plus probenecid	Tetracycline
Gonococcus (β-lactamase – producing)	Spectinomycin	Cefoxitin plus probenecid
Gram-negative rods		
Escherichia coli	Sulfonamide or ampicillin	Gentamicin or probenecid
Klebsiella sp	Gentamicin	Cefamandole
Enterobacter sp	Gentamicin	Cefamandole
Proteus mirabilis	Ampicillin	Gentamicin
Proteus vulgaris and others	Gentamicin or amikacin	Cefoxitin or chloramphenicol
Pseudomonas aeruginosa	Gentamicin plus carbenicillin	Polymyxin or colistimethate
Serratia sp	Co-trimoxazole and polymyxin	Gentamicin or amikacin
Haemophilus vaginalis	Metronidazole	Tetracycline
Chlamydiae *(Chlamydia trachomatis)*	Tetracycline	Erythromycin
Mycoplasmas *(Ureaplasma urealyticum)*	Erythromycin	Tetracycline

*Or other oral cephalosporin.
†Or amoxicillin.

tant to gentamicin or tobramycin respond to amikacin. In urinary tract infection caused by such resistant bacteria, amikacin, 5–8 mg/kg/d intramuscularly, provides urine levels sufficient to suppress the bacteria. Like all aminoglycosides, amikacin is nephrotoxic and ototoxic. Its levels should be monitored in patients with renal insufficiency.

Spectinomycin

This drug, related to aminoglycosides, is used only for treatment of penicillinase-producing gonococci. A single intramuscular injection of 2 g cures up to 95% of such gonorrhea. Pain at the injection site is significant.

Polymyxins

Polymyxin B and polymyxin E (colistin) are bactericidal for many gram-negative bacteria. Polymyxin B sulfate, 2.5 mg/kg/d, can be given intravenously in serious infections with resistant gram-negative organisms. Colistimethate (polymyxin E) produces little pain on intramuscular injection, and 2.5–5 mg/kg/d can be given to achieve very high levels in urine. *Pseudomonas* and *Serratia* are often susceptible.

In closed catheter drainage, mixtures of polymyxin B, 20 mg/L, plus neomycin, 40 mg/L, can be used for continuous irrigation to delay establishment of bacterial infection in the bladder. Polymyxins are bound and inactivated by purulent exudates and have no effect in deep tissue or organ infections. Their side-effects—dizziness, paresthesias, incoordination, and proteinuria—tend to

disappear upon cessation of the drug. Instillation of 300 mg or more of these drugs into the peritoneal cavity can result in respiratory arrest.

Erythromycins & Lincomycins

These drugs are active mainly against gram-positive bacteria and serve as substitutes for penicillins in allergic patients. Clindamycin is effective against anaerobic infections, particularly *Bacteroides fragilis*. It is given in doses of 300 mg orally or intravenously 2–4 times daily, but there is a substantial risk of developing antibiotic-associated colitis with prolonged use. There are few indications for these drugs in urology, although erythromycin diffuses well into the prostate.

URINARY ANTISEPTICS

Urinary antiseptics are drugs that exert antibacterial activity in the urine but have few or no systemic antibacterial effects. Their usefulness is limited to the treatment of urinary tract infections, and they rarely affect the microbial flora in other parts of the body.

Nitrofurantoin

Nitrofurans are inhibitory and can be bactericidal for both gram-positive and gram-negative bacteria in concentrations of 10–100 μg/mL. This is well within the range of concentrations achieved in the urine with the usual daily doses (100 mg 4 times daily by mouth). Disk sensitivity tests determine bacterial susceptibility in the urine. Most *Pseudomonas aeruginosa* and many indole-positive *Proteus* organisms are resistant to nitrofurantoin; however, there is no cross resistance between nitrofurantoin and other antimicrobials. In susceptible microbial strains, resistant mutants are very rare, and clinical resistance emerges slowly if at all. The activity of nitrofurantoin is enhanced at pH 5.5 or lower.

Nitrofurantoin is absorbed rapidly and completely after oral administration and is completely bound to protein in the bloodstream. The carrier protein is split off in the kidney, so the free drug can act in the urine. Excretion is by both glomerular filtration and tubular secretion. In the presence of renal failure, excretion is markedly reduced, and antibacterial drug levels in the urine are not reached. Thus, the drug is ineffective and toxic in uremia.

Nitrofurantoin, 400 mg daily for 7–10 days, can be effective in urinary tract infection. In chronic urinary tract infection, after initial suppression of the large bacterial population, 200 mg daily may be given for many weeks or months. In women subject to frequently recurring urinary tract infection, nitrofurantoin, 100 mg daily, is often effective prophylaxis.

The most frequent side-effects are gastrointestinal intolerance and allergic reactions ranging from rashes to pulmonary infiltrates. In glucose-6-phosphate dehydrogenase deficiency, hemolytic anemia or hepatic insufficiency may occur. Other side-effects (neuropathies, vasculitis) are rare.

Methenamine Salts of Organic Acids

Methenamine is absorbed readily after oral intake and is excreted into the urine. In acidic urine, methenamine liberates formaldehyde, which is antibacterial. Methenamine is usually administered as the salt of mandelic, sulfosalicylic, or hippuric acid. Each of these acids can be antibacterial by itself. The dosage of methenamine mandelate or sulfosalicylate is 1 g 4 times daily orally; that of mandelamine hippurate is 1 g twice daily orally.

The urinary pH must be 5.5 or lower to achieve antibacterial efficacy, and to permit a formaldehyde concentration of 100 μg/mL, the urine volume should be limited by fluid restriction to 1200 mL daily. This concentration of formaldehyde, however, may result in irritation of mucous membrane and even hematuria. Urine should be tested daily to ascertain that a suitably low pH is achieved. If necessary, methionine or ascorbic acid can be given to acidify the urine.

Methenamine drugs can be effective for suppression of bacteriuria in chronic infections, but they are less commonly effective in acute infections with very large bacterial populations. The efficacy of the 3 salts is similar, but the dosage of hippurate calls for fewer tablets to be swallowed daily. Gastrointestinal intolerance and dysuria or bladder pain are the commonest side-effects. Allergic reactions can occur. Laboratory tests with methenamine salts are meaningless, because the liberated formaldehyde is antibacterial.

Nalidixic Acid & Oxolinic Acid

In concentrations of 1–30 μg/mL, these and other synthetic organic acids inhibit many gram-negative bacteria both by making the urine acid and by inhibiting bacterial DNA synthesis. Because resistant variants (chromosomal mutants) emerge relatively commonly in susceptible populations, there is a substantial failure rate of these drugs during prolonged use in urinary tract infection. The drugs are absorbed rapidly after oral intake but are metabolized in a complex fashion so that only a small portion of active drug appears in the urine. With oral doses of 1 g 4 times daily, urine levels of active drug reach 20–200 μg/mL. For children, the dose is 30–60 mg/kg/d in 2–4 divided doses, but the drug is not recommended for young children. While no difference in efficacy of the 2 drugs can be demonstrated, individual patients may tolerate one drug better than the other. In several studies, the cure rate in acute urinary tract infection has been as high as with any other drug.

Prominent side-effects are gastrointestinal intolerance, hemolytic anemia in glucose-6-phosphate dehydrogenase deficiency, rashes, photosensitization, visual disturbances, dizziness, and restlessness. These drugs greatly increase the effect of oral anticoagulants.

Nalidixic acid in urine may give false-positive tests for glucose, but true hyperglycemia with glycosuria has also been observed.

•   •   •

References

Pathogenesis

Bahna SL, Torp KH: The sex variable in childhood urinary-tract infection. *Acta Paediatr Scand* 1975;**64**:581.

Bennett WM, Craven R: Urinary tract infections in patients with severe renal failure. *JAMA* 1976;**236**:946.

Brooker W, Aufderheide AC: Genitourinary tract infec-

tions due to atypical mycobacteria. *J Urol* 1980;**124**:242.

Cohen M: The first urinary tract infection in male children. *Am J Dis Child* 1976;**130**:810.

Cox CE: The urethra and its relationship to urinary tract infection: The flora of the normal female urethra. *South Med J* 1966;**59**:621.

Cox CE, Lacy SS, Hinman F Jr: The urethra and its relationship to urinary tract infection. 2. The urethral flora of the female with recurrent urinary infection. *J Urol* 1968;99:632.

Drew JH, Acton CM: Radiologic findings in newborn infants with urinary infection. *Arch Dis Child* 1976;51:628.

Edén CS, Janson GL, Lindberg U: Adhesiveness to urinary tract epithelial cells of fecal and urinary *Escherichia coli* isolates from patients with symptomatic urinary tract infections or asymptomatic bacteriuria of varying duration. *J Urol* 1979;122:185.

Elkins IB, Cox CE: Perineal, vaginal and urethral bacteriology of young women. 1. Incidence of gram-negative colonization. *J Urol* 1974;111:88.

Farkas A & others: Urinary prostaglandin E2 in acute bacterial cystitis. *J Urol* 1980;124:455.

Fowler JE, Latta R, Stamey TA: Studies of introital colonization in women with recurrent urinary infections. 8. Role of bacterial interference. *J Urol* 1977;118:296.

Heidrick WP, Mattingly RF, Amberg JR: Vesicoureteral reflux in pregnancy. *Obstet Gynecol* 1967;29:571.

Hinman F Jr: Bacterial elimination. *J Urol* 1968;99:811.

Hinman F Jr: Mechanism for the entry of bacteria and the establishment of urinary tract infection in female children. *J Urol* 1966;96:546.

Hodson CJ, Wilson S: Natural history of chronic pyelonephritic scarring. *Br Med J* 1965;2:191.

Hutch JA, Ayers RD, Noll LE: Vesicoureteral reflux as cause of pyelonephritis of pregnancy. *Am J Obstet Gynecol* 1963;87:478.

Jodal U: The immune response to urinary tract infections in childhood. 1. Serological diagnosis of primary symptomatic infection in girls by indirect hemagglutination. *Acta Paediatr Scand* 1975;64:96.

Klousia JW & others: Etiology of non-specific urethritis in active duty marines. *J Urol* 1978;120:67.

Kraft JK, Stamey TA: The natural history of symptomatic recurrent bacteriuria in women. *Medicine* 1977;56:55.

Krieger JN & others: Nosocomial epidemic of antibiotic-resistant *Serratia marcescens* urinary tract infections. *J Urol* 1980;124:498.

Lapides J: Mechanisms of urinary tract infection. *Urology* 1979;14:217.

Leadbetter G Jr, Slavin S: Pediatric urinary tract infections: Significance of vaginal bacteria. *Urology* 1974;3:581.

Meares EM Jr: Asymptomatic bacteriuria: Current concepts in management. *Postgrad Med* (Sept) 1977;62:106.

Michigan S: Genitourinary fungal infections. *J Urol* 1976;116:390.

Mooney JK, Mooney JS, Hinman F: The antibacterial effect of the bladder surface: An electron microscopic study. *J Urol* 1976;115:381.

Parsons CL & others: Role of surface mucin in primary antibacterial defense of bladder. *Urology* 1977;9:48.

Richards B, Cooke EM: Faecal and introital bacteria and urinary tract infection. *Br J Urol* 1979;51:317.

Roberts JA, Ricker P: Experimental pyelonephritis in the monkey. 6. Infection of infants versus adults. *Invest Urol* 1978;16:128.

Saxena SR, Laurance BM, Shaw DG: The justification for early radiological investigations of urinary-tract infection in children. *Lancet* 1975;2:403.

Shom SH, Parsons CL, Mulholland SG: Role of urothelial surface mucoprotein in intrinsic bladder defense. *Urology* 1977;9:526.

Stamey TA, Mihara G: Observations on growth of urethral and vaginal bacteria in sterile urine. *J Urol* 1980;124:461.

Stamey TA, Sexton CC: The role of vaginal colonization with enterobacteriaceae in recurrent urinary infections. *J Urol* 1975;113:214.

Stephens FD: Urologic aspects of recurrent urinary tract infection in children. *J Pediatr* 1972;80:725.

Tanagho EA, Miller ER: Abnormal voiding and urinary tract infection. *Int Urol Nephrol* 1972;4:165.

Turck M, Ronald AR, Petersdorf RF: Relapse and reinfection in chronic bacteriuria: The correlation between site of infection and pattern of recurrence in chronic bacteriuria. *N Engl J Med* 1968;278:422.

Uehling DT, Mizutani K, Balish E: Effect of immunization on bacterial adherence to urothelium. *Invest Urol* 1978;16:145.

Uehling DT, Mizutani K, Balish E: Inhibitors of bacterial adherence to urothelium. *Invest Urol* 1980;18:40.

Winberg J & others: Epidemiology of symptomatic urinary tract infection in childhood. *Acta Paediatr Scand* [*Suppl*] 1974;252:1.

Nonspecific Infections of the Kidneys

Abbate AD, Meyers J: Xanthogranulomatous pyelonephritis in childhood. *J Urol* 1976;116:231.

Bissada NK, Holder JC, Redman JF: Preoperative diagnosis of xanthogranulomatous pyelonephritis. *Urology* 1976;7:228.

Davidson AJ, Talner LB: Urographic and angiographic abnormalities in adult-onset acute bacterial nephritis. *Radiology* 1973;106:249.

Flynn JT & others: The underestimated hazards of xanthogranulomatous pyelonephritis. *Br J Urol* 1979;51:443.

Freedman LR: Chronic pyelonephritis at autopsy. *Ann Intern Med* 1967;66:697.

Gammill S & others: New thoughts concerning xanthogranulomatous pyelonephritis (X-P). *Am J Roentgenol* 1975;125:154.

Harris RE, Gilstrap LC III: Prevention of recurrent pyelonephritis during pregnancy. *Obstet Gynecol* 1974;44:637.

Hodson CJ: The radiological contribution toward the diagnosis of chronic pyelonephritis. *Radiology* 1967;88:857.

Hurwitz SR & others: Gallium-67 imaging to localize urinary-tract infections. *Br J Radiol* 1976;49:156.

Husain I, Pingle A, Kazi T: Bilateral diffuse xanthogranulomatous pyelonephritis. *Br J Urol* 1979;51:162.

Klugo RC & others: Xanthogranulomatous pyelonephritis in children. *J Urol* 1977;117:350.

Lee SE, Yoon DK, Kim YK: Emphysematous pyelonephritis. *J Urol* 1977;118:916.

Little PJ: The incidence of urinary infection in 5000 pregnant women. *Lancet* 1966;2:925.

Lohr JA & others: Prevention of recurrent urinary tract infections in girls. *Pediatrics* 1977;59:562.

Malek RS, Elder JS: Xanthogranulomatous pyelonephritis: Critical analysis of 26 cases and literature. *J Urol* 1978;119:589.

Palmer JM: Differential antibiotic excretion in unilateral structural pyelonephritis. *West J Med* 1974;120:363.

Saunders CD, Corriere JN Jr: The inability to diagnose chronic pyelonephritis on the excretory urogram in adults. *J Urol* 1974;111:560.

Silver TM & others: The radiological spectrum of acute pyelonephritis in adults and adolescents. *Radiology* 1976;**118**:65.

Still JL, Cotton D: Severe hypertension in childhood. *Arch Dis Child* 1967;**42**:34.

Thomas V, Shelokov A, Forland M: Antibody-coated bacteria in the urine and the site of urinary-tract infection. *N Engl J Med* 1974;**290**:588.

Tolia BM & others: Xanthogranulomatous pyelonephritis: Segmental or generalized disease? *J Urol* 1980;**124**:122.

Vlahos L & others: Unilateral emphysematous pyelonephritis. *Eur Urol* 1979;**5**:220.

Whalley PJ, Cunningham FG: Short-term versus continuous antimicrobial therapy for asymptomatic bacteriuria in pregnancy. *Obstet Gynecol* 1977;**49**:262.

Zinner SH, Kass EH: Long-term (10 to 14 years) follow-up of bacteriuria of pregnancy. *N Engl J Med* 1971;**285**:30.

Bacteremic Shock

Beller FK, Douglas GW: Thrombocytopenia indicating gram-negative infection and endotoxemia. *Obstet Gynecol* 1973;**41**:521.

Berk JL: Use of vasoactive drugs in the treatment of shock. *Surg Clin North Am* 1975;**55**:721.

Blaisdell FW: Pathophysiology of the respiratory distress syndrome. *Arch Surg* 1974;**108**:44.

Crowder JG, Gilkey GH, White AC: *Serratia marcescens* bacteremia: Clinical observations and studies of precipitin reactions. *Arch Intern Med* 1971;**128**:247.

Elin RJ & others: Lack of clinical usefulness of the limulus test in the diagnosis of endotoxemia. *N Engl J Med* 1975;**293**:521.

Feller I & others: Diagnosis and treatment of postoperative bacterial sepsis. *Surg Clin North Am* 1972;**52**:1391.

Gowen GF: Interpretation of central venous pressure. *Surg Clin North Am* 1973;**53**:649.

James PM Jr, Meyers RT: Central venous pressure monitoring: Misinterpretation, abuses, indications and a new technic. *Ann Surg* 1973;**175**:693.

Ledingham IM: Septic shock. *Br J Surg* 1975;**62**:777.

Lillehei RC & others: The pharmacologic approach to the treatment of shock. 1. Defining traumatic, septic, and cardiogenic shock. *Geriatrics* (July) 1972;**27**:73. 2. Diagnosis of shock and plan of treatment. *Geriatrics* (Aug) 1972;**27**:81.

Litton A: Gram-negative septicaemia in surgical practice. *Br J Surg* 1975;**62**:773.

McGovern VJ: The pathophysiology of gram-negative septicaemia. *Pathology* 1972;**4**:265.

McHenry MC, Hawk WA: Bacteremia caused by gram-negative bacilli. *Med Clin North Am* 1974;**58**:623.

Marcus AJ: Heparin therapy for disseminated intravascular coagulation. *Am J Med Sci* 1972;**264**:365.

Milligan GF & others: Pulmonary and hematologic disturbances during septic shock. *Surg Gynecol Obstet* 1974;**138**:43.

Myerowitz RL, Medeiros AA, O'Brien TF: Bacterial infection in renal homotransplant recipients. *Am J Med* 1972;**53**:308.

Preston FE & others: Intravascular coagulation and *E coli* septicaemia. *J Clin Pathol* 1973;**26**:120.

Roberts JM, Laros RK Jr: Hemorrhagic and endotoxic shock: A pathophysiologic approach to diagnosis and management. *Am J Obstet Gynecol* 1971;**110**:1041.

Robinson MRG & others: Bacteriaemia and bacteriogenic shock in district hospital urological practice. *Br J Urol* 1980;**52**:10.

Rodrigues RJ, Wolff WI: Fungal septicemia in surgical patients. *Ann Surg* 1974;**180**:741.

Rosen AJ: Shock lung: Fact or fancy? *Surg Clin North Am* 1975;**55**:613.

Rowe MI, Buckner DM, Newmark S: The early diagnosis of gram-negative septicemia in the pediatric surgical patient. *Ann Surg* 1975;**182**:280.

Schumer W: Steroids in the treatment of clinical shock. *Ann Surg* 1976;**184**:333.

Schumer W, Sperling R: Shock and its effect on the cell. *JAMA* 1968;**205**:215.

Shubin H, Weil MH: Bacterial shock. *JAMA* 1976;**235**:421.

Welch TR, Nogrady MB, Outerbridge EW: Roentgenologic sequelae of neonatal septicemia and urinary tract infection. *Am J Roentgenol* 1973;**18**:28.

Winslow EJ & others: Hemodynamic studies and results of therapy in 50 patients with bacteremic shock. *Am J Med* 1973;**54**:421.

Necrotizing Papillitis

Arger PH & others: Analgesic abuse nephropathy. *Urology* 1976;**7**:123.

Chrispin AR: Medullary necrosis in infancy. *Br Med Bull* 1973;**28**:233.

Desai S, Libertino JA, Dowd JB: Unilateral acute, fulminating renal papillary necrosis with *Escherichia* septicemia. *Urology* 1973;**2**:184.

Eckert DE, Jonutis AJ, Davidson AJ: The incidence and manifestations of urographic papillary abnormalities in patients with S hemoglobinopathies. *Radiology* 1974;**113**:59.

Flaster S, Lome LG, Presman D: Urologic complications of renal papillary necrosis. *Urology* 1975;**5**:331.

Freeland JP: Phenacetin nephritis. *Urology* 1975;**6**:37.

Goldberger LE, Talner LB: Analgesic abuse: A frequently overlooked cause of reversible renal failure. *Urology* 1975;**7**:728.

Heptinstall RH: Interstitial nephritis. *Am J Pathol* 1976;**83**:214.

Husband P, Howlett KA: Renal papillary necrosis in infancy. *Arch Dis Child* 1973;**48**:116.

Lalli AF: Renal papillary necrosis. *Am J Roentgenol* 1972;**114**:741.

Longacre AM, Popky GL: Papillary necrosis in patients with cirrhosis: A study of 102 patients. *J Urol* 1968;**99**:391.

Macklon AF & others: Aspirin and analgesic nephropathy. *Br Med J* 1974;**1**:597.

Murray RM: Analgesic nephropathy: Removal of phenacetin from proprietary analgesics. *Br Med J* 1972;**4**:131.

Murray T, Goldberg M: Chronic interstitial nephritis: Etiologic factors. *Ann Intern Med* 1975;**82**:453.

Pandya KK & others: Renal papillary necrosis in sickle cell hemoglobinopathies. *J Urol* 1976;**115**:497.

Parker RW, Shaw RE: Analgesic abuse in urological practice. *Br J Surg* 1975;**62**:298.

Poynter JD, Hare WSC: Necrosis in situ: A form of renal papillary necrosis seen in analgesic nephropathy. *Radiology* 1974;**111**:69.

Vordermark JS II, Modarelli RO, Buck AS: Torulopsis pyelonephritis associated with papillary necrosis. *J Urol* 1980;**123**:96.

Wainscoat JS, Finn R: Possible role of laxatives in analgesic nephropathy. *Br Med J* 1974;**4**:697.

Renal Abscess

Anderson KA, McAninch JW: Renal abscesses: Classification and review of 40 cases. *Urology* 1980;**16**:333.

Craven JD & others: Acute renal carbuncle: The importance of preoperative angiography. *J Urol* 1974;**111**:727.

Goldman SM & others: Renal carbuncle: The use of ultrasound in its diagnosis and treatment. *J Urol* 1977;**118**:525.

Khashu BL, Seery WH, Rothfeld SH: Nonstaphylococcal bacteria in renal cortical abscess. *Urology* 1976;**7**:256.

Koehler PR: The roentgen diagnosis of renal inflammatory masses: Special emphasis on angiographic changes. *Radiology* 1974;**112**:257.

Koehler PR, Nelson JA: Arteriographic findings in inflammatory mass lesions of the kidney. *Radiol Clin North Am* 1976;**14**:281.

Malgieri JJ, Kursh ED, Persky L: The changing clinicopathological pattern of abscesses in or adjacent to the kidney. *J Urol* 1977;**118**:230.

Pederson JF, Hancke S, Kristensen JK: Renal carbuncle: Antibiotic therapy governed by ultrasonically guided aspiration. *J Urol* 1973;**109**:777.

Rives RK, Harty JI, Amin M: Renal abscesses: Emerging concepts of diagnosis and treatment. *J Urol* 1980;**124**:446.

Schiff M Jr & others: Antibiotic treatment of renal carbuncle. *Ann Intern Med* 1977;**87**:305.

Timmons JW, Perlmutter AD: Renal abscess: A changing concept. *J Urol* 1976;**115**:299.

Perinephric Abscess

Hopkins GB, Hall RL, Mende CW: Gallium-67 scintigraphy for the diagnosis and localization of perinephric abscesses. *J Urol* 1976;**115**:126.

Love L, Baker D, Ramsey R: Gas-producing perinephric abscess. *Am J Roentgenol* 1973;**119**:783.

Meyers MA & others: Radiologic features of extraperitoneal effusions. *Radiology* 1972;**104**:249.

Simpkins KC, Barraclough NC: Renal cortical abscess, perinephritis and perinephric abscess in diabetes. *Br J Radiol* 1973;**46**:433.

Thorley JD, Jones SR, Sanford JP: Perinephric abscess. *Medicine* 1974;**53**:441.

Nonspecific Infections of the Bladder

Alexander AR, Morrisseau PM, Leadbetter GW Jr: Urethral-hymenal adhesions and recurrent post-coital cystitis: Treatment by hymenoplasty. *J Urol* 1972;**107**:597.

Anderson RU, Hatami-Tehrani G: Monitoring for bacteriuria in spinal cord-injured patients on intermittent catheterization: Dip-slide culture technique. *Urology* 1979;**14**:244.

Bailey RR & others: Urinary-tract infection in nonpregnant women. *Lancet* 1973;**2**:275.

Bass HN: "Bubble bath" as an irritant to the urinary tract of children. *Clin Pediatr (Phila)* 1968;**7**:174.

Berkson BM, Lome LG, Shapiro I: Severe cystitis induced by cyclophosphamide: Role of surgical management. *JAMA* 1973;**225**:605.

Cicmanec JF, Evans AT: Classification of urinary tract infections by biotype identification of pathogens. *J Urol* 1980;**124**:68.

Corriere JN Jr, Wise MF: Acute cystitis in young women: Diagnosis and treatment. *Urology* 1973;**1**:453.

Fair WR, McClennan BL, Jost RG: Are excretory urograms necessary in evaluating women with urinary tract infection? *J Urol* 1979;**121**:313.

Fair WR & others: Urinary tract infections in children. 1. Young girls with non-refluxing ureters. *West J Med* 1974;**121**:366.

Hawtry CE, Williams JJ, Schmidt JD: Cystitis emphysematosa. *Urology* 1974;**3**:612.

Helin I, Okmian L: Haemorrhagic cystitis complicating cyclophosphamide treatment in children. *Acta Paediatr Scand* 1973;**62**:497.

Kirk D & others: Hibitane bladder irrigation in the prevention of catheter-associated urinary infection. *Br J Urol* 1979;**51**:528.

Lapides J & others: Followup on unsterile, intermittent self-catheterization. *J Urol* 1974;**111**:184.

Lewis EL, Griffith TH: Recurring cystourethritis in women: Is an effective therapy available? *J Urol* 1973;**110**:544.

Mufson MA & others: Cause of acute hemorrhagic cystitis in children. *Am J Dis Child* 1973;**126**:605.

Powell NB & others: Allergy of the lower urinary tract. *J Urol* 1972;**107**:631.

Vosti KL: Recurrent urinary tract infections: Prevention by prophylactic antibiotics after sexual intercourse. *JAMA* 1975;**231**:934.

Acute Cystitis

Hashida Y, Gaffney PC, Yunis EJ: Acute hemorrhagic cystitis of childhood and papovavirus-like particles. *J Pediatr* 1976;**89**:85.

Mufson MA, Belshe RB: A review of adenoviruses in the etiology of acute hemorrhagic cystitis. *J Urol* 1976;**115**:191.

Sellin M & others: Micrococcal urinary-tract infections in young women. *Lancet* 1975;**2**:570.

Chronic Cystitis

See references listed under Nonspecific Infections of the Kidneys.

Nonspecific Infections of the Prostate Gland

Blacklock NJ: Anatomical factors in prostatitis. *Br J Urol* 1974;**46**:47.

Dabhoiwala NF, Bye A, Claridge M: A study of concentrations of trimethoprim-sulfamethoxazole in the human prostate gland. *Br J Urol* 1976;**48**:77.

Drach GW: Problems in diagnosis of bacterial prostatitis: Gram-negative, gram-positive and mixed infections. *J Urol* 1974;**111**:630.

Drach GW: Trimethoprim/sulfamethoxazole therapy of chronic bacterial prostatitis. *J Urol* 1974;**111**:637.

Fair WR: Diffusion of minocycline into prostatic secretion in dogs. *Urology* 1974;**3**:339.

Fair WR, Couch J, Wehner N: Prostatic antibacterial factor: Identity and significance. *Urology* 1976;**7**:169.

Hensle TW, Prout GR Jr, Griffin P: Minocycline diffusion into benign prostatic hyperplasia. *J Urol* 1977;**118**:609.

Kohnen PW, Drach GW: Patterns of inflammation in prostatic hyperplasia: Histologic and bacteriologic study. *J Urol* 1979;**121**:755.

Litvak AS & others: Cefazolin and cephalexin levels in prostatic tissue and sera. *Urology* 1976;**7**:497.

Madsen PO, Kjaer TB, Baumueller A: Prostatic tissue and fluid concentrations of trimethoprim and sulfamethoxazole: Experimental and clinical studies. *Urology* 1976;**8**:129.

Mann S: Prostatic abscess in the newborn. *Arch Dis Child* 1960;**35**:396.

Meares EM Jr: Prostatitis syndromes: New perspectives about old woes. *J Urol* 1980;**123**:141.

Mitchell RJ, Blake JRS: Spontaneous perforation of prostatic abscess with peritonitis. *J Urol* 1972;**107**:622.

Mobley DF: Erythromycin plus sodium bicarbonate in chronic bacterial prostatitis. *Urology* 1974;**3**:60.

Mobley DF: Semen cultures in the diagnosis of bacterial prostatitis. *J Urol* 1975;**114**:83.

Morrisseau PM, Phillips CA, Leadbetter GW Jr: Viral prostatitis. *J Urol* 1970;**103**:767.

Murnahan GF & others: Chronic prostatitis: An Australian view. *Br J Urol* 1974;**46**:55.

Nishimura T, Mobley DF, Carlton CE Jr: Immunoglobulin A in split ejaculates of patients with prostatitis. *Urology* 1977;**9**:186.

O'Dea MJ, Hunting DB, Greene LF: Non-specific granulomatous prostatitis. *J Urol* 1977;**118**:58.

Oosterlinck W, Defoort R, Renders G: The concentration of sulfamethoxazole and trimethoprim in human prostate gland. *Br J Urol* 1975;**47**:301.

Pai MG, Bhat HS: Prostatic abscess. *J Urol* 1972;**108**:599.

Smart CJ, Jenkins JD: The role of transurethral prostatectomy in chronic prostatitis. *Br J Urol* 1973;**45**:654.

Stamey TA, Mears EM Jr, Winningham DG: Chronic bacterial prostatitis and the diffusion of drugs into prostatic fluid. *J Urol* 1970;**103**:187.

Taylor EW & others: Granulomatous prostatitis: Confusion clinically with carcinoma of the prostate. *J Urol* 1977;**117**:316.

Towfighi J & others: Granulomatous prostatitis with emphasis on the eosinophilic variety. *Am J Clin Pathol* 1972;**58**:630.

Nonspecific Infections of the Male Urethra

Bennett AH, Kundsin RB, Shapiro SR: T-strain mycoplasmas, the etiologic agent of non-specific urethritis: A venereal disease. *J Urol* 1973;**109**:427.

Burns DC & others: Isolation of *Chlamydia* from women attending a clinic for sexually transmitted disease. *Br J Vener Dis* 1975;**51**:314.

Felman YM, Nikitas JA: Nongonococcal urethritis. *JAMA* 1981;**245**:381.

Furness G, Evangelista AT: Infection of a nonspecific urethritis patient and his consort with a pathogenic species of nonspecific urethritis corynebacteria, *Corynebacterium genitalium*, n. sp. *Invest Urol* 1976;**14**:202.

Helmy N, Fowler W: Intensive and prolonged tetracycline therapy in non-specific urethritis. *Br J Vener Dis* 1975;**51**:336.

Hobson D & others: Simplified method for diagnosis of genital and ocular infections with chlamydia. *Lancet* 1974;**2**:555.

Holmes KK & others: Etiology of nongonococcal urethritis. *N Engl J Med* 1975;**292**:1199.

Jacobs NF Jr, Kraus SJ: Gonococcal and nongonococcal urethritis in men: Clinical and laboratory differentiation. *Ann Intern Med* 1975;**82**:7.

McChesney JA & others: Acute urethritis in male college students. *JAMA* 1973;**226**:37.

McCormack WM & others: The genital mycoplasmas. *N Engl J Med* 1973;**288**:78.

Marshall S: The effect of bubble bath on the urinary tract. *J Urol* 1965;**93**:112.

Meares EM Jr: Infectious urethritis in men and women. *West J Med* 1975;**123**:436.

Oriel JD & others: Chlamydial infection of the male urethra. *Br J Vener Dis* 1976;**52**:46.

Vinson RK, Koff SA: Intermittent catheterization in treatment of acute purulent urethritis. *J Urol* 1977;**117**:251.

Nonspecific Infections of the Epididymis

Berger RE & others: Clinical use of epididymal aspiration cultures in management of selected patients with acute epididymitis. *J Urol* 1980;**124**:60.

Berger RE & others: Etiology, manifestations and therapy of acute epididymitis: Prospective study of 50 cases. *J Urol* 1979;**121**:750.

Gierup J, Von Hedenberg C, Österman A: Acute nonspecific epididymitis in boys: A survey based on 48 consecutive cases. *Scand J Urol Nephrol* 1975;**9**:5.

Kiviat MD, Shurtleff D, Ansell JS: Urinary reflux via the vas deferens: Unusual cause of epididymitis in infancy. *J Pediatr* 1972;**80**:476.

Koff SA: Altered bladder function and non-specific epididymitis. *J Urol* 1976;**116**:589.

Lawrence D, Mishkin F: Radionuclide imaging in epididymo-orchitis. *J Urol* 1974;**112**:387.

Miller HC: Local anesthesia for acute epididymitis. *J Urol* 1970;**104**:735.

Smith DR: Treatment of epididymitis by infiltration of the spermatic cord with procaine hydrochloride. *J Urol* 1941;**46**:74.

Wilson SK, Hagan KW, Rhamy RK: Epididymectomy for acute and chronic disease. *J Urol* 1974;**112**:357.

Nonspecific Infections of the Testis & Scrotum

Biswas M & others: Necrotizing infection of scrotum. *Urology* 1979;**14**:576.

Chilton CP, Smith PJB: Steroid therapy in the treatment of a granulomatous orchitis. *Br J Urol* 1979;**51**:404.

Fauer RB & others: Clinical aspects of granulomatous orchitis. *Urology* 1978;**12**:416.

Lyon RP, Bruyn HB: Treatment of mumps epididymoorchitis. *JAMA* 1966;**196**:736.

Riggs S, Sanford JP: Viral orchitis. *N Engl J Med* 1962;**266**:990.

Utz JP, Houk VN, Alling DW: Clinical and laboratory studies of mumps. 4. Viruria and abnormal renal function. *N Engl J Med* 1964;**270**:1283.

Antimicrobial Treatment of Urinary Tract Infections

Appel GB, Neu HC: The nephrotoxicity of antimicrobial agents. (3 parts.) *N Engl J Med* 1977;**296**:663, 722, 784.

Bailey RR, Koutsaimanis KG: Oral administration of a new carbenicillin in the treatment of urinary tract infection. *Br J Urol* 1972;**44**:235.

Bailey RR & others: Prevention of urinary-tract infection with low-dose nitrofurantoin. *Lancet* 1971;**2**:1112.

Balsdon MJ & others: *Corynebacterium vaginale* and vaginitis: A controlled trial of treatment. *Lancet* 1980;**1**:501.

Bennett WM & others: Guidelines for drug therapy in renal failure. *Ann Intern Med* 1977;**86**:754.

Bobrow SN, Jaffe E, Young RC: Anuria with acute tubular necrosis associated with gentamicin and cephalothin. *JAMA* 1972;**222**:1546.

Bodner SJ, Koenig MG: Clinical and in vitro evaluation of cephapirin: A new parenteral cephalosporin. *Am J Med Sci* 1972;**263**:43.

Böse W & others: Controlled trial of co-trimoxazole in children with urinary tract infection. *Lancet* 1974;**2**:614.

Brusch JL & others: An in vitro and pharmacological comparison of amoxicillin and ampicillin. *Am J Med Sci* 1974;**267**:41.

Burton JR & others: Acute renal failure during cephalothin therapy. *JAMA* 1974;**229**:679.

Calderwood SB, Moellering RC Jr: Common adverse effects of antibacterial agents on major organ systems. *Surg Clin North Am* 1980;**60**:65.

Carling PC & others: Nephrotoxicity associated with cephalothin administration. *Arch Intern Med* 1975;**135**:797.

Carvajal HF & others: Infections of the urinary tract. In: *Antimicrobial Therapy*, 3rd ed. Kagan BM (editor). Saunders, 1980.

CDC recommended treatment schedules 1979. [Gonorrhea.] *MMWR* 1979;**28**:13.

Cederberg Ä & others: Nalidixic acid in urinary tract infections with particular reference to the emergence of resistance. *Scand J Infect Dis* 1974;**6**:259.

Chodak GW, Plaut ME: Systemic antibiotics for prophylaxis in urologic surgery: Critical review. *J Urol* 1979;**121**:695.

Cosgrove MD, Morrow JW: Ampicillin versus trimethoprim/sulfamethoxazole in chronic urinary tract infection. *J Urol* 1974;**111**:670.

Craig WA, Kunin CM: Trimethoprim-sulfamethoxazole: Pharmacodynamic effects of urinary pH and impaired renal function. *Ann Intern Med* 1973;**78**:491.

Dean R, Herlihy E, McGuire EJ: Accuracy of antimicrobial disk sensitivity testing in urinary tract infections. *J Urol* 1978;**120**:80.

Dorfman LE, Smith JP: Sulfonamide crystalluria: A forgotten disease. *J Urol* 1970;**104**:482.

Fair WR & others: Three-day treatment of urinary tract infections. *J Urol* 1980;**123**:717.

Fillastre JP & others: Acute renal failure associated with combined gentamicin and cephalothin therapy. *Br Med J* 1973;**2**:396.

Freeman RB & others: Long-term therapy for chronic bacteriuria in men: US Public Health Service Cooperative Study. *Ann Intern Med* 1975;**83**:133.

Gary NE & others: Gentamicin-associated acute renal failure. *Arch Intern Med* 1976;**136**:1101.

Geddes AM & others: Cefoxitin: A hospital study. *Br Med J* 1977;**1**:1126.

Gleckman RA: Trimethoprim-sulfamethoxazole vs ampicillin in chronic urinary tract infections: A double-blind multicenter cooperative controlled study. *JAMA* 1975;**233**:427.

Govan DE & others: Management of children with urinary tract infections: The Stanford experience. *Urology* 1975;**6**:273.

Gower PE, Tasker PRW: Comparative double-blind study of cephalexin and co-trimoxazole in urinary tract infections. *Br Med J* 1976;**1**:684.

Grieco MH: Use of antibiotics in the elderly. *Bull NY Acad Med* (March) 1980;**56**:197.

Handbook of Antimicrobial Therapy. Med Lett Drug Ther, 1980.

Harrison LH: Treatment of complicated urinary tract infections with amikacin: Comparison of low and high dosage. *Urology* 1977;**10**:110.

Hausman MS: Treatment of urinary infections with cefa-

droxil: Controlled comparison of high-compliance oral dosage regimens. *Urology* 1980;**15**:40.

Hodges GR, Perkins RL: Carbenicillin indanyl sodium oral therapy of urinary tract infections. *Arch Intern Med* 1973;**131**:679.

Hodges GR, Saslaw S: Experiences with cefazolin: A new cephalosporin antibiotic. *Am J Med Sci* 1973;**265**:23.

Hulbert J: Gram-negative urinary infection treated with oral penicillin G. *Lancet* 1972;**2**:1216.

Jawetz E: Synergism and antagonism among antimicrobial drugs. *West J Med* 1975;**123**:87.

Jones RB & others: Cefoxitin in the treatment of gonorrhea. *Sex Transm Dis* 1979;**6**:239.

Khan AJ & others: Amikacin pharmacokinetics in the therapy of childhood urinary tract infection. *Pediatrics* 1976;**58**:873.

Klastersky J & others: Comparative clinical study of tobramycin and gentamicin. *Antimicrob Agents Chemother* (Feb) 1974;**5**:133.

Klastersky J & others: Effectiveness of the carbenicillin/cephalothin combination against gram-negative bacilli. *Am J Med Sci* 1973;**265**:45.

Kluge RM & others: The carbenicillin-gentamicin combination against *Pseudomonas aeruginosa. Ann Intern Med* 1974;**81**:584.

Koch-Weser J & others: Adverse reactions to sulfisoxazole, sulfamethoxazole, and nitrofurantoin. *Arch Intern Med* 1971;**128**:399.

Kunin CM: *Detection, Prevention and Management of Urinary Tract Infections*, 3rd ed. Lea & Febiger, 1978.

Kursh ED, Mostyn EM, Persky L: Nitrofurantoin pulmonary complications. *J Urol* 1975;**113**:392.

Lacey RW & others: Trimethoprim-resistant coliforms. *Lancet* 1972;**1**:409.

Landes RR: Long-term low dose cinoxacin therapy for prevention of recurrent urinary tract infections. *J Urol* 1980;**123**:47.

Laxdal T, Hallgrimsson J: The "grey toddler": Chloramphenicol toxicity. *Arch Dis Child* 1974;**49**:235.

Lohr JA & others: Prevention of recurrent urinary tract infections in girls. *Pediatrics* 1977;**59**:562.

McCracken GH Jr: Clinical pharmacology of gentamicin in infants 2 to 24 months of age. *Am J Dis Child* 1972;**124**:884.

McCracken GH Jr: Pharmacological basis for antimicrobial therapy in newborn infants. *Am J Dis Child* 1974;**128**:407.

McCracken GH Jr, Eichenwald HF: Antimicrobial therapy: Therapeutic recommendations and a review of the newer drugs. 2. The clinical pharmacology of the newer antimicrobial agents. *J Pediatr* 1974;**85**:451.

McHenry MC & others: Gentamicin dosages for renal insufficiency. *Ann Intern Med* 1971;**74**:192.

Margileth AM & others: Urinary tract infections: Office diagnosis and management. *Pediatr Clin North Am* 1976;**23**:721.

Maxwell D & others: Ampicillin nephropathy. *JAMA* 1974;**230**:586.

Miller H, Phillips E: Antibacterial correlates of urine drug levels of hexamethylenetetramine and formaldehyde. *Invest Urol* 1970;**8**:21.

Milman N: Renal failure with gentamicin therapy. *Acta Med Scand* 1974;**196**:87.

Moellering RC, Swartz MN: The newer cephalosporins. *N Engl J Med* 1976;**294**:24.

Nilsson S: Long-term treatment with methenamine hippurate in recurrent urinary tract infection. *Acta Med Scand* 1975;**198**:81.

Paisley JW, Smith AL, Smith DH: Gentamicin in newborn infants. *Am J Dis Child* 1973;**126**:473.

Pasternak DP, Stephens BG: Reversible nephrotoxicity associated with cephalothin therapy. *Arch Intern Med* 1975;**135**:599.

Paulson DF, White RD: Trimethoprim-sulfamethoxazole and minocycline-hydrochloride in treatment of culture-proved bacterial prostatitis. *J Urol* 1978;**120**:184.

Phillips ME & others: Tetracycline poisoning in renal failure. *Br Med J* 1974;**2**:149.

Pollock AA & others: Amikacin therapy for serious gram-negative infection. *JAMA* 1977;**237**:562.

Rahal JJ: Antibiotic combinations: The clinical relevance of synergy and antagonism. *Medicine* 1978;**57**:179.

Regamey C, Gordon RC, Kirby WMM: Cefazolin vs cephalothin and cephaloridine. *Arch Intern Med* 1974;**133**:407.

Reyes MP, Palutke M, Lerner AM: Granulocytopenia associated with carbenicillin: Five episodes in two patients. *Am J Med* 1973;**54**:413.

Rosenthal SL: Aminoglycoside antibiotics: Selected aspects of antibacterial activity and pharmacology. *NY State J Med* 1975;**75**:535.

Ross RR Jr, Conway GF: Hemorrhagic cystitis following accidental overdose of methenamine mandelate. *Am J Dis Child* 1970;**119**:86.

Sanders WE Jr, Johnson JE III, Taggart JG: Adverse reactions to cephalothin and cephapirin: Uniform occurrence on prolonged intravenous administration of high doses. *N Engl J Med* 1974;**290**:424.

Schachter J: Chlamydial infections. (3 parts.) *N Engl J Med* 1978;**298**:428, 490, 540.

Seneca H: Indanyl carbenicillin in chronic recurrent urinary tract infections. *J Urol* 1973;**110**:249.

Seneca H, Uson A, Peer P: Cephalexin in urinary tract infections. *J Urol* 1972;**107**:832.

Siegel WH: Unusual complication of therapy with sulfamethoxazole-trimethoprim. *J Urol* 1977;**117**:397.

Smith CR & others: Double-blind comparison of the nephrotoxicity and auditory toxicity of gentamicin and tobramycin. *N Engl J Med* 1980;**302**:1106.

Stamey TA: Resistance to nalidixic acid: A misconception due to underdosage. *JAMA* 1976;**236**:1857.

Stamey TA, Govan DE, Palmer JM: The localization and treatment of urinary tract infections: The role of bactericidal urine levels as opposed to serum levels. *Medicine* 1965;**44**:1.

Taylor-Robinson D, McCormack WM: The genital mycoplasmas. (2 parts.) *N Engl J Med* 1980;**302**:1003, 1063.

Toivonen S & others: Comparison of ampicillin and nalidixic acid in the treatment of urinary infections caused by E coli. *Acta Med Scand* 1974;**195**:181.

Verma S, Kieff E: Cephalexin-related nephropathy. *JAMA* 1975;**234**:618.

Vosti KL: Recurrent urinary tract infections: Prevention by prophylactic antibiotics after sexual intercourse. *JAMA* 1975;**231**:934.

Wallerstein RO & others: Statewide study of chloramphenicol therapy and fatal aplastic anemia. *JAMA* 1969;**208**:2045.

Weinstein AJ: Newer antibiotics: Guidelines for use. *Postgrad Med* (Oct) 1976;**60**:75.

Whelton A & others: Carbenicillin concentrations in normal and diseased kidneys. *Ann Intern Med* 1973;**78**:659.

Wilkowske CJ & others: Serratia marcescens. *JAMA* 1970;**214**:2157.

Wise GJ, Kozinn PJ, Goldberg P: Flucytosine in management of genitourinary candidiasis: 5 years of experience. *J Urol* 1980;**124**:70.

Wormser GP, Keusch GT: Trimethoprim-sulfamethoxazole in the United States. *Ann Intern Med* 1979;**91**:420.

Specific Infections of the Urinary Tract | 13

Donald R. Smith, MD

TUBERCULOSIS

Tubercle bacilli may invade one or more (or even all) of the organs of the genitourinary tract and cause a chronic granulomatous infection which shows the same characteristics as tuberculosis in other organs. Urinary tuberculosis is a disease of young adults (60% of patients are between the ages of 20 and 40) and is a little more common in males than in females.

Etiology

The infecting organism is *Mycobacterium tuberculosis,* which reaches the genitourinary organs by the hematogenous route from the lungs. The primary site is often not symptomatic or apparent.

The kidney and possibly the prostate are the primary sites of tuberculous infection in the genitourinary tract. All other genitourinary organs become involved either by ascent (prostate to bladder) or descent (kidney to bladder; prostate to epididymis). The testis may become involved by direct extension from epididymal infection.

Pathogenesis (Fig 13–1)

A. Kidney and Ureter: When a shower of tubercle bacilli hits the renal cortex, the organisms may be destroyed by normal tissue resistance. Evidence of this is commonly seen in autopsies of persons who have died of tuberculosis; only scars are found in the kidneys. However, if enough bacteria of sufficient virulence become lodged in the kidney and are not overcome, a clinical infection is established.

Tuberculosis of the kidney progresses slowly; it may take 15–20 years to destroy a kidney in a patient having good resistance to the infection. As a rule, therefore, there is no renal pain and little or no clinical disturbance of any type until the lesion has involved the calices or the pelvis, at which time pus and organisms may be discharged into the urine. It is only at this stage that symptoms (of cystitis) are manifested. The infection then proceeds to the pelvic mucosa and the ureter, particularly its upper and vesical ends. This may lead to stricture and back pressure (hydronephrosis).

As the disease progresses, a caseous breakdown of tissue occurs until the entire kidney is replaced by cheesy material. Calcium may be laid down in the reparative process. The ureter undergoes fibrosis and tends to be shortened and therefore straightened. This change leads to a "golf-hole" (gaping) ureteral orifice, typical of an incompetent valve.

B. Bladder: Vesical irritability develops as an early clinical manifestation of the disease as the bladder is bathed by infected material. Tubercles form later, usually in the region of the involved ureteral orifice, and finally coalesce and ulcerate. These ulcers may bleed. With severe involvement, the bladder becomes fibrosed and contracted; this leads to marked frequency. Ureteral reflux or stenosis and, therefore, hydronephrosis may develop. If contralateral renal involvement develops later, it is probably a separate hematogenous infection.

C. Prostate and Seminal Vesicles: The passage of infected urine through the prostatic urethra will ultimately lead to invasion of the prostate and one or both seminal vesicles. There is no local pain.

On occasion, the primary hematogenous lesion in the genitourinary tract is in the prostate. Prostatic infection can extend to the bladder and descend to the epididymis.

D. Epididymis and Testis: Tuberculosis of the prostate can extend along the vas or through the perivasal lymphatics and affect the epididymis. Because this is a slow process, there is usually no pain. If the epididymal infection is extensive and an abscess forms, it may rupture through the scrotal skin, thus establishing a permanent sinus, or it may extend into the testicle.

Pathology

A. Kidney and Ureter: The gross appearance of the kidney with moderately advanced tuberculosis is often normal on its outer surface, although it is usually surrounded by marked perinephritis. Usually, however, there is a soft, yellowish localized bulge. On section, the involved area is seen to be filled with cheesy material (caseation). Widespread destruction of parenchyma is evident. In otherwise normal tissue, small abscesses may be

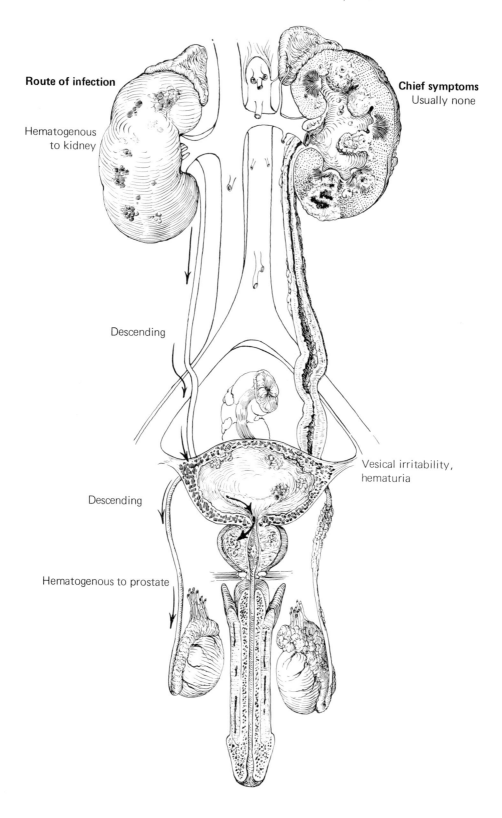

Figure 13–1. Pathogenesis of tuberculosis of the urinary tract.

seen. The walls of the pelvis, calices, and ureter may be thickened, and ulceration appears frequently in the region of the calices at the point at which the abscess drains. Ureteral stenosis may be complete, causing "autonephrectomy." Such a kidney is fibrosed and functionless. Under these circumstances, the bladder urine may be normal and symptoms absent.

Microscopically, the caseous material is seen as an amorphous mass. The surrounding parenchyma shows fibrosis with tissue destruction, small round cell and plasma cell infiltration, and epithelial and giant cells typical of tuberculosis. Acid-fast stains will usually demonstrate the organisms in the tissue. Similar changes can be demonstrated in the wall of the pelvis and ureter.

In both the kidney and ureter, calcification is common. It may be macroscopic or microscopic. Such a finding is strongly suggestive of tuberculosis but, of course, is also observed in bilharzial infection. Secondary renal stones occur in 10% of patients.

In the most advanced stage of renal tuberculosis, the parenchyma may be completely replaced by caseous substance or fibrous tissue. Perinephric abscess may develop, but this is rare.

B. Bladder: In the early stages, the mucosa may be inflamed, but this is not a specific change. The bladder is quite resistant to actual invasion. Later, tubercles form and can be seen easily, especially through the cystoscope, as white or yellow raised nodules surrounded by a halo of hyperemia. With severe vesical contracture, reflux may occur.

Microscopically, the nodules are typical tubercles. These break down to form deep, ragged ulcers. At this stage the bladder is quite irritable. With healing, fibrosis develops that involves the muscle wall.

C. Prostate and Seminal Vesicles: Grossly, the exterior surface of these organs may show nodules and areas of induration from fibrosis. Areas of necrosis are common. In rare cases, healing may end in calcification. Large calcifications in the prostate should suggest tuberculous involvement.

D. Spermatic Cord, Epididymis, and Testis: The vas deferens is often grossly involved; fusiform swellings represent tubercles. The epididymis is enlarged and quite firm. It is usually separate from the testis, although occasionally it may adhere to it. Microscopically, the changes typical of tuberculosis are seen. Tubular degeneration may be marked.

The testis is usually not involved except by direct extension of an abscess in the epididymis.

Clinical Findings

Tuberculosis of the genitourinary tract should be considered in the presence of any of the following situations: (1) chronic cystitis that refuses to respond to adequate therapy, (2) the finding of pus without bacteria in a methylene blue stain or culture of the urinary sediment, (3) gross or microscopic hematuria, (4) a nontender, enlarged epididymis with a beaded or thickened vas, (5) a chronic draining scrotal sinus, or (6) induration or nodulation of the prostate and thickening of one or both seminal vesicles (especially in a young man). A history of present or past tuberculosis elsewhere in the body should cause the physician to suspect tuberculosis in the genitourinary tract when signs or symptoms are present.

The diagnosis rests upon the demonstration of tubercle bacilli in the urine (acid-fast stain, culture). The extent of the infection is determined by (1) the palpable findings in the epididymides, vasa deferentia, prostate, and seminal vesicles; (2) the renal and ureteral lesions as revealed by excretory urograms; (3) involvement of the bladder as seen through the cystoscope; (4) the degree of renal damage as measured by loss of function; and (5) the presence of tubercle bacilli in one or both kidneys.

A. Symptoms: There is no classic clinical picture of renal tuberculosis. Most symptoms of this disease, even in the most advanced stage, are vesical in origin (cystitis). Vague generalized malaise, fatigability, low-grade but persistent fever, and night sweats are some of the nonspecific complaints. Even vesical irritability may be absent, in which case only proper collection and examination of the urine will afford the clue. Active tuberculosis elsewhere in the body is found in less than half of patients with genitourinary tuberculosis.

1. Kidney and ureter–Because of the slow progression of the disease, the affected kidney is usually completely asymptomatic. On occasion, however, there may be a dull ache in the flank. The passage of a blood clot, secondary calculi, or a mass of debris may cause renal and ureteral colic. Rarely, the presenting symptom may be a painless mass in the abdomen.

2. Bladder–The earliest symptoms of renal tuberculosis may arise from secondary vesical involvement. These include burning, frequency, and nocturia. Hematuria is occasionally found and is of either renal or vesical origin. At times, particularly in a late stage of the disease, the vesical irritability may become extreme. If ulceration occurs, suprapubic pain may be noted when the bladder becomes full.

3. Genital tract–Tuberculosis of the prostate and seminal vesicles usually causes no symptoms. The first clue to the presence of tuberculous infection of these organs is the onset of a tuberculous epididymitis.

Tuberculosis of the epididymis usually presents as a painless or only mildly painful swelling. An abscess may drain spontaneously through the scrotal wall. A chronic draining sinus should be regarded as tuberculous until proved otherwise. In rare cases, the onset is quite acute and may simulate an acute nonspecific epididymitis.

B. Signs: Evidence of extragenital tuberculosis

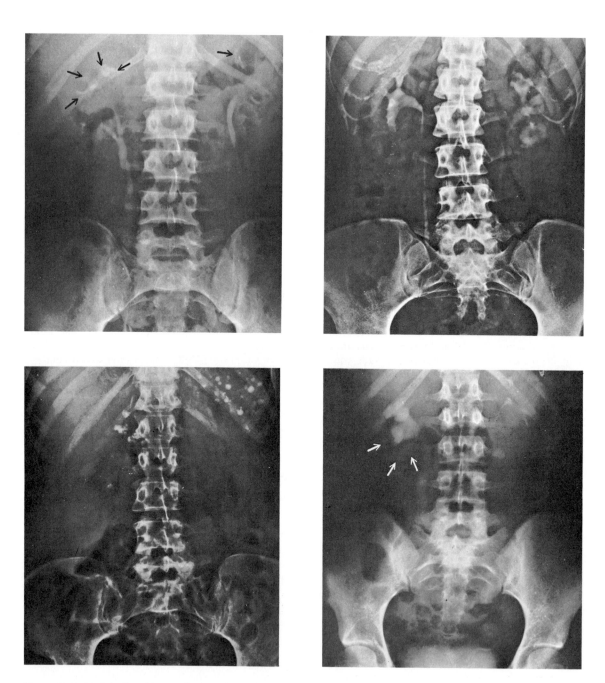

Figure 13–2. Radiologic evidence of tuberculosis. *Above left:* Excretory urogram showing "moth-eaten" calices in upper renal poles. Calcifications in upper calices; right upper ureter is straight and dilated. *Below left:* Plain film showing calcifications in right kidney, adrenals, and spleen (tuberculosis of right kidney and Addison's disease). *Above right:* Excretory urogram showing ulcerated and dilated calices on the left. *Below right:* Excretory urogram. Dilatation of calices; upper right ureter dilated and straight. Arrows point to poorly defined parenchymal abscesses.

may be found (lungs, bone, lymph nodes, tonsils, intestines).

1. Kidney–There is usually no enlargement or tenderness of the involved kidney.

2. External genitalia–A thickened, nontender, or only slightly tender epididymis may be discovered. The vas deferens often is thickened and beaded. A chronic draining sinus through the scrotal skin is almost pathognomonic of tuberculous epididymitis. In the more advanced stages, the epididymis cannot be differentiated from the testis upon palpation. This may mean that the testis has been directly invaded by the epididymal abscess.

Hydrocele occasionally accompanies tuberculous epididymitis. The "idiopathic" hydrocele should be tapped so that underlying pathologic changes, if present, can be evaluated (epididymitis, testicular tumor). Involvement of the penis and urethra is rare.

3. Prostate and seminal vesicles–These organs may be normal to palpation. Ordinarily, however, the tuberculous prostate shows areas of induration, even nodulation. The involved vesicle is usually indurated, enlarged, and fixed. If epididymitis is present, the ipsilateral vesicle usually shows changes as well.

C. Laboratory Findings: Proper urinalysis affords the most important clue to the diagnosis of genitourinary tuberculosis.

1. Persistent pyuria without organisms on culture or on the smear stained with methylene blue means tuberculosis until proved otherwise. Acid-fast stains done on the concentrated sediment from a 24-hour specimen are positive in at least 60% of cases. This must be corroborated by a positive culture.

About 15–20% of patients with tuberculosis have secondary pyogenic infection; the clue ("sterile" pyuria) is thereby obscured. If clinical response to adequate treatment fails and pyuria persists, tuberculosis must be ruled out by bacteriologic and roentgenologic means.

2. Cultures for tubercle bacilli from urine are positive in a very high percentage of cases of tuberculous infection. If positive, sensitivity tests should be ordered. In the face of strong presumptive evidence of tuberculosis, negative cultures should be repeated.

The blood count may be normal or may show anemia in advanced disease. The sedimentation rate is usually accelerated.

Tubercle bacilli may often be demonstrated in the secretions from an infected prostate. Renal function will be normal unless there is bilateral damage: as one kidney is slowly injured, compensatory hypertrophy of the normal kidney develops. It can also be infected with tubercle bacilli, or may become hydronephrotic from fibrosis of the bladder wall (ureterovesical stenosis) or vesicoureteral reflux.

If tuberculosis is suspected, perform the tuberculin test. A positive test, particularly in an adult, is hardly diagnostic; but a negative test in an otherwise healthy patient speaks against a diagnosis of tuberculosis.

D. X-Ray Findings: (Fig 13–2.) A chest film which shows evidence of tuberculosis should cause the physician to suspect tuberculosis of the urogenital tract in the presence of urinary signs and symptoms. A plain film of the abdomen may show enlargement of one kidney or obliteration of the renal and psoas shadows due to perinephric abscess. Punctate calcification in the renal parenchyma may be due to tuberculosis. Renal stones are found in 10% of cases. Calcification of the ureter may be noted, but this is rare (Fig 6–2). Small prostatic stones the size of grape seeds in the region of the pubic symphysis are ordinarily not due to tuberculosis, but large calcific bodies may be.

Excretory urograms can be diagnostic if the lesion is moderately advanced. The typical changes include (1) a "moth-eaten" appearance of the involved ulcerated calices, (2) obliteration of one or more calices, (3) dilatation of the calices due to ureteral stenosis from fibrosis, (4) abscess cavities that connect with calices, (5) single or multiple ureteral strictures, with secondary dilatation, with shortening and therefore straightening of the ureter, and (6) absence of function of the kidney, due to complete ureteral occlusion and renal destruction (autonephrectomy).

If the excretory urograms demonstrate gross tuberculosis in one kidney, there is no need to do a retrograde urogram on that side. In fact, there is at least a theoretical danger of hematogenous or lymphogenous dissemination resulting from the increased intrapelvic pressure. Retrograde urography may, however, be carried out on the unsuspected side as a verification of its normality. This is further substantiated if the urine from that side is free of both pus cells and tubercle bacilli.

E. Instrumental Examination: Thorough cystoscopic study is indicated even when the offending organism has been found in the urine and excretory urograms show the typical renal lesion. This will clearly demonstrate the extent of the disease. Cystoscopy may reveal the typical tubercles or ulcers of tuberculosis. Biopsy can be done if necessary. Severe contracture of the bladder may be noted. A cystogram may reveal ureteral reflux. A clean specimen of urine should also be obtained for further study.

Differential Diagnosis

Chronic nonspecific cystitis or pyelonephritis may mimic tuberculosis perfectly, especially since 15–20% of cases of tuberculosis are secondarily invaded by pyogenic organisms. If nonspecific infections do not respond to adequate therapy, a search for tubercle bacilli should be made. Painless epididymitis points to tuberculosis. Cystoscopic demonstration of tubercles and ulceration of the bladder wall means tuberculosis. Urograms are usually definitive.

Acute or chronic nonspecific epididymitis may be confused with tuberculosis, since the onset of tuberculosis is occasionally quite painful. It is rare to have palpatory changes in the seminal vesicles with nonspecific epididymitis, but these are almost routine findings in tuberculosis of the epididymis. The presence of tubercle bacilli in the urine is diagnostic. On occasion, only the pathologist can make the diagnosis by microscopic study of the surgically removed epididymis.

Amicrobic cystitis usually has an acute onset and is often preceded by a urethral discharge. "Sterile" pyuria is found, but tubercle bacilli are absent. Cystoscopy may reveal ulcerations, but these are acute and superficial. Although urograms show mild hydroureter and even hydronephrosis, there is no ulceration of the calices as seen in renal tuberculosis.

Interstitial cystitis is typically characterized by frequency, nocturia, and suprapubic pain with vesical filling. The urine is usually free of pus. Tubercle bacilli are absent.

Multiple small renal stones or nephrocalcinosis seen by x-ray may suggest the type of calcification seen in the tuberculous kidney. In renal tuberculosis, the calcium is in the parenchyma, although secondary stones are occasionally seen.

Necrotizing papillitis, which may involve all of the calices of one or both kidneys or, rarely, a solitary calix, shows caliceal lesions (including calcifications) which simulate those of tuberculosis. Careful bacteriologic studies will fail to demonstrate tubercle bacilli.

Medullary sponge kidneys may show small calcifications just distal to the calices. The calices, however, are sharp, and no other stigmas of tuberculosis can be demonstrated.

In disseminated coccidioidomycosis, renal involvement may occur. The renal lesion resembles that of tuberculosis (Connor, Drach, & Bucher, 1975). Coccidioidal epididymitis may be confused with tuberculous involvement (Cheng, 1974).

Urinary bilharziasis is a great mimic of tuberculosis. Both present with symptoms of cystitis and often hematuria. Vesical contraction, seen in both diseases, may lead to extreme frequency. Schistosomiasis must be suspected in endemic areas; the typical ova are found in the urine; cystoscopic and urographic findings are definitive in differential diagnosis.

Complications

A. Renal Tuberculosis: Perinephric abscess may cause an enlarging mass in the flank. A plain film of the abdomen will show obliteration of the renal and psoas shadows. Renal stones may develop if secondary nonspecific infection is present. Uremia is the end stage if both kidneys are involved.

B. Ureteral Tuberculosis: Scarring with stricture formation is one of the typical lesions of tuberculosis and most commonly affects the juxtavesical portion. This may cause progressive hydronephrosis. Complete ureteral obstruction may cause complete nonfunction of the kidney (Feldstein, Sullivan, & Banowsky, 1975).

C. Vesical Tuberculosis: When severely damaged, the bladder wall becomes fibrosed and contracted. Stenosis of the ureters or reflux occurs, causing hydronephrotic atrophy.

D. Genital Tuberculosis: The ducts of the involved epididymis become occluded. If this is bilateral, sterility results. Abscess of the epididymis may rupture into the testis, through the scrotal wall, or both, in which case the spermatogenic tubules may slough out.

Treatment

Tuberculosis must be treated as a generalized disease. Even when it can be demonstrated only in the urogenital tract, one must assume activity elsewhere. (It is theoretically possible, however, for the primary focus to have healed spontaneously.) This means that basically the treatment is medical. Surgical excision of an infected organ, when indicated, is merely an adjunct to overall therapy.

A. Renal Tuberculosis: A strict medical regimen should be instituted.

The following combinations of drugs can be utilized. Their choice can be governed by the results of sensitivity tests. (1) Cycloserine, aminosalicylic acid (PAS), and isoniazid (INH). (2) Cycloserine, ethambutol, and isoniazid. (3) Rifampin, ethambutol, and isoniazid. The latter group is probably the most efficacious. The oral dose of each is as follows: cycloserine, 250 mg twice daily; PAS, 15 g in divided doses; INH, 300 mg; ethambutol, 1.2 g; rifampin, 600 mg. Sensitivity testing may indicate the use of streptomycin intramuscularly. Administer 1 g/d the first month, 1 g 3 times a week for the next month, and then 1 g twice a week. Since INH may cause peripheral neuropathy, give pyridoxine, 100 mg/d orally. Wechsler & Lattimer (1975) prefer the combination of INH, ethambutol, and cycloserine.

While most authorities advise appropriate medication for 2 years (or longer if cultures remain positive), Gow (1979) finds that a 6-month course of drugs is adequate. He recommends rifampin 600 mg, isoniazid 300 mg, pyrazinamide 1 g, and vitamin C 1 g daily for 2 months, followed by rifampin 900 mg, pyrazinamide 1.5 g, and vitamin C 1 g twice a week for 4 months.

If, after 3 months, cultures are still positive and gross involvement of the affected kidney is radiologically evident, nephrectomy should be considered. Gow (1979) recommends that nonfunctioning kidneys be removed after 1–2 months of medical therapy.

If bacteriologic and radiographic studies demonstrate bilateral disease, only medical treatment can be considered. The only exceptions are (1) severe sepsis, pain, or bleeding from one kidney (may require nephrectomy as a palliative or lifesaving measure); and (2) marked advance of the disease on one side and minimal damage on the other (consider removal of the badly damaged organ).

B. Vesical Tuberculosis: Tuberculosis of the bladder is always secondary to renal or prostatic tuberculosis; it tends to heal promptly when definitive treatment for the "primary" genitourinary infection is given. Vesical ulcers which fail to respond to this regimen may require transurethral electrocoagulation. Vesical instillations of 0.2% monoxychlorosene (Clorpactin) may also stimulate healing.

Should extreme contracture of the bladder develop, it may be necessary to divert the urine from the bladder or perform subtotal cystectomy and anastomose a patch of ileum or sigmoid to the remainder (ileocystoplasty, sigmoidocystoplasty) in order to afford comfort (Abel & Gow, 1978).

C. Tuberculosis of the Epididymis: This is never an isolated lesion; the prostate is always involved and usually the kidney as well. Only rarely does the epididymal infection break through into the testis. Treatment is medical. If after months of treatment an abscess or a draining sinus exists, epididymectomy is indicated.

D. Tuberculosis of the Prostate and Seminal Vesicles: Although a few urologists advocate removal of the entire prostate and the vesicles when they become involved by tuberculosis, the majority opinion is that only medical therapy is indicated. Control can be checked by culture of the semen for tubercle bacilli.

E. General Measures for All Types: Optimum nutrition is no less important in treating tuberculosis of the genitourinary tract than in the treatment of tuberculosis elsewhere. Bladder sedatives may be given for the irritable bladder.

F. Treatment of Complications: Perinephric abscess usually occurs when the kidney is destroyed, but this is rare. The abscess must be drained, and nephrectomy should be done either then or later to prevent development of a chronic draining sinus. Prolonged antimicrobial therapy is indicated. If ureterovesical stricture or reflux develops and causes progressive hydronephrosis of the uninvolved kidney, diversion of the urine by cutaneous ureterostomy, nephrostomy, or replacement of the diseased ureter with a segment of ileum may have to be done to prevent death from uremia. For this reason, serial excretory urograms are necessary even under medical treatment.

Prognosis

The prognosis varies with the extent of the disease and the organs involved, but the overall control rate is 98% at 5 years. The urine must be studied bacteriologically every 6 months during treatment and then every year for 10 years (Wechsler & Lattimer, 1975). Relapse will indicate the need for reinstitution of treatment. Nephrectomy is rarely necessary. In the healing process, ureteral stenosis or vesical contraction may develop. Appropriate surgical intervention may be necessary.

AMICROBIC (ABACTERIAL) CYSTITIS

Amicrobic cystitis is a rare disease of abrupt onset with a marked local vesical reaction. Although it acts like an infectious disease, bacterial search for the usual urinary pathogens is negative. It affects adult men and occasionally children, usually boys.

Etiology

The patient usually gives a history of recent sexual exposure. Mycoplasma and chlamydia organisms have been isolated or suspected as etiologic agents. An adenovirus has been isolated from the urine in children suffering from acute hemorrhagic cystitis.

Pathogenesis & Pathology

Whatever the source and identity of the invader, the disease is primarily manifested as an acute inflammation of the bladder. Vesical irritability is severe and is often associated with terminal hematuria. The mucosa is red and edematous, and superficial ulceration is occasionally seen. A thin membrane of fibrin often lies upon the wall. Similar changes may be noted in the posterior urethra. The renal parenchyma is not involved, although the pelvic and ureteral mucosa may show mild inflammatory changes. Some dilatation of the lower ureters is apt to develop. This may be due to an inflammatory reaction about the ureteral orifices, for these changes regress after successful treatment.

Microscopically, there is nothing specific about the reaction. The mucosa and submucosa are infiltrated with neutrophils, plasma cells, and eosinophils. Submucosal hemorrhages are common; superficial ulceration of the mucosa may be noted.

Clinical Findings

A. Symptoms: All symptoms are local. Urethral discharge, which is usually clear and mucoid but which may be purulent, may be the initial symptom in men. Symptoms of acute cystitis come on abruptly. Urgency, frequency, and burning may be severe. Terminal hematuria is not uncommon. Suprapubic discomfort or even pain may be noted; it is most apt to be present as the bladder fills and is relieved somewhat by voiding. There is no fever or malaise.

B. Signs: Some suprapubic tenderness may be found. Urethral discharge may be profuse or scanty, and purulent or thin and mucoid. The prostate is usually normal to palpation. Massage is contraindicated during the acute stage of urinary tract infection. When done later, infection is usually not present.

C. Laboratory Findings: Some leukocytosis may develop. The urine is grossly purulent and may contain blood as well. Stained smears reveal an absence of bacteria. Routine cultures are uniformly negative. In a few cases, mycoplasma and TRIC agent have been identified, but the significance of this is not yet clear. Search for tubercle bacilli is not successful.

Urethral discharge reveals no bacteria. Renal function is not impaired.

D. X-Ray Findings: Excretory urograms may demonstrate some dilatation of the lower ureters, but these changes regress completely when the disease is cured. The bladder shadow is small because of its markedly diminished capacity. Cystograms may reveal reflux.

E. Instrumental Examination: Cystoscopy is not indicated in acute inflammation of the bladder. It has been done, however, when the diagnosis was obscure and tuberculosis suspected. In such cases it reveals redness and edema of the mucosa. Superficial ulceration may be noted. Bladder capacity is markedly diminished. Biopsy of the wall shows nonspecific changes.

Differential Diagnosis

Tuberculosis causes symptoms of cystitis, which, however, usually come on gradually and become severe only in the stage of ulceration. A painless, nontender enlargement of an epididymis suggests tuberculosis. Although both tuberculosis and amicrobic cystitis produce pus without bacteria, thorough laboratory study will demonstrate tubercle bacilli only in the former. On cystoscopy the tuberculous bladder may be studded with tubercles. The ulcers in this disease are deep and of a chronic type. The changes in amicrobic cystitis are more acute; ulceration, if present, is superficial. Excretory urograms in tuberculosis may show "moth-eaten" calices typical of infection with acid-fast organisms.

Nonspecific (pyogenic) cystitis may mimic amicrobic cystitis perfectly, but pathogenic organisms are easily found on a smear stained with methylene blue or on culture.

Cystitis secondary to chronic nonspecific prostatitis occasionally produces pus without bacteria. The findings on rectal examination, the pus in the prostatic secretion, and the response to antibiotics point to the proper diagnosis.

Vesical neoplasm may ulcerate, become infected, and bleed; hence it may mimic amicrobic cystitis. Bacteriuria, however, will be found. In case of doubt, cystoscopy is indicated.

Interstitial cystitis may be accompanied by severe symptoms of vesical irritability. However, it usually affects women past the menopause, and urinalysis is entirely negative except for a few red cells. Cystoscopy should be diagnostic.

Complications

Amicrobic cystitis is usually self-limited. Rarely, secondary contracture of the bladder develops. Under these circumstances, vesicoureteral reflux may be noted.

Treatment

A. Specific Measures: One of the tetracyclines or chloramphenicol, 1 g/d orally in divided doses for 3–4 days, is said to be curative in 75% of cases. Streptomycin, 1–2 g/d intramuscularly for 3–4 days, may be tried. Neoarsphenamine is also effective and appears to be the drug of choice, but arsenicals are hard to find. The first dose is 0.3 g intravenously; subsequent dosage is 0.45 g intravenously every 3–5 days for a total of 3–4 injections.

Penicillin and the sulfonamides are without effect.

In the cases reported in children, cure occurred spontaneously.

B. General Measures: Bladder sedatives are usually of little help if symptoms are severe. Analgesics or narcotics may prove necessary to combat pain. Hot sitz baths may relieve spasm.

Wettlaufer (1976) recommends the instillation of a 0.1% solution of sodium oxychlorosene (Clorpactin WCS-90).

Prognosis

The prognosis is excellent.

CANDIDIASIS

Candida albicans is a yeastlike fungus that is a normal inhabitant of the respiratory and gastrointestinal tracts and the vagina. The intensive use of potent modern antibiotics is apt to disturb the normal balance between normal and abnormal organisms, thus allowing fungi such as candida to overwhelm an otherwise healthy organ. The bladder and, to a lesser extent, the kidneys have proved vulnerable; candidemia has been observed.

The patient may present with vesical irritability or symptoms and signs of pyelonephritis. Fungus balls may be passed spontaneously. The diagnosis is made by observing mycelial or yeast forms of the fungus microscopically in a properly collected urine specimen. The diagnosis may be confirmed by culture. Excretory urograms may show caliceal defects and ureteral obstruction (fungus masses).

Vesical candidiasis usually responds to alkalinization of the urine with sodium bicarbonate. A urinary pH of 7.5 is desired; the dose is regulated by the patient, who checks the urine with indicator paper. Should this fail, amphotericin B should be instilled via catheter 3 times a day. Dissolve 100 mg of the drug in 500 mL of 5% dextrose solution.

If there is renal involvement, irrigations of the renal pelvis with a similar concentration of amphotericin B are efficacious. In the presence of systemic manifestations or candidemia, flucytosine (Ancobon) is the drug of choice. The dose is 100 mg/kg/d orally in divided doses given for 1 week. In the face of serious involvement, give 600 mg intravenously on the first day and then shift to the oral form of the drug. Grüneberg & Leaky (1976) recommend nifuratel, a nitrofuran antibiotic, which they claim is superior to flucytosine. The recommended dose is 400 mg 3 times daily for 1 week. The dose must be modified in the face of renal impairment. The drug is more active in acid urine. Amphotericin B (Fungizone) has the disadvantages of requiring parenteral administration and being highly nephrotoxic. It is given intravenously in a dosage of 1–5 mg/d in divided doses dissolved in 5% dextrose. The concentration of the solution should be 0.1 mg/mL.

ACTINOMYCOSIS

Actinomycosis is a chronic granulomatous disease in which fibrosis tends to become marked and spontaneous fistulas are the rule. On rare occasions, the disease involves the kidney, bladder, or testis by hematogenous invasion from a primary site of infection. The skin of the penis or scrotum may become involved through a local abrasion. The bladder may also become diseased by direct extension from the appendix, bowel, or oviduct.

Etiology
Actinomyces israelii (A bovis).

Clinical Findings
There is nothing specifically pathognomonic about the symptoms or signs in actinomycosis. The microscopic demonstration of the organisms, which are visible as yellow bodies called "sulfur granules," makes the diagnosis. If persistently sought for, these may be found in the discharge from sinuses or in the urine. Pollock & others (1978) recommend aspiration biopsy performed by a thin needle. They found that in addition to the discovery of sulfur granules, both Gram's Stain and a modified Ziehl-Neelsen Stain were useful in diagnosis. Definitive diagnosis is established by culture.

Urographically, the lesion in the kidney may resemble tuberculosis (eroded calices) or tumor (space-occupying lesion).

Treatment
Clindamycin is probably the drug of choice. Initially, it should be administered either intramuscularly or intravenously. The daily dose is 1.2–2.7 g in divided doses. Parenteral therapy may be required for 2 or more months, after which 1 g a day may be given by mouth. Penicillin G is also effective. Give 10–20 million units a day for 1 month and then switch to oral penicillin V in similar dosage for 3–6 months or longer. Surgical removal of the infected organ is usually indicated.

Prognosis
Removal of the involved organ (eg, kidney or testis) may be promptly curative. Drainage of a granulomatous abscess may cause the development of a chronic draining sinus. Chemotherapy is helpful.

TRICHOMONIASIS IN THE MALE

Etiology
Trichomonas vaginalis is the most common cause of vaginitis; about 15% of women harbor the organism. It is found not infrequently in the urethra and prostate in men and in the bladder in both sexes. It is transmitted to men by sexual intercourse. The sexual partners of all women with trichomoniasis should be examined for trichomonads.

Clinical Findings
A. Symptoms and Signs: Men harboring the organism may suffer from some degree of urethral itching and discharge which may be thin or purulent, scanty or profuse; at times there is frequency and burning on urination. There are usually, however, no symptoms at all.

B. Laboratory Findings:

1. Urethral discharge, wet preparation–The discharge should be mixed immediately with 1–2 mL of saline or Trichomonas solution and studied microscopically. In about 10% of those whose sexual partners harbor the protozoon, motile trichomonads (about the size of pus cells) are seen. A dried smear should be stained with methylene blue to study the bacterial flora as well, since secondary infection with pyogenic bacteria is common.

2. Urethral scrapings will reveal the organisms microscopically in 75% of cases. Dark-field examination may prove helpful.

3. Urine, wet preparation–The sediment of a centrifuged specimen of urine should be studied for the motile organisms. This is successful in 25% of patients.

4. Prostatic secretion–Motile trichomonads may be discovered in the secretion obtained by prostatic massage.

5. Culture of semen, prostatic secretion, or urethral discharge–If the wet preparations are negative, a suitable culture medium should be inoculated, incubated for 48 hours at 37 C, and examined microscopically. With this technic, 90% of men whose sexual partners are infected with *Trichomonas vaginalis* will have a positive culture.

6. Urethral discharge stained by the Papanicolaou technic often reveals the organism.

Treatment

Once the diagnosis has been made, a condom should be used during intercourse until treatment has been successful.

Metronidazole (Flagyl), 400 mg orally twice a day, should be administered for 7 days. Davidson finds that giving 1 g for 2 days in divided doses is also efficacious. Dykers (1978) reported equally good results giving 2 g as a single dose to both the patient and his sexual partner. Nitrimidazine (Naxogin), 250 mg twice a day for 6 days, is equally effective, as is flunidazole, 200 mg 3 times a day for 5 days.

Prognosis

Most trichomonad infections respond promptly to metronidazole or nitrimidazine. Vigorous treatment of the man's sexual partner is imperative.

SCHISTOSOMIASIS
(Bilharziasis)
Mohamed M. Al-Ghorab, MB, ChB, DS, MCh

Schistosomiasis, caused by a blood fluke, is a disease of warm climates. It is estimated that in its 3 forms it affects about 350 million people. Whereas *Schistosoma mansoni* is widely distributed in Africa, South and Central America, Pakistan, and India, and *Schistosoma japonicum* is found in the Far East, *Schistosoma haematobium (Bilharzia haematobia)* is limited to Africa, especially along its northern coast, Saudi Arabia, Israel, Jordan, Lebanon, and Syria.

Schistosomiasis is on the increase in endemic areas because of the construction of modern irrigation systems that provide favorable conditions for the intermediate host, a certain freshwater snail. This disease principally affects the urogenital system, especially the bladder, ureters, seminal vesicles, and, to a lesser extent, the male urethra and prostate gland. Because of emigration of people from endemic areas the disease is being seen with increasing frequency in both Europe and the USA. Infection with S mansoni and S japonicum mainly involves the colon.

Etiology

In endemic areas, humans are infected when they come in contact with larva-infested water in canals, ditches, or irrigation fields during swimming, bathing, or farming procedures. The skin is penetrated by fork-tailed larvae, the cercariae, which lose their tails and penetrate deep under the skin. They are then termed schistosomules. They cause allergic skin reactions that are more intense in people infected for the first time. These schistosomules enter the general circulation through the lymphatics and the peripheral veins and reach the lungs. If the infection is massive, they may cause pneumonitis. After passing through the pulmonary circulation, they go to the left side of the heart and are pumped into the general circulation. Those worms that reach the vesicoprostatic plexus of veins survive and mature, whereas those that go to other areas die.

Pathogenesis

The adult worm, a digenetic trematode, lives in the prostatovesical plexus of veins. The male is about 10×1 mm in size, is folded upon itself, and carries the long, slim 20×0.25 mm female in its "schist," or gynecophoric canal. In the smallest peripheral venules, the female leaves the male and partially penetrates the venule to lay her eggs in the subepithelial layer of the affected viscus, usually in the form of clusters that form tubercles. The ova are only rarely seen within the venules; they are almost always in the subepithelial or interstitial tissues. The female returns to the male, which carries her to other areas to repeat the same process.

The living ova, by a process of histolysis and helped by contraction of the detrusor muscle, penetrate the overlying urothelium, pass into the cavity of the bladder, and are extruded outside the body with the urine. If these ova reach fresh water, they hatch, and the contained larvae, ciliated miricidia, find a specific freshwater snail that they penetrate. There they form sporocysts that ultimately form the cercariae that leave the snail hosts and pass into fresh water to once again infect any human being and continue their life cycle in the human host.

Pathology

The fresh ova excite little tissue reaction when they leave the human host promptly through the urothelium. It is the contents of the ova trapped in the tissues and death of the organisms that cause a severe local reaction, with infiltration of round cells, monocytes, eosinophils, and giant cells. These early reactions are manifested as tubercles, nodules, and polyps that are later replaced by fibrous tissue that causes contraction of different parts of the bladder and strictures of the ureter. Fibrosis and massive deposits of eggs in subepithelial tissues interfere with the blood supply of the area and cause chronic bilharzial ulcerations. Epithelial metaplasia is common, and squamous cell carcinoma is a frequent sequela in these cases. Secondary infection of the urinary tract is a common complication and is difficult to overcome. The trapped dead ova become impregnated with calcium salts and form sheets of subepithelial calcified layers in the ureter, bladder, and seminal vesicles.

Clinical Findings

A. Symptoms: Penetration of the skin by the cercariae causes certain allergic reactions, with cutaneous hyperemia and itching. During the stage of generalization or invasion, the patient complains of malaise, fatigue and lassitude, low-grade fever, excessive sweating, headache, backache, etc. When the ova are laid in the bladder wall and begin to be extruded, the patient complains of terminal, slightly painful hematuria that is occasionally profuse. This may remain the only complaint for a long time until complications set in, when vesical symptoms become exaggerated and progressive. Increasing frequency, suprapubic and back pain, urethralgia, profuse hematuria, pyuria, and necroturia are likely to occur, with secondary infection, ulceration, or malignancy. Renal pain may be due to ureteral stricture, vesicoureteral reflux, or secondary stones obstructing the ureter. Fever, rigor, tox-

emia, and uremia are manifestations of renal involvement.

B. Signs: In early uncomplicated cases there are essentially no clinical findings. Later, a fibrosed, pitted bilharzial involvement of the glans penis, urethral stricture or fistula, or a perineal fibrous mass may be found. A suprapubic bladder mass or a renal swelling may be felt abdominally. Rectal examination may reveal a fibrosed prostate, an enlarged seminal vesicle, or a thickened bladder base.

C. Laboratory Findings: Urinalysis usually reveals the terminal-spined dead or living ova, blood and pus cells, and bacteria. Malignant squamous cells may be seen. The hemogram usually

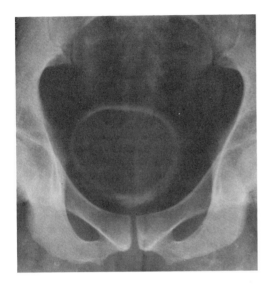

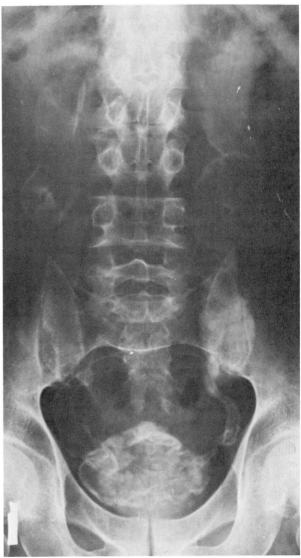

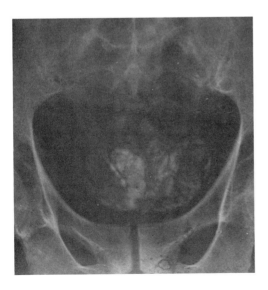

Figure 13–3. Schistosomiasis. Plain films. *Above left:* Extensive calcification in the wall of a contracted bladder. *Right:* Extensive calcification of the bladder and both ureters up to the renal pelves. The ureters are dilated and tortuous. *Below left:* Extensive calcification of seminal vesicles and ampullae of vasa.

shows leukocytosis with eosinophilia and hypochromic normocytic anemia. Serum creatinine and blood urea nitrogen measurements may demonstrate some degree of renal impairment.

D. X-Ray Findings: A plain film of the abdomen may show areas of grayness in the flank (enlarged hydronephrotic kidney) or in the bladder area (large tumor). Opacifications (stones) may be noted in the kidney, ureter, or bladder. Linear calcification may be seen in the ureteral and bladder walls (Fig 13–3). Punctate calcification of the ureter (ureteritis calcinosa) and a honeycombed calcification of the seminal vessels may be obvious (Fig 13–3).

Excretory urograms may show either normal or diminished renal function and varying degrees of dilatation of the upper urinary tracts (Fig 13–4). These changes include hydronephrosis, dilated and tortuous ureters, ureteral strictures, or a small contracted bladder having a capacity of only a few milliliters (Fig 13–4). Gross irregular defects of the bladder wall represent cancer (Fig 13–4).

Retrograde urethrography may reveal a bilharzial urethral stricture. Cystograms often reveal vesicoureteral reflux, particularly if the bladder is contracted.

E. Instrumental Examination: Urethral calibration with a sound may reveal stricture formation.

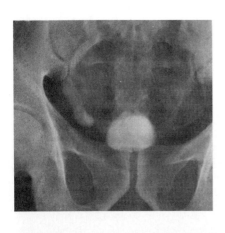

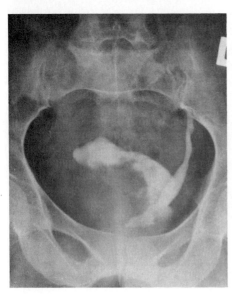

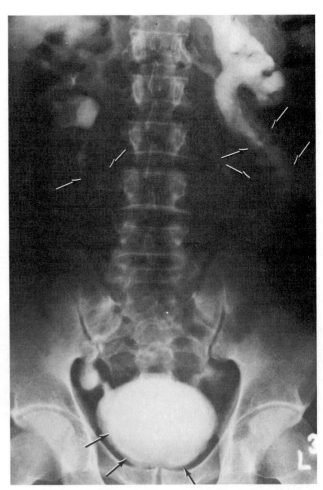

Figure 13–4. Schistosomiasis. *Above left:* Excretory urogram showing markedly contracted bladder. Lower right ureter dilated probably secondary to vesicoureteral reflux. *Right:* Excretory urogram at 2 hours showing a fairly normal right kidney. The upper ureter is distorted. Arrows point to calcified wall. The lower ureter is quite abnormal. The calices and pelvis of the left kidney are dilated, but the kidney shows atrophy secondary to nonspecific infection. The upper ureter is dilated and displaced by elongation due to obstruction. Arrows show calcification. Linear calcification can be seen in the periphery of the lower half of the bladder wall (arrows). *Below left:* Nodular squamous cell carcinoma of the bladder. Dilated left lower ureter probably secondary to obstruction by tumor. Nonvisualization of the right ureter caused by complete occlusion.

Cystoscopy may show fresh conglomerate, grayish tubercles surrounded by a halo of hyperemia, old calcified yellowish tubercles, sandy patches of mucous membrane, and a lusterless ground-glass mucosa that lacks the normal vascular pattern. Other obvious lesions include bilharzial polyps, chronic ulcers on the dome that bleed when the bladder is deflated (weeping ulcers), vesical stones, malignant lesions, stenosed or patulous ureteric orifices, and a distorted, asymmetric trigone. All are signs of schistosomal infestation.

Differential Diagnosis

Bilharzial cystitis is unmistakable in endemic areas. The presence of schistosoma ova in the urine, together with radiographic and cystoscopic findings, usually confirms the diagnosis. Nonspecific cystitis usually responds to medical treatment unless there is a complicating factor. Tuberculous cystitis may mimic bilharzial cystitis; the detection of the tubercle bacillus, together with the radiographic picture, is confirmatory, but tuberculosis may occur in a bilharzial bladder. Vesical calculi and malignancy should be diagnosed by thorough urologic examination, although both conditions are common in association with bilharzial bladder. Complications of schistosomiasis are the result of fibrosis, which may be extreme and which causes contraction of the bladder neck as well as the bladder itself. It also causes strictures of the urethra and ureter that are usually bilateral. Vesicoureteral reflux is a frequent sequela. Secondary persistent infection and stone formation usually complicate the picture still further. Squamous cell tumors of the bladder are common. They are seen as early as the second or third decade and are much more common in males than females.

Treatment

The medical treatment of early and uncomplicated cases is quite satisfactory, but repeated infections usually occur and require repeated courses of medical therapy.

A. Specific Measures:

1. Tartar emetic (antimony potassium tartrate) is extensively used in many endemic areas for massive treatment of the population. However, it is rather toxic. The drug is given intravenously as a 2% solution in saline or distilled water. Care should be taken not to allow leakage of the drug into the tissues, or necrosis may result. The initial dose is 30 mg, which is increased gradually by 30 mg increments until the maximum dose of 150 mg is reached. The total dose for an adult is 2 g. The injections are given every other day or twice a week.

2. Stibocaptate (antimony sodium dimercaptosuccinate, Astiban) is thought by many to be the drug of choice and is less toxic than tartar emetic, particularly in children. The recommended total dose is 30–50 mg/kg body weight. It is given as a 10% solution intramuscularly. Because the injection is painful, a local anesthetic, eg, 1% lidocaine, can be added. The total dose is divided into 5 equal parts and administered once a week.

Other useful antimony drugs include antimony lithium thiomalate (Anthiomaline), antimony sodium gluconate (Triostam), and antimony pyrocatechol sodium disulfonate (Fuadin, stibophen).

3. Trichlorfon (Bilharcid, metrifonate), a non-antimony compound, is given orally in doses of 7–10 mg/kg body weight. A total of 3 such doses is given at 2-week intervals. The drug affords a high cure rate and low toxicity and has few side-effects. It is useful in mass treatment.

B. General Measures: Antibiotics or urinary antiseptics are needed to overcome or control secondary infection. Supportive treatment in the form of iron, vitamins, and a high-calorie diet is indicated in selected cases.

C. Complications: Treatment of the complications of schistosomiasis of the genitourinary tract makes demands on the skill of the physician. Juxtavesical ureteral strictures require resection of the stenotic segment with ureteroneocystostomy. If the ureter is not long enough to reimplant, a tube of bladder may be fashioned, turned cephalad, and anastomosed to the ureter. Should the ureter be widely dilated, it must be tailored to approach normal size. Vesicoureteral reflux requires a suitable surgical repair. A contracted bladder neck may need transurethral anterior commissurotomy or a suprapubic Y-V plasty.

A chronic "weeping" bilharzial bladder ulcer necessitates partial cystectomy. The contracted bladder is treated by enteroplasty (placing a segment of bowel as a patch on the bladder), preferably with an isolated portion of sigmoid colon. This procedure, which significantly increases vesical capacity, is remarkably effective in lessening the severity of symptoms associated with contracted bladder. Preoperative vesicoureteral reflux may disappear.

The most dreaded complication, squamous cell carcinoma, requires total cystectomy with supravesical urinary diversion if the lesion is deemed operable. Unfortunately, late diagnosis is the rule.

Prognosis

With energetic treatment, mild and early cases of schistosomiasis are not likely to result in severe damage to the urinary tract. On the other hand, massive repeated infections undermine the function of the urinary tract to such an extent that patients are disabled and become chronic invalids whose life spans are shortened by 1 or 2 decades.

In many endemic areas, attempts have been made to control the disease by mass treatment of patients, proper education, mechanization of agriculture, and various methods of eradication or control of the snail population. All these efforts have failed to be fully effective.

FILARIASIS

Filariasis is endemic in the countries bordering the Mediterranean, in South China and Japan, the West Indies, and the South Pacific islands, particularly Samoa. Limited infection, as seen in American soldiers during World War II, gives an entirely different clinical picture than the frequent reinfections usually encountered among the native population.

Etiology

Wuchereria bancrofti is a threadlike nematode about 0.5 cm or more in length which lives in the human lymphatics. In the lymphatics the female gives off microfilariae, which are found, particularly at night, in the peripheral blood. The intermediate host (usually a mosquito), biting an infected person, becomes infested with microfilariae which develop into larvae. These are in turn transferred to another human being, in whom they reach maturity. Mating occurs, and microfilariae are again produced. *Brugia malayi*, a nematode, acts in a similar fashion.

Pathogenesis & Pathology

The adult nematode in the human host invades and obstructs the lymphatics; this leads to lymphangitis and lymphadenitis. In long-standing cases, the lymphatic vessels become thickened and fibrous; there is a marked reticuloendothelial reaction.

Clinical Findings

A. Symptoms: In mild cases (few exposures), the patient suffers recurrent lymphadenitis and lymphangitis with fever and malaise. Not infrequently, inflammation of the epididymis, testis, scrotum, and spermatic cord occurs. These structures then become edematous, boggy, and at times tender. Hydrocele is common. In advanced cases (many exposures), obstruction of major lymph channels may cause chyluria and elephantiasis.

B. Signs: Varying degrees of painless elephantiasis of the scrotum and extremities develop as obstruction to lymphatics progresses.

C. Laboratory Findings: Chylous urine may look normal if minimal amounts of fat are present, but, in an advanced case or following a fatty meal, it is milky. On standing, the urine layers: the top layer is fatty, the middle layer is pinkish, and the lower layer is clear. In the presence of chyluria, large amounts of protein are to be expected. Hypoproteinemia is found, and the albumin:globulin ratio is reversed. Both white and red cells are found. The fat will be dissolved by chloroform; the urine will therefore become clear.

Marked eosinophilia is the rule in the early stages. Microfilariae may be demonstrated in the blood, which should preferably be drawn at night. The adult worm may be found by biopsy. Skin and complement fixation tests are highly successful in diagnosis.

D. Cystoscopy: Following a fatty meal, endoscopy may differentiate between unilateral and bilateral cases by observing the efflux of milky urine from the ureteral orifices.

E. X-Ray Findings: Retrograde urography and lymphangiography may reveal the renolymphatic connections in patients with chyluria.

Prevention

In endemic areas, mosquito abatement programs must be intensively pursued.

Treatment

A. Specific Measures: Diethylcarbamazine (Hetrazan) is the drug of choice, but it is toxic (Nelson, 1979). The dose is 3 mg/kg orally 3 times daily for 21 days. This drug kills the microfilariae but not the adult worms. Several courses of the drug may be necessary. Antibiotics may be necessary to control secondary infection.

B. General Measures: Prompt removal of recently infected patients from the endemic area almost always results in regression of the symptoms and signs in early cases.

C. Surgical Measures: Elephantiasis of the scrotum may require surgical excision.

D. Treatment of Chyluria: Mild cases require no therapy. Spontaneous cure results in 50% of cases (Ohyama, Saita, & Miyasato, 1979). If nutrition is impaired, the lymphatic channels may be sealed off by irrigating the renal pelvis with 2% silver nitrate solution. Should this fail, renal decapsulation and resection of the renal lymphatics should be performed (Yu, Leong, & Ong, 1978).

Prognosis

If exposure has been limited, resolution of the disease is spontaneous, and the prognosis is excellent. Frequent reinfection may lead to elephantiasis of the scrotum or chyluria.

ECHINOCOCCOSIS
(Hydatid Disease)

Involvement of the urogenital organs by hydatid disease is relatively rare in the USA. It is common in Australia, New Zealand, South America, Africa, Asia, the Middle East, and Europe, especially where sheep are raised.

Etiology

The adult tapeworm (*Echinococcus granulosus*) inhabits the intestinal tracts of carnivorous animals, especially dogs. Its eggs pass out with the feces and may be ingested by such animals as sheep, cattle, pigs, and occasionally humans. Larvae from these eggs pass through the intestinal wall of the various intermediate hosts and are disseminated throughout the body. In humans, the liver is principally involved, but about 3% of infected humans develop echinococcosis of the kidney.

If a cyst of the liver should rupture into the peritoneal cavity, the scoleces (tapeworm heads) may directly invade the retrovesical tissues, thus leading to the development of cysts in this area.

Clinical Findings

If renal hydatid disease is closed (not communicating with the pelvis), there may be no symptoms until a mass is found. If communicating, there may be symptoms of cystitis, and renal colic may occur as cysts are passed from the kidney. Eosinophilia is the rule (Ferreira & Rangel, 1979). X-ray films may show calcification in the wall of the cyst (Fig 13–5), and urograms often reveal changes typical of a space-occupying lesion. Angiography reveals lucent masses. Needle aspiration will reveal chocolate-colored fluid containing scoleces and hooklets. The finding of scoleces and hooklets in the urine is pathognomonic. A positive skin sensitivity test (Casoni) is suggestive. Complement fixation tests are positive in 90% of cases.

Retroperitoneal (perivesical) cysts may cause symptoms of cystitis, or acute urinary retention may develop secondary to pressure. The presence of a suprapubic mass may be the only finding. It may rupture into the bladder and cause hydatiduria, which establishes the diagnosis.

Treatment

Nephrectomy is generally the treatment of

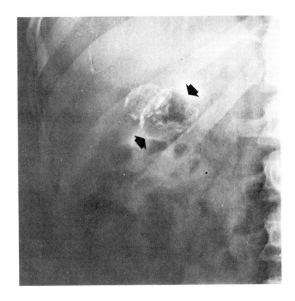

Figure 13–5. Hydatid disease, right kidney. Plain film showing 2 calcified hydatid cysts.

choice for renal hydatid disease, although aspiration and marsupialization have also been recommended. Retroperitoneal cysts are best treated by marsupialization and curettage.

Prognosis

Echinococcosis of the kidney usually has a good prognosis. The problem presented by perivesical cysts is more troublesome. After surgical intervention, drainage may be prolonged. It must be remembered, too, that involvement of other organs, especially the liver, is usually present.

● ● ●

References

Tuberculosis

Abel BJ, Gow JG: Results of caecocystoplasty for tuberculous bladder contracture. *Br J Urol* 1978;**50**:511.

Bjørn-Hansen R, Aakhus T: Angiography in renal tuberculosis. *Acta Radiol* [*Diagn*] (*Stockh*) 1971;**11**:167.

Bowersox DW & others: Isoniazid dosage in patients with renal failure. *N Engl J Med* 1973;**289**:84.

Cheng SF: Bilateral coccidioidal epididymitis. *Urology* 1974;**3**:362.

Conner WT, Drach GW, Bucher WC Jr: Genitourinary aspects of disseminated coccidioidomycosis. *J Urol* 1975;**113**:82.

Ehrlich RM, Lattimer JK: Urogenital tuberculosis in children. *J Urol* 1971;**105**:461.

Feldstein MS, Sullivan MJ, Banowsky LH: Ureteral involvement in genitourinary tuberculosis: Review of 20 cases encountered over three years. *Urology* 1975;**6**:175.

Gow JG: Genitourinary tuberculosis: A 7-year review. *Br J Urol* 1979;**51**:239.

Griffith DP, Saccomani MN, Johnson CF: Sensitivity studies in bacteriologic diagnosis of urinary tuberculosis. *Urology* 1975;**6**:182.

Kollins SA & others: Roentgenographic findings in urinary tract tuberculosis: A 10-year review. *Am J Roentgenol* 1974;**121**:487.

Narayana AS, Kelly DG, Duff FA: Tuberculosis of the penis. *Br J Urol* 1976;**48**:274.

Pagani JJ, Barbaric ZL, Cochran ST: Augmentation enterocystoplasty. *Radiology* 1979;**131**:321.

Simon HB & others: Genitourinary tuberculosis: Clinical features in a general hospital population. *Am J Med* 1977;**63**:410.

Symes JM, Blandy JP: Tuberculosis of the male urethra. *Br J Urol* 1973;**45**:432.

Wechsler M, Lattimer JK: An evaluation of the current

therapeutic regimen for renal tuberculosis. *J Urol* 1975;113:760.

Amicrobic (Abacterial) Cystitis

Hewitt CB, Stewart BH, Kiser WS: Abacterial pyuria. *J Urol* 1973;109:86.

Moore T, Parker C, Edwards EC: Sterile non-tuberculous pyuria. *Br J Urol* 1971;43:47.

Numazaki Y & others: Acute hemorrhagic cystitis in children: Isolation of adenovirus type II. *N Engl J Med* 1968;278:700.

Candidiasis

Grüneberg RN, Leaky A: Treatment of candidal urinary tract infection with nifuratel. *Br Med J* 1976;2:908.

Hamory BH, Wenzel RP: Hospital-associated candiduria: Predisposing factors and review of the literature. *J Urol* 1978;120:444.

Kozinn PJ & others: Advances in the diagnosis of renal candidiasis. *J Urol* 1978;119:184.

Michigan S: Genitourinary fungal infections. *J Urol* 1976;116:390.

Schönebeck J: Studies on Candida infection of the urinary tract and on the antimycotic drug 5-fluorocytosine. *Scand J Urol Nephrol* 1972;Suppl 11.

Schönebeck J, Segerbrand E: *Candida albicans* septicaemia during first half of pregnancy successfully treated with 5-fluorocytosine. *Br Med J* 1973;4:337.

Wise GJ, Goldberg P, Kozinn PJ: Genitourinary candidiasis: Diagnosis and treatment. *J Urol* 1976;116:778.

Actinomycosis

Crosse JEW, Soderdahl DW, Schamber DT: Renal actinomycosis. *Urology* 1976;7:309.

Fass RJ & others: Clindamycin in the treatment of serious anaerobic infections. *Ann Intern Med* 1973;78:853.

Pollock PG & others: Rapid diagnosis of actinomycosis by thin-needle aspiration biopsy. *Am J Clin Pathol* 1978;70:27.

Sarosdy MF, Brock WA, Parsons CL: Scrotal actinomycosis. *J Urol* 1979;121:256.

Trichomoniasis in the Male

Davidson F: Short-term high-dose metronidazole for vaginal trichomoniasis. *J Obstet Gynecol Br Commonw* 1973;80:368.

Dykers JR: Single-dose metronidazole for trichomonal vaginitis: Patient and consort. *Am J Obstet Gynecol* 1978;132:579.

Lumsden WHR, Robertson DHH, McNeillage GJC: Isolation, cultivation, low temperature preservation, and infectivity titration of *Trichomonas vaginalis*. *Br J Vener Dis* 1966;42:145.

McClean AN: Nitrimidazine (Naxogin) compared with metronidazole (Flagyl) in the treatment of trichomonal vaginitis. *Br J Vener Dis* 1972;48:69.

Summers JL, Ford ML: The Papanicolaou smear as a diagnostic tool in male trichomoniasis. *J Urol* 1972;107:840.

Schistosomiasis (Bilharziasis)

Al-Ghorab MM: Radiological manifestations of genitourinary bilharziasis. *Clin Radiol* 1968;19:100.

Al-Ghorab MM: Ureteritis calcinosa: A complication of bilharzial ureteritis and its relation to primary ureteric stone formation. *Br J Urol* 1962;34:33.

Al-Ghorab MM, El-Badawi AA, Effat H: Vesico-ureteric reflux in urinary bilharziasis: A clinico-radiological study. *Clin Radiol* 1966;17:41.

El-Bolkainy MN & others: Carcinoma of the bilharzial bladder: Diagnostic value with urine cytology. *Urology* 1974;3:319.

Farid Z & others: Symptomatic, radiological, and functional improvement following treatment of urinary schistosomiasis. *Lancet* 1967;2:1110.

Ghoneim MA, Ashamallah A, Khalik MA: Bilharzial strictures of the ureter presenting with anuria. *Br J Urol* 1971;43:439.

Ghoneim MA & others: Staging of the carcinoma of bilharzial bladder. *Urology* 1974;3:40.

Hanafy MH, Youssef TK, Saad MS: Radiographic aspects of (bilharzial) schistosomal ureter. *Urology* 1975;6:118.

Khafagy MM, El-Bolkainy MN, Mansour MA: Carcinoma of the bilharzial urinary bladder. *Cancer* 1972;30:150.

Wagenknecht LV: Carcinoma of bilharzial bladder and urogenital bilharziasis (author's translation). *Urologe (A)* 1974;13:59.

Young SW & others: Urinary tract lesion of *Schistosoma haematobium* with detailed radiographic consideration of the ureter. *Radiology* 1974;111:81.

Zahran MM & others: Bilharziasis of urinary bladder and ureter: Comparative histopathologic study. *Urology* 1976;8:73.

Filariasis

Crane DB, Wheeler WE, Smith MJV: Chyluria. *Urology* 1977;9:429.

Iturregui-Pagán Jr, Fortuño RF, Noy MA: Genital manifestation of filariasis. *Urology* 1976;8:207.

Lang EK, Redetzki JE, Brown RL: Lymphangiographic demonstration of lymphaticocalyceal fistulas causing chyluria (filariasis). *J Urol* 1972;108:321.

Nelson GS: Current concepts in parasitology: Filariasis. *N Engl J Med* 1979;300:1136.

Ohyama C, Saita H, Miyasato N: Spontaneous remission of chyluria. *J Urol* 1979;121:316.

Yu HHY, Leong CH, Ong GB: Chyluria: Result of surgical treatment in 50 cases. *J Urol* 1978;119:104.

Yu HHY, Ngan H, Leong CH: Chyluria: A 10-year follow-up. *Br J Urol* 1978;50:126.

Echinococcosis (Hydatid Disease)

Amir-Jahed AK & others: Clinical echinococcosis. *Ann Surg* 1975;182:541.

Baltaxe HA, Fleming RJ: The angiographic appearance of hydatid disease. *Radiology* 1970;97:599.

Birkhoff JD, McClennan BL: Echinococcal disease of the pelvis: Urologic complication, diagnosis and treatment. *J Urol* 1973;109:473.

Diamond HM & others: Echinococcal disease of the kidney. *J Urol* 1976;115:742.

Ferreira AM, Rangel AJR: Hydatid cyst of the kidney: 8 cases. *Br J Urol* 1979;51:345.

Haines JG & others: Echinococcal cyst of the kidney. *J Urol* 1977;117:788.

Urologic Aspects of Venereal Diseases in the Male | 14

Donald R. Smith, MD

GONORRHEA

Gonorrhea is primarily a urethral infection. If untreated it is a self-limiting disease, the bacteria dying out as a rule within 6 months. Infection does not confer immunity against reinfection.

Antibiotics have diminished the incidence of gonorrhea, but it is still the most common reportable infectious disease in the USA. Fortunately, disabling complications (prostatitis, epididymitis, urethral stricture, endocarditis, and arthritis) are now relatively rare.

Neisseria gonorrhoeae is almost without exception transmitted through sexual contact. The organisms are kidney-shaped and arranged as diplococci with their relatively flat surfaces apposed. They are gram-negative and are typically located within the neutrophils, although they are frequently found extracellularly as well. Other pyogenic cocci (eg, staphylococci) are also located intracellularly at times, but these can usually be differentiated morphologically from gonococci by Gram's stain or culture.

Prepubertal gonorrhea is being reported with increasing frequency, mostly in girls in association with sexual abuse (Meek, Askari, & Belman, 1979).

The pathologic findings consist mainly of diffuse infiltration of the tissues by neutrophils, lymphocytes, and plasma cells.

Clinical Findings

A. Symptoms: The first symptom of gonorrhea is a purulent urethral discharge, which usually appears 2–10 days after sexual exposure. There is usually some burning on urination, and urethral itching is common. Frequency, urgency, and nocturia do not occur unless the posterior urethra and prostate become involved (rare with antibiotic therapy).

B. Signs: The purulent urethral discharge is yellow or brown. The meatus is red and edematous, and its lips are everted. The urethra may be thickened and tender. The inflammation is mucosal and submucosal.

Prostatic massage and urethral instrumentation are contraindicated during the acute phase of the disease. If severe urinary symptoms are present and urinary obstruction supervenes, palpation of the prostate may show it to be swollen, hot, and tender (acute prostatitis).

C. Laboratory Findings: The urethral discharge should first be examined, unstained and in saline, for trichomonads. Examination of smears stained with Gram's stain and methylene blue should be done in order to establish a bacteriologic diagnosis. If microscopic study reveals the typical intracellular gram-negative diplococci, cultures are not necessary. If discharge is unobtainable, the first part of the urine should be centrifuged and the sediment treated as urethral discharge.

When the infection is limited to the anterior urethra, only the first portion of the urine is cloudy. If posterior urethritis develops, the entire stream becomes purulent. Gonococci are then found in the stained sediment of the midstream specimen.

In equivocal cases, cultures of the purulent discharge are necessary. This is particularly true in the diagnosis of pharyngeal and rectal involvement. Because gonococci die rapidly on drying, specimens must be cultured promptly on special media (chocolate blood agar) in an atmosphere of 10% CO_2.

Asymptomatic gonorrhea is common in men who have had sexual contact with women with proved infection. Such men should have cultures made. This is best done by urethral swab or urethral scrapings with a loop. Culture of the first 10 mL of urine passed is also a rewarding diagnostic procedure.

Differential Diagnosis

Chlamydial urethritis ("nonspecific" or nongonococcal urethritis, NGU) and trichomonal urethritis cause the same symptoms as gonorrhea, although the discharge in the latter is usually more purulent and profuse. Study of the discharge, both fresh and stained, demonstrates the etiologic organisms (Schachter, 1978).

NGU is now one of the commonest venereal diseases (42% of the venereal diseases in Seattle are NGU). There are a large number of possible complications. Treatment is with tetracyclines given orally as for gonorrhea.

Complications

Most complications are local (periurethral) and

prostatic. They are rare but may still occur if the diagnosis is missed or if improper treatment (without antibiotics) is instituted. Periurethritis may develop and may lead to abscess formation; in the healing process, periurethral fibrosis will cause stricture (Osoba & Alausa, 1976). Posterior urethritis and prostatitis occur if the disease process extends beyond the external sphincter. Symptoms of cystitis may occur at this stage, and all of the urine passed is purulent. The infection may then descend to the epididymis, causing a very painful swelling of that organ.

Gonorrheal arthritis is occasionally observed as a complication of bacteremia, which may be manifested by typical cutaneous lesions. Acute polyarthritis may develop, and monarticular disease with effusion may be seen. These usually respond promptly with definitive antibiotic therapy. Meningitis and endocarditis are quite rare. Of more importance is involvement of the rectum and pharynx in homosexual men (Klein & others, 1977). Gonococcal ophthalmia neonatorum is on the increase.

Prevention

Contacts known to have been exposed to gonorrhea should be treated as though they have the disease (see below).

Treatment

The gonococcus is very sensitive to most antibiotics, although there is some evidence that it is becoming increasingly resistant to penicillin. Some gonococci produce penicillinase. At least 90% of patients respond promptly to the proper drug given in adequate dosage. The discharge usually disappears in 12 hours, and complications seldom develop. In about 10–15% of patients, a scanty, thin discharge will remain following treatment. This usually disappears within a few days, particularly when treated with tetracycline.

Proof of cure rests on the absence of gonococci in whatever discharge remains or in the washings from the urethra (the first portion of the voided urine). If gonococci are absent, culture of the first portion of a urine specimen should then be done. If this is negative for gonococci, cure has been established. If the infective bacteria have not been eradicated by one antibiotic, another drug or combination of drugs should be used. Since syphilis may also have been contracted simultaneously, serologic tests for syphilis must be done in 3 weeks and then after 3, 6, 12, and 24 months.

A. Specific Measures: (As recommended by the USPHS.) Aqueous procaine penicillin, 4.8 million units intramuscularly in 2 divided doses given with 1 g of probenecid by mouth, cures over 90% of cases. Oral penicillins are also effective. A single dose of ampicillin, 3.5 g orally, simultaneously with probenecid, also results in a high cure rate. For patients in whom penicillin or ampicillin with pro-

benecid is contraindicated, give spectinomycin hydrochloride (Trobicin) intramuscularly as a single dose, 2 g for men and 4 g for women. The tetracyclines also cure 90% of infected persons and have the added advantage of combating *Chlamydia*, whose presence in the gonorrheal patient is apt to cause persistence of a scanty discharge even though the gonococcal infection has been cured. Kristensen & From (1975) noted an excellent response to trimethoprim-sulfamethoxazole (Bactrim, Septra). They recommend 5 tablets followed in 8 hours by 5 more tablets *(caution!)*.

Meek, Askari, & Belman (1979) make the following recommendations for treating the prepubertal child: In the uncomplicated case, give aqueous procaine penicillin G, 100,000 units/kg intramuscularly, plus probenecid, 25 mg/kg orally. In the face of complications, they suggest the same daily dose in 4 divided doses intravenously for 7 days. As an alternative, the same penicillin, same dose, can be given in 2 divided doses intramuscularly for 7 days.

B. General Measures: Response to the antibiotics is so prompt that general measures are not necessary. Sexual intercourse should be avoided until cure has been established.

C. Treatment of Complications: Complications are exceedingly rare. If any of the following develops, more extensive antibiotic therapy is indicated: acute prostatitis, acute epididymitis, periurethral abscess, cystitis, and arthritis. Urethral stricture requires urethral dilatations.

Prognosis

The prognosis is excellent if gonorrhea is diagnosed early and treated properly.

THE PRIMARY PENILE LESION OF SYPHILIS

Syphilis is caused by infection with *Treponema pallidum*, a distinctive spirochete. It makes its appearance about 2–4 weeks after sexual exposure. A painless papule or pustule develops on the glans, corona, foreskin, shaft, or even the pubic area or on the scrotum and breaks down to form an indurated, punched-out ulcer. The lesion may be so small and transient that it may be missed.

Microscopically, the tissues are heavily infiltrated with small round cells and plasma cells. Some proliferation of the intimal linings of the blood vessels develops. Neutrophils may be numerous if secondary infection occurs.

Clinical Findings

A. Symptoms and Signs: The patient usually presents himself because of the appearance of a painless penile sore 2–4 weeks after sexual contact. The ulcer is relatively deep, has indurated edges and a clean base, and is not painful on pressure. Without treatment, spontaneous healing is slow.

Discrete, enlarged inguinal lymph nodes may be palpable. They are not tender unless the primary lesion has become infected by pyogenic organisms, which occurs very rarely.

B. Laboratory Findings: The diagnosis is made by finding the pathogenic spirochetes in the serous discharge from the ulcer on darkfield examination. Serologic tests for syphilis may remain negative for 1–3 weeks or longer after the appearance of the chancre.

Differential Diagnosis (Table 14–1)

The primary penile lesions of chancroid, lymphogranuloma venereum, granuloma inguinale, gangrenous and erosive balanitis, and herpes simplex may resemble the chancre of syphilis. All penile ulcers must be considered syphilitic until proved otherwise. *Borrelia refringens* may be present and is most difficult to distinguish from *T pallidum* in the dark field.

Erythroplasia of Queyrat (see p 318) may resemble a chancre. Darkfield examination and biopsy will clarify the diagnosis.

Complications

Urologic complications of syphilis are rare. They include gummas of the testis and neurogenic (neuropathic) bladder due to neurosyphilis.

Prevention

Give benzathine penicillin G, 2.4 million units intramuscularly in one dose.

Treatment

Give 2.4 million units of procaine penicillin G with 2% aluminum monostearate into the buttocks and then 1.2 million units intramuscularly every other day for a total dose of 4.8 million units. Other satisfactory regimens include (1) benzathine penicillin G, 1.2 million units in each gluteal muscle, or (2) procaine penicillin G, 600,000 units intramuscularly daily for 8 days.

Prognosis

The prognosis is excellent. Relapse is rare and requires more intensive penicillin therapy. The blood serology of the patient should, however, be rechecked every 6 months for 3 years after treatment. The spinal fluid should be examined to rule out central nervous system syphilis, which requires more intensive treatment.

The patient should be cautioned not to have sexual intercourse until cure has been obtained.

CHANCROID
(Soft Chancre)

Chancroid is a common venereal disease whose primary ulcer may simulate the chancre of syphilis or lymphogranuloma venereum. It is usually accompanied by inguinal adenitis. The highest incidence occurs in men with long foreskins who practice poor hygiene.

The infecting organism is *Haemophilus ducreyi*, a short, nonmotile, gram-negative streptobacillus which usually occurs in chains. It is found with difficulty on stained smear; cultures are more successful. The incubation period is 1–5 days.

Macroscopically, one or several small penile ulcers are present. Biopsy of chancroid shows endothelial proliferation without much fibroplasia in the midzone; the deeper tissues are diffusely infiltrated with small round cells and plasma cells. These findings are considered to be diagnostic.

Inguinal adenitis, usually unilateral, develops in about 50% of cases. Progression is rapid, although the lesion may resolve spontaneously or go on to suppuration and spontaneous evacuation.

Clinical Findings

A. Symptoms: A few days after sexual exposure, one or more painful, dirty-appearing ulcers may be noted. They enlarge gradually. In 2 or 3 weeks, large, tender inguinal lymph nodes appear. These may suppurate and drain spontaneously. About 50% of patients have fever to 39 C (102.2 F), malaise, and headache.

B. Signs: The ulcer is rarely more than 1–2 cm in diameter. It is usually shallow and has irregular edges. The base is friable and bleeds easily. On occasion it may become very extensive and destructive.

C. Laboratory Findings: Diligent search of a smear stained with Gram's stain shows *H ducreyi* in 50% of cases. Culture, if available, is more successful. Skin tests (Ducrey test) are positive in about 75% of cases. Biopsy is diagnostic in all cases. Tests for other venereal ulcers should be done to establish or rule out the possibility of double infections: (1) darkfield examination for spirochetes (syphilis and erosive balanitis), (2) complement fixation (lymphogranuloma venereum), (3) search for "Donovan bodies" (granuloma inguinale), and (4) serologic tests for syphilis.

Differential Diagnosis (Table 14–1)

Chancroid must be differentiated from other ulcerative lesions of the external genitalia.

Complications

Secondary infection with *Borrelia refringens* and fusiform bacilli may cause marked destruction of tissue, but this is not common. Phimosis or paraphimosis may develop during the healing stage.

Prevention

Thorough washing of the genitalia with soap and water after sexual intercourse, or any of the antibiotics which are useful in treatment, will prevent the disease.

Treatment

A. Specific Measures: Even in the bubo stage, response to the tetracyclines is excellent. The optimum dose is 0.5 g every 6 hours for 7 days. The sulfonamides, 4 g/d for 10 days, are only slightly less effective. For those that are resistant to this treatment, give kanamycin, 500 mg intramuscularly twice a day for 7–14 days, depending on the response. Penicillin is without effect.

B. General Measures: Cleanliness is of the greatest importance. The parts should be washed regularly with bland soap and water. Oils and greases are contraindicated.

C. Treatment of Complications: If the symbiotic infection of fusiform bacilli and spirochetes complicates the picture, penicillin should be used in addition, although the antibiotics which are administered for the chancroidal infection will probably overcome these infections also. If phimosis or paraphimosis develops, surgical correction may be necessary. During the acute stage, only a dorsal slit is indicated. Later, circumcision can be done. Aspiration of fluctuant inguinal nodes may be necessary.

Prognosis

With proper antibiotic therapy, the prognosis for immediate cure is excellent.

LYMPHOGRANULOMA VENEREUM
(Lymphopathia Venereum)

Lymphogranuloma venereum is an infectious venereal disease caused by *Chlamydia trachomatis*, immunotypes L1, L2, L3. The disease is characterized by a transient genital lesion followed by lymphadenitis and at times, in the female, rectal stricture. In men, because of the anatomy of the lymphatics, the inguinal and subinguinal nodes become matted, and, although many resolve, the majority undergo suppuration and form multiple sinuses.

Microscopically, the lesion shows acute and subacute inflammation. There is nothing specific or diagnostic in its appearance. The lymph nodes show abscesses and heavy infiltration with neutrophils. Hyperplasia of lymphoid elements then takes place and plasma cells appear. In the late stages of the disease, the capsular areas become fibrotic; the centers are necrotic.

Clinical Findings

A. Symptoms and Signs: The penile lesion develops 30–60 days after sexual exposure; it heals spontaneously and rapidly and thus is often not seen. This lesion may be papular or vesicular, although only a superficial erosion may occur. A few days or weeks later, painful enlargement of inguinal nodes develops; because the primary lesion is so often missed, this may be the initial symptom. Later, the matted nodes usually break down,

whereupon multiple sinuses develop. At the stage of bubo formation, constitutional symptoms are present. These include chills, fever, headache, generalized joint pains, and nausea and vomiting. Skin rashes are frequent.

Rectal stricture is a late manifestation of the disease in females. If present, it can usually be palpated. It tends to be annular in type and may almost close the lumen. When this has developed, a change in bowel habits is evident.

B. Laboratory Findings: The white blood cell count may reach 20,000/μL during the stage of lymph node invasion. Anemia may also develop. The sedimentation rate is accelerated. Serum proteins (globulin) are increased. Complement fixation tests, if positive, are almost pathognomonic for present or past lymphogranuloma venereum. These tests cannot differentiate reliably between infection caused by any member of the chlamydia group of organisms. The serologic test for syphilis may give a weak false-positive reaction. This is usually transient, however.

Differential Diagnosis (Table 14–1)

All penile ulcers should be regarded as of syphilitic origin until proved otherwise; darkfield examinations for *T pallidum* and serologic studies are essential. Lymphogranuloma venereum must be suspected in any rectal stricture in a female.

Complications

Untreated or late cases may develop multiple sinuses from involved lymph nodes. Elephantiasis of the genitalia can occur if lymphatic drainage is severely obstructed. Occasionally in women (rarely in men), proctitis and rectal stricture may occur. Stricture sometimes becomes manifest years after the initial infection.

Prevention

Washing the genitals with soap and water immediately after sexual exposure is a successful preventive measure. One of the tetracycline group of antibiotics given for 1–2 days immediately after exposure may be a useful means of prophylaxis.

Treatment

A. Specific Measures: The tetracyclines are effective even in the stage of bubo formation. The usual dose is 0.5–1 g every 6 hours for a total dose of 15–30 g. These antibiotics are also reported to be moderately effective in relieving the anorectal stricture. They do not affect the fibrous tissue, however; their value probably lies in controlling bacterial activity and suppressing secondary infection, thus reducing edema associated with the inflammation.

Sulfonamides, 4 g/d for 3–4 weeks, although they probably have little effect upon the causative agent, control secondary infection.

Streptomycin and penicillin are not effective.

B. Treatment of Complications: Aspiration of

fluctuant inguinal nodes is indicated. Draining sinuses may have to be excised. Rectal stenosis may require surgical measures.

Prognosis

The prognosis is excellent. Only the late complications seen in old cases present difficulties (genital elephantiasis and rectal stricture).

GRANULOMA INGUINALE

Granuloma inguinale is a chronic venereal infection of the skin and subcutaneous tissues of the genitalia, perineum, or inguinal regions. The incubation period is 2–3 months.

The infective agent is *Calymmatobacterium granulomatis*, a bacterium related to *Klebsiella pneumoniae* (Friedländer's bacillus). It grows with difficulty on artificial media containing egg yolk or in the yolk sac of the chick embryo.

The ulcer does not excite a constitutional reaction and does not involve the lymph nodes or lymphatics.

The microscopic picture shows nonspecific infection, with necrosis of the skin and small abscesses. In the deeper portions there is an infiltration of plasma cells, giant cells, neutrophils, and large monocytes; the cytoplasm of the monocytes contains numerous "Donovan bodies," the intracellular stage of the etiologic organism.

Clinical Findings

A. Symptoms and Signs: The first sign of the disease is an elevation on the skin of the genitals or adjacent skin (commonly the groin), which finally breaks down. This moderately painful superficial ulcer gradually spreads and can become quite extensive. The base of the ulcer is covered by pink granulation tissue which bleeds easily. There is a more or less purulent discharge, particularly if secondary infection develops.

B. Laboratory Findings: Identification of the "Donovan body" in large monocytes on a stained smear makes the diagnosis. Scrapings from the base of the lesion are placed on a slide, fixed in air, and stained. Wright's and Giemsa's staining technics are both adequate.

In case of doubt, biopsy may be done. The bacteria take up hematoxylin as well as silver salts.

Complement fixation and skin sensitivity tests are not dependable and not readily available.

Differential Diagnosis

See Table 14–1.

Complications

Secondary infection may cause deep ulceration and tissue destruction. Sinuses may result. Marked phimosis may occur in advanced cases, even to the point of urinary obstruction. Other venereal diseases may be present at the same time.

Prevention

The use of a condom does not prevent perigenital inoculation. Thorough washing with soap immediately after contact will often prevent infection. Tetracycline antibiotics given for several days following contact may afford protection.

Treatment

A. Specific Measures: The tetracyclines and chloramphenicol have proved curative in a high percentage of cases. Dosage is 1 g/d in divided doses for 7–14 days.

Streptomycin is also effective. The dose is 1 g/d intramuscularly for 10 days.

B. Treatment of Complications: Secondary infection is effectively combated in most instances by the drug used to cure the primary disease. If fusiform bacilli and spirochetes (*Borrelia refringens*) are present, penicillin may be used also.

Prognosis

There are no serious complications, and antibiotics are quite efficient in treatment. The prognosis is excellent.

EROSIVE & GANGRENOUS BALANITIS

This is one of the less common penile lesions, presumably of venereal origin. A long foreskin is almost a necessary prerequisite to the development of the lesion, since the infecting organisms are anaerobic. Poor local hygiene also contributes to the establishment of the disease. The lesion ulcerates progressively and proceeds to gangrene of the glans and at times even of the shaft of the penis. The incubation period is 3–7 days.

The infecting organisms are a spirochete (*Borrelia refringens*) and a gram-negative bacillus (vibrio) acting in symbiosis. Both organisms are stained by the common dyes.

Microscopic examination of a biopsy specimen shows nothing specific; the picture is one of acute inflammation. Neutrophilic and small round cell infiltration is extensive.

Clinical Findings

A. Symptoms: The patient complains of local pain, a profuse, foul discharge, and, if the foreskin can be retracted, a progressive ulcerative lesion of the glans, foreskin, or shaft of the penis. In acute cases, chills, fever, and marked malaise may develop. Burning on urination is common and is caused by the inflammatory reaction in and about the urinary meatus.

B. Signs: The ulceration usually starts in the region of the corona under a tight, unclean prepuce. The ulcer gradually spreads and produces a foul,

Table 14–1. Differential diagnosis of genital ulcers.

	Syphilitic Chancre	Chancroid	Lymphogranuloma Venereum	Granuloma Inguinale	Erosive and Grangrenous Balanitis	Herpes Progenitalis	Epithelioma
Etiology	T pallidum	H ducreyi (Ducrey's bacillus)	Chlamydia trachomatis immunotypes L1, L2, L3	Calymmatobacterium granulomatis	Vibrio and spirochete (Borrelia refringens)	Herpesvirus type 2	. . .
Incubation time	2–4 weeks	3–10 days	3–21 days	2–3 months	3–7 days	Unknown (often recurrent)	. . .
Early lesion	Enlarging papule that finally ulcerates	Macule → papule, then formation of ulcer	Transient, usually not seen. Papule or macule heals rapidly.	Superficial ulcer of skin	Single or multiple ulcerations that fuse and spread	Multiple superficial vesicles on the foreskin or glans	May appear as small ulcer
Advanced local lesion	Ulcer becomes deep and edges indurated. Heals spontaneously.	Ulcer gradually spreads. May become extensive. Multiple lesions.	None	Becomes serpiginous and may spread widely	Ulcers become deep and painful. May spread rapidly. Profuse foul discharge.	Vesicles may coalesce and form superficial ulcer that heals spontaneously	May become large and destructive
Local pain	Absent unless secondarily infected	Very painful	None	Little	Very painful	Slight local burning or itching	None unless secondarily infected
Involvement of inguinal lymph nodes	Discrete, rubbery, nontender	In 50% of cases, nodes are enlarged and tender. May suppurate.	In almost all cases in 2–8 weeks after primary sore. Matted, tend to break down. Multiple sinuses.	None	Discrete, only mildly tender	None	Metastases usually unilateral. Painless.
Definitive diagnosis	T pallidum on darkfield examination. Serology.	Skin test, stained smear or culture, biopsy	Complement fixation test	Stained organisms in scrapings from ulcer or biopsy	Spirochetes and fusiform bacilli on darkfield examination or stained smear	Isolation of virus	Biopsy

often profuse discharge. The accompanying edema may prevent retraction of the foreskin; a dorsal slit may be necessary before the lesion can be observed. As the disease progresses, the invasion of the penile tissue goes deeper, and if it is not treated by appropriate means, portions of the penis may become gangrenous. In extreme cases the entire penis and even the scrotum may be destroyed.

C. Laboratory Findings: The finding of many spirochetes and fusiform bacilli in a smear is strongly suggestive, but it must be remembered that other ulcerative venereal lesions can be secondarily invaded by these organisms.

Differential Diagnosis

See Table 14–1.

Complications

If the disease is untreated, severe damage may occur to the penis and adjacent structures. If the infection is mild or is aborted by appropriate means, some fibrosis of the foreskin may occur. Contracture of this tissue leads to phimosis.

In elderly men, the fulminating form of this disease is to be feared, as overwhelming sepsis is often rapidly fatal.

Prevention

Proper hygienic care of the redundant foreskin will prevent the disease, but circumcision is definitive. This is a disease of filth and neglect.

Treatment

A. Specific Measures: Penicillin is the drug of choice; 0.6–1.2 million units/d for 5–7 days usually suffice. The tetracyclines are also effective; the dosage is 2 g/d in divided doses for 5–7 days.

B. General Measures: If response to antibiotics is not prompt, dorsal slit of the prepuce may be indicated for purposes of hygiene and because aerobic conditions discourage the organisms. Mild soap and water or hydrogen peroxide soaks are helpful and will combat the malodorous discharge.

C. Treatment of Complications: Plastic procedures on a badly damaged organ may be necessary. Circumcision is indicated if phimosis develops.

Prognosis

If diagnosed and treated early, the prognosis is excellent. Superficial loss of skin is replaced spontaneously with surprisingly little scar. Neglected patients may, however, suffer severe local tissue destruction.

● ● ●

References

General

King A, Nicol C: *Venereal Diseases*, 3rd ed. Williams & Wilkins, 1975.

Nicholas L: *Sexually Transmitted Diseases*. Thomas, 1973.

Symposium on venereal diseases. *Med Clin North Am* 1972;**56**:1055. [Entire issue.]

Wisdom A: *Color Atlas of Venereology*. Year Book, 1973.

Gonorrhea

Barrett-Connor E: The prophylaxis of gonorrhea. *Am J Med Sci* 1975;**269**:4.

Corman LC & others: The high frequency of pharyngeal gonococcal infection in a prenatal clinic population. *JAMA* 1974;**230**:568.

Feng WC, Medeiros AA, Murray ES: Diagnosis of gonorrhea in male patients by culture of uncentrifuged first-voided urine. *JAMA* 1977;**237**:896.

Handsfield HH, Hodson WA, Holmes KK: Neonatal gonococcal infection. 1. Orogastric contamination with *Neisseria gonorrhoeae*. *JAMA* 1973;**225**:697.

Harris JRW, McCann JS, Mahony JDH: Gonococcal arthritis: A common rarity. *Br J Vener Dis* 1973;**49**:42.

Klanica J, Stejskalová M: Direct immunofluorescent test for the detection of gonorrhea. *Br J Vener Dis* 1976;**52**:33.

Klein EJ & others: Anorectal gonococcal infection. *Ann Intern Med* 1977;**86**:340.

Kohen DP: Neonatal gonococcal arthritis: Three cases and review of literature. *Pediatrics* 1974;**53**:436.

Kristensen JK, From E: Trimethoprim-sulfamethoxazole in gonorrhoea: A comparison with pivampicillin combined with probenecid. *Br J Vener Dis* 1975;**51**:31.

Meek JM, Askari A, Belman AB: Prepubertal gonorrhea. *J Urol* 1979;**122**:532.

Nussbaum M, Scalettar H, Shenker IR: Gonococcal arthritis-dermatitis (GADS) as a complication of gonococcemia in adolescents. *Clin Pediatr (Phila)* 1975;**14**:1037.

Osoba AO, Alausa O: Gonococcal urethral stricture and watering-can perineum. *Br J Vener Dis* 1976;**52**:387.

Penicillinase-producing gonococci. (Editorial.) *Br Med J* 1976;**2**:963.

Perera PM, Lim KS: Asymptomatic urethral gonorrhoea in men. *Br Med J* 1975;**3**:415.

Sayeed ZA & others: Gonococcal meningitis. *JAMA* 1972;**219**:1730.

Schachter J: Chlamydial infections. (3 parts.) *N Engl J Med* 1978;**298**:428, 490, 540.

Tanowitz HB, Adler JJ, Chirito E: Gonococcal endocarditis. *NY State J Med* 1972;**72**:2782.

Thompson TR, Swanson RE, Wiesner PJ: Gonococcal ophthalmia neonatorum: Relationship of time of infection to relevant control measures. *JAMA* 1974;**228**:186.

Venereal Disease Control Center, Center for Disease Control: Treatment of gonococcal infections: Recommendations of the U.S. Public Health Service. *Urology* 1979;**13**:689.

Wheeler JK, Heffron WA, Williams RC Jr: Migratory arthralgias and cutaneous lesions as confusing initial manifestations of gonorrhea. *Am J Med Sci* 1970;**260**:150.

Wiesner PJ & others: Clinical spectrum of pharyngeal gonococcal infection. *N Engl J Med* 1973;**288**:181.

Primary Penile Lesion of Syphilis

Desmond FB: The diagnosis of infectious syphilis. *NZ Med J* 1971;**73**:135.

Fluker JL: Syphilis. *Practitioner* 1972;**209**:605.

Nicolis G, Loucopoulos A: Cephalothin in the treatment of syphilis. *Br J Vener Dis* 1974;**50**:270.

Penicillin in the treatment of syphilis. (Editorial.) *Br Med J* 1973;**2**:259.

Schroeter AL & others: Treatment for early syphilis and reactivity of serologic tests. *JAMA* 1972;**221**:471.

Syphilis: Recommended treatment schedules, 1976. Recommendations established by the Venereal Disease Control Advisory Committee, Center for Disease Control, Atlanta, Georgia. *Ann Intern Med* 1976;**85**:94.

Youmans JB: Syphilis and other venereal diseases. *Med Clin North Am* 1964;**48**:573.

Chancroid

Alergant CD: Chancroid. *Practitioner* 1972;**209**:624.

Marmar JL: The management of resistant chancroid in Vietnam. *J Urol* 1972;**107**:807.

Lymphogranuloma Venereum

Abrams AJ: Lymphogranuloma venereum. *JAMA* 1968;**205**:199.

McLelland BA, Anderson PC: Lymphogranuloma venereum: Outbreak in a university community. *JAMA* 1976;**235**:56.

Stewart DB: The gynecologic lesions of lymphogranuloma venereum and granuloma inguinale. *Med Clin North Am* 1964;**48**:773.

Granuloma Inguinale

Davis CM: Granuloma inguinale. *JAMA* 1970;**211**:632.

Lal S, Nicholas C: Epidemiological and clinical features in 165 cases of granuloma inguinale. *Br J Vener Dis* 1970;**46**:461.

Ribeiro J: Granuloma inguinale. *Practitioner* 1972;**209**:628.

15 | Urinary Stones

Donald R. Smith, MD

Urinary lithiasis is one of the most common diseases of the urinary tract. It occurs more frequently in men than in women, is rare in children and blacks, and often shows a familial predisposition.

If a stone is not obstructive, it is not apt to cause injury or symptoms. If it blocks a urinary passage (eg, the ureteropelvic junction), it leads to severe symptoms and renal damage. Since stones tend to recur, a patient with a nonobstructive stone may later form a stone that will cause obstruction; for this reason, investigation of the cause of the first stone is of importance in the prevention of later renal injury.

RENAL STONE*

Etiology

All the causes of renal stone formation are not known, but in most cases multiple factors are involved. An adequate stone analysis is the key to an understanding of the pathogenetic mechanisms involved. In the USA, two-thirds of all renal stones are composed of either calcium oxalate or mixtures of calcium oxalate and calcium phosphate in the form of hydroxyapatite. Pure apatite or brushite (calcium hydrogen phosphate dihydrate) stones are very rare. Magnesium ammonium phosphate (struvite) accounts for 15% of all stones and occurs almost exclusively in patients who have urinary tract infections with urea-splitting organisms and persistently alkaline urine. Uric acid and cystine stones account for about 10% (Broadus & Thier, 1979). Miscellaneous stones are composed of xanthine, silicates, or matrix and occasionally of artifacts brought in by patients as "kidney stones."

Calculous disease is often seen in infants and children, particularly primary vesical stones, which occur in India, Indonesia, the Middle East, and parts of China (Remzi, 1978). In the USA, most stones in young people are either due to a metabolic defect (eg, cystinuria) or are secondary to infection, which is often caused by congenital anomalies or

*Portions of the section on renal stone are contributed by Felix O. Kolb, MD.

occurs following urinary diversion. Most stones in children are renal. (Reiner, Kroovand, & Perlmutter, 1979; Noronha, Gregory, & Duke, 1979; Sinno, Boyce, & Resnick, 1979.)

The following factors are known to influence the formation and growth of uroliths:

A. Hyperexcretion of Relatively Insoluble Urinary Constituents:

1. Calcium–(Normal urinary excretion of calcium on a low-calcium diet [no milk or cheese for 4 days] is 100–175 mg/24 h.) On regular diets, normal females excrete less than 250 mg/24 h and males less than 300 mg/24 h. The major calcium foods are milk and cheese. Hypercalciuria may be seen in some adults who drink a quart or more of milk per day. It has been shown that the lactose in milk and dietary protein causes increased absorption of calcium from the gut (Smith, Van Den Berg, & Wilson, 1978).

Prolonged immobilization (spinal cord injury, fractures, poliomyelitis) and certain bone diseases (eg, metastatic cancer, myeloma, Paget's disease) cause hypercalciuria. Under these circumstances, calcium excretion may reach 450 mg/d or more.

Primary hyperparathyroidism causes hypercalciuria and hyperphosphaturia as well as hypercalcemia and hypophosphatemia. Two-thirds of these patients have renal stones.

Idiopathic hypercalciuria occurs most commonly in males. Serum calcium is normal and serum phosphorus is decreased. Even on a low-calcium intake, patients may excrete as much as 500 mg of calcium in 24 hours. This may reflect increased absorption of calcium from the gut or defective renal tubular reabsorption of calcium (Maggio Jr & others, 1979).

Hypervitaminosis D may so increase absorption of calcium from the intestine that urinary excretion of the ion may reach pathologically high levels.

Renal tubular acidosis causes hyperexcretion of calcium and a relatively fixed urinary pH inappropriate for the degree of acidosis, since the formation of ammonia and titratable acidity is defective.

2. Oxalate–Although oxalate is the major component of two-thirds of all renal stones, hyperoxaluria as a cause of lithiasis is relatively rare. Cabbage, rhubarb, spinach, tomatoes, celery, black tea, and cocoa contain large amounts of oxalate.

Ingestion of excessive amounts of ascorbic acid and certain fruit juices (eg, orange juice) may also increase urinary oxalate excretion. Restriction of these foods usually has limited effect in prevention of oxalate stones, because the major source of oxalate is endogenous, and dietary oxalate is usually poorly absorbed.

Primary hyperoxaluria is a rare, often lethal genetic disorder affecting the metabolism of glyoxylic acid, which forms oxalate rather than soluble end products. It is an important cause of nephrolithiasis and nephrocalcinosis in children. Acquired forms of hyperoxaluria include pyridoxine deficiency, ethylene glycol poisoning, methoxyflurane anesthesia, and small bowel disease with hyperabsorption of dietary oxalate (Gregory, Park, & Schoenberg, 1977).

3. Cystine–Cystinuria is a hereditary disease that is uncommon except in infants and children. Only a small percentage of patients with cystinuria form stones. Other amino acids (ornithine, lysine, and arginine) are lost simultaneously; however, these are quite soluble and do not form stones. The loss of these amino acids is due to a defect in renal tubular reabsorption.

4. Uric acid–Many patients with gout form uric acid calculi, particularly when under treatment for arthritis; most of these patients have elevated blood uric acid levels and increased urinary uric acid excretion. However, gout is not a necessary condition for stone formation. Uric acid crystalluria and stones may form when there is rapid tissue breakdown, eg, in the chemotherapeutic treatment of leukemia, polycythemia, and carcinoma; therefore, it is important to maintain an alkaline dilute urine when treating these diseases. The concomitant administration of allopurinol (Zyloprim) should also be considered.

Many uric acid stone formers have normal serum and urinary uric acid levels but show a consistently low urinary pH. This may be caused by decreased tubular formation of ammonia. Patients with chronic diarrheal states or with ileostomies also have strongly acid urines and may form uric acid stones. Elevated serum uric acid is often observed secondary to thiazide diuretic therapy, but this can be controlled by giving allopurinol. Recent evidence suggests that there is a relationship between the concentration of sodium urate and the tendency to calcium oxalate precipitation (Coe, 1977).

5. Xanthine–A rare cause of renal stone is associated with lack of xanthine oxidase and very low uric acid levels. Recently, a few cases have been observed after the use of allopurinol in the hyperuricemia of leukemia or Lesch-Nyhan syndrome.

6. Drug-induced stones–In rare cases, the long-term use of magnesium trisilicate in the treatment of peptic ulcer leads to the formation of radiopaque silicon stones. Patients receiving allopurinol may form oxypurinol stones (Stote, 1980), but this is also rare. Triamterene stones have been recently described (Ettinger, 1979).

7. Matrix stones–These are rare radiolucent "stones" formed in heavily infected urinary tracts.

8. Factitious stones–A variety of artifacts (seed, sand) may be presented by emotionally disturbed patients as having been passed as "kidney stones." It is important to analyze *all* stones passed, especially those from patients who are known to have previously passed stones.

B. Physical Changes That Occur in the Urine:

1. Increased concentration of salts and organic compounds–This may be due to low fluid intake; to excessive water losses in febrile diseases, in hot climates, or in occupations causing excessive perspiration; or to excessive water losses due to vomiting and diarrhea.

2. Urinary magnesium/calcium ratio–This appears to have some influence on stone formation. Acetazolamide (Diamox) causes hypercalciuria and a decrease in the ratio and is related to an increased incidence of stone formation. The thiazides, which appear to help prevent recurrences of stone, cause an increase in the ratio.

3. Urinary pH–The mean urinary pH is 5.85. It is influenced by diet, by ingestion of acid or alkaline medications (eg, in treatment of peptic ulcer), and by the use of acetazolamide in the treatment of glaucoma. The latter causes an increase in urinary pH. Urea-splitting bacteria—usually *Proteus mirabilis*—make the urine strongly alkaline (pH 7.5+) by liberating ammonia. The inorganic salts are less soluble in an alkaline medium (calcium phosphate forms at a pH of 6.6 or higher, and magnesium ammonium phosphate precipitates at a pH of 7.2 or higher). Organic substances (eg, cystine, uric acid) are least soluble at a pH below 7.0 (maximum insolubility, pH 5.5).

4. Colloid content–It has long been claimed that the colloids in the urine allow the inorganic salts to be held in a supersaturated state. Recent work has tended to negate this theory.

5. "Good" and "evil" urine–Howard (1970) found that some types of urine promote while others prevent stone formation. When rachitic rat cartilage is placed in "good" urine, calcification does not occur. In "evil" urine, the cartilage becomes calcified. "Evil" urine, however, becomes "good" urine following the oral administration of 3–6 g/d of phosphate with enhanced urinary excretion of pyrophosphate and polyphosphates. The use of aluminum hydroxide gels that absorb phosphate in the gut is therefore probably contraindicated if an attempt is being made to prevent calcium stone formation.

Other protective substances that act as crystal inhibitors must exist, eg, citrate, amino acids, magnesium, etc, since the crystalloids normally excreted in urine would precipitate in water. Most of these substances have not yet been isolated.

C. A Nidus (Core or "Nucleus") Upon Which Precipitation Occurs: Randall observed that calcific plaques ("Randall's plaques") are commonly seen on the renal papillae. He believed that they develop as a result of injury to cells of the collecting tubule secondary to infection elsewhere. Randall postulated that when the overlying mucosa finally ulcerates, the calcification acts as a nidus to which the insoluble substances in the urine can adhere. Vermeulen & others (1967) have verified this observation.

Some investigators believe that most stones develop by precipitation of crystals (eg, calcium oxalate) on an organic matrix formed of amino acids and carbohydrates, but support for the primary role of matrix in initiating stone disease is lacking. Other masses that can act as nidi include blood clots, clumps of epithelial or pus cells, or even bacteria.

Necrotic ischemic tissue and foreign bodies may encourage the precipitation of relatively insoluble substances. Tissues of this sort may be caused by neoplasms, retained necrotic papillae, or ulceration of mucous membranes by infection.

D. Structural Anomalies, Including Obstruction and Medullary Sponge Kidney: These disorders may be complicated by stones that form secondary to stasis or infection of urine in the dilated collecting tubules, but associated metabolic disorders (eg, hyperparathyroidism) must be considered (Rao & others, 1977).

Pathology

The size and position of the stone govern the development of secondary pathologic changes in the urinary tract. The obstruction caused by a small stone lodged in the ureteropelvic junction or in the ureter may slowly destroy a kidney (Fig 10–5), whereas a relatively large stone may be so placed as to cause little renal damage.

Infection is a common complication of an obstructing renal stone because of the stasis that it causes. The very presence of such a foreign body seems to decrease the local resistance to hematogenous infection. The parenchymal ischemia caused by local pressure from an enlarging staghorn stone may progressively damage a kidney, but the major cause of progressive renal damage is the renal infection that caused the stone to form.

The Physical Characteristics of Urinary Calculi (Fig 15–1)

(1) Calcium phosphate stones (often mixed with magnesium ammonium phosphate) may be soft or hard; they are usually yellow or brown (sometimes dark), often form staghorn masses, and are frequently laminated. They are readily seen on x-ray films; the lamination, if present, is clearly visible.

(2) Magnesium ammonium phosphate stones are usually yellow and somewhat friable. Staghorn formation is common. On radiograms, their density lies between that of calcium oxalate and cystine. Lamination may be noted if calcium oxalate or phosphate is also present.

(3) Calcium oxalate stones ("jackstones," "mulberry stones") are usually small, rough, and hard. Staghorn formation is rare. Spicules radiating from a central core can often be seen on x-rays.

(4) Cystine stones are smooth and light yellow or yellow-brown. They have a waxy appearance and are usually multiple and bilateral. They may enlarge quite rapidly, sometimes coalescing to

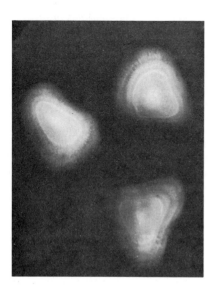 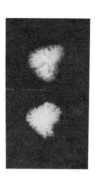 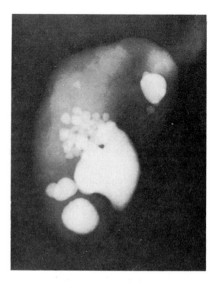

Figure 15–1. X-ray appearance of stones. *Left:* Calcium phosphate, laminated. *Center:* Calcium oxalate, spiculated. *Right:* Cystine, homogeneous. (Reproduced, with permission, from Albright & Reifenstein: *Parathyroid Glands and Metabolic Bone Disease.* Williams & Wilkins, 1948.)

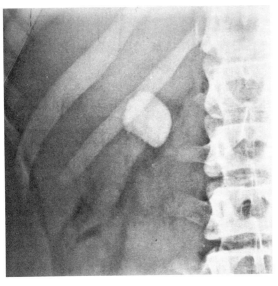
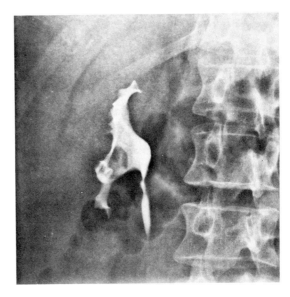

Figure 15–2. Cystine and uric acid stones. ***Left:*** Plain film showing homogeneous, mildly opaque stone, typically cystine. ***Right:*** Excretory urogram showing uric acid stone as "negative" shadow because radiopaque medium is more dense than the stone.

form staghorn calculi. Although their density is relatively low, they can be identified on a roentgenogram as homogeneous, slightly opaque, smoothly rounded bodies (Fig 15–2). They sometimes contain calcium salts and may then show some lamination.

(5) Uric acid crystals can precipitate in the renal parenchyma. The stones formed from these crystals in the renal pelvis are usually small and hard, varying in color from yellow to reddish-brown. They may be multiple. If they are composed of pure uric acid crystals, they cannot be seen on plain x-ray films. On excretory urograms, they are present as "negative" shadows (Fig 15–2).

Radiopacity

Radiopacity is directly related to the density of the stone compared to that of water (Table 15–1).

Clinical Findings

A. Symptoms: If the stone is free and obstructs a calix or the ureteropelvic junction, there will be

Table 15–1. Stone density as related to degree of radiopacity.

	Density	Degree of Radiopacity
Calcium phosphate	22.0	Very opaque
Calcium oxalate	10.8	Opaque
Magnesium ammonium phosphate	4.1	Moderately opaque
Cystine	3.7	Slightly opaque
Uric acid	1.4	Nonopaque
Xanthine	1.4	Nonopaque

dull flank pain due to parenchymal and capsular distention and colic due to hyperperistalsis and smooth muscle spasm of calices and pelvis; total hematuria; nausea and vomiting; and abdominal distention from paralytic ileus. Chills, high fever, and vesical irritability are due to infection.

The history should include a survey of fluid intake, diet (amount of milk, cheese), drugs (alkalies, analgesics, acetazolamide, vitamin D), periods of immobilization, previous passage of stones, and the presence of gout. There may be a family history of stone formation due to hereditary hyperoxaluria, hypercalciuria, cystinuria, hyperuricemia, or renal acidosis.

If the stone is still submucosal (Randall's plaque) or adherent to the parenchyma, there are no symptoms. The same is usually true of a small stone trapped in a minor calix.

Staghorn calculus may be asymptomatic even if infection is present. Symptoms are most apt to be gastrointestinal and may simulate gallbladder disease, peptic ulcer, or less specific enteric syndromes. Urologic symptoms may include mild back or flank pain, hematuria, and those due to infection (chills, fever, increased renal pain, and symptoms of cystitis).

B. Signs: Tenderness in the costovertebral angle or over the kidney may or may not be present. Acute renal infection may cause more definite findings. If marked hydronephrotic atrophy has occurred as a result of prolonged ureteral obstruction, a mass in the flank may be seen, felt, or percussed. Some muscle rigidity over the kidney may be found, and rebound tenderness may be elicited, particularly if acute infection is present. Abdominal distention and diminished peristalsis usually accompany acute renal colic.

C. Laboratory Findings:

1. Blood count–The white blood count may be increased due to complicating infection. If renal function is not adequate, anemia may be found.

2. Urinalysis–Protein may be noted because of the presence of hematuria. Pus cells and bacteria may be seen. Oxalate bodies are often observed in hyperparathyroidism, renal tubular acidosis, and hyperoxaluria. Calcium phosphate casts suggest hypercalciuria.

If the pH of the urine is higher than 7.6, urea-splitting organisms must be present, for the kidneys cannot produce urine in this range of alkalinity. Such a finding strongly suggests that the stones are composed of magnesium ammonium phosphate. Fixation of the pH at 6.0–6.5 is compatible with renal tubular acidosis. Consistently low pH is a common cause of the formation of uric acid calculi.

A search should be made for crystals in the sediment; the type may afford a clue to the type of stone (Fig 5–2). Cystine and uric acid crystals may be precipitated by adding a few drops of glacial acetic acid (which lowers the pH to about 4.0) to a test tube of urine that is then refrigerated. Cystine crystals resemble benzene rings; uric acid crystals are typically amber-brown.

A simple chemical screening test for cystine is as follows: To 5 mL of urine made alkaline with ammonium hydroxide, add 2 mL of 5% sodium cyanide and let stand for 5 minutes. Add a few drops of fresh 5% sodium nitroprusside. A deep purplish-red color means hypercystinuria. The definitive diagnosis and proper treatment rest upon quantitative estimation of the amounts of alpha-aminonitrogen and cystine excreted in 24 hours. Normal excretion is about 1 mg/lb (up to 150 mg/24 h) of alpha-aminonitrogen and 50–180 mg of cystine in a like period. Mild cystinurics excrete 200–400 mg of cystine; moderate cystinurics excrete 400–1000 mg; and those with a severe tubular defect, up to 3000 mg/d.

The Sulkowitch test should be done, in conjunction with specific gravity determination, on all patients with urinary stone. If strongly positive (especially if the urine is dilute), hypercalciuria is present. A positive test should be repeated after milk and cheese have been withdrawn for 4 days. If the test is still strongly positive, quantitative calcium determinations should be done.

After 4 days on a diet free of milk and cheese, the amount of calcium excreted in the urine in 24 hours should be determined. More than 175 mg of calcium per 24 hours suggests hyperparathyroidism or idiopathic hypercalciuria unless some obvious cause for calcium excess is found (eg, immobilization). The finding of hyperphosphaturia is compatible with a renal phosphate leak and strongly suggests hyperparathyroidism when hypercalcemia and hypercalciuria are found. Some patients with

mild hyperparathyroidism may not have hypercalciuria.

A 24-hour urine specimen should be subjected to a quantitative test for oxalate. (This test, however, is not generally available.) The upper limit of normal is 50 mg. Levels as high as 200–300 mg/24 h may be encountered in primary hyperoxaluria. Normal uric acid excretion is 300–600 mg/24 h.

A test for the presence of urea-splitting bacteria is performed by incubating noninfected acid urine overnight with a few drops of the infected urine. If the pH increases, urea-splitting organisms are present.

3. Renal function tests–The PSP may be normal even in the presence of bilateral staghorn stones or in chronic unilateral obstruction due to stone. Acute obstruction at the ureteropelvic junction may suddenly depress the PSP to two-thirds of normal. The complication of renal infection may also interfere with renal function. Urine culture and sensitivity tests are therefore mandatory.

A serum creatinine or urea nitrogen determination is indicated if the PSP is less than 30% in one-half hour. Unless the patient is dehydrated, elevation of either substance indicates decreased renal function.

4. Blood chemistry studies–Fasting serum calcium and phosphorus should be determined on 3 occasions. Serum proteins should also be estimated, since almost half of the calcium is normally un-ionized and bound to protein. If serum proteins are decreased but total calcium is normal, an increase in ionized calcium is indicated. This can be estimated by the use of a nomogram or by direct measurements, eg, with the Orion electrode. Hypercalcemia with hypophosphatemia strongly suggests primary hyperparathyroidism, but normal serum phosphate is found in 60% of patients. Estimation of serum chloride concentration may prove helpful in the differential diagnosis of hypercalcemia. It is above 102 mEq/L in hyperparathyroidism and below this figure in other conditions producing hypercalcemia (eg, cancer of the breast).

Hypercalcemia is most commonly seen in association with osteolytic or disseminated malignant disease, especially cancers of the breast and lung, multiple myeloma, leukemia, and sarcoidosis, but serum phosphate is usually normal. These conditions rarely cause renal stones unless associated with hyperparathyroidism.

Determination of the tubular reabsorption of phosphate (TRP) may prove helpful in the diagnosis of hyperparathyroidism when minimal hypercalcemia and normal blood phosphate levels are obtained. The normal range of tubular reabsorption of phosphate is about 90–95% with low phosphate intake and 75–85% with high phosphate intake. In hyperparathyroidism the values range from 40–80%, demonstrating the typical phosphate leak. Radioimmunoassay of parathyroid hormone is be-

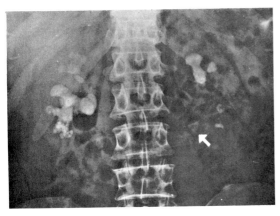 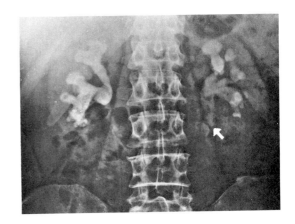

Figure 15–3. Bilateral staghorn calculi and left upper ureteral stone. *Left:* Plain film. Arrow points to ureteral stone. *Right:* Excretory urogram showing bilateral impaired function.

coming increasingly available. If elevated with serum calcium levels to above 10.7 mg/dL, the diagnosis of hyperparathyroidism is strongly suggested. Measurements of urinary nephrogenous cAMP are now available for the rapid diagnosis of hyperparathyroidism.

Serum alkaline phosphatase is increased in hyperparathyroidism only if bone disease (eg, osteitis fibrosa cystica) is present.

Elevated serum uric acid (normal is 2–6 mg/dL) is found in 50% of uric acid stone formers.

If plasma or serum bicarbonate is decreased, acidosis is present. Such a finding might be the clue to the cause of hypercalciuria and stone formation, because when renal tubular damage is advanced, the inability to generate NH_4^+ results in failure to reabsorb Na^+ and Ca^{2+}, which are then excreted as cations (fixed base). Low bicarbonate in the presence of high serum chloride is compatible with renal tubular acidosis or severe chronic renal insufficiency. An ammonium chloride load test will bring out latent cases of renal tubular acidosis. Electrophoretic analysis of the serum will point to sarcoidosis or myeloma as the cause of hypercalcemia.

D. X-Ray Findings: At least 90% of renal stones are radiopaque and are readily visible on a plain film of the abdomen unless they are small or overlie bone. It is necessary to differentiate renal stone from calcified mesenteric lymph nodes, calcium in rib cartilage, gallstones, phleboliths (which are seen in the region of the bladder or lower ureters), and solid medication (pills) present in the intestinal tract. Because the plain film is 2-dimensional, it has only presumptive value except in the case of a staghorn stone, which is never confused with other findings (Fig 15–3).

The morphology of the stone may give a clue to its chemical nature (Fig 15–1).

Bone disease may be discovered in the hands, ribs, spine, pelvis, or femoral heads. This may suggest the cause of hypercalciuria (eg, hy-

perparathyroidism, metastatic carcinoma, Paget's disease). X-rays of the long bones and skull may also show changes typical of these disorders (Fig 15–4). The pathognomonic sign of hyperparathyroidism is cortical subperiosteal resorption in the phalanges.

Excretory urograms are necessary because they accurately localize the calcific shadow unless the kidney is without function or unless it is acutely blocked by a stone (Fig 15–3). Oblique views may also be helpful. If a urogram is not obtained but the

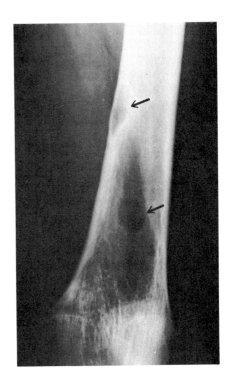

Figure 15–4. Osteitis fibrosa cystica with hyperparathyroidism. Note cystic changes in femur (arrows).

kidney shadow becomes dense (nephrogram, Fig 15–9), acute obstruction of a good kidney has probably occurred. If the stone is nonopaque, the films will demonstrate obstruction (dilatation), and the stone may appear as a darker area ("negative" shadow) in the renal pelvis (Fig 15–2). Excretory urograms also measure renal function, which is helpful in judging definitive treatment.

If function is poor, retrograde urograms may be needed.

E. Ultrasonography: Employing ultrasound, Edell & Zegel (1978) were able to distinguish between opaque and nonopaque stones.

F. Computed Tomography: This technic has proved useful in the diagnosis of nonopaque stones (Segal & others, 1978; Tessler & Ghazi, 1979).

G. Renal Scan: If the excretory urograms imply poor renal function, isotope studies may prove helpful in further assessing this factor (see Chapter 8). If the damage is irreversible, the ^{203}Hg scan will show little uptake by the tubules while the scintillations afforded by ^{131}I will be minimal. ^{99m}Tc will reveal poor vascularity. Such findings might indicate the need for nephrectomy rather than nephrolithotomy.

H. Instrumental Examination: Cystoscopy for diagnostic purposes is seldom necessary if the excretory urograms are satisfactory. Ureteral catheterization may prove helpful in localizing infection and measuring renal function. Such studies in conjunction with retrograde urograms may be the deciding factor in choosing between pyelolithotomy or nephrectomy.

I. Examination of Stone: Crystallographic examination of previously passed stones and examination of stones removed or passed are useful in establishing the cause of stone formation, especially in differentiating "primary" (metabolic) stones from "secondary" stones (eg, stones formed due to infection).

Differential Diagnosis

Acute pyelonephritis may start with acute and severe renal pain, thus mimicking a renal stone lodged at the ureteropelvic junction. Pus and bacteria are found in the urine, although it must be remembered that infection may be a complication of renal stone. Urograms will decide the issue. Chronic infection may be associated with little or no back pain and a few if any vesical symptoms. Urinalysis and radiographic study will settle the diagnosis.

Renal tumor may sometimes simulate stone, particularly if a blood clot causes obstruction (pain, hematuria). Urography will establish the diagnosis.

A tumor of the renal pelvis or calix can cause renal colic and hematuria. A space-occupying lesion on the urogram may be confused with a nonopaque stone (Figs 15–2 and 18–9). A CT scan and cytologic examination of the urine sediment will be helpful in differential diagnosis, but at times the diagnosis is made at the operating table.

Renal tuberculosis may be painful and, if associated with bleeding, may mimic renal stone. A plain abdominal x-ray may show calcium deposits in the renal shadow. Stone complicates tuberculosis in 10% of cases. A "sterile" pyuria and a suspicion of tuberculosis on urography suggest the diagnosis. Demonstration of acid-fast bacilli is diagnostic.

Papillary necrosis may be confused with renal stone, because sloughed papillae that are not passed tend to undergo peripheral calcification, thus giving the radiographic appearance of a uric acid stone containing an outer shell of calcium. The history, diminished renal function, pyuria, and the typical radiographic appearance of papillitis should make the diagnosis (Fig 12–5).

Infarction of the kidney, commonly secondary to a cardiac lesion, usually occurs without pain or gross hematuria; if the infarction is massive, however, renal pain and microscopic or even gross hematuria may be produced. Evidence of a cardiac lesion (eg, subacute infective endocarditis, atrial fibrillation) should suggest the possibility of infarction. Excretory urograms will show lack of secretion, and angiography will reveal arterial occlusion.

Complications

The presence of a stone lowers resistance to bacterial invasion. This is particularly true if the stone is obstructive. Calculi complicated by infection may cause pyonephrosis and ultimate complete destruction of the kidney, which becomes a cavity containing stones and purulent material only.

Obstruction of the ureter at the ureteropelvic junction leads to hydronephrosis, which can ultimately destroy the parenchyma of the kidney. Obstruction of a calix causes hydrocalicosis and focal renal damage. Complicating infection contributes to further injury.

Although an enlarging staghorn stone may cause some renal damage because of the pressure it exerts on the parenchyma, the major effect on kidney function is caused by pyelonephritis.

The rare epidermoid carcinoma of the renal pelvis is almost always associated with an infected kidney containing a stone.

Prevention

Patients who have formed stones should be managed prophylactically in an attempt to prevent recurrences. The measures indicated depend upon the type of stone formed in the past. If a stone is unavailable for analysis, its composition may be surmised from the following data: (1) x-ray density and morphology of stones in the urinary tract, (2) types of crystals in the urine, (3) positive test for urinary alpha-aminonitrogen and cystine crystals, and (4) abnormalities in blood chemistry (calcium, phosphorus, uric acid).

A. General Measures: Stone-formers must

maintain a high urine volume to keep solutes well diluted. Fluids should be taken at bedtime so that nocturia will occur; on waking, more water should be taken. This will prevent relative nocturnal dehydration. Infection should be treated with appropriate antibiotics; obstruction and stasis should be eliminated by surgery; and recumbency should be avoided.

The physician should ask patients if they are "vitamin addicts." They may be taking vitamin D, as well as mineral preparations that include considerable calcium. Calcium stone-formers should maintain an acid urine and should be asked about overuse of alkalies or milk for gastric distress.

B. Specific Measures: Prophylactic treatment specific for the various types of stones is as follows:

1. Calcium stones–If caused by primary hyperparathyroidism, the parathyroid glands should be explored and hyperfunctioning lesions resected.

a. Diet–Eliminate excessive intake of milk, cheese, and other dairy products if hypercalciuria is discovered. A low carbohydrate intake may be of value.

b. Urinary pH–Calcium phosphate and magnesium ammonium phosphate stones form most readily in neutral or alkaline urine. The pH of the urine should be kept below 6.0. It can be tested by the patient with Nitrazine paper. Cranberry juice; ascorbic acid, 1 g 4 times a day; and sodium or potassium acid phosphate are the most efficient acidifiers. In renal tubular acidosis, alkali should be given in the form of sodium and potassium citrate; this will dramatically reduce the output of urinary calcium.

c. Phosphates–According to Howard (1970), stone-formers manufacture "evil" urine. This effect can be negated by the administration of 2.5 g of neutral sodium (or potassium) phosphate (Na_2HPO_4) daily in divided doses. Sodium (or potassium) acid phosphate, 4–6 g/d, is also effective. The potassium salts are preferable; Neutra-Phos and K-Phos Neutral are commercially available preparations. Enough should be given to furnish 1–2 g of phosphate. If possible, urinary phosphate excretion should be increased to 1500–2000 mg/24 h. Cellulose phosphate may be of value for hypercalciuric patients who absorb calcium excessively (Pak, Delea, & Bartter, 1974). However, this expensive drug is not generally available and may lead to hyperoxaluria.

d. Diuretics–Yendt (1976) has observed that the administration of a benzothiadiazine diuretic (eg, hydrochlorothiazide [HydroDiuril], 50 mg twice a day) decreases the amount of calcium in the urine by half in patients with idiopathic hypercalciuria. Potassium supplements must be given if hypokalemia is induced. Long-term studies on the use of thiazides have shown that small stones may be flushed out and that recurrent calcium stones are prevented. This is the treatment of choice if urinary tract infection is present and phosphate therapy is contraindicated, since the tendency to triple phosphate stone formation is enhanced in an infected alkaline urine. If thiazides induce hyperuricemia, allopurinol (Zyloprim) must be added. Coe (1977) has reported that this combined program is most effective in preventing recurrent calcium nephrolithiasis.

2. Hyperoxaluria–There is no entirely effective method for decreasing the amount of oxalate in the urine in hyperoxaluria. Foods high in oxalate should be eliminated from the diet, especially in patients with ileitis or shunts. Pyridoxine in large doses may be helpful. Phosphate therapy (see above) may be useful unless renal function is impaired. Thiazides are useful agents that may decrease both urinary calcium and oxalate while increasing magnesium and citrate.

The administration of magnesium oxide, 150 mg 3 times a day, may control recurrence of oxalate stones. It does not diminish the level of urinary excretion; however, the magnesium may combine with oxalate, thus forming a more soluble complex. Marked restriction of calcium is contraindicated, since calcium combines with dietary oxalates in the gut, thus preventing absorption. Following intestinal shunts in those patients who have recurrent calcium oxalate stones, measures to prevent steatorrhea and administration of large amounts of calcium paradoxically reduce stone formation by binding oxalate and reducing hyperoxaluria.

3. Metabolic stones (uric acid, cystine)–Keep the pH at 7.0 or higher, thereby increasing the solubility of these substances (up to 100%). This can sometimes be done with an alkaline-ash diet (high in vegetable and fruit content, low in protein), but added alkalies are usually needed (give 50% sodium citrate solution, 1–2 tsp 4 times daily or oftener as needed, or a mixture of sodium and potassium bicarbonate). The patient can follow urinary pH with paper indicators. A low-purine diet may be prescribed for the uric acid stone-former. Allopurinol (Zyloprim), a xanthine oxidase inhibitor, decreases the endogenous production of uric acid and therefore has proved very effective in preventing recurrence of uric acid calculi. The dose is 300–600 mg/24 h. Toxic reactions (rash, fever, liver enzyme abnormalities, etc) may occur and must be watched for. In a rare patient with Lesch-Nyhan syndrome and an occasional patient with leukemia, allopurinol therapy may lead to xanthine stone formation. The use of allopurinol in patients with calcium stones who also have either hyperuricemia or hyperuricosuria has recently been advocated but has not yet been properly evaluated. The combined use of thiazides and allopurinol seems more rational, but the toxicity of either agent may thereby be enhanced.

In severe cystinurics (over 1200 mg/24 h), a low-methionine diet may be necessary in order to decrease the amount of endogenous cystine, but this diet is not very palatable. If the above measures fail to decrease the urinary cystine to safe levels, penicillamine (Cuprimine) should be added to the regimen. This preparation (30 mg/kg/d in divided doses) usually reduces the amount of cystine in the urine to 100 mg or less per day. Pyridoxine, 50 mg/d, should also be given. Stone formation ceases; some stones may dissolve. Skin rashes are not uncommon but can be controlled by corticosteroids, which are given for a few weeks and then withdrawn. Other more serious reactions, such as nephrosis, have been observed with penicillamine. Since the drug is expensive and also toxic, the lowest dose (1 g/d or less in divided doses) should be tried, combined with forced fluids, alkalinization, and a low-methionine diet. Less toxic and possibly cheaper preparations (acetylcysteine and mercaptopropionylglycine) are under investigation.

4. Urease inhibitors–Recently, use of urease inhibitors such as acetohydroxamic acid has been proposed as a potentially effective means of treatment of magnesium ammonium phosphate stone formers.

5. Methylene blue–Methylene blue has not proved effective for treatment or prevention of renal calculi.

6. Aluminum hydroxide–Although aluminum hydroxide gels had been advocated for the prevention of phosphate calculi, long-term studies have shown that hypercalciuria and osteomalacia are produced and that the low phosphate content of urine may promote calcium oxalate and calcium phosphate stone formation. These gels may be of value in triple phosphate stone-formers and in patients with renal stones who have progressive renal impairment.

C. Mixed Stones: If the patient forms more than one type of stone and the prophylactic regimens interfere with each other, it is best to determine which is the primary stone and direct prophylactic measures against that type.

Treatment

A. Conservative Measures:

1. No surgery is necessary in the following cases–

a. Randall's plaque requires no treatment as long as it remains submucosal. However, it may become free and pass down the ureter, causing obstruction.

b. A small stone trapped in a minor calix and causing few if any symptoms and no renal damage is best ignored.

c. In the elderly poor-risk patient, a coralline stone is best left alone unless it causes significant symptoms. In younger individuals, removal of such stones should be considered, since their primary cause (urea-splitting organisms) cannot be eradicated as long as the stone (containing embedded bacteria) remains. After nephrolithotomy, the renal infection can usually be treated successfully with antibiotics (eg, ampicillin).

d. Stones due to renal tubular acidosis should be treated conservatively even if multiple, since they may pass spontaneously with adequate medical treatment (alkalies).

2. Combating infection–This is of particular importance if the bacteria are urea-splitting, for they encourage the progression of calcium phosphate or magnesium stone formation. Unfortunately, this is often not successful unless the stone is removed.

3. Attempts at dissolution–Chemical dissolution of renal stones requires indwelling ureteral catheters for constant "through-and-through" irrigation with hemiacidrin (Renacidin) or with G (or M) solution (see p 240) and is usually mechanically impracticable. Sand and stone fragments occlude the catheters and cause acute obstruction. This may lead to exacerbation of pyelonephritis, and bacteremia and renal cortical abscesses may result.

With the increased use of the percutaneous technic for anterograde urography, it has become feasible to place a small catheter in the renal pelvis so that intermittent or continuous instillations can be used. Spataro, Linke, & Barbaric (1978) report success in dissolving uric acid stones by irrigating with 0.1-M solution of sodium bicarbonate and giving additional baking soda orally. Gordon, Carrion, & Politano (1978) report similar results irrigating with tromethamine THAM, which has a pH of 7.84. Smith (1979) dissolved cystine stones with a saline solution of acetylcysteine and sodium bicarbonate; Crissey & Gittes (1979) found tromethamine-E, with a pH of 10.2, to be equally effective. Dretler, Pfister, & Newhouse (1979) successfully dissolved infection stones with hemiacidrin. The urine should be sterilized before institution of this therapy.

Some uric acid stones may dissolve on allopurinol (Zyloprim) therapy. Cystine stones may disappear when penicillamine (Cuprimine) is administered.

B. Surgical Measures: Removal of the stone is indicated if it is obstructive and causes undue pain or progressive renal damage or if the infection complicating a stone cannot be eradicated.

The problem of the staghorn stone is more serious. In the younger individual, conservative management never eradicates the underlying infection (usually urea-splitting organisms). Because this can only lead to progressive stone growth and further renal damage in patients with a reasonable life expectancy, nephrolithotomy should be done (Resnick & Boyce, 1980; James & others, 1980). After removal of the major portion of the stone, it is not uncommon for fragments to be left in the calices. These can be discovered by intraoperative nephroscopy (direct vision of the pelves and calices) (Gittes, 1979) or by ultrasound scanning. Fragments can be removed through the nephroscope. If this is not successful, coagulum pyelolithotomy can be done using cryoprecipitate, thrombin, and calcium chloride (Fisher, Sonda III, & Diokno, 1980;

Marshall, Lyon, & Scott Jr, 1978). The mixture is introduced through a catheter placed in the pelvis. A strong clot forms in which the calculi are embedded. The clot is then gently removed.

If these more conservative measures fail, a small tube should be left in the kidney, and Renacidin irrigations should be done during the postoperative period. In most cases, the residual fragments will be dissolved. The tube is then removed. Intensive antibiotic therapy both before and after surgery is mandatory. Ampicillin is the most useful drug (Feit & Fair, 1979). Persistence of infection usually leads to stone recurrence.

If the lower calices contain infection stones, partial nephrectomy should be considered (Coleman & Witherington, 1979; Leach & Lieber, 1980). In cases where renal stones are constantly being passed and multiple ureterotomies are required, some urologists advise replacing the entire ureter with a segment of ileum whose diameter will allow free passage of the stones to the bladder (Boxer & others, 1979).

Prognosis

The recurrence rate of renal stone is significant, and the prognosis must therefore be guarded. The patient must be carefully followed for months or even years. The real danger from renal stone is not the pain but the kidney destruction caused by obstruction and infection. The recently introduced chemical forms of treatment (phosphates, thiazides, allopurinol, penicillamine) appear to have materially reduced the recurrence rates and have altered the prognosis favorably. The highest incidence of recurrent renal stones is in males ages 40–60. Thereafter, a spontaneous lowering of recurrences has been observed.

NEPHROCALCINOSIS*

Nephrocalcinosis is a precipitation of calcium in the tubules, parenchyma, and, occasionally, in the glomeruli of the kidney. The presence of nephrocalcinosis often signifies that primary or secondary impairment of renal function has occurred. It is therefore a more serious disease than calculus. Nephrocalcinosis and calculus formation may exist together. Passage of sand or gravel is common.

Etiology & Pathogenesis

Hyperparathyroidism is a common cause of nephrocalcinosis with hypercalcemia. Hypercalciuria with hypercalcemia may be due to hyperparathyroidism; hypervitaminosis D, particularly when accompanied by a high calcium intake or sarcoidosis; acute osteoporosis due to immobiliza-

---

*The section on nephrocalcinosis is contributed in part by Felix O. Kolb, MD.

tion, especially in children; metastatic malignancy involving bone; or hyperthyroidism.

Hypercalciuria without hypercalcemia is most often idiopathic but may be caused by chronic renal insufficiency, particularly that due to chronic pyelonephritis, glomerulonephritis, or polycystic kidney disease, all of which are sometimes accompanied by calcific deposits in the kidneys. Hyperchloremic acidosis (eg, renal tubular acidosis) resulting from loss of the power of the tubules to elaborate ammonia leads to excretion of calcium as well as potassium and sodium. The hypercalciuria contributes to the precipitation of calcium salts.

Nephrocalcinosis without hypercalciuria is usually due to excessive intake of milk and soluble alkalies, particularly in the treatment of peptic ulcer. It is also observed in hyperoxaluria and in association with structural anomalies, eg, medullary sponge kidney.

Pathology

The kidneys may be grossly normal or there may be obvious changes such as medullary sponge kidneys that suggest advanced renal disease (eg, hydronephrosis, chronic pyelonephritis). Calcific deposits in the tubules are seen microscopically. Primary tubular or glomerular lesions may also be noted.

Metastatic calcification is not uncommonly found in many other organs, including the skin, lungs, stomach, spleen, pancreas, cornea, thyroid, and around the joints.

Clinical Findings

A. Symptoms: There are no symptoms that suggest nephrocalcinosis, although patients at times pass stones and sand. The complaints are those of the primary disease (eg, primary hyperparathyroidism or renal insufficiency). In childhood, there may be lack of normal growth and bone changes suggestive of rickets.

B. Signs: The physical examination is usually negative. Signs of the primary cause may be found, as follows: (1) parathyroid adenoma or hyperplasia, (2) metastatic calcifications around the joints or in the cornea ("band keratopathy") as viewed with a slitlamp, (3) punched-out lesions in the fingertips (sarcoidosis), (4) pseudofractures (osteomalacia), (5) bilateral renal masses (polycystic kidneys), (6) dwarfism, or (7) renal osteodystrophy.

C. Laboratory Findings: Anemia may be noted in advanced renal disease. The urinary pH is fixed between 6.0–6.5 in renal tubular acidosis. Pus and bacteria are found in the urine in association with chronic renal infection. Casts and protein are constant findings in glomerulonephritis. Calcium phosphate casts may be seen. The Sulkowitch test is strongly positive in states of hypercalciuria; it may be positive with secondary parathyroid hyperplasia as well. In advanced renal disease, hypocalciuria may be seen.

Renal function tests will demonstrate some impairment of function whether the primary cause of the calcification is renal or not. Nitrogen retention is common.

Hypercalcemia and hypophosphatemia are to be expected in primary hyperparathyroidism. In chronic renal disease (with secondary hyperparathyroidism), the serum calcium may be low or normal and the phosphate normal or elevated.

Hyperchloremic acidosis (low blood pH) and hypokalemia accompany renal tubular acidosis.

Serum alkaline phosphatase will be elevated if nephrocalcinosis is accompanied by bone disease (osteitis, osteomalacia, etc).

Urinary oxalate levels are elevated in hyperoxaluria and oxalosis.

D. X-Ray Findings: A plain film of the abdomen will show the pathognomonic parenchymal calcifications (Fig 15–5). These consist of minute calcific densities with a linear arrangement in the region of the renal papillae and radiating outward from the calices. If renal function is not seriously impaired, excretory urograms will show that the calcium is in the renal parenchyma and not in the calices, although true stones may be present as well. These films may reveal changes compatible with atrophic pyelonephritis or hydronephrosis. X-rays of bones may show osteitis fibrosa

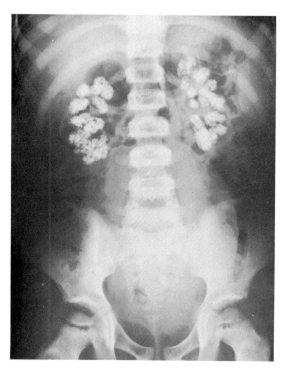

Figure 15–5. Nephrocalcinosis. Plain film showing parenchymal calcification in both kidneys. Large globular soft tissue shadow (greatly distended bladder) in midline extending from pelvis to level of lower poles of kidneys. It has displaced the bowel to the flanks.

generalisata and the soft tissue calcification of "renal rickets" (renal osteodystrophy).

Differential Diagnosis

Renal stones are usually discrete and lie in the calices or pelvis.

In renal tuberculosis, renal calcification is also parenchymal but tends to be related to the pericaliceal zones. Furthermore, the calcification is punctate rather than striated. Pus cells and tubercle bacilli are present, and excretory urograms will usually show the mucosal ulcerations or abscess cavities of tuberculosis.

Medullary sponge kidneys may develop multiple small calculi in their dilated cystic collecting tubules (Fig 22–10). Renal function is usually normal. Metabolic defects may coexist (Stella & others, 1973). Excretory urograms help in the differentiation.

Complications

Calcification secondary to extrarenal disease (eg, hyperparathyroidism) often causes minimal impairment of renal function. The calcium deposits secondary to preexisting renal disease cause more damage. If stones form and cause obstruction—particularly if there is secondary infection due to the obstruction—further renal injury occurs.

Treatment

A. Specific Measures: Treat the primary cause of the disease (eg, remove the parathyroid adenoma or hyperplastic glands, relieve obstruction, and treat urologic infection).

B. General Measures: Discontinue vitamin D and give a low-calcium diet (eliminate dairy products, especially milk and cheese), encourage mobilization, and force fluids. If osteomalacia is present, vitamin D and calcium may have to be given in spite of nephrocalcinosis. If hypercalciuria is present, thiazide therapy may be useful, but electrolytes must be carefully monitored.

If renal function is reasonably good and hyperchloremic (renal tubular) acidosis exists, replace base to decrease hypercalciuria: Give a 50% solution of sodium or potassium citrate (or a combination of both), 4–8 mL 4 times daily. Sodium bicarbonate, 4 g 4 times daily, can be given in orange juice or water. The goal is alkalinization (pH of 7.0–7.5) of the urine. Additional potassium is also indicated. At times the degree of nephrocalcinosis decreases with alkali treatment of renal tubular acidosis.

Prognosis

If the nephrocalcinosis is secondary to primary renal disease, the prognosis is poor although life can be prolonged significantly with adequate treatment. If the renal calcification has developed because of extrarenal disease and if renal function is fairly good, correction of the underlying disease may terminate the progression of kidney damage. Frequently, however, the outlook is poor even in these instances. Nephrocalcinosis with calcium oxalate deposits will recur in primary hyperoxaluria even after successful renal transplantation.

URETERAL STONE

Ureteral stones originate in the kidney. Gravity and peristalsis both contribute to spontaneous passage into and down the ureter.

Ureteral stones are seldom completely obstructive; they are usually spiculated, so that urine can flow around them. Occasionally, a stone will remain lodged in a ureter for many months without harming the kidney. Partial obstruction is usually present, however, and causes dilatation of the ureter and renal pelvis proximal to the stone. In the early phase, this dilatation is due more to distention than to "hydronephrosis," which implies definite renal damage. If the stone passes within a few days, there is no evidence of renal injury. However, if the stone is definitely obstructive and is allowed to remain for weeks or months, irreparable damage to the renal parenchyma can occur (Fig 6–4). A stone is apt to be arrested at the narrowest points in the ureter (Fig 15–6). If infection complicates the urinary stasis, further renal damage results.

Clinical Findings

A. Symptoms: Pain is usually abrupt in onset and becomes severe within minutes (Fig 15–7). There are 2 types of pain: (1) radiating, colicky, agonizing pain (from hyperperistalsis of the smooth muscle of the calices, pelvis, and ureter); and (2) the rather constant ache in the costovertebral area and flank (from obstruction and capsular tension). The radiation of pain at times suggests the position of the stone. If the stone is high in the ureter, the colic may radiate to the testicle. As the stone nears the bladder, the pain may spread to the scrotum or appear in the vulva. This is due to the common innervation of these organs and the lower ureter. At times the pain comes on more slowly and may be felt more anteriorly. It may occasionally be quite mild. In these instances, the diagnosis may not at first be obvious.

Gastrointestinal symptoms are commonly associated with stone in the ureter. Nausea and vomiting almost always occur, and abdominal distention due to paralytic ileus is always present. These symptoms may be so severe that the renal and ureteral pain may be overshadowed and an intraperitoneal lesion sought (eg, bowel obstruction, ruptured peptic ulcer, cholelithiasis, or acute appendicitis).

Gross hematuria is observed in about one-third of cases; small clots may be passed.

Even in the absence of infection, symptoms of

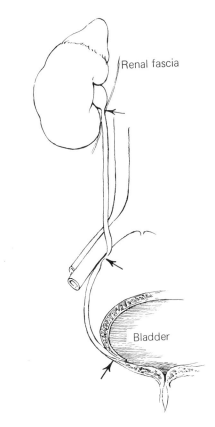

Figure 15–6. Points of ureteral narrowing. The ureter is narrow at 3 points: (1) at the ureteropelvic junction, (2) at the point where the ureter crosses over the iliac vessels, and (3) in the ureterovesical zone. A stone that passes the ureteropelvic junction has an excellent chance, therefore, of continuing the whole distance. If it becomes arrested, it is usually in the lower 5 cm of the ureter.

urgency and frequency may develop when the stone approaches the bladder.

Existing chronic renal infection may be exacerbated by the ureteral obstruction. Chills and fever with increased back pain may be noted. It is not common for stone to be complicated by acute (new) infection unless it is introduced by instrumentation. If this does occur, however, chills, fever, and sepsis are to be expected.

B. Signs: The patient is usually in agony, pacing the floor rather than lying quietly in bed (as a patient with peritoneal irritation is apt to do). Nothing affords relief. The skin may be cold and clammy, and there may be other signs of mild shock. There is marked tenderness in the costovertebral angle and flank. Fist percussion posteriorly causes severe pain. Spasm of the abdominal muscles on the affected side is to be expected.

Fever indicates that infection is a complicating feature. The abdomen is distended, tympanitic, and quiet on auscultation. The ipsilateral testis may be hypersensitive if the stone is in the upper ureter.

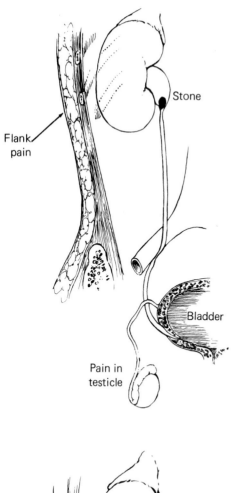

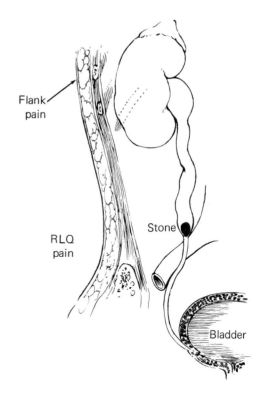

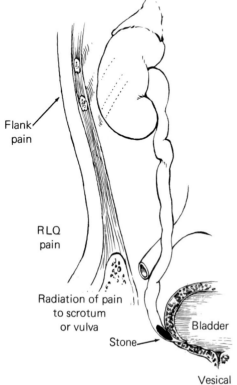

Figure 15–7. Radiation of pain with various types of ureteral stone. *Above left:* Ureteropelvic stone. Severe costovertebral angle pain from capsular and pelvic distention; acute renal and ureteral pain from hyperperistalsis of smooth muscle of calices, pelvis, and ureter, with pain radiating along the course of the ureter (and into the testicle, since the nerve supply to the kidney and testis is the same). The testis is hypersensitive. *Above right:* Midureteral stone. Same as above but with more pain in the lower abdominal quadrant. *Left:* Low ureteral stone. Same as above, with pain radiating into bladder, vulva, or scrotum. The scrotal wall is hyperesthetic. Testicular sensitivity is absent. When the stone approaches the bladder, urgency and frequency with burning on urination develop as a result of inflammation of the bladder wall around the ureteral orifice.

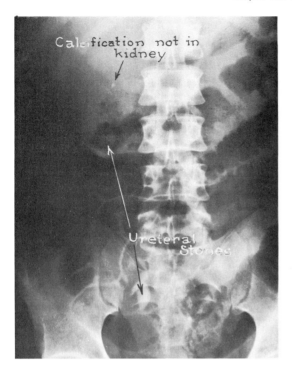

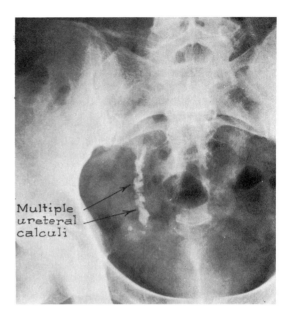

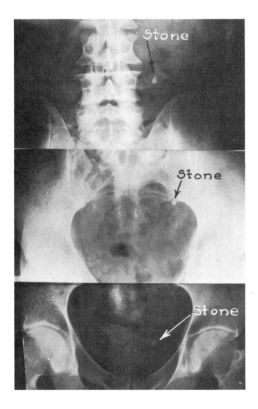

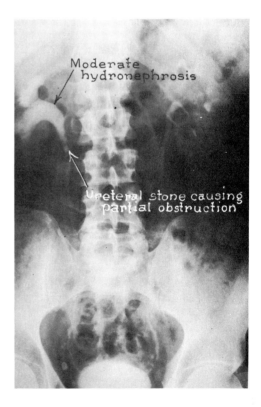

Figure 15–8. Radiograms showing ureteral stones. *Above left:* Two stones in right ureter, mildly radiopaque: cystine. *Above right:* Multiple stones, right ureter. *Below left:* Plain films showing progress of stone down ureter. *Below right:* Stone in upper right ureter causing moderate obstruction.

It may be retracted. The scrotal skin may be hyperesthetic if the stone lies low. A juxtavesical ureteral stone may at times be felt vaginally.

C. Laboratory Findings: They are the same as for renal stone (see p 226).

D. X-Ray Findings: A plain film of the abdomen may demonstrate a calcific body in the region of the ureter. This constitutes merely presumptive grounds for the diagnosis, however, for the shadow may be a phlebolith or some other intra-abdominal calcification.

Amar (1979) has noted that the phleboliths are in the bladder wall. Plain films taken both before and after urination will reveal their movement. He also pointed out that a calculus in the lower ureter is best seen on the plain film when the bladder is full.

Excretory urograms are invaluable (Fig 15–8). The ureterogram places the calcification in the ureter and usually demonstrates dilatation of the ureter above the stone. It also reveals the degree of obstruction. On occasion, no "dye" may enter the renal pelvis or ureter because of the obstruction but a marked density of the renal shadow occurs (nephrogram effect) (Fig 15–9). This is evidence of good kidney function and acute ureteral obstruction. The acute ureteral obstruction may cause extravasation of the radiopaque fluid in the region of the renal hilum. This finding in itself is rarely of consequence.

In the case of a nonopaque stone, a "negative" gray or black shadow is seen within the white area of the ureter. This may be difficult to differentiate from ureteral tumor or blood clot. A CT scan may make the differentiation (Alter, Peterson, & Plautz, 1979). If a small stone is lodged in the intramural ureter or if one has just been passed, the ipsilateral interureteric ridge becomes edematous, thus casting a "negative shadow" (Fig 15–9, right) (Wisoff & Parsavand, 1961).

The diagnosis of ureteral stone is established when, in both the anteroposterior and oblique views, the suspicious shadow can be seen hugging the cystoscopically placed ureteral catheter. This is necessary only if excretory urograms fail to visualize the ureter.

E. Instrumental Examination: Cystoscopy and ureteral catheterization are seldom needed for the diagnosis of ureteral stone. Instrumental examination should be avoided unless a proper conclusion cannot be drawn otherwise. No matter how careful one is, instrumentation always carries bacteria from the urethra into the urinary tract. Infection introduced in this way unnecessarily complicates the problem.

Differential Diagnosis

Passage of crystals down the ureter may occur during treatment or an exacerbation of gout or in oxaluria after excessive ingestion of foods high in oxalate content. Symptoms and signs are the same as those seen in stone, and hematuria is just as common. X-ray examination is usually normal. The presence of many crystals in the urine may explain the colic.

A tumor of the kidney or renal pelvis may bleed, and a clot or piece of necrotic tumor tissue may pass down the ureter. This will simulate ureteral stone perfectly. Excretory urograms should demonstrate a space-occupying lesion in the kidney and a "negative" shadow in the ureter. Retrograde urograms may then be indicated for more definitive diagnosis.

Ureteral tumor is often obstructive and may cause colic. Hematuria is common. X-ray visualiza-

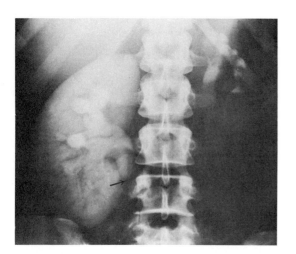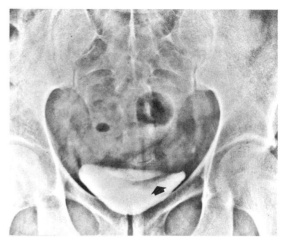

Figure 15–9. Ureteral stone. *Left:* "Nephrogram" caused by acute ureteral obstruction. Marked density of renal parenchyma with moderate hydronephrosis. Arrow points to nonopaque (uric acid) stone. Left kidney is contracted and scarred from previous infections. *Right:* Patient has just passed left ureteral calculus. Note secondary edema of left intravesical ureter as indicated by arrow and a second stone in the left ureter just above the bladder.

tion of the urinary tract should make the diagnosis.

Obstructive chronic lesions of the ureter may cause severe recurrent pain. These include congenital ureteral stenosis and extraureteral obstructions such as may be caused by lymph nodes containing cancer. A careful history and physical examination and excretory urograms should lead to the correct diagnosis.

Acute pyelonephritis may start so abruptly and the pain may be so acute as to suggest stone. The finding of pyuria and bacteriuria with normal urograms should establish the diagnosis.

Acute gallbladder disease (stone or infection) may be confused with ureteral stone if severe pain is referred to the back. A history of dyspepsia or jaundice can help in differentiation; however, renal and ureteral stones also cause gastrointestinal symptoms. Red cells in the urine suggest urinary stone. Cholecystograms and urography should settle the matter.

An aneurysm of the abdominal aorta may cause pain suggestive of left renal colic. Palpation of the aneurysm, the presence of a bruit, the absence of hematuria, and normal excretory urograms will differentiate the two. Aortography is definitive.

A sloughed papilla passing down the ureter may simulate ureteral stone. Urinalysis shows evidence of infection. Excretory urograms will reveal the changes typical of papillary necrosis.

Complications

The major complication of ureteral stone is obstruction, usually only partial. Permanent renal damage is rare except in the case that remains undiagnosed or is inadequately treated. Bilateral ureteral calculi may cause anuria, in which case drainage of the kidney by ureteral catheters or immediate removal of the stones must be accomplished.

Infection may gain a foothold in the presence of obstruction, but it is usually introduced by the cystoscopist in attempts to remove the stone. Drainage by either catheter or surgical attack is indicated in addition to appropriate antibiotic therapy.

Prevention

See p 228.

Treatment

A. Specific Measures: About 80% of stones that reach the ureter can pass spontaneously and should always be allowed to do so as long as complications do not develop. Antispasmodics may be helpful. Physical activity should be encouraged and adequate fluid intake maintained to increase ureteral peristalsis. A stone small enough to pass down the ureter will have no difficulty traversing the urethra.

Cystoscopic manipulation (Drach, 1978), electronic lithotripsy (Raney, 1978), or operation (ureterolithotomy) is necessary if the stone is too large to pass spontaneously. Stones up to 0.5 cm in diameter and even a few up to 1 cm in diameter may pass without surgical or cystoscopic assistance. Farkas & Firstater (1979) were able to "milk" 6 of 7 stones into the bladder by vaginal manipulation. The onset of infection may require removal of the obstructing agent before sepsis can be controlled. If periodic excretory urograms show progressive hydronephrosis or if pain remains intense and incapacitating, removal of the stone is indicated.

Smith & others (1979) advise percutaneous nephrostomy under fluoroscopic vision in selected cases for attempts to dissolve ureteral stones.

B. General Measures: Morphine or a similar opiate given intravenously is necessary to control pain. Morphine sulfate, 8 mg intravenously, or a comparable drug in the same relative strength should be given immediately and repeated in 5 minutes if relief has not been obtained. Pain can usually be controlled thereafter by subcutaneous injection. Initial subcutaneous morphine, even in doses of 30 mg, is not adequate for relief of pain of this degree. Elliot & others (1979) recommend butorphanol, 4 mg intramuscularly, which has low addictive qualities.

Atropine, 0.8 mg subcutaneously, is the antispasmodic of choice. Methantheline bromide (Banthine), 0.1 g intravenously, will usually relieve the pain; unfortunately, it may paralyze bladder action for some hours as well. Other antispasmodics can be given by mouth, but their efficacy is questionable.

Heat to the flank or a hot bath is often helpful as an adjunct to drug analgesia.

Prognosis

About 80% of stones that enter the ureter will pass spontaneously in a few days or weeks. If the effect of the stone upon the kidney is evaluated at intervals with excretory urograms, the physician will be able to intervene as necessary in order to prevent kidney damage.

VESICAL STONE

Primary vesical stones in children (mostly males) are rare in the USA but occur commonly in northwest India, Indonesia, the Middle East, and parts of China. It would appear that the affected children have diets low in protein and phosphate. They tend to be dehydrated because of hot weather and diarrhea, both of which are common in these countries. Most stones are composed of ammonium acid urate (Thalut & others, 1976).

Secondary vesical stone develops as a complication of other urologic disease; 95% occur in men. The most common cause of secondary vesical stone is infection of residual urine with urea-splitting organisms (eg, *Proteus*). This partial urinary retention may be due to prostatic or bladder neck obstruction, cystocele, or neurogenic bladder. Stagnation

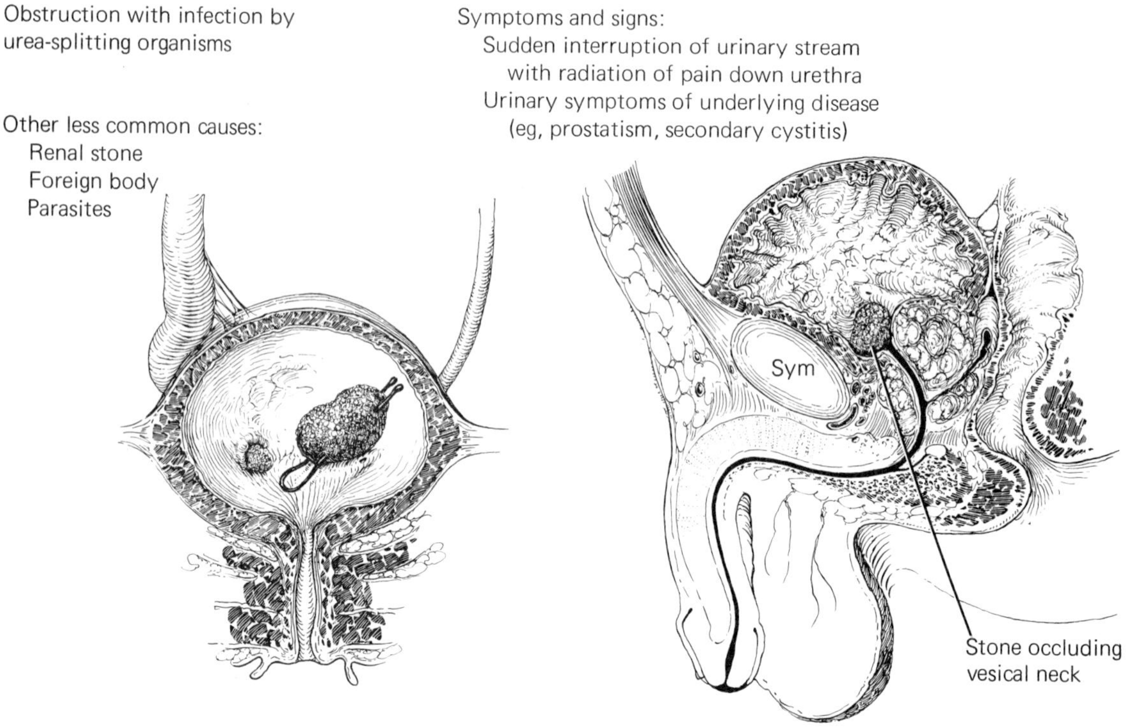

Obstruction with infection by
urea-splitting organisms

Symptoms and signs:
  Sudden interruption of urinary stream
    with radiation of pain down urethra
  Urinary symptoms of underlying disease
    (eg, prostatism, secondary cystitis)

Other less common causes:
  Renal stone
  Foreign body
  Parasites

Sym

Stone occluding
vesical neck

Figure 15–10. Genesis and symptoms and signs of vesical calculus.

is particularly marked in vesical diverticula; stones are often found when diverticula are present (Fig 15–11).

A stone that passes through the ureter into the bladder usually passes on through the urethra. If obstruction or urinary stasis is present, the stone may remain in the bladder and act as a nidus for precipitation of more urinary salts.

A markedly inflamed or ulcerated bladder may predispose to stone formation. This is seen in vesical schistosomiasis and following irradiation of the bladder.

Foreign bodies occasionally are introduced into the bladder, particularly in women (see Chapter 28). These include nonabsorbable sutures, candles, nail files, chewing gum, and even crochet hooks. They may act as nidi for the precipitation of calcific deposits (Fig 15–10). Infection complicates the picture and hastens calculus formation, particularly if the bacteria are urea-splitters.

Prolonged use of an indwelling catheter may permit the formation of calcium encrustations that may become dislodged when the catheter is removed.

Pathology

Vesical stones may be single or multiple. If single, they are ovoid; if multiple, they often are faceted (Fig 15–11). In addition to the infection that is uniformly present with secondary stones, inflammation of the bladder is increased.

Most vesical stones are radiopaque (calcium phosphate, calcium oxalate, or ammonium magnesium phosphate), but some are radiolucent (uric acid). Even calcium stones are at times invisible on a plain film. This may be due to the presence of large amounts of matrix.

Clinical Findings

A. Symptoms: Symptoms of chronic urinary tract obstruction or stasis and infection occur in most cases, for these are the common causes of vesical stone. There may be a history of introduction of a foreign body into the bladder or prolonged vesical catheter drainage. The male patient may complain of sudden interruption of the urinary stream associated with pain radiating down the penis when the stone rolls over the bladder neck. He may be unable to void except in certain positions that cause the stone to move off the bladder neck. Considerable hematuria may be noted, although this can also occur with pure obstruction or infection.

B. Signs: Only giant calculi can be felt suprapubically. The bladder may be visible, palpable, or percussible if there is a great deal of residual urine. Palpation of the urethra may reveal a thickening compatible with stricture. Rectal examination may demonstrate a relaxed anal sphincter (neurogenic bladder) or an enlarged or hard (cancerous) prostate. Cystocele may be noted.

C. Laboratory Findings: The urine is almost

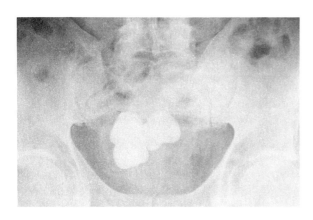
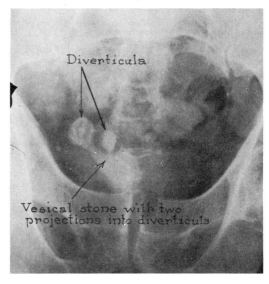

Figure 15–11. Vesical stones. *Left:* Plain film showing multiple-faceted stones. *Right:* Plain film showing dumbbell-shaped stone in bladder, with projections into diverticula.

always infected with secondary stones. Blood cells are commonly found. Excretion of PSP may be depressed because of chronic obstruction. A flattened curve (first and second half-hour specimens about equal in amount) suggests residual urine.

D. X-Ray Findings: Vesical stones are usually visible on a plain film (Fig 15–11). The exceptions are those formed of uric acid. They must be differentiated from calcified ovaries and fibroids. Oblique films are usually helpful. Excretory urograms may show back pressure changes in the kidneys, and a film taken after voiding may reveal residual urine. Diverticula may be noted. Stones will be localized in the excretory or retrograde cystograms.

The presence of a vesical calculus may cause vesicoureteral reflux, particularly in children. Removal of the stone usually relieves this abnormality.

E. Instrumental Examination: The attempt to pass a catheter or sound may lead to the diagnosis of urethral stricture. Successful passage of a catheter after urination allows estimation of the degree of obstruction and stasis by recovering residual urine. The positive diagnostic step of "sounding" for stone may be accomplished by passing a sound into the bladder. The definitive "click" of the instrument on the stone can readily be heard or felt. Cystoscopy usually visualizes the stone or stones and the obstructive lesion with its secondary vesical changes (Fig 10–1).

Differential Diagnosis

A pedunculated tumor of the bladder can suddenly occlude the vesical orifice, thereby simulating vesical stone. Cystoscopy will make the differentiation.

Extravesical calcifications on x-rays of the vesical region may appear to be in the bladder but are actually in the veins, omental fat pads, ovaries, or fibroids of the uterus. Cystoscopy will help in differentiation.

Complications

A primary stone will eventually lead to infection. If infection is present, it will be worsened by the presence of the calculus, which in turn will defeat attempts to sterilize the urine.

Vesicoureteral reflux is commonly associated with vesical calculi. Removal of the calculi may cause spontaneous cessation of the reflux.

A small vesical concretion may pass down the urethra and become lodged there (Paulk & others, 1976). This may cause complete urinary obstruction (Fig 15–12).

Prevention

Stasis and infection, whether primary or secondary, must be eradicated.

Treatment

A. Specific Measures:

1. Cystoscopy and surgical removal–

a. Transurethral route–Small stones can be removed by cystoscopic manipulation; large ones can be crushed (litholapaxy) and the fragments washed out (Hadley, Barnes, & Rosenquist, 1977). If the patient has an obstructing prostate that can be removed by transurethral resection, both procedures may be undertaken at the same time.

Stones can be cracked by an instrument called an electrohydraulic lithotrite. This instrument is passed transurethrally into the bladder, filled with

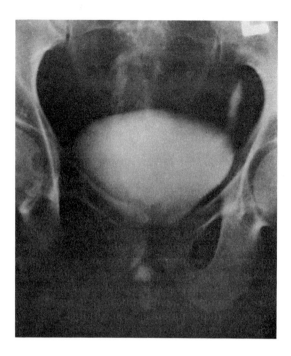

Figure 15–12. Excretory urogram showing multiple stones lodged in urethra. (Courtesy of MM Al-Ghorab.)

water, and its tip pressed against the stone. An electric charge is delivered, breaking up the stone (El Fahiq & Wallace, 1978).

b. Suprapubic route–Stones that are too large for transurethral removal or crushing are removed by this route. Suprapubic prostatectomy may also be done.

2. Chemical dissolution–This is usually successful, but it fails to treat the cause of the stone formation. It may be indicated if the patient refuses surgery or cystoscopic removal or is considered to be an unwarranted surgical risk.

In the dissolution of calcium and magnesium ammonium phosphate calculi, excellent results are obtained with Renacidin (an irrigating solution consisting of citric acid and D-gluconic acid). Thirty mL of 10% solution are instilled, and the catheter is clamped for 30–60 minutes. This is repeated 4–6 times a day. A continuous drip through a 3-way Foley catheter may also be used.

Calcium salts and magnesium ammonium phosphate are highly soluble in citric acid. Suby and Albright have evolved buffered solutions of this compound:

"Solution G" (pH 4.0)

Citric acid (monohydrated)	32.25
Magnesium oxide (anhydrous)	3.84
Sodium carbonate (anhydrous)	4.37
Water, qs ad	1000.0

If this solution proves irritating, the amount of sodium carbonate can be increased to 8.74 g ("solution M," which has a pH of 4.5).

In order to dissolve organic matrix, 0.05% pepsin should be added to the solution. The resulting mixture can be sterilized by passing it through a Millipore filter.

Through an indwelling catheter, 60–100 mL of solution G (or M) are introduced into the bladder. The fluid is retained for one-half hour, and the bladder is then drained. This procedure is repeated several times at intervals of 1–2 hours.

These solutions may fail with markedly radiopaque (hard) stones. They have no effect on uric acid or cystine stones.

In order to prevent precipitation of calcium salts on an indwelling catheter, Rollins & Finlayson (1973) recommend the use of 65 mg of methylene blue 4 times a day by mouth.

B. General Measures: Analgesics for pain and antibiotics for control of infection are used for relief of distressing symptoms until the stone can be removed and its cause eliminated.

C. Treatment of Complications: Infection cannot be eradicated until the stone and the cause of the obstruction are removed. Urethral stone may be extracted transurethrally or pushed back into the bladder and then extracted or crushed (Paulk & others, 1976).

Prognosis

The rate of recurrence of vesical stone is low if the primary cause (obstruction) is successfully treated.

PROSTATIC CALCULI

Prostatic calculi are seldom clinically important except that they cause indurated areas in the prostate that may be mistaken for carcinomas. They are common in association with benign prostatic

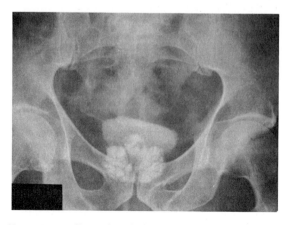

Figure 15–13. Prostatic calculi seen in typical locations behind the pubic symphysis.

hyperplasia. Rarely, in younger persons, they may be secondary to advanced but healing tuberculous prostatitis. They are also seen in ochronosis.

Prostatic calculi are formed of desquamated epithelial cells that finally acquire a shell of calcium. They average about 1–2 mm in diameter and are brown to black in color. They are situated between the hypertrophied adenoma and the surgical capsule. Therefore, on enucleation of the prostate or complete transurethral prostatectomy, they tend to be extruded.

On a plain film they are situated in the region of the pubic symphysis (Fig 15–13).

● ● ●

References

General

Boyce WH, Resnick MI: Biochemical profiles of stone-forming patients: A guide to treatment. *J Urol* 1979;**121**:706.

Coe FL: *Nephrolithiasis—Pathogenesis and Treatment.* Year Book, 1978.

Drach GW, Perin R, Jacobs S: Outpatient evaluation of patients with calcium urolithiasis. *J Urol* 1979;**121**:564.

Pak CYC & others: Evaluation of calcium urolithiasis in ambulatory patients: Comparison of results with those of inpatient evaluation. *Am J Med* 1978;**64**:979.

Peterson LJ, Hruska KA: The benefits of evaluation of the patients with recurrent or multiple calcium stones. *J Urol* 1979;**121**:766.

Pyrah LN: *Renal Calculus.* Springer-Verlag, 1979.

Renal Stone

Bordier P & others: On the pathogenesis of so-called idiopathic hypercalciuria. *Am J Med* 1977;**63**:398.

Boxer RJ & others: Replacement of the ureter by small intestine: Clinical application and results of the ileal ureter in 89 patients. *J Urol* 1979;**121**:728.

Broadus AE, Thier SO: Metabolic basis of renal-stone disease. *N Engl J Med* 1979;**300**:839.

Carswell GF & others: Experience with the radioimmunoassay for parathyroid hormone in the diagnosis of primary hyperparathyroidism. *J Urol* 1978;**119**:175.

Coe FL: Treated and untreated recurrent calcium nephrolithiasis in patients with idiopathic hypercalciuria, hyperuricosuria, or no metabolic disorder. *Ann Intern Med* 1977;**87**:404.

Coe FL, Parks JH, Moore ES: Familial idiopathic hypercalciuria. *N Engl J Med* 1979;**300**:337.

Coleman CH, Witherington R: A review of 117 partial nephrectomies. *J Urol* 1979;**122**:11.

Cook JH III, Lytton B: Intraoperative localization of renal calculi during nephrolithotomy by ultrasound scanning. *J Urol* 1977;**117**:543.

Crissey MM, Gittes RF: Dissolution of cystine ureteral calculus by irrigation with tromethamine. *J Urol* 1979;**121**:811.

Dahlberg PJ & others: Clinical features and management of cystinuria. *Mayo Clin Proc* 1977;**52**:533.

Dretler SP, Pfister RC, Newhouse JH: Renal-stone dissolution via percutaneous nephrostomy. *N Engl J Med* 1979;**300**:341.

Dunegan LJ & others: Primary hyperparathyroidism: Preoperative evaluation and correlation with surgical findings. *Am J Surg* 1974;**128**:471.

Earnest DL: Perspectives on incidence, etiology, and treatment of enteric hyperoxaluria. *Am J Clin Nutr* 1977;**30**:72.

Edell S, Zegel H: Ultrasonic evaluation of renal calculi. *AJR* 1978;**130**:261.

Ekburg M, Jeppsson J-O, Denneberg T: Penicillamine treatment of cystinuria. *Acta Med Scand* 1974;**195**:415.

Ettinger B, Kolb FO: Inorganic phosphate treatment of nephrolithiasis. *Am J Med* 1973;**55**:32.

Ettinger B & others: Triamterene-induced nephrolithiasis. *Ann Intern Med* 1979;**91**:745.

Feit RM, Fair WR: The treatment of infection stones with penicillin. *J Urol* 1979;**122**:592.

Fisher CP, Sonda LP III, Diokno AC: Use of cryoprecipitate coagulum in extracting renal calculi. *Urology* 1980;**15**:6.

Gibbons RP: Use of water-pik and nephroscope. *Urology* 1974;**4**:605.

Gittes RF: Nephroscopy. *Urol Clin North Am* 1979;**6**:555.

Gordon MR, Carrion HM, Politano VA: Dissolution of uric acid calculi with THAM irrigation. *Urology* 1978;**12**:393.

Gregory JG, Park KY, Schoenberg HW: Oxalate stone disease after intestinal resection. *J Urol* 1977;**117**:631.

Griffith DP, Moskowitz PA, Carlton CE Jr: Adjunctive chemotherapy of infection-induced staghorn calculi. *J Urol* 1979;**121**:711.

Hautmann R & others: Mercaptopropionylglycine: A progress in cystine stone therapy. *J Urol* 1977;**117**:628.

Howard JE: Tried, true, and new ways to treat and prevent kidney stones. *Res & Staff Physician* (Dec) 1970;**16**:67.

James R & others: Anatrophic nephrolithotomy for removal of staghorn or branched calculi. *Urology* 1980;**15**:108.

Joekes AM, Rose GA, Sutor J: Multiple renal silica stones. *Br Med J* 1973;**1**:46.

Kleeman CR & others: Kidney stones. (Clinical conference.) *West J Med* 1980;**132**:313.

Kolb FO: Non-operative management of renal calculi. *GU (The Journal of Genitourinary Medicine)* 1979;**1**:29.

Leach GE, Lieber MM: Partial nephrectomy: Mayo Clinic experience, 1957–1977. *Urology* 1980;**15**:219.

Lund HT: Primary hyperparathyroidism in childhood. *Acta Paediatr Scand* 1973;**62**:317.

Maggio AJ Jr & others: The role of vitamin D in idiopathic hypercalciuria. *J Urol* 1979;**122**:147.

Mahmood P, Morales PA: Extended pyelolithotomy (Gil Vernet's pyelotomy). *J Urol* 1973;**109**:772.

Mall JC, Collins PA, Lyon ES: Matrix calculi. *Br J Radiol* 1975;**48**:807.

Marshall S, Lyon RP, Scott MP Jr: Further simplifications for coagulum pyelolithotomy. *J Urol* 1978;**119**:588.

Marshall V & others: The natural history of renal and ureteric calculi. *Br J Urol* 1975;**47**:117.

Miki M, Inaba Y, Machida T: Operative nephroscopy with

fiberoptic scope: Preliminary report. *J Urol* 1978;**119**:166.

Muldowney FP & others: Serum ionized calcium and parathyroid hormone in renal stone disease. *Q J Med* 1976;**45**:75.

Nemoy NJ, Stamey TA: Use of hemiacidrin in management of infection stones. *J Urol* 1976;**116**:693.

Noronha RFX, Gregory JG, Duke JJ: Urolithiasis in children. *J Urol* 1979;**121**:478.

Pak CYC, Delea CS, Bartter FC: Successful treatment of recurrent nephrolithiasis (calcium stones) with cellulose phosphate. *N Engl J Med* 1974;**290**:175.

Parks J, Coe F, Favus M: Hyperparathyroidism in nephrolithiasis. *Arch Intern Med* 1980;**140**:1479.

Prien EL Sr, Gershoff SF: Magnesium oxide-pyridoxine therapy for recurrent calcium oxalate calculi. *J Urol* 1974;**112**:509.

Reiner RJ, Kroovand RL, Perlmutter AD: Unusual aspects of urinary calculi in children. *J Urol* 1979;**121**:480.

Remzi D: Urolithiasis in infancy. *Urology* 1978;**15**:248.

Resnick MI, Boyce WH: Bilateral staghorn calculi: Patient evaluation and management. *J Urol* 1980;**123**:338.

Robertson WG & others: Risk factors in calcium stone disease of the urinary tract. *Br J Urol* 1978;**50**:449.

Royle G, Smith JC: Recurrence of infected calculi following postoperative renal irrigation with stone solvent. *Br J Urol* 1976;**48**:531.

Segal AJ & others: Diagnosis of nonopaque calculi by computed tomography. *Radiology* 1978;**129**:447.

Sherer JF Jr: Cryoprecipitate coagulum pyelolithotomy. *J Urol* 1980;**123**:621.

Sherwood LM: Idiopathic hypercalciuria: A mixed bag of stones. (Editorial.) *J Lab Clin Med* 1977;**90**:951.

Sierakowski R & others: The frequency of urolithiasis in hospital discharge diagnoses in the United States. *Invest Urol* 1978;**15**:438.

Sinno K, Boyce WH, Resnick MI: Childhood urolithiasis. *J Urol* 1979;**121**:662.

Smith AD: Dissolution of cystine calculi by irrigation with acetylcysteine through percutaneous nephrostomy. *Urology* 1979;**13**:422.

Smith LH, Van Den Berg CJ, Wilson DM: Current concepts in nutrition: Nutrition and urolithiasis. *N Engl J Med* 1978;**298**:87.

Spataro RF, Linke CA, Barbaric ZL: The use of percutaneous nephrostomy and urinary alkalinization in the dissolution of obstructing uric acid stones. *Radiology* 1978;**129**:629.

Stote RM & others: Oxypurinol nephrolithiasis in regional enteritis secondary to allopurinol therapy. *Ann Intern Med* 1980;**92**:384.

Tessler AN, Ghazi MR: Case profile: Computerized tomographic assistance in diagnosis of radiolucent calculi. *Urology* 1979;**13**:672.

Thomas WC Jr: Clinical concepts of renal calculus disease. *J Urol* 1975;**113**:423.

Vermeulen CW & others: The renal papilla and calculogenesis. *J Urol* 1967;**97**:573.

Wallace MR, MacDiarmid J, Reeder J: Exacerbation of nephrolithiasis by a carbonic anhydrase inhibitor. *NZ Med J* 1974;**79**:687.

Welshman SG, McGeown MG: Urinary citrate excretion in stone-formers and normal controls. *Br J Urol* 1976;**48**:7.

Yendt ER, Cohanim M: The management of the patient with calcium stones. *Br J Urol* 1976;**48**:507.

Nephrocalcinosis

Buckalew VM & others: Hereditary renal tubular acidosis: Report of 64 member kindred with variable clinical expression including idiopathic hypercalciuria. *Medicine* 1974;**53**:229.

Courey WR, Pfister RC: The radiographic findings in renal tubular acidosis: Analysis of 21 cases. *Radiology* 1972;**105**:497.

Farrell RM, Horwith M, Muecke EC: Renal tubular acidosis and nephrocalcinosis: Diagnosis and clinical management. *J Urol* 1974;**111**:429.

Fletcher RF, Jones JH, Morgan DB: Bone disease in chronic renal failure. *Q J Med* 1963;**32**:321.

Hirschman GH & others: Renal tubular acidosis: Practical guides to diagnosis and treatment. *Clin Pediatr (Phila)* 1976;**15**:645.

Malek RS, Kelalis PP: Nephrocalcinosis in infancy and childhood. *J Urol* 1975;**114**:441.

Morris CR Jr, Sebastian A, McSherry E: Renal acidosis. *Kidney Int* 1972;**1**:2322.

Nash MA & others: Renal tubular acidosis in infants and children: Clinical course, response to treatment, and prognosis. *J Pediatr* 1972;**80**:738.

O'Regan PFB, Joekes AM: Primary hyperoxaluria. (Editorial.) *J R Soc Med* 1980;**73**:541.

Rao DS & others: Primary hyperparathyroidism: A cause of hypercalciuria and renal stones in patients with medullary sponge kidney. *JAMA* 1977;**237**:1353.

Stanbury SW, Lumb GA: Parathyroid function in chronic renal failure: A statistical survey of the plasma biochemistry in azotemic renal osteodystrophy. *Q J Med* 1966;**35**:1.

Stella FJ & others: Medullary sponge kidney associated with parathyroid adenoma: A report of 2 cases, *Nephron* 1973;**10**:332.

Vazquez AM: Nephrocalcinosis and hypertension in juvenile primary hyperparathyroidism. *Am J Dis Child* 1973;**125**:104.

Young JD Jr, Martin LG: Urinary calculi associated with incomplete renal tubular acidosis. *J Urol* 1972;**107**:170.

Ureteral Stone

Alter AJ, Peterson DT, Plautz AC Jr: Non-opaque calculus demonstrated by computerized tomography. *J Urol* 1979;**122**:699.

Amar AD: Improved radiographic visualization of calculus in distal ureter. *Urology* 1979;**14**:420.

Arnaldsson Ö, Holmlund D: Defects in the urographic contrast medium above and below a ureteric calculus. *Acta Radiol [Diagn] (Stockh)* 1971;**11**:26.

Bose TK, Shaw RE: Transperitoneal ureterolithotomy. *Br J Urol* 1975;**47**:613.

Drach GW: Stone manipulation: Modern usage and occasional mishaps. *Urology* 1978;**12**:286.

Elliot JP & others: Butorphanol and meperidine compared in patients with acute ureteral colic. *J Urol* 1979;**122**:455.

Farkas A, Firstater M: Transvaginal milking of lower ureteric stones into the bladder. *Br J Urol* 1979;**51**:193.

Kettlewell M & others: Spontaneous extravasation of urine secondary to ureteric obstruction. *Br J Urol* 1973;**45**:8.

O'Boyle PJ, Gibbon NOK: Vaginal ureterolithotomy. *Br J Urol* 1976;**48**:231.

Raney AM: Electrohydraulic ureterolithotripsy: Preliminary report. *Urology* 1978;**12**:284.

Smith AD & others: Percutaneous nephrostomy in the

management of ureteral and renal calculi. *Radiology* 1979;**133**:49.

Walsh A: An aggressive approach to stones in the lower ureter. *Br J Urol* 1974;**46**:11.

Wisoff CP, Parsavand R: Edema of the interureteric ridge: A useful Roentgen sign. *Am J Roentgenol* 1961;**86**:1123.

Vesical Stones

Aurora AL, Taneja OP, Gupta DN: Bladder stone disease of childhood. 1. An epidemiological study. 2. A clinicopathological study. *Acta Paediatr Scand* 1970;**59**:177, 385.

El Fahiq S, Wallace DM: Ultrasonic lithotriptor for urethral and bladder stones. *Br J Urol* 1978;**50**:255.

Hadley HL, Barnes RW, Rosenquist RC: Tactile litholapaxy: Safe and efficient. *Urology* 1977;**9**:263.

Mulvaney WP, Henning DC: Solvent treatment of urinary calculi: Refinements in technique. *J Urol* 1962;**88**:145.

Paulk SC & others: Urethral calculi. *J Urol* 1976;**116**:436.

Rollins R, Finlayson B: Mechanism of prevention of calcium oxalate encrustation by methylene blue and demonstration of the concentration dependence of its action. *J Urol* 1973;**110**:459.

Taneja OP: Pathogenesis of ureteric reflux in vesical calculus disease of childhood: A clinical study. *Br J Urol* 1975;**47**:623.

Thalut K & others: The endemic bladder stones of Indonesia: Epidemiology and clinical features. *Br J Urol* 1976;**48**:617.

Prostatic Calculi

Eykyn S & others: Prostatic calculi as a source of recurrent bacteriuria in the male. *Br J Urol* 1974;**46**:527.

Gawande AS, Kamat MH, Seebode JJ: Giant prostatic calculi. *Urology* 1974;**4**:319.

Meares EM Jr: Infection stones of prostate gland: Laboratory diagnosis and clinical management. *Urology* 1974;**4**:560.

Sutor DJ, Wooley SE: The crystalline composition of prostatic calculi. *Br J Urol* 1974;**46**:533.

16 | Injuries to the Genitourinary Tract

Jack W. McAninch, MD

EMERGENCY DIAGNOSIS & MANAGEMENT

About 10% of all injuries seen in the emergency room involve the genitourinary system to some extent. Many of them are subtle and difficult to define and require great diagnostic expertise. Early diagnosis is essential to prevent serious complications.

Initial assessment should include control of hemorrhage and shock along with resuscitation as required. Resuscitation may require intravenous lines and a urethral catheter. In men, before the catheter is inserted, the urethral meatus should be examined carefully for the presence of blood. Once the intravenous lines are established, if any suspicion of renal or ureteral injury is entertained, contrast material should be injected intravenously for later x-ray study.

The history should include a detailed description of the accident. In cases involving gunshot wounds, the type and caliber of the weapon should be determined, since high-velocity projectiles cause much more extensive damage.

The abdomen and genitalia should be examined for evidence of contusions or subcutaneous hematomas, which might indicate deeper injuries to the retroperitoneum and pelvic structures. Fractures of the lower ribs are often associated with renal injuries and pelvic fractures with bladder and urethral injuries. Diffuse abdominal tenderness is consistent with perforated bowel, free intraperitoneal blood or urine, or retroperitoneal hematoma. As an aid to diagnosis of intraperitoneal injuries, a small catheter inserted percutaneously into the abdomen followed by irrigation will help detect free intraperitoneal blood.

Initial radiographic studies should be done in the trauma unit, if possible, before moving the patient. Plain films of the abdomen will disclose early excretion of contrast material injected at the time intravenous lines were inserted. Lower rib fractures, vertebral body and transverse process fractures, and pelvic fractures may be associated with severe urinary tract injuries. Early extravasation of contrast material may be noted with renal, ureteral, or bladder injuries.

Special Examinations

When genitourinary tract injury is suspected on the basis of the history and physical examination, additional studies are required to establish its extent.

A. Catheterization and Assessment of Injury: Assessment of the injury should be done in an orderly fashion, so that accurate and complete information is obtained.

1. Catheterization–Blood at the urethral meatus in men indicates urethral injury; catheterization should not be attempted if blood is present, but retrograde urethrography should be done immediately. If no blood is present at the meatus, a urethral catheter can be carefully passed to the bladder to recover urine; microscopic or gross hematuria indicates urinary system injury. If catheterization is traumatic despite the greatest care, the significance of hematuria cannot be determined, and other studies must be done to investigate the possibility of urinary system injury.

2. Excretory urography–Immediately after intravenous lines have been established and the resuscitation process has begun, 150 mL of contrast material can be injected intravenously by push technic. As hypotension is overcome and renal perfusion improves, plain abdominal films will permit adequate visualization of the kidneys. This technic allows evaluation of renal injuries without undue delay before emergency operations, if indicated. If renal injury seems likely from the urogram, nephrotomography should be done immediately. In most cases, it is not necessary to inject more contrast medium, since adequate contrast remains and tomography will give additional information regarding parenchymal injuries.

3. Retrograde cystography–Filling of the bladder with contrast material is essential to establish whether bladder perforations exist. At least 250 mL of contrast medium should be instilled for full vesical distention. A film should be obtained with the bladder filled and a second one after the bladder has emptied itself by gravity drainage. These 2 films will establish the degree of bladder injury as well as the size of the surrounding pelvic hematomas.

4. Urethrography–A small (12F) catheter can

be inserted into the urethral meatus and 3 mL of water placed in the balloon to hold the catheter in position. After retrograde injection of 20 mL of contrast material, the urethra will be clearly outlined on film, and extravasation in the deep bulbar area in case of straddle injury—or free extravasation into the retropubic space in case of prostatomembranous disruption—will be visualized.

5. Arteriography–Arteriography may help define renal parenchymal and renal vascular injuries. It is also useful in the detection of persistent bleeding from pelvic fractures for purposes of embolization with Gelfoam or autologous clot.

6. Computed tomography–CT scan can help in assessing size and extent of retroperitoneal hematomas and of renal parenchymal trauma. It is a noninvasive test that gives accurate and fast information when excretory urography does not adequately establish the degree and extent of renal injury.

B. Cystoscopy and Retrograde Urography: These studies are seldom necessary, since information can be obtained by less invasive technics.

INJURIES TO THE KIDNEY

Renal injuries are the most common injuries of the urinary system. The kidney is well protected by heavy lumbar muscles, vertebral bodies, ribs, and the viscera anteriorly. Fractured ribs and trans-verse vertebral processes may penetrate the renal parenchyma or vasculature. Most injuries occur from automobile accidents or sporting mishaps, chiefly in men and boys. Kidneys with existing pathologic conditions such as hydronephrosis or malignant tumors are more readily ruptured from mild trauma.

Etiology (Fig 16–1)

Blunt trauma directly to the abdomen, flank, or back is the most common mechanism, accounting for 80–85% of all renal injuries. Trauma may result from motor vehicle accidents, fights, falls, and contact sports. Vehicle collisions at high speed may result in major renal trauma from rapid deceleration and cause major vascular injury. Gunshot and knife wounds cause most penetrating injuries to the kidney; any such wound in the flank area should be regarded as a cause of renal injury until proved otherwise. Associated abdominal visceral injuries are present in 80% of renal penetrating wounds.

Pathology & Classification (Fig 16–2)

A. Early Pathologic Findings: Lacerations from blunt trauma usually occur in the transverse plane of the kidney. This mechanism of injury is thought to consist of force transmitted from the center of the impact to the renal parenchyma. In injuries from rapid deceleration, the kidney moves upward or downward, causing sudden stretch on the renal pedicle and sometimes complete or partial avulsion. Acute thrombosis of the renal artery may

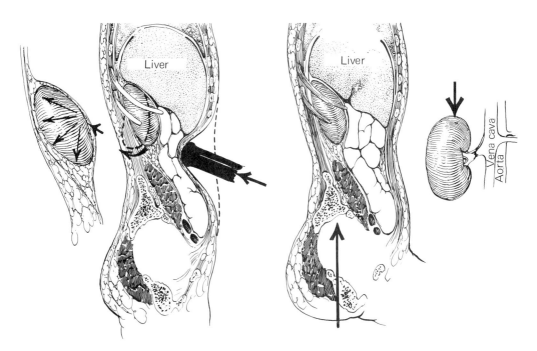

Figure 16–1. Mechanisms of renal injury. *Left:* Direct blow to abdomen. Smaller drawing shows force of blow radiating from the renal hilum. *Right:* Falling on buttocks from a height (contrecoup of kidney). Smaller drawing shows direction of force exerted upon the kidney from above. Tear of renal pedicle.

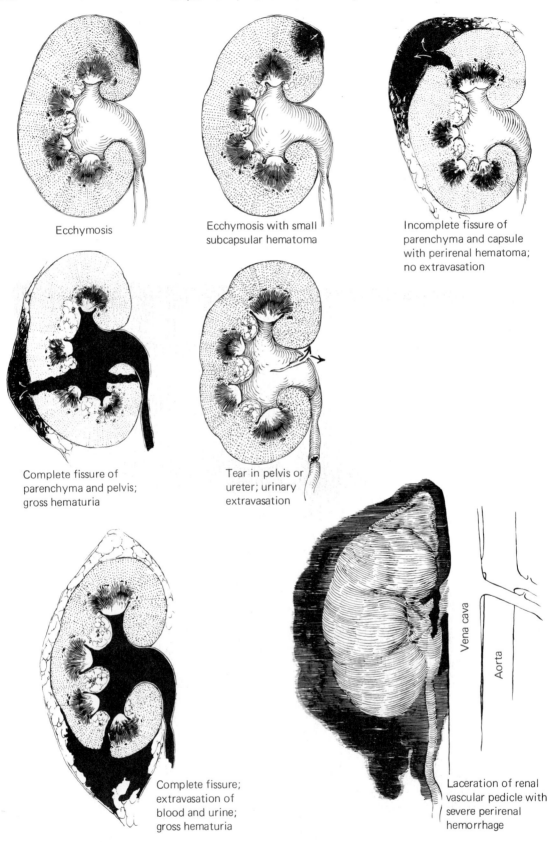

Figure 16–2. Types and degrees of renal injury.

occur as an intimal tear from rapid deceleration injuries owing to the sudden stretch.

Pathologic classification of renal injuries is as follows:

1. Minor renal trauma–(85% of cases.) Renal contusion or bruising of the parenchyma is the most common lesion. Subcapsular hematoma in association with contusion is also noted. Superficial cortical lacerations are also considered minor trauma. These injuries rarely require surgical exploration.

2. Major renal trauma–(15% of cases.) Deep corticomedullary lacerations may extend into the collecting system, resulting in urine extravasation in the perirenal space. Large retroperitoneal and perinephric hematomas accompany these deep lacerations. Multiple lacerations may cause complete destruction of the kidney. Laceration of the renal pelvis from blunt trauma is rare.

3. Vascular injury–(About 1% of all blunt trauma cases.) Vascular injury of the renal pedicle is rare but may occur, usually from blunt trauma. There may be total avulsion of the artery and vein or partial avulsion of the segmental branches of these vessels. Stretch on the main renal artery without avulsion may result in renal artery thrombosis. Vascular injuries are difficult to diagnose and result in total destruction of the kidney unless the diagnosis is made promptly.

B. Late Pathologic Findings: (Fig 16–3)

1. Urinoma–Deep lacerations that are not repaired may result in persistent urinary extravasation, late complications of a large perinephric renal mass and, eventually, hydronephrosis and abscess formation.

2. Hydronephrosis–Large hematomas in the retroperitoneum and associated urinary extravasation may result in perinephric fibrosis engulfing the ureteropelvic junction, causing hydronephrosis. Follow-up excretory urography is indicated in all cases of major renal trauma.

3. Arteriovenous fistula–Arteriovenous fistulas may occur after penetrating injuries but are not common.

4. Renal vascular hypertension–The blood flow in nonviable tissue from injury is compromised, which results in renal vascular hypertension in about 1% of cases. Fibrosis from surrounding trauma has also been reported to constrict the renal artery and cause renal hypertension.

Clinical Findings

Microscopic or gross hematuria following trauma to the abdomen indicates injury to the urinary tract. It bears repeating that stab or gunshot wounds to the flank area should alert the physician to possible renal injury whether or not hematuria is present. About 30% of cases of renal vascular injury are not associated with hematuria. These cases are almost always due to rapid deceleration accidents and are an indication for intravenous urography.

The degree of renal injury does not correspond to the degree of hematuria, since gross hematuria may occur in minor renal trauma and only mild hematuria in major trauma. The presence of hematuria demands evaluation.

A. Symptoms: There is usually visible evidence of abdominal trauma. Pain may be localized to one flank area or over the abdomen. Associated

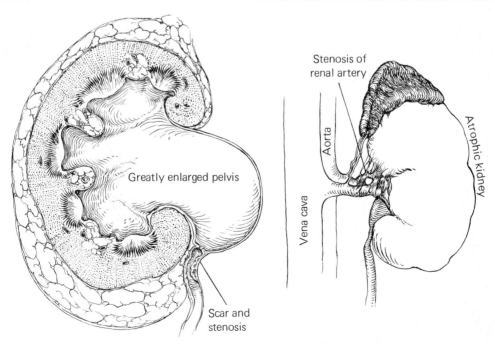

Figure 16–3. Late pathologic findings in renal trauma. *Left:* Ureteropelvic stenosis with hydronephrosis secondary to fibrosis from extravasation of blood and urine. *Right:* Atrophy of kidney caused by injury (stenosis) of arterial blood supply.

injuries such as ruptured abdominal viscera or multiple pelvic fractures also cause acute abdominal pain and may obscure the history of renal injury. Catheterization will usually reveal hematuria. Retroperitoneal bleeding may cause abdominal distention, ileus, and nausea and vomiting.

B. Signs: Initially, shock or signs of high blood loss from heavy retroperitoneal bleeding may be noted. Ecchymosis in the flank or upper quadrants of the abdomen is often noted. Lower rib fractures are frequently found. Diffuse abdominal tenderness may be found on palpation; an "acute abdomen" indicates free blood in the peritoneal cavity. A palpable mass may represent a large retroperitoneal hematoma or perhaps urinary extravasation. If the retroperitoneum has been torn, free blood may be noted in the peritoneal cavity but no palpable mass will be evident. The abdomen may be distended, and bowel sounds may be absent.

C. Laboratory Findings: Microscopic or gross hematuria is usually present. The hematocrit may be normal initially but will drop when serial studies are done. This finding represents persistent retroperitoneal bleeding and development of a large retroperitoneal hematoma. Persistent bleeding may require operation.

D. Staging and X-Ray Findings: Staging of renal injuries allows a systematic approach to these problems. Adequate studies help define the extent of injury and dictate appropriate management. For example, blunt trauma to the abdomen associated with gross hematuria and a normal urogram requires no additional renal studies; however, nonvisualization of the kidney will require immediate arteriography to determine whether renal vascular injury exists. Ultrasonography and retrograde urography are of little use initially in the evaluation of renal injuries.

Staging begins with excretory urography as soon as the intravenous lines are established and resuscitation has begun. This procedure avoids the delay involved in requesting a plain film of the abdomen but does not deprive the examiner of information obtained on the plain film, ie, bone fracture, free air, and displaced bowel. The urogram should establish the presence or absence of both kidneys, clearly define the renal outlines and cortical borders, and outline the collecting systems and ureters (Fig 16–4).

Nephrotomography is indicated if the urogram does not fully define the extent of injury. Tomograms outline the cortical borders and establish the presence of cortical lacerations, intrarenal hematomas, and areas of poor vascular perfusion. Excretory urography combined with tomography will adequately stage 85% of renal injuries.

Arteriography defines major arterial and parenchymal injuries when previous studies have not fully done so. Arterial thrombosis and avulsion of the renal pedicle are best diagnosed by arteriography and are indicated when the kidney is not

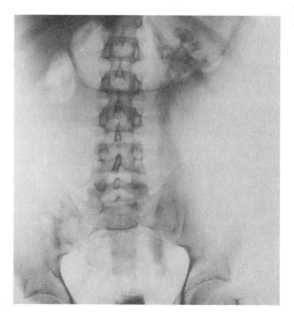

Figure 16–4. Blunt renal trauma to left kidney demonstrating extravasation on intravenous urogram.

visualized on the excretory urogram (Fig 16–5). The major causes of nonvisualization on an excretory urogram are total pedicle avulsion, arterial thrombosis, severe contusion causing vascular spasm, and absence of the kidney (either congenital or from operation).

Computed tomography (CT scan) is proving to be an effective means of staging renal trauma. This noninvasive technic provides excellent definition of parenchymal lacerations, clearly defines extravasation, shows extension of perirenal hematoma, defines nonviable renal tissue, and outlines surrounding organs such as pancreas, liver, and major vessels (Fig 16–6).

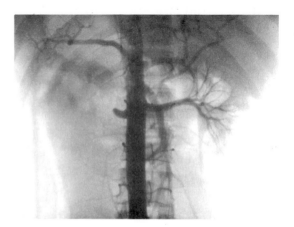

Figure 16–5. Arteriogram following blunt abdominal trauma shows typical findings of acute renal artery thrombosis of left kidney.

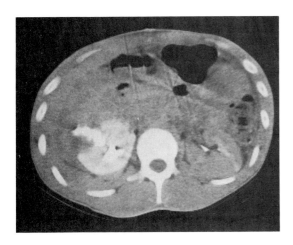

Figure 16–6. CT scan of right kidney following knife stab wound. Laceration with urine extravasation is seen. Large right retroperitoneal hematoma is present.

Radionuclide renal scans have been used in staging renal trauma. However, in emergency management, this technic is less sensitive than arteriography or CT scan.

Differential Diagnosis

Trauma to the abdomen and flank areas is not always associated with renal injury. In such cases, there is no hematuria, and the results of excretory urography are normal.

Complications

A. Early Complications: Hemorrhage is perhaps the most important immediate complication of renal injury. Heavy retroperitoneal bleeding may result in rapid exsanguination. Patients must be observed closely, with careful monitoring of blood pressure and hematocrit. Complete staging must be done early. The size and expansion of palpable masses must be carefully monitored. Bleeding will cease spontaneously in 80–85% of cases. Persistent retroperitoneal bleeding or heavy gross hematuria may require early operation.

Urinary extravasation from renal fracture may show as an expanding mass (urinoma) in the retroperitoneum. These collections are prone to abscess formation and sepsis. A resolving retroperitoneal hematoma may cause slight fever (38.3 C [101 F]), but higher temperatures suggest infection. A perinephric abscess may form, resulting in abdominal tenderness and flank pain. Prompt operation is indicated.

B. Late Complications: Hypertension, hydronephrosis, arteriovenous fistula, calculus formation, and pyelonephritis are important late complications. Careful monitoring of blood pressure for several months is necessary to watch for hypertension. At 3–6 months, a follow-up excretory urogram

should be obtained to be certain that perinephric scarring has not caused hydronephrosis or vascular compromise; renal atrophy may occur from vascular compromise and will be detected by follow-up urography.

Heavy late bleeding may occur 1–4 weeks after injury.

Treatment

A. Emergency Measures: The objectives of early management are prompt treatment of shock and hemorrhage and complete resuscitation and evaluation of associated injuries.

B. Surgical Measures:

1. Blunt injuries–Minor renal injuries from blunt trauma account for 85% of cases and do not usually require operation. Bleeding stops spontaneously with bed rest and hydration. Cases in which operation is indicated include those associated with persistent retroperitoneal bleeding, urinary extravasation, evidence of nonviable renal parenchyma, and renal pedicle injuries (15% of all renal injuries). Aggressive preoperative staging allows complete definition of injury before operation.

2. Penetrating injuries–Penetrating injuries should be surgically explored. A rare exception to this rule is when staging has been complete and only minor parenchymal injury, with no urinary extravasation, is noted. In 80% of cases of penetrating injury, associated organ injury requires operation; thus, renal exploration is only an extension of this procedure.

C. Treatment of Complications: Retroperitoneal urinoma or perinephric abscess demands prompt surgical drainage. Malignant hypertension requires vascular repair or nephrectomy. Hydronephrosis may require surgical correction or nephrectomy.

Prognosis

With careful follow-up, most renal injuries have an excellent prognosis, with spontaneous healing and return of renal function. Follow-up excretory urography and monitoring of blood pressure will ensure detection and appropriate management of late hydronephrosis and hypertension.

INJURIES TO THE URETER

Ureteral injury is rare but may occur, usually during the course of a difficult pelvic surgical procedure or as a result of gunshot wounds. Rapid deceleration accidents may avulse the ureter from the renal pelvis. Endoscopic basket manipulation of ureteral calculi may also result in injury. Injury to the intramural ureter during transurethral resections also occurs.

Etiology

Large pelvic masses (benign or malignant) may

displace the ureter laterally and engulf it in reactive fibrosis. This may lead to ureteral injury during dissection, since the organ is anatomically malpositioned. Inflammatory pelvic disorders may involve the ureter in a similar way. Extensive colon carcinomas may invade areas outside the colon wall and directly involve the ureter; thus, resection of the ureter may be required along with resection of the tumor mass. Devascularization may occur with extensive pelvic lymph node dissections or after radiation therapy to the pelvis for pelvic malignancies. In these situations, ureteral fibrosis and subsequent stricture formation may develop along with ureteral fistulas.

Endoscopic manipulation of a ureteral calculus with a stone basket may result in ureteral perforation or avulsion. Passage of a ureteral catheter beyond an area of obstruction may perforate the ureter. This is usually secondary to the acute inflammatory process in the ureteral wall and surrounding the calculus.

Pathogenesis & Pathology

The ureter may be inadvertently ligated and cut during difficult pelvic surgery. The postoperative course in such cases is usually sepsis and severe renal damage. A partially divided ureter unrecognized at operation will induce urinary extravasation and subsequent buildup of a large urinoma, which will usually lead to ureterovaginal or ureterocutaneous fistula formation. Intraperitoneal extravasation of urine can also occur, causing ileus and peritonitis. After partial transection of the ureter, some degree of stenosis and reactive fibrosis develops, with concomitant mild to moderate hydronephrosis.

Clinical Findings

A. Symptoms: If the ureter has been completely or partially ligated during operation, the postoperative course is usually marked by fever of 38.3–38.8 C (101–102 F) as well as flank and lower quadrant pain. Such patients often experience paralytic ileus with nausea and vomiting. If ureterovaginal or cutaneous fistula develops, it usually does so within the first 10 postoperative days. Bilateral ureteral injury will be manifested by postoperative anuria.

Ureteral injuries from external violence should be suspected in patients who have sustained stab or gunshot wounds to the retroperitoneum. The mid portion of the ureter seems to be the most common site of penetrating injury. There are usually associated vascular and other abdominal visceral injuries.

B. Signs: The acute hydronephrosis of a totally ligated ureter will result in severe flank pain and abdominal pain with nausea and vomiting early in the postoperative course and with associated ileus. Signs and symptoms of acute peritonitis may be present if there is urinary extravasation into the peritoneal cavity. Watery discharge from the wound or vagina may be identified as urine by examination of a small sample of the discharge for creatinine, which will be many times the serum concentration, and by intravenous injection of 10 mL of indigo carmine, which will appear in the urine as dark blue.

C. Laboratory Findings: Ureteral injury from external violence is manifested by microscopic hematuria in 90% of cases. Urinalysis and other laboratory studies are of little use in diagnosis when injury has occurred from other causes. Serum creatinine usually remains normal except in bilateral ureteral obstruction.

D. X-Ray Findings: Diagnosis is by excretory urography. A plain film of the abdomen may demonstrate a large area of increased density in the pelvis or in an area of retroperitoneum where injury is suspected. After injection of contrast material, delayed excretion is noted with hydronephrosis. Partial transection of the ureter will result in more rapid excretion, but persistent hydronephrosis is usually present and contrast extravasation at the site of injury will be noted on delayed films (Fig 16–7).

In acute injury from external violence, the excretory urogram usually appears normal, with very mild fullness down to the point of extravasation at the ureteral transection.

Retrograde ureterography will demonstrate the exact site of obstruction or extravasation.

E. Ultrasonography: Ultrasonography will outline hydroureter or urinary extravasation as it develops into a urinoma and is perhaps the best means of ruling out ureteral injury in the early postoperative period. It has the advantage of being noninvasive and rapid.

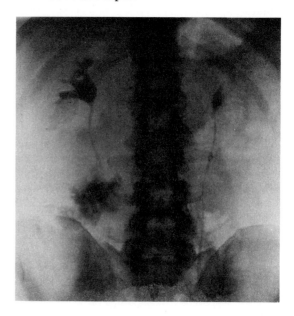

Figure 16–7. Stab wound of right ureter shows extravasation on intravenous urogram.

F. Radionuclide Scanning: Radionuclide scanning will demonstrate delayed excretion on the injured side, with evidence of increasing counts owing to accumulation of urine in the renal pelvis. Its great benefit, however, is to assess renal function after surgical correction.

Differential Diagnosis

Postoperative bowel obstruction and peritonitis may cause symptoms similar to those of acute ureteral obstruction from injury. Fever, "acute abdomen," and associated nausea and vomiting following difficult pelvic surgery are definite indications for screening sonography or excretory urography to establish whether or not ureteral injury has occurred.

Deep wound infection must be considered postoperatively in patients with fever, ileus, and localized tenderness. The same findings are consistent with urinary extravasation and urinoma formation.

Acute pyelonephritis in the early postoperative period may also result in findings similar to those of ureteral injury. Sonography is normal, and urography shows no evidence of obstruction.

Drainage of peritoneal fluid through the wound from impending evisceration may be confused with ureteral injury and urinary extravasation. The creatinine concentration of the transudate will be similar to that of serum, whereas urine will contain very high creatinine levels.

Complications

Ureteral injury may be complicated by stricture formation with resulting hydronephrosis in the area of injury. Chronic urinary extravasation from unrecognized injury may lead to formation of a large retroperitoneal urinoma. Pyelonephritis from hydronephrosis and urinary infection may require prompt proximal drainage.

Treatment

Prompt treatment of ureteral injuries is required. The best opportunity for successful repair is in the operating room when the injury occurs. If the injury is not recognized until 10–14 days after the event and no infection, abscess, or other complications exist, immediate reexploration and repair is indicated. Proximal urinary drainage by percutaneous nephrostomy or formal nephrostomy should be considered if the injury is recognized late or in patients with significant complications making immediate reconstruction unsatisfactory. The goals of ureteral repair are to achieve complete debridement, a tension-free spatulated anastomosis, watertight closure, ureteral stenting (in selected cases), and retroperitoneal drainage.

A. Lower Ureteral Injuries: Injuries to the lower third of the ureter allow several options in management. The procedure of choice is reimplantation into the bladder combined with a psoas-hitch procedure to minimize tension on the ureteral anastomosis. An antireflux-type procedure should be done when possible. Primary ureteroureterostomy can be utilized in lower third injuries when the ureter has been ligated without transection. Adequate ureteral length is usually available for this type of anastomosis. Bladder tube flap can be utilized when greater ureteral length is lost.

Transureteroureterostomy may be utilized in lower third injuries if extensive urinoma and pelvic infection have developed. This procedure allows anastomosis and reconstruction in an area away from the pathologic processes.

B. Mid Ureteral Injuries: Mid ureteral injuries usually result from external violence and are best repaired by primary ureteroureterostomy or transureteroureterostomy.

C. Upper Ureteral Injuries: Injuries to the upper third of the ureter are best managed by primary ureteroureterostomy. If there is extensive loss of the ureter, autotransplantation of the kidney can be done as well as bowel replacement of the ureter.

D. Stenting: Most anastomoses after repair of ureteral injury should be stented. The preferred technic is to insert a silicone internal stent through the anastomosis before closure. These stents are "double-J'd" to prevent their migration in the postoperative period. After 3–4 weeks' healing, stents can be endoscopically removed from the bladder. The advantages of internal stenting are maintenance of a straight ureter with a constant caliber during early healing; the presence of a conduit for urine during healing; prevention of urinary extravasation and maintenance of urinary diversion; and easy removal.

Prognosis

The prognosis for ureteral injury is excellent if the diagnosis is made early and prompt corrective surgery is done. Delay in diagnosis worsens the prognosis because of infection, hydronephrosis, abscess, and fistula formation.

INJURIES TO THE BLADDER

Bladder injuries occur most often from external force and are often associated with pelvic fractures. (About 15% of all pelvic fractures are associated with concomitant bladder or urethral injuries.) Iatrogenic injury may result from gynecologic and other extensive pelvic procedures as well as from hernia repairs and transurethral operations.

Pathogenesis & Pathology (Fig 16–8)

The bony pelvis protects the urinary bladder very well. When the pelvis is fractured by blunt trauma, fragments from the fracture site may perforate the bladder. These perforations usually result in extraperitoneal rupture. If the urine is infected,

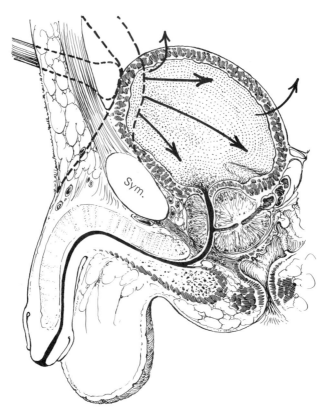

Figure 16–8. Mechanism of vesical injury. A direct blow over the full bladder causes increased intravesical pressure. If the bladder ruptures, it will usually rupture into the peritoneal cavity.

extraperitoneal bladder perforations may result in deep pelvic abscess and severe pelvic inflammation.

When the bladder is filled to near capacity, a direct blow to the lower abdomen may result in bladder disruption. This type of disruption ordinarily is intraperitoneal. Since the reflection of the pelvic peritoneum covers the dome of the bladder, a linear laceration will allow urine to flow into the abdominal cavity. If the diagnosis is not established immediately and if the urine is sterile, no symptoms may be noted for several days. If the urine is infected, immediate peritonitis and acute abdomen will develop.

Clinical Findings

Pelvic fracture often accompanies bladder rupture. The diagnosis of pelvic fracture can be made initially in the emergency room by lateral compression on the bony pelvis, since the fracture site will show crepitus and be painful to the touch. Lower abdominal and suprapubic tenderness is usually present. Pelvic fracture and suprapubic tenderness with acute abdomen suggest intraperitoneal bladder disruption.

A. Symptoms: There is usually a history of lower abdominal trauma. Blunt injury is the usual cause. Patients ordinarily are unable to urinate, but

when spontaneous voiding occurs, hematuria is usually present. Most patients complain of pelvic or lower abdominal pain.

B. Signs: Heavy bleeding associated with pelvic fracture may result in hemorrhagic shock, usually from venous disruption of pelvic vessels. Evidence of external injury from a gunshot or stab wound in the lower abdomen should make one suspect bladder injury, manifested by marked tenderness of the suprapubic area and lower abdomen. Acute abdomen will indicate intraperitoneal bladder rupture. A palpable mass in the lower abdomen usually represents a large pelvic hematoma. On rectal examination, landmarks may be indistinct because of large pelvic hematoma.

C. Laboratory Findings: Catheterization usually is required in patients with pelvic trauma but not if bloody urethral discharge is noted. Bloody urethral discharge indicates urethral injury, and a urethrogram is necessary before catheterization. When catheterization is done, gross or, less commonly, microscopic hematuria is usually present. Urine taken from the bladder at the initial catheterization should be cultured to determine whether infection is present.

D. X-Ray Findings: A plain abdominal film will generally demonstrate pelvic fractures. There may be haziness over the lower abdomen from

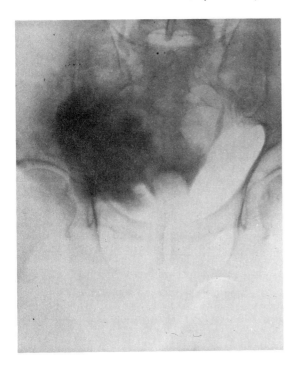

Figure 16–9. Extraperitoneal bladder rupture. Extravasation seen outside the bladder in the pelvis on cystogram.

blood and urine extravasation. An intravenous urogram should be obtained to establish whether kidney and ureteral injuries are present.

Bladder disruption will be shown on cystography. The bladder should be filled with 300 mL of contrast material and a plain film of the lower abdomen obtained. Contrast medium should then be allowed to drain out completely, and a second film of the abdomen should be obtained. The drainage film is extremely important, because it will demonstrate areas of extraperitoneal extravasation of blood and urine that may not appear on the filling film (Fig 16–9). With intraperitoneal extravasation, free contrast medium will be visualized in the abdomen, highlighting bowel loops (Fig 16–10).

E. Instrumental Examination: If urethral injury is suspected (bloody discharge), a urethrogram should be obtained before any attempt is made to catheterize the patient. If there is no evidence of urethral injury, catheterization can be safely accomplished.

Cystoscopy is not indicated, since bleeding and clot obscure visualization and prevent accurate diagnosis.

Differential Diagnosis

Abdominal trauma with hematuria may cause injury to the kidney and ureter as well as the bladder. A urogram is indicated for all patients with trauma-related hematuria. Associated injuries to the pelvic vessels and bowel should also be considered.

The urethra may be injured in association with the bladder; this possibility should be considered in any patient with blunt trauma and pelvic fractures. Urethrography will demonstrate disruption of the urethra.

Complications

A pelvic abscess may develop from extraperitoneal bladder rupture; if the urine becomes infected, the pelvic hematoma becomes infected too.

Intraperitoneal bladder rupture with extravasation of urine into the abdominal cavity will cause delayed peritonitis.

Partial incontinence may result from bladder injury when the laceration extends into the bladder neck. Meticulous repair may assure normal urinary control.

Treatment

A. Emergency Measures: Shock and hemorrhage should be treated.

B. Surgical Measures: A lower midline abdominal incision should be made. As the bladder is approached in the midline, a pelvic hematoma, which is usually lateral, should be avoided. Entering the pelvic hematoma can result in increased bleeding from release of tamponade and in infection of the hematoma, with subsequent pelvic abscess. The bladder should be opened in the midline and carefully inspected. After repair, a suprapubic cystostomy tube is usually left in place to ensure complete urinary drainage and control of bleeding.

1. Extraperitoneal rupture–Extraperitoneal rupture should be repaired intravesically. As the bladder is opened in the midline, it should be carefully inspected and lacerations closed from within.

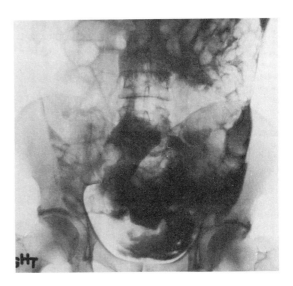

Figure 16–10. Intraperitoneal bladder rupture. Cystogram shows contrast surrounding loops of bowel.

Polyglycolic acid or chromic absorbable sutures should be used.

Extraperitoneal bladder lacerations occasionally extend into the bladder neck and should be repaired meticulously. Fine absorbable sutures should be used to ensure complete reconstruction, so that the patient will have urinary control after injury. Such injuries are best managed with indwelling urethral catheterization and suprapubic diversion.

Peritoneotomy should be done and the intraabdominal fluid inspected before completing the procedure. If abdominal fluid is bloody, complete abdominal exploration should be done to rule out associated injuries.

2. Intraperitoneal rupture–Intraperitoneal bladder ruptures should be repaired via a transperitoneal approach after careful transvesical inspection and closure of any other perforations. The peritoneum must be closed carefully over the area of injury. The bladder is then closed in separate layers by absorbable suture. All extravasated fluid from the peritoneal cavity should be removed before closure. At the time of closure, care should be taken that the suprapubic cystostomy is in the extraperitoneal position.

3. Pelvic fracture–Stable fracture of the pubic rami is usually present. In such cases, the patient can be ambulatory within 4–5 days without damage or difficulty. Unstable pelvic fractures requiring external fixation have a more protracted course.

4. Pelvic hematoma–There may be heavy uncontrolled bleeding from rupture of pelvic vessels even if the hematoma has not been entered at operation. At exploration and bladder repair, packing the pelvis with laparotomy tapes often controls the problem. If bleeding persists, it may be necessary to leave the tapes in place for 24 hours and operate again to remove them. Embolization of pelvic vessels with Gelfoam or skeletal muscle under angiographic control is useful in controlling persistent pelvic bleeding.

C. Medical Measures: The patient whose cystogram shows only a small degree of extravasation can be managed by placing a urethral catheter into the bladder, without operation or suprapubic cystostomy. Careful observation is necessary because of the potential for pelvic hematoma infection.

Prognosis
With appropriate treatment, the prognosis is excellent. The suprapubic cystostomy tube can be removed within 10 days, and the patient can usually void normally. Patients with lacerations extending into the bladder neck area may be temporarily incontinent, but full control is usually regained. At the time of discharge, urine culture should be done to determine whether catheter-associated infection requires further treatment.

INJURIES TO THE URETHRA

Urethral injuries are uncommon and occur most often in men, usually associated with pelvic fractures or straddle-type falls. They are rare in women.

Various parts of the urethra may be lacerated, transected, or contused. Management varies according to the level of injury. The urethra can be separated into 2 broad anatomic divisions: the posterior urethra, consisting of the prostatic and membranous portions; and the anterior urethra, consisting of the bulbous and pendulous portions.

1. INJURIES TO THE POSTERIOR URETHRA

Etiology (Fig 16–11)
The membranous urethra passes through the urogenital diaphragm and is the portion of the posterior urethra most likely to be injured. The urogenital diaphragm contains most of the voluntary urinary sphincter. It is attached to the pubic rami inferiorly, and when pelvic fractures occur from blunt trauma, the membranous urethra is sheared from the prostatic apex at the prostatomembranous junction.

Pathogenesis & Pathology
Injuries to the posterior urethra commonly occur from blunt trauma and pelvic fractures. The urethra usually is sheared off just proximal to the urogenital diaphragm, and the prostate is displaced superiorly by the developing hematoma in the periprostatic and perivesical spaces.

Clinical Findings
A. Symptoms: Patients usually complain of lower abdominal pain and inability to urinate. A history of crushing injury to the pelvis is usually obtained.

B. Signs: Blood at the urethral meatus is the single most important sign of urethral injury. The importance of this finding cannot be overemphasized, because an attempt to pass a urethral catheter may result in infection of the periprostatic and perivesical hematoma and conversion of an incomplete laceration to a complete one. The presence of blood at the external urethral meatus indicates that immediate urethrography is necessary to establish the diagnosis.

Suprapubic tenderness and the presence of pelvic fracture will be noted on physical examination. A large developing pelvic hematoma may be palpated. Perineal or suprapubic contusions are often noted. Rectal examination may reveal a large pelvic hematoma with the prostate displaced superiorly. Rectal examination can be misleading, however, because a tense pelvic hematoma may resemble the prostate on palpation. Superior displace-

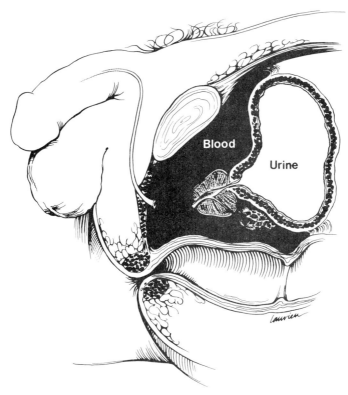

Figure 16–11. Injury to the posterior (membranous) urethra. The prostate has been avulsed from the membranous urethra secondary to fracture of the pelvis. Extravasation occurs above the triangular ligament and is periprostatic and perivesical.

ment of the prostate does not occur if the puboprostatic ligaments remain intact. Partial disruption of the membranous urethra (currently 10% of cases) is not accompanied by prostatic displacement.

C. Laboratory Findings: Anemia due to hemorrhage may be noted. Urine cannot usually be obtained initially, since the patient should not void and catheterization should not be attempted.

D. X-Ray Findings: Fractures of the bony pelvis are usually present. A urethrogram (20–30 mL of contrast material) will show the site of extravasation at the prostatomembranous junction. Ordinarily, there is free extravasation of contrast material into the perivesical space (Fig 16–12). Incomplete prostatomembranous disruption will be seen as minor extravasation, with a portion of contrast material passing into the prostatic urethra and bladder.

E. Instrumental Examination: The only instrumentation involved should be for urethrography. Catheterization or urethroscopy should not be done, because these procedures pose an increased risk of hematoma and infection and further damage to partial urethral disruptions.

Differential Diagnosis

Bladder rupture may be associated with posterior urethral injuries. An intravenous urogram should be considered part of the assessment. De-

layed films should be obtained to demonstrate the bladder and note extravasation. Cystography cannot be done preoperatively, since a urethral catheter should not be passed. Careful evaluation of the bladder at operation is necessary.

The anterior portion of the urethra may be injured as well as the prostatomembranous urethra.

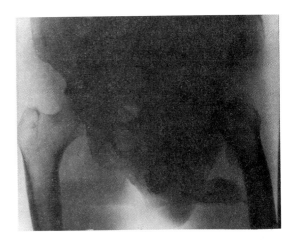

Figure 16–12. Ruptured prostatomembranous urethra shows free extravasation on urethrogram.

Complications

Stricture, impotence, and incontinence as complications of prostatomembranous disruption are among the most severe and debilitating mishaps that result from trauma to the urinary system.

Stricture following primary repair and anastomosis occurs in about half of cases. If the preferred transpubic approach with delayed repair is used, the incidence of stricture can be reduced to about 10%.

The incidence of impotence after primary repair is 30–80% (mean, about 50%). This can be reduced to 10–15% by suprapubic drainage with delayed urethral reconstruction.

Incontinence in primary reanastomosis is noted in one-third of patients. Delayed reconstruction reduces the incidence to less than 5%.

Treatment

A. Emergency Measures: Shock and hemorrhage should be treated.

B. Surgical Measures: Urethral catheterization should be avoided.

1. Immediate management–Initial management should consist of suprapubic cystostomy to provide urinary drainage. A midline lower abdominal incision should be made, care being taken to avoid the large pelvic hematoma. The bladder and prostate are usually elevated superiorly by large periprostatic and perivesical hematomas. The bladder will often be distended by a large volume of urine accumulated during the period of resuscitation and operative preparation. The urine is often clear and free of blood, but gross hematuria may be present. The bladder should be opened in the midline and carefully inspected for lacerations. If a laceration is present, the bladder should be closed with absorbable suture material and a cystostomy tube inserted for urinary drainage. This approach involves no urethral instrumentation or manipulation. Suprapubic cystostomy is maintained in place for about 3 months. This allows resolution of the pelvic hematoma, and the prostate and bladder will slowly return to their anatomic positions.

Incomplete laceration of the posterior urethra will heal spontaneously, and the suprapubic cystostomy can be removed within 2–3 weeks. The cystostomy tube should not be removed before voiding cystourethrography shows that no extravasation persists.

2. Urethral reconstruction–Reconstruction of the urethra after prostatic disruption can be undertaken within 3 months, assuming there is no pelvic abscess or other evidence of persistent pelvic infection. Before reconstruction, a combined cystogram and urethrogram should be done to determine the exact length of the resulting urethral stricture. This stricture usually is 1–2 cm long and situated immediately posterior to the pubic bone. The preferred approach is transpubic urethroplasty with direct excision of the strictured area and anastomosis of the bulbous urethra directly to the apex of the prostate. A 16F silicone urethral catheter should be left in place along with a suprapubic cystostomy. Catheters are removed within a month, and the patient is then able to void (Fig 16–13).

3. Immediate urethral realignment is preferred by some surgeons. Direct suture reconstruction of the prostatomembranous disruption in the acute injury is extremely difficult. Persistent bleeding and surrounding hematoma create technical problems. The incidence of stricture, impotence, and incontinence appears to be higher than with immediate cystostomy and delayed reconstruction.

C. General Measures: After delayed reconstruction by a transpubic approach, patients are allowed ambulation by the fifth postoperative day. No abnormality in gait or persistent pain due to removal of the pubic bone will be noted.

D. Treatment of Complications: Approximately 1 month after the delayed transpubic reconstruction, the urethral catheter can be removed and a voiding cystogram obtained through the suprapubic cystostomy tube. If the cystogram shows a patent area of reconstruction free of extravasation, the suprapubic catheter can be removed; if there is extravasation or stricture, suprapubic cystostomy should be maintained. A follow-up urethrogram should be obtained within 2 months to watch for stricture development.

Stricture, if present, is usually very short, and direct vision urethrotomy offers easy and rapid cure.

The patient may be impotent for several months after delayed repair. Impotence is permanent in about 10% of cases. Implantation of a penile prosthesis is indicated if impotence is still present 2 years after reconstruction (see Chapter 35).

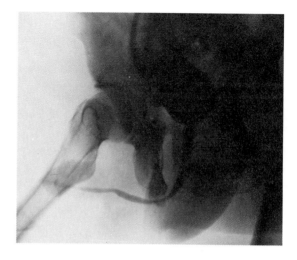

Figure 16–13. Delayed repair of urethral injury. Normal voiding urethrogram after transpubic repair of stricture 3 months following prostatomembranous urethral disruption.

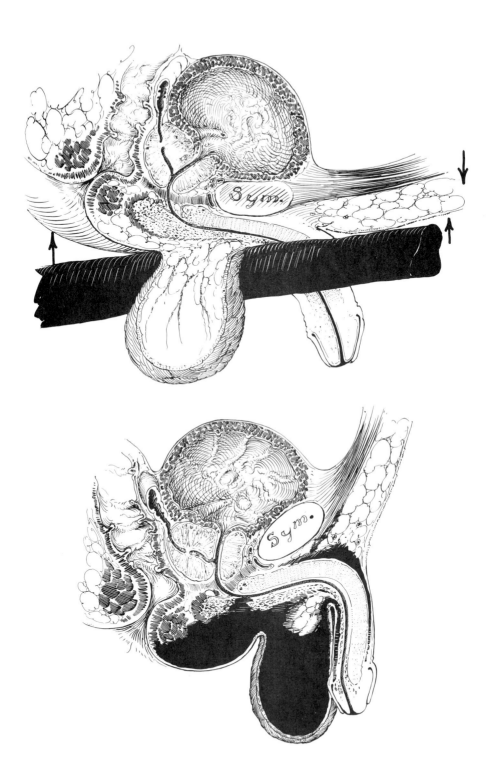

Figure 16–14. Injury to the bulbous urethra. *Above:* Mechanism: Usually a perineal blow or fall astride an object; crushing of urethra against inferior edge of pubic symphysis. *Below:* Extravasation of blood and urine enclosed within Colles' fascia (Fig 1–8).

Incontinence seldom follows transpubic reconstruction. If present, it will usually resolve slowly.

Prognosis

If complications can be avoided, the prognosis is excellent. Urinary infections ultimately resolve with appropriate management.

2. INJURIES TO THE ANTERIOR URETHRA

Etiology (Fig 16–14)

The anterior urethra is that portion distal to the urogenital diaphragm. Straddle injury may cause laceration or contusion of the urethra. Self-instrumentation or iatrogenic instrumentation may cause partial disruption.

Pathogenesis & Pathology

A. Contusion: Contusion of the urethra is a sign of crush injury without urethral disruption. Perineal hematoma usually resolves without complications.

B. Laceration: A severe straddle injury may result in laceration of part of the urethral wall, allowing extravasation of urine. If the extravasation is unrecognized, it may extend into the scrotum, along the penile shaft, and up to the abdominal wall. It is limited only by Colles' fascia and often results in sepsis, infection, and serious morbidity.

Clinical Findings

A. Symptoms: There is usually a history of a fall, and in some cases a history of instrumentation. Bleeding from the urethra is usually present. There is local pain into the perineum and sometimes massive perineal hematoma. If voiding has occurred and extravasation is noted, sudden swelling in the area will be present. If diagnosis has been delayed, sepsis and severe infection may be present.

B. Signs: The perineum is very tender, and a mass may be found. Rectal examination reveals a normal prostate. The patient usually has a desire to void, but voiding should not be allowed until assessment of the urethra is complete. No attempt should be made to pass a urethral catheter, but if the patient's bladder is overdistended, percutaneous suprapubic cystostomy can be done as a temporary procedure.

When presentation of such injuries is delayed, there is massive urinary extravasation and infection in the perineum and the scrotum. The lower abdominal wall may also be involved. The skin is usually swollen and discolored.

C. Laboratory Findings: Blood loss is not usually excessive, particularly if secondary injury has occurred. The white count may be elevated with infection.

D. X-Ray Findings: A urethrogram, with instillation of 15–20 mL of contrast material, will

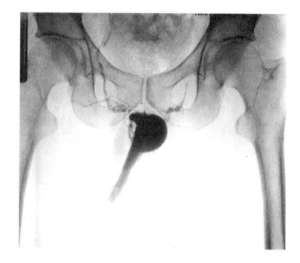

Figure 16–15. Ruptured bulbar (anterior) urethra following straddle injury. Extravasation on urethrogram.

demonstrate extravasation and the location of injury (Fig 16–15). The contused urethra will show no evidence of extravasation.

E. Instrumental Examination: If there is no evidence of extravasation on the urethrogram, a urethral catheter may be passed into the bladder. Extravasation is a contraindication to further instrumentation at this time.

Differential Diagnosis

Partial or complete disruption of the prostatomembranous urethra may occur if pelvic fracture is present. Urethrography will usually demonstrate the location and extent of extravasation and its relationship to the urogenital diaphragm.

Complications

Heavy bleeding from the corpus spongiosum injury may occur in the perineum as well as through the urethral meatus. Pressure applied to the perineum over the site of the injury usually controls bleeding. If hemorrhage cannot be controlled, immediate operation is required.

The complications of urinary extravasation are chiefly sepsis and infection. Aggressive debridement and drainage are required if there is infection.

Stricture at the site of injury is a common complication, but surgical reconstruction may not be required unless the stricture significantly reduces urinary flow rates.

Treatment

A. General Measures: Major blood loss usually does not occur from straddle injury. If heavy bleeding does occur, local pressure for control, followed by resuscitation, is required.

B. Specific Measures:

1. Urethral contusion–The patient with urethral contusion shows no evidence of extravasation, and the urethra remains intact. After urethrography, the patient is allowed to void; and if the voiding occurs normally, without pain or bleeding, no additional treatment is necessary. If bleeding persists, urethral catheter drainage can be done.

2. Urethral lacerations–Instrumentation of the urethra following urethrography should be avoided. A small midline incision in the suprapubic area readily exposes the dome of the bladder so that a suprapubic cystostomy tube can be inserted, allowing complete urinary diversion while the urethral laceration heals. If only minor extravasation is noted on the urethrogram, a voiding study can be performed within 7 days after suprapubic catheter drainage to search for extravasation. In more extensive injuries, one should wait 2–3 weeks before doing a voiding study through the suprapubic catheter. Healing at the site of injury may result in stricture formation. Most of these strictures are not severe and do not require surgical reconstruction. Removal of the suprapubic cystostomy catheter may be done if no extravasation is documented. Follow-up with documentation of urinary flow rates will show whether there is urethral obstruction from stricture.

3. Urethral laceration with extensive urinary extravasation–After major laceration, urinary extravasation may involve the perineum, scrotum, and lower abdomen. Drainage of these areas is indicated. Suprapubic cystostomy for urinary diversion is required. Infection and abscess formation are common, requiring antibiotic therapy.

4. Immediate repair–Immediate repair of urethral lacerations can be done, but the procedure is difficult and the incidence of stricture is high.

C. Treatment of Complications: Strictures at the site of injury may be extensive and require delayed reconstruction.

Prognosis

Urethral stricture is a major complication but in most cases does not require surgical reconstruction. If, when stricture resolves, urinary flow rates are poor and urinary infection and urethral fistula are present, reconstruction is required.

INJURIES TO THE PENIS

Disruption of the tunica albuginea of the penis can occur during sexual intercourse. At presentation, the patient has penile pain and hematoma. This injury should be surgically corrected.

Gangrene and urethral injury may be caused by obstructing rings placed around the base of the penis. These objects must be removed without causing further damage. Penile amputation is seen occasionally, and in a few patients the penis can be surgically replaced successfully by microsurgical technics.

Total avulsion of the penile skin occurs from machinery injuries. Immediate debridement and skin grafting are usually successful in salvage.

Injuries to the penis should suggest possible urethral damage, which should be investigated by urethrography.

INJURIES TO THE SCROTUM

Superficial lacerations of the scrotum may be debrided and closed primarily. Blunt trauma may cause local hematoma and ecchymosis, but these injuries resolve without difficulty. One must be certain that testicular rupture has not occurred.

Total avulsion of the scrotal skin may be caused by machinery accidents or other major trauma. The testes and spermatic cords are usually intact. It is important to provide coverage for these structures: this is best done by immediate surgical debridement and by placing the testes and spermatic cords in the subcutaneous tissues of the upper thighs. Later reconstruction of the scrotum can be done with a skin graft or thigh flap.

INJURIES TO THE TESTIS

Blunt trauma to the testis causes severe pain and often nausea and vomiting. Lower abdominal tenderness may be present. A hematoma may surround the testis and make delineation of its margin difficult. Ultrasonography can be used as an aid to better define the organ. If rupture has occurred, the sonogram will delineate the injury, which should be repaired.

●　●　●

References

Emergency Diagnosis & Management

Baker RJ: Newer techniques in evaluation of injured patients. *Surg Clin North Am* 1975;**55**:31.

Baker WNW, Mackie DB, Newcombe JF: Diagnostic paracentesis in the acute abdomen. *Br Med J* 1967;**3**:146.

Kaufman JJ, Brosman SA: Blunt injuries of the genitourinary tract. *Surg Clin North Am* 1972;**52**:747.

Lucey DT, Smith MJV: Initial diagnosis and management of urinary tract injuries. *Clin Med* 1973;**80**:17.

Orkin LA: The diagnosis of urological trauma in the presence of other injuries. *Surg Clin North Am* 1953;**33**:1473.

Richter MW & others: Radiology of genitourinary trauma. *Radiol Clin North Am* 1973;**11**:593.

Injuries to the Kidney

Carlton CE Jr, Scott R Jr, Goldman M: The management of penetrating injuries of the kidney. *J Trauma* 1968;**8**:1071.

Cass AS, Ireland GW: Comparison of the conservative and surgical management of the more severe degrees of renal trauma in multiple injured patients. *J Urol* 1973;**109**:8.

Cass AS, Ireland GW: Management of renal injuries in the severely injured patient. *J Trauma* 1972;**12**:516.

Cosgrove MD, Mendez R, Morrow JW: Traumatic renal arteriovenous fistula: Report of 12 cases. *J Urol* 1973;**110**:627.

Fay R & others: Renal artery thrombosis: A successful revascularization by autotransplantation. *J Urol* 1974;**111**:572.

Glenn JF, Harvard BM: The injured kidney. *JAMA* 1960;**173**:1189.

Kazman MH, Brosman SA, Cockett ATK: Diagnosis and early management of renal trauma: A study of 120 patients. *J Urol* 1969;**101**:783.

Lang EK: Arteriography in assessment of renal trauma. *J Trauma* 1975;**15**:553.

McAninch JW: Acute renal artery thrombosis from blunt trauma. *Urology* 1975;**6**:74.

Mahoney SA, Persky L: Intravenous drip nephrotomography as an adjunct in the evaluation of renal injury. *J Urol* 1968;**99**:513.

Mendez R: Renal trauma. *J Urol* 1977;**118**:698.

Morrow JW, Mendez R: Renal trauma. *J Urol* 1970;**104**:649.

Persky L, Forsythe WE: Renal trauma in childhood. *JAMA* 1962;**182**:709.

Peters PC, Bright TC III: Blunt renal injuries. *Urol Clin North Am* 1977;**4**:17.

Radwin HM, Fitch WP, Robison JR: A unified concept of renal trauma. *J Urol* 1976;**116**:20.

Schencker B: Drip infusion pyelography: Indications and applications in urological roentgen diagnosis. *Radiology* 1964;**83**:12.

Scholl AJ, Nation EF: Injuries of the kidney. Chap 20, p 785, in: *Urology*, 3rd ed. Vol 1. Campbell MF, Harrison JH (editors). Saunders, 1970.

Scott R Jr, Carlton CE Jr, Goldman M: Penetrating injuries of the kidney: An analysis of 181 patients. *J Urol* 1969;**101**:247.

Scott R Jr, Selzman HM: Complications of nephrectomy: Review of 450 patients and a description of a modifica-

tion of the transperitoneal approach. *J Urol* 1966;**95**:307.

Skinner DG: Traumatic renal artery thrombosis: A successful thrombectomy and revascularization. *Ann Surg* 1973;**177**:264.

Woodruff JF Jr & others: Radiologic aspects of renal trauma with emphasis on arteriography and renal isotope scanning. *J Urol* 1967;**97**:184.

Injuries to the Ureter

Carlton CE Jr, Guthrie AG, Scott R Jr: Surgical correction of ureteral injury. *J Trauma* 1969;**9**:457.

Carlton CE Jr, Scott R Jr, Guthrie AJ: The initial management of ureteral injuries: Report of 78 cases. *J Urol* 1971;**105**:335.

Ehrlich RM, Melman A, Skinner DG: The use of vesicopsoas hitch in urologic surgery. *J Urol* 1978;**119**:322.

Holden S & others: Gunshot wounds of the ureter: A 15 year review of 63 consecutive cases. *J Urol* 1976;**116**:562.

Liroff SA, Pontes JE, Pierce JM Jr: Gunshot wounds of the ureter: 5 year experience. *J Urol* 1977;**118**:551.

McAninch JW, Moore CA: Diagnosis and treatment of urologic complications of gynecologic surgery. *Am J Surg* 1970;**120**:542.

Stutzman RE: Ballistics and the management of ureteral injuries from high velocity missiles. *J Urol* 1977;**118**:947.

Injuries to the Bladder

Del Villar RG, Ireland GW, Cass AS: Management of bladder and urethral injury in conjunction with immediate surgical treatment of the severe trauma patient. *J Urol* 1972;**108**:581.

Montie J: Bladder injuries. *Urol Clin North Am* 1977;**4**:59.

Ochsner TC, Busch FM, Clark BG: Urogenital wounds in Vietnam. *J Urol* 1969;**101**:224.

Salvatierra O Jr: Vietnam experience in 252 urological war injuries. *J Urol* 1969;**101**:615.

Injuries to the Urethra

Allen TD: Transpubic approach for strictures of the posterior urethra superior to the urogenital diaphragm. *Urol Clin North Am* 1977;**4**:95.

Bredael JJ & others: Traumatic rupture of the female urethra. *J Urol* 1979;**122**:560.

Cass AS, Godec CJ: Urethral injury due to external trauma. *Urology* 1978;**11**:607.

Coffield KS, Weems WL: Experience with management of posterior urethral injury associated with pelvic fracture. *J Urol* 1977;**117**:722.

Colapinto V, McCallum RW: Injury to the posterior urethra in fractured pelvis: A new classification. *J Urol* 1977;**118**:575.

DeWeerd JH: Immediate realignment of posterior urethral injury. *Urol Clin North Am* 1977;**4**:75.

Gibson GR: Impotence following fractured pelvis and ruptured urethra. *Br J Urol* 1970;**42**:86.

Gibson GR: Urologic management and complications of fractured pelvis and ruptured urethra. *J Urol* 1974;**111**:353.

Glassberg KI & others: Partial tears of the prostatomembranous urethra in children. *Urology* 1979;**13**:500.

Glassberg KI & others: The radiographic approach to injuries of the prostatomembranous urethra in children. *J Urol* 1979;**122**:678.

Johanson B: Reconstruction of male urethral strictures. *Acta Chir Scand [Suppl]* 1953;**176**:1. [Entire issue.]

McAninch JW: Traumatic injuries to the urethra. *J Trauma* 1981;**21**:291.

McRoberts JW, Ragde H: The severed canine posterior urethra: A study of two distinct methods of repair. *J Urol* 1970;**104**:724.

Malloy TR, Wein AJ, Carpiniello L: Transpubic urethroplasty for prostatomembranous urethral disruption. *J Urol* 1980;**124**:359.

Morehouse DD, MacKinnon KJ: Management of prostatomembranous urethral disruption: 13 year experience. *J Urol* 1980;**123**:173.

Morehouse MD, MacKinnon KJ: Urological injuries associated with pelvic fractures. *J Trauma* 1969;**9**:479.

Moulonguet A: Ruptures traumatiques de l'urethra postérieur. *J Urol Nephrol* 1965;**71**:1.

Peltier LF: Complications associated with fractures of the pelvis. *J Bone Joint Surg [Am]* 1965;**47**:1060.

Persky L: Childhood urethral trauma. *Urology* 1978;**11**:603.

Pokorny M, Pontes JE, Pierce JM Jr: Urological injuries associated with pelvic trauma. *J Urol* 1979;**121**:455.

Pontes JE, Pierce JM Jr: Anterior urethral injuries: Four years of experience at the Detroit General Hospital. *J Urol* 1978;**120**:563.

Raffa J, Christensen NM: Compound fractures of the pelvis. *Am J Surg* 1976;**132**:282.

Trunkey DD & others: Management of pelvic fractures in blunt traumatic injury. *J Trauma* 1974;**14**:912.

Waterhouse K, Laugani G, Patil U: The surgical repair of membranous urethral strictures: Experience with 105 consecutive cases. *J Urol* 1980;**123**:500.

Injuries to the Penis

Engelman ER & others: Traumatic amputation of the penis. *J Urol* 1974;**112**:774.

Fleming JP: Reconstruction of the penis. *J Urol* 1970;**104**:213.

Flowerdew R, Fishman IJ, Churchill BM: Management of penile zipper injury. *J Urol* 1977;**117**:671.

Kendall AR, Karafin L: Repair of the denuded penis. *J Urol* 1967;**98**:484.

Mears EM Jr: Traumatic rupture of the corpus cavernosum. *J Urol* 1971;**105**:407.

Mendez R, Kiely WF, Morrow JW: Self-emasculation. *J Urol* 1972;**107**:981.

Shiraki IW, Trichel BE: Traumatic dislocation of the penis. *J Urol* 1969;**101**:186.

Stuppler SA & others: Incarceration of penis by foreign body. *Urology* 1973;**2**:308.

Tuerk M, Weir WH Jr: Successful replantation of a traumatically amputated glans penis. *Plast Reconstr Surg* 1971;**48**:499.

Injuries to the Scrotum

Millard R Jr: Scrotal construction and reconstruction. *Plast Reconstr Surg* 1966;**33**:10.

Injuries to the Testis

Merricks JW, Papiernak FB: Traumatic rupture of the testicle. *J Urol* 1970;**103**:77.

Redman JF, Rountree GA, Bissada NK: Injuries to scrotal contents by blunt trauma. *Urology* 1976;**7**:190.

Schulman CC: Traumatic rupture of the testicle: An underestimated pathology. *Urol Int* 1974;**29**:31.

Sethi RS, Singh W: Traumatic dislocation of testes. *J Urol* 1967;**98**:501.

Talarico RD, Clark JC: Nonpenetrating testicular rupture. *Urology* 1973;**1**:365.

17 | Immunology of Genitourinary Tumors

J. Vivian Wells, MD, FRACP, FRCPA, & H. Hugh Fudenberg, MD

The classic therapeutic approaches to cancer have been surgery, radiotherapy, and chemotherapy. In addition, for about the last 50 years, there have been sporadic attempts to influence the outcome of tumors by manipulating immunologic mechanisms. The rapid expansion of knowledge about immunology in recent years has been accompanied by increased interest in the role of immunology in the development and progress of cancer. This chapter briefly outlines immunologic concepts as they relate to the cause, diagnosis, treatment, and prognosis of genitourinary tumors.

IMMUNOLOGIC CONCEPTS OF ONCOGENESIS

The concept of "immunologic surveillance" against cancer was developed independently by Burnet and Thomas in the early 1960s. They proposed that an important function of the normal immune system is to recognize mutant or aberrant patterns in the body—such as malignant cells—and eliminate them. This implied the existence of foreign antigenic determinants on tumor cells, their recognition by the immune system of the host, and the development of effector mechanisms to destroy or neutralize these cells. A considerable body of evidence has accumulated to support this hypothesis.

Tumor-Associated Antigens (TAAs)

Tumor-associated antigens (TAAs) have been demonstrated in a wide variety of tumors in experimental animals—both those arising spontaneously and those induced by viral, chemical, or physical carcinogens. The term tumor-specific transplantation antigens was used in studies of inbred strains of animals with tumors induced by chemical carcinogens, eg, methylcholanthrene (MCA). The tumor in each animal appeared to have individually unique or specific antigens. Later studies in these animals suggest that they also contain TAAs that exhibit weak cross-reactivity between different animals. MCA-induced bladder tumors show weakly cross-reacting TAAs in both rats and mice, and MCA-induced rat bladder papil-

Abbreviations Used in This Chapter	
AFP	Alpha-1-fetoprotein
BCG	Bacillus Calmette-Guérin
CEA	Carcinoembryonic antigen
DHSR	Delayed hypersensitivity reaction
DNCB	Dinitrochlorobenzene
HLA	Human leukocyte antigen
MCA	Methylcholanthrene
MER	Methanol-extractable residue
MIF	Migration inhibitory factor
PAP	Prostatic acid phosphatase
PBL	Peripheral blood lymphocytes
PHA	Phytohemagglutinin
PPD	Purified protein derivative
RNA	Ribonucleic acid
TAA	Tumor-associated antigen
TF	Transfer factor
UCEA	Urinary carcinoembryonic antigen

lomas and carcinomas share TAAs. Animals with virus-induced tumors have easily detectable cross-reacting TAAs.

TAAs have been clearly demonstrated in a variety of human tumors, including neuroblastoma, melanoma, osteogenic sarcoma, leukemia and lymphoma, cerebral tumors (eg, meningioma), hepatoma, nasopharyngeal carcinoma, ovarian carcinoma, breast carcinoma, lung carcinoma, genitourinary tumors, etc. The genitourinary tumors include renal adenocarcinoma, nephroblastoma, transitional cell carcinoma of the genitourinary tract—including carcinoma of the bladder—and carcinoma of the prostate.

Comparisons with studies of TAAs in animal models led to the theory that human genitourinary tumors such as nephroblastoma are of viral origin, whereas bladder carcinoma is chemically induced. Multiple factors may also be involved in the etiology of genitourinary tumors in humans. Bladder tumors in workers handling benzidine compounds are thought to be due to carcinogens, but such tumors are more prevalent in workers with low concentrations of the serum complement component properdin. Virologic studies have tended to incriminate herpesviruses, especially in prostatic carcinoma. Renal adenocarcinoma can be induced in animals by chemical, viral, or physical agents, but the cause in humans is still unknown. This is unfortunate, since malignant renal tumors comprise 1.2% of all human cancers (not including skin cancers), and adenocarcinoma is clearly the most common malignant renal tumor (89%).

TAAs have not yet been isolated and characterized for the great majority of tumors. A putative soluble TAA has been isolated from human renal cell carcinoma. TAAs appear mainly on the membrane of affected cells; attempts at purification are complicated by the presence of various normal membrane components. Detection of TAAs thus has been based on their ability to elicit immune responses in the tumor-bearing host.

Immune Responses to TAAs

TAAs elicit immunologic responses from both components of the immune system: humoral and cellular. Humoral immunity is mediated by circulating antibodies or immunoglobulins secreted by plasma cells that develop from B cells (bursa- or bone marrow-derived lymphocytes). Cellular immunity is mediated by T cells (thymus-derived). Humoral responses to TAAs are therefore evaluated by a variety of methods used to detect antitumor antibodies. Cellular responses to TAAs are detected by appropriate tests for cell-mediated immunity. These are discussed below in the section on immunologic diagnosis of tumors. It should be emphasized here, however, that the 2 components—humoral immunity and cellular immunity—have varying degrees of importance and interrelationships during different stages of tumor development in any individual patient.

IMMUNOLOGIC METHODS IN TUMOR DIAGNOSIS

These may be divided into 3 broad areas: general diagnostic considerations, specific immunodiagnosis, and detection of tumor markers.

General Diagnostic Considerations

Although many of the procedures outlined below require sophisticated laboratory technics and experienced personnel, evaluation of histologic sections of tumor tissue is of great help in estimating prognosis. For example, infiltration of breast tumor tissue by immunologically competent cells favorably affects life span and response to chemotherapy. Regardless of clinical stage, patients whose urologic tumors are heavily infiltrated with plasma cells, lymphocytes, and eosinophils survive much longer than the average. It is therefore important that these simple histologic evaluations be performed.

In addition to standard methods of tumor diagnosis—eg, x-rays, radionuclide scanning, and biopsy—a general assessment of the patient's immunologic status should be made:

A. Humoral Immunity: Electrophoresis of serum proteins and measurement of serum immunoglobulin levels are usually not helpful unless the patient has an associated monoclonal gammopathy, but a test of the patient's antibody response to primary immunization may be of value. For example, the antibody response to immunization with monomeric flagellin antigen from *Salmonella adelaide* was depressed significantly in patients with active cancer compared with sick but not cancerous control patients. A significant correlation was found between the degree of depression and overall survival. Antibody responses in patients with clinically cured cancer were significantly greater than those in hospital controls and in patients with active cancer but even so were less marked than responses in healthy subjects.

B. Cellular Immunity: There are 5 principal methods of measuring cellular immunity in patients: (1) delayed hypersensitivity skin reactions (DHSR), (2) in vitro transformation of peripheral blood lymphocytes (PBL), (3) elaboration of MIF and other cellular mediators, (4) measurement of "active" and total T cells in peripheral blood, and (5) cytotoxicity.

The first 3 tests are performed with standard specific antigens, eg, PPD, mumps antigen, and streptokinase-streptodornase. Significant abnormalities are usually found in more advanced cancers where the diagnosis is already obvious and the abnormalities signify the generally altered immunologic status of the patient.

Peripheral blood T cells spontaneously bind sheep red blood cells to form a rosette; approximately 70–80% of normal human PBLs are rosette-forming T cells. Normal persons have 28 ± 6.8% "active" T cells as measured by a different rosetting technic. A lower percentage of "active" T rosette cell count may be present in patients with tumors before metastases develop or in patients with viral infections. This test gives no information about type or site of tumor.

Specific Diagnosis

These methods detect immune responses to a specific TAA.

A. Humoral Responses: These tests include immunofluorescence, complement fixation, immune cytolysis, and immunodiffusion.

Immunofluorescence testing is widely used to demonstrate serum antibodies in patients with tumors. Antibody specificities determine whether they react only with autologous tumor, autologous tumor and metastases from the primary tumor, tumors of the same histologic type in other patients, or long-term cultures of malignant cells of the same histologic type. Immunofluorescence methods have also been used to label antisera prepared in animals against TAAs, eg, human nephroblastoma.

B. Cellular Responses: The methods consist of lymphocyte-mediated cytotoxicity, in vitro stimulation of PBL by TAA, release of mediators from PBL, and DHSR to TAA.

The latter 3 methods refer to responses to the specific TAA for a particular type of tumor and not to general immune responses. They require the preparation of TAA from the tumor under study.

In cytotoxicity studies, PBL from the patient are tested for their ability to inactivate or kill labeled tumor cells in vitro. This method has been used to study renal carcinoma, nephroblastoma, and transitional cell carcinoma of the bladder. Such studies have been facilitated by the recent availability of long-term cell line cultures established from prostatic carcinoma, transitional cell carcinoma, and renal cell carcinoma. In each case, cell-mediated immunity was demonstrable, but in bladder carcinoma, some studies have demonstrated non-T cell-mediated cytotoxicity.

Recently, a significant association was reported between a histocompatibility marker (HLA-B7) and a reduced level of spontaneous cell-mediated cytotoxicity to renal carcinoma cells. Further studies are under way to characterize the nature of genetic control of the immune responses to genitourinary tumors in humans.

Tumor Markers

This imprecise term denotes any chemical or biologic factor that identifies a tumor. The TAAs discussed above are specific tumor markers that are (by definition) not found in normal tissues. Other antigens found in very small amounts in fetal, normal, or diseased but nonmalignant tissues are markedly elevated in some malignant tissues. The oncofetal antigens are included in this heterogeneous group. We shall discuss the 3 best-known types found in urologic tumors: carcinoembryonic antigen (CEA), alpha-1-fetoprotein (AFP), and prostatic acid phosphatase (PAP).

A. Carcinoembryonic Antigen (CEA): Gold and his colleagues in Montreal in the mid 1960s extracted a glycoprotein substance from human colonic carcinomas and prepared antisera against it. They found material with the same antigenic characteristics in fetal tissues, and it was therefore called CEA. The association of CEA with gastrointestinal cancer has now been fully documented, and extensive studies have shown that CEA is also associated with a variety of other cancers (including genitourinary tumors) and nonmalignant diseases. Many different technics have been employed to measure CEA, but those used most frequently show a plasma level of less than 2.5 ng/mL in over 98% of normal subjects. Slight to moderate increases in CEA are found with a variety of inflammatory diseases—eg, pancreatitis, ulcer-

Table 17–1. Plasma CEA levels.
(Normal: < 2.5 ng/mL)

Diseases	% Increase (> 2.5 ng/mL)
Gastrointestinal	
Carcinoma of colon, rectum	72–95
Carcinoma of pancreas	63
Colorectal polyposis	9–19
Diverticulitis	21
Respiratory	
Carcinoma of lung	72–76
Chronic bronchitis and emphysema	25–35
Carcinoma of breast	47–67
Genitourinary	
Carcinoma of kidney	35
Carcinoma of bladder	33
Carcinoma of prostate	40
Carcinoma of cervix	42
Carcinoma of ovary	35
Testicular tumors	33

ative colitis—and cancers. Markedly increased levels (> 40 ng/mL) are quite likely to be associated with cancer, especially carcinoma of the colon, pancreas, breast, or lung. Table 17–1 lists some data on the incidence of CEA in various conditions.

The degree of plasma CEA elevation is proportionate to the mass of the tumor and not its histologic type or parent tissue. The routine CEA test is not specific for any tumor and is therefore not suitable for screening tests. The principal current applications of CEA testing are in monitoring therapy and estimating prognosis. In a patient with a tumor and a markedly elevated plasma CEA, complete removal of the tumor will cause CEA levels to fall to normal, generally within 14 days. An intermediate but still increased CEA level following tumor removal indicates residual primary tumor tissue or the presence of secondary deposits. Patients who have had complete surgical removal of tumor and a fall to normal CEA levels can be monitored at regular intervals of 3–6 months. A rising plasma CEA level in such a patient suggests local recurrence of the tumor, growth of secondary deposits, or the unlikely development of a CEA-secreting tumor de novo.

CEA has the following properties:

> Molecular weight: 200,000
> Sedimentation rate: 7S–8S
> Carbohydrate/protein ratio: 6:1 to 1:1
> Sialic acid content: markedly variable
> N-Acetylglucosamine content: high
> N-Acetylgalactosamine content: trace
> Polydispersion on gel electrophoresis

Demonstration in normal and neoplastic tissues of trace amounts of molecules showing cross-reactivity with CEA signifies that antigenic determinants are shared. It appears likely that there exist several similar molecules or a family of CEA molecules with slight antigenic and structural differences.

When human prostate epithelial cells are cultured in vitro, the culture medium around the cells contains elevated levels of CEA (or a CEA-like substance). Very low levels of CEA have been found in the medium from cultures of prostate fibroblasts, other genitourinary tumors, melanoma cells, and nontumor tissues.

Urinary CEA. Measurement of CEA levels in the urine in male subjects showed that 95% had less than 35 ng of CEA per milliliter of urine. A survey of patients with urothelial tumors of all stages showed that 52% had increased urinary CEA levels. Urinary CEA elevations are specific for urothelial carcinomas (if infection is ruled out), since urinary CEA levels are normal in prostatic and colorectal cancer even if plasma levels are raised with the latter tumors. Urinary CEA is elevated with the latter tumors only if they directly invade the urinary tract. The urinary CEA level is influenced by the size of the tumor mass and not by its histologic characteristics. The incidence of positive tests and the amount of urinary CEA are increased with increasing tumor mass and therefore with tumor stage. Thus, urinary CEA levels were increased in 33% of stage T1 tumors and 79% of stage T4 tumors. Successful surgery for bladder carcinoma leads to a fall to normal levels of urinary CEA; a return of increased levels indicates local recurrence, the development of metastases, or a new primary tumor in another site.

Because the component studied in urine may have slight but definite antigenic and structural differences from CEA prepared from colon cancer tissue, it has been designated urinary carcinoembryonic antigen (UCEA). A test specific for UCEA has not yet been devised.

Measurements of both plasma and urinary CEA are of value in assessing the results of treatment of urothelial tumors and in detecting local or distant recurrences.

B. Alpha-1-Fetoprotein (AFP): Serum levels of AFP are high in the fetus but low in adult animals and humans. High levels are also found with certain tumors such as hepatoma (72–95%) and embryonic tumors (13–75%). Serum AFP levels are increased in teratocarcinoma or embryonal cell carcinoma of the gonad (45–75%) and in choriocarcinoma (13%). The serum AFP level is normal in seminoma and other gonadal tumors, nephroblastoma, etc. Sensitive technics are now available that can measure slightly increased levels of serum AFP in a small proportion of patients with nonmalignant conditions such as infectious hepatitis.

Measurements of serum AFP and human chorionic gonadotropin (hCG) have proved helpful in monitoring therapy and determining prognosis in patients with testicular tumors.

C. Prostatic Acid Phosphatase (PAP): Measurement of PAP in blood by standard methods has been of limited value, since it was elevated in only 60–75% of patients with prostatic carcinoma and documented bony metastases. The problem is that the antigens used in the tests have been prostate-specific but not prostatic cancer-specific. While there is often a significant association between the extent of initial elevation of PAP and survival, not all patients show this prognostic association, nor do the changes in their serum PAP levels necessarily accurately reflect tumor load and clinical response to treatment. Newer, more sensitive automated radioimmunoassays for PAP may increase its contribution to the management of patients with prostatic carcinoma.

IMMUNOLOGIC FACTORS IN PROGNOSIS

Many examples in both animals and humans confirm the view that changes in general immunologic status influence both the development and course of malignant disease. Analysis of cases reported to the Immunodeficiency Cancer Registry shows that patients with primary immunodeficiency have a far greater risk of developing cancer (2–10%) than normal subjects. This is most significant when their short life span is considered. Patients receiving immunosuppressive therapy after renal allotransplantation have a significantly higher risk of developing cancer, especially the less common types. Cancer in patients with severe immune system impairment generally carries a poor prognosis. One special example is the known association between the use of the cytotoxic immunosuppressive agent cyclophosphamide and bladder carcinoma.

Some forms of cancer treatment can be severely immunosuppressive, eg, radiotherapy and chemotherapy, with effects that may be counterproductive to the main goal of cure.

Serial blood lymphocyte counts in patients with bladder cancer may have some prognostic usefulness. One study of 34 patients disclosed—as expected—a marked decline in lymphocyte counts after radiotherapy. The lymphocyte counts returned to pretherapy levels within 3 years following radiotherapy in patients who remained clinically well for 5 years. Patients with recurrent or residual tumors, however, had lymphocyte counts that did not reach pretherapy levels within 3 years of therapy.

Specific Immune Responses & Clinical Stages

Specific responses to TAAs occur during the life of a tumor in a host, as outlined above. The relative balance between cellular and humoral responses is probably the major factor in determining the overall outcome of a tumor in immunologic terms.

Lymphocytes from patients with actively growing in vivo tumors were shown by means of in vitro tests to be cytotoxic for the patient's own tumor or a tumor of the same type from other patients. This disparity between in vivo and in vitro findings was postulated to be due to factors that "blocked" in vivo the cytotoxic effect of lymphocytes against tumor cells. Blocking of this sort can occur for 2 principal reasons:

(1) **Blocking factor:** IgG antibody-antigen complexes (probably in antigen excess) have now been detected in such patients; these complexes bind to the tumor cells (apparently without damaging them) and prevent the cytotoxic lymphocytes from attaching to the tumor cells via the TAAs.

(2) **Circulating TAAs:** When large tumor masses are present, membrane-bound TAAs may be released into the circulation as soluble glycoproteins. These eventually bind to the surface of specific lymphocytes, and this makes it impossible for the lymphocytes to bind to TAAs on tumor cells in the main tumor mass.

These mechanisms lead to in vivo growth of the tumor, since the specific cellular response to the tumor is blocked by the serum blocking factors.

The degree of lymphocyte cytotoxicity in bladder cancer varies with the course of the disease. A strong response generally indicates a good prognosis, especially after radiotherapy. The absence of cytotoxicity may have 2 entirely different interpretations: (1) at least temporary cure of the tumor, or (2) extensive tumor growth, metastasis, and a very bad prognosis.

A second major finding is that serum from some patients with tumors can reverse the "blocking" activity of serum found in patients with growing tumors. This "deblocking" activity due to "deblocking factors" is usually seen with regressing tumors. It has been proposed that this deblocking activity is due to the elimination of antigen-antibody complexes by additional antibody.

The serum from one patient with a transitional cell carcinoma of the bladder contained an IgG antibody that induced lymphocyte cytotoxicity against the tumor and did not require complement for this activity. The IgG antibody induced cytotoxicity in the lymphocytes from patients with or without bladder cancer, and the cytotoxicity was tumor-specific. It acted against transitional cell carcinoma but not against normal adult cells, normal embryonal cells, or nephroblastoma cells. The IgG antibody and TAA had to make contact before one could show this antibody-induced, noncomplement-dependent lymphocyte cytotoxicity for tumor cells.

Tests with TAAs for lymphocyte transformation and DHSR have also been performed in patients with cancer in various stages. Skin tests generally were positive in remission and negative in relapse. Remission induced by treatment was accompanied by restoration of a positive DHSR that was tumor-specific and not a response to antigens in general. Stimulation of lymphocytes by TAAs was found to be positive in equal numbers of patients in remission or in relapse. This lack of correlation between in vivo and in vitro tests of specific responses to TAAs has not yet been explained.

Studies on cytotoxicity against tumor cells have become very difficult to interpret since the discovery of cells that lack T and B cell determinants but are active against tumor cells; these are termed **killer** (K) cells. Furthermore, subjects with no detectable tumor may have natural killer (NK) cells active in vitro against tumor cells. The relevance of such cells to the etiology of tumors is still disputed.

These various opposing mechanisms resulting in tumor growth or tumor destruction may operate to different degrees in a given patient over the course of the illness, and this fact must be kept in mind when assessing the effects of therapy on the patient's immune system and pondering the form of immunotherapy to be employed.

GENERAL IMMUNOLOGIC CONSIDERATIONS IN TUMOR THERAPY

The greater the number of tumor cells of a given tumor injected into experimental animals, the shorter the survival of the host. This correlation between size of tumor and survival is apparently also true in humans. Unfortunately, in most patients, the tumor load is already great at the time of diagnosis. The aim of therapy, therefore, is rapid elimination of the tumor. This is accomplished if possible by surgical removal or radiotherapy. Chemotherapy is the method of choice with disseminated tumors. Cytotoxic drugs used for this purpose can be divided into 3 classes: (1) agents killing cells in all phases of the cell cycle irrespective of proliferative capacity (mechlorethamine, carmustine [BCNU], gamma irradiation); (2) agents killing cells in only one phase of the cell cycle (vinblastine, methotrexate); (3) agents killing cells in all phases of the cell cycle but closely correlated with the fraction of cells in the proliferative phase (fluorouracil, dactinomycin, cyclophosphamide).

Combination regimens of drugs have been used to kill maximal numbers of tumor cells. The use of surgery, radiotherapy, and chemotherapy is an important first stage in treatment, since the immune system is best suited to the elimination of small numbers of tumor cells rather than a large tumor mass. The presence of a large tumor indicates a failure in immunologic mechanisms.

An important feature of combination drug regimens is their suppressive effect on bone marrow cells and other rapidly dividing cells such as those of the gastrointestinal tract. Their immunosuppressive effect on lymphoid cells has led to a search for agents that stimulate the immune system.

IMMUNOTHERAPY

The methods used to stimulate the immune responses of patients with tumor are discussed under the headings of active, passive, and nonspecific immunotherapy.

Active Immunotherapy

Attempts are made to stimulate the patient's own immunity by one or more of the methods listed in Table 17–2. Animal experiments have confirmed the efficacy of many of these measures. Living tumor cells can be administered intradermally in small numbers that will not cause progressive tumor growth but will stimulate immunity. For obvious reasons, including ethical ones, living fresh tumor cells are generally not used in humans. Instead, tumor cells are administered after inactivation or, in many cases, modification. The various methods for modifying the tumor cells are directed toward increasing their immunogenicity, frequently by causing changes in membrane structure.

Another approach is to prepare subcellular components from the tumor cells and inject them into tumor-bearing subjects. These can be crude extracts of TAAs purified from membranes.

Finally, active immunity can be stimulated by the use of an adjuvant such as BCG. In humans, the available adjuvants are limited compared with the number that can be used in experimental animals.

The applications of these methods in humans have thus far been limited mainly to leukemias, malignant melanoma, and sarcomas. Remission maintenance in chronic granulocytic leukemia can be accomplished by the injection of inactivated tumor cells. This type of therapy has not yet been adequately studied in carcinomas and genitourinary tumors.

Passive Immunotherapy

This includes the administration of antitumor antisera, lymphocytes, or lymphocyte fractions to passively transfer immunity to tumor-bearing patients from normal subjects or subjects cured of cancer (Table 17–3).

A. Antitumor Antisera: Antisera prepared in animal species against various human tumors have generally yielded disappointing results when tested in tumor-bearing patients. They do not appear to be suitable for the elimination of a large tumor mass. The patient also tends to become sensitized to the foreign proteins in the antiserum, and this limits the treatment schedule.

Human plasma from 2 sources can be used to treat tumors. Normal subjects may be immunized with tumor extracts or TAAs and their plasma subsequently collected. Ethical considerations generally preclude widespread use of this approach. The other approach is to use plasma from patients who

Table 17–2. Active immunotherapy.

Whole tumor cell vaccines
  Living tumor cells
    Autologous
    Allogeneic
  Inactivated tumor cells
    Irradiation
    Mitomycin C
    Freezing and thawing
    Heat
  Modified tumor cells
    Carrier protein
    Chemical (iodoacetate)
    Neuraminidase
    Concanavalin A
Vaccines to subcellular components
  Crude cell extracts
  Isolated cell membranes
  Purified cell surface TAAs
Immune adjuvants
  Freund's adjuvant
  BCG
  MER (methanol-extractable residue of BCG)
  Corynebacterium parvum
  Levamisole

are in long-term remission or clinically "cured" (with or without treatment). Obviously, the plasma must be ABO compatible and negative for the serum hepatitis antigen (hepatitis B antigen). Careful serial monitoring of clinical and laboratory parameters is needed to make certain the treatment results in tumor destruction and not enhancement of tumor growth by blocking antibodies. A plasma donor must be selected who has an IgG "deblocking" antibody specific for the patient's tumor. If suitable donors are available, this type of therapy will undoubtedly be used more frequently in selected patients with genitourinary tumors.

Table 17–3. Passive immunotherapy.

Antitumor antisera
  Xenogeneic
  Allogeneic
Lymphocytes
  Xenogeneic
  Nonactivated lymphocytes
    Allogeneic cancer patients
    Normal identical twins or HLA-matched siblings
    Autologous lymphocytes grown in vitro
  Lymphocytes activated in vitro
    PHA
    TAAs
  Lymphocytes sensitized by cross transplantation of
    tumors
Extracts of sensitized cells
  Transfer factor
  Immune RNA

B. Lymphocytes: Lymphocytes from many sources have been administered to cancer patients to transfer passive immunity. This could circumvent the patient's own immunologic defects. Several studies have reported improvement in small numbers of selected patients with widespread disease.

1. Xenogeneic lymphocytes–The procedure consists of immunizing a selected animal against a particular tumor, harvesting lymphocytes from the animal after sensitization, and injecting these lymphocytes into the arterial blood supply of the patient's tumor. The pig has been selected as a suitable donor because it is easy to handle, is free of infection, and has a long continuous mesenteric lymph node chain. This approach was used in one study of 16 patients with advanced (stage T4) carcinoma of the bladder. Seven patients received significant benefit. The main disadvantages are that the foreign lymphocytes do not survive for long in the recipient and that readministration might cause serious anaphylactoid reactions.

2. Nonactivated lymphocytes–The donors of the lymphocytes may be patients with the same or another type of cancer, preferably in long-term remission. The main problem limiting the efficacy of this treatment is histoincompatibility. Genetic differences exist between lymphocytes of different subjects, and these lead to interactions between them and subsequent elimination of the foreign cells. This rejection phenomenon can be avoided by using lymphocytes from the patient's genetically identical normal twin. Most patients do not have an identical twin, however, and so a sibling must be found with the same HLA type as determined by serologic methods. Even if such a match is obtained, sensitization to the donor's cells usually occurs as a result of other genetic differences. A third method is to take the patient's own lymphocytes, grow them in vitro in short-term cultures, and then reinfuse them into the patient. The aim is to increase the cytotoxicity of the cells, eg, by removal of blocking factor. The results have been largely disappointing.

3. Activated lymphocytes–An alternative way of overcoming the problem of short survival of infused lymphocytes is to make them more effective in their active period by prior in vitro activation. Lymphocytes from any of the donors listed above can be stimulated in vitro by PHA or TAAs. The TAAs are usually provided by monolayers of long-term cultures of the specific tumor cells. After exposure, the lymphocytes are collected and infused into the patient.

4. Cross-transplantation of tumors–This complicated approach has certain problems, including ethical considerations. Patients with tumors are matched for tumor type and ABO and Rh groups. Tumor samples are exchanged between the patients and placed subcutaneously. After a period of time has elapsed to allow for "sensitization," plasma and leukocytes are exchanged between the patients. Reports of studies with small numbers of patients with advanced cancer have claimed complete regression in 3–5% and partial regression in 15–20%. The role of anti-HLA reactions and anti-TAA reactions in these cases has yet to be analyzed.

C. Extracts of Sensitized Lymphoid Cells: A persistent problem in long-term treatment with infusions of whole lymphocytes has been incompatibility from HLA and other antigens. Studies were therefore undertaken to eliminate tumors by using lymphoid cell extracts that do not have HLA specificity.

1. Transfer factor (TF)–TF is an extract of lymphocytes that transfers DHSR and other parameters of cellular immunity from a donor to a recipient. The mechanisms of this transfer are not yet clear. TF is a small dialyzable molecule with a molecular weight of about 7000. It is stable to repeated freezing and thawing, lyophilization, storage for over 5 years, and the action of DNase, RNase, and trypsin. It does not contain immunoglobulin or HLA antigens.

Administration of TF to a subject transfers DHSR in 1–7 days, and the effect may last up to a year. It also transfers the production of mediators of cellular immunity, eg, MIF. It does not lead to transfer of antigen-induced lymphocyte transformation. TF has been used with success in the clinical management of selected patients with defects in cellular immunity.

Trials are currently proceeding to assess the role of TF in certain types of cancer such as osteogenic sarcoma, malignant melanoma, and carcinoma of the breast. A major problem is the supply of donors, since TF must be obtained from the lymphocytes of human donors with proved cellular immunity against the specific type of tumor. Suitable donors are restricted to close household contacts who have demonstrable cellular immunity to the tumor, since "nonspecific" transfer factor is of no value and might even be deleterious. "Recovered" patients (free of disease for 5 years) almost always lack such immunity.

2. Immune RNA–The alternative approach is to prepare RNA extracts from lymphoid cells. This immune RNA can be prepared in animals, as it is not species-specific. One theoretic risk is the possibility of transferring RNA from oncogenic viruses in the immune RNA. Immune RNA has not yet been sufficiently tested in preliminary trials to ascertain whether it will have clinical applications.

Nonspecific Immunotherapy

This refers to use of the immune adjuvants listed in Table 17–2. The rationale appears to be general stimulation of the patient's immune system to control or eradicate a growing tumor. Animal studies have clearly confirmed the efficacy of some of these adjuvants under selected experimental conditions.

A. BCG: BCG can be administered to skin lesions such as metastatic nodules by direct injection or into noninvolved areas by scarification. Multiple BCG treatments are preferred for maximal effect. The status of the anergic patient is monitored by noting clinical progress, acquisition of DHSR to dinitrochlorobenzene (DNCB), and laboratory parameters such as tumor-specific lymphocyte cytotoxicity. Studies in malignant melanoma and other tumors have shown the immunopotentiating effect of BCG, and its clinical benefits were enhanced by simultaneous chemotherapy appropriate for disseminated solid tumors. One such study administered 6×10^8 viable units of fresh liquid Pasteur strain BCG by scarification on days 7, 12, and 17 of a course of chemotherapy. The regimen was repeated every 21 days if the patient's blood counts were acceptable. The appropriate chemoimmunotherapy courses for disseminated renal and bladder cancers have yet to be determined.

B. Levamisole: This drug is widely used in the treatment of roundworms and hookworms and is now known to stimulate a wide spectrum of immunologic functions. The administration of 150 mg of levamisole per day for 3 days to anergic patients with cancer restored DHSR. Patients were tested for DHSR to DNCB and PPD. Trials are in progress to see if levamisole, alone or in combination with antitumor chemotherapy, has any effect on the clinical course of disseminated malignant disease.

C. Interferon: This protein, a product of activated T cells (and perhaps other cells as well), inhibits viral replication. Trials with interferon preparations in human osteosarcoma (presumably a virally induced tumor) and other tumors had promising results, but interferon therapy must still be considered experimental.

CONCLUSION

There is a substantial body of evidence showing that some defect in immune surveillance permits the development of cancers or at least hampers their eradication. It is clear that various facets of a subject's immune response to a developing tumor play crucial roles in determining the outcome ("seed and soil" relationship).

The aim of immunotherapy is to stimulate the immune system to destroy an established tumor, prevent its recurrence, and prevent the development of a new tumor. Unfortunately, we cannot yet predict with certainty the effects of specific immunization in an individual patient. Both humoral and cellular immunity can be stimulated by a particular regimen, which may lead to enhancement of tumor growth by blocking antibodies rather than tumor destruction by cytotoxicity, or to the production of deblocking antibodies rather than blocking antibodies. Further studies with active immunization and passive transfer for genitourinary tumors are required. In the meantime, disseminated tumors are being studied with a combination of chemotherapy and immunotherapy with adjuvants (BCG or levamisole). If suitable donors were to become available, future therapy might involve plasma infusions with tumor-specific deblocking antibody and injection of tumor-specific TF. At present, these procedures remain experimental ones not generally available.

● ● ●

References

Allison AC: Immunological surveillance of tumours. *Cancer Immunol Immunother* 1977;**2**:151.

Bennington JL: Cancer of the kidney: Etiology, epidemiology and pathology. *Cancer* 1973;**32**:1017.

Bolhuits RLH: Cellular microcytotoxicity in a human bladder cancer system: Analysis of in vitro lymphocyte-mediated cytotoxicity against cultured target cells. *Cancer Immunol Immunother* 1977;**2**:245.

Dmochowski L & others: Virologic and immunologic studies of human prostatic carcinoma. *Cancer Chemother Rep* 1975;**59**:17.

Eidinger D: Immunotherapy for genitourinary cancer. Page 289 in: *Immunotherapy of Human Cancer*. Raven Press, 1978.

Elhilali MM & others: Critical evaluation of lymphocyte functions in urological cancer patients. *Cancer Res* 1976;**36**:132.

Elliott AY & others: Properties of cell lines established from transitional cell cancers of the human urinary tract. *Cancer Res* 1977;**37**:1279.

Fahey JL & others: Immunotherapy and human tumor immunology. *Ann Intern Med* 1976;**84**:107.

Frost P & others: Immunology of prostatic carcinoma: An overview. *Semin Oncol* 1976;**3**:107.

Golub SH & others: Correlation of in vivo and in vitro assays of immunocompetence in cancer patients. *Cancer Res* 1974;**34**:1833.

Grigor KM & others: Serum alpha-1-foetoprotein levels in 153 male patients with germ cell tumours. *Br J Cancer* 1977;**35**:52.

Guinan P & others: Immunologic considerations of carcinoma of the prostate. *Prog Exp Tumor Res* 1974;**19**:353.

Hamilton JM: Renal carcinogenesis. *Adv Cancer Res* 1975;**22**:1.

Hammarstrom S & others: K cell mediated lysis of cultured colon carcinoma and urinary bladder carcinoma cells induced by monospecific antisera against carcinoembryonic antigen (CEA) and two CEA-related normal glycoproteins. *Int J Cancer* 1977;**19**:756.

Hellstrom KE, Hellstrom I: The role of cell-mediated immunity in control and growth of tumors. Page 233 in: *Clinical Immunobiology*. Vol 2. Bach FH, Good RA (editors). Academic Press, 1974.

Herberman RB & others: Natural killer cells: Characteristics and regulation of activity. *Immunol Rev* 1979;**44**:43.

Holmes EJ: Crystalloids of prostatic carcinoma: Relationship to Bence-Jones crystals. *Cancer* 1977;**39**:2073.

Horton AW, Bingham EL: Risk of bladder tumors among benzidine workers and their serum properdin levels. *J Natl Cancer Inst* 1977;**58**:1225.

Javadpour N, Scardino PT: Recent advances in immunobiology of genitourinary cancer. *Urology* 1977;**9**:377.

Kjaer M, Christensen N: Ability of renal carcinoma tissue extract to induce leukocyte migration inhibition in patients with nonmetastatic renal carcinoma: Correlation with clinical and histopathological findings. *Cancer Immunol Immunother* 1977;**2**:41.

Laurence DJR, Neville AM: Foetal antigens and their role in the diagnosis and clinical management of human neoplasms: A review. *Br J Cancer* 1972;**26**:335.

Moore M, Robinson N: Cell-mediated cytotoxicity in carcinoma of the human urinary bladder. *Cancer Immunol Immunother* 1977;**2**:233.

Neville AM & others: Aspects of the structure and clinical role of the carcinoembryonic antigen (CEA) and related macromolecules with particular reference to urothelial carcinoma. *Br J Cancer* 1973;**28**(Suppl 1):198.

Ohtsuki Y & others: Virus-like particles in a case of human prostate carcinoma. *J Natl Cancer Inst* 1977;**58**:1493.

O'Toole C: A chromium isotope release assay for detecting cytotoxicity to human bladder carcinoma. *Int J Cancer* 1977;**19**:324.

O'Toole C, Unsgaard B: Clinical status and rate of recovery of blood lymphocyte levels after radiotherapy for bladder cancer. *Cancer Res* 1979;**39**:840.

Pape G & others: Characterization of cytolytic effector cells in peripheral blood of healthy individuals and cancer patients. 1. Surface markers and K cell activity after separation of B cells and lymphocytes and Fc-receptors by column fractionation. 2. Cytotoxicity to allogeneic or autochthonous tumor cells in tissue culture. *J Immunol* 1977;**118**:1919, 1925.

Perlmann P: Cellular immunity: Antibody-dependent cytotoxicity (K-cell activity). *Clin Immunobiol* 1976;**3**:107.

Prehn RT: Immunological surveillance: Pro and con. Page 191 in: *Clinical Immunobiology*. Vol 2. Bach FH, Good RA (editors). Academic Press, 1974.

Proceedings of the American Cancer Society's National Conference on Urologic Cancer, Los Angeles, April 4–6, 1979. *Cancer* 1980;**45**(Suppl 2):1735. [Entire issue.]

Salmon SE: Immunotherapy of cancer: Present status of trials in man. *Cancer Res* 1977;**37**:1245.

Schacter B & others: HLA-B7 association with low spontaneous cell-mediated cytotoxicity (Sp-CMC) to renal cell carcinoma cell lines. *Transplant Proc* 1977;**9**:1849.

Torti FM, Carter SK: The chemotherapy of prostatic adenocarcinoma. *Ann Intern Med* 1980;**92**:681.

Waksman BH: Immunoglobulins and lymphokines as mediators of inflammatory cell mobilization and target cell killing. *Cell Immunol* 1976;**27**:309.

Wall RL, Clausen KM: Carcinoma of the urinary bladder in patients receiving cyclophosphamide. *N Engl J Med* 1975;**293**:271.

Williams RD & others: Production of carcinoembryonic antigen by human prostate epithelial cells in vitro. *J Natl Cancer Inst* 1977;**58**:1115.

Wright GL & others: Isolation of a soluble tumor-associated antigen from human renal cell carcinoma by gradient acrylamide gel electrophoresis. *Cancer Res* 1977;**137**:4228.

Zeigel RF & others: A status report: Human prostatic carcinoma, with emphasis on potential for viral etiology. *Oncology* 1977;**34**:29.

Zimmerman R, Wahren B, Edsmyr F: Assessment of serial CEA determinations in urine of patients with bladder carcinoma. *Cancer* 1980;**46**:1802.

Tumors of the Genitourinary Tract | 18

Donald R. Smith, MD

Neoplasms of the prostate gland, bladder, and kidney are among the most common abnormal growths that afflict the human body. They are often silent, so that diagnosis may not be possible until quite late. Tumors of the testis are highly malignant and afflict young men. Neoplasms of the ureter, urethra, penis, scrotum, epididymis, and seminal vesicle are rare.

Adrenal tumors are discussed in Chapter 21.

MANIFESTATIONS OF UROGENITAL TRACT NEOPLASMS

Hematuria

Gross or microscopic hematuria is common when ulceration of a vesical, ureteral, or renal pelvic neoplasm occurs or when a renal parenchymal tumor breaks through the pelvic lining. It is seen often with benign prostatic hypertrophy, in which case bleeding is usually from dilated veins in the region of the bladder neck. Symptoms of prostatism plus hematuria do not, therefore, necessarily mean prostatic cancer; in fact, bleeding from the malignant prostate does not occur until the tumor grows through the mucosa of the bladder or urethra.

Pain

A. Renal Pain: Renal carcinoma can incite pain in the costovertebral angle (from renal capsular distention) if the tumor bleeds into its own substance. Renal and ureteral colic may occur if a blood clot or a mass of cells passes down the ureter. This type of pain is caused by hyperperistalsis of the pelvis or ureter.

B. Ureteral Pain: Ureteral tumors (rare) usually cause ureteral obstruction and occasionally colic.

C. Vesical Pain: Ulceration of a vesical tumor predisposes to midtract (bladder) infection, which causes symptoms of cystitis. With extravesical extension, constant suprapubic pain that increases with urination may be experienced.

D. Low Back Pain: Pain low in the back with radiation down one or both legs in an elderly man strongly suggests metastases to the pelvis and lumbar spine from cancer of the prostate. Local

(perineal) pain is seldom a symptom of neoplasia of the prostate.

E. Testicular Pain: Testicular neoplasm typically causes little or no pain, but if spontaneous bleeding occurs into the tumor it can mimic painful lesions (eg, torsion of the spermatic cord, acute epididymitis).

Dysuria

Hesitancy, impaired caliber and force of the urinary stream, and terminal dribbling are most commonly caused by benign prostatic hypertrophy, but cancer of the prostate produces the same difficulties. A tumor of the bladder on or near the internal vesical orifice may cause similar symptoms. Cystoscopy is therefore necessary in all cases of bladder neck obstruction.

Tumor of the urethra causes progressive diminution of the urinary stream. A palpable urethral mass suggests tumor or stricture. Biopsy may be needed for positive differentiation.

Skin Lesions

Tumors or ulcers of the penile and scrotal skin may be benign or malignant but can be caused by infection. If there is the slightest doubt, a specimen should be obtained for pathologic study.

Palpable Mass

A. Renal Mass: Renal tumors frequently present no symptoms other than the discovery of a tumor mass by the patient or the doctor. Neoplasms can be confused with simple renal cysts, polycystic kidney, hydronephrosis, cyst of the pancreas, or an enlarged spleen.

B. Abdominal Mass: An intra-abdominal mass near the umbilical region should suggest metastases to the preaortic lymph nodes from tumor of the testis. A suprapubic midline mass may represent a dilated (obstructed) bladder or may be caused by gastrointestinal or gynecologic tumor. It is not common for a vesical neoplasm to be palpable suprapubically except on bimanual (abdominorectal or abdominovaginal) examination under anesthesia.

C. Prostatic Mass: When the prostate is diffusely stony-hard and fixed, it is almost certainly cancerous, but a hard area in the gland may pose a

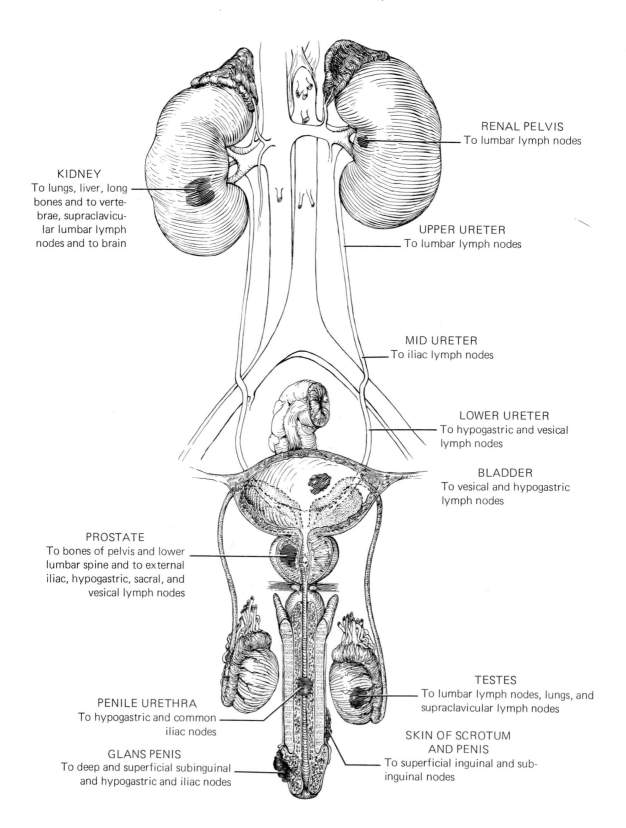

Figure 18–1. Sites of tumor origin and metastases in the male.

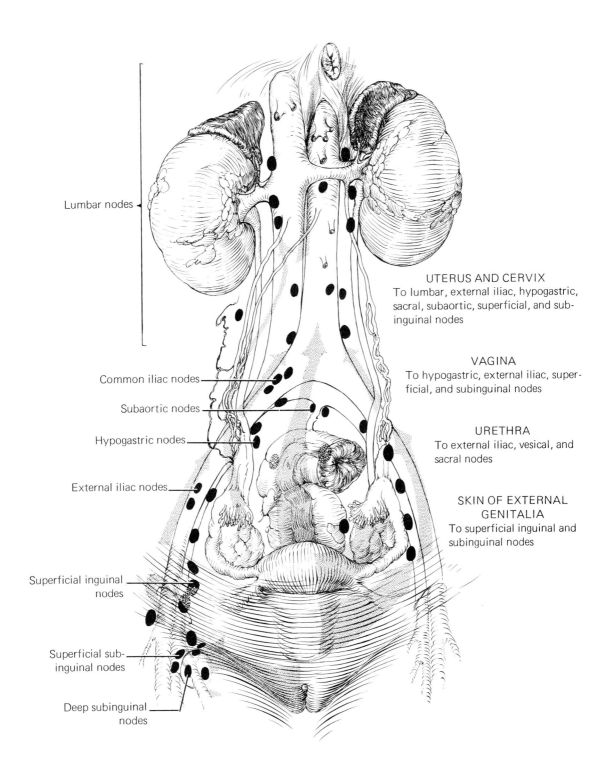

Figure 18–2. Sites and routes of tumor metastases in the female.

problem in differential diagnosis. The possibilities include early cancer, fibrosis from chronic infection, prostatic calculi, granulomatous prostatitis, and tuberculosis. At times the differentiation can only be made by biopsy.

D. Testicular Mass: A painless, firm testis should be regarded as neoplastic until proved otherwise. Gummas may cause induration, but they are rare; serologic tests will be helpful in differentiation.

Fever

Tumors of the kidney may excite no symptoms other than fever. Tumors of the urinary organs may also cause obstruction and be complicated by sepsis.

Hypertension

Hypertension is noted in about half of patients with Wilms's tumor, in some with renal adenocarcinoma, and in patients with juxtaglomerular adenomas.

Anemia

With advanced cancer in any urologic organ, anemia is to be expected even in the absence of blood loss. This is particularly true with prostatic malignancy, when bone marrow may be extensively involved.

Erythrocytosis

Erythrocytosis occurs in association with 4% of renal cancers, including Wilms's tumor. It may also be noted with certain benign renal lesions.

Urinalysis

In most individuals with vesical neoplasms and transitional cell tumors of the ureter or renal pelvis, the urinary sediment stained with methylene blue will reveal round (transitional) epithelial cells; therefore, the presence of these cells should always arouse suspicion of tumor. Cytologic examination of urine sediment using Papanicolaou technics is discussed in Chapter 5.

SYMPTOMS & SIGNS OF METASTASES

Tumors of the genitourinary tract often cause no local symptoms or definite signs. Clinical manifestations may arise only from metastases.

Central nervous system. Tumors of the kidney or prostate may metastasize to the central nervous system. The first symptoms may therefore be neurologic.

Lungs. Tumors of the kidney, prostate, and testis often spread to the lungs. Pleuritic pain may suggest secondary pleural involvement.

Liver. Renal tumors frequently metastasize to the liver, which then becomes enlarged and nodu-

lar. If compression of the common duct occurs, jaundice will be noted.

Lymph nodes. Enlargement of the left supraclavicular lymph nodes may be the only finding in cancer of the kidney or testis. Palpable para-aortic abdominal masses in a young man may mean tumor of the testis. Edema of one or both legs may develop from compression of the iliac vessels by masses of lymph nodes containing tumor cells from cancer of the prostate or bladder (Figs 18–1 and 18–2).

Bones. Metastasis to the skeletal system is most common from cancer of the prostate and kidney. This may cause pain in the bone, spontaneous fracture, or neurologic manifestations due to metastasis to the spine.

TUMORS OF THE RENAL PARENCHYMA

BENIGN TUMORS

From the clinical standpoint, benign tumors of the kidney are rare. However, small adenomas are often seen at autopsy. Their cells resemble those of the adult renal tubule. There is evidence that these adenomas are the source of the carcinomas of the renal parenchyma that are seen quite frequently in the adult.

Benign tumors of the renal parenchyma include adenomas, hemangiomas, carcinoid tumors, fibromas, endometriosis, lipomas, myomas, and neurofibromas. Most of these are 1–2 cm in diameter.

Large tumors of this type do occur with signs and symptoms similar to those described under carcinoma; it is almost impossible to differentiate these from the malignant variety by urographic means. Therefore, the kidney must be removed.

Angiomyolipoma (Hamartoma)

This tumor appears in 3 forms: (1) unilateral single tumor without stigmas of tuberous sclerosis; (2) multiple and bilateral hamartomas in patients showing widespread connective tissue defects; and (3) so-called fetal hamartoma or mesoblastic nephroma.

A. Angiomyolipoma, Single and Unilateral: These benign tumors are made up of fat, smooth muscle, and blood vessels. Grossly, the tumor resembles adenocarcinoma of the kidney, from which it must be differentiated. Most occur in women between ages 40 and 60 years. The first symptoms are often due to sudden spontaneous perirenal hemorrhage (Stavorovsky & others, 1979). The patient usually develops severe flank pain, an enlarging flank mass, and, in many cases, gross hematuria. Shock due to exsanguination is common.

On the plain abdominal film, areas of lucency

may be noted in the tumor, which displaces and distorts calices. Evidence of a large perinephric mass (blood) may be noted. Infusion urography shows increased vascularity, yet there are areas of lucency in the tumor if the content of fat is significant. These films ordinarily are suggestive of hamartoma but not diagnostic. CT scanning will show multiple quite lucent areas (more so than with cyst) representing fat. Enhancement of the nephrogram will show no increase in their density. The caliceal deformity will be evident. This technic would appear to be diagnostic. Selective renal angiography shows multiple small aneurysms and, in the early phase, a fine network of tortuous vessels. Areas of lucency are seen. Although it had been reported that renal vessels in patients with hamartoma failed to go into spasm after infusion of epinephrine (thus mimicking adenocarcinoma), Jander & Tonkin (1979) did observe spasm in their 6 cases. On late films, little venous and sinusoidal vascularity is noted. This is in contradistinction to the findings with cancer. Whorls of contrast material similar to those seen in uterine myomas are observed. Angiography is not definitive, and ultrasonography and CT scan may therefore be needed to enhance the diagnosis by more clearly demonstrating the presence of fat (Bush, Freeny, & Orme, 1979).

In the absence of bilateral disease or the stigmas of tuberous sclerosis, immediate nephrectomy may be necessary, but selective renal arterial embolization should be considered (Moorehead, Fritzsche, & Hadley, 1977).

B. Tuberous Sclerosis: This syndrome is characterized by the presence of multiple and bilateral renal hamartomas, miscellaneous cutaneous lesions including "adenoma sebaceum," mental retardation, epilepsy, tumorlike swellings of the retina, and various mixed tumors in the brain, heart, and lungs.

There are usually no symptoms directly related to the kidneys. The presence of other signs of tuberous sclerosis may lead to excretory urography or infusion nephrotomography, which reveals large kidneys containing many lucent areas, thus mimicking polycystic renal disease. CT scan, sonography (see Angiomyolipoma, above), or angiography will, however, show that the areas of lucency are compatible with fat rather than cyst. Angiography will reveal the vascular nature of these lesions.

Surgical treatment should be conservative. If spontaneous bleeding occurs, watchful waiting and blood replacement may be the treatment of choice in the hope that the hemorrhage will cease. If it does not, either renal artery embolization or partial nephrectomy should be done if feasible.

With the involvement of so many organ systems, the prognosis is guarded. Progression of growth of the renal lesions may lead to renal insufficiency.

C. Renal Fetal Hamartoma, Mesoblastic Nephroma: These benign tumors are seen in the first

few weeks or months of life. Until recently, they were diagnosed as Wilms's tumors. The mass consists of fetal mesenchymal tissue, largely hamartomatous and leiomyomatous elements. Therefore, they have also been considered fibrosarcomas and leiomyomas (Berdon, Wigger, & Baker, 1973).

The tumor presents as a mass in the flank. Excretory urograms show changes typical of a space-occupying lesion. Angiography may fail to differentiate these tumors from Wilms's tumors, although areas of lucency due to fat may be noted. Some neovascularity may be seen. If the angiogram does not reveal the fat content, a CT scan or sonography may do so.

Since Wilms's tumor is very rarely present at birth, fetal hamartoma should be suspected in this age group. Preoperative radiotherapy should not be given without a positive biopsy diagnosis. Treatment for these benign tumors consists of nephrectomy only.

Juxtaglomerular Cell Adenoma (Hemangiopericytoma)

These relatively rare, small, benign tumors secrete renin and therefore cause severe hypertension. Urinary aldosterone levels are elevated; plasma renin, particularly from the renal vein of the involved kidney, is elevated, and hypokalemia is found. The lesion may be depicted on selective renal angiograms. The effect of nephrectomy is dramatic (Phillips & Mukherjee, 1972).

Oncocytoma

Renal oncocytoma is a benign tumor heretofore confused with adenocarcinoma. About 30 cases have been reported (Morales, Wasan, & Bryniak, 1980). Reappraisal of several series of adenocarcinomas revealed that about 5% were actually oncocytomas. The tumor is well circumscribed and uniformly tannish-brown, with a central scar devoid of necrosis or hemorrhage (Yu & others, 1980). It is thought to arise from cells of the proximal tubules. Angiography reveals a typical "spoke wheel" pattern (Ambos & others, 1978). If the diagnosis can be established at operation, simple enucleation should be considered rather than nephrectomy.

ADENOCARCINOMA (Grawitz's Tumor; Hypernephroma)

About four-fifths of renal neoplasms are adenocarcinomas, and two-thirds of these occur in men. More than 150 cases have been reported in children (Abrams & others, 1979). Because adenocarcinomas produce symptoms relatively late, the prognosis is only fair.

Etiology

There has been considerable disagreement

over the origin of adenocarcinomas. Grawitz thought they arose from intrarenal adrenal rests, and the term "hypernephroma" was coined to describe them. The leading opinion now, however, is that they arise from cells of the renal tubules or from the benign adenomas. This theory is based on the histologic findings. Some of these tumors secrete hormones. Among those reported are parathyroid-like hormone, gonadotropins, ACTH, erythropoietin, placental lactogen, prolactin, enteroglucagon, insulinlike activity, and prostaglandin A, an antihypertensive substance. Altaffer & Chenault (1979) suggest, therefore, that tests for all of these substances be done when renal adenocarcinoma is suspected.

Pathogenesis & Pathology

Adenocarcinoma usually arises in one of the renal poles. As the neoplasm expands, it compresses adjacent renal tissue and displaces calices, blood vessels, and the pelvis, which then become distorted and tend to surround the mass. It is this characteristic that leads to urographic diagnosis. Multiple adenocarcinomas are often found in patients suffering from Lindau's disease (Fill, Lamiell, & Polk, 1979) (see Chapter 22).

The renal veins and even the vena cava are frequently invaded. This may be associated with the nephrotic syndrome or hepatic dysfunction. At times a column of tumor extends into the right heart. Occlusion of the renal vein may cause marked dilatation of the perirenal vessels and varicocele. As enlargement increases, intraperitoneal organs may be displaced (eg, stomach, intestines, spleen) or the diaphragm elevated. The tumor may invade adjacent muscle or organs (eg, duodenum, diaphragm).

Adenocarcinoma usually has a well-defined fibrous capsule. On section, the tumor is yellow and often contains zones of hemorrhage or necrosis. It produces a definite expansion of the kidney. Calcification may develop and may be visible on x-ray film.

Microscopically, varying patterns of cells may be seen even in the same tumor. In general, the cells resemble renal tubule cells and have small eccentric nuclei and an abundant clear cytoplasm. At times the cytoplasm may be more opaque and granular. A papillary or even anaplastic pattern may be seen. Tumors with well-differentiated clear cells seem to offer the best prognosis.

Most visceral metastases occur by way of the bloodstream. The liver, lungs, contralateral kidney, and long bones (and occasionally the brain and adrenal glands) may be affected. Lumbar lymph nodes about the renal pedicle may become involved, and enlarged left supraclavicular nodes are occasionally seen. The kidney is involved secondarily by metastases from other organs in 7.6% of cases. The bronchus is the most common primary site.

Rarely, metastases (usually pulmonary) may regress following nephrectomy, but this is usually only temporary (Freed, Halperin, & Gordon, 1977).

Staging of the Tumor

While a number of classifications paralleling the prognosis have been offered, the one suggested by Robson, Churchill, & Anderson (1969) seems most useful.

Stage A: Tumor confined to kidney.
Stage B: Perirenal spread confined within the perirenal fascia.
Stage C: Local spread.
  1. Renal vein or inferior vena cava.
  2. Local lymph nodes.
  3. Both vascular and lymphatic involvement.
Stage D: Advanced disease.
  1. Adjacent organs other than the adrenals.
  2. Distant metastases.

While the stage can often be judged only at the operating table, the use of sonography, CT scanning, and measurement of levels of tumor markers has significantly increased the accuracy of preoperative staging.

Futter, Collins, & Walsh (1979), and Bracken & Jonsson (1979) find that angiography is of little help in staging these tumors.

Clinical Findings (Boxer & others, 1979)

A. Symptoms: Gross total hematuria is the most common symptom and is usually not accompanied by pain. It occurs in two-thirds of patients. Pain may be the initial symptom but is usually a late manifestation. It may be of the dull type felt in the back, resulting from back pressure from ureteral compression, perirenal extension, or hemorrhage into the substance of the kidney; or it may be colicky if a clot or mass of tumor cells passes down the ureter.

Occasionally a patient may discover a mass in the flank in the absence of other symptoms. Gastrointestinal complaints resembling the syndromes of peptic ulcer or gallbladder disease may be the only subjective manifestations. These are caused by reflex action or by displacement or invasion of intraperitoneal organs. Unexplained low-grade fever may be the only symptom.

Symptoms from metastases may also occur as the first manifestations of renal tumor. These include unexplained loss of weight, increasing weakness, and anemia. Bone pain, spontaneous fracture, pulmonary difficulties, or a mass in the left side of the neck (Virchow's nodes) may be the presenting complaint.

B. Signs: A mass is often discovered in the flank. It must be pointed out, however, that the kidneys lie rather high, particularly on the left side. In an obese or muscular person, considerable enlargement can be present and still defy detection. Fixation may mean local invasion. Involvement of the vena cava by tumor or thrombosis may cause the development of dilated veins on the abdominal wall. An acute hydrocele or varicocele may develop as a rare and late sign if the spermatic vein is occluded. This is most apt to occur on the left side because this vein drains into the left renal vein.

Arteriovenous fistulas are occasionally observed in association with renal adenocarcinoma. This is suggested in the presence of cardiomegaly, diastolic hypertension, and a systolic murmur and bruit over the mass. The diagnosis is made on angiography.

A few cases of hypertension caused by renin secretion by the tumor have been reported (Hollifield & others, 1975). The picture is that of secondary aldosteronism.

Metastatic signs are varied and may be the presenting manifestations of the illness. A palpable mass in the left supraclavicular region may mean metastases to lymph nodes. Physical examination of the lung fields may reveal no pathologic changes even though metastases are present. Tenderness or even a palpable mass may be found over bone involved by tumor. Edema of the legs may be secondary to neoplastic involvement of the vena cava. The liver is a common site of metastases, in which case it may be enlarged and nodular. Ascites may be found. Loss of weight may be marked.

C. Laboratory Findings: Gross or microscopic hematuria is the cardinal finding, and even a few red cells must be explained. Erythrocytosis with an increased plasma erythropoietin level occurs in 3–4% of patients. Anemia may be present in advanced disease. Total renal function is usually not impaired, for even the involved kidney retains some function and bilateral renal cancer is rare. The sedimentation rate is usually accelerated. Hypercalcemia with secondary effects on muscle, heart, and brain may be noted; parathyroid hormone can be extracted from the tumor. A few tumors have been found that secrete ACTH. This has led to a cushingoid appearance. Elaboration of gonadotropins causes gynecomastia in the male. One tumor was found to elaborate prostaglandin A. Only after the tumor was removed did hypertension develop.

The presence of a hypernephroma may cause hepatic insufficiency as shown by tests of liver function. Removal of the tumor causes the test results to return to normal (Boxer & others, 1979).

D. X-Ray Findings (Clayman, Williams, & Fraley, 1979): A plain film of the abdomen often shows an enlarged kidney; a definite bulge of its contour is significant. The incidence of cystic or curvilinear calcification is 7% (Sniderman & others, 1979). The psoas margin may be obscured if a solid tumor overlies the muscle. If the tumor is a cyst, the psoas margin may be visible through it. The renal shadow may be displaced in any direction, depending upon the location of the tumor. A low left kidney

in particular must not be ignored. Osteolytic metastases may be noted on bone x-rays.

Excretory urograms usually show a filling defect caused by a space-occupying lesion (Fig 18–3). Calices are bent, elongated, or otherwise distorted by the enlarging tumor. On rare occasion the ureter may be compressed, and hydronephrosis may develop. If considerable renal tissue is destroyed by tumor, visualization may be poor. If the renal vein is involved, no excretion of dye may be seen; this is a bad prognostic sign.

Infusion angionephrotomograms almost always reveal increased opacification of a tumor, because of its increased vascularity. This technic may also show separation of the renal capsule from the parenchyma, which might be caused by bleeding from a small cortical tumor. Selective angiography will make the diagnosis.

Renal angiography, particularly the selective type, produces a dense renal shadow owing to the presence of contrast material in the renal vessels and tubules and therefore may reveal a bulge of the renal outline, indicating tumor. Late films may show pooling of the opaque material within the tumor, which occurs because of the tumor's great vascularity (Fig 18–3). A cyst will cast no shadow at all.

Some tumors are relatively avascular, which makes diagnosis doubtful. The infusion of epinephrine just before the radiopaque medium is instilled will cause marked spasm of the arterioles of normal renal tissue but not of the vessels in a tumor. The most striking feature is the typical neovascularity. In some cases, numerous arteriovenous aneurysms cause early opacification of the renal vein, which leads to diastolic hypertension and an audible bruit heard over the kidney.

Hellekant & Nyman (1979) recommend that at the time of renal angiography, celiac angiograms should be done also. This is apt to reveal previously unrecognized metastases (eg, to the liver).

Inferior venacavography or, better, selective renal phlebography may show tumor extension into the renal vein or vena cava. Selective renal phlebography may also help in the definitive diagnosis of a poorly vascularized tumor (Braedel & others, 1979).

A chest film may demonstrate the typical nodular metastases (Fig 18–4). A gastrointestinal series or barium enema may reveal displacement of the stomach or bowel if the renal mass is large.

Osteographic survey, particularly of the long bones, may demonstrate osteolytic metastases or pathologic fracture.

E. Ultrasonography: B-scan sonography differentiates between cyst and tumor in 95% of cases (Clayman, Williams, & Fraley, 1979).

F. Computed Tomography (CT Scan): Renal tumor has a density comparable to that of the kidney (Fig 18–5). Following the intravenous injection of a bolus of radiopaque fluid, the normal parenchyma

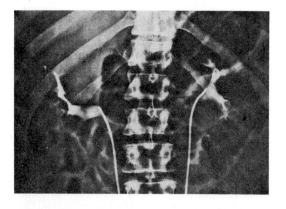
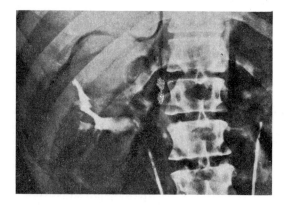
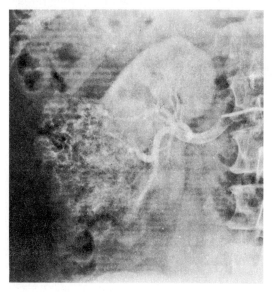
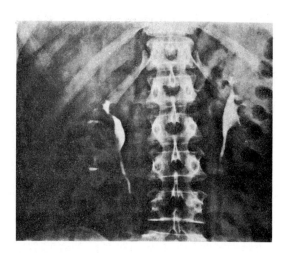

Figure 18–3. Adenocarcinoma of the kidney. *Above left:* Retrograde urogram showing lateral displacement of upper pole of right kidney and elongation and distortion of upper calices (carcinoma). Left urogram normal. *Above right:* Same patient. Retrograde urogram combined with pneumogram shows extent of mass and its relation to calices. Normal right adrenal. *Below left:* Selective renal angiogram showing marked neovascularity of mass in lower portion of right kidney typical of malignant tumor. *Below right:* Excretory urogram. Distortion of the pelvis, middle and lower calices of right kidney. Space-occupying lesion (adenocarcinoma). The left kidney is normal.

becomes quite dense, whereas only a slight increase in density is noted in the tumor.

G. Isotope Scanning: A rectilinear scan, using ^{203}Hg, will reveal a "cold" area where functioning parenchyma has been replaced by a mass, which is a finding with cyst, also. The gamma camera will show a negative shadow with both ^{203}Hg and ^{131}I, but with ^{99m}Tc, which portrays the vasculature of the kidney, the tumor area will show normal or increased perfusion (Fig 8–2), whereas a cyst will show none. A bone scan may reveal osseous metastases (Fig 8–9).

Preoperative liver scanning should also be performed, since metastasis to this site is common. Raghavaiah (1978) has pointed out, however, that false-positive scans may be caused by extrinsic compression by the primary tumor.

H. Percutaneous Needle Puncture: If the differential diagnosis between cyst and tumor is still equivocal, a needle can be passed into the mass under fluoroscopic or ultrasonic control. Tumor cell-free clear fluid implies a cyst; bloody fluid suggests tumor. The needle may deliver a piece of tissue that can be subjected to pathologic examination.

I. Instrumental Examination: If the patient has gross hematuria when first seen, immediate cystoscopy is indicated to demonstrate its source. Postponing this procedure almost guarantees the loss of this valuable information, since renal tumors tend to bleed intermittently. Retrograde urograms are rarely necessary (Fig 18–3).

J. Urinary Cytology: The Papanicolaou technic has been applied to the urinary sediment but

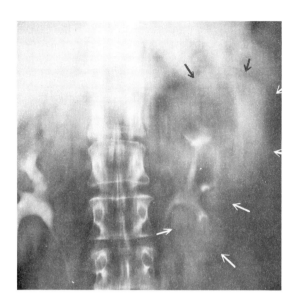
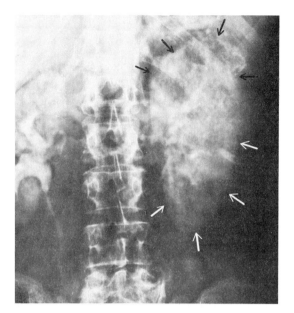
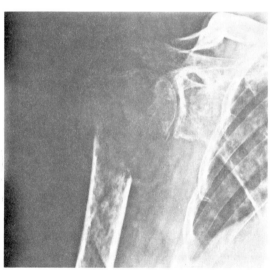
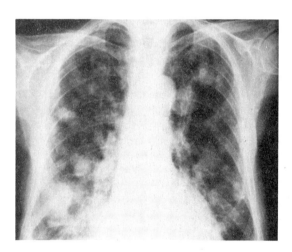

Figure 18–4. Adenocarcinoma of the kidney. *Above left:* Excretory urogram with tomography showing marked expansion of upper pole and elongated upper calix, left kidney. *Above right:* Infusion urogram, same patient, showing pooling of radiopaque fluid in cancer of upper pole, left kidney. *Below left:* Osteolytic metastases to humerus. *Below right:* Metastases to lung. Note typical "cannonball" lesions.

rarely proves helpful with adenocarcinoma.

K. Tumor Markers: At present, tumor markers for renal adenocarcinoma are not nearly as definitive as those for vesical, prostatic, and testicular neoplasms. Sufrin & others (1977) tested for plasma renin and serum erythropoietin in 57 patients with adenocarcinoma. Elevation of renin was found in 37%. These patients proved to have tumors both of high grade and advanced stage. Thus, a positive test was of prognostic significance. Elevated serum erythropoietin was present in 63% of the series, but this had no prognostic usefulness.

Both tests have a significant number of false negatives.

The serum polyamines may be increased also, but they are not specific for this tumor. Urinary levels of the polyamines, as in some nonurologic tumors, may be increased in these patients, and if so, may prove valuable in following response to treatment.

Plasma or urinary carcinoembryonic antigen is present in perhaps half of these tumors, but it is not specific for renal adenocarcinoma. However, if it is present before treatment has been started, the

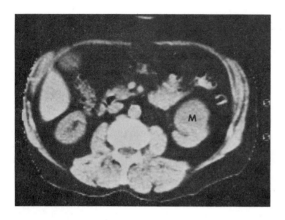

Figure 18–5. Left renal carcinoma. Mass (M) arising from anterior aspect of left kidney has a density similar to that of adjacent normal renal parenchyma, indicating it is not a simple cyst.

levels of carcinoembryonic antigen will reflect the response to therapy.

Differential Diagnosis

Hydronephrotic kidney may be accompanied by pain, a mass, and hematuria. Gross bleeding, however, is rare. Urography will establish the diagnosis.

Polycystic kidney disease may also present with hematuria and a renal mass, but total renal function is usually impaired even though only one kidney is large enough to be felt. Hypertension is common with polycystic disease. Renal angiography, ultrasonography, CT scan, or a technetium scan should differentiate the 2 lesions.

Simple cyst of the kidney may cause flank pain and may be palpable, but gross or even microscopic hematuria is unusual. Tumors are often associated with an increased sedimentation rate; cysts are not. Tumor and cyst both occupy space in the kidney, and so urograms of both may be similar. Cysts tend to be more extrinsic; solid tumors are prone to occupy the deeper renal tissues. If the renal mass overlies the psoas, the muscle is apt to be obliterated by a solid tumor but may be visible through a cyst. Infusion nephrotomograms (Fig 6–5) or angiograms (Fig 18–3) will usually make the differentiation: a cyst fails to opacify; a tumor becomes unusually dense.

CT scans may be the most definitive diagnostic step. A cyst is usually quite round and has a thin capsule that is well demarcated from the renal parenchyma. A tumor shows a density comparable to that of the kidney itself. It is poorly demarcated from the kidney (Fig 22–4). Following density enhancement with an intravenous injection of radiopaque solution, a cyst does not opacify. A tumor does to a small degree. Evidence of metastases to regional lymph nodes or liver may be noted (Fig 18–6).

If the radiographic diagnosis is cyst, this can be further confirmed if necessary by passing a needle into the mass. The fluid recovered should be analyzed for fat, whose absence confirms the diagnosis of cyst, and subjected to cytologic examination. Radiopaque fluid is then introduced and appropriate films taken (Fig 22–5). Differentiation may be possible only at surgery (Murphy & Marshall, 1980).

Renal tuberculosis can cause renal pain, a palpable mass, and gross hematuria, but symptoms of vesical irritability and pyuria are usually present. Acid-fast bacteria can almost always be demonstrated by culture. Cystoscopy may reveal tuberculous cystitis, and urograms should make an unequivocal differentiation.

A stone in the kidney or ureter can cause renal pain and hematuria, but the pain is often more acute. Roentgenograms should differentiate between stone and tumor.

Ureteral or renal pelvic tumor may mimic renal tumor, causing renal pain and often a palpable hydronephrotic kidney. Gross hematuria may also be present. Urinary cytology and urography will clearly differentiate the two.

Adrenal or other extrarenal tumor (pancreatic pseudocyst) may present a palpable mass (either the tumor or a displaced kidney), but hematuria and pain are unusual. Most adrenal tumors are functional and cause definite signs and symptoms (eg, hirsutism, amenorrhea, obesity). Pheochromocytoma and neuroblastoma elaborate increased amounts of vanilmandelic acid in the urine. Urography and other studies will show a mass displacing a kidney whose calices are normal.

Rheumatoid granuloma may present with gross hematuria. Excretory urograms reveal a space-occupying lesion that is shown to be avascular by angiography. The patient will have a high serum titer for rheumatoid arthritis (Ziegler & Albukerk, 1978).

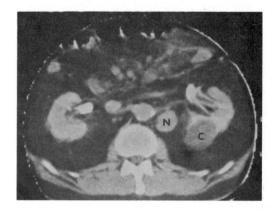

Figure 18–6. Enlarged retroperitoneal lymph node. Single enlarged lymph node (N) lies between left kidney, left psoas muscle, and the aorta. Left renal cyst (C) is also present. Lateral deviation of left ureter was present on urogram.

Chronic pyelonephritis often causes renal pain and hematuria, but such kidneys are not enlarged. Symptoms of cystitis are often noted. The finding of pus and bacteria in the urine is suggestive. Urography should establish the diagnosis.

The xanthogranulomatous pyelonephritic kidney usually does not show function on excretory urograms, but retrograde urograms reveal a distorted caliceal system not unlike that seen with tumor. Angiography will usually make the differentiation. Ballesteros, Faus, & Gironella (1980) were able to diagnose xanthogranulomatosis by finding foam cells in a spun specimen of urine prepared for cytologic examination.

Tumors of the bladder usually cause hematuria. Excretory urograms will show an absence of caliceal distortion, although hydronephrosis may be present if a ureteral orifice is partially occluded. The cystogram or urogram may show a defect consistent with tumor (Fig 18–12). Cystoscopy will reveal the growth.

A kidney deformed by scarring due to infarction or multiple attacks of acute pyelonephritis may develop focal areas of renal compensatory hypertrophy that, with expansion, may deform the calices, thus simulating tumor (Fig 18–7) (Carty, Short, & O'Connell, 1975). A similar picture may be caused by a very large column of Bertin that may resemble a tumor on excretory urography. An infusion nephrotomogram using abdominal compression will show the mass to be more dense than the surrounding parenchyma. It extends to the capsule and is seen between the upper and middle calices. Angiography will fail to show the neovascularity of cancer.

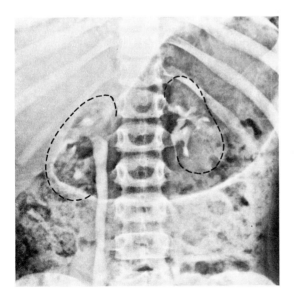

Figure 18–7. Renal pseudotumor. Bilateral healed pyelonephritis secondary to vesicoureteral reflux. Localized compensatory hypertrophy in lower pole of left kidney displaces calices, suggesting presence of space-occupying lesion.

Renal lymphoma or Hodgkin's disease may lead to deformity of the calices. The tumors are usually bilateral and multiple. Evidence of lymphoma elsewhere is helpful in differential diagnosis. Angiography may be helpful, but Hodgkin's tumor may be very vascular.

Complications

The complications of adenocarcinomas are largely related to local invasion or distant metastases. A few patients develop hydronephrosis from ureteral compression, hypertension from interference with the blood supply to the organ, or arteriovenous fistula. Occlusion of the renal vein by tumor may cause findings compatible with the nephrotic syndrome. Rarely, hematuria may be severe enough that death from exsanguination is a threat.

Treatment

A. Radical Nephrectomy: If there are no demonstrable metastases, radical nephrectomy, including removal of the perirenal fat and regional lymph nodes, should be performed. If extension of the tumor into the renal vein or vena cava has been demonstrated or is found at surgery, the vessels should be opened and the tumor removed (Clayman, Gonzales, & Fraley, 1980; Madayag & others, 1979; Cummings & others, 1979). Following nephrectomy, in the absence of metastases, levels of erythropoietin, renin, and carcinoembryonic antigen will fall to normal. Hepatic function will improve, hypercalcemia will be less severe, and hypertension may be relieved. If metastases develop, the levels of tumor markers will again rise. In a few patients, pulmonary metastases may regress following nephrectomy, but they usually reappear in a few months.

Many authors now recommend transcatheter renal arterial embolization 1–7 days before nephrectomy, which facilitates the procedure. Blood loss is decreased, and the secondary perinephric edema simplifies the dissection. Tumor cell dissemination during the operation may be prevented. The only sequelae are flank pain, fever, and nausea for 1–2 days (Mee & Heap, 1978; Singsass, Chopp, & Mendez, 1979).

Renal arterial occlusion by embolization or balloon should also be considered if life-threatening gross hematuria persists.

In the case of bilateral tumors or cancer in a solitary kidney, partial nephrectomy should be considered (Schiff, Bagley, & Lytton, 1979; Stigsson, Ekelund, & Karp, 1979). Graham & Glenn (1979) suggest simple enucleation of the tumors in such cases. They report survivals of up to 5 years.

B. X-Ray Therapy: Adenocarcinomas of the kidney and their metastases are usually radioresistant. Most authorities feel that x-ray therapy is therefore not indicated either preoperatively or postoperatively, but a few authors disagree (Rubin & others, 1975).

C. Chemotherapy: See p 333.

D. Follow-up Care: This includes abdominal palpation for tumor in the renal bed or an enlarging nodular liver, and a chest film. The patient should undergo abdominal angiography and bone scan yearly (Freed, Feldman, & Sprayragen, 1977). CT scan or sonography may reveal recurrence in the tumor bed or metastases to the liver (Bernardino, Green, & Goldstein, 1978; Bernardino & others, 1979).

Prognosis

Patel & Lavengood (1978) observed that the 5-year control rate with simple nephrectomy was 32%, whereas with radical removal it was 67%. Of the patients with metastases, 74% were dead within 1 year and 96% within 3 years. Radiotherapy was not effective. Recent improvements in chemotherapy may prove to be beneficial. The outlook for children is more encouraging.

NEPHROBLASTOMA
(Embryoma, Wilms's Tumor, Adenomyosarcoma)

Nephroblastoma of the kidney is a highly malignant mixed tumor. It is almost exclusively a disease of children under age 4 years; in this age group, it is third in incidence only to brain tumors and leukemia. It is the most common abdominal neoplasm in children. Ten percent are bilateral. The incidence is 1:10,000 live births. The literature contains reports of 167 adults with nephroblastoma (Babaian, Skinner, & Waisman, 1980).

Etiology

This tumor is considered by most investigators to be congenital and to arise from embryonal cells trapped in the kidney. About 6% are clinically present at birth, and these, if large, may cause dystocia.

Pathogenesis & Pathology

Wilms's tumor may arise in any portion of the kidney. It usually becomes quite large before it is discovered. Pain is not common. Hematuria is rare and late, for this tumor seldom breaks through the renal pelvis.

The tumor is usually large, pale, and lobulated. The surface of the kidney is usually covered by large, thin-walled veins. On cut section, the tissue is usually yellow or white and heterogeneous; hemorrhagic and cystic areas are often found. Microscopically, the major tissues are of connective tissue origin: muscle, cartilage, bone, and myxomatous or lipomatous tissue. The epithelial structures may be undifferentiated or may resemble renal tubules or even glomeruli. The term "adenomyosarcoma" has therefore been used to de-

scribe these tumors. Possibly half of them show abnormal chromosome sets.

If preoperative x-ray treatment has been given, the tumor may be small; in fact, the kidney may be only slightly enlarged. The entire tumor may be necrotic and hemorrhagic, although viable sarcoma and carcinoma cells are usually found microscopically. These primitive cells are quite radiosensitive.

The usual route of metastasis is through the bloodstream; the lungs, liver, and brain are most commonly involved. Regional lumbar lymph nodes may be affected.

The National Wilms's Tumor Study Group has devised the following clinical staging:

> *Stage A:* Tumor limited to the kidney, complete resection.
> *Stage B:* Tumor extending beyond the kidney, complete resection.
> *Stage C:* Residual tumor left in the abdomen.
> *Stage D:* Hematogenous metastases.
> *Stage E:* Bilateral tumors.

Clinical Findings

A. Symptoms: The most common symptom is a palpable mass in the flank, usually discovered by the child's parents. Rarely, pain may be experienced from local invasion or ureteral compression (hydronephrosis). Other symptoms include loss of weight, anorexia or vomiting from displacement or invasion of the enteric tract, and hematuria (unusual).

B. Signs: A palpable mass in the flank of a child under age 6 must be regarded as Wilms's tumor (or neuroblastoma of the adrenal) until proved otherwise. The mass does not transilluminate. An enlarged nodular liver strongly suggests that metastasis from the renal tumor has occurred. The lungs usually reveal no abnormal physical signs even though they contain metastases. Hypertension is found in 50% of children with embryoma of the kidney. Evidence suggests that these tumors secrete renin (Ganguly & others, 1973). The hypertension is usually relieved by removal of the involved organ. Weight loss is a prominent feature of the late stage of the disease. Hypospadias and cryptorchidism are not unusual. In 1–2% of cases, congenital aniridia has been observed. This is often associated with microcephaly, cataracts, glaucoma, and mental retardation. Hemihypertrophy is occasionally seen.

C. Laboratory Findings: Anemia may be present. Urinalysis is usually normal; the finding of red cells is unusual. Tests of total renal function are usually normal, for even the involved kidney usually retains some function.

D. X-Ray Findings:

1. Simple technics–A greatly enlarged renal shadow is usually evident on a plain film of the abdomen. There may be a rim of calcification around the periphery of the tumor. The bowel, as

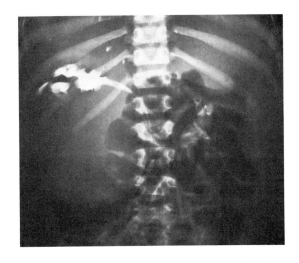

Figure 18–8. Wilms's tumor. *Left:* Excretory urogram showing large globular mass in right upper quadrant, with displacement and distortion of calices. Upper right ureter displaced over spine. *Below:* Bilateral embryomas as shown on angiography. *Left:* Early phase of left selective angiogram showing arcing of major renal arteries, vascular pooling, and typical tumor vessels. *Right:* Late phase of right selective angiogram showing vascular mass in upper pole.

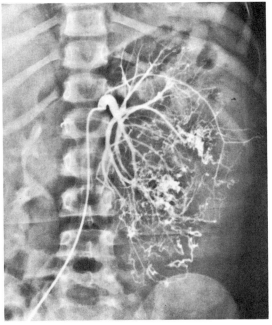

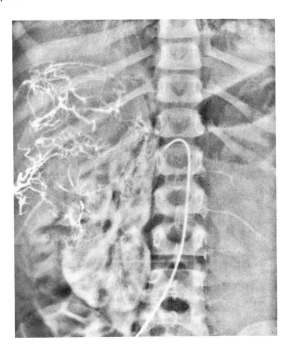

demonstrated by the gas pattern, may be displaced. There may be evidence of enlargement of the liver.

Excretory urograms usually show great distortion of the pelvis and calices on the involved side (Fig 18–8), although lack of excretion may occur secondary to ureteral occlusion or vascular invasion. Retrograde urograms are seldom needed.

A chest film may disclose metastases to the lungs.

2. Special radiographic studies–CT scans will show a mass with density equal to that of the normal renal tissue. A few areas of lucency may be noted. Following the intravenous instillation of radiopaque medium, a slight increase in density will be seen. Renal angiography will show the enlarged renal mass (Fig 18–8). Unlike adenocarcinoma, vascularity is sparse; zigzag arterioles are seen. There is no pooling of opaque medium, nor are arteriovenous

fistulas observed. The midstream study may show metastatic deposits in the liver. An inferior venacavogram may show compression or invasion of the cava or renal vein.

E. Isotope Scan: A bone scan may reveal osseous metastases. Hepatic scan may show tumor deposits.

F. Ultrasonography and CT Scan: These tests should differentiate between primary tumors of the adrenal or kidney and hydronephrosis.

G. Cytologic Examination: Papanicolaou studies are not helpful, since the tumor rarely breaks through the pelvic lining.

H. Tumor Markers: There are as yet no specific tumor markers for nephroblastoma, but many patients have high urinary lactate dehydrogenase levels. In such cases, continued elevation of the enzyme following nephrectomy or other definitive therapy implies the persistence of active tumor. Further work-up or intensive ancillary therapy is indicated.

Differential Diagnosis

Neuroblastoma of the adrenal medulla is an exceedingly malignant tumor that, for the most part, afflicts children under age 3. It usually presents as a mass in the flank, but since it metastasizes early and widely and by both lymphatics and blood vessels, the first symptoms may be caused by metastases. Neuroblastoma tends to invade the muscles of the back; it may therefore present a visible bulge in the costovertebral angle. Urography should permit differentiation. Neuroblastoma tends to displace the kidney; Wilms's tumors are intrinsic renal lesions and therefore distort the calices. Neuroblastomas frequently contain stippled calcification on the plain film, whereas 10% of Wilms's tumors exhibit peripheral crescent-shaped calcific deposits. Osseous metastases are frequently bilateral and almost symmetric, involving many bones. The urinary vanilmandelic acid level is increased with neuroblastoma but normal with Wilms's tumor.

Fetal hamartoma (congenital mesoblastic nephroma) is a benign tumor discovered during the first few months of life. On infusion urography and angiography, or on sonography and CT scan, lucent areas representing fat are seen. The vascular changes are typical of hamartoma.

Hydronephrosis may also cause a mass in the flank. It is usually softer than a tumor. It may transilluminate. If there is secondary infection, pyuria will be found. Urography or sonography is diagnostic.

Multicystic kidney seen in the newborn presents as a nodular mass in one flank and may, therefore, be confused with Wilms's tumor. This cystic kidney seldom secretes the radiopaque solution, but in a few cases it is visualized on infusion urography. The ureter is usually not connected to the mass; therefore, retrograde urography will not yield a urogram. Angiography or sonography may prove helpful, but the diagnosis may ultimately be possible only at operation.

Polycystic kidney disease may cause a palpable mass, although enlargement is usually bilateral. Renal function tests are depressed, and urograms show bilateral caliceal distortion. It must be remembered, however, that 10% of Wilms's tumors are bilateral. Renal angiography, sonography, or CT scan may be needed in case of doubt.

Complications

In addition to metastasizing, the tumor may occlude the renal vein and vena cava.

Treatment

A. Specific Measures:

1. Radiation therapy–Only if it is judged that the tumor is too large to allow nephrectomy readily should preoperative irradiation be administered. If the diagnosis is accurate, dramatic shrinkage of the mass should be observed. Following nephrectomy, radiotherapy to the tumor bed should be given if the tumor was invasive or if local lymph node metastases were found. In patients under age 1 year, there is some danger of damaging the vertebrae, leading to kyphosis or scoliosis.

2. Nephrectomy–The kidney and the contents of the perirenal fascia should be removed through a transperitoneal or thoracoabdominal incision as soon as the diagnosis is made. Preoperative embolization of the renal artery should be considered for large, necrotic hypervascular tumors (Danis & others, 1979). In bilateral renal involvement, some cures have been obtained by removal of one kidney and partial removal of the other. Bilateral nephrectomy followed by renal transplantation has its advocates (Penn, 1979).

3. Chemotherapy–This tumor has proved to be quite sensitive to dactinomycin, which should be started a few days before surgery and continued daily for 1 week and then at weekly intervals. Other dosage schedules have also been suggested. Other useful chemotherapeutic drugs include vincristine and doxorubicin. Multiple courses of dactinomycin should be given to control subsequent pulmonary metastases (see p 334).

B. Palliative Measures: If metastases are widespread—and particularly if they are discovered in bone or the brain—the prognosis appears to be hopeless, though radiotherapy and chemotherapy should not be withheld. Vincristine has been found useful under these circumstances. Instances have been reported in which resection of pulmonary and even hepatic metastases has led to cure (Wedemeyer & others, 1968).

C. Follow-Up Care: The patient should undergo palpation of the flank and periodic CT scan or sonography for evidence of local recurrence. Serial chest films are essential because pulmonary metastases are common.

Prognosis

In the absence of capsular extension, local lymph node involvement, and metastases, 80–90% of patients will be cured by combined treatment. Even if pulmonary lesions are present, cure is achieved in 50% of cases. Prognosis can also be estimated by considering the age of the child (the younger the better), the size of the primary tumor, the presence of local lymph node involvement, and the grade of the tumor (Green & Jaffe, 1979; Jereb & others, 1980).

SARCOMA

Sarcomas of the kidney are rare. They may be made up of smooth or striated muscle, fibroplastic tissue, bone, or fat. They may become quite large and fill the flank. Spread is usually by way of the bloodstream; the lungs and bones are commonly involved.

Morgan and Kidd (1978), in a review of 123 children diagnosed as having embryoma, found 9 instances of pure undifferentiated sarcoma. Metastases to bone were common (not so in Wilms's tumor), and the prognosis was poor.

The signs and symptoms are usually the presence of a mass and local pain. Hematuria is not common. Spontaneous perirenal hemorrhage may cause the first symptoms (pain, shock).

The diagnosis can be made with urographic evidence of a space-occupying renal lesion. The differential diagnosis between renal cancer and sarcoma can seldom be made even on angiography.

In the absence of metastases, nephrectomy is indicated unless lymphoblastoma is suspected, in which case radiation therapy should be used. The prognosis is quite poor for the entire group. The incidence of distant metastases and local recurrence after surgical extirpation is high.

TUMORS OF THE RENAL PELVIS & URETER

Histologically, the epithelial tumors of the renal pelvis and ureter resemble the tumors of the bladder. They may be benign but are usually malignant.

Although malignant tumors of the ureter arising from mesenchymal tissues have been described, they are rare and will therefore not be discussed here. Suffice it to say that clinically they mimic the more common epithelial growths and benign polyps.

TUMORS OF THE RENAL PELVIS

Most tumors arising from the caliceal or pelvic mucosa are papillary in type. They comprise about 10% of tumors of the kidney. Hematuria is usually the earliest symptom. Eighty percent are transitional cell tumors, most of which occur in men. Squamous cell carcinoma has an incidence of about 15%, with the majority of cases occurring in women. Adenocarcinomas and sarcomas are rare.

Etiology

The cause of the papillary growths is not known. Their tendency to "seed" in the ureter and bladder suggests that the mucosa generally is susceptible to such change. The rare epidermoid carcinoma is usually associated with chronic infection or stone; chronic inflammation may therefore play a part in its genesis.

The metabolites of tryptophan (alpha-aminophenols) are suspect as carcinogenic agents. For a discussion of this subject, see section on etiology of tumors of the bladder, p 289.

Numerous reports now incriminate phenacetin abuse as a cause of transitional tumors of the renal pelvis and ureter (Gaakeer & De Ruiter, 1979; Gonwa, Buckalew, & Corbett, 1979). Jackson & others (1978) did urinary cytologic studies on 98 patients with interstitial nephritis (analgesic nephropathy) and found 3 transitional tumors and 18 patients who were considered to be at risk for the development of such tumors.

Petković (1975) has observed a marked increase in the incidence of these tumors in Yugoslavia and other Balkan states during the past 20 years. He cites one area where their occurrence has increased by a factor of 100. In Taiwan, the incidence of transitional cell tumors of the renal pelvis is equal to that of adenocarcinoma (personal observation). An undiscovered carcinogen is suspected as the cause.

Pathogenesis & Pathology

These tumors may cause obstruction to calices or even the ureteropelvic junction, thereby causing renal pain and the changes associated with back pressure. The more malignant types tend to invade the parenchyma, thus simulating adenocarcinoma. Hematuria occurs earlier than in adenocarcinomas of the parenchyma. Similar tumors may also be found in the ureter and bladder, particularly near the ipsilateral ureteral orifice. It is therefore necessary to remove the kidney, ureter, and adjacent bladder wall when dealing with these growths. Most papillary tumors of the renal pelvis are malignant. Metastases are usually not widespread. The regional lumbar nodes may be involved.

Microscopically, these tumors show a central core of connective tissue that is covered by transitional epithelium. Invasion of the supporting stroma or mucosa or the finding of many cells in mitosis is evidence of malignancy, but at times it is difficult to draw the line between the malignant and benign types. Epidermoid cancers are invasive and highly malignant, and survival is rare. They are usually associated with severe chronic infection or lithiasis. They also spread to the regional lymphatics. Microscopic examination reveals the typical picture presented by squamous cell tumors seen elsewhere in the body.

Grabstald, Whitmore, & Melamed (1971) evolved the following staging for transitional cell tumors of the renal pelvis and ureter:

Stage A: Submucosal infiltration only.

Stage B: Muscular invasion without extension through the thin muscle wall of the calix, pelvis, or ureter.

Stage C: Invasion of the renal parenchyma or the peripelvic or periureteral fat.

Stage D: Extension outside the kidney or ureter into adjacent organs, regional lymph nodes, or distant metastases.

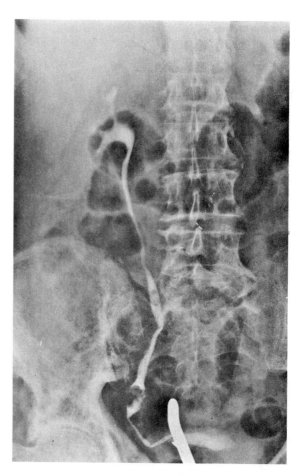

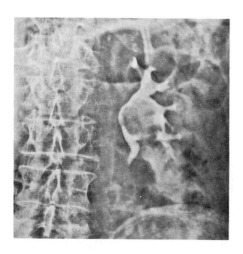

Figure 18–9. *Left:* Excretory urogram showing space-occupying lesion of left renal pelvis. Transitional cell carcinoma. *Right:* Retrograde urogram showing "negative" shadow caused by transitional cell carcinoma of the lower right ureter without evidence of obstruction.

Clinical Findings

A. Symptoms: Gross painless hematuria is the most common complaint of patients with renal pelvic tumor. Bleeding is at times quite profuse. Flank pain may be due to ureteral obstruction from the tumor; there may be ureteral colic from passage of clots.

B. Signs: Tenderness may be found over the kidney, particularly if ureteral obstruction has occurred or if infection has supervened. A palpably enlarged kidney is not common.

C. Laboratory Findings: Anemia can be marked if bleeding is profuse. Gross or microscopic hematuria is to be expected, but at intervals the urine may be free of red cells. Renal infection can result from obstruction or can be primary with epidermoid tumors, in which case pus and bacteria will be found in the urine. Renal function tests will be of little help; although the kidney may be gradually destroyed by the tumor, the other kidney will assume the lost function.

D. X-Ray Findings: A plain film of the abdomen will probably not be of much value, for the kidney is ordinarily not grossly enlarged. Excretory urograms, if good filling occurs, will show a space-occupying lesion in the pelvis (Fig 18–9) or a calix. A chest film should be taken routinely, although metastases to the lungs are not common.

Retrograde urography should reveal the filling defect. Secondary ureteral growths may also be demonstrated. Selective renal angiography usually reveals an enlarged pelviureteric artery, fine neo-vascularity, and often a tumor blush, but Goldman & others (1977) found the test accurate in only 60% of cases. Chew, Nouri, & Woo (1978) found that this technic was enhanced when epinephrine magnification angiography was used.

E. Instrumental Examination: Cystoscopy must be done immediately if and when gross bleeding is present; blood may be seen spurting from one ureteral orifice, which localizes the source of the bleeding. During cystoscopy, search must be made for "satellite" tumors on the bladder wall.

F. Cytologic Examination: The Papanicolaou technic or methylene blue smear of the urinary sediment is usually positive. The chances for a posi-

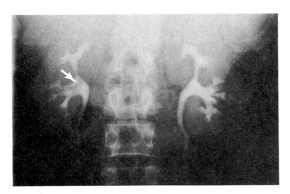

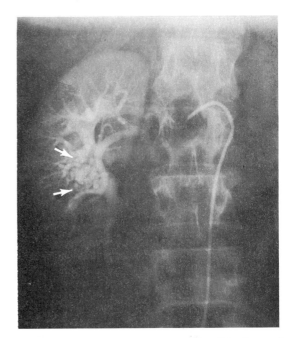

Figure 18–10. Renal hemangioma. *Left:* Excretory urogram showing filling defect in right renal pelvis. *Right:* Selective renal angiogram. Note multiple dilated arteries.

tive test are enhanced if the pelvic surface is brushed. Gill, Lu, & Bibbo (1979) observed no false-positive tests in 60 cases. Lang & others (1978) obtained brush biopsies by the percutaneous translumbar route.

G. Tumor Markers: Little has appeared in the literature as yet on this subject. One might expect markers to be similar to those encountered with vesical tumors (see p 293). It has been reported that about two-thirds of patients with renal pelvis tumors have elevated levels of urinary carcinoembryonic antigen (CEA); in these cases, serial estimates may help in choosing appropriate treatment, or they may suggest evidence of tumor elsewhere.

Differential Diagnosis

Adenocarcinoma of the kidney will cause hematuria. Such a tumor is apt to be palpable or may be visible on a plain film of the abdomen as an expansion of a portion of the kidney. Urograms will show the intrarenal nature of the growth. However, blood clots in the renal pelvis can mimic pelvic tumor. If a transitional cell tumor invades the parenchyma, it will simulate adenocarcinoma. Cytologic tests and angiography may make the differentiation.

A nonopaque renal stone may cause hematuria and renal pain. A mass may be palpable if hydronephrosis develops. Urograms will show a space-occupying lesion of the pelvis, but the outline of the negative (black) shadow (representing the stone) tends to be smoothly round or oval with stone and irregular (papillary) with tumor (Fig 15–2). With tumor, cytology is usually positive. Sonog-

raphy or CT scan will help in differentiation.

An opaque renal stone may be associated with an epidermoid carcinoma of the renal pelvis. Diagnosis under these circumstances may be difficult and may be possible only at the time of surgical exploration for the treatment of the calculus. Urinary cytology or sonography may help in differentiation.

Renal tuberculosis may mimic pelvic neoplasm. The urogram may show irregularity of the pelvic outline caused by ulceration. This might suggest tumor. The patient with urinary tract tuberculosis usually complains of vesical irritability and has "sterile" pyuria. Acid-fast organisms can be demonstrated in the urine.

Cholesteatoma of the renal pelvis comprises a mass of keratinized squamous cells. Urography shows an intrapelvic mass. The urine is loaded with squamous cells. Angiography reveals no evidence of tumor.

An ectopic or aberrant renal papilla projecting into the renal pelvis will show on urography as a space-occupying lesion. Selective angiography is definitive.

Hemangioma, an occasional cause of hematuria involving the renal pelvis or submucosal parenchyma, is usually too small to be seen on a urogram. A large hemangioma will present on the urogram as a space-occupying lesion of the pelvis. Renal angiography makes the diagnosis (Fig 18–10).

Complications

On rare occasion, hemorrhage may be so severe that embolization of the renal artery or emergency nephrectomy is necessary.

Hydronephrosis or hydrocalicosis may arise from progressive obstruction. Secondary infection may then develop.

Treatment

A. Specific Measures: Once the diagnosis has been made and evidence of metastasis ruled out, the kidney and all perinephric tissue, including regional lymph nodes, the ureter, and the periureteral portion of the bladder must be removed. This radical procedure is necessary because secondary ureteral and vesical tumors may be present or may develop later in the ureteral stump or bladder (Johansson & Wahlqvist, 1979). Retroperitoneal lymph node dissection should also be done (Skinner, 1978).

B. Palliative Measures: Even though metastases are demonstrated it may be advisable to remove the affected kidney if pain or infection from obstruction is severe or if bleeding is profuse.

Tumors of the renal pelvis have proved to be radioresistant. For a discussion of chemotherapy, see Transitional Cell Tumors, p 334.

C. Follow-Up Care: The patient should be seen periodically and examined by abdominal palpation to search for local recurrence and enlargement or nodulation of the liver. Serial chest films are indicated. Since vesical or contralateral pelvic tumors may develop, urinary cytology should be ordered.

Prognosis

The prognosis for the patient suffering from benign tumor is excellent. With low-grade malignancies the outlook is good (75% are alive after 5 years); it is fair to poor if the papillary tumor is undifferentiated (25% are alive after 5 years). Epidermoid carcinoma is almost always fatal within 1 year.

TUMORS OF THE URETER

Tumors of the ureter are rare; the majority are malignant and papillary in type. About two-thirds of them occur in men, and most are seen in the lower ureter.

Etiology

Although the cause of these tumors is not known, there is increasing evidence that carcinogens are involved (see section on etiology of tumors of the bladder, p 289). The incidence of this lesion is higher than normal in persons who habitually take large doses of phenacetin.

Pathogenesis & Pathology

Ureteral tumors may be primary or may be associated with similar tumors of the renal pelvis or bladder. Although they usually bleed, many of the symptoms are caused by ureteral obstruction (eg, renal and ureteral pain). Most involve the lower ureter.

These neoplasms are similar in all respects to those of the renal pelvis and bladder. Most are papillary; a few are sessile. Squamous cell carcinoma is rare. Benign fibrous polyps are occasionally seen (Debruyne & others, 1980). Endometriosis has been reported (Klein & Cattolica, 1979).

Transitional cell carcinomas range from a low to a high grade of malignancy. The most malignant show invasion of the stroma and ureteral wall by pleomorphic cells that have a marked tendency to metastasize to regional lymph nodes, lungs, and liver.

Metastatic tumors from other sources are occasionally seen. The primary sites include the uterus, colon, breast, and prostate (Babaian & others, 1979).

For staging classification, see tumors of the renal pelvis, p 285.

Clinical Findings

A. Symptoms: The most common symptom is hematuria, usually intermittent and sometimes quite profuse. There may be a dull pain over the kidney, caused by ureteral obstruction. Acute renal colic can occur from the passage of clots down the ureter. There may be symptoms of urinary tract infection (secondary to obstruction). These include fever, back pain, and vesical irritability.

B. Signs: Physical findings are usually absent. If the kidney has become hydronephrotic from ureteral obstruction, it may be palpable. If it is infected, it may be tender. An enlarged liver or a mass of lymph nodes (metastatic involvement) may be felt.

C. Laboratory Findings: Anemia may be found if bleeding is prolonged or severe. Gross or microscopic hematuria is usually present. Evidence of infection may be seen on urinalysis. Renal function is ordinarily not impaired unless the other kidney is also diseased.

D. X-Ray Findings: A plain film of the abdomen may show an enlarged renal shadow (hydronephrosis) secondary to ureteral obstruction. Excretory urograms will usually make the diagnosis. There is often dilatation of the urinary passages proximal to the obstructive tumor, and an intraureteral space-occupying lesion may be noted as the cause for the obstruction. An x-ray of the chest should be taken as soon as the diagnosis of ureteral tumor is made, since metastases may be found in the lungs.

A ureteral catheter passed up the ureter for urography often forms a loop at the site of the tumor. A retrograde urogram will demonstrate the lesion (Fig 18–9). Oblique views are often helpful.

E. Instrumental Examination: If the patient is actively bleeding, cystoscopy should be done immediately in order to locate the source of the hemorrhage. It must be done also to observe for "seeding" of secondary growths on the bladder wall. Occasionally the tumor can be seen protruding from the ureteral orifice.

Ureteral catheterization may cause considerable blood to drain from the catheter when it passes by the tumor. When its tip reaches the renal pelvis, the urine becomes clear: this may therefore be of diagnostic significance.

Kiriyama, Hironaka, & Fukuda (1976) have been very successful in procuring tumor tissue by means of the Dormia stone basket.

F. Cytologic Examination: Papanicolaou studies or a methylene blue smear of the urinary sediment often reveals abnormal transitional cells. Cytologic findings are more apt to be positive if ureteral brushing is done.

G. Tumor Markers: See Tumor Markers, p 287.

Differential Diagnosis

Ureteral calculus, if it is radiolucent, may cause the same symptoms and signs as ureteral tumor. The urogram in each case will show a "negative" (black) shadow in the ureter, with dilatation of the tract above it. Stone is suggested if a "grating" feeling is noted as a catheter is passed by it. Sonography (Arger & others, 1979) or CT scan should differentiate nonopaque stone from tumor. The correct diagnosis may be possible only at surgery.

Ureteral stenosis, often secondary to compression by masses of lymph nodes involved by cancer (eg, cervix), can mimic ureteral tumor. The discovery of a primary tumor will make the diagnosis. CT scans may reveal the involved nodes.

A blood clot from a renal stone, a sloughed papilla, renal adenocarcinoma, or pelvic tumor will also show as a "negative" shadow within the ureter. The urograms should make the differentiation. Air bubbles introduced through a ureteral catheter may cause some confusion.

Complications

Hydronephrosis is often found with ureteral tumor.

Because obstruction is usually present, infection may develop. The bacteriuria usually fails to clear despite appropriate medication; this should indicate the need for urography, which will demonstrate the tumor.

Treatment

A. Specific Measures: In the absence of demonstrable metastases, ureteronephrectomy and the resection of the periureteral bladder wall are necessary. When dealing with transitional cell tumors, if the lower ureter is left in, there is a 30% chance of recurrence of tumor in this segment (Strong & others, 1976). For benign or very low-grade tumors, sleeve resection of the involved ureteral segment with end-to-end anastomosis should

be considered (Babaian & Johnson, 1980).

B. Palliative Measures: Little can be accomplished if metastases are present, since these tumors are usually radioresistant. Ureteronephrectomy may be necessary to relieve pain due to the obstruction or to control otherwise intractable bleeding. It may also be indicated because of severe and persistent infection of the kidney. For chemotherapy, see Transitional Cell Tumors, p 334.

C. Follow-Up Care: Evidence of recurrence in the retroperitoneum and metastasis to the liver and lungs should be sought. Periodic cytologic examination of urine must be done to search for clues to the development of new transitional tumors in the other kidney, ureter, or bladder.

Prognosis

The prognosis in the benign type is excellent; with the malignant transitional cell carcinomas, it is only fair, particularly if they are invasive. The higher the grade, the poorer the outlook (Ghazi, Morales, & Al-Askari, 1979). Patients with squamous cell tumors or tumors that have involved the ureteral muscle and regional lymph nodes are rarely cured.

TUMORS OF THE BLADDER

Tumors of the bladder are the second most common of all genitourinary neoplasms. (Only prostatic tumors occur more frequently.) Seventy-five percent are found in men. Most are seen after age 50. Papillomatous growths submit readily to transurethral treatment if diagnosed early. Infiltrating (transitional cell) types constitute one of the most difficult of all urologic problems.

Etiology

It has long been established that prolonged exposure to certain industrial aromatic amines (eg, 2-naphthylamine, benzidine, 4-aminodiphenyl) may be associated with a high incidence of vesical neoplasm. Recent work suggests that the multiple transitional cell tumors involving the urinary tract (eg, renal pelvis, ureter, bladder) probably are caused by carcinogens, particularly tryptophan. This substance and the industrial amines listed above are metabolized to ortho-aminophenols by the liver, conjugated with sulfate or glucuronic acid, and excreted through the kidneys. These materials are attacked by hydrolytic enzymes (beta-glucuronidases), and orthophenols are liberated, some of which have been proved to be carcinogenic in dogs and mice. These carcinogens are found in increased concentration in the urine of patients harboring vesical tumors (Boyland, 1963). It is thought that many years of exposure to these

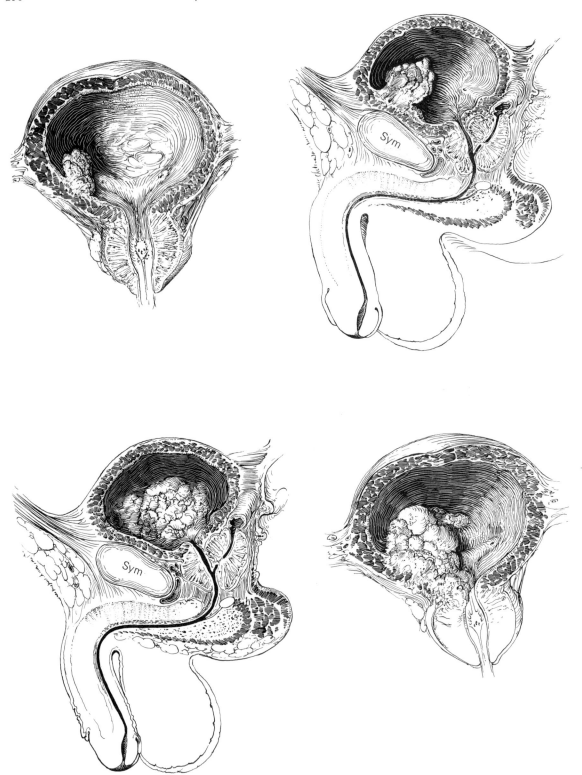

Figure 18–11. Transitional cell carcinomas of the bladder. **Above left:** Transitional cell (papillary) carcinoma with minimal invasion of the bladder wall. This is compatible with a grade II, stage A (T1) tumor. **Above right:** Larger, more invasive transitional cell carcinoma, probably grade II–III, stage B$_1$ (T2). **Below left:** More extensive transitional cell carcinoma involving the right ureteral orifice, compatible with grade III, stage B$_2$ (T3). **Below right:** Advanced large, invasive carcinoma of the bladder; occlusion of right ureteral orifice with extension into the bladder neck and prostate (grade IV, stage C [T4]).

carcinogens are necessary to stimulate the growth of these tumors.

There is evidence that the activity of urinary beta-glucuronidase is increased merely by forcing fluids and by the presence of vesical infection, even schistosomiasis. This substance is also found in increased amounts in the presence of other cancers, benign enlargement of the prostate, renal infection, renal cyst, and urolithiasis. Kallet & Lapco (1967) claim that this enzyme is elaborated by urologic epithelial cells that have been damaged; therefore, increases in urinary levels of beta-glucuronidase are of no diagnostic significance.

Smoking has been cited as a cause of the increased incidence of vesical neoplasm. It has recently been shown that smokers experience a 50% increase in carcinogenic metabolites of tryptophan excreted in the urine. On cessation of smoking, the levels return to normal. Rose & Wallace (1973) studied urinary chemiluminescence in both smokers and nonsmokers as well as in patients with vesical cancer. The latter showed the highest levels; smokers had the next highest levels; and nonsmokers had low levels. They found that ascorbic acid decreased this activity both in those who smoked and in those who did not.

A number of other physical agents have been implicated as causes of bladder cancer. Rathert, Melchior, & Lutzeyer (1975) incriminate phenacetin abuse; Howe, Burch, & Miller (1977) suspect artificial sweeteners (eg, saccharin); and Sadeghi, Behmard, & Vesselinovitch (1979) believe that opium is a potential carcinogen. Durkee & Benson (1980) and Fairchild and others (1979) suspect cyclophosphamide.

It is also well known that patients with severe vesical schistosomiasis have a high incidence of bladder cancer of the squamous type.

Pathogenesis & Pathology

It is customary to judge transitional cell vesical carcinomas in 2 ways: (1) the degree of differentiation of the cells, and (2) the depth of penetration of the tumor into the vesical wall or beyond (Fig 18–11).

A. The Grade and Stage of the Tumor:

1. Grade–The degree of cell differentiation.

Grade I tumors are quite well differentiated. The lamina propria is usually not involved. Most are relatively small, are papillary in type, and have a narrow base. These are curable by transurethral means but are radioresistant.

Grade II tumors are papillary in type, show less differentiation of their cells, and are apt to invade the lamina propria if not the detrusor muscle itself. They tend to be larger than the grade I tumors and have a wider connection with the bladder wall. They are often curable by transurethral resection. They do not respond too well to radiotherapy.

Grade III and IV neoplasms are poorly differ-

entiated, even anaplastic. They tend to be nodular rather than papillary, and as a rule are quite invasive. They respond poorly to transurethral removal but are sensitive to radiotherapy.

2. Stage–The degree of invasion. Two methods of staging vesical tumors are in vogue: the Jewett method, which is commonly used in the USA, and the international (UICC) system. The former uses letters O, A, B_1, B_2, C, and D, while the latter utilizes "T" numbers.

Stage O (T1S) is a papillary tumor or carcinoma in situ that has not invaded the lamina propria.

Stage A (T1) tumors have invaded the lamina propria but not the muscle of the vesical wall.

Stage B_1 (T2) neoplasms have extended into the superficial half of the detrusor muscle.

Stages B_2 and C (T3) tumors show deep muscle invasion or have grown through the entire bladder wall.

Stage D (T4) tumors have invaded peritoneum or adjacent organs.

Stage D_1 (NX) tumors have involved lymph nodes below the bifurcation of the aorta.

Stage D_2 (MX) tumors have metastasized to the periaortic nodes and distant organs.

B. Type and Location: Since 80% of vesical tumors arise on the base of the bladder, they may involve one or both ureteral orifices or the vesical neck. Hydroureteronephrosis and pyelonephritis are common complications. When tumors ulcerate, they bleed and often become infected.

Most growths are papillary in type and are malignant. They may be single or multiple; generalized papillomatosis is not uncommon. Generally speaking, the larger the tumor and the broader its base, the more malignant it is, and nodular tumors are more malignant than the papillary types.

In the male, secondary tumors may develop in the urethra.

After successful treatment of even the grade I and II types that are superficial (stages O [T1S] and A [T1]), there is a definite tendency for new tumors to develop elsewhere in the bladder. This suggests that the appearance of these tumors is in some way related to a generally increased susceptibility of the mucosa to neoplastic proliferation, perhaps in response to carcinogens. This is true also of the renal pelvic and ureteral transitional cell tumors.

Vesical neoplasms most commonly metastasize to the vesical, hypogastric, common iliac, and lumbar nodes. The bones, liver, and lungs are at times affected (Babaian & others, 1980).

Rarely, other types of vesical neoplasms may be encountered:

(1) Epidermoid carcinoma: About 5% of vesical neoplasms are of the squamous cell variety. These are ordinarily highly malignant (anaplastic), deeply invasive, and metastasize early. A high incidence of this tumor is observed in patients with vesical bilharziasis (see p 208).

(2) Adenocarcinoma is very rare (Kramer & others, 1979). It often arises in a urachal remnant (Ganguli, 1979).

(3) Rhabdomyosarcomas and leiomyosarcomas are quite rare. They occur most frequently in male children and adolescents. They infiltrate widely, metastasize early, and are usually fatal (Savir & Meiraz, 1980).

(4) Primary malignant lymphomas, carcinosarcomas, neurofibromas, hemangiomas, leiomyomas, and pheochromocytomas are rare. The latter may be associated with attacks of hypertension during voiding. Primary amyloidosis is rare (Caldemone & others, 1980).

(5) Cancers of the skin (melanoma), stomach, lung, and breast may metastasize to the bladder. Vesical invasion by endometriosis may occur.

Clinical Findings

A. Symptoms: Gross hematuria is the most common symptom. As with all tumors of the urinary tract, hematuria is usually intermittent. All bleeding, severe or mild, prolonged or transient, must be accounted for. If infection supervenes, symptoms of cystitis will usually be present. These include burning on urination, urgency, frequency, and nocturia. Symptoms of bladder neck obstruction may develop if the tumor encroaches on the internal orifice. These include hesitancy and decrease in force and caliber of the urinary stream. If there is perivesical extension, suprapubic pain may be constant and severe. Pain in the flank may be noted if the growth obstructs a ureteral orifice and produces hydronephrosis. This may be complicated by renal infection, which may cause increased pain and high fever. If metastases are present, if infection is severe, if both ureteral orifices become occluded, or if anemia has developed, the patient may complain of weakness and loss of weight.

B. Signs: In most cases nothing abnormal can be found on physical examination. Renal tenderness or enlargement may be present due to ureteral obstruction and infection. A suprapubic mass may be noted on rare occasion. This might be due either to a large cancer or to urinary retention caused by clots or invasion of the bladder neck by tumor. On vaginal examination a mass at the base of the bladder may be noted. Less often, rectal examination may reveal an invasive mass in the trigonal area. Bimanual palpation (abdominorectal or abdominovaginal) is of the greatest importance in feeling and estimating the size and extent as well as possible fixation, due to invasion of adjacent tissues, of the growth. This is best done under anesthesia. Signs of metastases may be noted. These include palpable abdominal masses (involved lymph nodes along the iliac vessels) and edema of one or both legs from occlusion of the iliacs.

C. Laboratory Findings: Anemia is not uncommon and may be from loss of blood, severe infection, or uremia caused by occlusion of both ureteral orifices by the growth. The urine may be very bloody, but between bouts of bleeding few if any red cells may be found. Pus and bacteria may also be noted. Renal function tests are usually normal unless there is bladder neck obstruction with residual urine or obstruction of both ureters.

D. X-Ray Findings: Excretory urograms are essential. Although they are usually normal, they may show the tumor itself (Fig 18–12), evidence of ureteral obstruction, or a primary tumor of the renal pelvis or ureter as a cause of the "primary" vesical growth. Retrograde cystograms may show the tumor if it is large enough. A "fractionated" cystogram may afford evidence of invasion of the tumor into the vesical wall. First, the vesical capacity is determined. This amount of diluted radiopaque medium is then prepared. One-fourth of this amount is then instilled into the bladder and an x-ray exposure made. The other three-fourths are successively instilled, and an x-ray exposure is then made on the same film. If the tumor is superficial, the vesical wall will fill symmetrically; in the presence of invasion, that portion of the wall will not expand. Vesical angiography may yield information concerning depth of infiltration of the tumor. It is quite accurate in revealing stage C (T3) tumors (Fig 18–12). CT scan may also give this information and may reveal enlarged metastatic lymph nodes as well as the more dense tumor surrounded by the less dense urine. Its rate of accuracy is 81% (Seidelmann & others, 1978). The study may be further enhanced by filling the bladder with air.

Lymphangiography alone has an accuracy rate of only 50% (Farah & Cerny, 1978). Sonography is of little value in estimating the stage of the tumor.

E. Instrumental Examination: Cystoscopy almost always reveals the tumor. Biopsy of the lesion should be routine. A few tumors may be missed by this means, but these can be visualized if the patient is given tetracycline for a few days before cystoscopy using ultraviolet illumination. The tetracycline causes fluorescence of the tumor.

Carcinoma in situ is often difficult to diagnose. The mucosa shows some erythema and has a granular and velvety appearance. This lesion leads to vesical contraction. In case of doubt, multiple biopsies are indicated.

F. Cytologic Examination: Papanicolaou preparations or the simpler methylene blue stain of fresh urinary sediment will almost always reveal transitional cells shed from the tumor (Rife, Farrow, & Utz, 1979). Well-differentiated tumors shed round cells of rather uniform size with large nuclei. When anaplastic tumors are present the urinary sediment usually reveals large epithelial cells (often in clumps) with very large dark staining nuclei (see Chapter 5). Holmquist (1980) has suggested a simple technic for urine cytologic study in which a 1% solution of toluidine blue is prepared and diluted times 15. One drop added to the urinary sediment clearly defines cell morphology.

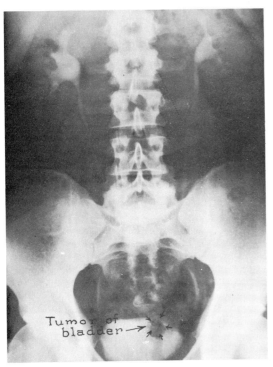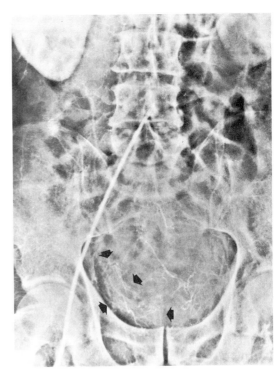

Figure 18–12. Tumors of the bladder. *Left:* Excretory urogram showing space-occupying lesion (transitional cell carcinoma) on the left side of the bladder; the upper tracts are normal. *Right:* Vesical angiogram, delayed film, showing increased vascularity of a deeply invasive transitional carcinoma grade IV, stage C, right vesical wall. Some of these vessels are presumed to be typical of tumor.

Trott & Edwards (1973) have suggested the following technic: 50 mL of normal saline are instilled into the bladder via the cystoscope or catheter. The solution is washed back and forth 3 times and then fixed for cytologic examination. They have found this method significantly superior to a similar study of the voided urine.

In those cases where tumor or carcinoma in situ is suspected and routine cytology is negative, Morales, Marriott, & Connolly (1975) suggest that the vesical mucosa be thoroughly scraped with the resectoscope loop and the washings obtained subjected to cytologic study.

This procedure is also useful in the follow-up of these patients and as a screening test for those exposed to chemical carcinogens. Suspicious cells (carcinoma in situ) may be noted months before a tumor can be discovered cystoscopically.

G. Tumor Markers: Guinan & others (1974) found that 60–70% of patients with vesical cancer had increased levels of urinary or plasma carcinoembryonic antigen. Following definitive therapy, these levels dropped but rose again when recurrence or metastases developed. Betkerur and others (1980) found this test of little value because there were too many false negatives. They did find that urinary immunoglobulins (IgG and IgA) are significantly elevated in patients with bladder carcinoma.

Young, Hammond, & Middleton (1979) studied the blood group antigens (A, B, O) on the cell surface. Patients without an antigen later developed invasive tumors, whereas those with an antigen did not.

Wajsman & others (1978), using a rapid immunoassay kit, studied the fibrinogen degradation products in patients with vesical cancer and in normal controls. Thirty-two percent of those with low-grade tumors had increased levels of these substances. When combined with urinary cytologic tests, this procedure disclosed evidence of early cancer in 80%.

Lamb (1967) noted that aberrations in chromosome count and structural abnormalities are apt to be seen in the undifferentiated tumors. Superficial tumors that have normal chromosomes are noninvasive. This is of some clinical importance, since what may appear to be a low-grade growth will probably recur and become invasive if its chromosome analysis is abnormal. Javadpour (1980) finds the combination of the specific red cell adherence test (SRCA) and chromosome analysis most helpful in predicting the natural history of superficial vesical tumors.

Differential Diagnosis

Renal or ureteral tumors also cause hematuria. Urograms will demonstrate the renal or ureteral lesion. Palpation or a plain abdominal film may reveal an enlarged kidney. It must be remembered that tumors of the renal pelvis or ureter may "seed" to the bladder wall, and the "primary" vesical neoplasm may really be "secondary."

Endometriosis occasionally involves the bladder. Bleeding and vesical irritability may be most marked at the menses. Cystoscopically, the lesion is bluish in color and looks like a vascular tumor. Pelvic examination usually reveals signs of other sites of involvement.

Acute nonspecific infections of the bladder may cause hematuria when the source is the prostate. A tumor often becomes infected. Differentiation depends upon cystoscopy.

Benign prostatic hypertrophy commonly causes hematuria, often initial or terminal. Cystoscopy is necessary in the differential diagnosis.

Tuberculosis of the urinary tract often causes bleeding. A "sterile" pyuria is usually found, and tubercle bacilli can be demonstrated by special technics. Excretory urograms will be negative for tumor but may show evidence of caliceal ulceration. Again, cystoscopy will establish the diagnosis.

Renal, ureteral, or vesical stones may mimic tumor, but a plain film or excretory urogram will usually demonstrate them.

Acute hemorrhagic nephritis in an adult may require differentiation from tumor. The urinary findings (casts), hypertension, and edema should lead to the proper diagnosis. In case of doubt, cystoscopy is indicated.

Tumors of the cervix or bowel may invade the bladder. Demonstration of the primary tumor and a biopsy of the vesical lesion should settle the diagnosis.

Complications

Secondary infection of the bladder is common when the tumor ulcerates. It may be severe. Renal infection is not uncommon when ureteral obstruction ensues. Urinary retention may develop if the tumor invades the bladder neck.

Hydronephrosis due to ureteral occlusion is common. If it is bilateral, uremia supervenes. This is the most common cause of death.

Hemorrhage may become a problem. If it is intractable, dilute standard 40% formalin 1:10 in sterile water to make a 4% solution that can be instilled via catheter to fill the bladder. Drain the bladder after 15 minutes and then irrigate with normal saline or with 10% alcohol followed by saline. Catheter drainage is maintained for the next few days. This procedure is highly successful, though occasionally it must be repeated. A cystogram must be done before initiating this treatment; if vesicoureteral reflux is demonstrated, formalin is contraindicated.

If hemorrhage does not cease following this procedure, transcatheter embolization of the hypogastric arteries should be considered (Carmi-

gnani & others, 1980; Lang & others, 1979). Chan, Bracken, & Johnson (1979) recommend a single dose of 1000 rads to the pelvis for intractable hemorrhage or bilateral ureterovesical obstruction.

Prevention

Employment in aniline dye factories should be restricted to 3 years, during which time periodic urinary Papanicolaou studies and cystoscopy are indicated. The clinical significance of endogenous carcinogenic agents has not been established. Schlegel & others (1970) have adduced evidence that the administration of ascorbic acid, 0.5 g 3 times a day, may prevent the formation of vesical tumors through neutralization of urinary carcinogens. Rose (1972) has found that giving large doses of pyridoxine decreases tryptophan metabolites in the urine. It seems worthwhile, therefore, to prescribe these drugs for those patients in whom the diagnosis has been made.

Treatment

There is still considerable disagreement about the proper treatment of vesical neoplasms. Certainly the low-grade superficial tumors lend themselves well to transurethral resection. For the more malignant and invasive tumors, the physician must choose between radiotherapy and radical surgery or a combination thereof.

A. Surgical Measures: Most single or multiple papillomas are best treated by transurethral resection, care being taken to "saucerize" deeply into the wall of the bladder in order to remove the base of the tumor completely. This procedure will cure many of the papillary carcinomas (eg, stage O, A, B_1 [T1S, T1, T2], grade I, II). However, if the tumor has deeply invaded the vesical muscle (stage B_2 [T3], C [T3]), this method will usually fail.

Partial (segmental) cystectomy has its proponents, particularly for tumors that lie on the lateral walls or dome of the bladder. Schoborg, Sapolsky, & Lewis (1979) found that when this procedure was used for grade III and IV tumors that were rated as stage A, all patients suffered recurrence, and the 5-year survival rate was only 40%. Partial cystectomy was more successful with grade I and II tumors rated as stage A; only 28% of patients suffered recurrence, and 86% were alive at 5 years. Merrell, Brown, & Rose (1979) used partial cystectomy for 54 patients with stage B_1–B_2 tumors, with a 5-year survival rate of 57%.

Total cystectomy (with removal of the prostate) is often practiced for the treatment of papillomatosis and many of the more undifferentiated invasive tumors. Diversion of the urinary stream presents a problem. Ureterosigmoidostomy results in urinary continence but frequently causes ureteral obstruction or reflux with hydronephrosis and renal infection. Many of these patients die of renal insufficiency rather than of cancer. A few will develop symptomatic hyperchloremic acidosis from absorption of the chloride ions in the urine. Hypokalemia may occur. The administration of potassium citrate will usually correct these electrolytic defects. The most popular method of urinary diversion today is anastomosis of the ureters to an isolated loop of ileum (or sigmoid), with one end of this loop brought to the skin to act as a conduit. Renal complications and electrolyte problems are minimized.

Most urologists advocate radical pelvic node dissection in conjunction with the cystectomy. Since similar tumors may develop in the urethra in both men and women, urethrectomy—particularly in the male—should be done (Faysal, 1980).

B. Radiation Therapy: In general, the more undifferentiated the tumor the more radiosensitive it is. It is therefore most useful in the grade III–IV, stage B_2 (T3) and C (T3) lesions. There is mounting evidence that radiotherapy in this type of neoplasm offers at least as good a control rate as radical surgery without the mortality associated with the latter. The optimal dose is 6000 rads given over a period of 6 weeks or more. This is compatible with the maintenance of good vesical function. If, after irradiation, viable tumor is still demonstrable, cystectomy can be considered. Good palliation can be obtained by radiotherapy alone when the tumor is deemed inoperable. Five-year survival rates of 12–25% have been reported in this group (Fish & Fayos, 1976; Birkhead, Conley, & Scott, 1976). There has been recent enthusiasm for use of radiotherapy (4500 rads) followed by planned cystectomy 1–2 months later. Peeples & others (1979) used preoperative radiotherapy followed by radical cystectomy; no tumor could be found in the bladder by the pathologist. Miller (1977) observed a 5-year survival rate of 14% with x-ray alone, 25% with cystectomy and postoperative irradiation, and 48% with preoperative radiotherapy and cystectomy. The present consensus is heavily in favor of preoperative irradiation (2000–4000 rads) followed by cystectomy and pelvic lymph node dissection (Whitmore Jr, 1980).

Until recently, it was thought that squamous cell tumors had a poor prognosis, but both Johnson & others (1976) and Richie & others (1976) have reported 5-year survival rates of 34–48% when combined therapy was used.

Hewitt & others (1972) advocate the use of intracavitary radium for treatment of superficial low-grade tumors and carcinoma in situ. They report a control rate of better than 50% for these lesions at 5 years.

C. Chemotherapy: Palliation of advanced high-grade vesical neoplasms with parenteral anticancer drugs has been reported. These include 5-fluorouracil, mitomycin C, bleomycin, methotrexate, and hydroxyurea. Ogata, Migita, & Nakamura (1973) have infused mitomycin C via the internal iliac artery. Merrin & Beckley (1978) report promising results with parenteral doxorubicin and cyclophosphamide. Peters & O'Neill (1980) adminis-

tered cis-diamminedichloroplatinum (cisplatin) to 8 patients with metastatic transitional cell carcinoma. Both subjective and objective improvement was noted. Nakazono & Iwata (1978) injected 10–20 mg of doxorubicin into the tumor 1–2 times per week, with a 78% success rate.

The instillation by catheter of 60 mg of thiotepa dissolved in 30–60 mL of normal saline was suggested by Veenema, Romas, & Fingerhut (1974) in the treatment of superficial low-grade papillomas. Four to 6 weekly treatments should be given, followed by instillations every month for 6–10 months. Similar therapy is indicated if new tumors appear following transurethral resection of a low-grade superficial neoplasm. Gavrell & others (1978) advise instillations of thiotepa in the postoperative period following transurethral resection of tumors. This may change the nature of the mucosa; the appearance of new tumors may cease. Before each instillation, a white cell and platelet count should be obtained. If the white count is less than 4000 or the platelets below 10,000/μL, treatment should be deferred until the hemogram shows improvement.

British urologists have had considerable experience with instillations of triethylene glycol diglyceridyl ether (etoglucide). Since it is poorly absorbed through the vesical wall, blood dyscrasia has not been observed. Inject 100–200 mL of a 1% solution (in distilled water) via catheter. Remove the catheter and instruct the patient to retain the drug for at least an hour. This instillation is repeated every week for 12 weeks, then every month for a year, and then every 3 months. If the response is poor, a 2% solution should be used.

Bracken & others (1980) treated 43 patients with small stage O–A tumors with weekly instillations of mitomycin C, 30 mg in 30 mL of water. After 8 treatments, they observed a complete response in 49% and a partial response in 30%. Mishina & others (1975) had similar success. They recommend instillation of 20 mg in 20 mL of water 3 times a week for a total of 20 procedures. No bone marrow depression was observed.

Lamm & others (1980) have used parenteral BCG immunotherapy for superficial bladder tumors. They felt that this lessened the recurrence rate.

Symes & others (1978) used intra-arterial infusions of tumor-immune pig lymph node cells to treat 24 patients who developed recurrent tumors after radical radiation therapy. Remission was noted in 11 patients, and in 3 patients the tumors disappeared.

D. Other Methods of Therapy: Helmstein (1972) advocates the utilization of a hydrostatic technic in the treatment of the more malignant tumors, though England & others (1973) found that only the stage A (T1) tumors responded. Under anesthesia, a balloon is placed in the bladder transurethrally and filled with water until the intravesical pressure approaches the systolic blood pressure.

This pressure is maintained for 5½–7 hours. A catheter is left in place for a few days. Tumor necrosis is caused by the ischemic effect of the balloon pressing on the tumor. It is too early to accurately judge its efficacy.

Reuter (1972) claims achievement of good results with transurethral freezing (cryosurgery) of vesical tumors.

E. Rhabdomyosarcoma: Although this tumor offers a poor prognosis, some cures have been reported recently when triple therapy was utilized (Bartholomew & others, 1979). This consists of prostatocystectomy, x-ray therapy, and chemotherapy (dactinomycin and vincristine).

Follow-Up Care & Prognosis

The superficial, well-differentiated tumors may recur, or new papillomas may appear. Constant vigilance, with periodic cystoscopy and urinary cytologic examination, is therefore necessary for at least 3 years. New tumors may also be well controlled by transurethral means, but if they tend to recur they are apt to become progressively invasive and of higher grade. Cystectomy or radiation therapy must then be considered.

Prognosis with any vesical tumor varies, in general, with the stage (invasion) and grade (differentiation). The best results are obtained by transurethral resection of the grade I–II, stage O (T1S), A (T1), and B$_1$ (T2) tumors. Cystectomy cures about 15–25% of grade III–IV, stage B$_2$ (T3) and C (T3) lesions, with an accompanying mortality rate from the operation of 5–15%. Radiotherapy for the same serious neoplasms offers a control rate of 15–25% at 5 years. When the combination of preoperative radiotherapy plus radical prostatocystectomy is utilized, the 5-year control rate approaches 35–50%.

If lymphangiography shows involvement of lymph nodes bilaterally, the prognosis is poor. Even with unilateral involvement the control rate is 6% at 5 years (Turner & others, 1976).

Few if any cures of rhabdomyosarcoma are achieved during the first year of life. Possibly 15–25% can be controlled in those that develop in childhood.

TUMORS OF
THE PROSTATE GLAND

The prostate is the urologic organ most often affected by benign or malignant neoplasm. Cancer of this organ is almost as common as malignancy of the lung or gastrointestinal tract.

The danger from adenomatous hypertrophy is not from the lesion per se but from the effects of obstruction: hydronephrosis and renal infection. The same is true, to a large extent, of prostatic cancer, although metastases may contribute to the death rate.

BENIGN PROSTATIC
HYPERPLASIA (OR HYPERTROPHY)

There is some debate about the cause of the prostatic enlargement. One group believes that the obstructing tissue represents hyperplasia of the periurethral glands, with compression of the true prostatic tissue peripherally to form the "surgical capsule." Thus, "prostatectomy" is not prostatectomy at all. The hyperplastic periurethral glandular tissue is removed; the prostate is not. Others believe that the prostatic lobes lying proximal to the verumontanum (the 2 lateral and subcervical lobes) undergo hyperplasia but in addition are invaded by the periurethral glands, thus giving the fibromuscular tissue its often striking glandular component. If this be true, then prostatectomy is accomplished. The latter theory is favored (Hutch & Rambo, 1970).

Benign prostatic hyperplasia causes progressive obstruction to the flow of urine and, in the later stages, causes back pressure in the kidneys (hydronephrosis) and contributes to the establishment of infection in the urinary tract.

Etiology

Some enlargement begins to develop in most men by age 50. The majority have palpable evidence of hyperplasia by age 60. Not all have symptoms of obstruction, however, nor is the hyperplasia necessarily progressive.

The cause of this disease is not entirely clear, although its relationship to hormonal activity is borne out by much experimental and clinical evidence. Animal investigation shows that prostatic obstruction is common in aging male dogs, but this does not develop if the animal has been previously castrated. Orchiectomy causes atrophy of the gland and therefore terminates the elaboration of prostatic fluid. Dogs with Sertoli cell (estrogen) tumors of the testis do not develop prostatic hyperplasia.

Previous castration also seems to prevent prostatic hypertrophy in men. However, administration of estrogens or even castration has little if any effect upon the gross size of the enlarged gland, although some atrophy of the epithelial structures may be noted microscopically. The administration of estrogens or androgens has little effect upon the amount of acid phosphatase elaborated by the gland.

Certainly androgens per se cannot be blamed for this hyperplasia, for the disease occurs at a time when the androgenic activity of the organism is decreasing. Therefore, an imbalance between androgens and estrogens may be the causative factor. It is not clear why hyperplasia of the prostate develops in some men and not in others and affects different individuals in varying degrees.

Pathogenesis

(See Chapter 10.)

The enlarged gland produces its harmful effects by obstructing the bladder neck and by upsetting the mechanisms that force open and funnel the vesical orifice. Djurhuus, Hansen, & Nerstrom (1975) performed urethral pressure profiles in men with prostatic enlargement. Pressures were high throughout the length of the gland. After prostatectomy, the pressure was limited to the distal prostatic urethra. Bates, Arnold, & Griffiths (1975) carried out similar studies. Attempts at urination caused increased resistance at the bladder neck.

A. Changes in the Bladder:

1. Early–As the degree of obstruction increases, the vesical detrusor undergoes compensatory hypertrophy in order to overcome the increasing urethral resistance. The muscle wall may become more than 2 cm thick. This power of compensation varies. One patient with a markedly obstructive gland may have few symptoms, whereas another may have great difficulty with a milder obstruction. There is therefore little relationship between the size of the gland and the severity of symptoms.

As compensatory hypertrophy develops, the following take place:

a. Trabeculation of the bladder wall–Taut, intertwined hypertrophic muscle bundles raise the mucosa.

b. Hypertrophy of the trigone and intereteric ridge.

c. Diverticula–As the intravesical voiding pressure rises (as it must to overcome increased urethral resistance), the mucosal layer may be forced between the muscle fibers and may finally balloon into the perivesical fat. It may then grow to large size. The diverticulum has no muscular wall and therefore cannot empty itself; the urine it contains easily becomes infected.

2. Late–In many men the power for further vesical compensation becomes exhausted when the muscle can no longer hypertrophy, and decompensation occurs. Urine is then retained in the bladder in increasing amounts, and symptoms may become severe. With chronic urinary retention, the hitherto thickened bladder wall may become markedly attenuated and atonic.

B. Changes in the Ureter and Kidney: With secondary hypertrophy of the trigonal-ureteral complex, there is increased downward traction on the intramural ureteral segments, thus increasing resistance to urine flow. This is further aggravated when there is significant residual urine, which causes further stretching and, therefore, pull on the intramural ureter. This leads to progressive proximal dilatation and is the common cause of hydroureteronephrosis and its accompanying impaired renal function. Significant residual urine leading to chronic vesical distention may cause a

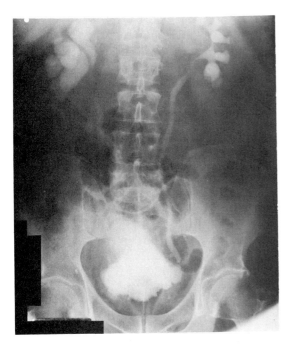 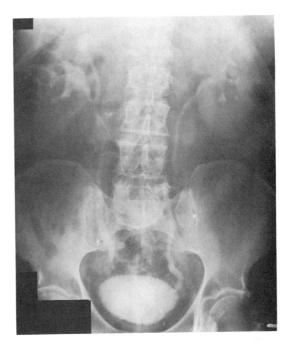

Figure 18–13. Benign prostatic hypertrophy. *Left:* Preoperative 1-hour excretory urogram showing bilateral hydronephrosis and a heavily trabeculated bladder. *Right:* Postoperative excretory urogram revealing regression of hydronephrosis. Bladder now of normal contour.

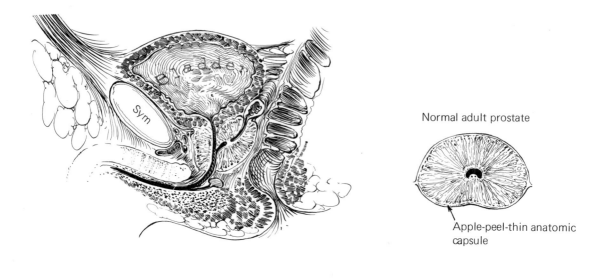

Normal adult prostate

Apple-peel-thin anatomic
capsule

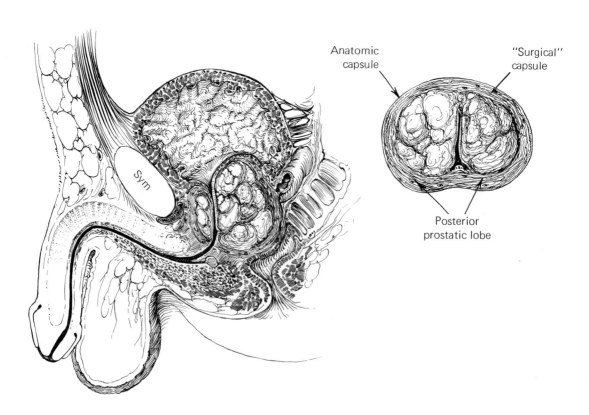

Anatomic
capsule

"Surgical"
capsule

Posterior
prostatic lobe

Figure 18–14. Pathogenesis of benign prostatic hyperplasia. *Above:* Normal bladder and prostate. Inset shows normal prostate (containing prostatic urethra) and thin fibrous anatomic capsule. *Below:* Enlarged prostate enclosed by a relatively thick "surgical" capsule composed of the posterior prostatic lobe.

vesicorenal reflex that is manifested by diminution of renal urinary secretion. In either case, catheter drainage or prostatectomy, by relieving trigonal stretch and allowing resolution of the trigonal hypertrophy, causes the hydroureteronephrosis to recede (Fig 18–13).

In a few advanced cases of prostatic enlargement, the ureterovesical "valves" may become incompetent. This not only hurts the kidney hydrodynamically but encourages the development and perpetuation of pyelonephritis.

C. Infection: In the presence of vesical residual urine or ureterovesical reflux, the urologic defense against infection is defeated. Some such patients develop cystitis that is, in all probability, secondary to a preexisting prostatitis. It is possible, however, that impaired urethral washout secondary to the obstruction may allow abnormal ascent of urethral flora.

If the organisms split urea (eg, *Proteus*), vesical stones may form. If vesicoureteral reflux develops, pyelonephritis ensues. The renal lesion is the important complication of prostatic obstruction.

Pathology (Fig 18–14)

The prostate in the young adult may be compared to an apple; its true capsule is thin and intimately attached to the underlying secretory tissue. For this reason, intracapsular enucleation of the young man's prostate is impossible. The enlarged gland, on the other hand, is more like an orange. It has a thick "surgical" capsule (the peripherally compressed extraurethral prostate) that is poorly connected to the central obstructing tissue; this permits easy "shelling out" of the hyperplastic prostatic lobes, leaving the "surgical" capsule behind. It should be noted that the posterior prostatic lobe is left as part of this surgical capsule. Since it is in this lobe that carcinoma develops, intracapsular or transurethral prostatectomy is not prophylactic against cancer developing later.

There are 3 lobes that commonly undergo hyperplasia: the 2 lateral lobes and the subcervical lobe. At times only the lateral lobes enlarge. Again, a fairly pure subcervical lobe hyperplasia is seen. In this instance, rectal examination may reveal a prostate of normal size, for this lobe cannot be felt. Very commonly, all 3 enlarge together. The gland becomes elongated and the lobes tend to herniate through the bladder neck; intravesical protrusion may be marked. Under these circumstances the true size of the gland, as judged by rectal palpation, will not be revealed.

On section, the adenomatous pattern is usually obvious; multiple nodules are noted. The "surgical" capsule is composed of atrophic true extraurethral (posterior lobe) prostatic tissue that has been compressed and displaced to the periphery. It may be 2–5 mm in thickness. This capsule is poorly connected to the hyperplastic lobes, which therefore may be easily enucleated.

Microscopically, the hyperplasia affects glandular, muscular, and fibrous tissue in varying degrees. The epithelial cells are of the tall columnar type. They may pile up into a papillary pattern. There are no mitoses.

Clinical Findings

Benign prostatic enlargement seldom causes significant symptoms before age 50. The complaints are referable to the obstruction and may be increased by infection. Rectal examination may or may not reveal prostatic enlargement. Urinary infection may be present. The PSP may be depressed because of incomplete emptying of the bladder (residual urine); back pressure on the kidneys will cause true impairment of renal function. Cystoscopy will reveal hypertrophy of the prostate and secondary changes in the bladder wall.

A. Symptoms: (The physiologic explanation for the obstructive symptoms is discussed in Chapter 10.) In the early stages, the patient may notice that if the bladder becomes too full there is a little hesitation in starting the stream and some loss of force and caliber of the stream. Later, the symptoms are more persistent and severe.

1. Bladder symptoms–Hesitancy in starting the stream may be marked. Considerable straining may be necessary. Because of the increased urethral resistance, decrease in caliber of the bladder neck, and derangement of the normal mechanisms that open the bladder neck, the stream is small and lacks force. This will be worse if the urge to urinate must be put off, for the smooth muscle of the bladder becomes overstretched and loses tone. Toward the end of urination the stream tends to diminish gradually and may end as a mere dribble. Frequency (both day and night) develops, depending on the degree of irritability of the bladder and the amount of residual urine; the greater this amount is, the smaller the working capacity of the organ. If infection complicates the picture, all of the above symptoms are increased. The inflammatory edema of the prostate or bladder neck will increase the degree of obstruction and will cause more residual urine, thereby further increasing frequency. Infection diminishes vesical capacity, further increasing the degree of frequency. Hematuria is not uncommon. It may be due to rupture of dilated veins at the bladder neck which are apt to develop with straining. Acute urinary retention may develop suddenly in a patient who has had few premonitory symptoms. At other times it occurs after some months or years of increasing symptoms of prostatism. The patient then experiences marked suprapubic pain and marked urgency; he is miserable until relieved by catheterization.

2. Renal symptoms–The hydronephrosis secondary to prostatic obstruction is usually painless unless it becomes infected. In a few men with vesicoureteral reflux, renal pain may be experienced during the act of voiding. In the advanced stage of the disease, symptoms of uremia may be noted: somnolence, vomiting, diarrhea, and loss of weight.

B. Signs: A visible mass low in the midline of the abdomen may be seen, felt, or percussed. In acute retention, it is quite tender. In chronic urinary retention, the bladder may be so flabby that only percussion will reveal it. On rectal examination the prostate may or may not be enlarged. One lobe may be larger than the other. The surface is usually smooth; it may be firm (fibromuscular) or unduly soft and boggy (adenomatous). Areas of induration (suggesting cancer) should be sought.

It should be mentioned that the degree of obstruction is measured not by rectal examination but by the severity of the symptoms and the amount of residual urine.

Unless acute urinary infection is present or the patient is verging on complete urinary retention, the gland should be massaged. If prostatitis is discovered or if the gland is found to be overfull of secretion, conservative treatment (massage, antimicrobial drugs) may afford some relief from obstructive symptoms. Tenderness over a kidney may indicate renal infection. The maximum intravesical voiding pressure is significantly increased; voiding flow rate is reduced. Hypertension may be found. It may be caused by renal back pressure (ischemia).

C. Laboratory Findings: Urinalysis may reveal an otherwise completely silent complicating infection (pus, bacteria). Measurement of renal function by the PSP test is a very important step in examination. It also indirectly estimates the presence or absence of residual urine. If the PSP is 50% or more at 30 minutes after injection and the urine volume is small, total renal function is normal and

there can be no significant residual urine. If it is only 25%, either residual urine is present or renal function is depressed. Determine the serum creatinine. If it is normal, then the man's kidneys must have excreted 60% of the dye. The residual urine would therefore have to be about equal to the volume of urine passed at one-half hour (see p 50). The passage of a catheter immediately after voiding will accurately measure the degree of retention.

D. X-Ray Findings: A plain film of the abdomen and excretory urograms may show complicating calculi. Often, hydroureteronephrosis is portrayed (Fig 18–13). This is usually caused by hypertrophy and chronic stretch of the trigone, which applies increased occlusive pull on the intravesical ureteral segments. Intravesical encroachment of the prostate and even ureteral reflux may be revealed on urethrography and cystography (Fig 18–15). The bladder may be raised well above the upper edge of the symphysis if the gland is significantly elongated. In this age group, a postvoiding film is mandatory to reveal the amount of urinary retention. Pinck, Corrigan, & Jasper (1980) believe that all preprostatectomy patients should have excretory urograms, since silent lesions might otherwise be missed. However, Bauer, Garrison, & McRoberts (1980) have concluded that such studies reveal so little unsuspected significant disease that, except when investigating a complaint of hematuria or evidence of renal disease, they are not worth the expense.

E. Instrumental Examination: The amount of urine retained after voiding is a measure of the degree of decompensation of the bladder. This can be ascertained by passing a catheter to the bladder immediately after voiding, by PSP test, or by noting

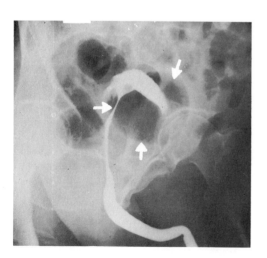
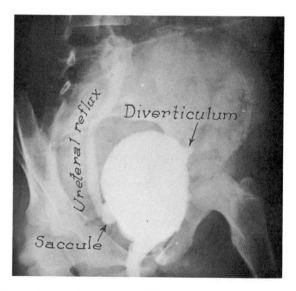

Figure 18–15. Benign prostatic hypertrophy. *Left:* Cystourethrogram. Thick radiopaque material seen in urethra and spreading over superior surface of greatly enlarged intravesical prostate. Arrows outline bladder filled with air. *Right:* Lateral voiding cystourethrogram showing diverticulum of the bladder ("Hutch" saccule; see Fig 11–6) and vesicoureteral reflux. Postoperative prostatectomy.

the amount of residual urine on the postvoiding film obtained with the urograms.

Cystoscopy or panendoscopy will show the degree of enlargement of the prostatic lobes and the secondary changes in the bladder wall (eg, trabeculation, diverticula, infection) and will also reveal complications such as vesical stone or incidental neoplasm.

F. Sonography: Transrectal sonograms of the prostate will reveal its size most accurately (Watanabe & others, 1977).

Differential Diagnosis

The neurogenic bladder also causes difficulty with urination and a low maximum voiding flow rate. There is often a history of spinal cord or peripheral nerve injury. Diabetic neuropathy may be present. Tranquilizers (eg, diazepam) lead to vesical atony. Neurologic examination may reveal definite abnormality (particularly perianal anesthesia), and the anal sphincter may be found to be atonic (relaxed). A cystometrogram is helpful. The bethanechol supersensitivity test (originally described by Lapides) is definitive (Melzer, 1972). With 100 mL of water in the bladder, intravesical pressure is estimated. A subcutaneous injection of 2.5 mg of bethanechol chloride (Urecholine) is given. If, after 30 minutes, the intravesical pressure has risen 15 cm of water or more, the test is positive for vesical atonicity. Cystoscopy may show little in the way of obstruction. A positive serologic test for syphilis of blood or spinal fluid may be suggestive. Herpes zoster involving the sacral spinal ganglia has caused urinary retention in a few patients.

Abrams (1980) investigated 60 patients who, following prostatectomy, still had symptoms suggesting obstruction. He found that 50 of them suffered from urgency or stress incontinence, an atonic detrusor, or impaired urethral sphincter mechanisms. Only 10 had prostatic obstruction from residual prostatic tissue. This points up the need for a careful neurologic examination and urodynamic studies before prostatectomy.

Ganglionic blocking agents and parasympatholytic drugs in the treatment of peptic ulcer and hypertension, as well as tranquilizers, weaken the power of detrusor contraction, causing symptoms simulating vesical neck obstruction. In a man with moderate prostatism, such drugs may cause urinary retention.

Contracture of the vesical neck caused by chronic prostatitis (rare) mimics the symptoms of benign enlargement perfectly. A fibrous or nodular prostate is to be expected, and its secretion will contain pus. Cystoscopy will settle the diagnosis.

Cancer of the prostate will be suggested by the finding of a hard gland. Besides the obstructive symptoms, lumbosacral backache with pain radiating down one or both legs suggests metastases to the bony pelvis or extension along the perineural lymphatics. If the disease is extensive, the serum acid phosphatase is increased. Serum alkaline phosphatase is elevated when the tumor has metastasized to bone. Osteoblastic metastases to the pelvic bones usually mean prostatic cancer. Biopsy of the prostate is definitive.

Acute prostatitis will cause obstructive symptoms, but this disease is acute, is associated with marked febrile response, and often occurs in young individuals. Pyuria is always found. Rectal examination will reveal an enlarged prostate that is hot, exquisitely tender, and often fluctuant (abscess).

Urethral stricture also causes obstruction to urinary flow. A history of complicated gonorrhea (now rare) or perineal trauma should suggest the possibility. Urethral discharge, pyuria, and infection in the prostatic secretion usually accompany this abnormality. Urethral exploration with catheter or sound or urethrography makes the diagnosis.

Sarcoma of the prostate is rare and affects younger men and boys. Symptoms are those of obstruction. A large, soft or firm mass is felt in the prostatic area.

Vesical stone will be suggested by sudden interruption of the urinary stream accompanied by pain radiating down the penis. It will be revealed by radiography or cystoscopy.

Complications

Obstruction may lead to infection. This may involve the bladder, kidneys, and the prostate itself. From the latter, epididymitis may develop. Stones may form in the bladder.

The obstruction may cause vesical diverticula. Hydronephrosis may occur from hypertrophy of the trigone or when a ureterovesical "valve" gives way. At times, hematuria may be brisk.

Treatment

Since benign prostatic hyperplasia is not necessarily a progressive disease, conservative therapy should be used where applicable. The problem is to decide which patients can be treated in this manner and which require surgery. Criteria for operation vary, but the following seem feasible: (1) Impaired renal function due to the obstruction corroborated by excretory urography. (This indication is hardly debatable.) (2) A degree of symptoms that so upsets the patient that he requests relief. This will vary, since one man may be distressed at urinating 3 times during the night, whereas another may not be particularly inconvenienced by nocturia of 6 times.

A. Conservative Measures: Regular intercourse is the best means of combating prostatic congestion. If necessary, this may be replaced or augmented by 3 or 4 prostatic massages given at intervals of 14 days. At times, improvement is striking.

Prostatitis should be treated by prostatic massage (once a week for 3 weeks) and antimicrobial drugs that are active in the prostate. These include trimethoprim-sulfamethoxazole and minocycline.

If pyuria is present, antimicrobials may give considerable relief. The choice of drug will depend upon the organism found. If there is a great deal of residual urine, drug therapy will probably not be successful.

To protect vesical tone, the patient should be conditioned to avoid excessive intake of fluids in a short period of time. Rapid distention of the bladder may cause the hypertrophic muscle to lose its tone and lead to sudden exacerbation of symptoms or even acute retention. The patient should be cautioned about the diuretic effect of alcohol (Richmond, 1974), which, combined with the volume of fluid taken, may lead to retention despite the fact that symptoms up to that time had been moderate. In fact, such an episode is the most common cause of acute urinary retention. For the same reason, the patient should void as soon as he feels the urge to do so, thus preventing the bladder from becoming overdistended.

The use of antiandrogen therapy (estrogens or orchiectomy) may have some beneficial effect upon benign prostatic hypertrophy, but the cost to the patient (impotence) is too high.

Men who are given testosterone for other reasons may notice improvement in their obstructive symptoms from increased vesical tone. Care should be taken to determine that the patient does not have cancer of the gland, because androgen therapy will hasten its growth. The administration of cyproterone acetate has given some encouraging results in the treatment of benign enlargement. Although hydroxyprogesterone caproate has been reported to be effective in some cases, Meiraz & others (1977) observed no such effect. Paulson & Kane (1975) utilized medrogestone and found that on a dose of 15 mg twice a day, most subjects experienced an increased urine flow rate.

Catheterization is mandatory for acute retention. If the patient is still unable to void spontaneously, and particularly if there have been few antecedent symptoms, a catheter should be left in place for 2–4 days. Thus, prostatic congestion is relieved, vesical tone is reestablished, and fairly normal voiding may return. If catheterization by any means is impossible, cystostomy must be performed. After a few days, the power of spontaneous urination may be restored. A permanent indwelling catheter (or cystostomy) may occasionally be indicated in the debilitated patient.

B. Surgery: There are 4 operations in vogue at present, but it is impossible to state the indications for each. The choice of operation is a personal matter for the surgeon.

Transurethral prostatectomy is most often used. Some surgeons remove only a small amount of tissue; others perform what is essentially a complete intracapsular removal. The latter method is to be preferred, since only this can compete with the results obtained by open surgery. The mortality

rate is about 1–2%, and the urinary result is good in most instances. Potency is maintained, and hospitalization is relatively short (Chilton & others, 1978).

Suprapubic transvesical prostatectomy is still the most popular open method of removal of the hypertrophied tissue. Its mortality rate is 1–3%. The urinary result is excellent, probably more consistently so than with the transurethral method. Potency is maintained.

Retropubic extravesical prostatectomy has a mortality rate of 1–2%. The urinary result is excellent. Potency is maintained.

Perineal prostatectomy involves little risk, but impotence may result. Finkle, Finkle, & Finkle (1975) believe that impotence can be decreased by encouragement and reassurance. There may be some delay in regaining normal control; in a few patients, urgency incontinence persists. Rectourethral fistula has an incidence of 1–3% and is most distressing. Surgical repair is indicated.

Cryosurgery. Some enthusiasm for this method of treatment is being evinced for the poor-risk patient. The instrument is passed down the urethra, with the freezing unit placed in the prostatic urethra. Liquid nitrogen is circulated through the probe until the temperature in the prostatic capsule reaches 0–10 C (32–50 F). This leads to death and slough of the obstructing tissue. Blood loss is usually minimal. The result in possibly 10% of patients is less than optimal.

Möhring, Pfitzmaier, & Panis-Hoffman (1975) found that transurethral prostatectomy gives superior results. Cryosurgery should be reserved for the poor-risk patient.

C. Follow-Up Care: Periodic urinalysis with stained smear or culture should be done postoperatively. Healing should be complete after 2 months, at which time an appropriate antibiotic should clear any residual infection.

Prognosis

Most patients can be given considerable relief by conservative means. If on follow-up their symptoms increase or renal function, as measured by the PSP test, begins to diminish, surgical intervention is indicated.

CARCINOMA OF THE PROSTATE

Carcinoma of the prostate is rare before age 60 and increases in frequency thereafter, probably afflicting 25% of men in the eighth decade, though Rullis, Shaeffer, & Lilien (1975), in a series of autopsies in men over age 80 years, found that two-thirds had prostatic cancer. The disease is rare in Orientals but more common in blacks, Maoris, white New Zealanders, and Scandinavians. There is a significant familial incidence, which suggests a genetic component. Multiple cancers are common in these patients. It metastasizes principally to the bones of the pelvis and the pelvic lymph nodes. Ureteral obstruction, with secondary renal injury, may develop from direct extension, compression by pelvic nodes, intramural metastases, or hypertrophy of the trigone secondary to the vesical neck obstruction.

Three instances of the elaboration of adrenocorticotropin have been reported. These patients presented with hypokalemic acidosis, diabetes, psychosis, and hypertension (Newmark, Dluhy, & Bennett, 1973).

Etiology

The true cause of prostatic carcinoma is not known, but it is quite clear that its growth is strikingly influenced by sex hormones. The adult prostate is the major site of elaboration of acid phosphatase. In advanced prostatic cancer, particularly when it has metastasized to bone, two-thirds of patients will have markedly increased amounts of this enzyme in the blood (Catalona & Scott, 1978).

The administration of androgens usually increases the rate of growth of this tumor and increases the acid phosphatase level in the serum. Estrogen therapy (or orchiectomy) slows the growth of these tumors and maintains the amount of acid phosphatase in the blood at a normal level. Determination of the amount of acid phosphatase in the serum or bone marrow is therefore an index of the extent of the tumor; it also indicates the degree of success of antiandrogen therapy.

Heshmat & others (1975) found a statistically significant correlation between previous gonococcal infection and the development of prostatic cancer.

Pathogenesis & Pathology (Fig 18–16)

Adenocarcinoma of the prostate is usually associated coincidentally with benign prostatic hyperplasia but does not develop from it. Most malignancies originate in the posterior lobe in the surgical capsule (compressed peripheral prostatic tissue), although a few may be found within the hyperplastic benign prostatic lobes. These latter tumors are usually very small ("occult" or "academic" cancers, stage A) and apparently are often completely removed by intracapsular enucleation of the enlarged gland.

The initial lesion is usually a firm area on the posterolateral surface. It gradually spreads in the capsule (posterior lobe) and involves the hyperplastic tissue as well. The seminal vesicles then become involved. Later, the tumor may extend through the urethral mucosa or bladder wall; the external sphincter may be invaded. The rectal wall is singularly immune; only rarely does the tumor invade Denonvilliers' fascia (Fry, Amin, & Harbrecht, 1979).

The cancer spreads in the perineural lymphatics. The vesical, sacral, external iliac, and lumbar lymph nodes then become involved. The left supraclavicular node is occasionally affected. When the seminal vesicles are involved, 80% of patients will have invasion of the pelvic nodes.

Metastases also occur by way of the veins, particularly through the vertebrals. This mechanism accounts for the predilection of this tumor for the bones of the pelvis, heads of the femurs, and the lower lumbar spine. Other bones, including the skull, are occasionally involved. Spread to the skin and viscera (eg, lungs, liver) is also seen. Infiltration of the bone marrow is particularly common.

Grossly, cancers of the prostate are white or yellow. They may be quite hard, if fibrous; or merely firm, if more cellular. Multiple zones of cancer are not uncommon. Rarely, a tumor may be medullary and so soft as to simulate abscess.

On microscopic study, the tissue may be largely epithelial or may be scirrhous. The epithelial elements may assume a papillary pattern or may be anaplastic. Invasion of the stroma is usually obvious. Mitoses are common. Invasion of perineural sheaths is an outstanding feature but is not necessarily of prognostic importance.

After antiandrogen therapy, retrogressive changes may be marked. The gland becomes smaller and assumes a more normal consistency. This change may be marked within 3 months after therapy is instituted. Obstructive symptoms regress to some extent. Microscopically, the malignant cells have become smaller and stain more darkly. The cytoplasm becomes scanty. The number of these cells is markedly diminished. Similar changes occur in metastatic tumors.

A few transitional cell carcinomas arising from the epithelium of the ducts have been reported. They are highly malignant, cause osteolytic metastases, and are usually hormonally independent. Kopelson & others (1978) reported positive cytologic findings in 9 of their 10 cases. The tumors seem to respond poorly to radical surgery. Radiation therapy is indicated. Squamous cell cancer is rare (Mott, 1979). Lymphomatous infiltration is occasionally seen.

Adenocarcinoma of the prostate is staged as follows:

1. *Stage A:* Rectal examination and serum acid phosphatase levels are normal. The tumor is found incidentally in tissue removed in the treatment of benign prostatic hypertrophy. These tumors are confined to the prostate.

a. A_F, focal carcinoma.

b. A_1, carcinoma involving only one lobe.

c. A_2, multifocal or diffuse carcinoma. Most tumors of this stage seem to have a low biologic potential, yet it might be wise to vigorously treat those that are extensive (A_2), poorly differentiated, or found in a young man.

2. *Stage B:* These comprise prostates containing indurated areas. Serum acid phosphatase is normal.

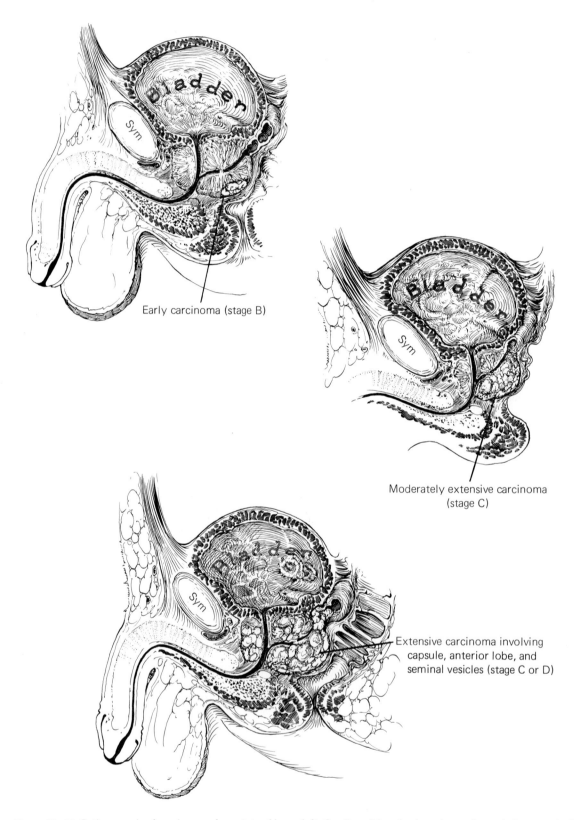

Early carcinoma (stage B)

Moderately extensive carcinoma
(stage C)

Extensive carcinoma involving
capsule, anterior lobe, and
seminal vesicles (stage C or D)

Figure 18–16. Pathogenesis of carcinoma of prostate. *Above left:* Small, well-localized carcinoma in posterior aspect of prostate, easily felt on rectal examination. *Above right:* Extension of carcinoma into posterior half of prostate. *Below:* Advanced carcinoma of prostate; trabeculation of bladder wall.

a. B_N, a solitary nodule no more than 1.5 cm in diameter.

b. B_1, involvement of most of one lobe; lymph node metastases found in 10–20%.

c. B_2, diffuse involvement of both lobes; lymph node metastases present in 15–40%.

3. *Stage C:* Tumor extends through prostatic capsule. No metastases. Acid phosphatase usually normal. Lymph node involvement in 40–80%.

4. *Stage D:* Metastatic prostatic carcinoma. Serum acid phosphatase is elevated in 70% of this group.

Prognosis is also influenced by the grade of the tumor. The undifferentiated tumor is much more aggressive than the well-differentiated one.

Clinical Findings

A. Symptoms: The presenting symptoms in 75% of men with prostatic malignancy are from obstruction to the flow of urine, infection, or both. They are similar to those described in the discussion of benign prostatic enlargement.

1. Bladder symptoms–These include hesitancy and straining to initiate the stream, loss of force and caliber of the stream, terminal dribbling, frequency with nocturia, symptoms of infection of the bladder, and urinary retention. Localized tumors unassociated with benign hyperplasia provoke no symptoms at all.

2. Symptoms due to metastases–One out of 20 patients have their first symptoms from metastases. Metastatic spread causes the following: pain in the lumbosacral region, which may radiate into the hips or down the legs; anemia and loss of weight; and hematuria late in the course of the disease when the bladder or urethra is invaded. Symptoms of renal insufficiency may be due to obstruction of the ureteral orifices by the primary tumor or by hypertrophy of the trigonal muscle, or to compression of the ureters by masses of iliac lymph nodes involved by metastatic cancer.

B. Signs: Rectal examination is the most important step in the diagnosis of cancer of the prostate. The early lesion is difficult to differentiate from certain benign conditions that cause areas of induration. A cancerous nodule is usually not raised above the surface of the gland. There is a sudden change in consistency between it and surrounding tissue (Fig 4–2). Diagnosis may not be possible without biopsy.

The more advanced lesion is usually stony-hard, and the gland is fixed. It may be nodular. The seminal vesicles may be indurated. Occlusion of the rectum by surrounding growth is very rare.

Other signs of prostatic cancer include an enlarged, nodular liver, pathologic fracture from metastasis (including sudden paraplegia from collapse of a vertebral body), and an enlarged, hard left supraclavicular node.

C. Laboratory Findings: Anemia may be extreme in the later stages, when bone marrow is replaced by tumor; hemorrhage and infection will also contribute to this. Urinalysis may or may not show infection. Red cells may be present.

In the early stages of obstruction, renal function is unimpaired. Later, if the ureters are occluded or if obstruction is so marked that renal back pressure develops, the PSP may be depressed because of renal impairment, residual urine, or both; serum creatinine or blood urea nitrogen may be increased. Raskin, McLain, & Medsger (1973) found hypocalcemia (below 8.6 mg/dL) in 16% and hypercalcemia in 9% of their patients.

D. X-Ray Findings: Excretory urograms may show (1) hydronephrosis with dilated ureters caused by hypertrophy of the trigone and leading to functional ureterovesical obstruction, (2) ureteral obstruction from metastases to pelvic lymph nodes, or (3) direct invasion by the primary tumor (Fig 18–18). A chest film may show metastases to the hilar nodes, lungs, or ribs. A plain film of the abdomen may reveal typical osteoblastic metastases from prostatic cancer (Fig 18–17); common sites are the pelvic bones, lumbar spine, and femoral heads. CT scan of the pelvis may reveal extraprostatic extension even including enlarged metastatic lymph nodes (Fig 18–19) (Bonney, Chiu, & Culp, 1978).

E. Scanning Technics: Although ^{85}Sr and ^{18}F bone scans have been widely used, ^{99m}Tc polyphosphate is probably the radiopharmaceutical of choice, since it has a relatively short half-life (see Chapter 8). The scan is much more sensitive than osteography in demonstrating metastases. A liver scan can be done, but metastases here are rare.

F. Instrumental Examination: Passage of a catheter immediately after voiding will measure the amount of residual urine. Cystoscopy will usually

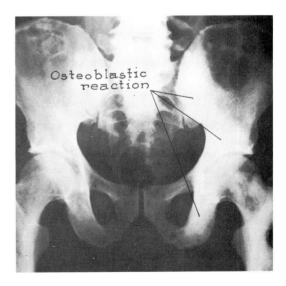

Figure 18–17. Metastases to bone from carcinoma of the prostate. Plain film of pelvis showing osteoblastic metastases to the lumbar vertebrae, ilium, ischium, and left femur.

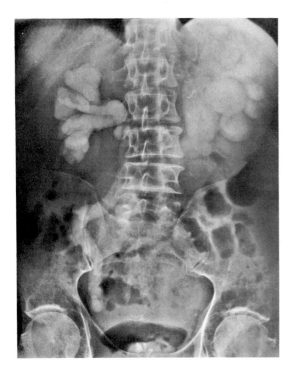
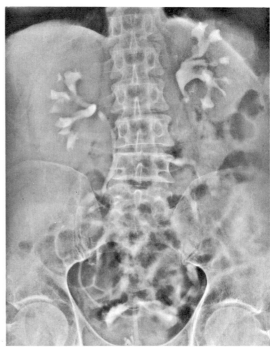

Figure 18–18. Cancer of prostate. *Left:* Excretory urogram at 75 minutes showing bilateral hydroureteronephrosis. *Right:* Fifteen-minute urogram after 3 months of diethylstilbestrol. Significant reduction of obstruction.

show nonspecific vesical changes from obstruction (eg, trabeculation, diverticula, infection). Only very late will invasion of the bladder be seen. Obstruction of the prostatic urethra will be evident. The gland may be found to be relatively fixed on movement of the instrument.

G. Cytologic Examination: Papanicolaou technics are of no value in the early stages. By the time malignant cells can be demonstrated in prostatic secretion, the diagnosis is usually quite evident clinically.

H. Biopsy: If the lesion is extensive, a positive diagnosis can be made on pathologic studies of tissue removed by transurethral resection. In early cases (limited to the capsule), this method fails. Needle biopsy (Rhind, 1980) or aspiration (Kohler & others, 1977) through the perineum or transrectally is a very useful procedure for establishing the diagnosis of cancer. With a very small nodule, a negative biopsy may be in question because of the difficulty of being sure that the needle is indeed within the nodule. A few cases of implantation of tumor in the needle track have been reported, but this is rare. Fever may occur following the test.

Aspiration of bone marrow from the posterior iliac crest may reveal the extent of malignant spread more clearly than will either bone scan or radiogram. Epstein (1976) found that needle biopsy was 86% accurate, whereas aspiration was positive in 87% of cases. Use of the combined procedures had a 96% accuracy rate. However, some workers claim

to find few positive bone marrow biopsies in patients known to have lymph node metastases.

I. Lymphangiography: This procedure is increasingly used to seek evidence of metastases to the pelvic nodes even in those patients suspected of having grade B tumors. Positive nodes preclude radical prostatectomy, though a few urologists feel that radical pelvic node dissection may cure a few of these patients. Radiotherapists employ the latter

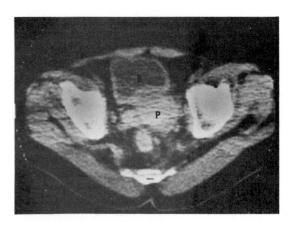

Figure 18–19. Prostatic carcinoma. Mass (P) posterior to thick-walled bladder (B) extends toward but does not involve lateral wall of pelvis. Differentiation of carcinoma from benign prostatic hypertrophy by CT scan alone has not been demonstrated.

technic before institution of therapy in order to better stage the tumor.

It is quite clear, however, that lymphangiography is associated with both false positives and false negatives. For this reason, lymphadenectomy is most often used for accurate staging of the tumor (Loening & others, 1977). Efremidis & others (1979) did lymphangiograms on 5 patients thought to have stage B cancer. Three were read as positive, and 2 were equivocal. However, fine needle aspiration of lymph nodes done under fluoroscopic control showed that all patients had metastatic disease (stage D). The choice of therapy was guided thereby.

J. Tumor Markers: Serum prostatic acid phosphatase determinations are important in the diagnosis, staging, and estimation of prognosis of prostatic cancer. When the cancer extends outside the prostatic capsule and metastases are present, about 70% of patients have elevated levels of this enzyme. This is considered to be pathognomonic of advanced disease whether metastases can be demonstrated or not, though a few patients without metastases or clinical extension locally may elaborate abnormal amounts of the enzyme (Chu & others, 1975). With antiandrogen therapy, the levels tend to revert to normal (Johnson & others, 1976).

Chu & others (1975) also found that urinary cholesterol and serum prostatic acid phosphatase levels were elevated in many patients. The determination of both gave more definitive information than determination of acid phosphatase alone: 86% versus 67%.

Kits for performing radioimmune assay for acid phosphatase are now available. Both serum and bone marrow estimates can be made (Farnsworth & others, 1980). Foti & Hershman (1979) found that simultaneous tests of serum and bone marrow acid phosphatase led to earlier diagnosis, were valuable in staging the tumor, and revealed evidence of subclinical lymphatic and bone marrow metastases (stage D). These tests were also used to monitor the effects of therapy.

Lee & others (1980) have reported on a fluorescent immunoassay for prostatic acid phosphatase, while Mooppan & others (1980) found that serial determinations of urinary hydroxyproline excretion were more sensitive in the diagnosis of osseous metastases than either osteograms or isotope scans.

Serum alkaline phosphatase will be elevated if there are bony metastases. This is a nonspecific reaction and merely reflects the amount of osteogenic activity in the body. After an initial further rise, it too tends to return to normal levels when hormonal treatment is instituted.

Differential Diagnosis

Benign prostatic hyperplasia can usually be differentiated by palpation of the prostate. CT scans alone cannot be used to differentiate between carcinoma and benign prostatic hypertrophy (Fig 18–19). Osteoblastic metastases in the pelvic bones as shown on x-ray or scan or an elevated serum or bone marrow acid phosphatase establishes the diagnosis of advanced cancer. At times only biopsy will clarify it.

Benign firm nodules may present difficulties in differential diagnosis. They may be caused by tuberculosis, chronic infection with fibrosis, granulomatous prostatitis, or calculi. The early cancerous nodule is usually not raised above the surface of the gland (Fig 4–2). The change in consistency from malignant to normal tissue is abrupt. Biopsy, however, is often necessary to make the diagnosis.

(1) Tuberculous nodules are often multiple. One or both seminal vesicles may be thickened. A nontender, thickened epididymis suggests tuberculosis. "Sterile" pyuria with the finding of tubercle bacilli establishes the diagnosis. Urograms may reveal the renal tuberculous lesion.

(2) The fibrous nodule associated with chronic prostatitis is usually raised above the surface of the gland. The induration gradually lessens as the palpating finger approaches normal tissue. Pus is found in the prostatic secretion. Biopsy, however, may be necessary.

(3) Granulomatous prostatitis will cause development of a hard, nodular prostate. A recent history of an acute prostatic infection can usually be elicited. Biopsy, however, may be needed for differentiation.

(4) Prostatic calculi often cause crepitation on palpation. An x-ray will usually reveal their presence just above or behind the symphysis. Occasionally a patient may have both calculi and cancer, however.

On a radiogram, Paget's disease may present a mottled area of increased density of the pelvic bones that must be differentiated from metastatic prostatic cancer. Although Paget's disease may cause a slight increase in serum acid phosphatase, it is less than 10 King-Armstrong units. Higher levels mean prostatic cancer. X-rays of the skull and long bones will show the typical lesion of Paget's disease. Rectal examination should settle the diagnosis.

Mastocytosis, a benign disease, may resemble the osteoblastic prostatic lesion.

Prolonged intake of fluoride (in drinking water) has been reported to cause osteosclerosis that simulates the x-ray appearance of osseous metastases from carcinoma of the prostate.

Complications

Obstruction of the prostatic urethra may cause the formation of vesical diverticula or stones. Infection is common.

Renal damage may be due to functional obstruction of the ureterovesical junction secondary to trigonal hypertrophy, invasion of the intramural portion of the ureters by tumor, or compression of the ureters at the pelvic brim by iliac nodes containing metastatic tumor. Infection may further impair renal function.

Edema of the legs—even of the genitalia—may occur as a result of pressure of involved iliac nodes upon the great vessels or blockage of lymph channels.

Spontaneous fractures can develop at the site of bony metastases. Sudden spinal cord compression is not uncommon and may require immediate laminectomy.

Prevention

At present, only 5% of men, when first seen by the urologist, have lesions that are amenable to cure by radical surgery or radiotherapy. In order that this percentage may be significantly increased, careful palpation of the prostate in all men over age 50 years is mandatory. Any suspicious induration requires a more extensive work-up.

Treatment

A. Surgical Measures:

1. Stage A–This is the tumor found by the pathologist examining prostatic tissue removed with a diagnosis of benign prostatic hypertrophy. Most seem to have low growth potential. Stage A_n requires observation only. Stage A_1—in a young man or if the cells are poorly differentiated—should be treated aggressively by radical surgery or radiotherapy. Men with stage A_2 tumors should be treated as having true carcinoma.

2. Stage B–If the clinician palpating an indurated nodule in the prostate of a well-preserved man under age 70 is unable to say that the patient does not have an early malignant tumor (and unless there is evidence of metastases to bone by x-ray or scan, elevations of serum or bone marrow prostatic acid phosphatase, or a positive bone marrow biopsy), radical prostatectomy should be considered. Needle biopsy (perineal or transrectal) can be done; or, on surgical exploration of the prostate, biopsy and frozen section can confirm the diagnosis. Curative surgery can then be done by either the perineal or retropubic route. The latter approach allows the surgeon to accurately stage the tumor by noting the presence or absence of pelvic lymph node metastases. This approach also permits pelvic lymphadenectomy (Golimbu & Morales, 1980). The entire prostate is removed, including the capsule, along with the seminal vesicles and a portion of the bladder neck. The remaining portion of the bladder neck is then anastomosed to the membranous urethra.

Prostatovesiculectomy will cure about 75% of these favorable stage A and B cases (Correa & others, 1977). Hodges, Pearse, & Stille (1979) summarized their 30-year experience with radical prostatectomy. In 3 series of patients, the 15-year survival rate was 15%, 26%, and 61%, with an average of 31%. Urinary control is usually normal, but impotence is to be expected, though Finkle,

Finkle, & Finkle (1975) believe that impotence is often of psychologic origin. Some advise giving estrogen for 3–6 months before radical prostatectomy is performed, feeling that overall control is thereby enhanced.

3. Stage C–Gill & others (1974) and Carson & others (1980) advise preoperative radiotherapy, radical retropubic prostatectomy, and pelvic lymph node dissection to convert stage C to stage B lesions. McCullough & Leadbetter (1972) practiced radical prostatectomy and pelvic lymph node dissection—even pelvic exenteration—for stage C disease. Combined radiotherapy and chemotherapy appears to be the present-day treatment of choice for stage C lesions.

4. Stage D–There is no surgical cure for these advanced cases. The following treatment methods can be tried: (1) chemotherapy, (2) radiotherapy to painful bony metastases or locally to relieve ureteral obstruction, and (3) antiandrogen therapy for pain.

B. Radiotherapy:

1. X-ray radiation–There is increasing (and justified) enthusiasm for radiation therapy in the management of stage B prostatic carcinoma. Clinicians who believe that stage B lesions should be subjected to radical prostatectomy give preoperative irradiation to patients with stage C tumors in the hope of cure and to those with stage D cancer for the purpose of palliation. The usual doses are 6000–7000 rads for cure and 4000–5000 rads for palliation. This regimen is extended over a period of 5–6 weeks. Proctitis, diarrhea, and urinary frequency are usually experienced toward the end of therapy, but chronic disability is rare. Impotence occurs in 30% of patients, probably as a result of obliteration of the arterioles to the corpora cavernosa. With this therapy, obstructive symptoms usually diminish, ureteral obstruction improves (Michigan & Catalona, 1977), and the prostate usually becomes smaller and softer.

Jazy & others (1979) report that for 116 patients with localized carcinoma, the 5-year survival rate following radiation therapy was 90% for stage A, 70% for stage B, and 40% for stage C. Bagshaw & others (1975) treated a group of patients with stage B disease. At 5 years, 70% were disease-free; at 10 years, 42% showed no signs of recurrence. In a group with extracapsular extension (stage C), 36% were well at 5 years and 29% seemed free of disease at 10 years. Resnick & others (1977) report that 55% of their grade C tumor patients appeared to be free of disease at 5 years. Most authors recommend that this group should be given estrogens as well.

Nachtscheim & others (1978) did prostatic biopsies on 50 patients following radiotherapy. Six of 17 stage A and B and 15 of 33 stage C tumors still had positive biopsies—35% and 45%, respectively. Kurth & others (1977) performed serial perineal biopsies on 53 patients following radiotherapy, noting sterilization in 43%. Radiotherapy, however, is certainly the treatment of choice for the more advanced lesions. For stage D tumors, antiandrogen therapy should also be used for pain from metastases.

In advanced stage D disease—particularly when pain is severe—half or total body irradiation should be considered (Epstein & others, 1979). This can be delivered as a single dose or in divided doses. Half body therapy is about 800 rads. Keen (1980) recommends 800–1000 rads to the lower half of the body followed 6 weeks later by 600 rads to the upper half. These authors claim good palliation.

2. Radioisotopes–Chan & Gutierrez (1976) and Carlton & others (1976) recommend the combination of interstitial radioactive gold implants (3000–4000 rads) in the prostate plus external irradiation (4000–5000 rads).

Whitmore & others (1974) injected ^{125}I into the suprapubically exposed prostate to allow for examination and biopsy of lymph nodes for accurate staging. There is considerable enthusiasm for this therapy. Fowler & others (1979) reported on 300 cases treated with this therapy; 68% were stage B (with negative pelvic lymph nodes) and 32% were stage C. There were only 2 deaths (0.67%); impotence was noted in only 7%. Lytton & others (1979) performed needle biopsies on 22 of 77 patients following treatment; half were positive. Schellhammer, Lagada, & El-Mahdi (1980) subjected 33 patients to ^{125}I therapy. Biopsies up to 18 months were negative in 57%; from 19 to 36 months, 73% were negative, which shows that sterilization continues at a slow rate following radiotherapy.

C. Antiandrogen Therapy: About 85% of prostatic cancers are androgen-dependent. These will show definite regression in size after a few weeks of antiandrogen therapy. The consistency of the gland tends to approach normal, the degree of urinary obstruction lessens, and bone pain disappears or decreases. The patient gains weight and strength, and anemia tends to correct itself. X-ray films often show healing of the metastatic lesions in bone. The price the patient must pay for this palliation includes impotence with loss of sexual desire, tender gynecomastia, and, at times, edema of the ankles. The edema can be controlled by restricted salt intake or the administration of furosemide (Kontturi & Sotaniemi, 1975). Painful gynecomastia can usually be prevented by directing x-ray therapy to the region of the areola before estrogen treatment is begun (Gagnon, Moss, & Stevens, 1979).

There is no doubt that this mode of therapy produces much comfort for patients who formerly suffered greatly. It is also true that the life of these patients is slightly prolonged.

Although antiandrogen therapy has a palliative effect on surgically incurable prostatic carcinoma, it has been shown that the administration of large doses of estrogen significantly increases the incidence of death from thromboembolic phenomena. Therefore, estrogens should be withheld until the patient develops symptoms or signs of metastases;

when this happens, estrogens can be expected to cause regression of metastases in most patients.

Considering the above, it is obvious why radiotherapy is widely utilized in the treatment of the more advanced carcinomas. Furthermore, some of these may be cured by such a method. This is not possible with antiandrogen therapy alone.

Antiandrogen therapy includes orchiectomy and medical neutralization of testicular (and adrenal) androgens. The latter may be accomplished in the following ways:

1. Estrogen medication–Diethylstilbestrol, 1 mg/d, has proved effective and does not seem to be associated with secondary thromboembolic disorders.

Prout & others (1976), however, find that 1 mg/d causes plasma testosterone levels to approach those of castration in only 50% of patients. They recommend that 3 mg/d be given. Other estrogens given in comparable dosage are equally efficient. A few clinicians advocate diethylstilbestrol, 5–100 mg/d for 3 months, and then 25 mg/d thereafter. Such large doses are of questionable value.

Therapy with massive doses of diethylstilbestrol diphosphate has been suggested for patients with extensive disease or for those who are no longer being controlled by the usual dose of estrogen. The drug is given intravenously, undiluted. The following dosage schedule has been recommended: 500 mg 3 times a day for 10 days, 500 mg 2 times a day for 10 days, and then a similar dose daily for the next 10 days followed by 500 mg every week. Possibly half of patients will experience significant improvement.

Smith, Walsh, & Goodwin (1973) note that cyproterone acetate also inhibits elaboration of testosterone and believe that it is superior to estrogens. Barnes & Ninen (1972) believe that in the treatment of stage B tumors the results of estrogen therapy rival those obtained by radical surgery.

Kjaer, Nilsson, & Madsen (1975) and Mittelman, Shukla, & Murphy (1976) recommend the use of estramustine phosphate for advanced prostatic cancer that no longer responds to other modes of treatment. The dose is 1 g/d in 3 divided doses. Both objective and subjective improvement was observed in some patients (Kadohama & others, 1978; Benson, Wear, & Gill, 1979). Sogani, Ray, & Whitmore (1975) administered flutamide in patients who became androgen-independent. The dose is 250 mg 3 times a day. Response was noted in about 30% of patients. Gee & Cole (1980) used orchiectomy and transurethral resection and believed their results to be as good as those obtained with radiotherapy or radical surgery.

2. Orchiectomy–Orchiectomy is similar in action to the administration of estrogens. Bone pain is relieved more promptly when this procedure is used. The combination of diethylstilbestrol and orchiectomy adds little to therapy. Both suppress plasma testosterone.

3. Medical adrenalectomy–This can be accomplished by the administration of cortisone (or an equivalent drug), 50 mg/d in divided doses. Salt must be restricted (0.3 g/d) and potassium added to the diet (3 g/d). This should be tried when the effectiveness of estrogen therapy begins to wane.

4. Surgical adrenalectomy–This rather rigorous procedure offers so little more relief than is afforded by cortisone that it is seldom indicated.

5. Hypophysectomy–Hypophysectomy has few advocates (West & Murphy, 1973), but 90-yttrium or cryosurgical hypophysectomy (Saglam, Wilson, & Seymour, 1970) has been shown to afford relief from diffuse bone pain in 75% of such patients when all other methods of therapy have been exhausted. Levin & others (1978) report significant relief with multiple injections of alcohol.

D. Transurethral Resection: If the degree of obstruction is severe or if antiandrogens or radiotherapy fails to afford much relief, transurethral resection of the prostate will be necessary. Since cancer of the prostate invades the hyperplastic tissue, there is no longer any cleavage plane that will permit intracapsular enucleation, as is ordinarily practiced for benign hyperplasia (eg, suprapubic prostatectomy).

E. Cryosurgery: This technic has been used in the poor-risk patient instead of transurethral resection, with some measure of successful relief of obstruction (Petersen & others, 1978). Gursel, Roberts, & Veenema (1973) have recorded relief of bone pain following prostatic cryosurgery. The implication is that the procedure enhances the immunologic response to the tumor. Other investigators failed to notice such an effect.

F. Testosterone and Radioisotope Therapy: If the tumor becomes androgen-independent and metastases to bone are widespread, some regression of pain may be obtained on the following regimen. Discontinue estrogens and steroids. Give testosterone, 100 mg/d for 17 days. Beginning on the sixth day of this course administer 1.8 mCi of ^{32}P per day orally or intravenously for 7 days. The latter should be followed by therapy with iron, vitamin B complex, and liver extract to maintain an adequate hemogram. Dicalcium phosphate will contribute to reossification of healing bone. Estrogen therapy should then be resumed. Such a course of therapy can be repeated. Johnson & Haynie (1977) noted a favorable response in two-thirds of their patients. Firusian, Mellin, & Schmidt (1976) noted an equally good response following intravenous injection of ^{89}strontium.

G. Testosterone Alone: When all else fails, the administration of testosterone alone can be tried. In most patients it increases existing pain, but in a few cases relief may be obtained. The mechanism for this effect is not clear.

H. Chemotherapy: There has recently been renewed interest in the use of various chemotherapeutic agents for palliation when other treatments fail. Schmidt & others (1979) report encouraging results with dacarbazine (imidazole carboxamide) followed by cyclophosphamide. Ihde (1980) reported partial responses using doxorubicin (Adriamycin) and cyclophosphamide. Merrin (1980) believes cisplatin to be the most effective agent, though renal toxicity is a threat. Soloway, Shippel, & Ikard (1979) used a combination of cyclophosphamide, doxorubicin, and fluorouracil, recording increased survival in 30% of patients. Chlebowski & others (1978) also used the 3 drugs together but concluded that cyclophosphamide alone was as efficacious as the combination. Mukamel, Nissenkorn, & Servadio (1980) noted good response to fluorouracil-cyclophosphamide (see also p 335).

Guinan & others (1979) used adjuvant immunotherapy in the form of BCG and found that treated patients survived 16½ months longer than those not treated.

I. Follow-Up Care: Following radical prostatectomy or radiotherapy, periodic rectal examination should be done to seek local recurrence. In these patients and in those receiving palliative treatment, it is essential to get serial chest films as well as osteograms of the pelvis and lumbar spine or isotope scans in a search for evidence of bony metastases. If the prostatic lesion is considered advanced, serum creatinine or blood urea nitrogen should be estimated. If these levels rise, excretory urograms should be obtained to seek ureteral obstruction that might require treatment.

Careful follow-up of tumor markers—ie, prostatic acid phosphatase and urinary hydroxyproline (for evidence of osseous metastases)—is necessary, since the concentrations of these substances reflect the mass of prostatic cancer cells in the body.

Prognosis

Of the 10% of men with prostatic carcinoma whose illness is diagnosed early enough so that radical surgery would offer a reasonable hope of cure, at least half are over age 70 years and may suffer from other infirmities of age. For this reason they are not good subjects for radical procedures, and most of them will live more comfortably and just as long with palliative treatment and will die of other causes. The cure rate for radical prostatectomy for stage B lesions is 60–70%. Radical radiotherapy offers a similar control rate. For stage C lesions, following radiotherapy, the control rate is about 50% at 5 years. When the effect of irradiation wears off, the physician still has a number of treatment modalities to offer.

SARCOMA OF THE PROSTATE

Sarcoma of the prostate is rare. Two-thirds of them are embryonal rhabdomyosarcomas, seen in young boys, and leiomyosarcomas, which occur in older men. The remainder are lymphomas. Most sarcomas grow rapidly; all are highly malignant. They may extend into the base of the bladder and finally occlude the urethra. They may compress the rectum and cause obstipation. These tumors metastasize by way of the lymphatics to the pelvic and lumbar lymph nodes. Venous spread may occur, in which case the lungs, liver, and bone may become involved.

Clinical Findings

A. Symptoms: Symptoms are largely those of urinary obstruction. Rectal obstruction may cause increasing constipation and symptoms of bowel obstruction.

B. Signs: Since these tumors often grow to large size, they may be felt suprapubically. Rectal examination reveals a very large mass in the prostatic area. It may be firm or may be soft enough to suggest abscess. Considerable residual urine is usually recovered upon catheterization.

C. X-Ray Findings: Cystograms or excretory urograms may show that the bladder has been lifted up by the tumor. A urethrogram will demonstrate the compression and elongation of the posterior urethra.

D. Instrumental Examination: Cystoscopy or panendoscopy will demonstrate the prostatic enlargement. Grapelike masses often fill the prostatic urethra and bladder neck in children.

Treatment & Prognosis

Only recently, with the utilization of combined therapy—cystoprostatectomy, postoperative radiotherapy, and chemotherapy—have a few cures been reported.

TUMORS OF THE SEMINAL VESICLES

About 30 cases of primary carcinoma of the seminal vesicles have been reported in the literature; sarcoma and benign lesions are even rarer. The tumors cause symptoms suggesting obstruction from an enlarged prostate. Bloody ejaculation may be noted. Rectal examination will reveal a mass above the prostate and involving one vesicle. Angiography reveals neovascularity. Radical extirpation of the lesion is indicated, but cure is rare.

TUMORS OF THE URETHRA

BENIGN TUMORS

Benign tumors of the urethra are not common in men or women. A few cases of congenital urethral polyps have been described. They are usually papillary and may be found anywhere between the bladder neck and the external orifice. The most distal tumors may be visible; the others may make their presence known by bloody spotting. If the tumor is large enough, symptoms of urinary obstruction may develop. If the tumor arises in the prostatic urethra, bleeding may be noted in the last portion of the urine. If the tumor is obstructive, infection is apt to be a complication. The diagnosis is made by biopsy. Transurethral electrocoagulation cures these lesions.

MALIGNANT TUMORS

Malignant tumors of the urethra are not common; they occur more often in women than in men. Those arising from the most distal portion of the urethra are epidermoid carcinomas. Those originating more proximally are of the transitional cell type, though a few adenocarcinomas have been reported. Tumors involving the region of the external meatus metastasize to the superficial and deep subinguinal lymph nodes. The more proximal tumors spread to the vesical, sacral, hypogastric, and external iliac nodes (Figs 18–1 and 18–2). They may infiltrate the vulva or vagina.

One of the most common groups of urethral tumors occurs in men who suffer from primary transitional cell tumors of the bladder (Stewart & others, 1978). About half involve the prostatic urethra and half the entire urethra.

If distal, in either men or women, these tumors may first present themselves as visible or palpable masses. Bloody discharge may be noted. Urinary obstruction may occur. The deeper tumors may be quite obstructive and are often complicated by infection. In men, they may be misdiagnosed and treated as urethral strictures. At times these tumors are complicated by periurethral abscesses that may lead to the formation of urinary fistulas.

The diagnosis is made by biopsy of the tumor, which is either palpated externally or seen directly by panendoscopy or on urethrograms (Fig 6–10).

Tumors of the distal urethra in women can often be cured by local excision, though Prempree, Wizenberg, & Scott (1978) recommend the insertion of radium needles or radiotherapy for the smaller tumors. Similar tumors in men require amputation of the penis proximal to the lesion. Radical inguinal node dissection (which includes the superficial and deep subinguinal and the superficial inguinal nodes) is indicated if the nodes are involved.

Cancer of the perineal urethra may require radical penectomy with the formation of a perineal urethral orifice. If the bulb is involved, prostatocystectomy must be performed as well and the urinary stream diverted. In the female, if the deep urethra or all of the urethra is involved, consideration should be given to radiotherapy followed by urethrocystectomy with urinary diversion.

Radiotherapy or surgical excision of small distal lesions offers a 5-year control rate of about 50%. The prognosis is poor for proximal tumors.

On the whole, these tumors are very malignant, and few cures are obtained in patients whose lesions involve the proximal urethra.

TUMORS OF
THE SPERMATIC CORD
& PARATESTICULAR TISSUES

More than 300 cases of tumors of the spermatic cord have been reported. Most are benign and are composed of connective tissue elements. The malignant tumors (eg, rhabdomyosarcoma, fibrosarcoma) spread by both the hematogenous and lymphatic routes. The latter is the most common. They involve the iliac and preaortic lymph nodes as well as the liver and lungs.

These tumors present palpable masses that may be associated with local pain. A blow to the area may bring the lesion to the attention of the patient. They must be differentiated from hernias, hydrocele of the cord, spermatocele, and testis tumor.

Benign tumors require orchiectomy with division of the cord at the internal inguinal ring just in case the pathologist should find a malignant focus. Sarcomas require a similar procedure. If no hematogenous spread can be demonstrated, radical retroperitoneal lymphadenectomy should be done. The latter operation has produced cures in some patients with positive nodes. An improved control rate has been reported following lymph node dissection, radiotherapy, and chemotherapy, particularly in children (Sogani, Grabstald, & Whitmore, 1978; Cromie, Raney, & Duckett, 1979).

TUMORS OF THE TESTIS

Most tumors of the testes are malignant. While most develop between ages 18 and 35 years, Osborn & Jeffrey (1976) have found over 650 instances of such tumors in childhood, the majority occurring during the first year of life. Most of these are embryonal carcinomas, benign teratomas, and teratocarcinomas. Seminomas are rare (Viprakasit & others, 1977). Tsuji & others (1973) report a high incidence of such new growths in Japanese children. Brosman (1979) reviewed 556 pediatric cases from the literature and his own experience. Germ cell tumors accounted for 424 (76%); of these, 86% were yolk sac carcinoma (the adult type of embryonal carcinoma was rare) and the remainder were teratomas. Nongerminal cell tumors (132) comprised 24% of all tumors. Of these, 16% were Sertoli cell tumors, 40% were Leydig cell tumors, and 58% were connective tissue tumors (eg, rhabdomyosarcoma). Most of those seen after age 60 years are reticulum cell sarcomas or Sertoli cell or interstitial cell tumors; only 25% arise from germ cells. Testis tumors account for about 0.5% of all malignancies in men and 4% of all tumors affecting the genitourinary tract. About 30 instances of bilateral tumors have been reported. Metastasis occurs relatively early. Some elaborate chorionic gonadotropins, and the prognosis in this type is poor. Retroperitoneal and mediastinal tumors without evidence of testicular involvement are occasionally seen (Das, Bochetto, & Alpert, 1975).

Testicular tumors are relatively rare in blacks.

Etiology
The cause of testicular tumors is not known. It may be significant, however, that they usually develop during the age of greatest sexual activity. Many authorities believe that the undescended testis, particularly in the pseudohermaphrodite, has a definite tendency to undergo carcinomatous change. Whether maldescent is the cause or whether some unknown factor causes both the lack of descent and tumor formation is not decided.

Pathogenesis & Pathology
A. Classification: Many classifications of tumor of the testis have been offered, most of them based upon morphology. Since about 30% of these tumors elaborate chorionic gonadotropin (Wilson & Woodhead, 1972), a morphologic-endocrine grouping is feasible.

1. Totipotent cell pattern–Most authorities agree that all of the teratomatous tumors of the testis, mixed or pure, arise from a totipotent cell that can develop in many directions. These cells have been likened to a twin of the host—a twin that develops in the host's own testis. Mixed tumors (teratomas) contain both mesenchymal and epithelial tissues. Fewer than 5% are benign, and most of those occur in children; the rest are malignant. The malignant epithelial cells may overgrow the other elements and appear as the only cell in the tumor unless serial sections are studied. However, one tumor frequently contains elements of 2 or even 3 of the common types.

a. Seminoma pattern (30%)–These tumors are made up of sheets of round epithelial cells with clear cytoplasm and large nuclei. Fibrous septa course through the tumor; these may be infiltrated with lymphocytes. Mitoses are common. Thirteen percent are chromatin-positive (female). The modal chromosome numbers are usually 50 or more. About 7% secrete chorionic gonadotropin.

b. Carcinoma pattern (40%)–This type tends to secrete chorionic gonadotropin and is often associated with hyperplasia of the interstitial cells. These tumors may therefore have arisen from primitive chorionic tissues. These embryonal epithelial cells may take on a papillary pattern. The cytoplasm is often granular. There is considerable variation in the size of the cells. Many mitoses are present. In some, syncytial cells are apparent; in others, the small Langhans' cells are seen. Typical choriocarcinoma may be observed (2% of all testis tumors); almost all secrete gonadotropin. Embryonal carcinoma is the most common tumor in this group. Thirty percent elaborate chorionic gonadotropins.

c. Teratoma pattern (25%)–These tumors contain numerous types of immature and mature mesenchymal and epithelial structures, including muscle, cartilage, nerve, and mucosa. One or more of these may predominate and present malignant change. These tumors may represent malformed embryos. The pure teratoma does not elaborate chorionic gonadotropin, so hyperplasia of Leydig cells is not seen. This hormone, however, is secreted in 37% of patients whose tumors contain embryonal carcinoma or choriocarcinoma. Abnormal chromosome patterns are seen in 32% of this group. Many have 50 or more chromosomes.

2. Interstitial cell tumors–More than 170 cases of Leydig cell tumors have been reported (Selvaggi & others, 1973). About 75% are seen after age 30; 90% are benign. They secrete an increased amount of estrogens; 17-ketosteroids are normal or low. When the tumor develops before puberty, macrogenitosomia occurs. About 20% of adults develop gynecomastia, and most are impotent and sterile. The malignant form metastasizes widely, but particularly to bone.

3. Sertoli cell tumors–These rare, usually benign tumors are feminizing. Gynecomastia is a cardinal finding.

4. Lymphoma and reticulum cell sarcoma–These tumor types are occasionally observed (Sussman & others, 1977). Leukemic infiltration has been reported.

5. Adrenal rests are occasionally seen.

6. Metastatic testis tumors–Tumors metastatic to the testis include tumors of the lung, prostate, and gastrointestinal tract and malignant melanoma (skin).

B. Chorionic Gonadotropins: These substances may be found in the urine in abnormal amounts in about 30% of patients with testicular tumors. The prognosis in those with positive hormone titers is relatively poor. Usually such tumors have a carcinomatous pattern. If a positive hormone test is found in what seems to be a seminoma or teratoma, further sectioning will often reveal tumor

of the carcinoma type (Javadpour, McIntire, & Waldmann, 1978). If the level of this hormone drops to normal after orchiectomy, the prognosis is improved. If, however, it rises again or if, after orchiectomy, it fails to drop, the presumption is that metastatic tumor is present. Clinically, these tumors must be considered choriocarcinomas even though typical cells cannot be found in the testis. At autopsy, many of these patients will be found to have the hemorrhagic metastases typical of choriocarcinoma.

C. Metastases: Except for choriocarcinoma, the major route for metastases is lymphatic. The lumbar and mediastinal nodes are most commonly involved. The left and occasionally the right supraclavicular nodes are at times affected. The lesion will spread to the superficial inguinal and subinguinal nodes only if the scrotum becomes invaded (and this is unusual) or if previous orchiectomy or hernioplasty has been performed. In 20% of cases with lymph node metastases, the abdominal (lumbar) lymph nodes on the side opposite the primary tumor will contain metastatic cancer. It is for this reason that lymph node dissection should be bilateral.

Masses of lumbar lymph nodes may displace the ureters or kidneys. Ureteral occlusion occasionally is observed. Bowel may also be displaced.

Metastases are also commonly found in the lungs and liver; other organs are involved less frequently. Probably 30–40% of the patients have metastases when they are first seen.

Staging of Germinal Cell Testicular Tumors

The following is the Walter Reed General Hospital staging system (Buck & others, 1972):

Stage A₁: Tumor confined to testis; no clinical or radiographic evidence of spread.

Stage A₂: Tumor confined to testis; no clinical or radiographic evidence of spread, but histologic evidence of metastases to iliac or para-aortic nodes seen at retroperitoneal lymphadenectomy.

Stage B: Clinical or radiographic evidence of metastases to nodes below the diaphragm; no demonstrable metastases above the diaphragm or to viscera.

Stage C: Clinical or radiographic evidence of metastases above the diaphragm or to viscera.

Pretreatment staging of these tumors is of great importance in choosing optimum treatment. This requires excretory urograms, whole lung tomograms, liver scan, and serum tumor markers. Sago & others (1978) gained little from the gallium scan, routine supraclavicular lymph node biopsy (unless palpable), or lymphangiography, which has an accuracy rate of only about 60% (Hutschenreiter, Alken, & Schneider, 1979). Both sonograms and CT scans are far more accurate than lymphangiography; Burney & Klatte (1979) believe that both tests should be used. Wettlaufer & Modarelli (1979) stress the need for biopsy of solitary pulmonary

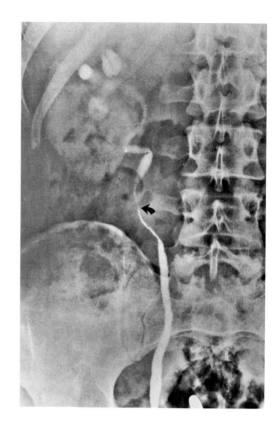

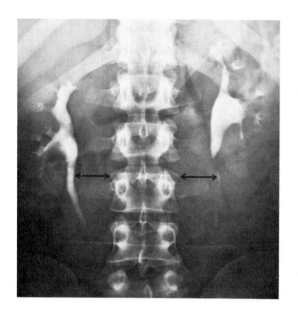

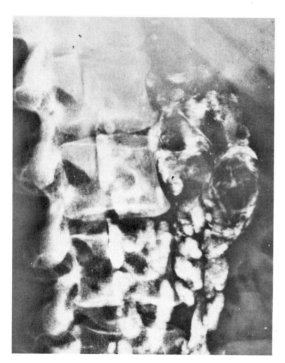

Figure 18–20. Carcinoma of the testis. *Above left:* Excretory urogram showing lateral displacement of both upper ureters by metastases to lumbar lymph nodes. *Above right:* Retrograde bulb ureterogram showing hydronephrosis and ureteral deviation at L4 secondary to metastases in right lumbar lymph nodes. (See Fig 6–14 for venacavogram on same patient.) *Left:* Lymphangiogram demonstrating enlarged lumbar lymph nodes involved by metastatic tumor.

nodules, citing 3 cases where lesions proved to be benign.

Clinical Findings

A painless lump in the testis must be regarded as tumor until proved otherwise. The common sites of metastases are the preaortic lymph nodes and the lungs. Gynecomastia suggests the presence of a functioning tumor and is a bad prognostic sign. About 10% of tumors produce this symptom. If carcinoma of the testis cannot be unequivocally ruled out, orchiectomy must be done immediately.

A. Symptoms: The most common presenting symptom is enlargement of the testis. It may be discovered quite by accident, or attention may be drawn to it because of mild discomfort caused by its weight. On rare occasion it can be quite painful if bleeding occurs into its own substance.

If the tumor is elaborating large amounts of chorionic gonadotropins, gynecomastia may be seen (Walsh, 1975). This change is also seen with Sertoli and Leydig cell tumors, both of which cause secretion of estrogen.

Symptoms from metastases include a supraclavicular or abdominal mass (lymph nodes), abdominal pain from bowel or ureteral obstruction, cough from metastases to the lung, and nonspecific symptoms of loss of weight and anorexia.

In the rare instance of a Leydig cell tumor, a preadolescent boy may undergo precocious development of sexual organs and secondary sex characteristics. The adult experiences no accentuation of sex characteristics; in fact, he is apt to become impotent. The boy with Sertoli cell tumor may develop a female escutcheon and gynecomastia.

B. Signs: The testis is usually definitely enlarged and diffusely involved. The tumor is ordinarily smooth and in general maintains the ovoid shape of the testis. It is firm and gives the sensation of abnormal weight. It does not transilluminate. Of the greatest importance is the fact that pressure on the organ fails to cause the typical sickening testicular discomfort. The epididymis can be distinguished from the testis in the early stages, but later it is lost in the mass. A very early tumor may present as a firm, nontender nodule embedded in the testis.

The spermatic cord is usually normal on palpation. It is rare for the scrotum to be involved except in the last stage of the disease unless previous orchiopexy, herniorrhaphy, or removal of the tumor through a scrotal incision has been done (Herr, Silber, & Martin, 1973). Hydrocele develops secondary to tumor in about 10% of cases. In such instances in young men, if adequate palpation of the testis cannot be done, the hydrocele must be aspirated.

Metastases without an evident primary source occurring in a young cryptorchid patient should suggest the possibility of tumor of that testis. A hard mass in the left supraclavicular area in a young man should be regarded as testicular malignancy until proved otherwise, since tumor of the testis is the most common malignancy in that age group. Gynecomastia should suggest the presence of a functioning testicular neoplasm. Metastases should be sought along the aorta; masses of involved lymph nodes are often palpable.

In the later stages, evidence of weight loss and even cachexia may be seen.

C. Laboratory Findings: The patient may be anemic if metastases are widespread. Urinalysis is of no help in diagnosis. Renal function is usually normal even though unilateral ureteral occlusion develops. An estimate of the level of urinary or serum chorionic gonadotropins should be done. Their presence means testicular tumor of the carcinoma type or choriocarcinoma and is a grave prognostic sign. A negative test has no diagnostic significance.

The 17-ketosteroids are normal or low with Leydig cell tumor. Urinary estrogens may be increased with both Leydig cell and Sertoli cell neoplasms.

D. X-Ray Findings: A chest film with tomograms may show evidence of metastases. Excretory urograms are indicated in all cases of testicular tumor; masses of carcinomatous lumbar nodes may displace the ureter or kidney (Fig 18–20) and may cause ureteral stenosis. Retrograde ureterograms (Fig 18–20) or venacavograms (Fig 6–14) may more clearly delineate an extraureteral mass. Lymphangiography is a good method for demonstrating lymph node metastases (Fig 18–20), although a number of false positives and a few false negatives have been observed. CT scans are proving to be quite accurate in depicting metastases to retroperitoneal lymph nodes. They are therefore of value in follow-up.

E. Ultrasonography: This is a very successful method for discovering retroperitoneal node involvement.

F. Biopsy: Though Buck & others (1972) recommended that stage B patients have bilateral supraclavicular node biopsy, Fowler, McLeod, & Stutzman (1979) gained little information from this procedure.

G. Isotope Scans: A liver scan should be ordered. Total body scanning with [67]gallium has been recommended by Bailey & others (1973) to discover lymph node or lung metastases. Paterson, Peckham, & McCready (1977) found it helpful with seminoma but of little value in teratoma.

H. Tumor Markers: Serum alpha-fetoprotein (AFP) and human chorionic gonadotropin (hCG) are excellent germ cell tumor-markers whose presence in increased amounts corroborates the diagnosis, contributes to the staging of the tumor, and monitors the response of the tumor to therapy. Javadpour (1980) reports that the combination of these 2 tests has markedly decreased staging errors. He found that stage B or C tumors have elevated markers following orchidectomy. If markers remain positive after retroperitoneal node dissection, the tumor is probably stage C. If the lymph nodes are free of tumor and the levels remain elevated, the tumor is stage C.

About 35% of nonseminomatous tumors will elaborate AFP and 38% will secrete hCG (Shultz & others, 1978). Skinner & Scardino (1980) found elevated levels of serum AFP or hCG (or both) in 94% of their patients, with no false positives observed. Seminomas, on the other hand, were found to be associated with increased hCG in only 7.6% of cases, and none were found to have increased AFP (Javadpour, McIntire, & Waldmann, 1978). These statistics are obviously important in choosing therapy.

While plasma carcinoembryonic antigen (CEA) is a nonspecific marker, if it is found to be elevated, serial estimates will show a parallel response to treatment (Javadpour, 1973).

Serum lactic dehydrogenase (LDH) is quite nonspecific, but Lieskovsky and Skinner (1980) found test results to be positive in 62% of stage B and 35% of stage C lesions. If positive, it can be used to estimate response to treatment.

Recently, a new marker has been investigated: pregnancy-specific β_1 glycoprotein (SP$_1$) (Javadpour, 1980). It is elevated in 10–50% of nonseminomatous tumors but is usually normal with seminoma. It arises in the syncytiotrophoblastic giant cells. Lange & others (1980) found SP$_1$ elevated in most patients with metastases in nonseminomatous tumors, which were usually also associated with increased levels of AFP and hCG.

Differential Diagnosis

A. Painless Scrotal Swellings: Hydrocele may be quite tense and even firm if the tunica vaginalis is thickened. It will transilluminate. Hydrocele, it must be remembered, develops secondary to some testicular malignancies. In case of doubt, aspirate the hydroceles of young men to afford adequate palpation of the testis.

A spermatocele is a free cystic mass lying above and behind the testis.

Tuberculosis of the epididymis may present itself as an enlargement, but palpation should show that the testis is separate from the mass. If the testis has become secondarily involved, differentiation may be more difficult. The diagnosis of tuberculosis will be enhanced by finding beading of the vas, induration of the prostate or seminal vesicles, and pus and tubercle bacilli in the urine.

Gumma is a very rare nontender testicular lesion that causes enlargement. A history of syphilis and a positive serologic test should suggest this diagnosis.

About 75 instances of epidermoid cyst of the testis have been reported. The correct diagnosis is made by the pathologist. Occasionally, other tumors may metastasize to the testes. The primary sites are the prostate, lung, gastrointestinal tract, and skin (melanoma).

B. Painful Scrotal Swellings: It is rare for testicular tumors to be exquisitely painful, but moderate discomfort is present in 40% of patients. Nonspecific epididymitis, if acute, is exceedingly painful. If this condition is seen early, it is obvious that only the epididymis is involved. After some hours, the entire testis becomes swollen. Pyuria and symptoms of lower tract infection are usually present. Chronic epididymitis should not be confusing, for the induration will involve the epididymis only.

Mumps orchitis is usually much more painful than tumor and is quite tender. Parotitis is almost always evident, and fever may be quite high.

Torsion of the spermatic cord is a disease of childhood, at which age tumor is unusual. Torsion is suggested if the epididymis can be felt anterior to the testis. Also, elevation of the testis onto the pubis increases the torsion and therefore the pain.

Complications

Complications arise from the metastases. Rarely, a ureter may become completely occluded by extrinsic pressure from involved lymph nodes.

Following bilateral retroperitoneal lymphadenectomy, most patients will produce no ejaculate with orgasm. This is caused by damage to the lumbar sympathetic trunks that govern seminal emission.

Treatment

If careful examination does not rule out testicular tumor, the testicle should be explored through a groin incision. If the diagnosis is still in doubt, biopsy can be done with a vascular clamp on the spermatic cord. Otherwise, orchidectomy is done at the level of the internal inguinal ring. The type of tumor governs the choice of treatment.

A. Germinal Tumors:

1. Seminoma–In the absence of evidence of metastases or if retroperitoneal node involvement is not bulky, irradiation is the treatment of choice and the response is excellent. In case of massive metastases to the retroperitoneal nodes (stage B$_3$) or other organs (stage C), Smith, de Kernion, & Skinner (1979) recommend preradiation chemotherapy using dactinomycin, vincristine, and cyclophosphamide. Radiotherapy is then directed to the retroperitoneum, mediastinum, and supraclavicular lymph nodes. If retroperitoneal nodes persist, these authors perform node dissection.

2. Nonseminoma–These tumors are not as radiosensitive as the seminomas, so other treatment methods must be employed. Bilateral retroperitoneal lymphadenectomy is recommended for stage A tumors, followed by radiotherapy to the same area. Edson (1979) gives dactinomycin both before and after lymph node resection and claims improved results. For stage B tumors, Donohue,

Einhorn, & Perez (1978) recommend dactinomycin before lymphadenectomy, while Edson (1979), Hendry & others (1980), and Oliver & others (1980) recommend triple drug therapy before giving radiotherapy to the retroperitoneum in stage C tumors. Useful drugs appear to be cisplatin, vinblastine, and bleomycin. These drugs are quite toxic, but many lives are saved with their use.

Lobectomy has been successfully employed in a few patients with isolated pulmonary metastases (Reed, Barry, & Hodges, 1976).

B. Nongerminal Tumors:

1. Interstitial cell (Leydig cell) tumor–Radical orchidectomy will suffice for the common benign form. Chemotherapy and retroperitoneal lymphadenectomy or even radiotherapy should be considered if the tumor proves to be malignant (Caldamone & others, 1979; Klippel & others, 1979).

2. Sertoli cell tumors–These are seldom malignant, so orchidectomy only is indicated (Weitzner, Aldridge, & Weems, 1979).

3. Lymphoma and reticulum cell sarcoma–Radiotherapy or chemotherapy is valuable if other sites of these tumors are found.

Follow-Up Care

Periodic abdominal palpation in search of masses of lymph nodes, liver enlargement, or nodular formation is essential. Examination for supraclavicular lymph node enlargement is also necessary, and serial chest films should be done. If the patient had elevated tumor markers before treatment was started, they should be measured periodically. If they remain normal, one can assume that no residual tumor is present. A later elevation is a worrisome sign that may suggest the need for adjuvant chemotherapy. Survey of the abdomen by CT scan (Lee & others, 1979) or ultrasonography may reveal enlarging lymph node masses.

Prognosis

During the last few years, the survival rate, particularly for the nonseminoma group, has significantly improved because of more sophisticated chemotherapy and the valuable information provided by tumor markers. Stage A seminoma has a survival rate of 97%; nonseminomatous tumors of similar grade have a rate close to 95%. Chemotherapy is making a real impact. Donohue, Einhorn, & Perez (1978), reporting a series of patients with nonseminoma tumors, recorded 100% survival for stage A, 68% survival for stage B, and 50% survival for stage C. Stoter & others (1979), treating advanced nonseminomas with triple drug therapy in 40 patients, noted complete remission in 60% and partial improvement in 28%. Three of their patients died as a consequence of the drugs.

Almost all patients with choriocarcinoma are dead within 2 years of diagnosis.

Ise & others (1976) treated 67 children with testis tumors. Most had metastases to lymph nodes, lungs, or bone. They reported long-term survival in 89% following orchiectomy, radiation therapy, and lymphadenectomy. Hopkins & others (1978) report even better results when chemotherapy was added to the regimen.

Hyperplasia of interstitial cells is a bad prognostic sign. The majority of these patients also have increased levels of urinary gonadotropins. The finding of chorionic gonadotropin in the urine is a serious sign. Most of these patients die within 2 years.

TUMORS OF THE EPIDIDYMIS

Tumors of the epididymis are quite rare, but most are benign (adenomatoid tumors). They may arise from epithelial or connective tissue structures. The malignant group spreads by lymphatics (same as testis) and veins and offers a poor prognosis. Tumors metastasizing to the epididymis are rare.

These tumors often present as painless enlargement, although mild discomfort may be felt. Hydrocele may be the only change present; this, of course, is also true of tumors of the testis. Aspiration of hydroceles is imperative if the testicle cannot be properly palpated.

These lesions must be differentiated from tuberculous or nonspecific epididymitis; this may prove impossible without surgical exploration.

Treatment consists of epididymectomy if one can be sure the lesion is benign (frozen section). Orchiectomy must be undertaken for cancer or sarcoma. X-ray therapy to regional lymph nodes is also indicated. The prognosis is poor for the malignant tumors.

TUMORS OF THE PENIS

Almost all tumors of the penis are of epithelial origin and almost always involve the prepuce or glans. They are similar in all respects to epitheliomas elsewhere on the body. A few sarcomas have been reported (Lue & others, 1980).

Etiology

There seems to be no doubt that the most common cause of cancer of the penis is chronic inflammation from infection of the foreskin and glans. In China, Africa, and Southeast Asia, 10–15% of all tumors are of the penis. On the other hand, the incidence is less than 5% where circumcision is the rule. Kuruvilla, Garlick, & Mammen (1971) note that the incidence of penile cancer is higher in Hindus than in Muslims. The latter practice circumcision; the former do not.

Pathogenesis & Pathology

Certain precancerous lesions can be recognized. Leukoplakia may rarely involve the penis. It consists of a white scaly lesion that causes some thickening of the skin. Microscopically, hyperplasia of the squamous cell layer is evident. There is no invasion of the subcutaneous tissue. Considerable small round cell infiltration is seen.

Erythroplasia of Queyrat is strictly a lesion of the penis. Its surface is ordinarily red and indurated and may ulcerate. On microscopic examination, considerable overdevelopment of the rete pegs is noted, yet their basement membranes remain intact. Mitoses are present, but the cells are fairly uniform in size. Some increase in vascularity is noticeable. It may respond to fluorouracil applied locally.

Bowen's disease (carcinoma in situ) may be found on any skin surface. A raised, indurated, red plaque may be noted; its center may be ulcerated. Microscopic study reveals anaplasia of epithelial elements, with considerable hyperplasia of the squamous cell layers and mitotic activity. The basement membrane, however, remains intact.

Epidermoid carcinoma of the penis is rarely found in a man who has been circumcised during infancy. The growth usually arises on the glans or the inner surface of the foreskin. It may first appear as a raised, red, firm plaque or as an ulcer. As it grows it may be proliferative or ulcerative. It is usually painless, although severe secondary infection may cause discomfort. Because of the tumor and the edema from infection, retraction of the prepuce may be impossible.

The microscopic picture in epidermoid carcinoma is the same as that of epidermoid cancer anywhere on the skin or mucous surfaces. Hyperkeratosis is prominent. Hyperplasia of the rete is marked, and mitoses are frequent. Invasion of the connective tissue is obvious. Metastases occur through lymph channels that drain to the superficial and deep subinguinal and superficial inguinal nodes; the iliac nodes may also become involved. Enlarged lymph nodes are commonly found in these patients; some are inflammatory and others contain metastatic tumor cells. Widespread metastases by way of veins are not common.

Among the rare growths reported are leiomyosarcoma, melanoma, Kaposi's sarcoma, and vascular tumors.

Tumors metastatic to the penis include the following primary sites: bladder, prostate, rectum, lung, nasopharynx, pancreas, and skin.

Staging of Tumors of the Penis

Stage A: Lesion limited to glans or foreskin.
Stage B: Tumor invading shaft or corpora cavernosa. No nodes involved.
Stage C: Tumor invading shaft. Operable lymph node involvement.
Stage D: Inoperable lymph nodes and distant metastases.

Clinical Findings

Neoplasms of the penis are usually epithelial and malignant. They involve the foreskin or glans and may be papillary or infiltrating. Metastases to the subinguinal and inguinal lymph nodes are common and imply a poor prognosis.

A. Symptoms: The patient may notice an enlarging warty growth or a spreading ulcer on the glans or foreskin. These lesions are usually painless unless secondary infection is marked. Tumors of the shaft are rare.

If the foreskin cannot be retracted, the patient may complain of local pain from infection; a foul, often bloody discharge emanating from the preputial pouch; and a firm lump in the region of the glans.

Masses in the inguinal region may be noted. They can be quite painful and tender if inflammatory, although this finding does not rule out the presence of metastases.

B. Signs: A papillary or ulcerating tumor may be seen. The latter type may be quite destructive. If tumor is suspected and the foreskin cannot be retracted, the prepuce should be slit dorsally.

Enlarged lymph nodes may be found both above and below the inguinal ligament. These can be due to metastases, infection, or both. In the advanced stage, these masses may be quite large and may ulcerate through the skin and bleed.

C. Laboratory Findings: Anemia may be evident in the later stages of the disease. Leukocytosis may be secondary to local infection. The urine bathing an unretractable foreskin will show pus, bacteria, and often red cells. Biopsy is necessary in all patients suspected of having tumors. This can usually be done under local anesthesia. A slit in the dorsal surface of the foreskin may be necessary to properly visualize the lesion.

D. X-Ray Findings: Lymphangiography may show metastases to the inguinal lymph nodes, but CT scanning is less invasive and probably more dependable.

E. Sonography: This is a noninvasive method of seeking pelvic node involvement.

Differential Diagnosis

Syphilitic chancre may simulate a small ulcerating epithelioma. Dark-field examination should reveal *Treponema pallidum.* In case of doubt, biopsy is indicated.

Chancroid can at times cause some confusion in diagnosis. It is ordinarily a rapidly spreading ulcerative lesion that is quite painful. Complement fixation tests or the finding of *Haemophilus ducreyi* on smears from the lesion is diagnostic.

Condylomata acuminata are soft warty growths

usually of venereal origin and probably caused by a virus. They are usually not invasive. If any doubt exists, biopsy should be done.

Complications

The common complications of tumors of the penis are infection of the tumor and inguinal adenitis, metastatic involvement to the ilioinguinal and iliac nodes, and, rarely, invasion of the urethra, with urinary obstruction.

Prevention

The evidence seems to be quite clear that circumcision in infancy will almost certainly prevent carcinoma of the penis in later life.

Treatment

Before treatment is instituted, a biopsy must be obtained and a positive diagnosis of cancer established.

A. The Local Lesion: Small lesions without evidence of metastases (stage A) can be destroyed by local excision or by x-ray or radium therapy. Salaverria & others (1979) use iridium-192 wire, with which they deliver 6000 rads to the tumor. More extensive lesions (stage B) may require partial amputation, though evidence is mounting that irradiation offers a comparable cure rate (50%). Amputation should be done at a level 2 cm proximal to the tumor. Local recurrence after amputation is rare.

B. The Inguinal and Subinguinal Lymph Nodes: If the primary lesion is small and no adenopathy is demonstrable (stage A), radical resection of the inguinal areas is not indicated. These wounds are often slow to heal, and considerable lymphedema of the area develops.

If a few metastatic inguinal nodes are evident (stage C) as judged by examination or biopsy and if the lymphangiogram shows no involvement of the iliac nodes, bilateral radical inguinal and subinguinal node dissection must be done because of the cross-connection between the 2 sides.

In the presence of advanced metastases, either local or general, excision of these nodes is valueless.

C. The Iliac Lymph Nodes: If lymphangiography or exploratory laparotomy reveals involvement of the iliac nodes, radical resection of these nodes should be considered.

D. X-Ray Therapy: Gursel & others (1973) found that lymph node dissection contributed little to their cure rates. They advise irradiation of the inguinal and subinguinal nodes should they be involved (stage C) and similar therapy to the deep pelvic nodes should laparotomy or lymphangiography reveal their involvement (stage D). Most authors, however, would only irradiate inoperable lymph nodes for palliation.

E. Chemotherapy: Bleomycin has been employed in advanced cases, but it is quite toxic and occasionally causes pulmonary fibrosis (De Kernion

& others, 1973). Encouraging results have been obtained with cisplatin (Sklaroff & Yagoda, 1979) and methotrexate (Skarloff & Yagoda, 1980).

Prognosis

When a small tumor is localized to the penis and there are no metastases (stage A), the 5-year control rate is 70–90%. If the tumor invades the penile shaft or corpora cavernosa (without lymph node involvement), the cure rate drops to about 70%. Should there be moderate lymph node spread, cure is obtained in only 30%. When there are distant metastases, the cure rate is zero.

TUMORS OF THE SCROTUM

Tumors of the scrotal skin are rare. Most of them arise from occupational exposure to various carcinogens, including soot, tars, creosote, and petroleum products. While a few benign tumors of the skin or subcutaneous tissues occur, most are epitheliomas. Also encountered are reticulum cell sarcoma, melanoma, rhabdomyosarcoma, leiomyosarcoma, and liposarcoma. They metastasize by lymphatic channels to the superficial inguinal and subinguinal nodes.

The diagnosis should be considered in any lesion of the scrotal skin in a man who gives a history of prolonged exposure to carcinogens. Biopsy is necessary if any doubt exists. Treatment consists of wide excision of the primary tumor. If a few inguinal metastases are noted, bilateral inguinal node dissection is indicated.

In the absence of lymph node metastasis, the cure rate is 50%. When lymph node spread is found, only 25% of patients survive.

RETROPERITONEAL EXTRARENAL TUMORS

Although these tumors and cysts are rare, they must be considered in the differential diagnosis of renal and suprarenal masses, since they present as masses in the flank. Most of these neoplasms arise from mesothelial tissues of the retroperitoneum and are therefore of connective tissue origin. They may be comprised of a single type of cell (eg, lipoma, fibroma) but more commonly are mixed tumors (eg, chondrolipomyxoma). Many are malignant (eg, lipomyxorhabdomyosarcoma). Others, for the most part, arise from the mesonephros and its duct and from the gonads. The cystic tumors are benign; the solid growths may be benign but are more often malignant. Even if benign, however, they tend to

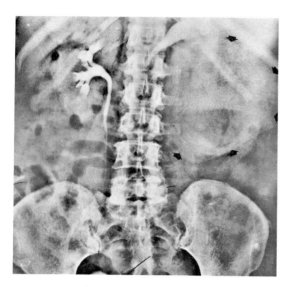 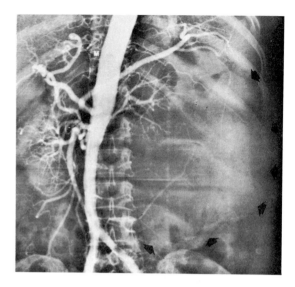

Figure 18–21. Retroperitoneal lipoma. *Left:* Excretory urogram showing large soft tissue mass in left upper quadrant displacing kidney superomedially. Right kidney is normal. *Right:* Renal angiogram, same patient, revealing large, relatively avascular mass in left abdomen. Left renal vasculature displaced medially and superiorly.

grow to large size and to surround and displace adjacent organs.

The most common finding is a painless mass in the flank. Gastrointestinal symptoms caused by displacement or invasion of intraperitoneal organs may also be noted. Edema of the legs may occur if the vena cava is occluded. A plain film of the abdomen may show a large soft tissue mass in the upper abdomen. The kidney may be displaced, yet its caliceal system is not distorted; this is a cardinal sign of retroperitoneal extrarenal tumor (Fig 18–21). Hydronephrosis may develop from ureteral compression. Gastrointestinal studies may reveal displacement of the stomach or colon. Renal tumors or cysts cause distortion of the pelvis and calices; extrarenal tumors ordinarily do not. CT scans and sonograms will show that the mass does not arise from the kidney but merely displaces it. A tumor will be more dense than a cyst. Angiography shows a relatively avascular mass whose blood supply is largely derived from the lumbar arteries.

Adrenal tumors are rarely large enough to be palpable. The x-ray findings are the same in both adrenal and retroperitoneal extrarenal tumors, but most adrenal tumors are associated with symptoms and signs of hyperfunction. Angiography, sonography, or CT scan will differentiate between the two.

An enlarged spleen may present as a mass in the left upper abdomen and at times can displace the kidney. Hematologic changes may accompany splenomegaly; findings elsewhere consistent with lymphoma may be helpful. Again, angiography, ultrasonography, or CT scan will make the diagnosis.

The main complication is displacement, envelopment, or invasion of adjacent organs (eg, spleen, stomach, liver, ureter, kidney, vena cava, and aorta).

Surgical removal of the cyst or tumor is the only method of cure. The solid tumors are difficult to remove in toto because of their penchant for invading and surrounding vital structures. Though these tumors are considered radioresistant, Duncan & Evans (1977) recommend radiation therapy following surgical excision. Binder, Katz, & Sheridan (1978) feel that if the tumor is large, preoperative irradiation might shrink it, making resection easier. In both cases, irradiation should be augmented by chemotherapy.

The prognosis after the excision of cysts is good. The recurrence rate after removal of the solid tumors is high even though the neoplasm is benign.

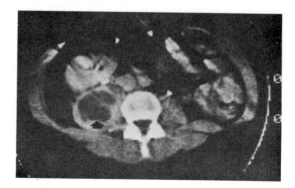

Figure 18–22. Right psoas abscess. Massive enlargement of right psoas muscle with lobulated low-density center (arrow) is characteristic of psoas abscess. Necrotic retroperitoneal neoplasm may present similar appearance.

CHEMOTHERAPY OF UROLOGIC MALIGNANCIES
Samuel D. Spivack, MD

The chemotherapy of urologic cancer exemplifies many of the recent advances in the field of oncology in general and also encompasses still unsolved problems. The number of effective chemotherapeutic agents has increased dramatically over the last 3 decades, and advances in supportive care have permitted more aggressive use of single agents and combinations. Interdisciplinary cooperative efforts among oncologists in the fields of surgery, radiotherapy, and chemotherapy are producing greater benefits than each discipline alone could offer. This discussion will consider current therapeutic approaches to urologic malignancy.

CLASSIFICATION OF TUMORS

Although the term tumor originally denoted any mass or swelling, it is now generally synonymous with neoplasm (a new pathologic growth of tissue). A neoplasm may be characterized as benign or malignant depending upon its histologic, gross, and clinical features. Malignant neoplasms usually show imperfect differentiation and structure atypical of the tissue of origin, an infiltrative growth pattern not contained by a true capsule, and relatively frequent and abnormal mitotic figures. Growth rarely ceases, although the rate of growth may be irregular, and many malignant tumors have a propensity for metastasis. Benign tumors generally lack these features, although they may be fatal as a result of impingement on other structures and impairment of function.

Neoplasms are classified according to their tissue of origin. Those derived from mesenchyme (muscle, bone, tendon, cartilage, fat, vessels, lymphoid, and connective tissue) are called sarcomas. Malignant tumors of epithelial origin are carcinomas and may be further classified, according to their histologic appearance, as adenocarcinomas (glandular) or squamous (epidermoid), transitional, or undifferentiated carcinomas. Tumors may be composed of one neoplastic cell type (although also containing nonneoplastic stromal elements such as blood vessels); may contain several neoplastic cell types of common derivation from the same germ cell layer (mixed tumors); or may derive from more than one embryonic germ cell layer (teratomas).

ETIOLOGIC FACTORS IN TUMOR FORMATION

Immunologic Disease & Cancer

Cancer as a sequela to immunologic derangements is thought to represent a failure of immune surveillance or ineffective immune control. Neoplasms are more common when cell-mediated immunity is impaired, and some tumors have a distinctly better prognosis when there is histologic evidence of lymphocytic infiltration of the tumor or regional nodes. Tumor-specific antigens are present in tumors induced in experimental animals by chemicals and viruses. Human colon cancer contains carcinoembryonic antigens capable of eliciting an immunologic response. Similar antigens have recently been found in Burkitt's lymphoma, malignant melanoma, neuroblastoma, and osteosarcoma. Serum "blocking factors" that impair lymphocyte-mediated tumor inhibition have been demonstrated in patients with progressive, uncontrolled neuroblastoma but not in patients whose disease is controlled. Immunologic manipulations aimed at reconstituting host immune defenses are now being investigated, although no specific form of "immunotherapy" has yet been established as effective in the prevention or treatment of human neoplasms.

Chemical Oncogenesis

One of the first documented associations between occupation and disease was made by Sir Percival Pott, who recognized that chimney sweeps were at increased risk of scrotal carcinoma induced by exposure to coal tar carcinogens. Chemical carcinogenesis induced by coal tars, aromatic amines, azo dyes, aflatoxins, or alkylators is a 2-stage phenomenon consisting of tumor initiation and subsequent neoplastic growth, with a variable but distinct latent period between these 2 stages. Carcinogenesis requires cell proliferation once the malignant initiation phase has occurred. Carcinogens are dose-dependent, additive, and irreversible. According to the Huebner hypothesis of oncogenesis, carcinogens may activate the "oncogene" or may modify host RNA in such a way that faulty "reverse transcription" occurs according to the Temin theory (see below).

Radiation Oncogenesis

Radiation oncogenesis is a complex process that appears to involve irreversible injury to chromosomes. The incidence of the spontaneous human neoplasms is increased by radiation, probably in proportion to the incidence of the spontaneous tumor in the population at risk. Chronic myelocytic leukemia, all forms of acute leukemia, malignant lymphomas, osteosarcoma, breast and lung carcinoma, and pancreatic, pharyngeal, thyroid, and colon carcinomas—the neoplasia that account for 85% of human cancer morbidity and mortality—are increased in populations exposed to radiation above background levels.

Viral Oncogenesis

The contention that viruses may cause cancer

in humans rests mainly on analogous reasoning from observations in other species, particularly laboratory animals. Of the oncogenic DNA viruses, a human herpesvirus of major interest is the Epstein-Barr (EB) virus, which was discovered by electron microscopy in cultured Burkitt's lymphoma cells and subsequently found in many isolates of Burkitt's lymphoma. EB virus has also been associated with nasopharyngeal carcinoma, but its causal role in that illness is far from certain. A herpesvirus has also been associated with cancer of the uterine cervix, since viral antibodies are present in more women with this cancer than in control populations.

Oncogenic RNA viruses (oncornaviruses) have recently been thought to cause some human cancers. An RNA tumor virus might produce a stable genetic trait if viral RNA served as the template for DNA synthesis and the DNA became integrated into the host genome, resulting in neoplastic transformation. This revolutionary concept challenged the classic Watson-Crick hypothesis that information flow was unidirectional from DNA → RNA → protein. This hypothesis became more tenable with the demonstration that "reverse transcriptase" existed in nearly all RNA viruses with oncogenic potential, in human lymphoblastic leukemia cells, and in viruslike C particles from human milk in patients with breast cancer and, to a lesser extent, in their seemingly normal relatives.

Two interesting theories of oncogenesis have recently been proposed on the basis of these data:

(1) Huebner's oncogene theory states that many (if not all) vertebrates contain the genetic information for producing C type RNA viruses. This information (virogene) is transmitted vertically from one generation to the next and from one cell to the daughter cells. A portion of the virogene is responsible for neoplastic transformation (oncogene) and is expressed in undifferentiated fetal cells but not in normal, mature nonproliferative cells. Exposure to a carcinogenic stimulus (x-ray, chemical, or tumor virus) and the host genotype itself determine whether activation of the oncogenome will occur. This theory is based on the idea that a regulatory switch mechanism controls a stable alteration in genotype.

(2) Temin's protovirus theory proposes that C particles originate from cellular genes which have incorporated a "protovirus" as a product of action of reverse transcriptase upon a cellular RNA template. Alterations or abnormal integrations of protovirus (due to changes in RNA, DNA, or the transcriptase) lead to oncogenesis.

The available evidence does not permit a clear choice between these 2 theories. Both have already broadened the conceptual role of viruses in oncogenesis and may have more general biologic import.

VALUE OF GRADING & STAGING IN MALIGNANT DISEASE

For most curable neoplasms, the first therapeutic attempt must be definitive if cure is to be achieved; this means that initial therapy must be radical enough to encompass and extirpate or sterilize all existing foci of disease. An accurate delineation of the stage and extent of disease is thus an important initial step in determining the most appropriate treatment for the patient.

Grading and staging of neoplasms are attempts to describe the degree of malignancy and the extent of its dissemination. Histologic grading determines the degree of anaplasia of tumor cells, varying from grade I (very well differentiated) to grade IV (undifferentiated). Grading has prognostic value in some tumors (transitional cell carcinoma of bladder, astrocytoma, and chondrosarcoma) but is of little predictive value in others (melanoma or osteosarcoma). Staging of cancer is based upon the extent of its spread rather than on histologic appearance and has been standardized for many cancers by use of the TNM system. T refers to the degree of local extension at the primary site, N to the clinical findings in regional nodes, and M to the presence of distant metastases. Some cancers are staged by clinical examination alone (eg, squamous cell carcinoma of the cervix), whereas for others (eg, transitional cell carcinoma of the bladder and adenocarcinoma of the colon) the stage is determined on the basis of findings in the resected surgical specimen. In both instances, there is an excellent correlation of stage with prognosis.

For many neoplasms, both the histologic grading and the clinical staging are relevant to the choice of treatment and prognosis.

THERAPY OF MALIGNANT DISEASES

SURGERY

Surgical excision is the most effective means of removing the primary lesion of most neoplasms. It also provides palliation of symptoms, as by the relief of intestinal obstruction in tumors that may be unresectable or may have already metastasized. A number of highly malignant tumors have been found to respond favorably to limited surgical excision combined with radiation therapy and chemotherapy.

Solitary Metastasis

Even though more than 80% of apparently solitary metastases are eventually found to be multiple, an occasional cure results from their excision. In patients with a solitary lung metastasis, lobectomy gives 5-year survival rates of 15–60% depending upon the tissue of origin, the histologic characteristics of the tumor, and the time of appearance of the metastasis. The best results have been achieved when the metastasis was discovered more than 2 years after treatment of the primary. Surgery is much less successful for solitary brain metastases from lung tumors. The prognosis for solitary bony and liver metastases is poor, but occasional cures have followed removal of metastases from hypernephroma, testicular and gynecologic neoplasms, various sarcomas, and occasional intestinal tumors.

Long-term palliation sometimes follows radiation therapy for metastases from certain radiosensitive tumors such as Wilms's tumor, seminoma, neuroblastoma, and some sarcomas.

Radiotherapy has also produced long-term survival in patients with metastases in neck nodes from an occult primary, presumably in the oropharynx or nasopharynx.

RADIATION THERAPY

Radiation therapy, alone or in conjunction with surgery or chemotherapy, may also serve as definitive treatment of certain malignant diseases. Local obstructions and inoperable masses are frequently and effectively controlled by radiation therapy.

IMMUNOTHERAPY

All forms of immunotherapy must be considered experimental at present, since none are of established efficacy as yet. Tumor immunotherapy may be active, stimulating the patient's own immune system to increased activity; or passive, in which case the therapeutic agents are passively transferred. Immunotherapy may be specific, attempting to enhance reactivity to the tumor-specific transplantation antigens (TSTA) of the patient's tumor; or nonspecific, attempting to generally enhance the patient's immune reactivity.

In experimental animals, growth of transplanted or virally induced tumors has been prevented by prior sensitization. Established (experimental) tumors have been eradicated by local immunotherapy (eg, intralesional BCG) but only rarely by systemic immunotherapy. Thus, immunotherapy is most likely to be effective when the patient is clinically free of tumor but the likelihood of recurrence is high—eg, after surgical removal of the primary lesion and metastases. It may also be effective during and following reduction of the tumor burden by radiotherapy with or without chemotherapy.

The decision to use immunotherapy must take into account the potential of all forms of manipulation of the immune system to increase tumor growth: the unanticipated appearance of enhancing antibodies, production of low levels of cellular immunity, or immunosuppression—any of these, which are only examples of many untoward events, could result in loss of control of the tumor.

BCG

BCG has been used most widely in the therapy of acute myelogenous leukemia (AML) and malignant melanoma. The results of several large controlled clinical trials with BCG are conflicting. Life may be slightly prolonged in patients with AML. In malignant melanoma, there does not seem to be any effect on visceral disease. In patients with primary melanoma or lymph node metastases, 2 studies with concurrent controls showed no effect of BCG; one study with historic controls showed a positive effect; and one study is still incomplete. At best, if BCG has an effect, it will be not more than a 20–25% decrease in recurrence rate.

BCG is not without risk. Aside from the possibility of producing accelerated tumor growth, fever and malaise are common. Administration of BCG by scarification results in a local reaction and scab formation not unlike that resulting from smallpox vaccination. More severe systemic reactions may occur in patients strongly sensitive to PPD, and 2 deaths have been reported.

Transfer Factor

Transfer factor is a dialyzable extract of leukocytes that enhances immune reactivity in the recipient when it is given by subcutaneous injection. It has been used in the therapy of immunodeficiency disease, infectious diseases, and cancer, mainly malignant melanoma and osteogenic sarcoma. In small groups of patients, transfer factor has resulted in tumor regression and prolonged survival in patients with a poor prognosis who were clinically free of tumor at the initiation of therapy. The use of transfer factor is still experimental.

Interferon

Interferon is a naturally occurring protein with physiologic regulatory functions and potent antiviral, antiproliferative, and immunomodulating properties. Clinical experience in treating viral and neoplastic diseases with interferon has been limited, owing to the small quantities of human leukocyte interferon available. Recent advances in genetic biosynthetic technology may soon make enough available for large-scale clinical trials. Preliminary evidence suggests that interferon can induce tumor regression in some patients with advanced breast carcinoma, multiple myeloma, and malignant lymphoma. Toxicity includes modest leukopenia and thrombopenia with fever and mild alopecia.

CHEMOTHERAPY

Scientific Basis of Chemotherapy

A. Selective Toxicity: The Qualitative Approach: A basic goal of cancer chemotherapy is the development of agents which have "selective toxicity" against replicating tumor cells but which at the same time spare replicating host tissues. Such an ideal drug has not yet been found, and only the hormones and asparaginase (and, to a lesser extent, mitotane [o,p'-DDD; Lysodren] and streptozocin*) approach this goal. Although these drugs have important side-effects, their toxicity is not primarily directed against normal replicating cells.

B. The Quantitative Kinetic Approach: Since in most instances qualitative metabolic differences between normal and neoplastic cells have not been discovered, the chemotherapist must plan according to quantitative differences in the proliferative kinetics of normal and neoplastic cell growth if tumor regression without major host toxicity is to be achieved. Early bacteriologists, in their study of germicidal agents, formulated the concept of "the logarithmic order of cell kill." According to this theory, any particular treatment will kill a certain fraction of cells *independently* of the total number of cells present (provided the growth rate is constant). Thus, "cure," in the sense of killing the last remaining tumor cells, is more readily achieved by drugs when the total tumor cell burden is small. For example, a drug that is 99% efficient kills 2 logs of cells regardless of the total number of cells present and will reduce a tumor cell population of 100 to a single remaining cell, whereas it will leave 10,000 remaining cells of an initial tumor cell number of 1 million.

The quantitative evaluation of drug effects on normal and neoplastic tissues was furthered by the development of an in vivo assay system to allow measurement of the dose-response relationship of a variety of agents against both neoplastic and normal hematopoietic stem cells. As a result of these experiments, at least 2 cell survival curves are generated. The first curve shows decimation of both normal and neoplastic cells to almost the same degree, whereas the other curve shows a much greater decimation of tumor cells than of normal stem cells. The selectivity of the agents in the second class was attributed to a differential effect of the agents, which attacked proliferating cells in the mitotic cycle while sparing resting cells not in mitotic division. Thus arose the classification of forms of therapy into (1) cell cycle–specific (CCS) agents, which attack only actively proliferating cells engaged in DNA synthesis and the mitotic cycle; and (2) cell cycle–nonspecific (CCNS) agents, which kill both normal and tumor cells regardless of their proliferative state.

The important implications of these data are borne out by evidence in experimental tumor systems and to some extent in humans: (1) Differences in sensitivity of normal hematopoietic precursors and neoplastic cells are a function of the difference in their proliferative states and not a result of any inherent qualitative biochemical differences between the 2 cell types. (2) Injured or "stimulated" marrow or normal tissue that is proliferating as rapidly as neoplastic tissue will be affected to the same extent as neoplastic tissue.

As a general rule, any tissue, normal or neoplastic, manifests an early logarithmic phase of exponential growth during which most cells are in active mitosis. When a certain bulk is achieved, there is a transition to a later "steady state" plateau phase of growth during which a lesser fraction of cells is in the proliferative cycle. To maximize the therapeutic effects of CCS antineoplastic agents, resting cells must be induced to enter the proliferative cycle without at the same time increasing normal tissue vulnerability. This implies a reduction of tumor bulk with a reentry from the plateau phase into the log phase of exponential growth. Methods for reducing tumor bulk presently include treatment by CCNS agents such as x-ray or mechlorethamine and removal of gross tumor masses at surgery, but these stratagems all too often have attendant toxicities.

Utilizing these concepts, Schabel has proposed an approach to "curative" sequential chemotherapy of advanced tumors using a CCNS agent followed by a CCS agent in repeated courses.

While this is an idealized approach to curative therapy, similar approaches have led to cure of laboratory-induced neoplasms, and such concepts form the basis for several successful new antileukemic regimens—particularly for childhood leukemia. Clearly, this approach will be furthered by a better understanding of human tumor cell kinetics in individual patients, by new knowledge about the dose, duration, and site of action of antitumor agents, by the development of new "marrow-sparing" agents, and by appropriately synergistic combinations of drugs as well as better means of measuring their effects on microscopic tumor deposits.

A new technic for growing tumor stem cells with clonogenic or colony-forming capability has recently been developed. The clonogenic cells are obtained from a fresh tumor biopsy specimen and can be grown in soft agar and tested against standard and new anticancer drugs for inhibition of clonogenicity. This technic may simplify the identification of clinically effective drugs. It is 99% accurate in predicting lack of clinical response, which suggests that the assay may be most useful in avoiding fruitless clinical trials. Further studies using the tumor stem cell assay will focus on the use of drug combinations. If the results of prospective studies follow the pattern predicted by this assay, the de-

*See Note to Reader on p 325.

sign of future trials and individual patient treatment will be radically altered from the present empiric approach.

Guidelines for the Institution of Cancer Chemotherapy

A. Establish the Diagnosis: A firm diagnosis of neoplastic disease must be made before treatment is started. This will usually (and preferably) include a histologic diagnosis, but in some instances the diagnosis may be based solely on analysis of exfoliative cytology. In rare instances, a biochemical parameter (eg, chorionic gonadotropin) in a consistent clinical setting may constitute a rationale for institution of therapy, although tissue diagnosis is always preferable. In emergency situations (eg, superior vena cava syndrome), it may be necessary to institute appropriate therapy without histologic or biochemical documentation; in such cases, appropriate diagnostic procedures are required after clinical stabilization has been achieved.

B. Delineate the Stage and Extent of Disease: This can frequently be achieved by correlating symptoms and the known natural history of the neoplasm with appropriate radiologic, chemical, and surgical staging data. The lymphomas are staged according to the modified Ann Arbor classification; many solid tumors are best staged by the TNM system.

C. Establish the Goal of Therapy: The histologic diagnosis and extent of the disease frequently define the goal of therapy as either curative or palliative with or without likelihood for prolongation of survival, and frequently determine the most appropriate treatment—surgery, radiotherapy, chemotherapy, or a combination of these.

Thus, the therapeutic objective should be based upon what can be accomplished by each mode of therapy. For example, the following disseminated cancers are curable by chemotherapy: most postgestational choriocarcinomas, many Wilms's tumors and seminomas, some childhood acute lymphoblastic leukemias, adult and childhood lymphomas, and some testicular carcinomas in young men. For other neoplasms, chemotherapy may afford significant palliation and prolongation of life, even in advanced stages of breast, endometrial, prostate, thyroid, and oat cell cancers and for acute leukemia, lymphomas, myeloma, and macroglobulinemia. Some patients with colon or gastric carcinoma, sarcomas, and head and neck tumors may be relieved of symptoms by chemotherapy, but survival cannot yet be prolonged. Most patients with disseminated melanoma and lung, renal, and pancreatic carcinoma are not objectively benefited by systemic chemotherapy.

D. Measure Antitumor Response: After treatment is started, serial observations of objectively measured parameters are essential to judge antitumor response (measurable mass, tumor product, or remote effect) and to monitor the toxicity of the treatment. For example, in the treatment of gestational trophoblastic disease, assay of chorionic gonadotropin measures a tumor product that correlates directly with the numbers of neoplastic cells,

---

Anticancer Drugs

Allopurinol (Zyloprim)
Aminoglutethimide* (Cytadren, Elipten)
Asparaginase (L-asparaginase, Elspar)
BCNU (see Carmustine)
Bleomycin (Blenoxane)
Busulfan (Myleran)
CCNU (see Lomustine)
Carmustine (bischloroethylnitrosourea, BCNU)
Chlorambucil (Leukeran)
Cisplatin (Platinol)
Cyclophosphamide (Cytoxan)
Cyproterone acetate
Cytarabine (Ara-C, Cytosar)
Dacarbazine (dimethyltriazeno imidazole carboxamide, imidazole carboxamide)
Dactinomycin (actinomycin D, Cosmegen)
Daunorubicin (daunomycin)
Doxorubicin (Adriamycin)
Estramustine phosphate* (Estracyt)
Fluorouracil (5-FU, Adrucil)
Flutamide*
Hexamethylmelamine
Lomustine (cyclohexylchloroethylnitrosourea, CCNU)
Mechlorethamine (nitrogen mustard, HN2, Mustargen)
Melphalan (phenylalanine mustard, L-sarcolysin, Alkeran)
Mercaptopurine (6-MP, Purinethol)
Methotrexate (amethopterin)
Methyl-CCNU (methylcyclohexylchloroethylnitrosourea)
Mithramycin (Mithracin)
Mitomycin (Mutamycin)
Mitotane (o,p'-DDD, Lysodren)
Nafoxidine*
Procarbazine (Matulane)
Streptozocin
Thioguanine (6-TG)
Tamoxifen* (Nolvadex)
Thiotepa (triethylenethiophosphoramide)
Vinblastine sulfate (Velban)
Vincristine sulfate (Oncovin)

*See Note to Reader, below.

Note to reader: Agents designated with an asterisk in the following discussion and in Table 18–2 are investigational and not generally available to the practicing physician. Further information concerning these agents may be obtained from the various regional or national cooperative cancer chemotherapy study groups or the National Cancer Institute.

and it also reveals subclinical amounts (10^6 cells or less) of tumor that require additional chemotherapy. The sensitivity of this assay is largely responsible for the 90% cure rate of trophoblastic disease. In contrast, a "complete clinical remission" of acute leukemia (a normal bone marrow) occurs with a tumor cell mass of 10^9; most solid tumors contain 10^{10}–10^{11} (10–100 g) of tumor cells before the mass can be detected clinically.

Currently useful markers for testicular tumors include the beta-subunit of human chorionic gonadotropin, carcinoembryonic antigen (CEA), and alpha-fetoprotein. A rising CEA titer measured serially may also predict in a nonquantitative manner the recurrence of progression of colonic carcinoma, and alpha-fetoprotein may indicate the presence of a hepatocellular carcinoma. Other tumor products—such as monoclonal paraproteins (myeloma, macroglobulinemia, occasional lymphomas), 5-hydroxyindoleacetic acid (carcinoid), and acid phosphatase (prostatic cancer)—and ectopic hormone production (oat cell carcinomas) may correlate positively with the presence and proliferation of specific neoplasms. Estrogen and progesterone receptors should be measured in tissue from breast carcinoma, since the findings predict responsiveness to hormone manipulations for metastatic disease. Radionuclide, CT, and ultrasound scanning provide serial noninvasive measurements of tumor response to therapy. Only rarely should a "second look" laparotomy be necessary to determine the status of a previously treated abdominal neoplasm.

E. Establish the Acceptable Drug Toxicity: The degree of toxicity that is acceptable depends on the probability and risks of achieving the therapeutic goal, other clinical characteristics of the individual patient, and the availability of supportive facilities to manage the anticipated toxicity.

F. Evaluate the Status of the Patient: The patient's subjective and functional status must always be considered in formulating and instituting a therapeutic program. Subjective symptoms of disease usually parallel objective parameters of progression or regression of the neoplasm. When this is not so, other factors such as unrecognized drug toxicity, unreliable parameters of tumor response, and the masking of disease progression by certain forms of therapy (eg, corticosteroids) must be considered. The Karnofsky performance index (Table 18–1) is useful for following the functional status of the patient and must be considered at least as valuable as objectively measurable parameters, especially when the goal of treatment is palliation.

The above considerations apply generally to cancer chemotherapy. Use of experimental drugs or treatment protocols may be considered if all of the following criteria are met: (1) Proved methods of effective therapy have been exhausted. (2) Data collection and dissemination of the information obtained will contribute toward answering the ques-

Table 18–1. Karnofsky performance index.

	%	
Able to carry on normal activity. No special care is needed.	100	Normal. No complaints. No evidence of disease.
	90	Able to carry on normal activity. Minor signs or symptoms of disease.
	80	Normal activity with effort. Some signs or symptoms of disease.
Unable to work. Able to live at home and care for most personal needs. A varying amount of assistance is needed.	70	Cares for self. Unable to carry on normal activity or to do active work.
	60	Requires occasional assistance but is able to care for most of his needs.
	50	Requires considerable assistance and frequent medical care.
Unable to care for self. Requires equivalent of institutional or hospital care. Disease may be progressing rapidly.	40	Disabled. Requires special care and assistance.
	30	Severely disabled. Hospitalization is indicated, although death is not imminent.
	20	Very sick. Hospitalization necessary.
	10	Moribund. Fatal processes progressing rapidly.
	0	Dead.

tions asked in the protocol. (3) The patient's human rights are fully protected, and informed consent has been obtained. (4) There is a reasonable expectation that the treatment will do more good than harm.

• • •

CHEMOTHERAPEUTIC AGENTS
(See Table 18–2.)

Chemotherapeutic Agents With Selective Toxicity

Only the adrenocortical hormones, sex hormones, and asparaginase have demonstrated a predictable **selective killing power of tumor cells** based on metabolically exploitable differences between neoplastic and normal tissue.

A. Glucocorticoids: The glucocorticoids exert a "lympholytic" effect that can repeatedly induce remission of acute lymphoblastic leukemia, especially in combination with vincristine. This lympholytic effect, which does not depend on the mitotic activity of the tumor, is also useful in chronic lymphocytic leukemia, lymphomas, and myeloma.

The adrenal corticosteroids are also beneficial for certain hormonally sensitive tumors such as breast and prostatic cancer. They improve cerebral edema accompanying brain tumors, palliate hemolytic anemias associated with chronic lymphocytic leukemia and the lymphomas, and correct hypercalcemia associated with various neoplasms. Their antineoplastic effects are less if given on an intermittent schedule; large daily doses for the shortest time necessary to produce the desired effect are preferred. Toxicity may be metabolic (hyperglycemia, sodium retention, potassium wasting), gastrointestinal (peptic ulceration), or immunosuppressive (increased susceptibility to infection). Myopathies, psychosis, hypertension, and osteoporosis are important side-effects of long-term administration.

B. Estrogens: The estrogenic steroids were used in the early 1940s for prostatic carcinoma and represented one of the first successful attempts at rational cancer chemotherapy. Shortly thereafter, estrogens were found useful in postmenopausal patients with breast cancer. Diethylstilbestrol, the most widely used estrogen, is potent, inexpensive, and effective when given orally but may cause gastrointestinal disturbance, fluid retention, feminization in males, and uterine bleeding. Its administration may cause hypercalcemia and "tumor flare" of disseminated breast carcinoma.

C. Synthetic Progestational Agents: These drugs are useful in pharmacologic doses for disseminated or uncontrolled carcinoma of the endometrium and occasionally for hypernephroma and breast cancer.

D. Androgens: The androgens are used principally in the treatment of disseminated breast cancer, especially in pre- and perimenopausal (1–4 years) women. They also have a role in the stimulation of erythropoiesis in anemic patients with several neoplastic and myelophthisic diseases. The toxic effects of androgens include excessive virilization of women, prostatism in men, and fluid retention; tumor flare and hypercalcemia occur occasionally. The halogenated androgens, which are effective when given orally, can produce cholestatic jaundice, although the parenteral nonhalogenated compounds do not do so.

E. Antihormones: Antiestrogens (nafoxidine* and tamoxifen* [Nolvadex]) are a new class of nonsteroidal agents that block estrogen receptor sites on tumor cells and antagonize estrogen stimulation of hormone-dependent tumors such as breast and possibly renal carcinoma. Nausea, hot flashes, and mild thrombocytopenia are toxicities of oral administration.

Antiandrogens include cyproterone acetate,* a steroidal congener that possesses potent progestational actions; and flutamide,* a nonsteroidal anilide that acts by inhibiting androgen binding and tumor tissue. These drugs may be of benefit in advanced prostatic carcinoma no longer responsive to hormonal manipulations that were effective in the past. No major toxicities are reported in a few small trials.

*See note to reader on p 325.

The Alkylators

The alkylators, whose prototype is mechlorethamine, react with nucleophilic substances within the cell to form cross-links at the guanine residues of parallel double DNA strands. With the possible exception of cyclophosphamide, the alkylators are cell cycle nonspecific and affect both resting and dividing cells; both normal and malignant cells are injured.

Mechlorethamine (nitrogen mustard, HN2, Mustargen) is the alkylator of choice in the treatment of Hodgkin's disease, either singly or in combination with other drugs. For Burkitt's lymphoma, cyclophosphamide may be curative, and it is also the agent of choice for undifferentiated small cell carcinoma of the lung. Cyclophosphamide has a unique role in childhood acute leukemia, in which other alkylators are ineffective. For most purposes, however, equivalent doses of the various alkylators produce equivalent responses, and there is cross-resistance among the various alkylators except for the nitrosoureas (see below). The choice of alkylators thus rests upon the desired route and mode of administration and variations in toxicity.

Chlorambucil (Leukeran) has had its major use in chronic lymphocytic leukemia, Hodgkin's disease, and Waldenström's macroglobulinemia. Its major advantage is its narrow spectrum of toxicity (hematopoietic only) and ease of administration (oral). **Phenylalanine mustard (melphalan)** is usually given for multiple myeloma, but this may be merely traditional; **busulfan (Myleran)** is customarily used in chronic myelocytic leukemia and in polycythemia vera; all alkylators are equally effective against ovarian carcinoma.

Mechlorethamine is a vesicant if extravasated. **Cyclophosphamide (Cytoxan)** and **thiotepa** are much less irritating if applied directly to tissues, because they must first be metabolized to the active form. The immediate effects of intravenous alkylator administration are nausea and vomiting beginning within 30 minutes and persisting for 8–10 hours; premedication with phenothiazine is preventive. The important delayed effects of alkylators are principally on rapidly proliferating tissues (hematopoietic, gonadal, skin, and gastrointestinal), with bone marrow suppression being the most prominent. In the marrow, cell necrosis begins at 12 hours; the nadir of blood count depression is at 7–10 days; and marrow regeneration time limits the administration of mechlorethamine to intervals of 4–6 weeks.

Several of the alkylators cause relatively characteristic adverse reactions. Examples are alopecia and hemorrhagic cystitis associated with cyclophosphamide and melanosis and pulmonary fibrosis with busulfan. All alkylators can cause hypospermia, menstrual irregularities, and fetal anomalies.

Thiotepa is discussed in Table 18–2.

The Nitrosoureas

BCNU, CCNU, and methyl-CCNU are cell cycle–nonspecific synthetic chemicals that act much like the classic alkylators but have several unique and exploitable properties, including lipid solubility and delayed onset of marrow suppression compared to the alkylators (see above). Moreover, there appears to be no cross-resistance with other alkylators. These drugs are effective in Hodgkin's disease but less so in non-Hodgkin's lymphomas; they appear promising for metastatic and primary central nervous system neoplasms because of their lipid solubility. BCNU is administered intravenously; CCNU and methyl-CCNU are given orally.

Structural Analogs (Antimetabolites)

The antimetabolites are specific cytotoxic agents closely related to substrates normally utilized by cells for metabolism and growth. The structural analogs interfere with nucleic acid synthesis to impair proliferation of normal and neoplastic cells. They are generally cell cycle–specific, with proliferating cells being more vulnerable to their effects than are resting cells.

A. Methotrexate: Methotrexate competitively inhibits dihydrofolate reductase; acquired resistance to methotrexate results from increased dihydrofolate reductase activity, since the rate of enzyme synthesis exceeds the rate of methotrexate uptake by resistant cells.

Methotrexate toxicity may be hematologic, gastrointestinal, hepatic, and dermatologic. These effects may be alleviated or prevented by the prompt (preferably within 1 hour, but no longer than several hours) administration of folinic acid (citrovorum factor). One treatment regimen has used folinic acid to "rescue" the marrow after administration of toxic doses, although it is not yet certain that the antitumor effect is more pronounced. Methotrexate may be administered orally, intramuscularly, intravenously, or intrathecally; it is bound to plasma protein and excreted in the urine. Hepatic or renal failure is a contraindication; leukopenia, thrombocytopenia, stomatitis, and gastroenteritis with diarrhea are the toxic side-effects that may require reduction in dosage.

Methotrexate can cure most cases of gestational choriocarcinoma. It has been used extensively in the treatment of epithelial neoplasia of the head and neck and is useful in breast cancer, testicular tumors, lung cancer, medulloblastomas, and other brain tumors.

B. Fluorouracil: Fluorouracil (5-FU) is a thymine analog that in vivo interferes with thymidylate synthetase, an enzyme involved in the formation of thymidylic acid, a DNA precursor. The agent is first metabolized to 2'-deoxy-5-fluorouridine. This compound itself is now available (as floxuridine; FUDR) for use by perfusion, but it has not been shown to have a clear advantage over fluorouracil.

Fluorouracil is metabolized principally in the liver. Its major toxicities include stomatitis, enteritis, and marrow suppression; significant atrophic dermatitis is occasionally reported; neurotoxicity is rare.

Fluorouracil has been most useful in breast and colonic adenocarcinoma, but it is also beneficial against pancreatic, gastric, ovarian, and prostatic cancer. The preferred schedule of administration is once weekly rather than the 4-day loading dose schedule initially advocated, since the latter is more toxic without being more effective. The dosage should be in the range of 15–20 mg/kg intravenously, weekly as tolerated.

Since antimetabolites such as methotrexate and fluorouracil act only on rapidly proliferating cells, they damage the cells of mucosal surfaces such as the gastrointestinal tract. Methotrexate has similar effects on the skin. These toxicities are at times more significant than those that have occurred in the bone marrow, and they should be looked for routinely when these agents are used.

Erythema of the buccal mucosa is an early sign of mucosal toxicity. If therapy is continued beyond this point, oral ulceration will develop. In general, it is wise to discontinue therapy if early oral ulceration appears. This symptom usually heralds the appearance of similar but potentially more serious ulceration at other sites lower in the gastrointestinal tract. Therapy can usually be reinstituted when the oral ulcer heals (within 1 week to 10 days). The dose of drug used may need to be modified downward at this point, with titration to an acceptable level of effect on the mucosa.

Cytotoxic Antibiotics

These agents, the first of which was dactinomycin, were isolated in the 1940s by Waksman from soil strains of bacteria of the *Streptomyces* class.

A. Dactinomycin: Dactinomycin (actinomycin D, Cosmegen) is an inhibitor of DNA-dependent synthesis of RNA by ribosomes. Its toxicities include hematopoietic suppression, ulcerative stomatitis, and gastroenteritis. It causes intense local tissue necrosis if extravasated. The drug is retained for a considerable time intracellularly, and acquired resistance is thought to correlate with poor cellular uptake or poor retention of the drug. The major use for dactinomycin is in sequential combination with radiation therapy for Wilms's tumor; "maintenance" long-term administration of the drug adds significantly to the salvage obtained with combinations of surgery, radiation therapy, and "adjuvant" short-term courses of the drug. Dactinomycin is of proved value in trophoblastic malignancy, soft tissue sarcomas, and testicular carcinoma, especially in combination with alkylators and antimetabolites. The optimal scheduling and combination of drugs with dactinomycin is not known, but the most customary has been in courses of several days at dosages of 15 μg/kg/d intravenously repeated after 2–4 weeks as toxicity allows.

B. Doxorubicin: Doxorubicin (Adriamycin) and daunorubicin are tumoricidal antibiotics that intercalate between adjacent base pairs of double-stranded DNA. Toxicity includes marrow suppression, alopecia, and mucositis. Severe local tissue necrosis occurs if the drug is extravasated. Doxorubicin is excreted mainly through the bile and must be used in reduced dosage in patients whose hepatic function is impaired. The anthracycline antibiotics doxorubicin and daunomycin both have a delayed cardiac toxicity. The problem is greater with doxorubicin, because this drug has a major role in the treatment of sarcomas, breast cancer, lymphomas, and certain other solid tumors; the use of daunorubicin is limited to the treatment of acute leukemias. Recent studies of left ventricular function indicate that some reversible changes in cardiac dynamics occur in most patients by the time they have received 300 mg/m^2. Serial echocardiographic measurements can detect these abnormalities. Echocardiographic measurement of left ventricular ejection fraction appears most useful in this regard. Alternatively, the left ventricular voltage can be measured serially on ECGs. Doxorubicin should not be used in elderly patients with significant intrinsic cardiac disease, and no patient should receive a total dose in excess of 550 mg/m^2. Patients who have had prior chest or mediastinal radiotherapy may be more prone to develop doxorubicin heart disease. ECGs should be obtained serially. The appearance of a high resting pulse may herald the appearance of overt cardiac toxicity. Unfortunately, toxicity may be irreversible or fatal at high dosage levels. At lower dosages (eg, 350 mg/m^2), the symptoms and signs of cardiac failure generally respond well to digitalis, diuretics, and cessation of doxorubicin therapy.

C. Mithramycin: Mithramycin (Mithracin) is useful in the treatment of hypercalcemia resistant to hydration and corticosteroids, and the dosage may be less than that required for tumoricidal activity although still within the toxic range. Its major usefulness is in embryonal cell carcinoma and other testicular tumors, and its toxicity includes marrow suppression, hepatic and gastrointestinal injury, and complex coagulopathies.

D. Bleomycin (Blenoxane): Bleomycin is an antitumor antibiotic that in clinical use as an anticancer drug is a mixture of various fractions differing in the amine moiety. The principal mode of action appears to be scission of DNA strands or inhibition of ligase, thus impairing cell division. The most serious toxic effects are pulmonary interstitial pneumonitis and fibrosis, which may be fatal and are usually dose-related, occurring with a cumulative dosage greater than 150 units/m^2 or less if given in conjunction with prior pulmonary radiation. Generally, older patients or those with preexisting lung disease are most susceptible. Bleomycin hypersensitivity pneumonitis with

eosinophilia may occur at any dosage and may respond favorably to corticosteroid administration—in contrast to fibrosing pneumonitis, for which steroids are not as effective.

Other bleomycin toxicities include anaphylactic and acute febrile reactions, stomatitis, and dermatitis with hyperpigmentation and desquamation of palms, soles, and pressure areas. The drug is marrow-sparing and may be administered by the intravenous, intramuscular, or subcutaneous routes, although the intravenous route is usual. Its major usefulness is in testicular neoplasia, squamous carcinomas, lymphomas, and cervical carcinoma.

E. Mitomycin: Mitomycin is a useful agent against gastric and pancreatic adenocarcinoma and shows promise against breast cancer.

The Plant Alkaloids

The plant alkaloids include the periwinkle (*Vinca rosea*) derivatives, vincristine and vinblastine, 2 closely related compounds with widely different toxicities and somewhat different spectra of activity. Both *Vinca* alkaloids are bound to cytoplasmic precursors of the mitotic spindle in S phase, with polymerization of the microtubular proteins that comprise the mitotic spindle.

A. Vinblastine: Vinblastine sulfate (Velban) is a major agent against Hodgkin's disease and testicular carcinoma and has lesser efficacy in the non-Hodgkin's lymphomas. The toxicity of vinblastine is primarily marrow suppression, but gastroenteritis, neurotoxicity, and alopecia also occur—the latter much less commonly than with vincristine. The drug is usually given once a week. Severe local ulceration may occur if the drug extravasates into the subcutaneous tissues.

B. Vincristine: Vincristine sulfate (Oncovin) is primarily neurotoxic and may induce peripheral, autonomic, and, less commonly, cranial neuropathies. The peripheral neuropathy can be sensory, motor, autonomic, or a combination of these effects. In its mildest form it consists of paresthesias ("pins and needles") of the fingers and toes. Occasional patients develop acute jaw or throat pain after vincristine therapy. This may be a form of trigeminal neuralgia. With continued vincristine therapy, the paresthesias extend to the proximal interphalangeal joints, hyporeflexia appears in the lower extremities, and significant weakness develops in the quadriceps muscle group. At this point, it is wise to discontinue vincristine therapy until the neuropathy has subsided somewhat. Peroneal weakness should be avoided lest symptomatic foot drop and impairment of gait occur.

Constipation is the most common symptom of the autonomic neuropathy that occurs with vincristine therapy. This symptom should always be dealt with prophylactically, ie, patients receiving vincristine should be started on stool softeners and mild cathartics when therapy is instituted. If this poten-

Table 18–2. Drugs useful in urologic malignancy.*

Agent	Route	Toxicity	Usual Adult Dose†	Specificity‡
Hormones				
Glucocorticoids	Orally. (IV and IM preparations also available.)	Sodium retention, potassium wasting, hyperglycemia, peptic ulcer, immunosuppression, hypertension, osteoporosis.	Prednisone: 1–2 mg/kg/d for brief intervals (< 6 weeks if possible); then maintain at minimal required daily dosage.	CCNS
Estrogens	Orally	Sodium retention, feminization, uterine bleeding, nausea and vomiting.	Diethylstilbestrol: 2.5–5 mg/d for prostate. Ethinyl estradiol: 1 mg/d.	CCNS
Progestogens	Orally, IM	Sodium retention.	Hydroxyprogesterone: 1 g 2–3 times weekly IM. Medroxyprogesterone: 200–600 mg orally twice weekly.	CCNS
Androgens	Orally, IM	Sodium retention, masculinization; cholestatic jaundice with oral preparations.	Testosterone propionate: 100 mg 2–3 times weekly. Fluoxymesterone: 10–40 mg/d orally. Calusterone: 200 mg/d orally.	CCNS
Antihormones				
Antiestrogens				
Tamoxifen* (Nolvadex)	Orally	Nausea, hot flashes.	20–60 mg/d.	CCNS
Nafoxidine*	Orally	Nausea, dermatitis; rarely, tumor flare.	60–180 mg/d.	CCNS
Antiandrogens				
Flutamide*	Orally	Gynecomastia; loss of male body hair.	750 mg–1.5 g/d.	CCNS
Cyproterone acetate*	Orally	Fluid retention.	200–300 mg/d.	CCNS
Hormone-alkylator complex				
Estramustine phosphate* (Estracyt)	Orally	Nausea and vomiting, phlebitis, mild marrow depression.	15 mg/kg/d as single dose.	Not known
Alkylators				
Mechlorethamine (nitrogen mustard, HN2, Mustargen)	IV, intracavitary	Nausea and vomiting, marrow depression, ulcer if extravasated, hypogonadism, fetal anomalies, alopecia.	0.4 mg/kg IV as single dose every 4–6 weeks; 0.4 mg/kg by intracavitary injection.	CCNS
Cyclophosphamide (Cytoxan)	IV, orally	Nausea and vomiting, marrow depression, alopecia, hemorrhagic cystitis.	40–60 mg/kg IV every 3–5 weeks; 5 mg/kg/d orally for 10 days, then 1–3 mg/kg/d as maintenance.	(?)CCNS
Chlorambucil (Leukeran)	Orally	Marrow depression, gastroenteritis.	0.1–0.2 mg/kg/d.	CCNS
Melphalan (phenylalanine mustard, Alkeran)	Orally	Marrow depression (occasionally prolonged), gastroenteritis.	0.25 mg/kg/d orally for 4 days every 6 weeks; 2–4 mg/d as maintenance.	CCNS
Thiotepa	IV, intracavitary	Marrow depression.	0.8 mg/kg IV as single dose every 4–6 weeks; 0.8 mg/kg by intracavitary injection.	CCNS
Nitrosoureas				
Carmustine (BCNU), lomustine (CCNU), methyl-CCNU	BCNU, IV; CCNU and methyl-CCNU, orally	Nausea and vomiting, prolonged marrow depression, local phlebitis.	BCNU: 75–100 mg/m² IV daily for 2 days every 4–6 weeks. CCNU: 130 mg/m² orally every 6 weeks. Methyl-CCNU: 200 mg/m² orally every 6 weeks.	CCNS
Structural analogs				
Methotrexate (amethopterin)	Orally, IV, intrathecally	Ulcerative mucositis, gastroenteritis, dermatitis, marrow depression, hepatitis, abortion.	20–40 mg IV twice weekly; 5–15 mg intrathecally weekly; 2.5–5 mg/d orally.	CCS
Fluorouracil (5-FU, Adrucil)	IV	Atrophic dermatitis, gastroenteritis, mucositis, marrow depression, neuritis.	15–20 mg/kg IV weekly for at least 6 weeks.	CCS
Dacarbazine	IV	Gastroenteritis, marrow depression, hepatitis, phlebitis.	150–250 mg/m²/d IV for 5 days every 4–6 weeks.	Not known

Table 18–2 (cont'd). Drugs useful in urologic malignancy.*

Agent	Route	Toxicity	Usual Adult Dose†	Specificity‡
Cytotoxic antibiotics Dactinomycin (actinomycin D, Cosmegen)	IV	Nausea and vomiting, stomatitis, gastroenteritis, proctitis, marrow depression, ulcer if extravasated, alopecia; radiation potentiator.	0.01 mg/kg/d for 5 days every 4–6 weeks.	CCS
Doxorubicin (Adriamycin)	IV	Alopecia, marrow depression, myocardiopathies, ulcer if extravasated; stomatitis.	1 mg/kg/wk; total cumulative dose should not exceed 550 mg/m^2.	CCNS
Mithramycin (Mithracin)	IV	Marrow depression, nausea and vomiting, complex coagulopathies, hepatotoxicity.	0.05 mg/kg IV every other day to toxicity or 8 doses per course.	Not known
Bleomycin (Blenoxane)	IV, IM, subcut	Allergic dermatitis, pulmonary fibrosis, fever, mucositis.	15 mg twice weekly; total cumulative dosage should not exceed 300 mg.	Not known
***Vinca* alkaloids** Vinblastine (Velban)	IV	Marrow depression, alopecia, ulcer if extravasated, nausea and vomiting, neuropathy.	0.1–0.2 mg/kg IV weekly.	CCS
Vincristine (Oncovin)	IV	Alopecia, neuropathy (peripheral and autonomic), ulcer if extravasated; rarely, marrow depression.	1.5 mg/m^2 weekly or less. No individual dosage should exceed 2 mg.	CCS
Miscellaneous agents Mitotane (o,p'-DDD, Lysodren)	Orally	Gastroenteritis, dermatitis, CNS abnormalities.	5–12 g daily orally.	Not known
Aminoglutethimide* (Cytadren, Elipten)	Orally	Gastroenteritis, dermatitis, somnolence.	1–1.5 g daily orally in 3–4 divided doses.	CCNS
Inorganic metallic salt Cisplatin	IV with mannitol diuresis	Nausea and vomiting, bone marrow depression, nephrotoxicity, ototoxicity.	1 mg/kg every 3 weeks IV, or 80 mg/m^2 IV every 3 weeks. Use lower dose when renal function is impaired.	CCNS

*See Note to Reader on p 325.
†Modifications of drug dosages: If white count is >4500 and platelet count > 150,000, give full dose; if white count is 3500–4500 and platelet count is 100–150 thousand, give 75% of full dose; if white count is 3000–3500 and platelet count is 75–100 thousand, give 50–75% of full dose; if white count is < 3000 and platelet count is < 75,000, give 0–25% of full dose.
‡CCS = cell cycle specific. CCNS = cell cycle nonspecific. See text.

tial complication is neglected, severe impaction may result in association with an atonic bowel.

More serious autonomic involvement can lead to acute intestinal obstruction with signs indistinguishable from those of an acute abdomen. Bladder neuropathies are uncommon but may be severe.

Alopecia occurs in 20% of patients, but hematologic suppression is unusual. The drug is extremely effective in inducing remissions in acute lymphoblastic leukemia, especially in combination with prednisone, and is quite active in all forms of lymphoma. It is one of the most effective agents against childhood tumors, choriocarcinoma, and various sarcomas. Because of its lack of significant overlapping toxicity with most other chemotherapeutic agents, vincristine is receiving wide use in combination with other agents. The optimal dosage and scheduling for this agent remain to be elucidated; weekly administration is customary but may not be the best regimen.

Miscellaneous Compounds

Mitotane (o,p'-DDD; Lysodren) is a DDT congener that may cause adrenocortical necrosis and therefore plays a useful role in reducing excessive steroid output in 70% of patients with adrenocortical carcinoma; in about 35%, an objective decrease in tumor mass is also recorded. Toxicities include dermatitis, gastroenteritis, and central nervous system abnormalities.

Aminoglutethimide* (Cytadren, Elipten) is a derivative of glutethimide, a sedative-hypnotic drug that causes adrenal insufficiency with chronic use. Aminoglutethimide blocks adrenal steroidogenesis by inhibiting the enzymatic conversion of cholesterol to pregnenolone, thus reducing mineralocorticoid, glucocorticoid, and sex steroid production. The "medical adrenalectomy" thus induced can be beneficial for breast and prostatic cancers, although the degree of benefit is not precisely defined as yet. Toxicities include somnolence, nausea and vomiting, and, occasionally, skin rash. Supplemental mineralocorticoids and glucocorticoids must be administered with aminoglutethimide.

*See note to reader on p 325.

Estramustine phosphate* (Estracyt) is a promising new compound that combines an estradiol and an alkylator. It is not yet clear whether this complex will prove to be superior to either agent used alone, but the approach may lead to similar combinations in the future. Toxicities of oral administration include nausea and vomiting, thrombophlebitis; and mild hematopoietic suppression.

Dacarbazine is a synthetic derivative of the triazene class that has both antimetabolite and alkylatorlike activity. Dacarbazine has significant activity against melanoma and, in combination with doxorubicin, against various sarcomas. Toxicities may include gastroenteritis, marrow depression, hepatitis, phlebitis, alopecia, ulcer if extravasated, and a flulike syndrome with myalgias.

Cisplatin (Platinol) is a member of a new class of heavy metal antitumor agents whose mechanism of action is unknown. Major acute toxicities may include severe vomiting and renal tubular necrosis, which may be minimized by careful hydration and mannitol administration to promote brisk diuresis during the infusion of cisplatin. Other toxicities include high-frequency ototoxicity and bone marrow suppression, with leukopenia, thrombocytopenia, and anemia. The drug is usually given as a 2-hour infusion in a covered bottle (because it is light-sensitive). Major uses include testicular, bladder, and ovarian carcinomas.

SURGICAL ADJUVANT CHEMOTHERAPY

It has been suggested that surgical or radiotherapeutic (cell cycle–nonspecific) measures that reduce tumor bulk and increase the growth fraction of a tumor might increase tumor sensitivity to chemotherapeutic agents (cell cycle–specific) without increasing marrow sensitivity. Thus, chemotherapeutic agents given after operation might improve results when there is no clinical evidence of residual disease but recurrence is statistically likely.

Adjuvant chemotherapy has been of documented worth in Wilms's tumor and neuroblastoma and may be of benefit in stage II–IIIB Hodgkin's disease in conjunction with radiation therapy. Adjuvant chemotherapy with high-dose methotrexate therapy followed by citrovorum (folinic acid) "rescue" or with doxorubicin has been shown to prolong the disease-free interval in childhood osteosarcoma after appropriate control of the primary lesion. Among other tumors that seem promising candidates for controlled studies of adjuvant chemotherapy are ovarian carcinoma, testicular tumors, and certain other soft tissue sarcomas.

Rhabdomyosarcoma in children can now be treated effectively by wide local excision (avoiding amputation) followed by irradiation and repeated

*See note to reader on p 325.

cyclic therapy with dactinomycin and vincristine.

Adjuvant chemotherapy after surgery for breast carcinoma is under intensive study.

LATE COMPLICATIONS OF CHEMOTHERAPY

The increasing effectiveness of chemotherapy in prolonging survival has meant that treated patients are often at increased risk of developing a second malignant growth. The most frequent second malignancy is acute myelogenous leukemia; other second drug- or radiation-associated malignancies are sporadic. Acute myelogenous leukemia has been observed in up to 2% of long-term survivors of Hodgkin's disease treated with radiotherapy and MOPP and in patients with ovarian carcinoma or myeloma treated with melphalan. Despite this problem, the risk/benefit ratio is strongly in favor of the initial therapeutic regimen. However, the risks of adjuvant alkylator therapy of stage I breast carcinoma may exceed benefits if the incidence of leukemia surpasses 2%. There is evidence that certain drugs (melphalan, procarbazine) are more carcinogenic or leukemogenic than other alkylators, such as cyclophosphamide, and other classes of drugs, such as antimetabolites.

INFUSION & PERFUSION THERAPY

Selective arterial infusion has been used to deliver higher concentrations of drugs to the tumor than could be tolerated by systemic administration. One worker gave fluorouracil by hepatic arterial infusion to 200 patients with hepatic metastases, most of whom had failed to respond to intravenous fluorouracil. About 60% of the patients objectively improved and survived an average of 8.7 months; nonresponders lived an average of 2.5 months.

Regional perfusion is an experimental technic that has given promising results in the following situations: (1) melanoma of an extremity perfused with mechlorethamine, phenylalanine mustard, or dacarbazine; (2) head and neck tumors perfused through the carotid artery with alkylators, fluorouracil, or methotrexate; and (3) hepatomas and metastatic adenocarcinoma in liver infused via the hepatic artery with fluorouracil and other drugs.

COMBINATION CHEMOTHERAPY

Combinations of drugs that block multiple biosynthetic pathways are given in an attempt to obtain a synergistic effect on the tumor. The drugs of a combination are selected to avoid overlapping toxicity. This approach has been of greatest value where no single agent is highly effective. Thus, vincristine plus prednisone or cytarabine plus thioguanine produce more complete remissions of acute leukemia than either agent alone, and toxicity is not enhanced. Survival is prolonged in proportion to the duration of remission, which documents the importance of achieving complete remission.

The treatment of testicular malignancies is representative of an era of chemotherapeutic and radiotherapeutic progress since the development in 1960 by Li and others of combination chemotherapy (chlorambucil, methotrexate, and dactinomycin) for patients with disseminated disease. Non-seminomatous testicular carcinomas have recently been treated successfully with varying combinations of bleomycin, vinblastine, and cisplatin. Samuels reported an overall 75% response rate, with a 45% complete remission rate, to a regimen of vinblastine and bleomycin. Einhorn and Donohue treated 50 patients with a triple combination of bleomycin, vinblastine, and cisplatin with 75% complete and 25% partial remissions. Toxicity was significant, but remissions lasted for 6 months to more than 30 months.

· · ·

EVALUATION & MANAGEMENT OF PATIENTS WITH AN UNKNOWN PRIMARY CARCINOMA

About 15% of cancer patients present with metastatic tumor of unknown primary site of origin. The most common sources are pancreas and lung. If the presenting metastasis is a squamous carcinoma, the primary is most often lung, but an occult nasal, oropharyngeal, or laryngeal primary may occasionally be treated with curative intent if evaluation reveals no dissemination beyond regional nodes.

For adenocarcinomas or undifferentiated carcinomas, an extensive search for the primary may be unrevealing until late in the course. The objectives of care are to palliate symptoms from metastases and diagnose the primary source, especially in the case of more treatable (often hormonally responsive) tumors such as those of breast, prostate, uterus, and thyroid. Extensive radiologic and endoscopic evaluation is justified in the search for a primary source of a solitary metastasis, but it usually produces little benefit for those with multiple dissemination sites; palliative therapy of symptoms caused by the metastases is usually more important. Unusual sites of metastatic presentation include the skin (usually from a lung, colon, or kidney primary), intraocular structures (usually from a female breast primary), and the lower female genital tract (usually from an ovarian or uterine primary).

THE PARANEOPLASTIC SYNDROMES

The paraneoplastic ("beyond tumor growth") syndromes (Table 18–3) may present bizarre signs and symptoms resembling primary endocrine, metabolic, hematologic, or neuromuscular disorders. These syndromes may be the first clue to the presence of certain tumors, the early diagnosis of which may favorably affect the prognosis. All too often, however, they are a manifestation of disseminated or advanced disease; even then, their palliation may provide more symptomatic relief than would reduction of tumor mass alone.

CHEMOTHERAPY OF SPECIFIC UROLOGIC MALIGNANCIES

Adrenal Cortical Carcinoma

In the past decade, mitotane (o,p'-DDD, Lysodren) has been used in the management of metastatic or functional adrenal cortical neoplasia. Mitotane produces a decrease in corticosteroid excretion in 70% of patients as a result of degeneration of the zona reticularis and zona fasciculata of the adrenal gland. Cushing's syndrome and virilism associated with hyperadrenocorticism are often palliated after 3–4 weeks of therapy, and in 35% of patients so treated, tumor regression occurs as well.

Aminoglutethimide* (Cytadren, Elipten) has also been useful for control of hypersecretion of corticosteroids because it inhibits adrenal synthesis through interference with the conversion of cholesterol to pregnenolone. The drug is beneficial when Cushing's syndrome is uncontrolled by mitotane or the toxicity of mitotane prohibits its use in doses large enough to be effective. However, aminoglutethimide is not cytotoxic against tumor tissue and does not reduce tumor bulk.

Neuroblastoma

Chemotherapy has not been very effective for this tumor but must be tried where disseminated disease makes surgical control impossible. Cyclophosphamide (Cytoxan), vincristine (Oncovin), and dacarbazine can be used. Recently, some success has been achieved where chemotherapy followed surgical excision of the tumor. Evans & others (1980) report very good results in children who had widespread metastases (but not to bone).

Renal Cell Carcinoma (Hypernephroma)

Metastatic renal cell carcinoma is not highly susceptible to cytotoxic chemotherapy, although favorable responses are reported in the treatment of pulmonary metastases with vinblastine (Velban), 0.1–0.2 mg/kg intravenously weekly, and with nitrosoureas such as lomustine (CCNU), 130 mg/m^2 orally every 6 weeks. A 25% remission rate was reported in one study of 135 patients treated with vinblastine, whereas nitrosourea produced remissions in only 9% of 79 patients. Other studies have shown little effectiveness for these agents.

*See note to reader on p 325.

Bloom (1973) suggests that hormonal therapy may be beneficial in renal cell carcinoma. He observed that stilbestrol implants in male hamsters sometimes produced renal carcinomas and adenomas and that removal of the pellets altered the growth of induced tumors, as did the administration of testosterone or progesterone. Clinically, less than 15% of patients so treated show an objective response to pharmacologic doses of progesterone (Depo-Provera, Megace) or testosterone, but individual very good responses and relatively mild toxicity make this treatment worthy of consideration when a 1- to 2-month trial administration can be evaluated. Antiestrogens (tamoxifen* [Nolvadex], nafoxidine*) have not yet been definitively evaluated but may also be of benefit in some patients whose tumor tissue is assay-positive for estrogen or progesterone receptors. According to one recent study, a 15% response rate was obtained with antiestrogen therapy as compared to a 5% response rate with progestogens.

Although there are reports of rare instances of regression of pulmonary metastases after nephrectomy to remove the primary neoplasm, this procedure is not likely to be of significant benefit for disseminated disease. If symptoms referable to the primary tumor are present (eg, pain, hematuria), nephrectomy may be justified for local control.

The sometimes unusual clinical behavior of metastatic renal carcinoma suggests that host immune factors may be operative, but there is no documentation of significant benefit from any type of immunotherapy except in anecdotal cases.

Wilms's Tumor (Nephroblastoma)

The treatment of Wilms's tumor is a singular example of the benefits of adjuvant chemotherapy and of multimodal forms of combined treatment, including sequential therapy with surgery, radiation therapy, and chemotherapy with curative intent, even where metastatic disease is present. Nephrectomy alone cures 20% of children with localized Wilms's tumor; the addition of radiation therapy to the tumor bed after nephrectomy increases the cure rate to 47%; and the addition of multiple courses of dactinomycin as adjuvant treatment has increased the overall cure rate to 80%. Furthermore, half of children who develop multiple pulmonary metastases may be curable by the use of bilateral whole lung radiation therapy combined with chemotherapy using dactinomycin and possibly vincristine. The combination of dactinomycin and vincristine may be more effective than either drug used alone in this previously fatal cancer. Doxorubicin is also a useful drug for patients who fail to respond to dactinomycin with or without vincristine. Metastases solely to the lungs appear to have a distinctly better prognosis than liver, brain, or bone metastases.

The optimum dosage schedules and duration of therapy are not known with certainty, but recommended regimens are as follows:

(1) Dactinomycin, 15 mg/kg intravenously daily for 5 days, or 600 μg/m^2 intravenously every other day for 4 doses, beginning as soon as the diagnosis is established and continuing within 24 hours after surgery, followed by multiple courses at 6 weeks and 3, 7, 9, 12, and 15 months thereafter.

(2) Vincristine, 1.5 mg/m^2 intravenously weekly for 6 weeks beginning postoperatively, followed by 2 doses (4 days apart) of 1.5 mg/m^2 intravenously, repeated every 3 months for 15 months. No single dose of vincristine should exceed 2 mg.

Transitional Cell Tumors

Renal pelvis and ureteral tumors, which are uncommon, are biologically related to urothelial tumors arising in the bladder. Chemotherapy has not generally been effective for the palliation of such neoplasms, but newer drugs such as doxorubicin and cisplatin, reportedly useful for bladder carcinoma, may also be of some benefit for other urothelial malignancies.

Bladder carcinomas are a histologically and biologically heterogeneous group whose aggressiveness and prognosis are related to the stage and grade of tumor. For a further discussion of staging and grading, see p 291.

Up to two-thirds of selected patients with multiple small superficial papillary tumors show a favorable response to thiotepa, 60 mg instilled into the bladder in 60 mL of sterile water and retained for 2 hours. One-third may achieve a complete remission, which can be maintained with 30- to 60-mg instillations every 4–6 weeks. Adverse effects include marrow suppression and cystitis.

Doxorubicin is one of the most useful drugs for palliation of advanced bladder cancer. DeKernion has reported an overall response rate of 23% in 235 patients with objective regressions of skin, liver, lung, and nodal metastases occurring within 1 month and lasting up to 5 months. Fluorouracil is one of the most carefully studied drugs for treatment of bladder cancer, with an overall response rate of 35% in 74 patients; cisplatin showed a 35% response rate lasting up to 5 months but had more significant toxicity. Mitomycin may also be a useful agent, especially when instilled intravesically.

Immunotherapy has not yet been a significant treatment for bladder carcinoma, although data suggest that patients with bladder cancer have altered cellular and humoral immune responses.

Combined regimens of cyclophosphamide, doxorubicin, and cisplatin are more effective than single agents in small series, but the response rate in large numbers of patients is not yet determined.

Adjuvant chemotherapy of high-risk invasive bladder carcinoma has been proposed, and studies are under way; definitive results have not yet been

*See note to reader on p 325.

reported from a randomized trial now being conducted.

Bladder Sarcomas

Bladder sarcomas may respond temporarily to combination chemotherapy with doxorubicin and dacarbazine in up to 40% of adults treated as follows: Doxorubicin, 60 mg/m^2 intravenously on day 1, and dacarbazine, 250 mg/m^2 intravenously on days 1 through 5, with the cycle repeated every 22 days unless toxicity prohibits.

Childhood rhabdomyosarcomas of the lower urinary tract, bladder, and vagina can be controlled, with achievement of a 5-year remission in half of patients, by a cooperative effort with surgery, where feasible, in conjunction with radiation therapy and combination adjuvant chemotherapy consisting of dactinomycin and vincristine. Twenty percent of children with clinical evidence of metastases are curable by aggressive combined therapy with 3 drugs (dactinomycin, vincristine, and cyclophosphamide) in conjunction with radiation therapy. Drugs are given in 3-month cycles for 1–2 years, as in the VAC regimen of Wilbur: vincristine, 2 mg/m^2 intravenously weekly for 12 weeks (maximum, 2 mg/dose); dactinomycin, 0.075 mg/kg/course intravenously over 5 days (maximum, 0.5 mg/d) every 3 months for 5 courses; and cyclophosphamide, 2.5 mg/kg orally daily for 2 years.

Prostatic Carcinoma

Disseminated symptomatic or rapidly progressive prostatic carcinoma should be considered for palliative therapy even though no increase in survival can be documented by controlled studies. Eighty percent of patients receiving hormonal therapy or orchiectomy experienced both subjective and objective benefit of symptoms. The era of hormonal antineoplastic therapy began when Huggins and associates observed improvement following androgenic hormone suppression or treatment with estrogens in such patients. Hormonal therapy is discussed on p 309.

Also noteworthy is the recent development of the antiandrogens (flutamide* and cyproterone acetate*) and of the estradiol-alkylator complex estramustine phosphate* (Estracyt). Estramustine* has been extensively studied in Europe, where a response rate of 38% has been reported in over 200 patients with advanced prostatic carcinoma following intravenous administration. Oral estramustine* is reported to yield a 22% response rate, according to Mittelman, Shukla, & Murphy (1976).

Chemotherapy of prostatic carcinoma that has not responded to endocrine therapy has been moderately effective, with responses of approximately 35% reported for fluorouracil, cyclophosphamide, and doxorubicin as single agents. Such therapy was superior to secondary palliative hormonal manipu-

lations after failure of orchiectomy or estrogen therapy. Other effective single agents include cisplatin and dacarbazine in small series.

Patients who respond to chemotherapy fare better in terms of pain palliation, and their overall survival rate is 1½ times to twice that of nonresponders. Combinations of drugs may yield higher response rates, with doxorubicin plus cyclophosphamide or cisplatin apparently one of the most effective combinations; however, the numbers of patients so treated are too small and follow-up periods too brief to justify any statements about the duration of benefit. Full dosage of these cytotoxic agents is often not possible because of extensive previous radiation therapy to marrow-bearing areas of bone or because of bone marrow infiltration by the tumor. Hypercalcemia is sometimes a complication of prostatic carcinoma with extensive bony involvement.

Testicular Neoplasms

The treatment of testicular malignancies exemplifies the progress made in chemotherapy and radiotherapy since 1960, when Li and others developed combination chemotherapy (chlorambucil, methotrexate, and dactinomycin) for patients with disseminated disease. Friedman & Purkayastha (1960) showed that relatively low doses of radiation may be curative for seminoma when metastases to the neck and mediastinum are present.

Metastases contain pure seminomatous elements in two-thirds of cases, and these are usually radiosensitive; in one-fourth of cases, the metastatic tissue type is embryonal carcinoma, implying that apparently "pure" seminomas may in fact contain combinations of germ cell elements, including chorionic tissue in 9% and teratomatous elements in 4%. Alkylators such as melphalan and chlorambucil have been reported to be effective in 90% of cases; in instances where combined elements are documented, dactinomycin, cisplatin, vinblastine, and bleomycin in various combinations may be the drugs of choice.

The presence of nonseminomatous elements in a testicular tumor is suggested by finding alpha-fetoprotein or beta-hCG tumor markers in serum as determined by radioimmunoassay or in tumor tissue as determined by immunocytochemical technics.

The beta-subunit of hCG is unique and specific to the hCG molecule and does not give false-positive radioimmunoassays with elevated levels of LH or other stimulating hormones. Up to 60% of nonseminomatous germ cell tumors of the testis are associated with initially high serum hCG levels, which return to normal with effective therapy. A persistently elevated or rising level implies the presence of active disease.

Alpha-fetoprotein elevation indicates an element of embryonal carcinoma in a testicular tumor.

*See note to reader on p 325.

Seventy percent of testicular neoplasms have elevation of alpha-fetoprotein by sensitive radioimmunoassay technics; persistent elevation implies recurrent or progressive tumor. One or the other marker is elevated in as many as 90% of patients with nonseminomatous testicular tumors, whereas less than 10% of pure seminomas produce these markers. CEA (carcinoembryonic antigen) has also been reported to be a product of testicular germ cell neoplasms but is not as tissue-specific as hCG and alpha-fetoprotein.

Nonseminomatous testicular carcinomas have recently been treated successfully with varying combinations of bleomycin, vinblastine, and cisplatin. Samuels (1975) reports an overall 75% response rate, with a 45% complete remission rate, to a regimen of vinblastine, 0.2 mg/kg intravenously daily on days 1 and 2; and bleomycin, 30 units infused in 1000 mL of 5% glucose and water over 24 hours on day 2 and for 5 additional days.

Courses are repeated every 3–4 weeks for 3 or 4 cycles depending upon the degree and duration of toxicity. Side-effects include severe leuukopenia (80%), thrombocytopenia (40%), and stomatitis (100%). Anemia and pneumonitis due to bleomycin occur in a lower percentage of patients. Median duration of response was 34 weeks.

The Memorial Sloan-Kettering program of therapy consists of continuous intravenous infusion of bleomycin, 0.5 units/kg daily for 7 days, combined with cisplatin, 1 mg/kg intravenously on day 7. Responses were observed in 11 of 16 patients who were resistant to previous weekly bleomycin and vinblastine or dactinomycin therapy. Responses lasted 2–7 months, and toxicity was predominantly mucosal, with one-third of patients also having transient nephrotoxicity and ototoxicity due to platinum.

Einhorn, Furnas, & Powell (1976) used a triple combination of bleomycin, vinblastine, and cisplatin with 100% success in 20 patients, 15 of whom achieved complete remission with a median duration of 9 months (range 6–18 months). This regimen is as follows: vinblastine, 0.2 mg/kg intravenously on days 1 and 2 every 3 weeks; bleomycin, 30 units intravenously weekly for 12 weeks; and cisplatin, 20 mg/m^2 intravenously daily on days 1–5 every 3 weeks.

If a complete remission is not achieved after 4 courses of combination chemotherapy, surgical excision of residual disease should be considered if feasible. This means wedge resection of a solitary pulmonary nodule or multiple nodules confined to a single lobe of the lung and resection of persistent abdominal masses detected by CT scanning or palpation. Occasionally, pathologic examination of resected tissue reveals only necrotic fibrous tissue or benign mature teratomas.

Aggressive chemotherapy should be undertaken only by a clinician experienced in the use of the drugs involved, since major toxicities may ensue

and require skillful supportive care. Cisplatin causes moderate to severe nausea and vomiting in nearly all patients and requires vigorous intravenous hydration before and during administration to avoid significant nephrotoxicity. Many patients experience a 25–50% reduction in creatinine clearance when compared with a baseline pretreatment value. Granulocytopenia with sepsis is a major manifestation of the hematologic toxicity of the 3 drugs, and the use of aminoglycoside antibiotics may cause further deterioration of renal function. Anemia and thrombocytopenia are frequently observed also, but are usually less severe than granulocytopenia. Other toxicities include weight loss, high-frequency hearing loss, fever, alopecia, myalgias, and pulmonary manifestations of bleomycin toxicity.

Mithramycin has been useful as a single agent, with a 36% response rate when used in embryonal carcinoma, or in various combinations; and doxorubicin is also reportedly a useful agent, with a 20% response rate.

It is apparent that the use of these aggressive chemotherapeutic combination regimens can achieve significant disease control for relatively long durations, but they may also carry the risk of major toxicity and must be given by knowledgeable clinicians experienced in their administration and in a setting where adequate supportive facilities are available.

Penile Carcinoma

Penile carcinoma with massive inguinal or pelvic nodal metastases refractory to radiation therapy and beyond the scope of surgery may, on occasion, be successfully treated with bleomycin with or without methotrexate, although the contributions of chemotherapy have not been well defined for this malignancy.

PAIN PALLIATION IN CANCER

Malignant disease may cause pain by obstruction of a hollow viscus, by destruction of the supporting architecture of weight-bearing bones, by infiltration of nerve roots or plexuses by tumor, and by infiltrative growth within a closed compartment such as periosteum, fascia, or a visceral capsule. Pain can sometimes be controlled by decreasing tumor bulk with radiation therapy, surgery, and chemotherapy. Radiation therapy is most effective for bony metastases; surgery may bypass an obstruction of bowel or biliary tract; regional intraarterial chemotherapy can reduce liver pain of hepatic metastases in 50–70% of selected patients.

All too often, however, these measures are only temporarily or partially effective, and nonspecific symptomatic treatment of pain is required. Aspirin and acetaminophen are the most effective nonnarcotics and, combined with codeine, are useful for ambulatory patients. Narcotic analgesics such as morphine or hydromorphone (Dilaudid) are often required in terminal malignancy; the fear of producing drug addiction should never prevent their administration to such patients. In patients with persistent or recurrent pain, a regular schedule of administration at 3- to 4-hour intervals may afford better palliation than larger doses at less frequent intervals.

Neurosurgical and anesthetic measures are appropriate in patients who have not responded to other palliative measures or who have neuroanatomically localized pain that can be eradicated without producing major neurologic dysfunction. Dorsal rhizotomy is appropriate for segmental somatic pain of thoracoabdominal dermatomes but would be a poor choice for pain in an extremity because of the concomitant loss of sensory function resulting from the procedure. Percutaneous cordotomy is an effective procedure for unilateral pain located in segments lower than the upper thoracic area. Thalamotomy may be useful in control of head and facial pain, as may tractotomy (trigeminal or spinal thalamic). Somatic nerve and autonomic plexus blocks may be useful when a more effective surgical procedure is refused or otherwise unavailable.

BACTERIAL SEPSIS IN CANCER PATIENTS

Infection is the cause of death in 60–75% of patients with leukemia or lymphoma and 40–50% of patients with solid tumors. In some instances, this is due to impaired host defense mechanisms (leukemia, lymphoma, myeloma); in others, it is due to the myelosuppressive and immunosuppressive effects of cancer therapy or progressive malignancy with cachexia.

In patients with acute leukemia or granulocytopenia (granulocyte count $< 600/\mu$L), infection is a medical emergency, and fever is virtually pathognomonic of infection, usually with gram-negative organisms, in these patients.

Appropriate cultures (eg, blood, sputum, urine, cerebrospinal fluid) should always be obtained before starting therapy; however, one usually cannot await the results of these studies before beginning bactericidal antibiotic therapy. Gram's stains may clearly demonstrate the presence of a predominant organism.

In the absence of granulocytopenia and in non-leukemic patients, the empiric combination of a cephalosporin type antibiotic and tobramycin has been very beneficial for patients with acute bacteremia. This therapy has a very broad spectrum, however, and therefore must be used judiciously and should always be replaced by the most appropriate antibiotics as soon as culture data become

available. The combination of cephalosporin and kanamycin is ineffective against *Pseudomonas* infection. In the current era of intensive chemotherapy of cancer, *Pseudomonas* bacteremia is now the most frequent infection in granulocytopenic patients and is all too often fulminant and fatal within 72 hours. Prompt institution of combination therapy with tobramycin and ticarcillin may offer the best chance of cure. Because of drug interactions, these 2 compounds cannot be mixed but must be administered separately. This combination is less effective against *Escherichia coli* sepsis and should not be used for that purpose. Initial treatment of febrile patients with acute leukemia or granulocytopenia should consist of 3 drugs: cephalothin, tobramycin, and ticarcillin. If a causative organism is isolated, the combination is replaced with the best agent or agents; otherwise, the combination is continued until the infection has resolved.

Granulocyte transfusions have recently been proved to have significant value for granulocytopenic cancer patients with sepsis; however, until recently, complex procurement procedures limited their availability. Untreated patients with chronic myelogenous leukemia can serve as excellent granulocyte donors for cancer patients with granulocytopenia. Although collection is ideally carried out with a blood cell separator, simple leukapheresis technics may also be of value with chronic myelogenous leukemia donors. Use of normal donors requires a blood cell separator or filtration-leukapheresis device. Optimal use of normal granulocyte transfusion appears to require at least 4 daily transfusions (in addition to antibiotics) to localize infection.

PALLIATION OF LOCAL COMPLICATIONS OF NEOPLASIA

Effusions

At least half of all patients with lung or breast cancer will develop a pleural effusion at some time during their illness. Ascites is a common complication of ovarian carcinoma. Lymphomas may be associated with chylous or nonchylous effusion of either or both sites. One-fourth of all effusions are neoplastic in origin, and where pulmonary infarction is unlikely, most bloody effusions are from neoplasm. The diagnosis in malignant pleural effusions can be established by cytologic study of the fluid and pleural biopsy with the Cope needle.

Diuretics may be sufficient to control neoplastic ascitic effusions. However, when recurrent accumulations of fluid cause dyspnea, abdominal distention, or pericardial tamponade, palliative control should be attempted.

A. Pleural Effusions: Control of pleural effusions is best achieved by obliteration of the pleural space with sclerosing agents such as mechlorethamine or tetracycline. Up to 90% of pleural effusions can be palliated with this technic. Criteria for obliteration and details of procedure should be decided upon by experienced personnel only.

B. Ascitic Effusions: Ascites is generally best treated by attempting to control the underlying disease, usually ovarian carcinoma or malignant lymphoma. Mechlorethamine frequently induces chemical peritonitis. Thiotepa and bleomycin do not have a vesicant action on tissues and are thus more gentle.

C. Pericardial Effusions: Pericardial effusions are best treated by irradiation except when previous radiotherapy has included the proposed field or when the effusion is due to a radioresistant tumor. Impending tamponade must always be anticipated and treated by pericardiocentesis, creation of a pericardial window, or pericardiectomy. If needle pericardiocentesis is performed for a malignant effusion, thiotepa may be instilled into the pericardial cavity (in systemic doses) at the termination of the procedure. Mechlorethamine should not be used, since it induces too severe an inflammatory response.

Obstructions & Lytic Lesions of Bone

A. Caval Obstruction: Superior vena caval obstruction is a medical emergency that should be treated by a combination of chemotherapy and radiotherapy. It is characterized by venous congestion and distention of tributaries of the superior vena cava, and thus presents clinically as edema of the face and arms—frequently associated with dyspnea and the hazard of cerebral venous thrombosis or cerebral edema. The syndrome may occur with various diseases affecting the mediastinum, but neoplastic disease—especially bronchogenic carcinoma and the malignant lymphomas—is by far the most common cause. Although a biopsy should be obtained whenever possible, this should not delay the start of therapy. Thoracic surgery or mediastinoscopy should not be performed, since such intervention increases morbidity and mortality rates. Treatment should be started as soon as the clinical syndrome is recognized and consists of diuretics, corticosteroids, and maintenance of the upright posture. An intravenous alkylator should be given through an unobstructed vein (eg, femoral vein) and radiotherapy begun immediately. Cyclophosphamide or thiotepa is preferable to mechlorethamine, since the former agents induce less vomiting. Venography or sodium pertechnetate Tc 99m scanning will demonstrate large collateral veins and a block to the flow of contrast material into the right heart. Although the underlying carcinoma is usually incurable when this condition develops, emergency therapy may provide substantial palliation.

B. Bony Lytic Lesions: Palliation of metastases to weight-bearing bones is best achieved by irradiation. If pathologic fracture is impending, prophylactic fixation can minimize morbidity, especially in areas such as the femoral neck that are susceptible to considerable stress. Prolonged bed rest should be avoided whenever possible, for in addition to the usual complications, patients with bony disease are prone to develop hypercalcemia, and this tendency is accentuated by immobilization. Supportive bracing is often a useful adjunct for vertebral involvement.

Metabolic Complications of Neoplasia

A. Hypercalcemia Associated With Neoplastic Disease: Hypercalcemia occurs most commonly with myeloma, breast carcinoma, and lung carcinoma and is occasionally seen in patients with prostatic carcinoma, lymphomas, and leukemia. It has also been reported with a wide variety of metastatic or disseminated neoplasms. Symptoms include confusion, somnolence, nausea and vomiting, constipation, dehydration with polyuria, and general clinical deterioration that can easily be mistaken for progressive disease or direct neurologic involvement by tumor. The true nature of this metabolic complication may easily be overlooked, resulting in hypercalcemic death secondary to cardiac, neurologic, and renal toxicity. Hypercalcemia may be due to elaboration of a parathyroid hormone-like substance by tumor (lung carcinoma), to osteolytic sterols (as secreted by breast tumors), or to increased bone resorption by invasion and neoplastic destruction of bone (as in myeloma).

The mainstay of therapy to reduce calcium is hydration with isotonic saline (to promote a diuresis of 2–3 L/24 h) in addition to appropriate tumoricidal therapy, mobilization of the bedridden, institution of a low-calcium diet devoid of dairy products, and appropriate treatment of bacterial infections. If the patient was receiving androgens or estrogens for breast carcinoma, they should be withdrawn. Chelating agents such as sodium citrate promote renal excretion of calcium, and potent diuretics such as furosemide or ethacrynic acid also inhibit calcium resorption by the renal tubule. These measures, however, may not be appropriate in patients with impaired renal function or congestive heart failure or may not be sufficient of themselves, and other measures such as glucocorticoids (prednisone, 60–100 mg/d) may be required. The corticosteroids appear to act by reducing calcium resorption from bone. Oral phosphate is often rapidly effective, but intravenous phosphates are too hazardous to be recommended. Mithramycin, 25 μg/kg intravenously, is a prompt and effective agent for marked hypercalcemia. It may be the drug of choice where vigorous hydration is not possible because of renal failure or fluid overload; preexisting pancytopenia is a relative contraindication. A rapid fall in serum calcium concentration will also be produced by salmon calcitonin, 4 MRC units/kg intramuscularly every 12 hours, when it is used in conjunction with other measures discussed above.

B. Hyperuricemia in Neoplastic Disease: Hyperuricemia is a potentially lethal result of high nucleic acid turnover associated with some malignancies—especially after effective cytotoxic therapy. Uric acid nephropathy is related to intraluminal precipitation of uric acid in the distal renal tubule and collecting duct, with progressive intrarenal obstruction and failure. This sequence of events can often be avoided by maintaining satisfactory hydration and alkalinization of the urine to pH 7.0 by oral sodium bicarbonate (6–12 g/d) or by giving acetazolamide (Diamox) (0.5–1 g/d). Although allopurinol does not replace these measures, the preventive use of this drug (300–800 mg/d) should be considered in patients with leukemia, lymphomas, and myeloproliferative disorders. If mercaptopurine is being given, the dose must be reduced to one-fourth to one-third of usual when allopurinol is started. In addition to the above measures, peritoneal dialysis or hemodialysis may be required to treat established urate uropathy.

NUTRITIONAL SUPPORT IN CANCER PATIENTS

Many patients with malignant disease eat and digest a normal diet but nevertheless continue to lose weight. Superimposed pain or therapeutic ministrations such as chemotherapy, radiation therapy, or surgery may lead to anorexia and inanition. The quickest and safest way to improve nutrition in the cachectic patient is by intravenous hyperalimentation, but this is appropriate only when the patient appears likely to benefit from further antineoplastic therapy.

PSYCHOLOGIC SUPPORT OF THE PATIENT WITH NEOPLASTIC DISEASE

The physician who undertakes primary management of a patient with neoplastic disease assumes an obligation that may extend from initial diagnosis to terminal care. Because of the wide variations in the clinical course of the disease, this period may be brief or extend over many years. During this time, the physician must coordinate various methods of therapy. However, among the major palliative benefits offered by the physician will be rapport with the patient and family based upon skillful treatment, effective and honest communication, and humane care and consideration. Such a relationship can support hope despite the statistical unlikelihood of long survival, because the patient's anxieties and fears are usually of abandonment, dependency, pain, and loss of individuality or of dignity rather than of impending death.

HOME CARE OF THE PATIENT WITH ADVANCED CANCER

Some patients with advanced cancer and their families may prefer that the terminal phase of illness be spent in the home, with its comforts and access to relatives and friends. Careful assessment of the patient's physical and emotional needs must be considered by the physician before discharge from the hospital. It is important to ensure a smooth transition to home care by obtaining in advance all required equipment and supportive assistance. Home care is not appropriate for all patients but must be individually determined. The physician in charge should ideally be the coordinator of all supportive personnel—including visiting nurses, the dietitian, home health aides, priests and ministers, and medical social workers—rather than delegating this responsibility to others who do not have an established therapeutic relationship with the patient and family. In many instances, the guidance thus provided is more significant and more beneficial than the specialized technical therapies discussed throughout this chapter. Quality of care is best secured by acting upon the principle that much can yet be done for the patient even when little can be done against the neoplasm.

● ● ●

References

General

Proceedings of The American Cancer Society's National Conference on Urologic Cancer. *Cancer* 1973;**32**:1017.

Benign Tumors of the Renal Parenchyma

Ambos MA & others: Angiographic patterns in renal oncocytomas. *Radiology* 1978;**129**:615.

Bagley D & others: Renal angiomyolipoma: Diagnosis and management. *Urology* 1980;**15**:1.

Berdon WE, Wigger HJ, Baker DH: Fetal renal hamartoma: A benign tumor to be distinguished from Wilms' tumor. *Am J Roentgenol* 1973;**118**:18.

Bissada NK & others: Tuberous sclerosis complex and renal angiomyolipoma: Collective review. *Urology* 1975; **6**:105.

Bush WH Jr, Freeny PC, Orme BM: Angiomyolipoma: Characteristic images by ultrasound and computed tomography. *Urology* 1979;**14**:531.

Cass AS: Large renal adenoma. *J Urol* 1980;**124**:281.

Conn JW, Bookstein JJ, Cohen EL: Renin-secreting juxtaglomerular-cell adenoma: Preoperative clinical and angiographic diagnosis. *Radiology* 1973;**106**:543.

Evins SC, Varner W: Renal adenoma: A misnomer. *Urology* 1979;**13**:85.

Fois A, Pindinelli CA, Berardi R: Early signs of tuberous sclerosis in infancy and childhood. *Helv Paediatr Acta* 1973;**28**:313.

Ghazi MR, Brown JS, Warner RS: Carcinoid tumor of kidney. *Urology* 1979;**14**:610.

Hajdu SI, Koss LG: Endometriosis of the kidney. *Am J Obstet Gynecol* 1970;**106**:314.

Horton WA, Wong V, Eldridge R: Von Hippel-Lindau disease: Clinical and pathological manifestations in nine families with 50 affected members. *Arch Intern Med* 1976;**136**:769.

Jander HP, Tonkin IL: Epinephrine-enhanced renal angiography in the diagnosis of hamartoma (angiomyolipoma): A reevaluation. *Radiology* 1979;**132**:61.

Loening S, Richardson JR Jr: Papillary cystadenoma of kidney. *Urology* 1973;**1**:593.

Moorehead JD, Fritzsche P, Hadley HL: Management of hemorrhage secondary to renal angiolipoma with selective arterial embolization. *J Urol* 1977;**117**:122.

Morales A, Wasan S, Bryniak S: Renal oncocytomas: Clinical, radiological and histological features. *J Urol* 1980;**123**:261.

Mouded IM & others: Symptomatic renal angiomyolipoma: Report of 8 cases, 2 with spontaneous rupture. *J Urol* 1978;**119**:684.

Peters HJ, Nuri M, Münzenmaier R: Hemangioendothelioma of the kidney: A case report and review of the literature. *J Urol* 1974;**112**:723.

Phillips G, Mukherjee TM: A juxtaglomerular cell tumour: Light and electron microscopic studies of a reninsecreting kidney tumour containing both juxtaglomerular cells and mass cells. *Pathology* 1972;**4**:194.

Sood S, Mancini AA, Kropp K: Tuberous sclerosis: Emphasis on the angiographic findings. *J Urol* 1975;**114**:185.

Stanley RJ & others: Cavernous hemangioma of the kidney. *Am J Roentgenol* 1975;**125**:862.

Stavorovsky M & others: Rupture of a renal angiomyolipoma (hamartoma). *Postgrad Med J* 1979;**55**:840.

Walker D, Richard GA: Fetal hamartoma of the kidney: Recurrence and death of a patient. *J Urol* 1973;**110**:352.

Yu GSM & others: Renal oncocytoma: Report of five cases and review of literature. *Cancer* 1980;**45**:1010.

Adenocarcinoma

Abrams HJ & others: Renal carcinoma in adolescents. *J Urol* 1979;**121**:92.

Altaffer LF III, Chenault OW Jr: Paraneoplastic endocrinopathies associated with renal tumors. *J Urol* 1979;**122**:573.

Ballesteros JJ, Faus R, Gironella J: Preoperative diagnosis of renal xanthogranulomatosis by serial urinary cytology: Preliminary report. *J Urol* 1980;**124**:9.

Bernardino ME, Green B, Goldstein HM: Ultrasonography in the evaluation of post-nephrectomy renal cancer patients. *Radiology* 1978;**128**:455.

Bernardino ME & others: Computed tomography in the evaluation of post-nephrectomy patients. *Radiology* 1979;**130**:183.

Bosniak MA & others: Epinephrine-enhanced renal angiography in renal mass lesions: Is it worth performing? *AJR* 1977;**129**:647.

Boxer RJ & others: Nonmetastatic hepatic dysfunction associated with renal carcinoma. *J Urol* 1978;**119**:468.

Boxer RJ & others: Renal carcinoma: Computer analysis of 96 patients treated by nephrectomy. *J Urol* 1979;**122**:598.

Bracken B, Jonsson K: How accurate is angiographic staging of renal carcinoma? *Urology* 1979;**14**:96.

Braedel HU & others: Renal phlebography in diagnosis of poorly vascularized renal malignancies. *Urology* 1979;**13**:91.

Carty AT, Short MD, O'Connell MEA: The diagnosis of renal pseudotumor. *Br J Urol* 1975;**47**:495.

Chu TM & others: Plasma carcinoembryonic antigen in renal cell carcinoma patients. *J Urol* 1974;**111**:742.

Chuang VP & others: Arterial occlusion in the management of pain from metastatic renal carcinoma. *Radiology* 1979;**133**:611.

Clayman RV, Gonzales R, Fraley EE: Renal cell cancer invading the inferior vena cava: Clinical review and anatomical approach. *J Urol* 1980;**123**:157.

Clayman RV, Williams RD, Fraley EE: The pursuit of the renal mass. *N Engl J Med* 1979;**300**:72.

Cole AT & others: The place of bone scan in the diagnosis of renal cell carcinoma. *J Urol* 1976;**114**:364.

Cummings KB & others: Intraoperative management of renal cell carcinoma with supradiaphragmatic caval extension. *J Urol* 1979;**122**:829.

Donaldson JC & others: Metastatic renal cell carcinoma 24 years after nephrectomy. *JAMA* 1976;**236**:950.

Doust VL, Doust BD, Redman HC: Evaluation of ultrasonic B-mode scanning in the diagnosis of renal masses. *Am J Roentgenol* 1973;**117**:112.

Fill WL, Lamiell JM, Polk NO: The radiographic manifestations of von Hippel-Lindau disease. *Radiology* 1979;**133**:289.

Fitzer PM: Newly recognized findings on bone scanning in patients with renal cell adenocarcinoma. *Urology* 1975;**6**:435.

Forbes GS, McLeod RA, Hattery RR: Radiographic manifestations of bone metastases from renal carcinoma. *AJR* 1977;**129**:61.

Freed SZ, Feldman JA, Sprayragen S: Follow-up of patients after nephrectomy for renal cell carcinoma. *Urology* 1977;**9**:500.

Freed SZ, Halperin JP, Gordon M: Idiopathic regression of metastases from renal cell carcinoma. *J Urol* 1977;**118**:538.

Futter NG, Collins JP, Walsh WG: Inaccuracies in angiographic staging of renal cell carcinoma. *Urology* 1979;**14**:629.

Gibbons RP, Bush WH Jr, Burnett LL: Needle tract seeding following aspiration of renal cell carcinoma. *J Urol* 1977;**118**:865.

Gittes RF, McCullough DL: Bench surgery for tumor in solitary kidney. *J Urol* 1975;**113**:12.

Golde DW & others: Gonadotropin-secreting renal carcinoma. *Cancer* 1974;**33**:1048.

Gorder JL, Stargardter FL: Pancreatic pseudocysts simulating intrarenal masses. *Am J Roentgenol* 1969;**107**:65.

Graham SD Jr, Glenn JF: Enucleative surgery for renal malignancy. *J Urol* 1979;**122**:546.

Green WM & others: "Column of Bertin": Diagnosis by

nephrotomography. *Am J Roentgenol* 1972;**116**:714.

Gross M, Minkowitz S: Ureteral metastasis from renal adenocarcinoma. *J Urol* 1971;**106**:23.

Guinan PD & others: Carcinoembryonic antigen test in renal cell carcinoma. *Urology* 1975;**5**:185.

Hattery RR: Computed tomography of renal abnormalities. *Radiol Clin North Am* 1977;**15**:401.

Hellekant C, Nyman U: Routine celiac angiography in patients with renal cell carcinoma. *J Urol* 1979;**122**:17.

Hollifield JW & others: Renin-secreting clear cell carcinoma of the kidney. *Arch Intern Med* 1975;**135**:859.

Javadpour N: Tumor markers in urologic cancer. *Urology* 1980;**16**:127.

Klugo RC, Farah RN, Cerny JC: Renal malignant histiocytoma. *J Urol* 1974;**112**:727.

Klugo RC & others: Aggressive vs conservative management of stage IV renal cell carcinoma. *J Urol* 1977;**118**:244.

Krieger JN & others: Calcified renal cell carcinoma: A clinical, radiographic and pathologic study. *J Urol* 1979;**121**:575.

Kvartstein B, Lindemann R, Mathisen W: Renal carcinoma with increased erythropoietin production and secondary polycythemia. *Scand J Urol Nephrol* 1973;**7**:178.

Lange PH: Immunologic testing of patients with genitourinary malignancies. *Urol Clin North Am* 1979;**6**:587.

Levine E & others: Comparison of computed tomography and ultrasound in abdominal staging of renal cancer. *Urology* 1980;**16**:317.

Lubensky JD, Gangai MP: The hypercalcemia of genitourinary malignancy. *J Urol* 1979;**121**:259.

McAninch JW, Stutzman RE: Avascular renal adenocarcinoma: Variations and characteristics. *Urology* 1977;**9**:212.

Madayag MA & others: Involvement of the inferior vena cava in patients with renal cell carcinoma. *Radiology* 1979;**133**:321.

Marshall FF, Walsh PC: Extrarenal manifestations of renal cell carcinoma. *J Urol* 1977;**117**:439.

Mee AD, Heap SW: Pre-operative balloon occlusion of the renal artery for radical nephrectomy. *Br J Urol* 1978;**50**:153.

Merrin C & others: Chemotherapy of advanced renal cell carcinoma with vinblastine and CCNU. *J Urol* 1975;**113**:21.

Montie JE & others: The role of adjunctive nephrectomy in patients with metastatic renal cell carcinoma. *J Urol* 1977;**117**:272.

Morales A, Kiruluta G, Lott S: Hormones in the treatment of metastatic renal cancer. *J Urol* 1975;**114**:692.

Murphy JB, Marshall FF: Renal cyst versus tumor: A continuing dilemma. *J Urol* 1980;**123**:566.

Patel NP, Lavengood RW: Renal cell carcinoma: Natural history and results of treatment. *J Urol* 1978;**119**:722.

Peterson LJ & others: Hormonal therapy in metastatic hypernephroma. *Urology* 1974;**4**:669.

Raghavaiah NV: False positive findings on liver scans in carcinoma of kidney. *Urology* 1978;**12**:733.

Robson CJ, Churchill BM, Anderson W: The results of radical nephrectomy for renal cell carcinoma. *J Urol* 1969;**101**:297.

Rubin P & others: Preoperative irradiation in renal cancer: Evaluation of radiation treatment plans. *Am J Roentgenol* 1975;**123**:114.

Sagel SS & others: Computed tomography of the kidney. *Radiology* 1977;**124**:359.

Sanford EJ & others: Preliminary evaluation of urinary polyamines in the diagnosis of genitourinary tract malignancy. *J Urol* 1975;**113**:218.

Schiff M Jr, Bagley DH, Lytton B: Treatment of solitary and bilateral renal carcinomas. *J Urol* 1979;**121**:581.

Singsaas MW, Chopp RT, Mendez R: Preoperative renal embolization as adjunct to radical nephrectomy. *Urology* 1979;**14**:1.

Smith JC Jr & others: Renal venography in the evaluation of poorly vascularized neoplasms of the kidney. *Am J Roentgenol* 1975;**123**:552.

Sniderman KW & others: The radiologic and clinical aspects of calcified hypernephroma. *Radiology* 1979;**131**:31.

Sondag TJ & others: Hypernephromas with massive arteriovenous fistulas. *Am J Roentgenol* 1973;**117**:97.

Stigsson L, Ekelund L, Karp W: Bilateral concurrent renal neoplasms. *AJR* 1979;**132**:37.

Sufrin G & others: Hormones in renal cancer. *J Urol* 1977;**117**:433.

Sullivan M, Rösch J, Hodges CV: Angiographic infarction of a large hypernephroma with a tissue adhesive for control of hematuria. *J Urol* 1977;**118**:863.

Thomas ML, Lamb GHR: The value of large volume selective arteriophlebography of the renal veins in the preoperative assessment of renal carcinoma. *Br J Urol* 1979;**51**:78.

Wagle DG, Moore RH, Murphy GP: Secondary carcinomas of the kidney. *J Urol* 1975;**114**:30.

Warren MM, Utz DC, Kelalis PP: Concurrence of hypernephroma and hypercalcemia. *Ann Surg* 1971;**174**:863.

Wasko R: Regression of pulmonary metastases from renal carcinoma. *Urology* 1976;**7**:299.

Waters WB, Richie JP: Aggressive surgical approach to renal cell carcinoma: Review of 130 cases. *J Urol* 1979;**122**:306.

Wiley AL Jr & others: Combined intra-arterial actinomycin D and radiation therapy for surgically unresectable hypernephroma. *J Urol* 1975;**114**:198.

Ziegler P, Albukerk J: Rheumatoid granuloma of kidney. *Urology* 1978;**12**:85.

Zusman RM & others: Antihypertensive function of a renal-cell carcinoma: Evidence for a prostaglandin-A-secreting tumor. *N Engl J Med* 1974;**290**:843.

Embryoma

Babaian RJ, Skinner DG, Waisman J: Wilms' tumor in the adult patient: Diagnosis, management, and review of the world medical literature. *Cancer* 1980;**45**:1713.

Bishop HC & others: Survival in bilateral Wilms' tumor: Review of 30 National Wilms' Tumor Study cases. *J Pediatr Surg* 1977;**12**:631.

Boldt DW, Reilly BJ: Computed tomography of abdominal mass lesions in children. *Radiology* 1977;**124**:371.

Cassady JR, Jaffe N, Filler RM: The increasing importance of radiation therapy in the improved prognosis of children with Wilms' tumor. *Cancer* 1977;**39**:825.

Cox D: Chromosome constitution of nephroblastomas. *Cancer* 1966;**19**:1217.

D'Angio GJ & others: The treatment of Wilms' tumor: Results of the National Wilms' Tumor Study. *Cancer* 1976;**38**:633.

Danis RK & others: Preoperative embolization of Wilms' tumors. *Am J Dis Child* 1979;**133**:503.

Ehrlich RM & others: Wilms tumor, misdiagnosed

preoperatively: Review of 19 National Wilms Tumor Study I Cases. *J Urol* 1979;**122**:790.

Fraumeni JF, Glass AG: Wilms' tumor and congenital aniridia. *JAMA* 1968;**206**:825.

Ganguly A & others: Renin-secreting Wilms' tumor with severe hypertension: Report of a case and brief review of renin-secreting tumors. *Ann Intern Med* 1973;**79**: 835.

Green DM, Jaffe N: The role of chemotherapy in the treatment of Wilms' tumor. *Cancer* 1979;**44**:52.

Jenkin RDT & others: Wilms' tumour: Treatment of 113 patients from 1960 to 1971. *Can Med Assoc J* 1975;**112**:308.

Jereb B & others: Lymph node invasion and prognosis in nephroblastoma. *Cancer* 1980;**45**:1632.

Kenny GM & others: Erythropoietin levels in Wilms' tumor patients. *J Urol* 1970;**104**:758.

Kilton L, Matthews MJ, Cohen MH: Adult Wilms tumor: Report of prolonged survival and review of literature. *J Urol* 1980;**124**:1.

Lawler W, Marsden HB, Palmer MK: Wilms' tumor: Histologic variation and prognosis. *Cancer* 1975;**36**:1122.

Leape LL, Breslow NE, Bishop HC: The surgical treatment of Wilms' tumor: Results of The National Wilms' Tumor Study. *Ann Surg* 1978;**187**:351.

Lemerle J & others: Wilms' tumor: Natural history and prognostic factors: A retrospective study of 248 cases treated at the Institute Gustave-Roussy 1952–1967. *Cancer* 1976;**37**:2557.

Maurer HS & others: THe role of genetic factors in the etiology of Wilms' tumor: Two pairs of monozygous twins with congenital abnormalities (hemihypertrophy) and discordance for Wilms' tumor. *Cancer* 1979;**43**:205.

Penn I: Renal transplantation for Wilms tumor: Report of 20 cases. *J Urol* 1979;**122**:793.

Sanders RC: B-scan ultrasound in the management of abdominal masses in children. *JAMA* 1975;**231**:81.

Schwartz AD: Neuroblastoma and Wilms' tumor. *Med Clin North Am* 1977;**61**:1053.

Tank ES, Kay R: Neoplasms associated with hemihypertrophy, Beckwith-Wiedeman syndrome and aniridia. *J Urol* 1980;**124**:266.

Wedemeyer PP & others: Resection of metastases in Wilms' tumor: A report of three cases cured of pulmonary and hepatic metastases. *Pediatrics* 1968;**41**:446.

Sarcoma

Beccia DJ, Elkort RJ, Krane RJ: Adjuvant chemotherapy in renal leiomyosarcoma. *Urology* 1979;**13**:652.

Biggers R, Stewart J: Primary renal osteosarcoma. *Urology* 1979;**13**:674.

Kansara V, Powell I: Fibrosarcoma of kidney. *Urology* 1980;**16**:419.

Kotecha NM: Embryonal rhabdomyosarcoma of the kidney. *J Urol* 1977;**118**:325.

Morgan E, Kidd JM: Undifferentiated sarcoma of the kidney: A tumor of childhood with histopathologic and clinical characteristics distinct from Wilms' tumor. *Cancer* 1978;**42**:1916.

Rios JT: Renal liposarcoma with hypertension. *Urology* 1973;**1**:246.

Silber SJ, Chang CY: Primary lymphoma of kidney. *J Urol* 1973;**110**:282.

Tumors of the Renal Pelvis

Binder R & others: Aberrant papillae and other filling defects of the renal pelvis. *Am J Roentgenol* 1972;**114**:746.

Chew QT, Nouri MS, Woo BH: Small renal pelvic carcinomas: Value of epinephrine magnification angiography. *J Urol* 1978;**120**:243.

Gaakeer HA, DeRuiter HJ: Carcinoma of the renal pelvis following abuse of phenacetin-containing analgesic drugs. *Br J Urol* 1979;**51**:188.

Geerdsen J: Tumours of the renal pelvis and ureter: Symptomatology, diagnosis, treatment and prognosis. *Scand J Urol Nephrol* 1979;**13**:287.

Gill WB, Lu CT, Bibbo M: Retrograde brush biopsy of the ureter and renal pelvis. *Urol Clin North Am* 1979;**6**:573.

Goldman SM & others: Transitional cell tumors of the kidney: How diagnostic is the angiogram? *AJR* 1977;**129**:99.

Gonwa TA, Buckalew VM Jr, Corbett WT: Analgesic nephropathy and urinary tract carcinoma. *Ann Intern Med* 1979;**90**:432.

Grabstald H, Whitmore WF, Melamed MR: Renal pelvic tumors. *JAMA* 1971;**218**:845.

Homer MJ, Klein LA: Ultrasonic B-mode scanning for invasive transitional cell carcinoma of kidney. *Urology* 1975;**6**:650.

Jackson B & others: Urine cytology findings in analgesic nephropathy. *J Urol* 1978;**120**:145.

Johansson S, Wahlqvist L: A prognostic study of urothelial renal pelvic tumors: Comparison between the prognosis of patients treated with intrafascial nephrectomy and perifascial nephroureterectomy. *Cancer* 1979;**43**:2525.

Lang EK & others: Brush biopsy of pyelocalyceal lesions via a percutaneous translumbar approach. *Radiology* 1978;**129**:623.

Mancilla-Jimenez R, Stanley RJ, Blath RA: Papillary renal cell carcinoma: A clinical, radiologic, and pathologic study of 34 cases. *Cancer* 1976;**38**:2469.

Myrvold H, Fritjofsson Å, Magnusson P: Cholesteatoma of the renal pelvis. *Scand J Urol Nephrol* 1974;**8**:69.

Newman LB & others: Small round cell sarcoma of the renal pelvis: A case report. *J Urol* 1972;**108**:227.

Petkovic SD: Epidemiology and treatment of renal pelvic and ureteral tumors. *J Urol* 1975;**114**:858.

Pontes JE, Christensen LC, Pierce JM Jr: Angiographic aspects of tumors of renal pelvis and ureter. *Urology* 1976;**7**:334.

Poole-Wilson DS: Occupational tumours of the renal pelvis and ureter arising in dye-making industry. *Proc R Soc Med* 1969;**62**:93.

Raney AM: Detection of carcinoma of upper urinary tract with steerable brush biopsy. *Urology* 1979;**14**:77.

Skinner DG: Technique of nephroureterectomy with regional lymph node dissection. *Urol Clin North Am* 1978;**5**:253.

Summers JL, Keitzer A: Radiographic clue to the diagnosis of hemangioma of the kidney. *J Urol* 1972;**108**:852.

Tolia BM, Hajdu SI, Whitmore WF Jr: Leiomyosarcoma of the renal pelvis. *J Urol* 1973;**109**:974.

Vinocur C & others: Renal pelvic tumors in childhood. *Urology* 1980;**16**:393.

Wagle DC, Moore RH, Murphy GP: Squamous cell carcinoma of the renal pelvis. *J Urol* 1974;**111**:453.

Tumors of the Ureter

Arger PH & others: Ultrasonic assessment of renal transitional cell carcinoma: Preliminary report. *AJR* 1979;**132**:407.

Babaian RJ, Johnson DE: Primary carcinoma of the ureter. *J Urol* 1980;**123**:357.

Babaian RJ & others: Metastases from transitional cell carcinoma of urinary bladder. *Urology* 1980;**16**:142.

Babaian RJ & others: Secondary tumors of ureter. *Urology* 1979;**14**:341.

Banner MP, Pollack HM: Fibrous ureteral polyps. *Radiology* 1979;**130**:73.

Cancelmo JJ Jr & others: Tumors of the ureter: Problems in diagnosis. *Am J Roentgenol* 1973;**117**:132.

Cohen WM, Freed SZ, Hasson J: Metastatic cancer to the ureter: A review of the literature and case presentations. *J Urol* 1974;**112**:188.

Debruyne FMJ & others: Fibroepithelial polyp of ureter. *Urology* 1980;**16**:355.

Ghazi MR, Morales PA, Al-Askari S: Primary carcinoma of ureter: Report of 27 new cases. *Urology* 1979;**14**:18.

Kiriyama T, Hironaka H, Fukuda K: Six years of experience with retrograde biopsy of intraureteral carcinoma using the Dormia stone basket. *J Urol* 1976;**116**:308.

Klein RS, Cattolica EV: Ureteral endometriosis. *Urology* 1979;**13**:477.

Pontes JE, Christensen LC, Pierce JM Jr: Angiographic aspects of tumors of renal pelvis and ureter. *Urology* 1976;**7**:334.

Stiehm WD, Becker JA, Weiss RM: Ureteral endometriosis. *Radiology* 1972;**102**:563.

Strong DW & others: The ureteral stump after nephroureterectomy. *J Urol* 1976;**115**:654.

Takaha M, Nagata H, Sonoda T: Localized amyloid tumor of the ureter: Report of a case. *J Urol* 1971;**105**:502.

Tumors of the Bladder

Aquilina JN, Bugeja TJ: Primary malignant lymphoma of the bladder: Case report and review of literature. *J Urol* 1974;**112**:64.

Babaian RJ & others: Mixed mesodermal tumors of urinary bladder: Prognosis and management. *Urology* 1980;**15**:261.

Bartholomew TH & others: Changing concepts in management of pelvic rhabdomyosarcoma in children. *Urology* 1979;**13**:613.

Betkerur V & others: Screening tests for detection of bladder cancer. *Urology* 1980;**16**:16.

Birkhead BM, Conley JG, Scott RM: Intensive radiotherapy of locally advanced bladder cancer. *Cancer* 1976;**37**:2746.

Bladder cancer and smoking. *Br Med J* 1972;**1**:763.

Boyland E: *The Biochemistry of Bladder Cancer.* Thomas, 1963.

Bracken RB & others: Role of intravesical mitomycin C in management of superficial bladder tumors. *Urology* 1980;**16**:11.

Bryniak SR, Morales A, Challis T: Assessment of cavernous hemangioma of bladder by technetium-99-tagged albumin scan. *Urology* 1979;**13**:289.

Caldamone AA & others: Primary localized amyloidosis of urinary bladder. *Urology* 1980;**15**:174.

Carmignani G & others: Transcatheter embolization of the hypogastric arteries in cases of bladder hemorrhage from advanced pelvic cancers: Followup in 9 cases. *J Urol* 1980;**124**:196.

Caro DJ, Brown JS: Hemangioma of bladder. *Urology* 1976;**8**:479.

Chan RC, Bracken RB, Johnson DE: Single dose whole pelvis megavoltage irradiation for palliative control of hematuria or ureteral obstruction. *J Urol* 1979;**122**:750.

Chan RC, Johnson DE: Integrated therapy for invasive bladder carcinoma: Experience with 108 patients. *Urology* 1978;**12**:549.

Cooper EH, Williams RE: *The Biology and Clinical Management of Bladder Cancer.* Blackwell, 1975.

Cross RJ & others: Treatment of advanced bladder cancer with adriamycin and 5-fluorouracil. *Br J Urol* 1976;**48**:609.

Cummings KB & others: Segmental resection in the management of bladder carcinoma. *J Urol* 1978;**119**:56.

Davies JM, Somerville SM, Wallace DM: Occupational bladder tumour cases identified during ten years' interviewing of patients. *Br J Urol* 1976;**48**:561.

DeWeerd JH & others: Cystectomy after radiotherapeutic ablation of invasive transitional cell cancer. *J Urol* 1977;**118**:260.

Doctor VM, Phadke AG, Sirat MV: Pheochromocytoma of the urinary bladder. *Br J Urol* 1972;**44**:351.

Durkee C, Benson R Jr: Bladder cancer following administration of cyclophosphamide. *Urology* 1980;**16**:145.

El-Bolkainy MN: Cytology of bladder carcinoma. *J Urol* 1980;**124**:20.

England HR & others: Evaluation of Helmstein's distention method for carcinoma of the bladder. *Br J Urol* 1973;**45**:593.

Fairchild WV & others: The incidence of bladder cancer after cyclophosphamide therapy. *J Urol* 1979;**122**:163.

Falor WH: Chromosomes in noninvasive papillary carcinoma of the bladder. *JAMA* 1971;**216**:791.

Farah RN, Cerny JC: Lymphangiography in staging patients with carcinoma of the bladder. *J Urol* 1978;**119**:40.

Faysal MH: Urethrectomy in men with transitional cell carcinoma of the bladder. *Urology* 1980;**16**:23.

Fish JC, Fayos JV: Carcinoma of the urinary bladder: Influence of dose and volume irradiated on survival. *Radiology* 1976;**118**:179.

Fitzpatrick JM & others: Long-term follow-up in patients with superficial bladder tumours treated with intravesical epodyl. *Br J Urol* 1979;**51**:545.

Freiha FS: Complications of cystectomy. *J Urol* 1980;**123**:168.

Friedell GH & others: The pathogenesis of bladder cancer. *Am J Pathol* 1977;**89**:431.

Ganguli SK: Urachal carcinoma. *Urology* 1979;**13**:306.

Gavrell GJ & others: Intravesical thio-tepa in the immediate postoperative period in patients with recurrent transitional cell carcinoma of the bladder. *J Urol* 1978;**120**:410.

Ghoneim MA & others: Cystectomy for carcinoma of the bilharzial bladder: 138 cases 5 years later. *Br J Urol* 1979;**51**:541.

Glashan RW, Brown PR: Initial experience with Helmstein's treatment by a hydrostatic pressure technique in carcinoma of the bladder. *Br J Surg* 1974;**61**:466.

Goldstein AG: Metastatic carcinoma to the bladder. *J Urol* 1967;**98**:209.

Grossman HB: Current therapy of bladder carcinoma. *J Urol* 1979;**121**:1.

Guinan P & others: Urinary carcinoembryonic-like antigen levels in patients with bladder carcinoma. *J Urol* 1974;**111**:350.

Hall RR & others: Methotrexate treatment for advanced bladder cancer. *Br J Urol* 1974;**46**:431.

Helmstein K: Treatment of bladder carcinoma by a hydrostatic technique: Report on 43 cases. *Br J Urol* 1972;44:434.

Heney NM & others: Positive urinary cytology in patients without evident tumor. *J Urol* 1977;117:223.

Hewitt CB & others: Intercavitary radiation in the treatment of bladder tumors. *J Urol* 1972;107:603.

Holmquist ND: Detection of urinary cancer with urinalysis sediment. *J Urol* 1980;123:188.

Howe GR, Burch JD, Miller AB: Artificial sweeteners and human bladder cancer. *Lancet* 1977;2:578.

Javadpour N: Tumor markers in urologic cancer. *Urology* 1980;16:127.

Jensen A, Nissen HM: Neurofibromatosis of the bladder. *Scand J Urol Nephrol* 1976;10:157.

Johnson DE & others: Squamous cell carcinoma of the bladder. *J Urol* 1976;115:542.

Jones WA & others: Primary adenocarcinoma of bladder. *Urology* 1980;15:119.

Kallet HA, Lapco L: Urine beta glucuronidase activity in urinary tract disease. *J Urol* 1967;97:352.

Kramer SA & others: Primary non-urachal adenocarcinoma of the bladder. *J Urol* 1979;121:278.

Lamb D: Correlation of chromosome counts with histological appearances and prognosis in transitional-cell carcinoma of bladder. *Br Med J* 1967;1:273.

Lamm DL & others: Bacillus Calmette-Guérin immunotherapy of superficial bladder cancer. *J Urol* 1980;124:38.

Lang EK & others: Transcatheter embolization of hypogastric branch arteries in the management of intractable bladder hemorrhage. *J Urol* 1979;121:30.

Lindenauer SM, Cerny JC, Morley GW: Ureterosigmoid conduit urinary diversion. *Surgery* 1974;75:705.

Loening SA & others: Adenocarcinoma of the urachus. *J Urol* 1978;119:68.

Makhyoun NA: Smoking and bladder cancer in Egypt. *Br J Cancer* 1974;30:577.

Merrell RW, Brown HE, Rose JF: Bladder carcinoma treated by partial cystectomy: A review of 54 cases. *J Urol* 1979;122:471.

Merrin C, Beckley S: Adjuvant chemotherapy for bladder cancer with doxorubicin hydrochloride and cyclophosphamide: Preliminary report. *J Urol* 1978; 119:62.

Miller LS: Bladder cancer superiority of preoperative irradiation and cystectomy in clinical stages B_2 and C. *Cancer* 1977;39:973.

Mishina T & others: Mitomycin C bladder instillation therapy for bladder tumors. *J Urol* 1975;114:217.

Mohiuddin M, Kramer S, Strong G: Adjuvant "sandwich" radiation therapy for bladder cancer. *Urology* 1980;15:115.

Morales A, Marriott J, Connolly JG: The value of mechanical cell harvesting in diagnosis and prognosis of bladder tumor recurrence. *J Urol* 1975;114:220.

Mullin EM, Glenn JF, Paulson DF: Lesions of bone and bladder cancer. *J Urol* 1975;113:45.

Nakazono M, Iwata S: A preliminary study of chemotherapeutic treatment for bladder tumors. *J Urol* 1978;119:598.

Narayana AS & others: Sarcoma of the bladder and prostate. *J Urol* 1978;119:72.

Nevin JE & others: Advanced carcinoma of bladder: Treatment using hypogastric artery infusion with 5-fluorouracil, either as a single agent or in combination with bleomycin or Adriamycin and supravoltage radiation. *J Urol* 1974;112:752.

Nielsen HV, Thybo E: Epodyl treatment of bladder tumours. *Scand J Urol Nephrol* 1979;13:59.

Ogata J, Migita N, Nakamura T: Treatment of carcinoma of the bladder by infusion of the anticancer agent (Mitomycin C) via the internal iliac artery. *J Urol* 1973;110:667.

Peeples WJ & others: Pathological findings after preoperative irradiation for carcinoma of the urinary bladder. *Radiology* 1979;132:451.

Peters PC, O'Neill MR: Cis-diamminedichloroplatinum as therapeutic agent in metastatic transitional cell carcinoma. *J Urol* 1980;123:375.

Prout GR Jr: Bladder carcinoma and a TNM system of classification. *J Urol* 1977;117:583.

Rathert P, Melchior H, Lutzeyer W: Phenacetin: A carcinogen for the urinary tract? *J Urol* 1975;113:653.

Redman JF, McGinnis TB, Bissada NK: Management of neoplasms in vesical diverticula. *Urology* 1976;7:492.

Reid EC, Oliver JA, Fishman IJ: Preoperative irradiation and cystectomy in 135 cases of bladder cancer. *Urology* 1976; 8:247.

Reuter HJ: Endoscopic cryosurgery of prostate and bladder tumors. *J Urol* 1972;107:389.

Richie JP & others: Squamous carcinoma of the bladder: Treatment by radical cystectomy. *J Urol* 1976;115:670.

Rife CC, Farrow GM, Utz DC: Urine cytology of transitional cell neoplasms. *Urol Clin North Am* 1979;6:599.

Rogers PCJ, Howards SS, Komp DM: Urogenital rhabdomyosarcoma in childhood. *J Urol* 1976;115:738.

Romas NA & others: A new method for determination of urinary tryptophan metabolites in bladder carcinoma. *J Urol* 1975;114:223.

Rose DP: Aspects of tryptophan metabolism in health and disease: A review. *J Clin Pathol* 1972;25:17.

Rose GA, Wallace DM: Observations on urinary chemiluminescence of normal smokers and non-smokers and of patients with bladder cancer. *Br J Urol* 1973;45:520.

Rous SN: Squamous cell carcinoma of the bladder. *J Urol* 1978;120:561.

Sadeghi A, Behmard S, Vesselinovitch SD: Opium: A potential urinary bladder carcinogen in man. *Cancer* 1979;43:2315.

Savir A, Meiraz D: Malignant mesodermal (mesenchymal) tumors of bladder. *Urology* 1980;16:307.

Schlegel JU & others: The role of ascorbic acid in the prevention of bladder tumor formation. *J Urol* 1970;103:155.

Schoborg TW, Sapolsky JL, Lewis CW Jr: Carcinoma of the bladder treated by segmental resection. *J Urol* 1979; 122:473.

Seidelmann FE & others: Accuracy of CT staging of bladder neoplasms using the gas-filled method: Report of 21 patients with surgical confirmation. *AJR* 1978;130:735.

Shrom SH & others: Formalin treatment for intractable hemorrhagic cystitis. *Cancer* 1976;38:1785.

Skinner DG, Crawford ED, Kaufman JJ: Complications of radical cystectomy for carcinoma of the bladder. *J Urol* 1980;123:640.

Skor AB, Warren MM, Mueller EO Jr: Endometriosis of bladder. *Urology* 1977;9:689.

Soloway MS: Rationale for intensive intravesical chemotherapy for superficial bladder cancer. *J Urol* 1980; 123:461.

Sufrin G & others: Secondary involvement of the bladder in malignant lymphoma. *J Urol* 1977;118:251.

Susan LP, Marsh RJ: Phenolization of bladder in treatment of massive intractable hematuria. *Urology* 1975;5:119.

Sutton AP & others: Correlation of cytology and cystoscopy. *Urology* 1979;**13**:83.

Symes MO & others: Transfer of adoptive immunity by intra-arterial injection of tumor-immune pig lymph node cells. *Urology* 1978;**12**:398.

Théôret G & others: Inverted papilloma of urinary tract. *Urology* 1980;**16**:149.

Timmons JW Jr & others: Embryonal rhabdomyosarcoma of the bladder and prostate in childhood. *J Urol* 1975;**113**:694.

Trott PA, Edwards L: Comparison of bladder washings and urine cytology in the diagnosis of bladder cancer. *J Urol* 1973;**110**:665.

Troup CW, Thatcher G, Hodgson NB: Infiltrative lesion of the bladder presenting as gross hematuria in child with leukemia: Case report. *J Urol* 1972;**107**:314.

Turner AG & others: The value of lymphangiography in the management of bladder cancer. *Br J Urol* 1976;**48**:579.

Veenema RJ, Romas NA, Fingerhut B: Chemotherapy for bladder cancer. *Urology* 1974;**3**:135.

Wajsman Z & others: Further study of fibrinogen degradation products in bladder cancer detection. *Urology* 1978;**12**:659.

Weitzner S: Leiomyosarcoma of urinary bladder in children. *Urology* 1978;**12**:450.

Whitmore WF Jr: Integrated irradiation and cystectomy for bladder cancer. *Br J Urol* 1980;**52**:1.

Winterberger AR & others: Eight years of experience with preoperative angiographic and lymphographic staging of bladder cancer. *J Urol* 1978;**119**:208.

Young AK, Hammond E, Middleton AW Jr: Prognostic value of cell surface antigens in low grade, non-invasive, transitional cell carcinoma of bladder. *J Urol* 1979;**122**:462.

Benign Prostatic Hyperplasia

Abrams PH: Investigation of postprostatectomy problems. *Urology* 1980;**15**:209.

Bates CP, Arnold EP, Griffiths DJ: The nature of the abnormality of bladder neck obstruction. *Br J Urol* 1975;**47**:651.

Bauer DL, Garrison RW, McRoberts JW: The health and cost implications of routine excretory urography before transurethral prostatectomy. *J Urol* 1980;**123**:386.

Chilton CP & others: A critical evaluation of the results of transurethral resection of the prostate. *Br J Urol* 1978;**50**:542.

Djurhuus JC, Hansen RI, Nerstrom B: Urethral pressure profile in prostatic surgery: A preliminary report. *Scand J Urol Nephrol* 1975;**9**:87.

Finkle JE, Finkle PS, Finkle AL: Encouraging preservation of sexual function postprostatectomy. *Urology* 1975;**6**:697.

Goland M: *Normal and Abnormal Growth of the Prostate.* Thomas, 1975.

Hutch JA, Rambo ON Jr: A study of the anatomy of the prostate, prostatic urethra and the urinary sphincter system. *J Urol* 1970;**104**:443.

Izumi AK, Edwards J Jr: Herpes zoster and neurogenic bladder dysfunction. *JAMA* 1973;**224**:1748.

Lytton B, Kupfer DJ, Traurig AR: The vesicorenal reflex. *Invest Urol* 1967;**4**:521.

Meiraz D & others: Treatment of benign prostatic hyperplasia with hydroxyprogesterone-caproate. *Urology* 1977;**9**:144.

Melzer M: The urecholine test. *J Urol* 1972;**108**:728.

Merrill DC, Markland C: Vesical dysfunction induced by the major tranquilizers. *J Urol* 1972;**107**:769.

Michaels MM, Brown HE, Favino CJ: Leiomyoma of prostate. *Urology* 1974;**3**:617.

Mitchell ME & others: Control of massive prostatic bleeding with angiographic techniques. *J Urol* 1976;**115**:692.

Möhring K, Pfitzmaier N, Panis-Hoffman C: Cryosurgery of the prostate and transurethral resection in poor risk patients. *Urol Int* 1975;**30**:414.

Nicoll GA: Suprapubic prostatectomy: A comparative analysis of 525 consecutive cases. *J Urol* 1974;**111**:213.

Paulson DF, Kane RD: Medrogestone: A prospective study in the pharmaceutical management of benign prostatic hyperplasia. *J Urol* 1975;**113**:811.

Perrin P & others: Forty years of transurethral prostatic resections. *J Urol* 1976;**116**:757.

Pinck BD, Corrigan MJ, Jasper P: Pre-prostatectomy excretory urography: Does it merit the expense? *J Urol* 1980;**123**:390.

Richmond DE: Effects of alcohol on the kidney and blood electrolytes. *NZ Med J* 1974;**79**:561.

Scott WW, Wade JC: Medical treatment of benign nodular prostatic hyperplasia with cyproterone acetate. *J Urol* 1969;**101**:81.

Turner-Warwick R & others: A urodynamic view of prostatic obstruction and the results of prostatectomy. *Br J Urol* 1973;**45**:631.

Watanabe H & others: Mass screening program for prostatic disease with transrectal ultrasonography. *J Urol* 1977;**117**:746.

Zinman L, Flint LD, Libertino JA: Techniques of open prostatectomy. *Geriatrics* (Sept) 1974;**29**:107.

Carcinoma of the Prostate

Bagshaw MA & others: External beam radiation therapy of primary carcinoma of the prostate. *Cancer* 1975;**36**(Suppl):723.

Barnes RW, Ninan CA: Carcinoma of the prostate: Biopsy and conservative therapy. *J Urol* 1972;**108**:897.

Bärring NE & others: Interstitial irradiation of the pituitary gland with a ^{90}Sr-^{90}Y applicator having adjustable active length. *Acta Radiol* [*Ther*] (*Stockh*) 1969;**8**:294.

Benson RC, Wear JB, Gill GM: Treatment of stage D hormone-resistant carcinoma of the prostate with estramustine phosphate. *J Urol* 1979;**121**:452.

Bhanalaph T, Varkarakis MJ, Murphy GP: Current status of bilateral adrenalectomy for advanced prostatic carcinoma. *Ann Surg* 1974;**179**:17.

Blackard CE, Byar DP, Jordan WP Jr: Orchiectomy for advanced prostatic carcinoma. *Urology* 1973;**1**:553.

Bonney WW, Chill LC, Culp DA: Computed tomography of the pelvis. *J Urol* 1978;**120**:457.

Boxer RJ, Kaufman JJ, Goodwin WE: Radical prostatectomy for carcinoma of the prostate: 1951–1976. A review of 329 patients. *J Urol* 1977;**117**:208.

Carlton CE Jr & others: Radiotherapy in the management of stage C carcinoma of the prostate. *J Urol* 1976;**116**:206.

Carson CC III & others: Radical prostatectomy after radiotherapy for prostatic cancer. *J Urol* 1980;**124**:237.

Catalona WJ, Kadmon D, Martin SA: Surgical considerations in the treatment of intraductal carcinoma of the prostate. *J Urol* 1978;**120**:259.

Catalona WJ, Scott WW: Carcinoma of the prostate: A review. *J Urol* 1978;**119**:1.

Chan RC, Gutierrez AE: Carcinoma of the prostate: Its treatment by a combination of radioactive goldgrain implant and external irradiation. *Cancer* 1976;37:2749.

Chiu CL, Weber DL: Prostatic carcinoma in young adults. *JAMA* 1974;230:724.

Chlebowski RT & others: Cyclophosphamide (NSC 26271) versus the combination of adriamycin (NSC 123127), 5-fluorouracil (NSC 19893), and cyclophosphamide in the treatment of metastatic prostatic cancer: A randomized trial. *Cancer* 1978;42:2546.

Chu TM & others: Comparative evaluation of serum acid phosphatase, urinary cholesterol, and androgens in diagnosis of prostatic cancer. *Urology* 1975;6:291.

Cooper JF, Foti A, Herschman H: Combined serum and bone marrow radioimmunoassays for prostatic acid phosphatase. *J Urol* 1979;122:498.

Correa RJ Jr & others: Total prostatectomy for stage B carcinoma of the prostate. *J Urol* 1977;117:328.

Dias SM, Barnett RN: Elevated bone marrow acid phosphatase: The problem of false positives. *J Urol* 1977;117:749.

Dowlen LW Jr, Block NL, Politano VA: Complications of transrectal biopsy examination of the prostate. *South Med J* 1974;67:1453.

Efremidis SC & others: Post-lymphangiography fine needle aspiration lymph node biopsy in staging carcinoma of the prostate: Preliminary report. *J Urol* 1979;122:495.

Epstein LM & others: Half and total body radiation for carcinoma of the prostate. *J Urol* 1979;122:330.

Epstein NA: Prostatic biopsy: A morphologic correlation of aspiration cytology with needle biopsy histology. *Cancer* 1976;38:2078.

Epstein NA, Fatti LP: Prostatic carcinoma: Some morphological features affecting prognosis. *Cancer* 1976;37:2455.

Farnsworth WE & others: Comparative performance of three radioimmunoassays for prostatic acid phosphatase. *Urology* 1980;16:165.

Finkle JE, Finkle PS, Finkle AL: Encouraging preservation of sexual function postprostatectomy. *Urology* 1975;6:697.

Firusian N, Mellin P, Schmidt CG: Results of [89]strontium therapy in patients with carcinoma of the prostate and incurable pain from bone metastases: A preliminary report. *J Urol* 1976;116:764.

Fletcher JW & others: Radioisotopic detection of osseous metastases: Evaluation of ^{99m}Tc polyphosphate and ^{99m}Tc pyrophosphate. *Arch Intern Med* 1975;135:553.

Fowler JE Jr & others: Complications of [125]iodine implantation and pelvic lymphadenectomy in the treatment of prostatic cancer. *J Urol* 1979;121:447.

Fry DE, Amin M, Harbrecht PJ: Rectal obstruction secondary to carcinoma of the prostate. *Ann Surg* 1979;189:488.

Gagnon JD, Moss WT, Stevens KR: Pre-estrogen breast irradiation for patients with carcinoma of the prostate: A critical review. *J Urol* 1979;121:182.

Gee WF, Cole JR: Symptomatic stage C carcinoma of prostate. *Urology* 1980;15:335.

Gill WB & others: Radical retropubic prostatectomy and retroperitoneal lymphadenectomy following radiotherapy conversion of stage C to stage B carcinoma of the prostate. *J Urol* 1974;111:656.

Golimbu M, Morales P: Extended pelvic lymphadenectomy. *Urology* 1980;15:298.

Greene LF, O'Dea MJ, Dockerty MB: Primary transitional cell carcinoma of the prostate. *J Urol* 1976;116:761.

Greene LF & others: Prostatic adenocarcinoma of ductal origin. *J Urol* 1979;121:303.

Guinan PD & others: Adjuvant immunotherapy with bacillus Calmette-Guérin in prostatic cancer. *Urology* 1979;14:561.

Guinan PD & others: Immunostaging in carcinoma of prostate. *Urology* 1976;7:178.

Gursel EO, Roberts MS, Veenema RJ: Cryotherapy in advanced prostatic cancer. *Urology* 1973;1:392.

Hackler RH, Texter JH Jr: Evaluation and management of early stages of carcinoma of prostate. *Urology* 1980;15:329.

Heshmat MY & others: Epidemiologic association between gonorrhea and prostatic carcinoma. *Urology* 1975;6:457.

Hilaris BS & others: Radiation therapy and pelvic node dissection in the management of cancer of the prostate. *Am J Roentgenol* 1974;121:832.

Hodges CV, Pearse HD, Stille L: Radical prostatectomy for carcinoma: 30-year experience and 15-year survivals. *J Urol* 1979;122:180.

Ihde DC & others: Effective treatment of hormonally-unresponsive metastatic carcinoma of the prostate with adriamycin and cyclophosphamide: Methods of documenting tumor response and progression. *Cancer* 1980;45:1300.

Javadpour N: Tumor markers in urologic cancer. *Urology* 1980;16:127.

Jazy FK & others: Radiation therapy as definitive treatment for localized carcinoma of prostate. *Urology* 1979;14:555.

Johnson CD, Costa D, Castro JE: Acid phosphatase after examination of the prostate. *Br J Urol* 1979;51:218.

Johnson DE, Chalbaud R, Ayala AG: Secondary tumors of the prostate. *J Urol* 1974;112:507.

Johnson DE, Haynie TP: Phosphorus-32 for intractable pain in carcinoma of prostate. *Urology* 1977;9:137.

Johnson DE & others: Clinical significance of serum acid phosphatase levels in advanced prostatic carcinoma. *Urology* 1976;8:123.

Kadohama N & others: Estramustine phosphate: Metabolic aspects related to its action in prostatic cancer. *J Urol* 1978;119:235.

Kane RD, Paulson DF: Radioisotope bone scanning characteristics of metastatic skeletal deposits of prostatic adenocarcinoma. *J Urol* 1977;117:618.

Keen CW: Half body radiotherapy in the management of metastatic carcinoma of the prostate. *J Urol* 1980;123:713.

Kilduff JT, Ansell JS: Mastocytosis: A benign mimic of malignant osteoblastic metastases. *J Urol* 1973;110:104.

Kirk D, Hinton CE, Shaldon C: Transitional cell carcinoma of the prostate. *Br J Urol* 1979;51:575.

Kjaer TB, Nilsson T, Madsen PO: Effect of estramustine phosphate on plasma testosterone during treatment of carcinoma of prostate. *Urology* 1975;5:802.

Klein LA: Prostatic carcinoma. *N Engl J Med* 1979;300:824.

Kohler FP & others: Needle aspiration of the prostate. *J Urol* 1977;118:1012.

Kontturi MJ, Sotaniemi EO: Prevention of body fluid retention by furosemide during estrogen therapy of prostatic cancer. *J Urol* 1975;114:251.

Kopelson G & others: Periurethral prostatic duct carcinoma: Clinical features and treatment results. *Cancer* 1978;**42:**2894.

Kurth KH & others: Follow-up of irradiated prostate carcinoma by aspiration biopsy. *J Urol* 1977;**117:**615.

Lamb D: Correlation of chromosome counts with histological appearance and prognosis in transitional cell carcinoma of the bladder. *Br Med J* 1967;**1:**273.

Lee CL & others: Value of new fluorescent immunoassay for human prostatic acid phosphatase in prostate cancer. *Urology* 1980;**15:**338.

Levin AB & others: Chemical hypophysectomy for relief of bone pain in carcinoma of the prostate. *J Urol* 1978;**119:**517.

Loening SA & others: A comparison between lymphangiography and pelvic node dissection in the staging of prostatic cancer. *J Urol* 1977;**117:**752.

Lytton B & others: Results of biopsy after early stage prostatic cancer treatment by implantation of ^{125}I seeds. *J Urol* 1979;**121:**306.

McCullough DL, Leadbetter WF: Radical pelvic surgery for locally extensive carcinoma of the prostate. *J Urol* 1972;**108:**939.

Melicow MM, Uson AC: A spectrum of malignant epithelial tumors of the prostate gland. *J Urol* 1976;**115:**696.

Merrin CE: Treatment of previously untreated (by hormonal manipulation) stage D adenocarcinoma of prostate with combined orchiectomy, estrogen, and cis diamminedichloroplatinum. *Urology* 1980;**15:**123.

Michigan S, Catalona WJ: Ureteral obstruction from prostatic carcinoma: Response to endocrine and radiation therapy. *J Urol* 1977;**118:**733.

Mittemeyer BT, Cox HD: Modified radical retropubic prostatectomy. *Urology* 1978;**12:**313.

Mittleman A, Shukla SK, Murphy GP: Extended therapy of stage D carcinoma of the prostate with oral estramustine phosphate. *J Urol* 1976;**115:**409.

Mooppan MMU & others: Urinary hydroxyproline excretion as a marker of osseous metastasis in carcinoma of the prostate. *J Urol* 1980;**123:**694.

Morales A, Connolly JG, Bruce AW: Androgen therapy in advanced carcinoma of the prostate. *Can Med Assoc J* 1971;**105:**71.

Mott LJM: Squamous cell carcinoma of the prostate: Report of 2 cases and review of the literature. *J Urol* 1979;**121:**833.

Mukamel E, Nissenkorn I, Servadio C: Early combined hormonal and chemotherapy for metastatic carcinoma of prostate. *Urology* 1980;**16:**257.

Nachtscheim DA & others: Latent residual tumor following external radiotherapy for prostate adenocarcinoma. *J Urol* 1978;**120:**312.

Newmark SR, Dluhy RG, Bennett AH: Ectopic adrenocorticotropin syndrome with prostatic carcinoma. *Urology* 1973;**2:**666.

Petersen DS & others: Biopsy and clinical course after cryosurgery for prostatic cancer. *J Urol* 1978;**120:**308.

Prout GR Jr & others: Endocrine changes after diethylstilbestrol therapy: Effects on prostatic neoplasm and pituitary-gonadal axis. *Urology* 1976;**7:**148.

Raskin P, McLain CJ, Medsger TA Jr: Hypocalcemia associated with metastatic bone disease. *Arch Intern Med* 1973;**132:**539.

Resnick M & others: Radiation therapy for carcinoma of the prostate: 5-year follow-up. *J Urol* 1977;**117:**241.

Rhind JR: Prostatic biopsy. *Br Med J* 1980;**281:**722.

Robinson MRG, Shearer RJ, Fergusson JD: Adrenal suppression in the treatment of carcinoma of the prostate. *Br J Urol* 1974;**46:**555.

Rullis I, Shaeffer JA, Lilien OM: Incidence of prostatic carcinoma in the elderly. *Urology* 1975;**6:**295.

Saglam S, Wilson CB, Seymour RJ: Indications for hypophysectomy in diabetic retinopathy and cancer of the breast and prostate. *Calif Med* (Feb) 1970;**113:**1.

Schellhammer PF, Ladaga LE, El-Mahdi A: Histological characteristics of prostatic biopsies after [125]iodine implantation. *J Urol* 1980;**123:**700.

Schellhammer PF, Milsten R, Bunts RC: Prostatic carcinoma with cutaneous metastases. *Br J Urol* 1973;**45:**169.

Schmidt JD & others: Comparison of procarbazine, imidazole-carboxamide and cyclophosphamide in relapsing patients with advanced carcinoma of the prostate. *J Urol* 1979;**121:**185.

Schroeder FH, Belt E: Carcinoma of the prostate: A study of 213 patients with stage C tumors treated by total perineal prostatectomy. *J Urol* 1975;**114:**257.

Smith RB, Walsh PC, Goodwin WE: Cyproterone acetate in the treatment of advanced carcinoma of the prostate. *J Urol* 1973;**110:**106.

Sogani PC, Ray B, Whitmore WF Jr: Advanced prostatic carcinoma: Flutamide therapy after conventional endocrine treatment. *Urology* 1975;**6:**164.

Soloway MS, Shippel RM, Ikard M: Cyclophosphamide, doxorubicin hydrochloride and 5-fluorouracil in advanced carcinoma of the prostate. *J Urol* 1979;**122:**637.

Susan LP, Roth RB, Adkins WC: Regression of prostatic cancer metastasis by high doses of diethylstilbestrol diphosphate. *Urology* 1976;**7:**598.

Tannenbaum M: Sarcomas of the prostate gland. *Urology* 1975;**5:**810.

Tannenbaum M: *Urologic Pathology: The Prostate.* Lea & Febiger, 1977.

Veenema RJ, Gursel EO, Lattimer KK: Radical retropubic prostatectomy for cancer: A 20-year experience. *J Urol* 1977;**117:**330.

Veenema RJ & others: Bone marrow acid phosphatase: Prognostic value in patients undergoing radical prostatectomy. *J Urol* 1977;**117:**81.

Von Buedingen RP: Prevention of infection during transrectal biopsy of the prostate through double-glove technique. *Urology* 1976;**7:**296.

West CR, Murphy GP: Pituitary ablation and disseminated prostatic carcinoma. *JAMA* 1973;**225:**253.

Whitmore WF Jr & others: Implantation of ^{125}I in prostatic cancer. *Surg Clin North Am* 1974;**54:**887.

Sarcoma of the Prostate

Lemmon WT Jr, Holland JM, Ketcham AS: Rhabdomyosarcoma of the prostate. *Surgery* 1966;**59:**736.

Siegel J: Sarcoma of the prostate: A report of four cases and a review of current therapy. *J Urol* 1963;**89:**78.

Smith BH, Dehner LP: Sarcoma of the prostate gland. *Am J Clin Pathol* 1972;**58:**43.

Tumors of the Seminal Vesicles

Damjanov I, Apić R: Cystadenoma of seminal vesicles. *J Urol* 1974;**111:**808.

Goldstein AG, Wilson ES: Carcinoma of the seminal vesicle: With particular reference to the angiographic appearances. *Br J Urol* 1973;**45:**211.

Hajdu SI, Faruque AA: Adenocarcinoma of the seminal vesicle. *J Urol* 1968;**99:**798.

Smith BA Jr, Webb EA, Price WE: Carcinoma of the seminal vesicle. *J Urol* 1967;**97**:743.

Tumors of the Urethra

Bracken RB & others: Primary carcinoma of the female urethra. *J Urol* 1976;**116**:188.

Nellans RE, Stein JJ: Pedunculated polyp of posterior urethra. *Urology* 1975;**6**:474.

Prempree T, Wizenberg MJ, Scott RM: Radiation treatment of primary carcinoma of the female urethra. *Cancer* 1978;**42**:1177.

Ray B, Canto AR, Whitmore WF Jr: Experience with primary carcinoma of the male urethra. *J Urol* 1977;**117**:591.

Roller MF, Naranjo CA: Benign urethral polyp of prostatic urethra. *Urology* 1975;**6**:34.

Selikowitz SM, Olsson CA: Metastatic urethral obstruction. *Radiology* 1973;**107**:906.

Stewart PA & others: Urethral tumours. *Br J Urol* 1978;**50**:583.

Tumors of the Spermatic Cord & Paratesticular Tumors

Beall ME, Young IS: Spermatic cord rhabdomyosarcoma: Case report. *J Urol* 1977;**117**:807.

Cromie WJ, Raney RB Jr, Duckett JW: Paratesticular rhabdomyosarcoma in children. *J Urol* 1979;**122**:80.

Curnes JT, Pratt CB, Hustu HO: Five-year survival after disseminated paratesticular rhabdomyosarcoma. *J Urol* 1977;**118**:662.

Hoekstra HJ & others: Embryonal rhabdomyosarcoma of spermatic cord. *Urology* 1980;**16**:360.

Olney LE & others: Intrascrotal rhabdomyosarcoma. *Urology* 1979;**14**:113.

Reyes CV: Spermatic cord liposarcoma. *Urology* 1980;**15**:416.

Sogani PC, Grabstald H, Whitmore WF Jr: Spermatic cord sarcoma in adults. *J Urol* 1978;**120**:301.

Wacksman J, Case G, Glenn JF: Extragenital gonadal neoplasia and metastatic testicular tumor. *Urology* 1975;**5**:221.

Tumors of the Testis

Abell MR, Holtz F: Testicular and paratesticular neoplasms in patients 60 years of age and older. *Cancer* 1968;**21**:852.

Atkin NB: High chromosome numbers of seminomata and malignant teratomata of the testis: A review of data on 103 tumors. *Br J Cancer* 1973;**28**:275.

Bailey TB & others: A new adjunct in testis tumor staging: Gallium-67 citrate. *J Urol* 1973;**110**:307.

Bloom HJG, Hendry WF: Possible role of hormones in treatment of metastatic testicular teratomas: Tumor regression with medroxyprogesterone acetate. *Br Med J* 1973;**3**:563.

Bracken RB, Johnson DE, Samuels ML: Alpha fetoprotein determinations in germ cell tumors of the testis. *Urology* 1975;**6**:382.

Brosman SA: Testicular tumors in prepubertal children. *Urology* 1979;**13**:581.

Buck AS & others: Supraclavicular node biopsy and malignant testicular tumors. *J Urol* 1972;**107**:619.

Burke EF, Gilbert E, Uehling DT: Adrenal rest tumors of the testes. *J Urol* 1973;**109**:649.

Burney BT, Klatte EC: Ultrasound and computed tomography of the abdomen in the staging and management of testicular carcinoma. *Radiology* 1979;**132**:415.

Caldamone AA & others: Leydig cell tumor of testis. *Urology* 1979;**14**:39.

Caldwell WL: Why retroperitoneal lymphadenectomy for testicular tumor? *J Urol* 1978;**119**:754.

Catalona WJ: Tumor markers in testicular cancer. *Urol Clin North Am* 1979;**6**:613.

Cochran JS: The seminoma decoy: Measurement of serum human chorionic gonadotropin in patients with seminoma. *J Urol* 1976;**116**:465.

Collins DH, Pugh RCB: The pathology of testicular tumors. *Br J Urol* 1964;**36**(Suppl):1.

Cricco RP, Kandzari SJ: Secondary testicular tumors. *J Urol* 1977;**118**:489.

Das S, Bochetto JR, Alpert LI: Primary retroperitoneal seminoma: Report of a case and review of the literature. *Cancer* 1975;**36**:595.

DeKernion JB, Lupu AN: The response of metastatic retroperitoneal seminoma to chemotherapy. *J Urol* 1977;**117**:736.

De Klerk DP, Nime F: Adenomatoid tumors (mesothelioma) of testicular and paratesticular tissue. *Urology* 1975;**6**:635.

Donohue JP, Einhorn LH, Perez JM: Improved management of nonseminomatous testis tumors. *Cancer* 1978;**42**:2903.

Donohue RE & others: Supraclavicular node biopsy in testicular tumors. *Urology* 1977;**9**:546.

Earle JD, Bagshaw MA, Kaplan HS: Supervoltage radiation therapy of the testicular tumors. *Am J Roentgenol* 1973;**117**:653.

Edson M: Testis cancer: The pendulum swings: Experience in 430 patients. *J Urol* 1979;**122**:763.

Einhorn LH, Donohue JP: Improved chemotherapy in disseminated testicular cancer. *J Urol* 1977;**117**:65.

Fowler JE Jr, McLeod DG, Stutzman RE: Critical appraisal of routine supraclavicular lymph node biopsy in staging of testicular tumors. *Urology* 1979;**14**:230.

Gabrilove JL & others: Feminizing interstitial cell tumor of the testis: Personal observations and a review of the literature. *Cancer* 1975;**35**:1184.

Gehring GG, Rodriguez FR, Woodhead DM: Malignant degeneration of cryptorchid testes following orchiopexy. *J Urol* 1974;**112**:354.

Grabstald H: Germinal tumors of the testes. *CA* 1975;**25**:82.

Gulley RM, Kowalski R, Neuhoff CF: Familial occurrence of testicular neoplasms: A case report. *J Urol* 1974;**112**:620.

Hendry WF & others: The role of surgery in the combined management of metastases from malignant teratomas of testis. *Br J Urol* 1980;**52**:38.

Henry SC, Walsh PC, Rotner MB: Choriocarcinoma of the testis. *J Urol* 1974;**112**:105.

Herr HW, Silber I, Martin DC: Management of inguinal lymph nodes in patients with testicular tumors following orchiopexy, inguinal or scrotal operations. *J Urol* 1973;**110**:223.

Hessl JM: Orchioblastoma or infantile embryonal carcinoma: Pediatric testis tumor. *Urology* 1975;**5**:265.

Hopkins TB & others: The management of testicular tumors in children. *J Urol* 1978;**120**:96.

Hutschenreiter G, Alken P, Schneider HM: The value of sonography and lymphography in the detection of retroperitoneal metastases in testicular tumors. *J Urol* 1979;**122**:766.

Ise T & others: Management of malignant testicular tumors

in children. *Cancer* 1976;**37**:1539.

Javadpour N: Immunologic features of genitourinary cancer. *Urology* 1973;**2**:103.

Javadpour N: Improved staging for testicular cancer using biologic tumor markers: A prospective study. *J Urol* 1980;**124**:58.

Javadpour N: The National Cancer Institute experience with testicular cancer. *J Urol* 1978;**120**:651.

Javadpour N, McIntire KR, Waldmann TA: Human chorionic gonadotropin (HCG) and alpha-fetoprotein (AFP) in sera and tumor cells of patients with testicular seminoma: A prospective study. *Cancer* 1978;**42**:2768.

Johnson DE, Bracken RB, Blight EM: Prognosis for pathologic stage 1 non-seminomatous germ cell tumors of the testes managed by retro-peritoneal lymphadenectomy. *J Urol* 1976;**116**:63.

Johnson DE & others: Metastases from testicular carcinoma: Study of 78 autopsied cases. *Urology* 1976;**8**:234.

Kademian M, Wirtanen G: Accuracy of bipedal lymphangiography in testicular tumors. *Urology* 1977;**9**:218.

Kenny GM & others: Radiation therapy: Testicular tumors. *J Urol* 1974;**112**:495.

Keough B & others: Urinary gonadotropins in management and prognosis of testicular tumor. *Urology* 1975;**5**:496.

Klippel KF & others: Interstitial cell tumor of testis: A delicate problem. *Urology* 1979;**14**:79.

Koppikar DD, Sirat MV: A malignant Sertoli cell tumour of the testis. *Br J Urol* 1973;**45**:213.

Lange PH & others: Is SP1 a marker for testicular cancer? *Urology* 1980;**15**:251.

Lee JKT & others: Computed tomography in the staging of testicular neoplasms. *Radiology* 1979;**130**:387.

LeFevre RE & others: Testis tumors: Review of 125 cases at the Cleveland Clinic. *Urology* 1975;**6**:588.

Lieskovsky G, Skinner DG: Significance of serum lactic dehydrogenase in stages B and C non-seminomatous testis tumors. *J Urol* 1980;**123**:516.

Lindsay CM, Glenn JF: Germinal malignancies of the testis: Experience, management and prognosis. *J Urol* 1976;**116**:59.

Lo TCM, Son YH: Radiation therapy for testicular tumors metastasizing to the lungs. *Am J Roentgenol* 1976;**126**:475.

Lynch DF Jr & others: Sandwich therapy in testis tumor: Current experience. *J Urol* 1978;**119**:612.

Mahon FB Jr & others: Malignant interstitial cell testicular tumor. *Cancer* 1973;**31**:1208.

Maier JG, Mittlemeyer B: Carcinoma of the testis. *Cancer* 1977;**39**:981.

Markland C, Kedia K, Fraley EE: Inadequate orchiectomy for patients with testicular tumors. *JAMA* 1973;**224**:1025.

Martini N & others: Primary mediastinal germ cell tumors. *Cancer* 1974;**33**:763.

Morin LJ, Loening S: Malignant androblastoma (Sertoli cell tumor) of the testis: A case report with a review of the literature. *J Urol* 1975;**114**:476.

Nicholson TC, Walsh PC, Rotner MB: Lymphadenectomy combined with preoperative and postoperative cobalt 60 teletherapy in the management of embryonal carcinoma and teratocarcinoma of the testis. *J Urol* 1974;**112**:109.

Oliver RTD & others: Chemotherapy of metastatic testicular tumours. *Br J Urol* 1980;**52**:34.

Osborn DE, Jeffrey PJ: Testicular tumor in children: Report of 4 cases. *Urology* 1976;**7**:433.

Paterson AHG, Peckham MJ, McCready VR: Value of gallium scanning in seminoma of the testis. *Br Med J* 1977;**1**:1118.

Peterson LJ, Catalona WJ, Koehler RE: Ultrasonic localization of a non-palpable testis tumor. *J Urol* 1979;**122**:843.

Price EB Jr: Epidermoid cysts of the testis: A clinical and pathologic analysis of 69 cases from the testicular tumor registry. *J Urol* 1969;**102**:708.

Ramsey EW, Bowman DM, Weinerman B: The management of disseminated testicular cancer. *Br J Urol* 1980;**52**:45.

Ray B, Hajdu SI, Whitmore WF Jr: Distribution of retroperitoneal lymph node metastases in testicular germinal tumors. *Cancer* 1974;**33**:340.

Reed RR, Barry JM, Hodges CV: Testis tumor metastatic to lung: Twenty-two-year survivor. *Urology* 1976;**7**:302.

Sadough N & others: Bilateral germ-cell tumors of testis. *Urology* 1973;**2**:452.

Safer ML & others: Lymphangiographic accuracy in the staging of testicular tumors. *Cancer* 1975;**35**:1603.

Sago AL & others: Accuracy of preoperative studies in staging nonseminomatous germ cell testicular tumors. *Urology* 1978;**12**:420.

Samuels ML, Holoye PY, Johnson DE: Bleomycin combination chemotherapy in the management of testicular neoplasia. *Cancer* 1975;**36**:318.

Schultz H & others: Serum alpha-fetoprotein and human chorionic gonadotropin as markers for the effect of postoperative radiation therapy and/or chemotherapy in testicular cancer. *Cancer* 1978;**42**:2182.

Selvaggi FP & others: Interstitial cell tumor of the testis in an adult: Two case reports. *J Urol* 1973;**109**:436.

Sickles EA, Belliveau RE, Wiernik PH: Primary mediastinal choriocarcinoma in the male. *Cancer* 1974;**33**:1196.

Silvert MA, Gray CP: Reticulum cell sarcoma of testes. *Urology* 1976;**8**:395.

Skinner DG, Scardino PT: Relevance of biochemical tumor markers and lymphadenectomy in management of nonseminomatous testis tumors: Current perspective. *J Urol* 1980;**123**:378.

Slawson RG: Radiation therapy for germinal tumors of the testes. *Cancer* 1978;**42**:2216.

Smith RB, DeKernion JB, Skinner DG: Management of advanced testicular seminoma. *J Urol* 1979;**121**:429.

Smithers DW, Wallace DM, Austin DE: Fertility after unilateral orchidectomy and radiotherapy for patients with malignant tumours of the testis. *Br Med J* 1973;**4**:77.

Staubitz WJ & others: Surgical management of testis tumor. *J Urol* 1974;**111**:205.

Stoffel TJ, Nesbit ME, Levitt SH: Extramedullary involvement of the testes in childhood leukemia. *Cancer* 1975;**35**:1203.

Storm PB & others: Evaluation of pedal lymphangiography in staging non-seminomatous testicular carcinoma. *J Urol* 1977;**118**:1000.

Stoter G & others: Combination chemotherapy with cis-diammine-dichloro-platinum, vinblastine, and bleomycin in advanced testicular non-seminoma. *Lancet* 1979;**1**:941.

Sussman EB & others: Malignant lymphoma of the testis: A clinicopathologic study of 37 cases. *J Urol* 1977;**118**:1004.

Talerman S & others: Primary carcinoid tumor of the testis: Case report, ultrastructure and review of the literature. *Cancer* 1978;**42**:2696.

Tsuji I & others: Testicular tumors in children. *J Urol* 1973;**110**:127.

Viprakasit D & others: Seminoma in children. *Urology* 1977;**9**:568.

Walsh PC: The etiology of gynecomastia in patients with malignant testicular tumors. *Urol Dig* (July) 1975;**14**:8.

Ware SM, Al-Askari S, Morales P: Testicular germ cell tumors: Prognostic factors. *Urology* 1980;**15**:348.

Warikoo S, Gonick P: Testicular lymphoma. *Urology* 1975;**5**:261.

Weitzman SA, Carey RW: High dose cyclophosphamide as an adjunct to radiotherapy for advanced seminoma. *J Urol* 1977;**117**:613.

Weitzner S, Aldridge JE Jr, Weems WL: Sertoli cell tumor of testis. *Urology* 1979;**13**:87.

Wettlaufer JN, Modarelli RO: Thoracotomy in re-staging germinal testis tumors. *J Urol* 1979;**122**:845.

Wilson JM, Woodhead DM: Prognostic and therapeutic implications of urinary gonadotropin levels in the management of testicular neoplasm. *J Urol* 1972;**108**:754.

Wittes RE & others: Chemotherapy of germ cell tumors of the testes. 1. Induction of remissions with vinblastine, actinomycin D, and bleomycin. *Cancer* 1976;**37**:637.

Ytredal DO, Bradfield JS: Seminoma of the testicle: Prophylactic mediastinal irradiation versus periaortic and pelvic irradiation alone. *Cancer* 1972;**30**:628.

Tumors of the Epididymis

Broth G, Bullock WK, Morrow J: Epididymal tumors: 1. Report of 15 new cases including review of literature. 2. Histochemical study of the so-called adenomatoid tumor. *J Urol* 1968;**100**:530.

Farrell MA, Donnelly BJ: Malignant smooth muscle tumors of the epididymis. *J Urol* 1980;**124**:151.

Fisher ER, Klieger H: Epididymal carcinoma (malignant adenomatoid tumor, mesonephric, mesodermal carcinoma of epididymis). *J Urol* 1966;**95**:568.

Spark RP: Leiomyoma of epididymis. *Arch Pathol* 1972;**93**:18.

Viprakasit D, Tannenbaum M, Smith AM: Adenomatoid tumor of male genital tract. *Urology* 1974;**4**:325.

Wachtel TL, Mehan DJ: Metastatic tumors of the epididymis. *J Urol* 1970;**103**:624.

Williams G, Banerjee R: Paratesticular tumours. *Br J Urol* 1969;**41**:332.

Tumors of the Penis

Alexander LL & others: Radium management of tumors of penis. *NY State J Med* 1971;**71**:1946.

Almgard LE, Edsmyr F: Radiotherapy in treatment of patients with carcinoma of the penis. *Scand J Urol Nephrol* 1973;**7**:1.

Bachrach P, Dahlen CP: Metastatic tumors to the penis. *Urology* 1973;**1**:359.

Cabanas RM: An approach for the treatment of penile carcinoma. *Cancer* 1977;**39**:456.

DeKernion JB & others: Carcinoma of the penis. *Cancer* 1973;**32**:1256.

Fraley EE, Hutchens HC: Radical ilio-inguinal node dissection: The skin bridge technique. *J Urol* 1972;**108**:279.

Gursel EO & others: Penile cancer: Clinicopathologic study of 64 cases. *Urology* 1973;**1**:569.

Hayes CW, Clark RM, Politano VA: Kaposi's sarcoma of the penis. *J Urol* 1971;**105**:525.

Hoppmann HJ, Fraley EE: Squamous cell carcinoma of the penis. *J Urol* 1978;**120**:393.

Johnson DE, Ayala AG: Primary melanoma of penis. *Urology* 1973;**2**:174.

Kelley CD & others: Radiation therapy of penile cancer. *Urology* 1974;**4**:570.

Konigsberg HA, Gray GF: Benign melanosis and malignant melanoma of penis and male urethra. *Urology* 1976;**7**:323.

Kuruvilla JT, Garlick FH, Mammen KE: Results of surgical treatment of carcinoma of the penis. *NZ J Surg* 1971;**41**:157.

Lue TF & others: Fibrosarcoma of penis. *Urology* 1980;**15**:498.

McAninch JW, Moore CA: Precancerous penile lesions in young men. *J Urol* 1970;**104**:287.

Pratt RM, Ross RTA: Leiomyosarcoma of the penis. *Br J Surg* 1969;**56**:870.

Salaverria JC & others: Conservative treatment of carcinoma of the penis. *Br J Urol* 1979;**51**:32.

Sklaroff RB, Yagoda A: Cis-diamminedichloride platinum II (DDP) in the treatment of penile carcinoma. *Cancer* 1979;**44**:1563.

Sklaroff RB, Yagoda A: Methotrexate in the treatment of penile cancer. *Cancer* 1980;**45**:214.

Wajsman Z & others: Surgical treatment of penile cancer: A follow-up report. *Cancer* 1977;**40**:1697.

Williams RD, Blackard CE: Chemotherapy for metastatic squamous-cell carcinoma of penis: Combination of vincristine and bleomycin. *Urology* 1974;**4**:69.

Tumors of the Scrotum

El-Domeiri AA, Paglia MA: Carcinoma of the scrotum, radical excision and repair using ox fascia: Case report. *J Urol* 1971;**106**:575.

Kickham CJE, Dufresne M: An assessment of carcinoma of the scrotum. *J Urol* 1967;**98**:108.

Ray B, Huvos AG, Whitmore WF Jr: Unusual malignant tumors of the scrotum: Review of 5 cases. *J Urol* 1972;**108**:760.

Ray B, Whitmore WF Jr: Experience with carcinoma of the scrotum. *J Urol* 1977;**117**:741.

Tucci P, Haralambides G: Carcinoma of the scrotum: Review of literature and presentation of 2 cases. *J Urol* 1963;**89**:585.

Retroperitoneal Extrarenal Tumors

Binder SC, Katz B, Sheridan B: Retroperitoneal liposarcoma. *Ann Surg* 1978;**187**:257.

Damascelli B & others: Angiography of retroperitoneal tumors: A review. *Am J Roentgenol* 1975;**124**:565.

Duncan RE, Evans AT: Diagnosis of primary retroperitoneal tumors. *J Urol* 1977;**117**:19.

Kinne DW & others: Treatment of primary and recurrent retroperitoneal liposarcoma: Twenty-five year experience at Memorial Hospital. *Cancer* 1973;**31**:53.

Polsky MS & others: Retrovesical liposarcoma. *Urology* 1974;**3**:226.

Sadoughi N & others: Retroperitoneal xanthogranuloma. *Urology* 1973;**1**:470.

Smith EH, Bartum RJ Jr: Ultrasonic evaluation of pararenal masses. *JAMA* 1975;**231**:51.

Stephens DH & others: Computed tomography of the

retroperitoneal space. *Radiol Clin North Am* 1977;**15**:377.

Stephens DH & others: Diagnosis and evaluation of retroperitoneal tumors by computed tomography. *AJR* 1977;**129**:395.

CHEMOTHERAPY OF UROLOGIC MALIGNANCIES

General References

Bagshawe KD (editor): *Medical Oncology.* Blackwell, 1975.

Bodansky O: *Biochemistry of Human Cancer.* Academic Press, 1975.

Brodsky I, Kahn SB, Moyer JH: *Cancer Chemotherapy: Basic and Clinical Applications.* (Twenty-Second Hahnemann Symposium.) Grune & Stratton, 1972.

Carter SK & others: *Chemotherapy of Cancer.* Wiley, 1977.

Cline MJ, Haskell CM III: *Cancer Chemotherapy,* 3rd ed. Saunders, 1980.

Criss WE, Ono T, Sabine JR (editors): *Control Mechanisms in Cancer.* Raven Press, 1976.

Dunphy JE: On caring for the patient with cancer. *N Engl J Med* 1976;**295**:313.

Haskell CM: *Cancer Treatment.* Saunders, 1980.

Holland JF, Frei E III (editors): *Cancer Medicine.* Lea & Febiger, 1973.

Horton J, Hill GJ II (editors): *Clinical Oncology.* Saunders, 1977.

Jones SE, Salmon SE (editors): *Adjuvant Therapy of Cancer II.* Grune & Stratton, 1977.

Krakoff IH: Cancer chemotherapeutic agents. *CA* 1977;**27**:130.

Krakoff IH (editor): Symposium on medical aspects of cancer. *Med Clin North Am* 1971;**55**:525. [Entire issue.]

Lawrence W Jr, Terz JJ (editors): *Cancer Management.* Grune & Stratton, 1977.

Moss WT, Brand WN, Battifora H: *Radiation Oncology.* Mosby, 1979.

Munster AM (editor): *Surgical Immunology.* Grune & Stratton, 1976.

Nealon TF Jr (editor): *Management of the Patient With Cancer,* 2nd ed. Saunders, 1976.

Noskell CM: *Cancer Treatment.* Saunders, 1980.

Salmon SE: Cancer chemotherapy. Chap 45, pp 477–513, in: *Review of Medical Pharmacology,* 7th ed. Lange, 1980.

Van Der Veer LD Jr, Balini JA: Chemotherapy of gastrointestinal malignancy. *Am J Gastroenterol* 1980;**74**:40.

Veidenheimer MC (editor): Symposium on the care and treatment of the cancer patient. *Surg Clin North Am* 1967;**47**:557.

Etiologic Factors in Tumor Formation

Allen DW & others: Viruses and human cancer. *N Engl J Med* 1972;**286**:70.

Bast RC Jr & others: BCG and cancer. (2 parts.) *N Engl J Med* 1974;**290**:1413.

Gallo RC: RNA-dependent DNA polymerase in viruses and cells. *Blood* 1972;**39**:117.

Gofman JW, Tamplin AR: Radiation, cancer, and environmental health. *Hosp Pract* (Oct) 1970;**5**:91.

Ryser HJP: Chemical carcinogenesis. *N Engl J Med* 1971;**285**:721.

Smith RT: Possibilities and problems of immunologic intervention in cancer. *N Engl J Med* 1972;**287**: 439.

Zamcheck N & others: Immunologic evaluation of human digestive tract cancer: Carcinoembryonic antigens. *N Engl J Med* 1972;**286**:83.

Solitary Metastasis

Adkins PC & others: Thoracotomy on the patient with previous malignancy: Metastasis or new primary? *J Thorac Cardiovasc Surg* 1968;**56**:361.

Rubin P, Green J: *Solitary Metastases.* Thomas, 1968.

Immunotherapy

Gutterman JU & others: Leukocyte interferon-induced tumor regression in human metastatic breast cancer, multiple myeloma, and malignant lymphoma. *Ann Intern Med* 1980;**93**:399.

Munster AM (editor): *Surgical Immunology.* Grune & Stratton, 1976.

Smith RT: Possibilities and problems of immunologic intervention in cancer. *N Engl J Med* 1972;**287**:437.

Terry WD (editor): Symposium on immunotherapy in malignant disease. *Med Clin North Am* 1976;**60**:387. [Entire issue.]

Terry WD, Windhorst D (editors): *Immunotherapy of Cancer: Present Status of Trials in Man.* Vol 6 of: *Progress in Cancer Research and Therapy.* Raven Press, 1978. [Entire volume.]

Chemotherapy

Alberts DS: In-vitro clonogenic assay for predicting response of ovarian cancer to chemotherapy. *Lancet* 1980;**2**:340.

Bergevin PR, Tormey DC, Blom J: Guide to the use of cancer chemotherapeutic agents. *Mod Treat* 1972;**9**:185.

Bruce WR & others: Comparison of the sensitivity of normal hematopoietic and transplanted lymphoma colony-forming cells to chemotherapeutic agents administered in vivo. *J Natl Cancer Inst* 1966;**37**:233.

The choice of therapy in the treatment of malignancy. *Med Lett Drugs Ther* 1973;**15**:9.

DeVita VT: Cell kinetics and the chemotherapy of cancer. *Cancer Chemother Rep* 1971;**2**:23.

DeVita VT, Schein PS: The use of drugs in combination for the treatment of cancer. *N Engl J Med* 1973;**288**: 998.

Livingston RB, Carter SK: *Single Agents in Cancer Chemotherapy.* Plenum Press, 1970.

Rall DP (chairman): Design of more selective antitumor agents. *Cancer Res* 1969;**29**:2384.

Salmon SE (editor): Clinical correlation of drug sensitivity. Pages 265–285 in: *Cloning of Human Tumor Stem-Cells.* Liss, 1980.

Salmon SE & others: Quantitation of differential sensitivities of human-tumor stem-cells to anti-cancer drugs. *N Engl J Med* 1978;**298**:1231.

Skipper HE & others: Implications of biochemical, cytokinetic, pharmacologic, and toxicologic relationships in the design of optimal therapeutic schedules. *Cancer Chemother Rep* 1970;**54**:431.

Valeriote FA, Edelstein MB: The role of cell kinetics in cancer chemotherapy. *Semin Oncol* 1977;**4**:217.

Surgical Adjuvant Chemotherapy

Bonnadonna G & others: Combination chemotherapy as an adjuvant treatment in operable breast cancer. *N Engl J Med* 1976;**294**:405.

Fisher B & others: L-Phenylalanine mustard (L-PAM) in the management of primary breast cancer: A report of early findings. *N Engl J Med* 1975;**292**:117.

Fisher F & others: Surgical adjuvant chemotherapy in cancer of the breast: Results of a decade of cooperative investigation. *Ann Surg* 1968;**168**:337.

Jones SE, Salmon SE (editors): *Adjuvant Therapy of Cancer II.* Grune & Stratton, 1977.

Li MC & others: Chemoprophylaxis for patients with colorectal cancer. *JAMA* 1976;**235**:2825.

Mackman S, Curreri AR, Ansfield FS: Second look operation for colon carcinoma after fluorouracil therapy. *Arch Surg* 1970;**100**:527.

Infusion & Perfusion Therapy

Ansfield FJ & others: Intrahepatic arterial infusion with 5-fluorouracil. *Cancer* 1971;**28**:1147.

Freckman HA: Chemotherapy for metastatic colorectal liver carcinoma by intra-aortic infusion. *Cancer* 1971;**28**:1152.

Krementz ET, Creech O Jr, Ryan RF: Evaluation of chemotherapy of cancer by regional perfusion. *Cancer* 1967;**20**:834.

Combination Chemotherapy

Carbone PP, Davis TE: Medical treatment for advanced breast cancer. *Semin Oncol* 1978;**5**:417.

DeVita VT Jr, Serpick AA, Carbone PP: Combination chemotherapy in the treatment of advanced Hodgkin's disease. *Ann Intern Med* 1970;**73**:881.

DeVita VT Jr & others: Combination versus single agent chemotherapy: A review of the basis for selection of drug treatment of cancer. *Cancer* 1975;**35**:98.

Einhorn LH, Donohue J: Cis-diamminedichloroplatinum, vinblastine, and bleomycin combination chemotherapy in disseminated testicular cancer. *Ann Intern Med* 1977;**87**:293.

Greenspan EM: Combination cytotoxic chemotherapy in advanced disseminated breast carcinoma. *Mt Sinai J Med NY* 1966;**33**:1.

Li MC & others: Effects of combined drug therapy on metastatic cancer of the testis. *JAMA* 1960;**174**:1291.

Luce JK: Chemotherapy for lymphomas: Current status. Page 295 in: *Leukemia-Lymphoma.* Year Book, 1969.

Evaluation & Management of Patients With an Unknown Primary Carcinoma

Brady LW & others: Unusual sites of metastases. *Semin Oncol* 1977;**4**:59.

Nystrom JS & others: Identifying the primary site in metastatic cancer of unknown origin: Inadequacy of roentgenographic procedures. *JAMA* 1979;**241**:381.

Nystrom JS & others: Metastatic and histologic presentations in unknown primary cancer. *Semin Oncol* 1977;**4**:53.

Paraneoplastic Syndromes

Hall TC (editor): Paraneoplastic syndromes. *Ann NY Acad Sci* 1974;**230**:1. [Entire issue.]

Waldenström JG: *Paraneoplasia.* Wiley, 1978.

Neuroblastoma

Evans AE & others: A review of 17 IV-S neuroblastoma patients at the Children's Hospital of Philadelphia. *Cancer* 1980;**45**:833.

Renal Cell Carcinoma

Bloom HJG: Proceedings: Hormone-induced and spontaneous regression of metastatic renal cancer. *Cancer* 1973;**32**:1066.

Klippel KF, Altwein JE: Palliative Therapiemoglichkeiten beim metastasierten Hypernephrom. *Dtsch Med Wochenschr* 1979;**104**:28.

Lokich JJ, Harrison JH: Renal cell carcinoma: Natural history and chemotherapeutic experience. *J Urol* 1975;**114**:371.

Talley RW: Proceedings: Chemotherapy of adenocarcinoma of the kidney. *Cancer* 1973;**32**:1062.

Wilms's Tumor

Green DM, Jaffe N: Wilms' tumor: Model of a curable pediatric malignant solid tumor. *Cancer Treat Rev* (Sept) 1978;**5**:143.

Transitional Cell Tumors

Carter SK: Chemotherapy and genitourinary oncology. 1. Bladder cancer. *Cancer Treat Rev* (June) 1978;**5**:85.

Hahn RG: Bladder cancer treatment considerations for metastatic disease. *Semin Oncol* 1979;**6**:236.

Koontz WW Jr: Intravesical chemotherapy and chemoprevention of superficial, low grade, low stage bladder carcinoma. *Semin Oncol* 1979;**6**:217.

Prostatic Carcinoma

Mittelman A, Shukla SK, Murphy GP: Extended therapy of stage D carcinoma of the prostate with oral estramustine phosphate. *J Urol* 1976;**115**:409.

Torti FM, Carter SK: The chemotherapy of prostatic adenocarcinoma. *Ann Intern Med* 1980;**92**:681.

Testicular Neoplasms

Cvitkovic E & others: Bleomycin (BLEO) infusion with cis-platinum diammine dichloride (CPDD) as secondary chemotherapy for germinal cell tumors. (Abstract.) *Proc Am Assoc Cancer Res* 1975;**16**:273.

Einhorn LH, Donohue JP: Combination chemotherapy in disseminated testicular cancer. *Semin Oncol* 1979;**6**:87.

Einhorn LH, Furnas BE, Powell N: Combination chemotherapy of disseminated testicular carcinoma with cis-platinum diammine dichloride (CPDD), vinblastine (VLB), and bleomycin (BLEO). (Abstract.) *Proc Am Assoc Cancer Res* 1976;**17**:240.

Friedman M, Purkayastha MC: Recurrent seminoma: The management of late metastasis, recurrence, or a second primary tumor. *Am J Roentgenol* 1960;**83**:25.

Golbey RB, Reynolds TF, Vugrin D: The chemotherapy of metastatic germ cell tumors. *Semin Oncol* 1979;**6**:82.

Javadpour N: The value of biologic markers in the diagnosis and treatment of testicular carcinoma. *Semin Oncol* 1979;**6**:37.

Samuels ML: Continuous intravenous bleomycin therapy with vinblastine in testicular and extragonadal germinal tumors. (Abstract.) *Proc Am Assoc Cancer Res* 1975;**16**:112.

Pain Palliation in Cancer

Brechner VL, Ferrer-Buchner T, Allen GD: Anesthetic

measures in management of pain associated with malignancy. *Semin Oncol* 1977;4:99.

Catalano RB: The medical approach to management of pain caused by cancer. *Semin Oncol* 1975;2:379.

Bacterial Sepsis in Cancer Patients

Alavi JB & others: Randomized clinical trial of granulocyte transfusions and infection in acute leukemia. *N Engl J Med* 1977;**296**:706.

Dilworth JA, Mandell GL: Infections in patients with cancer. *Semin Oncol* 1975;2:349.

Herzig R & others: Successful granulocyte transfusion therapy for gram-negative septicemia: A prospectively randomized controlled study. *N Engl J Med* 1977;**296**:701.

Ketchel SJ, Rodriguez V: Acute infections in cancer patients. *Semin Oncol* 1978;**5**:167.

Wiernik PH: The management of infection in the cancer patient. *JAMA* 1980;**244**:185.

Palliation of Local Complications of Neoplasia

Davenport D & others: Radiation therapy in the treatment of superior vena caval obstruction. *Cancer* 1978;42:2600.

Lambert CJ: Treatment of malignant pleural effusions by closed trocar tube drainage. *Ann Thorac Surg* 1967;3:1.

Lenhard RE Jr (editor): Clinical case records in chemotherapy: The management of hypercalcemia complicating cancer. *Cancer Chemother Rep* 1971;**55**:509.

Levitt SH & others: Treatment of malignant superior vena caval obstruction. *Cancer* 1969;**24**:447.

Millburn L, Hibbs GG, Hendrickson FR: Treatment of spinal cord compression from metastatic carcinoma. *Cancer* 1968;**21**:447.

Perez CA, Bradfield JS, Morgan HC: Management of pathologic fractures. *Cancer* 1972;**29**:684.

Rubin P & others: Superior vena caval syndrome: Slow low dose versus rapid high dose schedule. *Radiology* 1963;**81**:388.

Nutritional Support in Cancer Patients

Copeland EM, Dudrick SJ: Cancer: Nutritional concepts. *Semin Oncol* 1975;2:329.

DeWys WD: Nutritional care of the cancer patient. *JAMA* 1980;**244**:374.

Psychologic Support of the Patient With Neoplastic Disease

Dunphy JE: Caring for the patient with cancer. *N Engl J Med* 1976;**295**:313.

Home Care of the Patient With Advanced Cancer

Rosenbaum EH: Principles of home care for the patient with advanced cancer. *JAMA* 1980;**244**:1484.

19 | Neuropathic Bladder Disorders

Emil A. Tanagho, MD

Normal vesical action depends upon an intact nerve supply. If either the sensory or motor nerves are interrupted, bladder function will be impaired. The type of abnormality is determined by the site and degree of the injury.

Spinal cord trauma secondary to vertebral fracture is the most common cause of neuropathic bladder dysfunction. Certain diseases (eg, tabes dorsalis, diabetes mellitus, multiple sclerosis) and cord tumors or herniated intervertebral disks also may cause abnormalities in micturition. Some congenital anomalies (myelomeningocele, spina bifida, sacral agenesis) are also associated with neuropathic bladder dysfunction. Cordotomy to relieve intractable pain may affect perception of the need for voiding; abdominoperineal resection of the rectum disturbs the innervation of the bladder and may be followed by at least temporary difficulty with urination. Parkinsonism and herpes zoster may cause a transient neurologic deficit.

NORMAL VESICAL FUNCTION

ANATOMY

Detrusor Muscle

The bladder wall is composed of a mesh of muscle fibers running in every direction except near the internal orifice, where they form 3 definite layers: internal longitudinal, middle circular, and external longitudinal. The outer layer extends down the whole length of the female urethra and to the distal end of the prostate but is circularly and spirally oriented; thus, it functions as the major involuntary sphincter. The middle circular detrusor muscle layer ends at the internal orifice of the bladder; it is most developed anteriorly. The internal component remains longitudinal and reaches the distal end of the urethra in the female and the end of the prostate in the male. These converging fibers cause a thickening that forms the so-called vesical neck, but anatomically there is no true sphincter at this point.

External Sphincters

A voluntary external sphincter mechanism formed of striated muscle lies between the fascial layers of the urogenital diaphragm. In the female it is maximally condensed around the middle third of the urethra (external to the external layer of urethral musculature), while in the male these fibers surround the distal portion of the prostate and the membranous urethra. The striated muscles of the pelvic floor (eg, levator ani) act as an indirect sphincter and contribute to sphincteric function.

Diaphragm & Abdominal Muscles

These play only secondary roles in micturition. Their contraction may further increase intravesical pressure.

Nerve Supply

The sacral portion of the spinal cord, which contains the center controlling micturition (S2–4), is housed within the vertebral bodies T12 to L1. Fractures in the region of the twelfth thoracic and first lumbar vertebrae or below lead to flaccid neuropathic bladder because they destroy the voiding reflex center or the pelvic nerves (or both). Injuries above this level cause a spastic type of neuropathic bladder because the upper motor neurons are damaged.

A. Motor Innervation: (Fig 19–1.)

1. To the detrusor–These nerves are part of the parasympathetic nervous system. They arise from S2–4 and reach the bladder wall through the pelvic nerves. The trigonal portion of the bladder, because of its different embryologic origin, is innervated by motor fibers from the thoracolumbar outflow (T11 to L2) of the sympathetic nervous system. In dogs, intravenously administered epinephrine causes contraction of the trigone, the function of which is 2-fold. First, its tone pulls downward upon the ureterovesical junctions, thus combating possible reflux; second, its contracture helps open the bladder neck just before the detrusor is activated. Interruption of the sympathetic pathways may denervate the genital ducts and cause loss of the power of emission.

2. To the external sphincter–The motor nerve

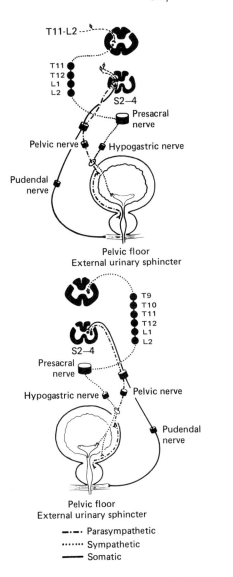

T11-L2

T11
T12
L1
L2

S2—4

Presacral
nerve

Pelvic nerve   Hypogastric nerve

Pudendal
nerve

Pelvic floor
External urinary sphincter

T9
T10
T11
T12
L1
L2

S2—4

Presacral
nerve

Hypogastric nerve   Pelvic nerve

Pudendal
nerve

Pelvic floor
External urinary sphincter

—·—· Parasympathetic
········· Sympathetic
———— Somatic

Figure 19–1. *Top:* Motor innervation of the bladder. *Bottom:* Sensory innervation of the bladder.

supply to the external sphincter and perineal muscles is somatic (voluntary) and reaches those structures through the pudendal nerves. Motor nerves also arise from S2–4. The motor fibers descend in the pyramidal tracts.

B. Sensory Innervation: Sensation from the urethra and bladder is returned to the central nervous system by fibers that travel with the sympathetic (T9 to L2), parasympathetic, and somatic (S2–4) nerves. The parasympathetic nerves carry the sensory stretch receptors. Sensations of touch, temperature, and pain are carried by sympathetic fibers. The sensory fibers ascend in the lateral spinothalamic tracts and fasciculus gracilis.

C. Voiding (Spinal) Reflex: The afferent and efferent fibers of the sacral portion of the cord (S2–4) form a simple spinal reflex arc that controls

vesical function. Its activity is under the voluntary control of the cerebral cortex through the mediation of suprasegmental connections.

PHYSIOLOGY

Neurophysiology

Urinary control is largely centered in the simple reflex reaction between the bladder and the sacral cord, which in turn is under the control of higher midbrain and cortical centers. The normal bladder is able to distend gradually to normal capacity (400 mL) without appreciable increase in intravesical pressure. At this point, sensations of fullness are transmitted to the sacral cord where, if voluntary (cerebral) control is lacking (as in infants), discharges through the motor side of the reflex arc cause powerful, sustained detrusor contraction and spontaneous involuntary urination. As myelinization and training of the young child progress, cerebral inhibitory functions suppress the sacral reflex and the individual voids when it is convenient to do so.

The urinary bladder is the only part of the urinary tract that is totally dependent on intact innervation to perform its function. It is made up of 3 main units that serve its functions as reservoir, as sphincteric mechanism, and as ureterovesical junction to prevent backflow of urine.

Reservoir. The principal features of the bladder as reservoir are (1) a normal capacity of 400–500 mL; (2) a sensation of distention noted when this capacity is reached; (3) the ability to accommodate various volumes within the vesical lumen without a change of intraluminal pressure; (4) the ability to contract and to sustain the contraction until completely empty; and (5) voluntary initiation or inhibition of contraction (despite the involuntary nature of the organ).

Sphincteric mechanism. In both males and females there are 2 sphincteric elements: one is the involuntary smooth muscle sphincter, commonly called the internal sphincter, which is a direct continuation of the detrusor musculature into the urethra. The other is a voluntary skeletal muscle sphincter derived from the musculature of the genitourinary diaphragm. (This voluntary sphincter is wrapped around the mid urethral segment in the female and the membranous urethra in the male.) The 2 mechanisms maintain control and function in concert with detrusor activity. The smooth sphincter, being a direct continuation of the detrusor muscle, has the same nerve supply and thus shares its various phases of activity. In the relaxed filling state of the bladder, this element is occlusive to the bladder outlet and generates a sustained closing pressure around the urethral tube to maintain continence. With bladder activity and voiding, the smooth sphincter shares in the contraction, and during this phase the sphincter opens up, permitting free urinary flow. The voluntary sphincter maintains a constant tonus that adds to the efficiency of the sphincteric element. The tonus can be augmented or increased whenever needed and decreased or abolished during voiding—thus appreciably lowering urethral resistance to again permit free flow of urine. Efficiency of the combined sphincteric units is indirectly increased by the integrity of the entire pelvic floor. Weakness of the pelvic floor might lessen closure efficiency of these 2 otherwise normal units.

Ureterovesical junction. The function of the ureterovesical junction is to prevent backflow of urine from the bladder to the upper urinary tract (reflux). A properly functioning ureterovesical junction will permit urine to flow freely from the ureter to the bladder but never in the reverse direction. The anatomic structure of the ureterovesical junction and the morphology of its musculature constitute an adaptable mechanism that will prevent reflux of urine from the bladder to the ureter regardless of bladder distention or detrusor activity. (See Chapter 11.) Resistance to the flow of urine is minimal in the absence of trigonal stretch (associated with bladder distention or residual urine) or trigonal hypertrophy. The combination of trigonal hypertrophy and stretch due to residual urine can significantly obstruct the flow of urine from the lower end of the ureter toward the bladder.

Vesical Physiology

Micturition is completely under voluntary control. Detrusor response to stretch can be inhibited, permitting the bladder to accommodate larger volumes, or detrusor contraction can be initiated whether at full capacity or not. Detrusor contraction is usually preceded by relaxation of the pelvic floor musculature, including the voluntary sphincter around the urethra. This appreciably reduces the efficiency of urethral closure and also leads to a drop in the vesical base, further minimizing urethral resistance.

Next, the trigone contracts, exerting increased pull on the ureterovesical junction and thus increasing ureteral occlusion. This prevents vesicoureteral reflux during the high intravesical pressure that develops with voiding. It also pulls the posterior portion of the bladder neck open, leading to its funneling. Only then do the detrusor fibers of the bladder contract, and intravesical pressure begins to rise. Because the vesical longitudinal muscles insert into the urethra, their contraction along with that of the trigone tends to pull the internal vesical meatus open, further contributing to funneling of the vesical outlet. The increased hydrostatic pressure (30–40 cm of water) exerted by the detrusor is directed down the urethra. Reciprocally, the urethral counterpressure drops, and voiding ensues. The detrusor maintains its contraction until complete emptying has occurred.

When the bladder is empty, the detrusor mus-cle relaxes, and the bladder neck is allowed to close; urethral and perineal muscle tone then return to normal. Finally, the trigone resumes its normal tone. The urinary stream can also be interrupted by voluntary contraction of the external sphincter. Detrusor muscle spasm then relaxes by reciprocal reflex action, and the bladder neck closes.

URODYNAMIC STUDIES

Cystometry—the urodynamic evaluation of the reservoir function of the lower urinary tract—has contributed much to our understanding of normal vesical function and aberrations resulting from interruption of nerve connections and leading to neuropathic bladder disorders. A normal cystometrogram is shown in Fig 19–2, with a water cystometer shown at the left. Gas cystometers are used today instead of water cystometers, but they are less informative and less reliable. Cystometrographic studies provide data about the presence of residual urine, total bladder capacity, the resting pressure within the bladder during the filling phase, the presence of uncontrolled, uninhibited detrusor contractions, the ability of the bladder to contract and to sustain a contraction, the sensory aspect of the perception of fullness and the desire to urinate, and the ability to inhibit detrusor activity voluntarily whenever it is perceived. Normal bladder capacity is about 400–500 mL. Normally, there is no residual urine, and resting bladder filling pressure is usually under 10–15 cm of water. At maximum capacity there is a slight rise in pressure, perceived as fullness, followed by detrusor contraction, which, if sustained, results in voiding with complete emptying. Voiding pressure is usually 20–40 cm of water.

Uroflowmetry. If detrusor contraction is properly harmonized with sphincteric activity, the result will be lowering of the outlet resistance and adequate flow rate. Normally, males deliver 20–25 mL/s and females between 25–30 mL/s. Any flow rate below 15 mL/s is highly suggestive of obstruction or dysfunction. A flow rate under 10 mL/s is definitely pathologic.

Urethral pressure profiles measure and record sphincteric activity by determining the efficiency of the sphincteric elements around the urethral canal. The anatomic distribution of these elements can distinguish the activity of the smooth and voluntary components, their anatomic and functional lengths along the sphincteric segment, and their magnitude. Pressure profiles detect any weakness or hyperactivity in either element (see Chapter 20).

The normal bladder can usually perceive the first injection of fluid through a catheter. The desire to void is felt initially when 100–200 mL of fluid have been instilled. As fluid is introduced, intravesical pressure remains fairly constant at 8–10 cm of

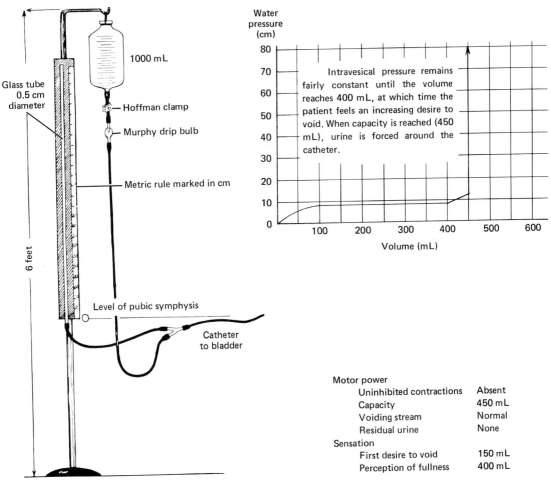

Motor power	
Uninhibited contractions	Absent
Capacity	450 mL
Voiding stream	Normal
Residual urine	None
Sensation	
First desire to void	150 mL
Perception of fullness	400 mL

Figure 19–2. Cystometry. *Left:* A simple water manometer. *Right:* Normal cystometrogram. As fluid is slowly introduced into the bladder, the detrusor gradually relaxes to accept increasing amounts of fluid without change in intravesical pressure. At a volume of 400 mL, the patient felt an urge to void. Shortly thereafter, an involuntary contraction of the detrusor occurred that was reflected in a sharp increase in intravesical pressure.

water. There are no sharp rises of pressure (uninhibited contractions) until 350–450 mL of fluid have been introduced, at which point a definite sensation of fullness (capacity) and distress is noted and the pressure increases sharply to 40–100 cm of water. This results in involuntary voiding around the catheter. If the catheter is withdrawn, the patient voids with a forceful, continuous stream. If bladder function is normal, there is no residual urine. The patient should be cautioned against voluntarily straining to void, because if straining occurs, the resulting intravesical pressure recorded by the manometer will be a summation of true intravesical pressure and intra-abdominal pressure.

More sophisticated methods have been developed to study intravesical pressure and urethral resistance during the resting phase and while voiding, but these methods are not generally available for clinical use. Measurement of intravesical pressure and urethral resistance yields more information of a dynamic nature. Urinary continence requires that urethral pressure exceed intravesical pressure. In the normal person, during voiding, intravesical pressure rises to 30–40 cm of water, exceeding urethral resistance, which drops reciprocally. If urethral resistance is high (eg, in benign prostatic hyperplasia or spasm of the striated periurethral muscles), voiding will require an abnormally high intravesical pressure. Should urethral resistance be low, even normal intravesical pressure or increased intra-abdominal pressure may be associated with incontinence.

ABNORMAL VESICAL FUNCTION

Neuropathic bladder disorders can be classified according to type of neurologic deficit (with common causes) as follows:

(1) Purely sensory (diabetes mellitus, tabes dorsalis).

(2) Purely motor (amyotrophic lateral sclerosis, occasionally parkinsonism).

(3) Mixed motor and sensory:

    (a) Acquired (tumors, trauma).

    (b) Congenital.

The main anatomic subdivisions are (1) upper motor neuron lesions (spastic bladder) and (2) lower motor neuron lesions (flaccid bladder).

The following descriptions assume that the upper and lower motor neuron lesions are complete, but it must be realized that many incomplete lesions occur. Mixed lesions are not uncommon.

The bladder and the lower extremities respond similarly to injury or disease, since their innervation arises from essentially the same segments of the spinal cord. Thus, an upper motor neuron (suprasegmental) lesion causes spasticity in both; a lower motor neuron (segmental or infrasegmental) lesion causes flaccidity. Any lesion that damages the sacral cord on either side of the arc (sensory or motor) causes flaccidity.

SPASTIC (REFLEX OR AUTOMATIC) NEUROPATHIC BLADDER
(Caused by Upper Motor Neuron Lesion)

This type of bladder disorder is caused by any lesion of the cord above the voiding reflex arc. Trauma is the most common cause, but the disorder may also be produced by tumor or multiple sclerosis. The lesion usually affects both the suprasegmental motor and sensory fibers (Fig 19–3). The sacral reflex arc remains intact, but the loss of conscious sensation and cerebral motor control lead to severe aberrations of function. This is potentially the most serious type of injury because the cord below the lesion is hyperirritable rather than "dead" and affects the bladder most adversely. For this reason, the incidence of renal damage is relatively high in this group. Injury to the pyramidal tracts deprives the bladder of cortical inhibition; uninhibited contractions then occur with filling, and vesical capacity is diminished. Voiding is interrupted, involuntary, and incomplete. Hypertrophy of the detrusor develops, often leading to vesicoureteral reflux. Trigonal hypertrophy may cause functional obstruction of the ureterovesical junctions. Dilatation of the bladder neck occurs. The external sphincter and perineal muscles become spastic (upper motor neuron lesion) and obstructive. This causes increased resistance to the flow of urine and results in an impaired stream and residual urine. If complete, the sensory lesion deprives the patient of the perception of vesical fullness.

In summary, the spastic neuropathic bladder is typified by (1) reduced capacity, (2) involuntary detrusor contractions, (3) high intravesical voiding pressure, (4) marked hypertrophy of the bladder

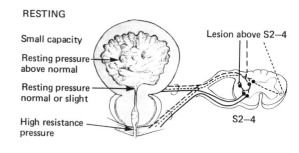

RESTING

Small capacity

Resting pressure above normal

Resting pressure normal or slight

High resistance pressure

Lesion above S2–4

S2–4

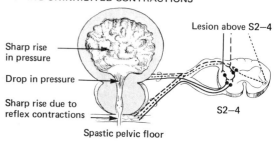

DURING UNINHIBITED CONTRACTIONS

Sharp rise in pressure

Drop in pressure

Sharp rise due to reflex contractions

Spastic pelvic floor

Lesion above S2–4

S2–4

Figure 19–3. Spastic (upper motor neuron) neuropathic bladder.

wall (trabeculation), and (5) spasm of the striated urinary sphincters (Fig 19–3).

UNINHIBITED NEUROPATHIC BLADDER
(Mild Spastic Neuropathic Bladder)

The uninhibited neuropathic bladder, a mild form of the spastic neuropathic bladder, may develop following cerebrovascular accident or arteriosclerotic degeneration in the spinal cord. A prolapsed intervertebral disk may cause this disorder. It may also occur as the first sign of multiple sclerosis or be associated with Parkinson's disease. A similar clinical picture is seen with the spastic type of psychosomatic bladder reaction (see Chapter 36). The lesion is centered either in the inhibitory centers of the cortex or in the pyramidal tracts (upper neuron). Minor lesions due to myelomeningocele or spina bifida may occasionally affect the suprasegmental motor fibers, in which case the cortical inhibition to the vesical stretch reflex is lost, and voiding may become precipitate and involuntary. Because all other mechanisms, including the sacral reflex arc, are normal, the sensation of fullness is retained, the stream is free, and there is no residual urine. Capacity is, however, diminished. The cystometrogram is diagrammed in Fig 19–5.

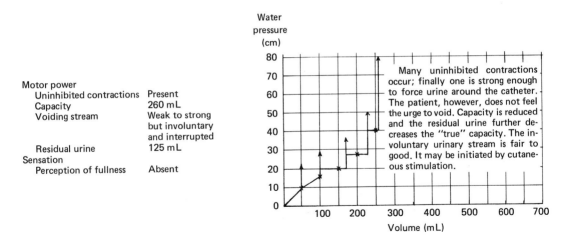

Motor power
    Uninhibited contractions Present
    Capacity 260 mL
    Voiding stream Weak to strong
        but involuntary
        and interrupted
    Residual urine 125 mL
Sensation
    Perception of fullness Absent

Many uninhibited contractions occur; finally one is strong enough to force urine around the catheter. The patient, however, does not feel the urge to void. Capacity is reduced and the residual urine further decreases the "true" capacity. The involuntary urinary stream is fair to good. It may be initiated by cutaneous stimulation.

Figure 19–4. Cystometric study of a typical case of complete spastic neuropathic bladder following recovery from spinal shock.

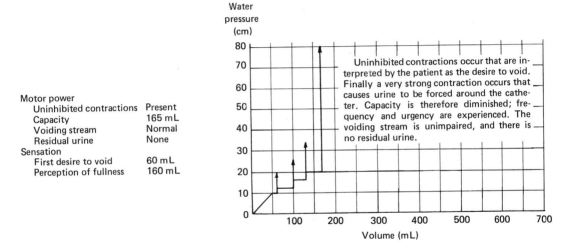

Motor power
    Uninhibited contractions Present
    Capacity 165 mL
    Voiding stream Normal
    Residual urine None
Sensation
    First desire to void 60 mL
    Perception of fullness 160 mL

Uninhibited contractions occur that are interpreted by the patient as the desire to void. Finally a very strong contraction occurs that causes urine to be forced around the catheter. Capacity is therefore diminished; frequency and urgency are experienced. The voiding stream is unimpaired, and there is no residual urine.

Figure 19–5. Cystometric study of a typical case of uninhibited neuropathic bladder.

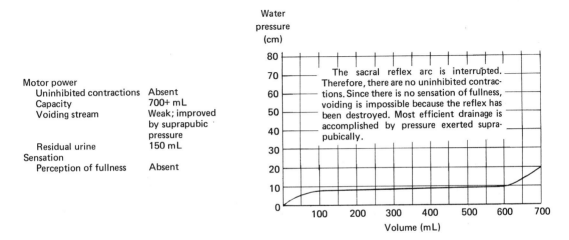

Motor power
    Uninhibited contractions Absent
    Capacity 700+ mL
    Voiding stream Weak; improved
        by suprapubic
        pressure
    Residual urine 150 mL
Sensation
    Perception of fullness Absent

The sacral reflex arc is interrupted. Therefore, there are no uninhibited contractions. Since there is no sensation of fullness, voiding is impossible because the reflex has been destroyed. Most efficient drainage is accomplished by pressure exerted suprapubically.

Figure 19–6. Cystometric study of a typical case of flaccid neuropathic bladder following recovery from spinal shock.

FLACCID (ATONIC, NONREFLEX, OR AUTONOMOUS) NEUROPATHIC BLADDER
(Caused by Lower Motor Neuron Lesion)

The most common cause of flaccid neuropathic bladder is trauma, although tumors, herniated intervertebral disks, tabes dorsalis, poliomyelitis, and certain congenital defects, including meningomyelocele, can affect the same centers. Tranquilizers may cause vesical atonicity, as do parasympathetic blocking agents. Vesical dysfunction arises when there is injury to the center of micturition in the cord (S2–4), cauda equina, or sacral roots or nerves (Fig 19–7), thereby interrupting the sacral reflex arc. Loss of the perception of fullness permits overstretching of the detrusor and atony of the muscle, and this further contributes to weak and inefficient detrusor contraction. Thus, capacity is increased and the amount of residual urine is often large. Mild to moderate trabeculation (hypertrophy) of the bladder wall develops, accompanied by dilatation of the vesical outlet. External sphincter and perineal muscle tone is usually diminished, as is typical of striated muscle when a lower motor neuron lesion is present. Voluntary urination does not occur, but fairly efficient emptying can be accomplished by increased intraabdominal and suprapubic (manual) pressure. The vesical (motor) paralysis that occurs occasionally in poliomyelitis usually clears quickly and spontaneously.

Myelomeningocele and spina bifida are associated with mild to severe vesical dysfunction, usually of the flaccid type, because the lesion affects the cauda equina and at times the sacral portion of the cord. Incontinence is the major symptom because of atony of the pelvic floor (external sphincter). Occasionally, in conjunction with somatic (external sphincter) flaccidity, there may be visceral (bladder) spasticity as well; this is a difficult combination to treat.

In summary, flaccid neuropathic bladder is typified by (1) large capacity, (2) no involuntary detrusor contractions, (3) low intravesical pressure, and (4) usually mild, but at times marked, trabeculation (hypertrophy) of the bladder wall and decreased tone of the external sphincter.

RECOVERY OF VESICAL FUNCTION AFTER SPINAL CORD INJURY

Initial Phase

A. Spinal Shock: Immediately following a severe injury to the spinal cord or cauda equina, no matter at what level, there is complete anesthesia and flaccid paralysis below the level of the lesion. Because the bladder is innervated from the lowest part of the spinal cord, it is similarly affected. Perception of fullness and detrusor contraction are absent. The bladder gradually fills until overflow incontinence occurs.

The cystometrogram (Fig 19–8) shows a very large bladder capacity, no involuntary detrusor contractions, and low intravesical pressure.

B. Recovery From Spinal Shock: Spinal shock may last for a period of a few weeks to 6 months or more (usually 2–3 months). The early clues to the return of reflex activity (upper neuron lesion) include movement of a toe, spontaneous spasm in a leg, return of sensation in some area, and spontaneous voiding around the indwelling catheter.

Cystometric studies (Fig 19–9) may demonstrate a large bladder capacity (but smaller than during the shock period), a few weak involuntary contractions of the detrusor, and the beginning of return of intravesical pressure (tone).

If the injury involves the cord above the sacral arc, anal sphincter tone and the bulbocavernosus reflex will return, usually much earlier than detrusor response.

The ice water test should be tried periodically. Ninety mL of saline solution at 3.3 C (38 F) should be introduced forcefully into the bladder through a straight catheter. If the catheter is immediately ejected, the reaction is "positive." If ejection does not occur, the catheter should be removed quickly; if the fluid is ejected within 1 minute, the test is also considered to be "positive." "Negative" responses occur during the stage of spinal shock. The "positive" reaction is one of the first to return with recovery if the sacral reflex arc is intact (upper neuron lesion). This test is therefore of value in differentiating an upper from a lower motor neuron lesion early in the recovery phase.

Final Phase

The condition of the bladder after spinal shock is over depends upon the level and extent of the lesion in the spinal cord.

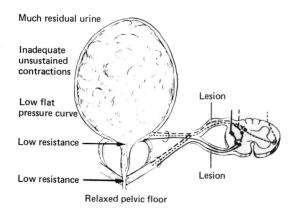

Much residual urine

Inadequate unsustained contractions

Low flat pressure curve

Low resistance

Low resistance

Lesion

Lesion

Relaxed pelvic floor

Figure 19–7. Flaccid (lower motor neuron) neuropathic bladder.

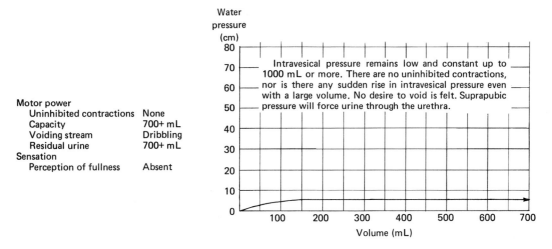

Motor power
Uninhibited contractions None
Capacity 700+ mL
Voiding stream Dribbling
Residual urine 700+ mL
Sensation
Perception of fullness Absent

Intravesical pressure remains low and constant up to 1000 mL or more. There are no uninhibited contractions, nor is there any sudden rise in intravesical pressure even with a large volume. No desire to void is felt. Suprapubic pressure will force urine through the urethra.

Figure 19–8. Stage of spinal shock. Cystometrogram showing flaccidity and lack of response of the bladder during the first few weeks or months after injury.

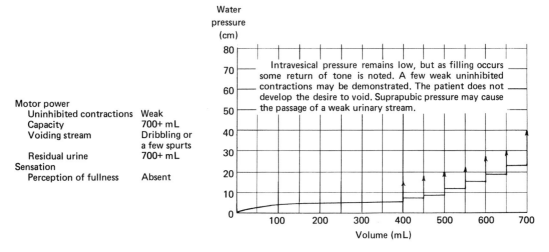

Motor power
Uninhibited contractions Weak
Capacity 700+ mL
Voiding stream Dribbling or a few spurts
Residual urine 700+ mL
Sensation
Perception of fullness Absent

Intravesical pressure remains low, but as filling occurs some return of tone is noted. A few weak uninhibited contractions may be demonstrated. The patient does not develop the desire to void. Suprapubic pressure may cause the passage of a weak urinary stream.

Figure 19–9. Stage of recovery of vesical function after severe injury to the spinal cord or cauda equina. Cystometrogram demonstrating the activity of the bladder with upper neuron lesion during the early stages of recovery from spinal shock.

A. Upper Motor Neuron (Suprasegmental) Lesion: Toward the end of the stage of spinal shock, more obvious evidence of reflex activity is observed: movement of an extremity; vigorous spasm of an extremity, often accompanied by voiding around the catheter; progressive return of sensation in one or more areas; and hyperactive peripheral reflex activity and muscle tone. On removal of the catheter, spontaneous though inefficient urination occurs.

Cystometry (Fig 19–4) will show the changes typical of a spastic neuropathic bladder: bladder capacity below normal (100–300 mL); forceful, involuntary detrusor contractions; and increased intravesical pressure.

B. Lower Motor Neuron (Segmental or Infrasegmental) Lesion: When spinal shock has cleared,

the following may occur: progressive return of sensation in some areas, hypoactive peripheral reflexes, and flaccid muscle tone. It is difficult to know when the patient is coming out of shock, for this phase of recovery resembles shock. On removal of the catheter, spontaneous urination does not occur. As capacity is reached, overflow dribbling develops. The bladder can be partially emptied by manual pressure over the bladder (Credé maneuver).

The usual reactions seen with the flaccid neuropathic bladder are shown on cystometric study (Fig 19–6): bladder capacity above normal (600–1000 mL), absence of uninhibited detrusor contractions, and decreased intravesical pressure.

SPECIFIC TYPES OF
NEUROPATHIC BLADDERS

The diagnosis of neuropathic bladder disorder depends upon a complete history and physical (including neurologic) examination and the application of such specialized urologic tests as cystoscopy, cystography, excretory urography, and cystometry, including determination of residual urine. These tests may have to be repeated several times as recovery progresses.

COMPLETE SPASTIC (REFLEX, AUTOMATIC) NEUROPATHIC BLADDER

This type of cord bladder is the result of a partial or complete transection of the cord above the sacral level (above the lumbar spine) following recovery from spinal shock. The common causes are trauma, tumor, and multiple sclerosis. Cerebral control is lacking; the bladder functions in conjunction with its sacral reflex arc. The principal findings are diminished bladder capacity, increased intravesical pressure, spasm (obstruction) of the external urinary sphincters, and involuntary contractions of the vesical muscle.

Clinical Findings

A. Symptoms: The severity of symptoms depends on the site and extent of the lesion. Urinary symptoms include involuntary urination, often frequent and scanty, which may occur with involuntary spasm of the extremities. True sensation of fullness is lacking, although vague lower abdominal sensations due to stretching of the overlying peritoneum may be felt. The major nonurologic symptoms are spastic paralysis and objective sensory changes.

B. Signs: Complete neurologic examination will establish the site of the lesion. The anal sphincter tone is normal or increased; the bulbocavernosus reflex is intact or hyperactive (upper motor neuron lesion). Palpation and percussion usually do not reveal a distended bladder, since the bladder automatically discharges a portion of its contents when the urine volume reaches 150–300 mL. Stimulation of the skin of the abdomen, thigh, or genitals may trigger or initiate voiding. Such stimulation may also cause involuntary contraction of the extremities. This is called trigger voiding and is used as a method of treatment.

If the lesion is in the upper thoracic or cervical cord, distention of the bladder (plugged catheter, cystometry, cystoscopy) may excite hyperactive autonomic reflexes, which include severe hypertension, bradycardia, and pilomotor and sudomotor responses above the neurologic level. Headache may be severe; the hypertension may cause a cerebrovascular accident. Patients reacting in this man-

ner should have an indwelling catheter open at all times. They are benefited by the administration of phenoxybenzamine hydrochloride (Dibenzyline), 10 mg orally twice a day. If instrumentation is necessary, spinal anesthesia or the administration of a ganglionic or postganglionic blocking agent will protect the patient from this reaction.

C. Laboratory Findings: Anemia may be found if infection of the urinary tract has been prolonged and poorly controlled. If secondary renal damage is severe and uremia has developed, anemia is to be expected. The urine is infected secondary to the indwelling catheter. Red cells may be found if calculi have developed. Renal function may be normal or impaired, depending on the efficacy of treatment and the absence of renal complications (hydronephrosis, pyelonephritis, calculosis).

D. X-Ray Findings: Excretory urograms and retrograde cystograms are essential, since renal complications (eg, calculi, hydronephrosis) are common. Urinary stones may be seen. A trabeculated bladder of small capacity is typical of this type of neuropathic bladder. Ureteral reflux may be noted on the cystogram (Fig 19–10), which will almost certainly show a dilated bladder neck. If the cause of the neuropathic abnormality is undetermined, a plain film may reveal fracture or disease (eg, metastases) of the spine above the first lumbar vertebra.

E. Instrumental Examination: Cystoscopy and panendoscopy usually show moderate to severe trabeculation of the bladder wall, vesical diverticula, and changes compatible with infection. Stones may be visualized. The bladder is often hyperirritable to instrumentation.

The site of the lesion and the type of cystometrogram are diagrammed in Figs 19–3 and 19–4. As fluid is introduced into the bladder, strong, uninhibited contractions are noted until a contraction of such strength develops that involuntary urination occurs around the catheter. Capacity is diminished to 100–300 mL, and significant amounts of residual urine are found (50–150 mL). Although a true sense of fullness is lacking, various auras may be experienced (eg, sweating, vague low abdominal pain, intense spasm of the legs) when capacity is reached.

The ice water test is positive.

UNINHIBITED NEUROPATHIC BLADDER
(Mild Spastic Neuropathic Bladder)

Incomplete lesions of the cortex or the pyramidal (motor) tracts may weaken or abolish cerebral restraint. The patient may have frequency and nocturia, and may suffer episodes of incontinence due to uncontrollable urgency. Brain tumors, multiple sclerosis, prolapsed lumbar disk, arteriosclerotic changes within the cord, and, at times, cerebrovascular accidents may be etiologic factors, but the cause is not always known. This type of reaction is

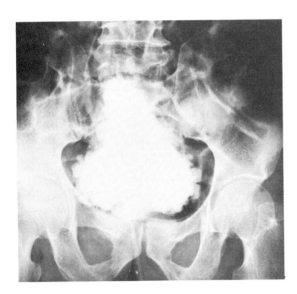 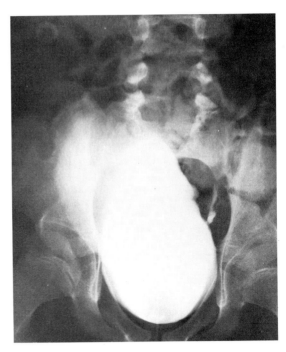

Figure 19–10. The spastic and flaccid neuropathic bladders as seen on cystography. *Left:* Spastic neuropathic bladder showing "Christmas tree" or "pine tree" effect. Heavy trabeculation, cellules, and small diverticula. *Right:* Flaccid neuropathic bladder showing oval-shaped bladder of large capacity in a boy 8 years old. The bladder, characteristically, is tipped to one side. Note severe spina bifida (myelomeningocele) and left ureteral reflux.

often found in patients suffering from anxiety (see Chapter 36). The symptoms and clinical findings in adults are similar to those seen in normal infants.

Clinical Findings

A. Symptoms: Frequency, nocturia, and urgency are the principal symptoms and are similar to those of cystitis. If symptoms are due to organic neurologic disorders (eg, cerebrovascular accident, brain tumor), characteristic symptoms of these lesions may be found.

B. Signs: The results obtained in general and neurologic examinations are normal unless primary central nervous system disease is present, in which case hyperreflexia and abnormal peripheral reflexes may be elicited (eg, multiple sclerosis).

C. X-Ray Findings: Some patients with multiple sclerosis may develop vesicoureteral reflux or ureterovesical obstruction. Urethrograms and cystograms are usually normal, but reflux may be seen.

D. Instrumental Examination: Cystoscopy and panendoscopy are normal, although some vesical irritability and diminished capacity may be demonstrated.

The type of cystometrogram is diagrammed in Fig 19–5. As the bladder is filled, strong, uninhibited contractions are noted; long before "normal" capacity is reached, involuntary urination occurs around the catheter. Perception of sensation is normal, and there is no residual urine.

FLACCID (ATONIC, NONREFLEX, OR AUTONOMOUS) NEUROPATHIC BLADDER

Injury to the sacral portion of the cord or to the motor or sensory roots of the cauda equina impairs the reflex arcs of the bladder. The common causes of this type of vesical reaction are trauma, tumors, tabes dorsalis, and congenital anomalies (eg, meningomyelocele). It may be seen following surgery in which the pelvic nerves are inadvertently injured (eg, abdominoperineal resection of the rectum). The bladder is also flaccid during the stage of spinal shock (Fig 19–8). This type of neuropathic bladder is characterized by large vesical capacity, low intravesical pressure, and the absence of involuntary detrusor contractions.

Clinical Findings

A. Symptoms: The patient complains of muscular paralysis and loss of peripheral sensation. The main urinary symptom is overflow incontinence. Suprapubic pressure may be required to initiate urination. Perception of fullness is absent.

B. Signs: Neurologic examination reveals evidence of a lower neuron lesion: absent or hypoactive peripheral reflexes, flaccid paralysis, absence of the bulbocavernosus reflex, and loss of anal sphincter tone. Sensation is diminished or absent. If perianal anesthesia alone is present, only one arm of the sacral reflex arc is damaged.

An overdistended bladder may be discovered on palpation or percussion. Pressure over the organ will cause passage of a stream of urine.

C. Laboratory Findings: Anemia may be noted, due either to chronic pyelonephritis or to uremia secondary to advanced renal damage (eg, infection, hydronephrosis, calculi). Pus cells and bacteria are found in the urine. Because of the amount of residual urine in the bladder, the PSP test must be performed with a catheter in place. Nitrogen retention may be associated with severe renal complications.

D. X-Ray Findings: A plain film of the abdomen may reveal a fracture of the lumbar spine or extensive spina bifida. Calcific shadows compatible with urinary stone may be visualized. Excretory urograms and retrograde cystograms should be performed routinely, since complications are common. These include vesical and renal calculi, renal scarring from pyelonephritis, and hydroureteronephrosis. However, the latter condition is usually less marked in these cases than when seen with the spastic neuropathic bladder because the incidence of ureteral reflux and functional ureterovesical obstruction is lower. The bladder will appear large on the urogram.

E. Instrumental Examination: Cystoscopy and panendoscopy, when performed some weeks after the injury, reveal mild to moderate trabeculation (hypertrophy) of the detrusor. Vesical capacity is increased, inflammatory changes may be present, and the bladder neck is usually dilated. Stones may be visualized. The patient may experience little discomfort with instrumentation because of loss of local sensation.

Cystography will show a bladder of increased capacity (Fig 19–10). Reflux of the radiopaque fluid to the kidneys may be demonstrated.

Urethrography may reveal some laxness of the external urinary sphincter (lower neuron lesion). The bladder neck is usually wide open.

The cystometrogram is diagrammed in Fig 19–6. Vesical capacity is increased, the intravesical pressure is decreased, and there are no uninhibited contractions. Even after abdominal pressure is used to expel the bladder contents, as much as 250 mL of urine may be retained.

F. Denervation Hypersensitivity Test: This test is performed by giving bethanechol chloride (Urecholine), 2.5 mg subcutaneously, and taking cystometric readings 10, 20, and 30 minutes later. A rise in intravesical pressure above 15 cm of water indicates detrusor denervation due to a lower motor neuron lesion. A normal response (under 10 cm of water) indicates a normal large-capacity bladder. No response indicates a large atonic bladder associated with myogenic damage.

The test is not applicable to patients with reduced bladder capacity, decreased compliance (sharp rise in pressure with bladder filling), or forceful contractions with voiding.

DIFFERENTIAL DIAGNOSIS OF NEUROPATHIC BLADDERS

The diagnosis of most cases of neuropathic bladder is obvious. Sacral nerve damage is evident, as judged by the bulbocavernosus reflex, anal sphincter tone, and perianal sensation. Too often the diagnosis of neuropathic bladder is made on very tenuous grounds.

Cystitis

Inflammations of the bladder, both nonspecific and tuberculous, cause frequency of urination and urgency, even to the point of incontinence. Pyuria and bacteriuria are found, although it must be remembered that the neuropathic bladder is usually secondarily infected because of the presence of residual urine or a retention catheter.

The cystometrogram of the inflamed bladder is similar to that of the uninhibited neuropathic bladder (Fig 19–5). However, with inflammation, symptoms will disappear after definitive antibiotic therapy, and the cystometrogram will be normal. If symptoms are not relieved following antibiotic therapy, a primary neurologic lesion should be sought (eg, multiple sclerosis).

Chronic Urethritis

Symptoms of frequency, nocturia, and burning on urination may be due to chronic inflammation of the urethra. The urine is not infected. Panendoscopy will often reveal urethral stenosis and signs of urethral inflammation. Neurologic and cystometric studies are normal.

Vesical Irritation Due to Psychic Disturbance

The patient gives a long history of periodic bouts of urinary frequency, usually occurring only in the morning. Comparable nocturia is absent. The symptoms are precipitated by anxiety. The urine is normal.

Cystometric studies reveal a hyperirritable bladder of diminished capacity. The pressure curve is similar to that seen with the uninhibited neuropathic bladder (Fig 19–5). If the patient's anxiety can be allayed, the intravesical pressure and vesical capacity may return to normal.

Interstitial Cystitis

The patient with interstitial fibrosis is almost always a woman over age 40 years. She complains of great frequency, nocturia, urgency, and suprapubic pain when the bladder reaches its markedly limited capacity (60–100 mL). The urinalysis is usually normal, and there is no residual urine. Cystometry usually shows a hypertonic detrusor reaction with some uninhibited contractions. The voiding pressure is usually quite high, and voiding is involuntary. Cystoscopy shows typical scarring; the mucosa is apt to split and bleed with vesical distention.

Cystocele

Relaxation of the pelvic floor following childbirth may cause some frequency, nocturia, and stress incontinence. Since residual urine is often present, infection may be demonstrated on urinalysis.

Pelvic examination usually reveals relaxation of the anterior vaginal wall and descent of the urethra and bladder when the patient strains to urinate. Cystoscopy will reveal similar findings.

Infravesical Obstruction

Congenital urethral valves or strictures and benign or malignant enlargements of the prostate usually cause impairment of the urinary stream. Hypertrophy (trabeculation) of the detrusor occurs, and residual urine accumulates. During this compensatory stage, bladder neck obstruction may resemble that of the spastic neuropathic bladder.

If decompensation occurs, the vesical wall becomes attenuated and atonic, and capacity may be markedly increased. Overflow incontinence may develop. The cystometrogram may be similar to that of the flaccid neuropathic bladder (Fig 19–6).

If the difficulty is nonneuropathic, the anal sphincter tone is normal and the bulbocavernosus reflex is intact. Peripheral sensation, motor power, and reflexes are normal. Cystoscopy and panendoscopy will reveal the local lesion causing the obstruction. Even though appropriately treated, the decompensated bladder may require prolonged catheter drainage before the vesical tone returns to normal.

COMPLICATIONS OF NEUROPATHIC BLADDER

The principal complications of neuropathic bladder are infection, hydronephrosis, and calculus formation. The primary factors that contribute to these complications are the presence of residual urine, ureteral reflux of urine, and confinement to bed. Sexual problems are common.

Incontinence in neuropathic disorders may be passive in flaccid lesions, resulting from extremely low outlet resistance; and active in spastic lesions—in spite of high outlet resistance—as a result of uninhibited detrusor contractions.

Infection

In neurovesical disease, the bladder loses the power to empty itself, making infection almost inevitable. With acute trauma to the spinal cord, the bladder is temporarily paralyzed and a retention catheter is therefore necessary. The introduction of an indwelling catheter always causes cystitis no matter what mechanical or medical measures are taken to prevent infection. The key to whether the kidneys will become involved is the ureterovesical junction. If the ureterovesical valves become incompetent, reflux of infected urine from the bladder reaches the kidneys. Valve incompetence may be caused by elevation of intravesical pressure from irrigations or expression of urine by the Credé maneuver, in which case these procedures must be discontinued.

If a large catheter is placed in the male bladder, periurethral abscess may ensue. This may rupture to the outside, producing a urinary fistula. If spontaneous drainage does not occur, urethral diverticulum may develop. Epididymitis secondary to prostatocystitis is not uncommon. The testis may become secondarily involved.

Hydronephrosis

Two mechanisms lead to back pressure on the kidney. Early in the course of the disorder, trigonal hypertrophy is compounded by stretch due to the variable volumes of residual urine; resistance at the ureterovesical junction induces progressive back pressure on the kidney and, ultimately, hydronephrosis. This condition can be relieved by continuous or intermittent bladder drainage.

Later, hydronephrosis is caused by decompression of the ureterovesical junction and reflux.

The incidence of vesicoureteral reflux, particularly in the patient with a spastic neuropathic bladder, is significant. The etiologic factor appears to be the trabeculation that develops in association with this bladder condition. Secondary hydroureteronephrosis is the rule. Hypertrophy of the trigone is associated with vesical trabeculation. This causes an abnormal pull upon the ureterovesical junction that may lead to functional obstruction and therefore proximal ureteral dilatation.

Calculus

A number of factors may contribute to stone formation in the bladder or kidneys. Bed rest and inactivity cause demineralization of the skeleton and therefore hypercalciuria. Recumbency also contributes to urinary stasis.

If the infection is due to urea-splitting bacteria, the urine remains alkaline, in which medium calcium is less soluble.

In order to "build up" the injured patient, the physician may mistakenly encourage the drinking of milk (thereby increasing the calcium intake and urinary output) and prescribe vitamin preparations including vitamin D. The latter only increases the efficiency of the bowel to absorb calcium into the bloodstream; increased urinary calcium excretion then occurs.

Renal Amyloidosis

Secondary amyloidosis of the kidneys is a common cause of death in patients with neuropathic bladder. Its incidence is highest in patients who have had decubitus ulcers or urethral infection.

Sexual Problems

Men who have suffered traumatic cord or cauda equina lesions experience varying degrees of sexual trouble. Those with upper motor lesions fare well; 95% will have psychic or reflex erections. In patients with complete lower neuron lesions, impotence occurs in 80%, but if the lesion is incomplete the incidence is 25%. The patient with an upper motor neuron defect has little chance of experiencing ejaculation or orgasm, although an incomplete lesion has a better prognosis.

TREATMENT OF NEUROPATHIC BLADDER

The treatment of any form of neuropathic bladder is aimed at maintaining a relatively good functional capacity, combating infection, controlling incontinence, and preserving renal function. Functional capacity is measured by the difference between true capacity and the amount of urine retained after voiding. The desirable interval between voidings should be at least 2 and preferably 3 hours.

Urinary continence should not be sought at the expense of vesical capacity or renal function. Few paralytics are so confident of their control that they appear in public without some type of collecting apparatus (Fig 19–12).

Treatment of Stage of Spinal Shock

Following severe injury to the spinal cord, the bladder is temporarily paralyzed. During the next few months it undergoes gradual improvement. If the sacral cord or cauda equina is damaged, the end result is a flaccid bladder. If the injury is higher, the bladder becomes spastic in type.

During spinal shock, when the bladder is paralyzed, some type of vesical drainage must be instituted immediately and then maintained.

It has become increasingly clear that the presence of a permanent indwelling catheter always leads to persistent bacteriuria. Intermittent catheterization prevents this complication in a high percentage of cases, but it requires intensive nursing care. If this is not possible, an indwelling catheter must be used.

Either a No. 16F Foley (balloon) or a No. 8 or 10F Gibbon (polythene) catheter can be used. The latter, because of its small size, may decrease the incidence of urethral complications (eg, periurethral abscess, urethral diverticulum). The Foley catheter in the male should be taped to the abdomen so that sharp angulation does not occur at the penoscrotal junction. It should be changed every week. The Gibbon catheter usually needs to be changed only once a month.

Some advocate the use of cystostomy rather than a urethral catheter, thus circumventing the often serious urethral and genital tract complications. Should these develop in association with urethral catheter drainage, cystostomy should be seriously considered; it will allow removal of the offending urethral catheter.

Bladder irrigation is sometimes desirable.

Cystograms and cystometrograms should be obtained periodically. If they reveal ureteral reflux or detrusor activity, continuous catheter drainage may be interrupted (see below).

In order to control infection, a fluid intake of at least 3000 mL/d must be maintained (200 mL of fluid every hour when awake). This reduces stasis and decreases the concentration of calcium in the urine. Renal and ureteral drainage are enhanced by raising the head of the bed, moving the patient frequently, and, above all, ambulating the patient in a wheelchair as early as possible. These measures lessen the incidence of acute pyelonephritis and renal and vesical calculosis. Sulfonamides or antibiotics should be vigorously administered if febrile reactions occur. Little is gained by prolonged prophylactic medication, since sterilization of the urine is impossible when a catheter is in place.

Prevention of calculosis requires a low-calcium diet (elimination of dairy products) containing no vitamin D. As mentioned above, early ambulation in a wheelchair reduces the incidence of calculosis. If hypercalciuria is demonstrated by periodic Sulkowitch tests, other prophylactic measures should be considered (see Chapter 15).

TREATMENT OF SPECIFIC TYPES OF NEUROPATHIC BLADDER

Once the specific type of neuropathic bladder is established (including the posttraumatic group after emergence from spinal shock), the following steps should be taken to attain optimum function.

Spastic Neuropathic Bladder

A. Patient With Large Bladder Capacity: To successfully train the spastic neuropathic bladder, patients must be able to wait 2–3 hours between involuntary voidings; should not leak during this period; and must be able to initiate voiding by manual stimulation or squeezing of the abdomen, genitalia, or thighs (trigger mechanism). Patients can do this by themselves unless they are quadriplegic.

B. Patient With Markedly Diminished Functional Vesical Capacity: If the functional capacity is only 50–100 mL, involuntary voidings may occur as often as every 15–30 minutes, and satisfactory bladder training cannot be attained (see cystometrogram in Fig 19–11). The alternatives are as follows:

1. Permanent retention catheter, cutaneous vesicostomy, cutaneous ureterostomy, ureteroileo-

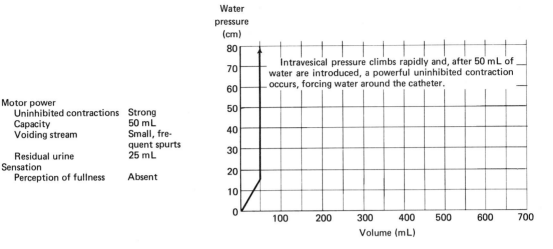

Motor power
Uninhibited contractions — Strong
Capacity — 50 mL
Voiding stream — Small, frequent spurts
Residual urine — 25 mL
Sensation
Perception of fullness — Absent

Water pressure (cm) / Volume (mL)

Intravesical pressure climbs rapidly and, after 50 mL of water are introduced, a powerful uninhibited contraction occurs, forcing water around the catheter.

Figure 19–11. Cystometrogram typical of severely spastic bladder.

cutaneous anastomosis, or cystostomy, particularly if ureteral reflux can be demonstrated on cystograms.

2. Urinal or other collecting apparatus constantly in place.

3. If low functional capacity is due to the retention of a large volume of urine, transurethral resection of the bladder neck may be undertaken. If this does not satisfactorily improve emptying power, transurethral destruction of the external sphincter may be necessary. This operation is quite efficacious in reducing the amount of residual urine. Since the patient will probably be incontinent, an external collecting device will be necessary.

4. If the true capacity is very low, and particularly if the patient suffers involuntary spasm of the extremities when voiding, the spastic bladder (and extremities) should be made flaccid.

If, despite catheter drainage, progressive hydroureteronephrosis develops, conversion of an upper motor to a lower motor neuron lesion may cause regression of the upper tract changes. Conversion can be accomplished by one of the following technics:

a. Subarachnoid injection of absolute alcohol–With the patient under spinal anesthesia, voiding should be stimulated manually. If this is successful, alcohol should be injected to destroy the conus and the cauda equina.

b. Anterior and posterior rhizotomy from T12 to and including S5 is also effective in converting the lesion to a lower neuron type.

c. Sacral neurotomy of S2–4 has an effect on the bladder similar to what can be achieved with alcohol injection or rhizotomy, but the results are not sufficient to eradicate annoying spasms of the extremities.

These procedures may have to be combined with resection of the bladder neck if stenosis of that structure is found.

5. Progressive upper tract deterioration may require urinary diversion.

C. Parasympatholytic Drugs: The quaternary ammonium amines methantheline bromide (Banthine), 50–100 mg 3–4 times daily orally, and propantheline bromide (Pro-Banthine), 15–30 mg 3–4 times daily orally, reduce vesical tone and thereby increase vesical capacity. Because of the prolonged nature of the disease, these agents have proved of little practical value except in patients with mildly spastic bladders (uninhibited neuropathic bladder).

Diokno & Lapides (1972) found that oxybutynin (Ditropan) has both analgesic and anticholinergic properties. It is effective in selected cases.

Flaccid Neuropathic Bladder

If the neurologic lesion is complete, volitional voiding cannot be accomplished without manual suprapubic pressure augmented, if possible, by abdominal and diaphragmatic contraction. If the lesion is incomplete, spontaneous voiding may occur, but the size and force of the stream are impaired, and residual urine remains in the bladder. Proper care of the flaccid bladder requires the following:

A. Bladder Training and Care: Voiding every 2 hours by the clock protects the bladder from overdistention, which the patient is unable to perceive, and preserves maximum tone.

Intermittent catheterization. Any patient with adequate bladder capacity can benefit from regular intermittent catheter drainage every 4–6 hours. This eliminates residual urine, helps to clear infection, and maintains the integrity of the ureterovesical junction. It simulates normal voiding and, if properly used, can be the answer to most of the problems of flaccid lesions. Intermittent catheterization has an excellent chance of rendering the urine sterile. Catheter drainage must be used for the patient who has ureteral reflux on cystography.

B. Surgery: Transurethral resection of the

bladder neck is indicated for hypertrophy or spasm, which causes the retention of a large volume of residual urine. At times this operation may fail to reduce residual urine to an amount that allows a proper interval between voidings, in which case transurethral incision of the external sphincter may be considered (Gibbon, 1973). This will require the use of a collection device.

C. Parasympathomimetic Drugs: The stable derivatives of acetylcholine are at times of value in initiating and increasing the efficiency of the contraction of the detrusor. They may therefore be helpful in the symptomatic treatment of the milder types of flaccid neuropathic bladder. Their usefulness may be gauged during cystometric study. When the bladder has been filled to a volume of 400 mL, the minimal recommended dose should be given subcutaneously. If intravesical pressure rises appreciably within a few minutes, the drug can be expected to be helpful clinically.

Bethanechol chloride (Urecholine) is the drug of choice. It is given either orally, 10–50 mg every 4–6 hours (the latter dose is usually necessary), or subcutaneously, 5–10 mg every 4–6 hours. Methacholine chloride (Mecholyl) is given orally, 0.2–0.4 g every 4–6 hours, or subcutaneously, 10–20 mg every 4–6 hours.

D. Implanted Electrodes: An attempt is being made to implant electrodes into the bladder wall that can be stimulated from an external source to achieve efficient detrusor action. Even more promising is the placement of electrodes in the sacral cord, where stimulation is more efficient than in the vesical wall. When perfected, this technic may prove to be an important step in the treatment of the flaccid bladder.

Scott, Bradley, & Timm (1973) have designed an implantable prosthetic sphincter. Results so far are encouraging.

Neuropathic Bladder Associated With Spina Bifida

Following the repair of meningocele or myelomeningocele, the cauda equina and sacral cord are apt to be involved by scar tissue. Patients usually have neuropathic vesical dysfunction that may be of the atonic or spastic type but is often of the mixed type (spastic bladder—upper motor neuron lesion; atony of the pelvic floor—lower neuron lesion).

The goals of therapy are to control incontinence and to preserve renal function.

A. Conservative Treatment: Lyon, Scott, & Marshall (1975) find that clean intermittent catheterization will afford a sterile urine in most cases. Parents can be taught to do this for the child; later, the patient can take over this function. It should be done 3–5 times a day. This will also control incontinence in many of these patients.

1. Mild symptoms–If there is occasional dribbling or some residual urine associated with lack of desire to void, the patient should try to void every 2 hours when awake. Manual suprapubic pressure will enhance the efficiency of emptying. An external condom catheter (Fig 19–12) will protect the male who still suffers small losses; the female with this complaint will require an indwelling catheter.

2. More severe symptoms–If true urinary incontinence associated with residual urine and ureteral reflux is found, the following steps should be taken.

a. Mostly atonic bladder–If reflux is demonstrable, self-catheterization 4 times a day may protect the upper urinary tract from deterioration and the complication of pyelonephritis. Ureteral reimplantation might be considered if all other factors are favorable. It should be followed by intermittent catheterization.

b. Mostly spastic bladder–The problem with patients in this category is more serious because the bladder is hypertonic and has a small capacity, but the external sphincter is atonic. Almost constant dribbling may result. In addition, a cystogram will reveal a heavily trabeculated bladder and, in many cases, reflux due to advanced hydroureteronephrosis. Lyon recommends the placement of an indwelling catheter for many months. In most instances, the bladder assumes a normal smooth contour and the hydroureteronephrosis subsides. The patient is then able to resume intermittent self-catheterization. With time, many of these children develop a more balanced bladder and may continue to improve. Continence may finally be gained. Urinary diversion will not be necessary in most of these patients. If vesicoureteral reflux persists, ureterovesicoplasty is highly successful once the bladder has smoothed out. Shochat & Perlmutter (1972) find that severe neonatal hydronephrosis may resolve after urethral dilatation.

B. Surgical Treatment: If significant residual urine is associated with considerable dribbling, transurethral resection of the bladder neck or division of the external sphincter will reduce the residual urine and will cure some of these children. A few may notice increased incontinence, however.

If the bladder is of the spastic type with diminished capacity, sacral nerve block, internal pudendal neurectomy, or selective neurectomy (S3) may improve capacity and stop ureteral reflux.

Stanton & Edwards (1973) have had good success after implanting a stimulator in the bladder. Candidates must have good upper tracts and adequate bladder emptying; must be free of vesicoureteral reflux, with good bladder capacity; and must have urethral incompetence.

If the refluxing patient suffers recurrent fever (pyelonephritis) despite the presence of an indwelling catheter, or if incontinence cannot be controlled, urinary diversion must be considered. The colonic conduit is the method of choice.

THE CONTROL OF URINARY INCONTINENCE

In the Hospital

Urinary incontinence is a distressing aspect of neurovesical dysfunction, particularly if the patient achieves a bladder that otherwise functions adequately. This difficulty is minimized in men under hospital conditions, for with close supervision and the ever-present urinal, the urine can usually be properly collected. Women have a greater problem because of the need for placement of the bedpan, and bedwetting may be frequent. Even an indwelling catheter does not guarantee dryness for the incontinent woman, since leakage around the catheter often occurs. No simple and satisfactory solution to this problem has yet been devised. Urinary diversion may be necessary.

After Discharge

When the time comes for discharge from the hospital, almost all men, even though they have achieved "excellent" bladder control, must wear a "condom catheter" (Fig 19–12). This consists of a condom with a catheter at the distal end for drainage of any urine unexpectedly lost. The catheter drains into a leg urinal. The condom may be secured to the penis by Elastoplast, cellulose tape, or cement.

A McGuire urinal (Fig 19–12) consists of a heavy condom incorporated into an athletic supporter. If there is considerable leakage of urine, the dependent end can be drained through a tube into a leg urinal.

Urethral compression by means of a Cunningham clamp is preferred by some patients. It may, however, lead to the development of a urethral diverticulum (Fig 19–13).

Recent Developments

Extensive research work is now being conducted in an attempt to find a feasible means of implanting an electrode in the sacral canal around one or more sacral nerve roots with the hope of controlling detrusor activity. There is a certain degree of selectivity in nerve fiber distribution between the detrusor muscle and the sphincter. One sacral root may be predominantly destined to innervate the detrusor muscle, whereas another might be primarily responsible for the sphincteric

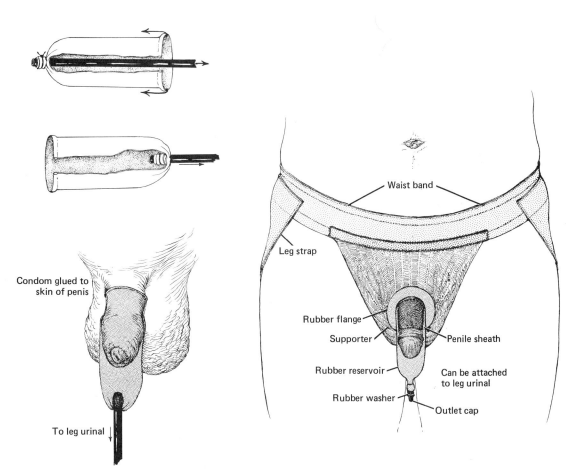

Figure 19–12. *Left:* Condom catheter. *Right:* McGuire urinal.

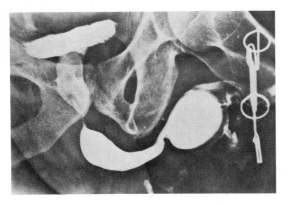

Figure 19–13. Urethral diverticulum. Atonic neuropathic bladder after transurethral resection. Diverticulum is a complication of prolonged use of a Cunningham clamp.

unit. Application of a chronically implantable electrode with a subcutaneous receiver around this particular root would make external stimulation feasible at will at set intervals, to initiate detrusor contraction and emptying. The same principle can be applied to the sacral root predominantly destined to control the sphincter so that continence may be maintained. These studies have proved to be highly successful in experimental animal models. However, their clinical application has not yet been implemented. It is anticipated that these technics will have important consequences in the management of neuropathic bladder and urinary incontinence as long as an intact reflex arc to the sacral roots and the spinal cord is present.

TREATMENT OF COMPLICATIONS

The most common and significant complications can be discovered by cystography, cystometry, cystoscopy, and excretory urography repeated at least once a year.

Hydronephrosis

Ureteral reflux, as shown by cystography, is an indication for an indwelling catheter. Over a period of months, the ureterovesical junction may again become competent. If, despite prolonged drainage, reflux persists, vesicoureteroplasty may be indicated in flaccid lesions with adequate bladder capacity, though it is difficult when severe vesical trabeculation and trigonal hypertrophy are present. Progressive hydroureteronephrosis, found on urography, may require nephrostomy or urinary diversion as a lifesaving measure.

Pyelonephritis

Bouts of renal infection must be treated by antimicrobials. Intermittent self-catheterization may render the urine sterile. If the pyelonephritis is associated with ureteral reflux, constant vesical drainage must be instituted. Urinary diversion should be considered.

Epididymitis

In acute epididymitis secondary to prostatitis initiated by the urethral catheter, prophylactic vasoligation is indicated during a quiescent period. Should this not suffice, removal of the urethral catheter and placement of a suprapubic tube or intermittent catheterization will be necessary.

Calculi

A. Vesical: Vesical calculi, diagnosed by x-ray or cystoscopy, can usually be washed out through an instrument or crushed and removed transurethrally. If they are large, suprapubic removal will be required.

B. Ureteral: These can usually be diagnosed by excretory urograms; if no radiopaque fluid is excreted, cystoscopy and the passage of a ureteral catheter may be necessary. Most ureteral stones can be removed cystoscopically. Operative removal may at times be required.

C. Renal: The diagnosis of renal calculi is made by radiography. If the calculus is obstructive, it must be removed; if not, conservative treatment is the rule, for the recurrence rate is high because of the presence of urea-splitting organisms in the kidney.

If stones form despite the prophylactic steps listed on p 366, an even more rigorous regimen should be instituted (Chapter 15).

PROGNOSIS

The greatest threat to the patient with a neuropathic bladder is progressive renal damage (pyelonephritis, calculosis, and hydronephrosis). Some degree of hydronephrosis is found in 25% of these patients; a few will die because of it unless appropriate treatment is instituted.

The quadriplegic patient presents a serious problem. If the bladder is spastic, voiding cannot be initiated by self-stimulation; if the bladder has been made flaccid, the patient is unable to exert suprapubic pressure. An indwelling catheter may be the best solution. Most paraplegics can eventually achieve comfortable bladder function, although many must continue to wear some type of collecting apparatus.

● ● ●

References

Al-Mefty O, Kandzari S, Fox JL: Neurogenic bladder and tethered spinal cord syndrome. *J Urol* 1979;**122**:112.

The American Academy of Pediatrics: Current approaches to evaluation and management of children with myelomeningocele. *Pediatrics* 1979;**63**:663.

Andersen JT, Bradley WE: Abnormalities of detrusor and sphincter function in multiple sclerosis. *Br J Urol* 1976;**48**:193.

Anderson RU: Non-sterile intermittent catheterization with antibiotic prophylaxis in acute and spinal cord injured male patient. *J Urol* 1980;**124**:392.

Awad SA & others: Treatment of uninhibited bladder with dicyclomine. *J Urol* 1977;**117**:161.

Bors E, Comarr AE: *Neurological Urology: Physiology of Micturition, Its Neurological Disorders and Sequelae.* University Park Press, 1971.

Bradley WE: Autonomic neuropathy and the genitourinary system. *J Urol* 1979;**119**:399.

Bradley WE, Andersen JT: Neuromuscular dysfunction of the lower urinary tracts in patients with lesions of cauda equina and conus medullaris. *J Urol* 1976;**116**:620.

Bradley WE & others: Neurology of micturition. *J Urol* 1976;**115**:481.

Brown BT, Carrion HM, Politano VA: Guanethidine sulfate in prevention of autonomic hyperreflexia. *J Urol* 1979;**122**:55.

Cardozo LD, Stanton SL: Objective comparison of effects of parenterally administered drugs in patients suffering from detrusor instability. *J Urol* 1979;**122**:58.

Comarr AE: Intermittent catheterization for the traumatic cord bladder patient. *J Urol* 1972;**108**:79.

Comarr AE: Sexual function among patients with spinal cord injury. *Urol Int* 1970;**25**:134.

Cosbie RJ, Gibbon NOK, Sham SG: Division of the external urethral sphincter in the neuropathic bladder: A twenty years' review. *Br J Urol* 1976;**48**:649.

Crane DB, Hackler RH: External sphincterostomy: Its effect on erections. *J Urol* 1976;**116**:316.

DeLaere KPJ & others: Prolonged bladder distension in management of unstable bladder. *J Urol* 1980;**124**:334.

Dermot OJ: An assessment of surgical treatment of vesical outlet obstruction in spinal cord injury: A review of 471 cases. *Br J Urol* 1976;**48**:657.

Diokno AC, Kass E, Lapides J: New approach to myelodysplasia. *J Urol* 1976;**116**:771.

Diokno AC, Koppenhoefer R: Bethanechol chloride in neurogenic bladder dysfunction. *Urology* 1976;**8**:455.

Diokno AC, Lapides J: Oxybutynin: A new drug with analgesic and anticholinergic properties. *J Urol* 1972;**108**:307.

Diokno AC, Vinson RK, McGillicuddy J: Treatment of severe uninhibited neurogenic bladder by selective sacral rhizotomy. *J Urol* 1977;**118**:299.

Engel RME, Schirmer HKA: Pudendal neurectomy in neurogenic bladder. *J Urol* 1974;**112**:57.

Fischer CP, Diokno A, Lapides J: Anticholinergic effects of dicyclomine hydrochloride in uninhibited neurogenic bladder dysfunction. *J Urol* 1978;**120**:328.

Flanigan RC, Kursh ED, Persky L: Thirteen year experience with ileal loop diversion in children with myelodysplasia. *Am J Surg* 1975;**130**:535.

Gibbon NOK: Division of external sphincter. *Br J Urol* 1973;**45**:110.

Gibbon NOK: Nomenclature of neurogenic bladder. *Urology* 1976;**8**:423.

Golji H: Experience with penile prosthesis in spinal cord injury patients. *J Urol* 1979;**121**:288.

Greenberg M, Gordon HL, McCutchen JJ: Neurogenic bladder in Parkinson's disease. *South Med J* 1972;**65**:446.

Grimes JH, Nashold BS, Anderson EE: Clinical application of electronic bladder stimulation in paraplegics. *J Urol* 1975;**113**:338.

Jacobs SC, Kaufman JM: Complications of permanent bladder catheter drainage in spinal cord injury patients. *J Urol* 1978;**119**:740.

Jeffs RD, Jonas P, Schillinger JF: Surgical correction of vesicoureteral reflux in children with neurogenic bladder. *J Urol* 1976;**115**:449.

Johnston JH, Farkas A: Congenital neuropathic bladder: Practicalities and possibilities of conservational management. *Urology* 1975;**5**:719.

Johnston JH, Shapiro SR, Thomas GG: Anti-reflux surgery in the congenital neuropathic bladder. *Br J Urol* 1976;**48**:639.

Jonas U, Jones LW, Tanagho EA: Spinal cord stimulation versus detrusor stimulation: A comparative study in six "acute" dogs. *Invest Urol* 1975;**13**:171.

Jonas U, Petri E, Kissel J: Effect of flavoxate on hyperactive detrusor muscle. *Eur Urol* 1979;**5**:106.

Jones DL, Moore T: The types of neuropathic bladder dysfunction associated with prolapsed lumbar intervertebral discs. *Br J Urol* 1973;**45**:39.

Kahan M, Goldberg PD, Mandel EE: Neurogenic vesical dysfunction and diabetes mellitus. *NY State J Med* 1970;**70**:2448.

Koff SA, DeRidder PA: Patterns of neurogenic bladder dysfunction in sacral agenesis. *J Urol* 1977;**118**:87.

Koff SA, Lapides J, Piazza DH: Association of urinary tract infections and reflux with uninhibited bladder contractions and voluntary sphincteric obstruction. *J Urol* 1979;**122**:373.

Kontturi M, Larmi TKI, Tuononen S: Bladder dysfunction and its manifestations following abdominoperineal extirpation of the rectum. *Ann Surg* 1974;**179**:179.

Koontz WW Jr, Smith MJV: Transurethral external sphincterotomy in boys with myelodysplasia. *J Urol* 1977;**117**:500.

Kursh ED, Freehafer A, Persky L: Complications of autonomic dysreflexia. *J Urol* 1977;**118**:70.

Lapides J & others: Further observations on self-catheterization. *J Urol* 1976;**116**:169.

Light K, Van Blerk PJP: Causes of renal deterioration in patients with meningomyelocele. *Br J Urol* 1977;**49**:257.

Linker DG, Tanagho EA: Complete external sphincterotomy: Correlation between endoscopic observation and the anatomic sphincter. *J Urol* 1975;**113**:348.

Lyon RP, Scott MP, Marshall S: Intermittent catheterization rather than urinary diversion in children with meningomyelocele. *J Urol* 1975;**113**:409.

MacGregor RJ, Diokno AC: Self-catheterization for decompensated bladder: A review of 100 cases. *J Urol* 1979;**122**:602.

McGuire EJ, Diddel G, Wagner F Jr: Balanced bladder function in spinal cord injury patients. *J Urol* 1977;**118**:623.

Manfredi RA, Leal JF: Selective sacral rhizotomy for the spastic bladder syndrome in patients with spinal cord injuries. *J Urol* 1968;**100**:17.

Merrill DC: Clinical experience with the Mentor bladder

stimulator. 3. Patients with urinary vesical hypotonia. *J Urol* 1975;**113**:335.

Mobley DF: Phenoxybenzamine in the management of neurogenic vesical dysfunction. *J Urol* 1976;**116**:737.

Morrow JW, Bogaard TP: Bladder rehabilitation in patients with old spinal cord injuries with bladder neck incision and external sphincterotomy. *J Urol* 1977;**117**:164.

Mulcahy JJ, James HE: Management of neurogenic bladder in infancy and childhood. *Urology* 1979;**13**:235.

Nanninga JB, Rosen J, O'Conor VJ Jr: Experience with transurethral external sphincterotomy in patients with spinal cord injury. *J Urol* 1974;**112**:72.

Nordling J, Meyhoff HH: Dissociation of urethral and anal sphincter activity in neurogenic bladder dysfunction. *J Urol* 1979;**122**:352.

Olsson CA, Siroky SB, Krane RJ: Phentolamine test in neurogenic bladder dysfunction. *J Urol* 1977;**117**:418.

Pearman JW: Urological follow-up of 99 spinal cord injured patients initially managed by intermittent catheterisation. *Br J Urol* 1976;**48**:297.

Pedersen E (editor): The neurogenic bladder. (Symposium.) *Acta Neurol Scand* 1966;**42**(Suppl 20):7. [Entire issue.]

Perkash I: Intermittent catheterization and bladder rehabilitation in spinal cord injury patients. *J Urol* 1975;**114**:230.

Perkash I: Problems of decatheterization in long-term spinal cord injury patients. *J Urol* 1980;**124**:249.

Piazza DH, Diokno AC: Review of neurogenic bladder in multiple sclerosis. *Urology* 1979;**14**:33.

Plunkett JM, Braren V: Clean intermittent catheterization in children. *J Urol* 1979;**121**:469.

Rabinovitch HH: Bladder evacuation in child with meningomyelocele. *Urology* 1974;**3**:425.

Raz S, Bradley WE: Neuromuscular dysfunction of the lower urinary tract. In: *Campbell's Urology.* Harrison JH & others (editors). Saunders, 1979.

Redman JF: Credé expression of the bladder: A sometimes useful maneuver. *J Urol* 1976;**116**:794.

Rosenblum R: Urological care of patients with acute spinal cord injury using tidal drainage. *J Urol* 1976;**116**:587.

Ross JC, Gibbon NOK, Sunder GS: Division of the external urethral sphincter in the neuropathic bladder: A twenty years' review. *Br J Urol* 1976;**48**:649.

Rossier AB, Ott R: Urinary manometry in spinal cord injury: A follow-up study. Value of cysto-sphincterometrography as an indicator for sphincterotomy. *Br J Urol* 1974;**46**:439.

Schoenberg HW, Guthrie J, Banno J: Urodynamic patterns in multiple sclerosis. *J Urol* 1979;**122**:648.

Schoenberg HW & others: Changing attitudes toward urinary dysfunction in myelodysplasia. *J Urol* 1977;**117**:501.

Schoenfeld L, Carrion HM, Politano VA: Erectile impotence: Complication of external sphincterotomy. *Urology* 1974;**4**:681.

Scott FB, Bradley WE, Timm GW: Treatment of urinary incontinence by implantable prosthetic sphincter. *Urology* 1973;**1**:252.

Shochat SJ, Perlmutter AD: Myelodysplasia with severe neonatal hydronephrosis: The value of urethral dilatation. *J Urol* 1972;**107**:146.

Siroky MB, Sax DS, Krane RJ: Sacral signal tracing: The electrophysiology of the bulbocavernosus reflex. *J Urol* 1979;**122**:661.

Smith AD, Sazama R, Lange PH: Penile prosthesis: Adjunct to treatment in patients with neurogenic bladder. *J Urol* 1980;**124**:363.

Stanton SL, Edwards L: Treatment of paediatric urinary incontinence by stimulator implant. *Br J Urol* 1973;**45**:508.

Tanagho EA: Meningomyelocele: Urologic considerations. *West J Med* 1974;**121**:292.

Tanagho EA, Meyers FH, Smith DR: The trigone: Anatomical and physiological considerations. 1. In relation to the ureterovesical junction. *J Urol* 1968;**100**:623.

Tanagho EA, Miller ER: Initiation of voiding. *Br J Urol* 1970;**42**:175.

Tarabulcy E: Neurogenic diseases of the bladder in the geriatric population. *Geriatrics* (Sept) 1974;**29**:123.

Texter JH Jr, Reece RW, Hranowsky N: Pentolinium in the management of autonomic hyperreflexia. *J Urol* 1976;**116**:350.

Thompson IM, Kirk RM, Dale M: Sacral agenesis. *Pediatrics* 1974;**54**:236.

Thompson IM, Lauvetz R: Oxybutynin in bladder spasm, neurogenic bladder, and enuresis. *Urology* 1976;**8**:452.

Van Gool JD & others: Measurement of intravesical and rectal pressures simultaneously with electromyography of anal sphincter in children with myelomeningocele. *Dev Med Child Neurol* 1976;**18**:287.

Wein AJ, Raezer DM, Benson GS: Management of neurogenic bladder dysfunction in the adult. *Urology* 1976;**8**:432.

Whitmore WF III, Fam BA, Yalla SV: Experience with anteromedian (12 o'clock) external urethral sphincterotomy in 100 male subjects with neuropathic bladders. *Br J Urol* 1978;**50**:99.

Yalla SV & others: Anteromedian external urethral sphincterotomy: Technique, rationale and complications. *J Urol* 1977;**117**:489.

Zinke H & others: Neurovesical vesical dysfunction in diabetes mellitus: Another look at vesical neck resection. *J Urol* 1974;**111**:488.

Urodynamic Studies | 20

Emil A. Tanagho, MD

Urodynamic study is becoming an important part of the evaluation of patients with voiding dysfunctions—dysuria, urinary incontinence, neuropathic disorders, etc. Formerly, the examiner simply observed the act of voiding, noting the strength of the urinary stream and drawing inferences about the possibility of obstruction of the bladder outlet. In the 1950s, it became possible to observe the lower urinary tract by fluoroscopy during the act of voiding; and in the 1960s, the principles of hydrodynamics were applied to lower urinary tract physiology. The field of urodynamics now has clinical applications in evaluating voiding problems resulting from lower urinary tract disease.

The nomenclature of the tests used in urodynamic studies is not yet settled, and the meanings of urodynamic terms are sometimes overlapping or confusing. In spite of these difficulties, however, urodynamic tests are extremely valuable. Symptoms elicited by the history or by physical, endoscopic, or even radiographic examination must often be further investigated by the technics so that therapy can be devised that is based on an understanding of the altered physiology of the lower urinary tract.

As is true of many high-technology testing procedures (eg, electrocardiography, electroencephalography), urodynamic tests have greatest clinical validity when their interpretation is left to the treating physician, who should either supervise the study or be responsible for correlating all of the findings into his or her own clinical observation.

FUNCTIONS RELEVANT TO URODYNAMICS & MODALITIES APPLICABLE TO EACH

Urodynamic study of the lower urinary tract can provide useful clinical information about the function of the urinary bladder, the sphincteric mechanism, and the voiding pattern itself.

Bladder function has been classically studied by cystography and active motion fluoroscopy. Urodynamic studies utilize cystometry. Conventional radiographic studies and urodynamic studies can of course be usefully combined.

Sphincteric function depends upon 2 elements: the smooth muscle sphincter and the voluntary sphincter. The activity of both elements can be recorded urodynamically by pressure measurements; the activity of the voluntary sphincter can be recorded by electromyography.

The act of voiding is a function of the interaction between bladder and sphincter, and the result is the **flow rate.** The flow rate is one major aspect of the total function of the lower urinary tract: It is generally recorded in millimeters per second as well as by total urine volume voided. The simultaneous recording of bladder activity (by intraluminal pressure measurements), sphincteric activity (by electromyography or pressure measurements), and flow rate will reveal interrelationships between the 3 elements. Each measurement may give useful information about the normality or abnormality of one specific aspect of lower urinary tract function. A more complete picture is provided by integrating all 3 lower tract elements in a simultaneously recorded comparative manner. This comprehensive approach may involve synchronous recordings of variable pressures, flow rate, volume voided, and electrical activity of skeletal musculature around the urinary sphincter (electromyography), along with fluoroscopic imaging of the lower urinary tract. The multiple pressures to be recorded are quite variable and usually include intravesical pressure, intraurethral pressure at several levels, intraabdominal pressure, and anal sphincter pressure as a function of muscular activity of the pelvic floor.

The technics of urodynamic study must be tailored to the needs of specific patients. Each technic has advantages and limitations depending upon the requirements of each study. In one patient, recording of a single parameter might be sufficient to establish the diagnosis and suggest appropriate therapy; in another, many more studies might be necessary.

PHYSIOLOGIC & HYDRODYNAMIC CONSIDERATIONS

URINARY FLOW RATE

Because urinary flow rate is the product of detrusor action against outlet resistance, a variation from the normal flow rate might reflect dysfunction of either. The normal flow rate from a full bladder is about 20–25 mL/s in men and 25–30 mL/s in women. These variations are directly related to the volume voided and the subject's age. Obstruction should be suspected in any adult voiding with a full bladder at a rate of less than 15 mL/s. A flow rate of less than 10 mL/s is considered definite evidence of obstruction. Occasionally, one encounters "supervoiders" with flow rates far above the normal range. This may signify low outlet resistance but is of less concern clinically than obstruction.

Outlet Resistance

Outlet resistance is the primary determinant of flow rate and varies according to mechanical or functional factors. Functionally, outlet resistance is primarily related to sphincteric activity, which is controlled by both the smooth sphincter and the voluntary sphincter. The smooth sphincter is rarely overactive in women; we have never seen an example of it in any of our urodynamic evaluations. Overactivity of the smooth sphincter is rarely seen in men but may occur in association with hypertrophy of the bladder neck due to neurogenic dysfunction or distal obstruction. However, such cases must be critically evaluated before this conclusion is reached.

Increased voluntary sphincter activity is not uncommon. It is often neglected as a primary underlying cause of increased sphincteric resistance. It is manifested either as lack of relaxation or as actual overactivity during voiding. The normal voluntary sphincter provides adequate resistance, along with the smooth sphincter, to prevent escape of bladder urine; if the voluntary sphincter does not relax during detrusor contraction, partial obstruction occurs. Overactivity of the sphincter, resulting in increased outlet resistance, is usually a neuropathic phenomenon. However, it can also be functional, resulting from irritative phenomena such as infection or other factors—chemical, bacterial, hormonal, or even more commonly and often not appreciated, psychologic.

Mechanical Factors

Mechanical factors resulting in obstruction to urine flow are the easiest to identify by conventional methods. In women, they may take the form of cystoceles, urethral kinks, or, most commonly, iatrogenic scarring, fibrosis, and compression from previous vaginal or periurethral operative procedures. Mechanical factors in men are well known to all urologists; the classic form is benign prostatic hypertrophy. Urethral stricture due to various causes and posterior urethral valves are other common causes of urinary obstruction in men, and there are many others.

Normal voiding with a normal flow rate is the product of both detrusor activity and outlet resistance. A high intravesical pressure resulting from detrusor contraction is not necessary to initiate voiding, because outlet resistance has usually dropped to a minimum. Sphincteric relaxation usually precedes detrusor contraction by a few seconds, and when relaxation is maximal, detrusor activity starts and is sustained until the bladder is empty.

Variations in Normal Flow Rate

The sequence just described is not essential for normal flow rates. The flow rate may be normal in the absence of any detrusor contraction if sphincteric relaxation is assisted by increased intra-abdominal pressure from straining. Persons with weak outlet resistance and weak sphincteric control can achieve a normal flow rate by complete voluntary sphincteric relaxation without detrusor contraction or straining. A normal flow rate can be achieved in spite of increased sphincteric activity or lack of complete relaxation if detrusor contraction is increased to overcome outlet resistance.

Because a normal flow rate can be achieved in spite of abnormalities of one or more of the mechanisms involved, recording the flow rate alone does not provide insight into the precise mechanisms by which it occurs. Distinction between patterns of flow can be difficult. For practical purposes, if the flow rate is adequate, with normal pattern and configuration of the flow curve recorded, these variations may not be significant clinically except in rare cases.

Nomenclature

The study of urinary flow rate itself is usually called **uroflowmetry**. The flow rate is generally identified as **maximum flow rate, average flow rate, flow time, maximum flow time** (the time elapsed before maximum flow rate is reached), and **total flow time** (the aggregate of flow time if the flow has been interrupted by periods of no voiding) (Fig 20–1). The **flow rate pattern** is characterized as continuous or intermittent, etc.

Pattern Measurement of Flow Rate

A normal flow pattern is represented by a bell-shaped curve (Fig 20–1). However, the curve is rarely completely smooth; it may vary within certain limits and still be normal. Flow rate can be determined by measuring a 5-second collection at the peak of flow and dividing the amount obtained by 5 to arrive at the average rate per second. This rough estimate is useful, especially if the flow rate is normal and the values are above 20 mL/s. Peak urine flow can also be measured quite easily with a Peakometer—a device employing a color indicator strip impregnated with urine to show maximum flow rate by changes in color against a predetermined scale. The Drake uroflowmeter is a plastic container with several chambers into which the patient voids; the maximum flow rate is determined by noting how many chambers contain urine.

In modern practice, the flow rate is more often

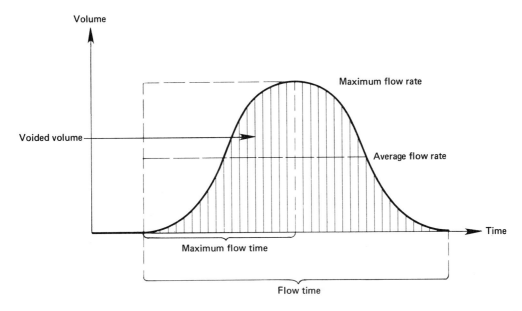

Figure 20–1. Uroflowmetry. Basic elements of maximum flow, average flow, total flow time, and total volume voided.

recorded electronically: The patient voids into a container on top of a measuring device that leads to a transducer, the weight being converted to volume and recorded on a chart in mL/s. Fig 20–2 is an example of such a recording from a normal man. The general bell-shaped curve is quite clear, and the tracing shows all of the parameters discussed above: total flow time, maximum flow time, maximum flow rate, average flow rate, and total volume voided. Occasional "supervoiders" can exceed the record limits, but this is usually not of clinical concern (Fig 20–3). The possible variation in the bell appearance is seen in Fig 20–4.

The overall appearance of the flow curve may disclose unsuspected abnormalities. In Fig 20–5, for example, flow time is greatly prolonged. Maximum flow rate may not be low, but the average flow rate is very low—though the maximum flow rate is at one time within the normal range. Such fluctuation in flow rate is most commonly related to variations in voluntary sphincter activity. In Fig 20–6, this pattern is extreme: Maximum flow rate never exceeds 15 mL/s and average flow rate is about 10 mL/s, which is indicative of obstruction. (Again, this fluctuation in pattern probably reflects sphincteric hyperactivity.)

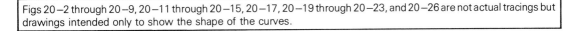

Figs 20–2 through 20–9, 20–11 through 20–15, 20–17, 20–19 through 20–23, and 20–26 are not actual tracings but drawings intended only to show the shape of the curves.

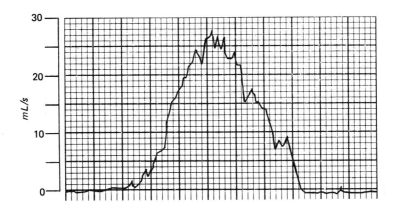

Figure 20–2. Classic normal flow rate, with peak of about 30 mL/s and average of about 20 mL/s.

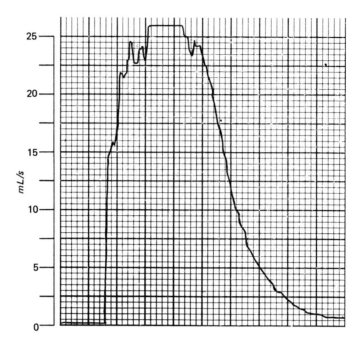

Figure 20–3. Flow rate of "supervoider." Maximum flow rate exceeds limits of chart. Writer shows fast build-up and complete bladder emptying of large volume of urine in very short period.

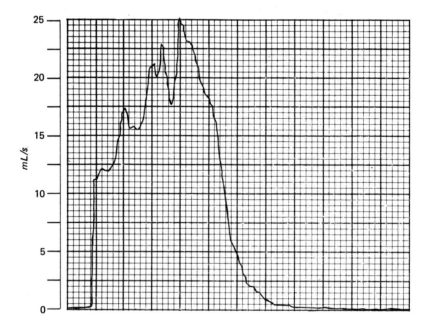

Figure 20–4. Normal flow rate but with some variation in appearance of curve. Note rapid pressure rise but progressive increase to maximum, then a sharp drop. Also fluctuation in ascending limb.

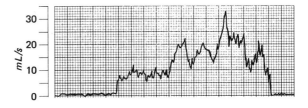

Figure 20–5. Rather low flow rate (not exceeding 10 mL/s), yet at one point peak reaching 30–32 mL/s. Note again fluctuation in flow.

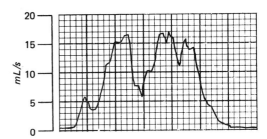

Figure 20–6. Very low flow rate of short duration, small volume. Note that maximum flow is not above 15 mL/s; however, flow average is less than 10 mL/s, and flow is almost completely interrupted in middle.

The flow rate pattern reveals a great deal about the forces involved. For example, if the patient is voiding without the aid of detrusor contractions—primarily by straining—this can be easily deduced from the flow rate. Fig 20–7 shows an example of intermittent voiding, primarily by straining, with no detrusor activity and at a rate that sometimes does not reach the usual peaks. With experience, one becomes expert at detecting the mechanism underlying abnormalities in flow rate. For example, in Fig 20–5, the maximum flow rate is in the normal range, the average flow rate is slightly low, and the curve has a general bell pattern, yet brief partial intermittent obstructions to flow can be readily interpreted as due to overactivity of the voluntary sphincter, a mild form of detrusor/sphincter dyssynergia (see below).

Flow rates in mechanical obstruction are totally different, classically in the range of 5 or 6 mL/s; flow time is greatly prolonged, and there is sustained low flow with minimal variation (Fig 20–8). Fig 20–9 shows a striking example of a patient with benign prostatic hypertrophy. No simultaneous studies are needed with such a pattern, since the pattern is obviously one of mechanical obstruction.

Reduced flow rate in the absence of mechani-

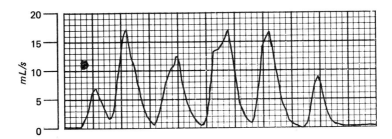

Figure 20–7. Classic flow rate due to abdominal straining with no detrusor activity. See effect of spurts of urine with complete interruption between them, since patient cannot sustain increased intra-abdominal pressure.

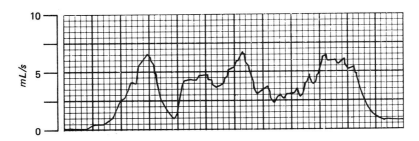

Figure 20–8. Flow rate in a case of urinary obstruction showing very low average flow rate (not above 5 or 6 mL/s). Prolonged duration of flow is associated with incomplete emptying.

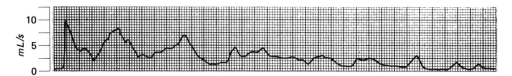

Figure 20-9. Classic low flow rate of bladder outlet obstruction (benign prostatic hypertrophy), markedly prolonged flow time, and fluctuation due to attempt at improving flow by increased intra-abdominal pressure.

cal obstruction is due to some impairment of sphincteric or detrusor activity. This is seen in a variety of conditions, eg, normal detrusor contraction with no associated sphincteric relaxation and normal detrusor contraction with sphincteric overactivity, which is more serious. These 2 entities are commonly referred to as **detrusor/sphincter dyssynergia.** If, with detrusor contraction, the sphincter does not relax and open up or (worse) if it becomes overactive, urine flow is obstructed, ie, flow rate is reduced and of abnormal pattern. Reduced flow rate may occur even with increased detrusor activity if the latter is not adequate to overcome sphincteric resistance.

So many variations are possible in the shape of the flow curve—no matter how accurately the flow is recorded in the patient's privacy or how often it is repeated to confirm abnormal findings—that it is beneficial to relate it to simultaneous recordings, such as of bladder pressure, pelvic floor electromyography, urethral pressure profile, or simply cinefluoroscopy. Nevertheless, by itself it can be one of the most valuable urodynamic studies undertaken to evaluate a specific type of voiding dysfunction. Flowmetry is not only of diagnostic value but is also valuable in follow-up studies and in deciding on treatment. In some cases, however, flowmetry alone does not provide enough data about the abnormality in the voiding mechanism. More information must then be obtained by evaluation of bladder function.

BLADDER FUNCTION

The basic features of normal bladder function are bladder capacity, sensation, accommodation, contractility, voluntary control, and response to drugs. All of them can be evaluated by cystometry. If all are within the normal range, bladder physiology can be assumed to be normal. Every evaluation of every entity has its own implication, and, before a definitive conclusion is reached, must be examined in the light of associated manifestations and findings.

Capacity, Accommodation, & Sensation

Cystometry can be done by either of 2 basic methods: (1) by physiologic filling with secreted urine and continuous recording of intravesical pressure throughout a voiding cycle—starting from an empty bladder and continuing until it is full, at which time the patient is asked to urinate; or (2) by filling the bladder with water and recording intravesical pressure against the volume introduced into the bladder. (Gas cystometry is now being used in some laboratories as a substitute for water cystometry. However, the results are so unreliable that the technic should be used only for preliminary screening. If gas cystometry reveals any abnormality, the results must be confirmed by water cystometry.)

With the first (physiologic filling) method, the assessment of bladder function is based on voided volume (assuming that the presence of residual urine has been ruled out). The second method permits accurate determination of the volume distending the bladder and of the pressures at each particular level of filling, yet it has inherent defects: Fluid is introduced rather than naturally secreted, and bladder filling occurs more rapidly than normal.

The cystometric curve obtained is the filling phase, which is recorded with progressive bladder filling and begins to show some change when the bladder reaches capacity. The first sensation of fullness and then the first desire to void are usually recorded during the filling phase. The curve itself, by relating the volume introduced to the pressure inside the bladder, shows bladder wall compliance to filling. A normal bladder has a capacity of 400–500 mL. The sensation of fullness becomes a desire to void when the bladder is filled to capacity. However, the bladder has a power of accommodation, ie, it can maintain an almost constant intraluminal pressure throughout its filling phase regardless of the volume of fluid present. This will directly influence compliance. As the bladder progressively accommodates larger volumes with no change in intraluminal pressure, the compliance values become higher (Compliance = Volume ÷ Pressure) (Fig 20–10).

Contractility & Voluntary Control

The bladder normally shows no evidence of contractility or activity during the filling phase. However, once it is filled to capacity and the desire to urinate is perceived by the subject, who then consciously allows urination to proceed, strong bladder contractions will occur and will be sustained until the bladder is empty. The individual can of course consciously inhibit detrusor contraction. Both of these aspects of voluntary detrusor

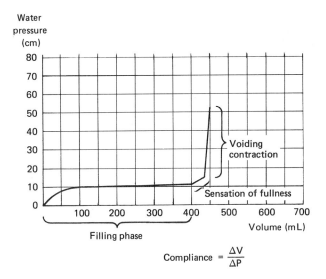

Figure 20–10. Cystometrogram of patient with normal bladder capacity. Note stable intravesical pressure during filling phase; slight rise at end of filling phase, indicating bladder capacity perceived as sense of fullness; and sharp rise at end (voiding contraction).

control must be assessed during cystometric study in order to rule out uninhibited bladder activity and to determine whether the patient can inhibit urination with a full bladder and initiate urination when asked to do so. The latter is occasionally difficult to verify clinically because of conscious inhibition by a patient who may be embarrassed by the unnatural circumstances.

Responses to Drugs

Drugs are being used with increasing frequency to evaluate detrusor function. They can help to diagnose underlying neuropathy and help determine whether drug treatment might be of value in individual cases. Study of the relationship of bladder capacity in a given patient to intravesical pressure and bladder contractility gives a rough evaluation of the patient's bladder function. Low intravesical pressure with normal bladder capacity might not be significant, whereas low pressure with a very large capacity might imply sensory loss or a flaccid lower motor neuron lesion, a chronically distended bladder, or a large bladder due to myogenic damage. High pressure (usually associated with reduced capacity) that rises rapidly with bladder filling is most commonly due to inflammation, enuresis, or reduced bladder capacity. However, uninhibited activity during this high-pressure filling phase might indicate neuropathic bladder or an upper motor neuron lesion.

The parasympathetic drug bethanechol chloride (Urecholine) is often used to assess bladder muscle function in patients with low bladder pressure associated with lack of detrusor contraction. No response to bethanechol suggests myogenic damage; a normal response indicates a bladder of

large capacity with normal musculature; and an exaggerated response indicates a lower motor neuron lesion. The test has so many variables that it must be done meticulously to give reliable results.

Testing with anticholinergics or muscle depressants may be of value in the evaluation of uninhibited detrusor contraction or increased bladder tonus and low compliance. Information obtained can be helpful in choosing drugs for treatment.

Recording of Intravesical Pressure

Intravesical pressure can be measured directly from the vesical cavity, either by a suprapubic approach or via a transurethral catheter. The pressure inside the bladder is actually a function of both intra-abdominal and intravesical pressure. Thus, true detrusor pressure is the pressure recorded from the bladder cavity minus intra-abdominal pressure. The point is important because variations in intra-abdominal pressure may influence the recorded intravesical pressure, which may then be mistaken for the force of detrusor contraction and not increased intra-abdominal pressure due to straining.

In clinical practice, it is not necessary to measure intra-abdominal pressure, since abdominal wall contraction can be observed during the course of cystometry. A notation in the patient's chart will serve to distinguish true detrusor contraction from possible overlap or increase in intra-abdominal pressure. When necessary—ie, in case of uncertainty and in order to be absolutely accurate—intra-abdominal pressure should be recorded simultaneously with intravesical pressure, since there is no other way to determine the true detrusor pressure. Intra-abdominal pressure is usually re-

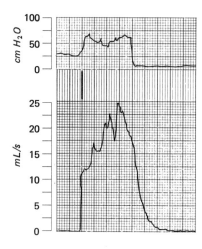

Figure 20–11. Simultaneous recording of voiding contraction and resulting flow rate. Note normal range of intravesical pressure during voiding phase as well as adequate normal flow rate (shown in Fig 20–4).

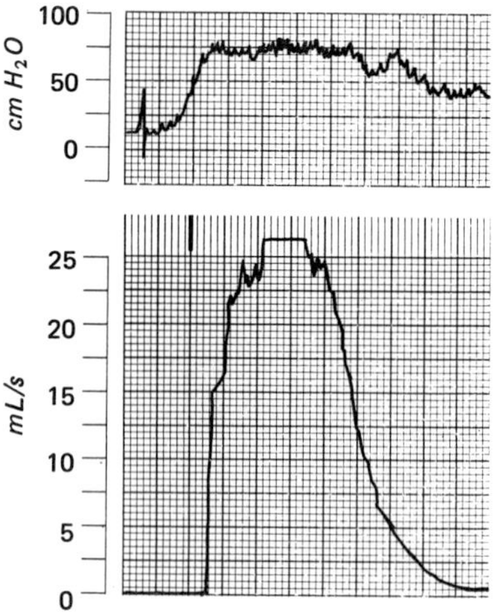

Figure 20–12. Recording of bladder pressure simultaneously with flow rate. Note slightly higher intravesical pressure with high flow rate which, at its maximum, is that of a supervoider (see Fig 20–3).

corded by a small balloon catheter inserted high in the rectum and connected to a separate transducer.

The most valuable part of the cystometric study is the determination of voiding activity or voiding contraction. The characteristics of intravesical pressure can be quite significant. Normally, voiding contractions are not high (20–40 cm of water); this magnitude of intravesical pressure is generally adequate to deliver a normal flow rate of 20–30 mL/s and completely empty the bladder if it is well sustained. A higher voiding pressure is indicative of possible increase in outlet resistance yet denotes an overactive, healthy detrusor musculature. Fig 20–11 shows a normal flow rate associated

with normal detrusor contraction at a magnitude of 20 cm of water that is well sustained and of short duration and results in complete bladder emptying.

The quality of bladder pressure can also be informative, even without simultaneous recording of flow rate. However, in such cases, it is preferable to record flow rate under normal circumstances. A well-sustained detrusor contraction, high at initiation and then well sustained at normal values, is seen in Fig 20–12. In Fig 20–13, the voiding pressure is too high—there is an element of sphincter dyssynergia triggering variations in voiding pressures and flow rate. Simultaneous recording of bladder and intra-abdominal pressures would pro-

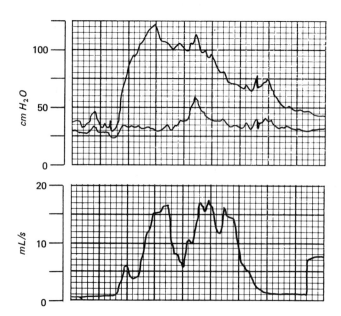

Figure 20–13. Simultaneous recording of flow rate and intra-abdominal pressure; intravesical pressure overlap in top recording. Note very high voiding pressure. However, flow rate is relatively low, with some interruption most likely due to sphincteric overactivity.

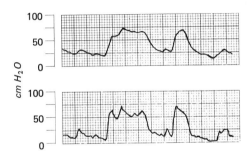

Figure 20–14. Simultaneous recording of intra-abdominal and intravesical pressures. If one considers only top recording of intravesical pressure, one might assume adequate detrusor contraction. Comparison with intra-abdominal pressure in lower recording shows that they are almost identical and that there is no detrusor contraction at all.

Table 20–1. Causes of reduced or increased bladder capacity. (Normal capacity in adults is 400–500 mL.)

Causes of reduced bladder capacity
Enuresis or incontinence
Bladder infections
Bladder contractions due to fibrosis (from tuberculosis, interstitial cystitis, etc)
Upper motor neuron lesions
Defunctionalized bladder
Postsurgical bladder
Causes of increased bladder capacity*
Sensory neuropathic disorders
Lower motor neuron lesions
Megacystis (congenital)
Chronic urinary tract obstruction

*Most such patients are women.

vide more information. As suggested above, the pressure curve of the intravesical pressure is not as accurate as may be required, and increased intra-abdominal pressure might be mistaken for detrusor action. This is illustrated in Fig 20–14: The bladder pressure appears to indicate good detrusor function; nevertheless, simultaneous recording of intra-abdominal pressure makes it clear that all of the apparent changes in vesical intraluminal pressure in fact represent variations in intra-abdominal pressure.

Fig 20–15 shows the 2 pressures recorded on the same chart, with the same channel, by having the writing pen share the time between 2 transducers—one recording intra-abdominal pressure while the other records intravesical pressure.

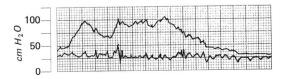

Figure 20–15. Simultaneous recording of a single channel for 2 parameters—intra-abdominal pressure and intravesical pressure. The difference between the 2 can be clearly seen as pure detrusor contraction.

A. Pathologic Changes in Bladder Capacity:

The normal bladder capacity of 400–500 mL can be reduced in a variety of disorders and lesions (Table 20–1). Some common causes are enuresis, urinary tract infection, contracted bladder, upper motor neuron lesion, and defunctionalized bladder. Reduced bladder capacity also occurs in association with some cases of incontinence and in postsurgical bladder. Increased bladder capacity is not uncommon in women who have trained themselves to retain large volumes of urine. Bladder capacity is increased also in sensory neuropathic disorders,

lower motor neuron lesions, and chronic obstruction from myogenic damage. It is important to relate bladder capacity to the vesical intraluminal pressure (Table 20–2). Slight variations in bladder capacity with no change in bladder pressure might be of less significance than the reverse. What is usually of greatest interest is the bladder with reduced capacity associated with normal pressure or, more significantly, with increased pressure, or the bladder with large capacity associated with decreased pressure.

B. Pathologic Changes in Accommodation:

Accommodation reflects intraluminal pressure in response to filling. In a bladder with normal power of accommodation—in which case the micturition center of the spinal cord is controlled by the central nervous system—intraluminal pressure will not vary with progressive bladder filling until capacity is reached. However, whenever detrusor tonicity is increased—or, in other words, when compliance is reduced—there will be progressive increase in intraluminal pressure and loss of accommodation; this usually occurs at smaller volumes and with reduced capacity. The patient being studied by cystometry

Table 20–2. Relationship between intravesical pressure and capacity in various diseases.

Low intravesical pressure
Normal capacity
Large capacity
Sensory deficits (diabetes mellitus, tabes dorsalis)
Flaccid lower motor neuron lesions
Large bladder (due to repeated stretching)
High intravesical pressure
Rapidly rising
Reduced capacity
Inflammation
Enuresis
Uninhibited contraction
Uninhibited neurogenic bladder
Upper motor neuron lesions

can always note the presence or absence of a sensation of fullness. One normally does not sense volumes in the bladder but only changes in pressure.

C. Pathologic Changes in Sensation: A slight rise in intraluminal pressure on cystometry signifies that the bladder is full to normal capacity and that the patient is perceiving it. This sign is usually absent in pure sensory neuropathy and in mixed sensory and motor loss. (Other sensations can be tested for in different ways; see Chapter 19.)

D. Pathologic Changes in Contractility: The bladder is normally capable of sustaining contraction until it is empty. Absence of residual urine after voiding usually denotes well-sustained contractions. Neuropathic dysfunction is usually associated with residual urine of variable amount depending on the type of dysfunction. Significant outlet resistance—mechanical or functional—is also a cause of residual urine.

Cystometric study may disclose complete absence of detrusor contractility due to motor or sensory deficits, or the patient may consciously inhibit detrusor activity (Table 20–3). Detrusor hyperactivity is shown as uninhibited activity, usually due to interruption of the neural connection between spinal cord centers and the higher midbrain and cortical centers.

Table 20–3. Variations in detrusor contractility in various diseases.

Normal contractions
  Normal volume
  Well sustained
Absent or weak contractions
  Sensory neuropathic disorders
  Conscious inhibition of contractions
  Lower motor neuron lesions
Uninhibited contractions
  Upper motor neuron lesions
  Cerebrovascular lesions

An integrated picture of bladder capacity, intraluminal pressure, and contractility serves as a general assessment of the basic physiologic mechanisms of the bladder. Low intravesical pressure in a patient with normal bladder capacity may have no clinical significance, whereas low pressure with a very large capacity may signify sensory loss or a flaccid lower motor neuron lesion, a chronically distended bladder, or a large bladder from myogenic damage. High pressure (usually associated with reduced capacity) that rises rapidly with bladder filling is most commonly associated with inflammation, enuresis, or actually reduced bladder capacity. However, uninhibited activity during the interval of rising pressure that occurs with bladder filling may indicate a neurogenic bladder or an upper motor neuron lesion.

SPHINCTERIC FUNCTION

Urinary sphincteric function can be evaluated either by recording the electromyographic activity of the voluntary component of the sphincteric mechanism or by recording the activity of both smooth and voluntary components by measuring the intraluminal pressure of the sphincteric unit. The latter method is called pressure profile measurement (profilometry).

Profilometry

The urethral pressure profile is determined by recording the pressure in the urethra at every level of the sphincteric unit from the internal meatus to the end of the sphincteric segment. Profilometry can be done by the gas or water perfusion technic, the membrane catheter technic, or the microtransducer catheter technic. The perfusion methods of urethral pressure profile recording were first introduced by Brown and Whitcomb. The catheter is perfused either with gas (usually CO_2) or with water or saline solution at a fixed flow rate. The measurement is actually that of the escaped pressure, which will permit the flow of either the gas or the fluid.

Gas profilometry requires a very high flow rate (120–150 mL/min) and is mentioned only to be condemned. The results are inaccurate, often misleading, and not reproducible, and the information it provides is extremely limited. **Water perfusion** requires much smaller flow rates of about 2 mL/min. It is much more accurate than gas profilometry, but the test lacks sensitivity and is less consistent, less reproducible, and less accurate than the 2 methods discussed below.

A. Membrane Catheter Technic: Membrane catheters used for recording pressure profiles usually have several channels, so that several parameters can be obtained simultaneously. Our current membrane catheter has 4 lumens and an outside diameter of 7F; 2 of its 4 lumens are open at the end—one for bladder filling and the other for recording bladder pressure; the 2 remaining ones—at 7 and 8 cm, respectively, from the catheter tip—are covered by a thin membrane with a small chamber underneath (Fig 20–16). The space under the membrane and the lumen connected to it are filled with fluid, free of any gas, and connected to a pressure transducer. The pressure under this membrane should be zero at the level of the transducer, so it can register any pressure applied to the membrane whatever its level at any particular time. The catheter also has radiopaque markers at 1-cm intervals starting at the tip, with a heavier marker every 5 cm; it also has a special marker showing the site of each membrane. The markers permit fluoroscopic visualization of the catheter and the membrane levels during the entire study.

B. Microtransducer Technic: This technic is as accurate as that of the membrane catheter. Two

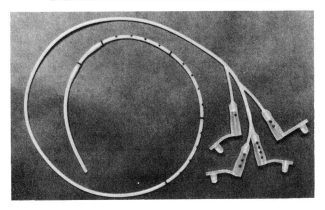

Figure 20–16. Membrane catheter showing radiopaque markers. Note 2 membrane chambers for urethral pressure measurements and 4 separate channels, each of which is connected to a separate ending—2 channels for urethral pressure recording, one for bladder pressure recording, and one for bladder filling. (Reproduced, with permission, from Tanagho EA, Jonas U: Membrane catheter: Effective for recording pressure in lower urinary tract. *Urology* 1977;10:173.)

microtransducers can be mounted on the same catheter, one at the tip for recording of bladder pressure and the other about 5–7 cm from the tip to record the urethral pressure profile as the catheter is gradually withdrawn from the bladder cavity to below the sphincteric segment.

Electromyographic Study of Sphincteric Function

Electromyography alone gives useful information about sphincteric function, but it is most valuable when done in conjunction with cystometry. There are several technics for electromyographic studies of the urinary sphincter—essentially by surface electrodes or by needle electrodes. Surface electrode recordings can be obtained either from the lumen of the urethra in the region of the voluntary sphincter or, preferably, from the anal sphincter by using an anal plug electrode. Recording via needle electrodes can be obtained from the anal sphincter; from the bulk of the musculature of the pelvic floor; or from the external sphincter itself, though the placement is difficult and the accuracy of the results is questionable.

Direct needle electromyography of the urethral sphincter provides the most accurate information. However, because the technic is difficult, simpler approaches are generally used. The anal sphincter is readily accessible for electromyographic testing, and testing of any area of the pelvic floor musculature will generally reflect the overall electrical activity of the pelvic floor, including the external sphincter. Electromyography is not a simple technic, and the assistance of an experienced electromyographer is probably essential. Electromyographic study makes use of the electrical activity which is constantly present within the pelvic floor and external urinary sphincter at rest and which increases progressively with bladder filling. If the bladder contracts for voiding, electrical activity ceases completely, permitting free flow of urine, and is resumed at the termination of detrusor contraction to secure closure of the bladder outlet (Fig 20–17). Electromyography is important in showing this effect and, along with bladder pressure measurement, can pinpoint the exact time of detrusor contraction. Persistence of electromyographic activity during the phase of detrusor contraction for voiding—or, even worse, its overactivity during that phase—interferes with the voiding mechanism and leads to incoordination between detrusor and sphincter (**detrusor/sphincter dyssynergia**). During the interval of detrusor contraction, both increased and absent electromyographic activity interfere with the free flow of urine, as can be shown by simultaneous recording of flow rate.

Electromyographic recording shows only the activity of the voluntary component of the urinary sphincteric mechanism, as well as pelvic floor func-

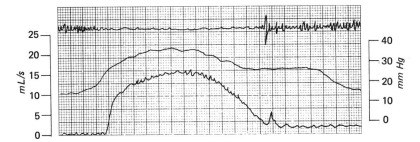

Figure 20–17. Simultaneous recording of bladder pressure and flow rate and electromyography of anal sphincter. With rise in bladder pressure for voiding, start of flow rate has a smooth, continuous, bell-shaped curve. Note also complete absence of electromyographic activity of the anal sphincter throughout the voiding act.

tion. More information is gained when it is recorded simultaneously with detrusor pressure or flow rate. However, it gives no information about the smooth component of the urinary sphincter.

Pressure Measurement for Evaluation of Sphincteric Function

The perfusion technics are adequate for screening purposes in patients with incontinence or functional obstruction. However, the membrane catheter and microtransducer technics give more detailed information.

The simple pressure profile obtained by the perfusion technic will evaluate the maximum pressure within the sphincteric segment, usually with the bladder empty and the patient supine. The pressure profile enables one to quantitate the maximum pressure within the urethra and, more importantly, the **maximum closure pressure,** ie, the difference between bladder pressure and urethral pressure. For that reason, simultaneous recording of bladder pressure will always give a more meaningful urethral pressure profile. It is the difference between the 2 pressures that is most important in evaluating the activity of the sphincteric unit and its responses to various factors.

A. Total Pressure and Closure Pressure: The urethral pressure profile recording will show the closure pressure along the entire length of the urethra from internal to external meatus. Two values are registered: the total pressure (ie, the pressure directly recorded within the urethral lumen) and the urethral closure pressure (ie, the difference between the intravesical pressure and the pressure in the urethral canal). The latter, of course, is the more important. The virtue of the multiple channel is that it can simultaneously record both pressures in both the membrane catheter and microtransducer technics (but not by perfusion technics). From the simplest pressure profile obtained via the membrane catheter or microtransducer, at least 4 distinct parameters can be determined (Fig 20–18): (1) the maximum pressure exerted around the sphincteric segment, (2) the net closure pressure of the urethra, (3) the distribution of this closure pressure along the entire sphincteric length, and (4) the exact functional length of the sphincteric unit and its relation to the anatomic length.

B. Distribution of Closure Pressure: As the catheter is withdrawn down the urethra, it will record the closure pressure at various levels along the entire length of the sphincteric segment.

C. Functional Length of the Sphincteric Unit: The functional length of the sphincteric unit is that portion with positive closure pressure, ie, where urethral pressure is greater than bladder pressure. The distinction between anatomic length and functional length is important. Regardless of the anatomic length, the effectiveness of the urethral sphincter may be limited to a shorter segment. In women, the normal pressure profile is rather low at

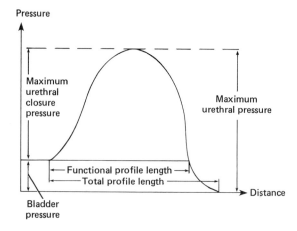

Figure 20–18. Urethral pressure profile and its components. Note functional length, anatomic length, and the shape of the profile, with maximum closure pressure in the middle segment of the urethra rather than at the level of the internal meatus. (Reproduced, with permission, from Bradley W: Cystometry and sphincter electromyography. *Mayo Clin Proc* 1976;**329**:335.)

the level of the internal meatus but builds up gradually until it reaches its maximum in the mid urethra, where the voluntary sphincter is concentrated; it slowly drops until it is at its lowest at the external meatus. With these measurements, it is clear that the anatomic and functional lengths of the normal urethra in women are about the same and that the maximum closure pressure is at about the center of the urethra—not at the level of the internal meatus. In adult men, the pressure profile is slightly different: The functional length is longer, and the maximum closure pressure builds up in the prostatic segment, reaches a peak in the membranous urethra, and drops as it reaches the level of the bulbous urethra (Fig 20–19). The entire functional length in men is about 6–7 cm; in women, it is about 4 cm.

Dynamic Changes in Pressure Profile

The usefulness of the pressure profile is enhanced by noting the sphincteric responses to various physiologic stimuli: (1) postural changes (supine, sitting, standing); (2) changes in intra-abdominal pressure (sharp increase with coughing; sustained increase with bearing down); (3) voluntary contractions of the pelvic floor musculature to assess activity of the voluntary sphincter; and (4) bladder filling. The latter test consists of making baseline recordings with both an empty bladder and a full bladder and comparing those values with recordings made under conditions of stress (coughing, bearing down) and voluntary contraction with an empty bladder and a full bladder.

A simple pressure profile is informative but does not provide data that will delineate and identify specific sites of sphincteric dysfunction. The

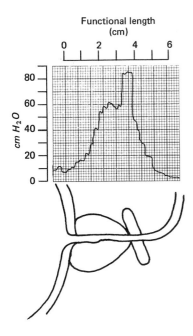

Figure 20–19. Normal male urethral pressure profile showing progressive rise throughout prostatic segment and peak being reached in membranous urethra. (Reproduced, with permission, from Tanagho EA: Membrane and microtransducer catheters: Their effectiveness for profilometry of the lower urinary tract. *Urol Clin North Am* 1979;**6**:110.)

advantage of a membrane catheter or microtransducer is that the pressure profile can be spread along a longer segment by slowing the process of withdrawal and speeding up the motion of the recording paper. Since the catheter can be held at different levels for any length of time, other parameters can be measured and their effects monitored. Response to stress (particularly when standing), response to bladder distention, response to changes in position, the effects of drugs, and the effects of nerve stimulation—all can be evaluated if needed. Bladder filling normally leads to increase in tonus of the sphincteric element, with some rise in closure pressure, especially when bladder filling approaches maximum capacity. Stress from coughing or straining also normally results in sustained or increased closure pressure (Fig 20–20). When the standing position is assumed, closure pressure is usually substantially increased (Fig 20–21). Testing for activity of the voluntary sphincter by the hold maneuver (asking the patient to actively contract the perineal muscles) shows a significant rise in urethral pressure (Fig 20–22). When all of these parameters are recorded concomitantly with in-

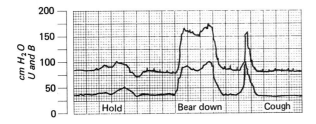

Figure 20–20. Simultaneous recording of intraurethral and intravesical pressures and of responses to coughing and bearing down. Rise in intravesical pressure as a result of increase in intra-abdominal pressure is associated with simultaneous rise in intraurethral pressure, maintaining a constant closure pressure.

Figure 20–21. Urethral pressure profile of normal woman in sitting and standing positions. Note marked improvement in closure pressure (in both functional length and magnitude) when patient stands up. (Reproduced, with permission, from Tanagho EA: Urodynamics of female urinary incontinence with emphasis on stress incontinence. *J Urol* 1979;**122**:200.)

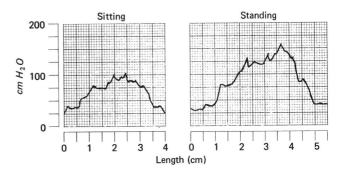

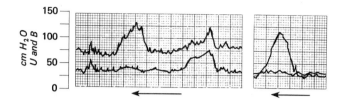

Figure 20–22. *Right:* Urethral pressure profile in normal range. *Left:* Main point of effect of hold maneuver is significant increase in closure pressure of urethra without change in bladder pressure—act of voluntary sphincter.

travesical pressure, they can be interrelated and the exact closure pressure at any given time can be ascertained.

The response to stress with the patient standing should usually be recorded also. Especially in cases of stress incontinence, weakness of the sphincteric mechanism may not be apparent with the patient sitting or supine but becomes clear when the patient stands up.

The effectiveness of drugs in increasing or reducing the urethral pressure profile can be tested also. Administering phenoxybenzamine (Regitine) and then recording the urethral pressure profile is an example. A rising pressure will establish the possible effectiveness of alpha-blockers as a means of increasing urethral resistance, with obvious implications for the management of urinary incontinence. Anticholinergic drugs such as propantheline bromide can be tested for possible use as detrusor depressants. Detrusor activity can be investigated by administering bethanechol chloride (Urecholine) along with simultaneous recordings of bladder and urethral pressures.

Characteristics of the Normal Pressure Profile (Fig 20–23)

The basic features of the ideal pressure profile are not easily defined. In women, the normal urethral pressure profile has a peak of 100–150 cm of water, and the closure pressure is in the range of 90–100 cm of water. Closure pressure is lowest at the level of the internal meatus, gradually builds up in the proximal 0.5 cm, and reaches its maximum about 1 cm below the internal meatus. It is sustained for another 2 cm and then starts to drop in the distal urethra. The functional length of a normal

adult female urethra is about 4 cm. The response to stress with coughing and bearing down is sustained or augmented closure pressure. Standing up also increases this pressure, with maximum rise in the mid segment. Nervous stimulation is rarely tested in normal subjects, but sacral root stimulation can reveal the closure pressure in the voluntary element of the sphincteric segment of the urethra.

Pressure Profile in Certain Pathologic Entities

A. Urinary Stress Incontinence: The classic pressure changes noted in this type of incontinence are as follows:

1. Low urethral closure pressure.

2. Short urethral functional length at the expense of the proximal segment.

3. Weak responses to stress.

4. Loss of urethral closure pressure with bladder filling.

5. Fall in closure pressure upon assuming the upright position.

6. Weak responses to stress in the upright position.

B. Urinary Urge Incontinence: The most pertinent pressure changes in this type of incontinence are normal or high closure pressures with normal responses to stress, normal responses to bladder filling, and normal responses when the upright position is assumed. Urge incontinence can result from any of the following mechanisms (Fig 20–24).

1. Detrusor hyperirritability, with active detrusor contractions overcoming urethral resistance and leading to urine leakage.

2. The exact reverse, ie, a constant detrusor pressure with no evidence of detrusor instability, but urethral instability in that urethral pressure

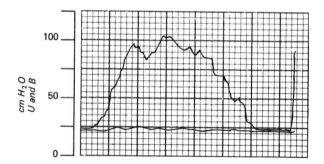

Figure 20–23. Recording of normal female urethral pressure profile, showing basic features and actual values, anatomic as well as functional length. (Reproduced, with permission, from Tanagho EA: Membrane and microtransducer catheters: Their effectiveness for profilometry of the lower urinary tract. *Urol Clin North Am* 1979;6:110.)

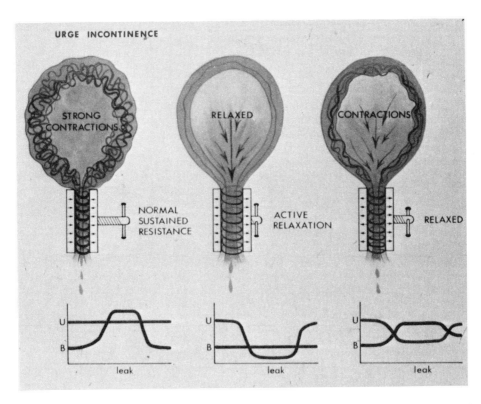

Figure 20–24. Three mechanisms of urinary urge incontinence. *A:* Normal sphincter activity exceeded by hyperactive detrusor. *B:* Normal detrusor, without any overactivity, yet unstable urethra with marked drop in urethral pressure leading to leakage. *C:* Most common combination—some rise in intravesical pressure due to detrusor hyperirritability associated with drop in urethral pressure due to sphincteric relaxation.

becomes less than bladder pressure, so that urine leakage occurs without any detrusor contraction.

3. A combination of the above (the most common form), ie, some drop in closure pressure and some rise in bladder pressure. In such cases, the drop in urethral pressure is often the initiating factor.

C. Combination of Stress and Urge Incontinence: In this common clinical condition, profilometry is used to determine the magnitude of each component, ie, whether primarily urge, primarily stress, or both equally. As a guide to treatment, profilometric studies sometimes show that stress incontinence precipitates urge incontinence. The stress elements initiate urine leakage in the proximal urethra, exciting detrusor response and sphincteric relaxation and ending with complete urine leakage. Once the stress components are corrected, the urge element disappears. This combination cannot be detected clinically.

D. Postprostatectomy Incontinence: After prostatectomy, there is usually no positive pressure in the entire prostatic fossa; minimal closure pressure at the apex of the prostate; and normal or greater than normal pressure within the voluntary sphincteric segment of the membranous urethra. It is the functional length of the sphincteric segment above the genitourinary diaphragm that determines the degree of incontinence. The magnitude of closure in the voluntary sphincteric segment has no bearing on the patient's symptoms. High pressure is almost always recorded within the voluntary sphincter, despite the common belief that what someone termed "iatrogenically induced incontinence" is due to damage to the voluntary sphincter—which is definitely not the case.

E. Detrusor/Sphincter Dyssynergia: In this situation, findings of cystometric studies are normal at the filling phase, with possible closure pressure above average. However, the pathologic entity becomes clear when the patient attempts to void: Detrusor contraction is associated with a simultaneous increase in urethral closure pressure instead of a drop in pressure. This is a direct effect of overactivity of the voluntary component, leading to obstructive voiding or low flow rate and frequent interruption of voiding. This phenomenon is commonly seen in supraspinal lesions. It can be encountered in several other conditions as well.

VALUE OF SIMULTANEOUS RECORDINGS

Measurement of each of the physiologic variables described above gives useful clinical information. A rise in intravesical pressure has greater significance when related to intra-abdominal pressure. The urine flow rate is more significant if recorded in conjunction with the total volume voided as well as with evidence of detrusor contraction. The urethral pressure profile is more significant when related to bladder pressure and to variations in intra-abdominal pressure and voluntary muscular activity. And for greatest clinical usefulness, all parameters must be recorded simultaneously, thus enabling the investigator to analyze the activity involved in each sequence.

A proper urodynamic study should at a minimum include recordings of bladder pressure, intra-abdominal pressure (true detrusor), urethral pressure or electromyography, flow rate, and, if possible, voided volume. For a complete study, the following are necessary: intra-abdominal pressure, intravesical pressure, urethral sphincteric pressure at various (usually 2) levels, flow rate, voided volume, anal sphincter pressure (as a function of pelvic floor activity), and electromyography of the anal or urethral striated sphincter. These physiologic data are recorded with the patient quiet as well as during activity—ie, voluntary increase in intra-abdominal pressure, or changes in the state of bladder filling, or voluntary contraction of perineal muscles, or, more comprehensively, an entire voiding act starting from an empty bladder to a completely full bladder to initiation of voiding and continuing until the bladder is empty.

The data derived from urodynamic study are descriptive of urinary tract function. Visualization of the lower urinary tract simultaneously with mul-

tiple recordings gives more precise information about the pathologic changes underlying the symptoms. By means of cinefluoroscopy, the examiner can observe the configuration of the bladder, bladder base, and bladder outlet during bladder filling (usually with radiopaque medium). The information obtained can then be correlated with the level of catheters, of pressure recordings, and changes in pelvic floor support during voiding. Combined cinefluoroscopy and pressure measurements thus represent the ultimate in urodynamic studies.

A model of such a urodynamic laboratory has been developed at the University of California School of Medicine. As shown in Fig 20–25, the patient sits in a specially designed toilet chair over a device for collecting urine and measuring flow rate. The patient faces the x-ray tube that receives the image of the bladder and bladder outlet, to be projected on a fluoroscopic screen. The pressure-recording catheters are connected to a set of transducers, in turn connected to a polygraph recording machine, on top of which a television camera is mounted. On a separate television monitor, the image of the pressure recording is combined with the image from the fluoroscopic monitor. A permanent record can be obtained by videotape or movie camera.

The product of such a study is then recorded on the chart as well as on motion picture film or videotape. Sound can usually be added to the film or the videotape to record the history as well as the examiner's observations and instructions during the study and to translate pressure measurements into

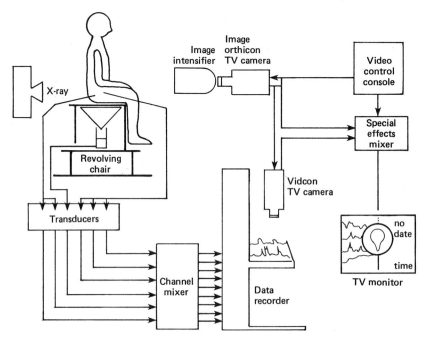

Figure 20–25. Urodynamic laboratory with specially designed toilet chair where patient sits between x-ray tube and image intensifier. A television camera records the fluoroscopic image, and a second camera picks up recordings from a polygraph machine to be projected onto one television monitor, photographed, and recorded on videotape.

sound so they can be followed from outside the examination room.

Several recording machines are available for urodynamic study. Some of them are simple, limited to one or 2 channels; more complex machines may have as many as 8 channels. Each type is designed to meet a particular need of the investigator or institution. The needs in private practice are quite different from those of a large institution or referral center for complex urologic problems, especially neuropathic dysfunctions. In our laboratory we have developed a series of pressure-recording units from a single-channel instrument to a 4-channel instrument. Every channel is capable of recording 2 parameters, so that the single-channel machine represents in reality 2 channels and the 4-channel machine represents eight. Pressure recordings are obtained with an 8-channel machine (Fig 20–26). Six such parameters are bladder pressure, 2 urethral pressures, rectal pressure, flow rate, and total volume voided; and 2 additional parameters (not shown) are anal sphincter pressure and electromyogram. The ability to use every channel to record 2 simultaneous parameters allows the

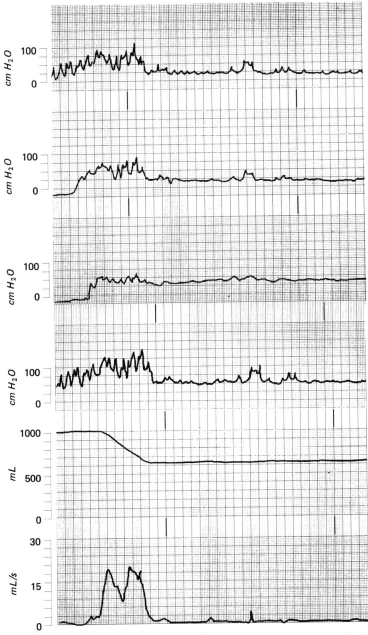

Figure 20–26. Simultaneous pressure recordings, showing bladder pressure followed by proximal urethral pressure, then midurethral pressure, then intra-abdominal pressure, and total volume voided as well as flow rate.

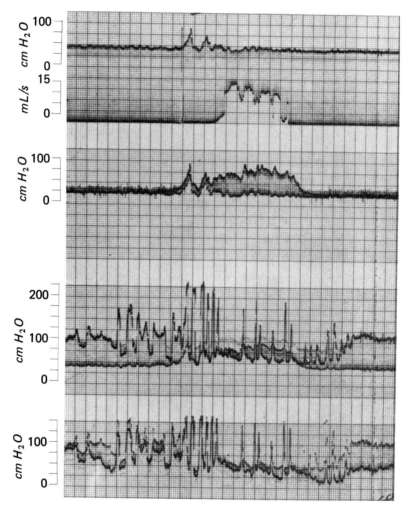

Figure 20–27. Eight parameters recorded on 4-channel unit, in which each pen is writing 2 parameters. *Top channel:* Flow rate and intra-abdominal pressure. *Second channel:* Combination of bladder pressure and intra-abdominal pressure, the difference between the 2 showing true detrusor contraction pressure. *Third channel:* Combination of bladder pressure and maximum urethral pressure, the difference between the 2 showing urethral closure pressure. *Bottom channel:* Anal sphincter pressure and midurethral pressure as a function of overall perineal activity. Any combination can be set on such a machine.

investigator to record intra-abdominal pressure and bladder pressure overlapped, so that the net detrusor pressure is recorded. Finally, anal sphincteric pressure and midurethral pressure are recorded so that the reflection of each on the other is also readily seen (Fig 20–27).

The complete recording machine has 4 channels and an attached set of transducers. Mounted on top of this machine is the television camera. In the upper left-hand corner, a readout indicates the volume of flow infused into the bladder during filling and the volume voided during emptying. Within the machine is a pump for infusion and bladder filling, with variable speeds—usually 25–50 mL/min—and a switch that can automatically limit the total volume infused (between 25 and 1000 mL, depending on the age of the patient and bladder capacity). Finally, there is an assembly for the recording of the volume voided, the flow rate, and, at the same time, the volume infused into the bladder. In a modification of the machine, a speaker is attached to one of the transducers to transform pressure into sound, so that any increase or decrease in pressure and any variation due to any activity can be amplified by the speaker, each in a different tone. The machine is portable and can be rolled anywhere, to a bedside or into an operating theater. It can also be attached to the cinefluoroscopic machine.

• • •

References

Urethra & Bladder

Abrams PH: Perfusion urethral profilometry. *Urol Clin North Am* 1979;6:103.

Abrams PH, Martin S, Griffiths DJ: The measurement and interpretation of urethral pressures obtained by the method of Brown and Wickham. *Br J Urol* 1978;50:33.

Andersen JT, Bradley WE: Urethral pressure profilometry: Assessment of urethral function by combined intraurethral pressure and EMG recording. *Urol Int* 1978;33:40.

Awad SA & others: Urethral pressure profile in female stress incontinence. *J Urol* 1978;120:475.

Bruschini H, Schmidt RA, Tanagho EA: Effect of urethral stretch on urethral pressure profile. *Invest Urol* 1977;15:107.

Bruschini H, Schmidt RA, Tanagho EA: The male genitourinary sphincter mechanism in the dog. *Invest Urol* 1978;15:288.

Bruskewitz R, Raz S: Urethral pressure profile using microtip catheter in females. *Urology* 1979;14:303.

Drutz HP, Mandel F: Urodynamic analysis of urinary incontinence symptoms in women. *Am J Obstet Gynecol* 1979;134:789.

Erlandson B-E, Fall M: Urethral pressure profile studies by two different microtip transducers and an open catheter system. *Urol Int* 1978;33:79.

Gershon CR, Diokno AC: Urodynamic evaluation of female stress urinary incontinence. *J Urol* 1978;119:787.

Gilmour RF & others: Analysis of the urethral pressure profile using a mechanical model. *Invest Urol* 1980;18:54.

Godec CJ, Cass AS: Comparison of pressure measurement in lower urinary and lower fecal pathways. *J Urol* 1980;123:58.

Graber P, Laurent G, Tanagho EA: Effect of abdominal pressure rise on the urethral profile: An experimental study on dogs. *Invest Urol* 1974;12:57.

Hakky SI: A new self-retaining catheter with triple microtip pressure transducer: The Baghdad modification. *Br J Urol* 1978;50:535.

Henriksson L, Andersson K-E, Ulmsten U: The urethral pressure profiles in continence and stress-incontinent women. *Scand J Urol Nephrol* 1979;13:5.

Henriksson L, Aspelin P, Ulmsten U: Combined urethrocystometry and cinefluorography in continent and incontinent women. *Radiology* 1979;130:607.

Hurt WG, Fantl JA: Direct electronic urethrocystometry. *Clin Obstet Gynecol* 1978;21:695.

Jonas U, Hohenfellner R: Which anatomical structures in fact achieve urinary continence? *Urol Int* 1978;33:199.

Jonas U, Klotter HJ: Study of three urethral pressure recording devices: Theoretical considerations. *Urol Res* 1978;6:119.

Lindstrom K, Ulmsten U: Some methodological aspects on the measurement of intraluminal pressures in the female urogenital tract in vivo. *Acta Obstet Gynecol Scand* 1978;57:63.

McGuire EJ, Brady S: Detrusor-sphincter dyssynergia. *J Urol* 1979;121:774.

Mayo ME, Ansell JS: Urodynamic assessment of incontinence after prostatectomy. *J Urol* 1979;122:60.

Meunier P, Mollard P: Urethral pressure profile in children: A comparison between perfused catheters and microtransducers, and a study of the usefulness of urethral pressure profile measurements in children. *J Urol* 1978;120:207.

Obrink A, Bunne G, Ingelman-Sundberg A: Pressure transmission to the preurethral space in stress incontinence. *Urol Res* 1978;6:135.

Obrink A, Bunne G, Ingelman-Sundberg A: The urethral pressure profile in urge incontinence before and after unilateral blockade of the inferior hypogastric plexus. *Urol Int* 1978;33:107.

Robertson JR: Gynecologic urology. 2. Gas urethroscopy with pressure studies. *Clin Obstet Gynaecol* 1978;5:39.

Rossier AB & others: Urodynamics in spinal shock patients. *J Urol* 1979;122:783.

Schmidt RA, Witherow R, Tanagho EA: Recording urethral pressure profile. *Urology* 1977;10:390.

Schmidt RA & others: Urethral pressure profilometry with membrane catheter compared with perfusion catheter systems. *Urol Int* 1978;33:345.

Tanagho EA: Interpretation of the physiology of micturition. Pages 18–45 in: *Hydrodynamics*. Hinman F Jr (editor). Thomas, 1971.

Tanagho EA: Membrane and microtransducer catheters: Their effectiveness for profilometry of the lower urinary tract. *Urol Clin North Am* 1979;6:110.

Tanagho EA: Neurophysiology of urinary incontinence. Pages 31–60 in: *Female Urinary Stress Incontinence*. Cantor EB (editor). Thomas, 1979.

Tanagho EA: Pathophysiology of incontinence: Anatomical and functional considerations. In: *Proceedings of Symposium of Myelomeningocele*. Cincinnati, 1976.

Tanagho EA: Urinary stress incontinence. *Urol Arch (Belgrade)* 1977;8:17.

Tanagho EA: Urodynamics of female urinary stress incontinence with emphasis on stress incontinence. *J Urol* 1979;122:200.

Tanagho EA: Vesicourethral dynamics. Pages 215–236 in: *Urodynamics*. Lutzeyer W, Melchior H (editors). Springer-Verlag, 1974.

Tanagho EA, Jonas U: Membrane catheter: Effective for recording pressure in lower urinary tract. *Urology* 1977;10:173.

Tanagho EA, Meyers FH, Smith DR: Urethral resistance: Its components and implications. 2. Striated muscle component. *Invest Urol* 1969;7:136.

Tanagho EA, Miller ER: Functional considerations of urethral sphincteric dynamics. *J Urol* 1973;109:273.

Teague CT, Merrill DC: Comparative study of air and water measurements of peak and stabilized static urethral pressures. *Urology* 1978;12:481.

Teague CT, Merrill DC: Laboratory comparison of urethral profilometry techniques. *Urology* 1979;13:221.

Toguri AG & others: Parameters of gas urethral pressure profiles: Part 1. *J Urol* 1979;122:195.

Ulmsten U, Hok B, Lindstrom K: Aspects of present and future possibilities for intraluminal pressure recordings in the urogenital tract. *Acta Pharmacol Toxicol (Kbh)* 1978;43:41.

van Gool JD, Schmidt RA, Tanagho EA: Development of reflex activity of detrusor and striated sphincter muscles in experimental paraplegia. *Urol Int* 1978;33:293.

Woodside JR, McGuire EJ: A simple inexpensive urodynamic catheter. *J Urol* 1979;122:788.

Yalla SV & others: Striated sphincter participation in distal passive urinary continence mechanisms: Studies in male subjects deprived of proximal sphincter mechanism. *J Urol* 1979;**122**:655.

Urinary Flow

Abrams P, Torrens M: Urine flow studies. *Urol Clin North Am* 1979;**6**:71.

Drach GW, Ignatoff J, Layton T: Peak urinary flow rate: Observation in female subjects and comparison to male subjects. *J Urol* 1979;**122**:215.

Drach GW, Layton TN, Binard WJ: Male peak urinary flow rate: Relationships to volume and age. *J Urol* 1979;**122**:210.

Kondo A, Mitsuya H, Torii H: Computer analysis of micturition parameters and accuracy of uroflowmeter. *Urol Int* 1978;**33**:337.

Koppler PJ, Bruijnes E: Experience with a newly developed automatic uroflowmeter. *Urol Int* 1979;**34**:114.

Nyman CR, Boman J, Gidlof A: Von Garrelts' uroflowmeter: A technical evaluation. *Urol Int* 1979;**34**:184.

Siroky MB, Olsson CA, Krane RJ: The flow rate nomogram. 1. Development. *J Urol* 1979;**122**:665.

Siroky MB, Olsson CA, Krane RJ: The flow rate nomogram. 2. Clinical correlation. *J Urol* 1980;**23**:208.

Stubbs AJ, Resnic MI: Office uroflowmetry using maximum flow rate purge meter. *J Urol* 1979;**122**:62.

Tanagho EA, McCurry E: Pressure and flow rate as related to lumen caliber and entrance configuration. *J Urol* 1971;**105**:583.

Electromyography

DiBenedetto M, Yalla SV: Electrodiagnosis of striated urethral sphincter dysfunction. *J Urol* 1979;**122**:361.

Girard R & others: Anal and urethral sphincter electromyography in spinal cord injured patients. *Paraplegia* 1978;**16**:244.

King DG: Anal stimulating electrodes in electromyography. *Urology* 1979;**13**:345.

King DG, Teague CT: Choice of electrode in electromyography of external urethral and anal sphincter. *J Urol* 1980;**124**:75.

Urodynamic Testing

Blaivas JG & others: Cystometric response to propantheline in detrusor hyperreflexia: Therapeutic implications. *J Urol* 1980;**124**:259.

Hinman F Jr: Urodynamic testing: Alternatives to electronics. *J Urol* 1980;**121**:256.

Tanagho EA: Urodynamics of female urinary incontinence with emphasis on stress incontinence. *J Urol* 1979;**122**:200.

Turner-Warwick R, Brown AD: A urodynamic evaluation of urinary incontinence in the female and its treatment. *Urol Clin North Am* 1979;**6**:203.

Turner-Warwick R, Milroy E: A reappraisal of the value of routine urological procedures in the assessment of urodynamic function. *Urol Clin North Am* 1979;**6**:63.

Webster GD, Older RA: Video urodynamics. *Urology* 1980;**16**:106.

Wein AJ & others: Effects of bethanechol chloride on urodynamic parameters in normal women and in women with significant residual urine volumes. *J Urol* 1980;**124**:397.

Disorders of the Adrenal Glands | 21

Peter H. Forsham, MD

Diseases of the adrenal glands are accompanied by characteristic physical changes secondary to hormonal alterations or by abdominal pressure or pain due to the size of the diseased glands. Diagnosis can be made by appropriate hormonal and localizing determinations (Fig 21–1).

DISEASES OF THE ADRENAL CORTEX

CUSHING'S SYNDROME

Cushing's syndrome or Cushing's disease is caused by overproduction of cortisol (hydrocortisone). The majority of cases (85%) are due to bilateral adrenocortical hyperplasia stimulated by overproduction of pituitary adrenocorticotropic hormone (corticotropin, ACTH). A few cases are due to an undifferentiated ectopic ACTH-producing tumor that may be found (in decreasing order of incidence) in the lungs, the bronchial tree, the kidneys, the islets of the pancreas, or the thymus. Adrenal adenoma is the cause in 10% of cases and adenocarcinoma in 5%. In children, tumors are the most common cause.

Pathophysiology

Overproduction of cortisol or closely related glucocorticoids by abnormal adrenocortical tissue leads to a protein catabolic state. This causes liberation of amino acids from muscle tissue; the acids are transformed into glucose and glycogen in the liver by glyconeogenesis. The resulting weakened protein structures (muscle and elastic tissue) cause a protuberant abdomen and poor wound healing, generalized muscle weakness, and marked osteoporosis, which is made worse by excessive urinary calcium loss and is irreversible in adults.

The protein catabolic state leads to a variety of secondary changes. Excess glucose is transformed largely into fat and appears in characteristic sites such as the abdomen, supraclavicular fat pads, and cheeks. There is a diabetic tendency, with an elevated fasting plasma glucose in 20% of cases and a diabetic glucose tolerance curve in 80%, yet with insulinoplethora in the majority of cases.

Destruction of most of the lymphoid tissue leads to impairment of the immune mechanisms, which makes these patients susceptible to repeated infections. Inhibition of fibroplasia by excess cortisol further interferes with wound healing and host defenses against infection.

Hypertension is present in 99% of cases. Although aldosterone is not usually elevated, cortisol itself exerts a hypertensive effect when present in excessive amounts and favors the formation of angiotensinogen by the liver, resulting in excess production of angiotensin, the most potent hypertensive agent known.

The moderate rise in serum sodium with a marked fall in serum potassium is due to an excess of cortisol and of the primary mineralocorticoid 11-deoxycorticosterone. The plasma bicarbonate is often elevated as a consequence of the low serum potassium.

An adrenal adenoma is stimulated to grow by the administration of ACTH in the same way as are hyperplastic adrenals. Adenocarcinoma of an adrenal gland, on the other hand, is independent of pituitary influence and does not respond to the administration of exogenous ACTH.

Pathology

The cells in adrenal hyperplasia resemble those of the zona fasciculata of the normal adrenal cortex. Frank adenocarcinoma reveals pleomorphism and invasion of the capsule or the vascular system or both (Fig 21–2). Local invasion may occur, and functional metastases are common to the liver, lungs, bone, or brain. Differentiation between adenoma and adenocarcinoma is sometimes difficult. The former is stimulated by the administration of exogenous ACTH, as reflected in an increased level of urinary or plasma hydroxycorticosteroids; this does not usually occur with adenocarcinoma.

In the presence of adenoma or malignant tumor, atrophy of the cortices of both adrenals occurs because the main secretory product of the tumor is cortisol, which inhibits the pituitary secretion of ACTH. Thus, although the tumor continues

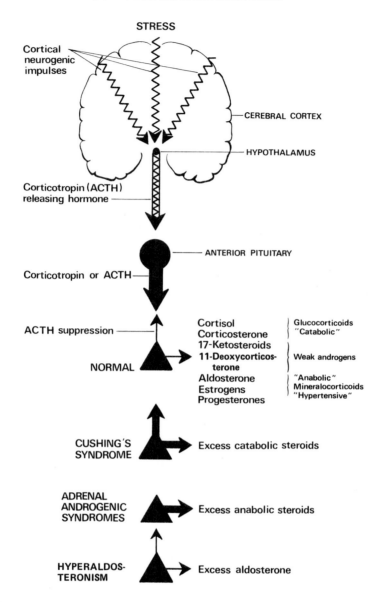

Figure 21-1. The hypothalamic pituitary-adrenocortical relationships in various adrenocortical syndromes.

to grow, the contralateral adrenal undergoes atrophy.

Clinical Findings

A. Symptoms and Signs: (Figs 21–3 and 21–4.) The presence of at least 3 of the following strongly suggests Cushing's syndrome:

1. Marked weakness, especially in the quadriceps femoris, making unaided rising from a chair difficult.

2. Obesity (with sparing of the extremities), moon face, and fat pads over the clavicles and the seventh cervical vertebra (buffalo hump). The abnormal distribution of fat is more characteristic of the disease than is the rise in body weight, which rarely exceeds 100 kg (220 lb).

3. Striae (red and depressed) over the abdomen and thighs. Festering ulcers of the skin may be present.

4. Irritability, difficulty in sleeping, and sometimes psychotic personality.

5. Hypertension (almost always present).

6. Osteoporosis (common), with back pain from compression fractures of the lumbar vertebrae as well as rib fractures.

7. In 80% of cases, a diabetic glucose tolerance curve is present, and in 20% there is an elevated fasting plasma glucose.

8. To a variable extent there are features of the adrenogenital syndrome in cases of Cushing's syndrome—least marked in the case of adenoma, most severe with carcinoma, and to an intermediate

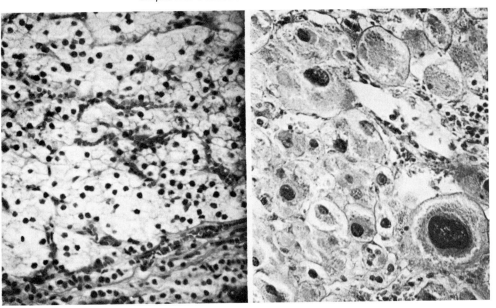

Figure 21–2. *Left:* Histologic appearance of a typical benign adenoma of the adrenal cortex made up of a large number of identical cells from the zona fasciculata removed from a 39-year-old woman with Cushing's syndrome. *Right:* Section of an adenocarcinoma removed from a 36-year-old woman with metastatic adenocarcinoma showing significant pleomorphism of the cells. Invasion of a large vein is not shown in this micrograph. Note that benign adenomas will occasionally have this appearance but without invasion of the bloodstream. (Reproduced, with permission, from Forsham PH: The adrenal cortex. In: *Textbook of Endocrinology,* 4th ed. Williams RH [editor]. Saunders, 1968.)

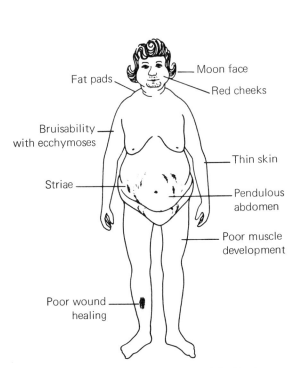

Figure 21–3. Drawing of a typical case of Cushing's syndrome showing the principal clinical features. (Reproduced, with permission, from Forsham PH: The adrenal cortex. In: *Textbook of Endocrinology,* 4th ed. Williams RH [editor]. Saunders, 1968.)

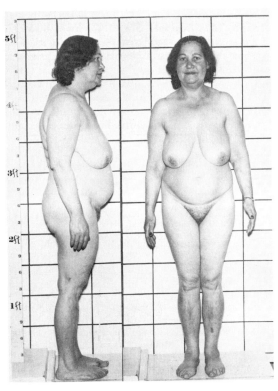

Figure 21–4. A case of Cushing's syndrome due to bilateral hyperplasia. Note the red moon face, receding hairline, buffalo hump over the seventh vertebra, protuberant abdomen, and inappropriately thin arms and legs. The combined adrenal weight was 20 g (as opposed to normal weight of 10 g).

degree with bilateral adrenocortical hyperplasia. They consist of recession of the hairline, hirsutism, small breasts, and generalized muscular over-development, with lowering of the voice. These relate to the excess of ketosteroids in general.

On the basis of the foregoing clinical findings alone, it is not possible to differentiate between bilateral adrenocortical hyperplasia, unilateral adenoma, and adenocarcinoma.

The most rapid onset is noted in cases caused by ectopic ACTH-producing tumor with high glucocorticoid output or those due to adrenal adenocarcinoma. In the case of adenoma or adenocarcinoma, the tumor may be palpable above the kidneys.

B. Laboratory Findings: The white count is elevated to the range of 12–20 thousand/μL. Eosinophils are few in number or absent. Polycythemia is present in over half of cases, with the hemoglobin ranging from 14–16 g/dL. Anemia, however, is found in association with ectopic ACTH-producing tumors in the lungs, pancreas, kidney, thymus, and other organs.

Blood chemical analyses are apt to show an increase in serum Na^+ and CO_2 and a decrease in serum K^+ (metabolic alkalosis). A diabetic glucose tolerance curve is usually found.

1. Specific tests for Cushing's syndrome–

a. Suppression of ACTH by dexamethasone– In normal individuals, the ACTH level is twice as high at night as in the late afternoon (Fig 21–5). In patients with cortical hyperplasia, this diurnal variation does not occur. In those with cortical tumors producing hydrocortisone, there is suppression of ACTH. Thus, if dexamethasone is given at 11 PM, ACTH is suppressed in normal persons but not in those with Cushing's syndrome. Dexamethasone is useful because it has 30 times the potency of hy-

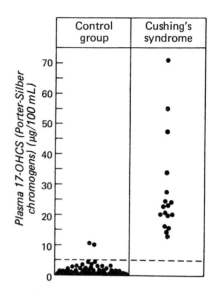

Figure 21–6. Results of the dexamethasone suppression test in obese individuals and patients with Cushing's syndrome. See text for procedure. 17-OHCS = 17-hydroxycorticosteroids. (Reproduced, with permission, from Pavlatos FC, Smilo RP, Forsham PH: A rapid screening test for Cushing's syndrome. *JAMA* 1965;**193**:720.)

drocortisone as an ACTH suppressant. It therefore can be used in such a small amount that it will have little effect upon the determination of circulating 17-hydroxycorticosteroids.

The procedure is to give 1–2 mg of dexamethasone by mouth at 11 PM with 0.2 g of pentobarbital to allay anxiety that might stimulate adrenocortical activity. Draw blood in the morning for measurement of plasma 11-hydroxycorticosteroids. If the level is below 5 μg/dL (normal is 5–20 μg/dL), Cushing's syndrome can be ruled out. If the value is above 10 μg/dL, Cushing's syndrome is present (Fig 21–6). A level in the range of 5–10 μg/dL is equivocal, and the test should be repeated.

Women taking birth control pills will have high plasma hydroxycorticosteroid levels because, as in pregnancy, the estrogen stimulates production of the cortisol-binding globulin. The pills must be withheld for at least 3 weeks before the dexamethasone suppression test, or a baseline plasma 17-hydroxycorticosteroid level must be obtained one morning shortly before the test. Normally, a greater than 50% suppression is observed, whereas in Cushing's syndrome a significantly smaller suppression is noted.

b. 24-Hour urinary free cortisol level– Measure the urinary free cortisol level in a 24-hour specimen of urine. A value above 120 μg establishes the diagnosis of Cushing's syndrome with near certainty. Obesity or hyperthyroidism does not raise normal levels.

c. 24-Hour urinary 17-hydroxycorticosteroids and 17-ketosteroids–These constituents must be

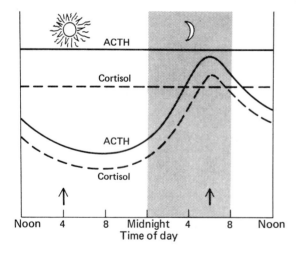

Figure 21–5. The circadian rhythm of ACTH and cortisol secretion that forms the basis of the dexamethasone suppression test for Cushing's syndrome.

Table 21–1. Normal "steroid" levels in plasma and urine.*

	Children	Adult Males	Adult Females
Plasma			
17-Hydroxycortico-steroids (μg/dL as cortisol)	5–20	5–20	5–20
Testosterone (ng/dL)	< 10	300–1200	30–120
Urine (mg/24 h as cortisol or dehydroepiandrosterone†)			
17-Hydroxycortico-steroids (per kg body weight)	0.02–0.04	6–10	4–8
17-Ketogenic ste-roids‡	0.03–0.05	8–12	6–10
Cortisol (free)	1 μg/kg	20–120	20–120
17-Ketosteroids	Low, but rises to normal adult levels during puberty	8–20	5–15
Pregnanetriol		0.5–3	0.5–2.5

*There may be wide variations with different technics and as done by different laboratories.

†Except as noted in the case of cortisol in second column.

‡This artificially derived entity is used in many laboratories in lieu of 17-hydroxycorticosteroids.

determined on a specimen collected for exactly 24 hours for comparison with normal levels (Table 21–1). This procedure, while not as diagnostic as a and b, does reveal the degree of androgenic excess in comparison with glucocorticoids by comparing their urinary excretory products. In Cushing's syndrome, both 17-hydroxycorticosteroids and 17-ketosteroids are elevated if adrenal hyperplasia or adenocarcinoma is present; with adenoma, 17-ketosteroids remain normal or low. Since 17-hydroxycorticosteroids vary with body weight, a high level in an obese patient is significant only if the value (in mg) exceeds the body weight in pounds × 0.06. In hyperthyroidism, high levels are noted in the presence of normal plasma levels.

2. Specific tests for differentiation of causes of Cushing's syndrome–

a. Plasma ACTH–If the diagnosis of Cushing's syndrome has been established, this test will differentiate between hyperplasia and tumor (Fig 21–7). Draw blood in the morning in a plastic syringe (glass absorbs ACTH). The blood must be stored in ice. The normal range for ACTH is 20–100 pg/mL. A higher value indicates hyperplasia; a lower level means that tumor is present. The highest levels are found in ectopic ACTH syndromes. Tests 1a and 2a together will give the exact and complete diagnosis of Cushing's syndrome.

b. ACTH administration–Give ACTH (eg, Cortrosyn), 0.25–0.5 mg subcutaneously. Collect blood at 1 and 2 hours for plasma hydroxycorticosteroid determinations. With adenoma, there is usually a rise; with carcinoma, there is not.

c. 11-Deoxycortisol–A marked increase in the concentration of this substance in the urine suggests adenocarcinoma.

C. X-Ray Findings and Special Examinations:

1. Localization of source of ACTH excess– When tests suggest bilateral adrenal cortical overactivity, and an elevated plasma level of ACTH is present, the source of ACTH must be identified. A possible source is a microadenoma of the pituitary gland. High resolution tomography of the sella turcica will best visualize sella wall irregularities that may be very small but compatible with adenoma. Rarely, an adenoma produces no radiologic findings. If an adenoma of the pituitary is not identified, a search should be made for an ectopic source of ACTH.

2. Localization of a tumor–Following good catharsis but without enemas, tomograms of the kidney area may reveal a mass on one side and adrenal atrophy on the other. This finding is typical of an adrenal tumor. With bilateral hyperplasia, 2 enlarged adrenal shadows are seen. However, this finding is not diagnostic, since perirenal fat may simulate adrenal enlargement.

CT scans are an excellent noninvasive method of localization of tumor (Dunnick & others, 1979). [131]I-19-iodocholesterol adrenal scan is the most reliable method for localizing a tumor. After giving iodine by mouth to protect the thyroid, a dose of ^{131}I-labeled cholesterol is given intravenously, and abdominal scans are taken 5 and 10 days later. A tumor will show a unilateral flush on one scan or the other, depending on its steroidogenic activity. A carcinoma will show the flush only on the earlier scan, because it rapidly discharges the hormonal steroids produced (Herwig & Sonda, 1979).

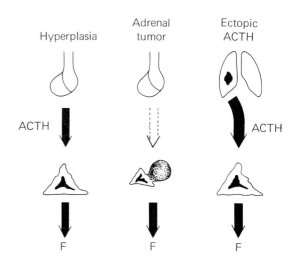

Figure 21–7. Schematic presentation of the pituitary-adrenal interrelationship in cases of hyperplasia, functional adrenocortical tumors, and ectopic ACTH syndrome. (Reproduced, with permission, from Forsham PH: The adrenal cortex. In: *Textbook of Endocrinology,* 4th ed. Williams RH [editor]. Saunders, 1968.)

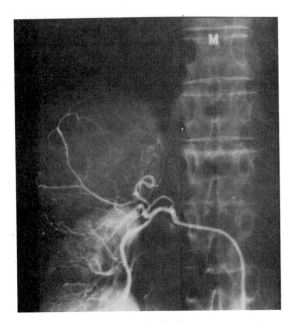
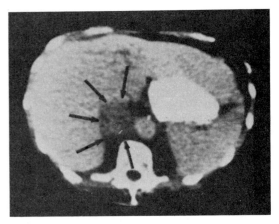
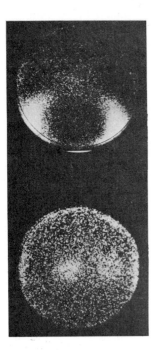
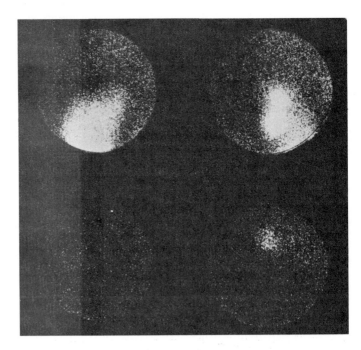

Figure 21–8. Localization of adrenal lesions. *Above left:* Selective arteriogram showing large right adrenal adenoma above the upper pole of the right kidney. *Above right:* CT scan showing right suprarenal pheochromocytoma localized between the vertebral column, the aorta, and the liver. *Below left:* Simultaneous renal (upper circle) and iodocholesterol adrenal (lower circle) scans showing bilateral adrenocortical hyperplasia. *Below right:* Posterior view of simultaneous renal (upper circles) and iodocholesterol adrenal (lower circles) scans showing right adrenal glucocorticoid-producing adenoma. The normal left adrenal is suppressed and therefore does not concentrate the isotope, giving a negative image on the scan.

Small changes in the wall of the sella turcica are most frequently the sign of a chromophobe or basophil microadenoma.

Differential Diagnosis

An adrenal cyst may present as a suprarenal mass with displacement of the kidney on tomography (Kearney & others, 1977). There is often some curvilinear calcification in its capsule (Ghandur-Mnaymneh, Slim, & Muakassa, 1979). A sonogram will reveal its nature. It is devoid of endocrinologic function.

A tumor or cyst of the upper pole of the kidney may appear to be a suprarenal mass, but excretory urograms will reveal the caliceal distortion of a space-occupying lesion while renal angiography will show its intrinsic nature.

Fluid in the cardiac end of the stomach may appear as a round opacity in the left suprarenal area on a plain x-ray film. It disappears on an upright film. Tomography is also conclusive. Rarely, the splenic shadow will simulate a left adrenal mass.

Enlargement of the liver or spleen may displace the kidney downward; this will be revealed by physical examination and tomography.

Complications

Hypertension may lead to cardiac failure or stroke. Diabetes may be a problem but is usually mild. Intractable skin or systemic infections are common. Compression fractures of osteoporotic vertebrae and rib fractures (often remarkably painless) may develop. Renal stones are not uncommon as a result of leaching of calcium from the bones. Gastric (stress) ulcer may become a problem. Psychosis is not uncommon. Chromophobe adenoma develops in up to 25% of treated patients and often preexists as a pituitary microadenoma in cases of bilateral hyperplasia.

Treatment

A. Bilateral Adrenocortical Hyperplasia: The total adrenocortical mass must be significantly reduced by the following methods: (1) An anterior pituitary tumor (Cushing's disease) that is producing a fixed or increased amount of ACTH should be removed. The best treatment for an ACTH-producing pituitary tumor is transsphenoidal microadenomectomy, which is not usually followed by any hypopituitarism. (2) A known or suspected basophilic or chromophobe pituitary tumor should be treated with 5000 rads of radiation delivered by linear accelerator or cobalt. The success rate with this treatment is 20–60%, though a 100% successful response is claimed when heavy particle irradiation (medical cyclotron) is delivered. Varying degrees of hypopituitarism may ensue. (3) Total bilateral adrenalectomy will produce Addison's disease, but this can be controlled by substitution therapy.

Total bilateral adrenalectomy is no longer recommended for the treatment of hyperplasia. In 5% of cases, ectopic adrenocortical tissue will lead to recrudescence of the disease. An undesirable consequence of total adrenalectomy is growth of a chromophobe pituitary adenoma in up to 25% of cases, leading to excessive ACTH secretion (Nelson's syndrome), though this may be prevented or slowed by irradiation of the pituitary.

1. Preoperative preparation—Because removal of the source of excessive cortisol will inevitably lead to temporary or permanent adrenal insufficiency, it is of the utmost importance to administer cortisol preoperatively and to continue substitution therapy after surgery to control Addison's disease. In the postoperative period, the dose is tapered downward until oral medication provides sufficient control.

2. Postoperative status—The patient feels moderately well following removal of the source of excess ACTH or adrenalectomy or while receiving a high dose of hydrocortisone in excess of the usual daily output of approximately 20 mg. When dosage approaches the maximum normal physiologic output, the patient may complain of nausea, abdominal pain resembling that of pancreatitis (which in fact may occur), and extreme weakness with the adrenocortical withdrawal syndrome. Thus, it is important to reduce the steroid substitution gradually over a period of several days. On the day of operation, 200 mg of cortisol are given; the dosage is then reduced gradually on successive days (150, 100, 80, 60, and 40 mg) until a maintenance dosage of 30 mg cortisol combined with 0.1 mg fludrocortisone is reached.

3. Follow-up—The status of adrenocortical secretion cannot be determined during substitution therapy, since one-third of administered cortisol appears in the urine. In order to obtain a valid measurement of 24-hour urinary 17-hydroxycorticosteroid levels, it is necessary to stop the usual cortisol replacement and give 1 mg of dexamethasone daily for 2 days while covering with additional sodium chloride.

Urinary 17-hydroxycorticosteroids or 17-ketogenic steroids should be measured at intervals of 3–6 months. The patient should cease taking cortisol temporarily and should be given 1 mg of dexamethasone orally on the day before and the day of the urine collection, along with a high sodium intake which will reveal any reactivation of residual cortical tissue. Plasma ACTH measurements, which are usually high when the patient is on standard replacement therapy, will be even higher with a chromophobe adenoma.

A plain film of the sella turcica (anteroposterior and lateral) or, better still, tomograms of the fossa, when compared with preoperative films, will reveal an expanding chromophobe tumor. This study should be done every 6 months until the patient has remained asymptomatic for 1 year, especially if increased melanin pigmentation occurs due to excess ACTH secretion.

B. Adenoma and Adenocarcinoma: Preoperative preparation is the same for bilateral hyperplasia, because removal of one adrenal and the invariable atrophy of the contralateral gland almost always result in immediate hypoadrenalism.

1. Surgical technic–Depending on the size of the tumor and the patient's body habitus, the lesion can be approached through the flank with resection of the eleventh or twelfth rib. For large tumors, a transthoracic transdiaphragmatic incision provides ideal exposure of the mass.

2. Postoperative treatment and follow-up– Because of atrophy of the contralateral adrenal, postoperative substitution therapy must encourage return of function of the atrophic gland. Hydrocortisone is given orally in a dosage of 10 mg 3 times daily initially and reduced within 2 weeks to 10 mg daily given at 7 or 8 AM. This may be necessary for 1 month to 2 years depending on the rate of recovery of the gland. Sodium supplementation is rarely necessary, since the atrophic adrenal usually produces sufficient aldosterone. Serial determinations of urinary 17-hydroxycorticosteroids and 17-ketosteroids can be used as tumor markers.

Prognosis

Treatment of hypercortisolism usually leads to disappearance of symptoms and many signs within days to weeks, but osteoporosis is usually quite irreversible in adults, whereas hypertension and diabetes often improve. Bilateral hyperplasia treated by pituitary adenomectomy has an excellent early prognosis, but long-range follow-up is not available. X-ray or heavy particle treatment leads to only slow normalization, which may take up to 2 years. Removal of an adenoma offers an excellent prognosis.

The outlook for the patient with adenocarcinoma is poor. The antineoplastic drug mitotane (o,p′-DDD; Lysodren) given in doses of up to 30 g orally daily reduces the symptoms and signs of Cushing's syndrome but does little to prolong survival, and nausea is usually troublesome. This drug in combination with fluorouracil has recently been shown to arrest metastases.

ADRENAL ANDROGENIC SYNDROMES

These conditions are more common in females. Congenital bilateral adrenal hyperplasia and tumors, both benign and malignant, may be observed. They all represent excessive or abnormal levels of androgen. In contrast to Cushing's syndrome, which is protein catabolic, the androgenic syndromes are strongly anabolic. In untreated cases, there is a marked recession of the hairline, increased beard growth, and excessive growth of pubic and sexual hair in general in both sexes. In the male, there is enlargement of the penis, usually with atrophic testes; in the female, enlargement of

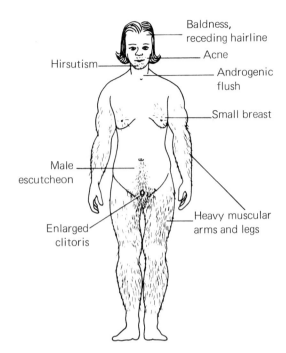

Figure 21–9. Clinical features of a full-blown case of virilism in a female with adrenogenital syndrome. (Reproduced, with permission, from Forsham PH: The adrenal cortex. In: *Textbook of Endocrinology,* 4th ed. Williams RH [editor]. Saunders, 1968.)

the clitoris occurs, with atrophy of the breasts and amenorrhea (Fig 21–9). Muscle mass increases and fat content decreases, leading to a powerful but trim figure. The voice becomes deeper, particularly in the female; this condition is irreversible, since it is due to enlargement of the larynx. The psyche of these patients is often deranged. In both sexes there is increased physical aggressiveness and libido.

1. CONGENITAL BILATERAL ADRENAL ANDROGENIC HYPERPLASIA

Pathophysiology

A congenital defect in certain adrenal enzymes results in the production of abnormal steroids (Fig 21–10), causing **pseudohermaphroditism** in females and **macrogenitosomia** in males. The enzyme defect is associated with excess androgen production in utero. In females, the müllerian duct structures (eg, ovaries, uterus, and vagina) will develop normally, but the excess androgen exerts a masculinizing effect on the urogenital sinus and genital tubercle, so that the vagina is connected to the urethra, which, in turn, opens at the base of an enlarged clitoris. The labia are often hypertrophied. Externally, the appearance is that of severe hypospadias with cryptorchidism.

The adrenal cortex secretes mostly anabolic and androgenic steroids, leading to various degrees

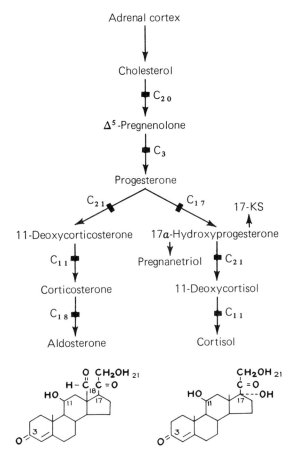

Figure 21–10. Deficiencies in hydroxylases and related enzymes in the adrenal cortex, giving rise to typical cases of adrenogenital syndrome.

of cortisol deficiency depending on the nature of the enzyme block. This increases the secretion of ACTH, which causes hyperplasia of both adrenal cortices. The cortices continue to secrete large amounts of inappropriate anabolic, androgenic, or hypertensive steroids. Absence or severe reduction of the usual tissue concentration of various enzymes—oxidases, hydrogenases, isomerases, or desmolases—accounts for blocks in the adrenocortical synthetic pathways (Fig 21–10).

A block at C_{20} with absence of 20,22-desmolase leads to the rare congenital lipoid adrenal hyperplasia with complete absence of any steroidal hormone production; the infant will die at an early age unless she receives full substitution therapy for life.

A block at C_3 with lack of 3β-hydroxydehydrogenase and isomerase prevents formation of progesterone, aldosterone, and cortisol. Dehydroepiandrosterone is produced in excess. This uncommon syndrome is characterized by hypotension, hypoglycemia, and male pseudohermaphroditism, with females showing unusual sexual development with hirsutism. There is variable melanin pigmentation.

A block at C_{21} with deficiency or absence of 21-hydroxylase does not allow for the transformation of 17α-hydroxyprogesterone to cortisol. This more common deficiency occurs in 2 forms: the salt-losing variety, with low to absent aldosterone, and the more frequent non–salt-losing type. Hirsutism, virilism, hypotension, and melanin pigmentation are common.

A block at C_{17} with lack of 17-hydroxylase occurs mostly in females and may not be discovered until adulthood. Findings include low cortisol with high ACTH, primary amenorrhea, and sexual infantilism, as neither the glucocorticoids nor the sex steroids are produced in adequate amounts. Rarely, there is male pseudohermaphroditism. Hypertension due to excess mineralocorticoids, notably 11-deoxycorticosterone, is characteristically present.

A block at C_{11} with lack of 11-hydroxylase prevents formation of cortisol and corticosterone and thus leads to a marked excess of ACTH, with deep melanin pigmentation. Unlike Addison's disease, there is hypertension due to excess 11-deoxycorticosterone. There are no marked sexual abnormalities.

A block at C_{18} with lack of an oxidase is exceedingly rare; 11-deoxycorticosterone will take over from aldosterone as the essential mineralocorticoid.

Increased androgenicity manifested by hirsutism and amenorrhea only rarely develops after puberty and seldom leads to virilism in middle age. This acquired mild enzyme abnormality of the adrenals is known as **benign androgenic overactivity of the adrenal cortices.**

Clinical Findings

A. Symptoms and Signs: In the newborn female, the appearance of the external genitalia resembles severe hypospadias with cryptorchidism. The male infant may appear quite normal at birth. The earlier in intrauterine life the fetus has been exposed to excess androgen, the more marked the anomalies.

In untreated cases, hirsutism, excess muscle mass, and, eventually, amenorrhea are the rule. Breast development is poor. In males, growth of the phallus is excessive. The testes are often atrophic because of inhibition of gonadotropin secretion by the elevated androgens. On rare occasion, hyperplastic adrenocortical rests in the testes make them large and firm. In most instances, there is aspermia after puberty.

In both males and females with androgenic hyperplasia, the growth rate is initially increased, so that they are taller than their classmates. At about age 9–10 years, premature fusion of the epiphyses caused by excess androgen causes termination of growth, so that these patients are short as adults. In both sexes, there is increased aggressiveness and libido that can cause social and disciplinary

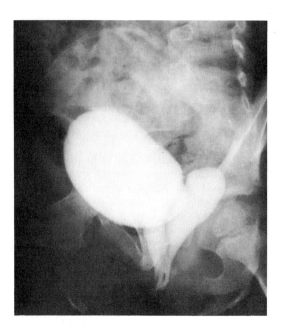

Figure 21–11. Urogenital sinus in congenital virilizing cortical hyperplasia. Oblique urethrogram showing connection of vagina with distal urethra. (Courtesy of F Hinman, Jr.)

problems, particularly in some boys.

B. Laboratory Findings: Urinary 17-ketosteroids are higher than normal for sex and age (Table 21–1). Urinary pregnanetriol is elevated early (this is a more sensitive test than measurement of 17-ketosteroid levels, since pregnanetriol is the precursor of the androgenic steroids). The most sensitive indicator of androgenic activity is elevation of plasma 17-hydroxyprogesterone, and this test is particularly useful in children. The buccal smear is positive for Barr bodies in females. Chromosome studies are normal.

C. X-Ray Findings: X-rays will reveal acceleration of bone age. A lateral cystourethrogram may show the vagina as well as the urethra and bladder (Fig 21–11).

D. Computed Tomography: This will usually show the hypertrophied adrenals.

E. Instrumental Examination: Urethroscopy may permit visualization of the point at which the vagina opens into the posterior wall of the urethra. The vaginal tract can often be entered and the cervix seen.

Differential Diagnosis

A number of congenital anomalies that affect the development of the external genitalia resemble adrenal androgenic syndrome. These include (1) severe hypospadias with cryptorchidism, (2) female pseudohermaphroditism of the nonadrenal type (caused by administration of androgens or progesta-

tional compounds during the pregnancy), (3) male pseudohermaphroditism, and (4) true hermaphroditism. These children show no hormonal abnormalities, however, and accelerated bone age and maturation do not occur.

Treatment

It is imperative to make the diagnosis early. Treatment of the underlying cause is medical, with the goal of suppressing excessive ACTH secretion, thus minimizing excess androgenicity. This is accomplished by giving the long-acting glucocorticoid dexamethasone, 0.5–1.5 mg orally at 11 PM every night, so that the adrenal cortex is suppressed at the time of its greatest activity, ie, 2–8 AM. In a severe case of salt-losing syndrome, fludrocortisone (0.05–0.3 mg, depending on severity and age) together with good salt intake is necessary to stabilize blood pressure and body weight.

After puberty, the vaginal opening can be surgically separated from the urethra and opened in the normal position on the perineum. If frequent clitoral erections occur, resection or, preferably, recession of the clitoris should be considered (Parrott, Scheflan, & Hester, 1980). Judicious administration of estrogens or birth control pills will feminize the figure in pseudohermaphrodites and improve their psyche considerably.

Prognosis

If the condition is recognized early and ACTH suppression is begun even before surgical repair of the genital anomaly, the outlook for normal linear growth and development is excellent. Delay in treatment will inevitably result in stunted growth and a propensity to coronary artery disease, with early death due to myocardial infarction. In some female pseudohermaphrodites, menses begin after treatment, and conception and childbirth can occur when the anatomic abnormalities are minimal or have been surgically repaired.

2. ADRENOCORTICAL TUMORS

The differentiation between hyperplasia (a medical problem) and adrenocortical tumor (a surgical problem) is done by means of the **dexamethasone suppression test.** The procedure is as follows: A 24-hour urine specimen is collected and 17-ketosteroids measured. An adult patient is then given dexamethasone, 2 mg orally 4 times a day. On the second day, a 24-hour urine specimen is also taken and the concentration of 17-ketosteroids is measured. If the second specimen contains less than half the 17-ketosteroids found in the first specimen, adrenal activity is suppressible and the condition is due to hyperplasia. Suppression does not occur when adrenal overactivity is due to tumor. Zaitoon & Mackie (1978) have reviewed the literature on adrenal cortical tumors in children.

Tumor localization can be accomplished by tomography, angiography, iodocholesterol scans, sonography, or CT scans (Fig 21–8). In these cases, there is no atrophy of the contralateral adrenal because there is no marked elevation of 17-hydroxycorticosteroids. Therefore, preoperative cortisol medication can be minimal, eg, 50 mg cortisol phosphate given just before induction of anesthesia. The tumor can readily be removed through the flank. In contrast to patients with Cushing's syndrome, hemostasis is easy to obtain, and wound healing is normal.

Adenocarcinoma is a highly malignant tumor that metastasizes to the liver, lungs, and brain. Successive determinations of urinary 17-ketosteroids as a tumor marker will reveal the completeness of the resection and the presence or later development of metastases. When metastases have occurred, hyperandrogenicity can be combated by giving up to 30 g of mitotane (*o,p'*-DDD; Lysodren) orally daily. Unfortunately, this drug only temporarily halts tumor growth, and fluorouracil (5-FU; Adrucil) is not successful either. X-ray treatment in large doses may postpone the inevitable death of these patients, and mitotane combined with fluorouracil may offer some help.

Prognosis

Removal of a benign adenoma is curative. Patients with adenocarcinoma rarely live more than 1 year after diagnosis—partly because diagnosis is delayed an average of 7 months after onset of symptoms.

THE HYPERTENSIVE, HYPOKALEMIC SYNDROME
(Primary Aldosteronism)

Excessive production of aldosterone, due mostly to aldosteronoma or to spontaneous bilateral nodular hyperplasia of the zona glomerulosa of the adrenal cortex, leads to the combination of hypertension, hypokalemia, nocturia, and rarely diabetes insipidus. Rarer causes for these are an adrenocortical aldosterone-producing carcinoma; a glucocorticoid-remediable ACTH excess syndrome; and indeterminate aldosteronism that in part appears to be due to an adenoma or hyperplasia. The low serum potassium may lead to muscular weakness with fully conscious collapse and postural hypotension due to baroreceptor paralysis, leading to syncope. A syndrome resembling diabetes insipidus may occur as a result of reversible damage to the renal collecting tubules. The alkalosis may produce tetany.

Pathophysiology

Excessive aldosterone, acting on most cell membranes in the body, produces typical changes in the distal renal tubule and the small bowel that

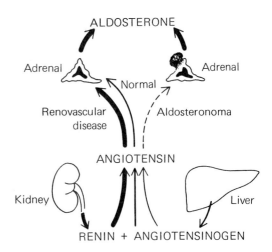

Figure 21–12. The angiotensin-aldosterone relationships in a case of aldosteronoma and hypertension due to renal vascular disease. (Reproduced, with permission, from Forsham PH: The adrenal cortex. In: *Textbook of Endocrinology,* 4th ed. Williams RH [editor]. Saunders, 1968.)

lead to urinary potassium loss and sodium reabsorption together with an increased renal hydrogen ion secretion. This results in potassium depletion, metabolic alkalosis, increased plasma sodium concentration, and hypervolemia. Potassium depletion affects baroreceptors, so that postural fall in blood pressure no longer results in reflex tachycardia. With low serum potassium, the concentrating ability of the kidney is lowered and the tubules no longer respond to the administration of vasopressin by increased reabsorption of water. Finally, impairment of insulin release secondary to potassium depletion increases carbohydrate intolerance in about 50% of cases.

Plasma renin and, secondarily, plasma angiotensin are depressed by excess aldosterone, presumably as a result of blood volume expansion (Fig 21–12). Early in the course of excess aldosterone production, there may be hypertension with a normal serum potassium. Later, potassium will be low as well, and this suggests the diagnosis.

Clinical Findings

A. Symptoms and Signs: Whereas adenoma predominates in females, bilateral nodular adrenal hyperplasia occurs predominantly in young males. Headaches are common, nocturia is invariably present, and rare episodes of paralysis occur with very low serum potassium levels. Numbness and tingling of the extremities are related to alkalosis that may lead to tetany. Hypertension is of varying severity. Orthostatic hypotension is common. Inappropriate control of vasomotor tone is usually demonstrable. Feel the pulse while the patient is standing. Then have the patient crouch and straighten up and take the pulse again. In a normal person, the pulse will be slower the second time; with hyperaldosteronism, it is not.

Ophthalmoscopic examination usually shows normal vessels inconsistent with the degree of hypertension. Unless acute heart failure is present, there is no edema. The Chvostek sign is often positive.

B. Laboratory Findings: Before the tests outlined below are done, one must ascertain that the patient is not taking oral contraceptives or other estrogen preparations, since these may increase renin and angiotensin levels and therefore aldosterone levels, thus raising the blood pressure artificially. Withdrawal of these medications for 1 week is mandatory. Diuretics must also be discontinued, since they lower blood volume and induce secondary aldosteronism and hypokalemia. Also, if the patient is taking a salt-restricted diet, aldosterone is normally elevated.

Before serum electrolytes are measured, the patient is loaded with 6 g of salt for at least 2 days. This will furnish exchangeable sodium in the distal tubule and allow potassium to exchange with sodium, thus clearly revealing the low serum potassium and electrolyte imbalance. Later, serum potassium must also be replenished because a very low level of this ion may artificially decrease the secretory rate of aldosterone.

In true aldosterone excess, serum sodium will be slightly elevated and CO_2 increased, whereas serum potassium will be very low, eg, 3 mEq/L or less. Urine and serum potassium determinations while the patient is receiving good sodium replacement provide a screening test. Potassium wasting is considered to be established if the urinary potassium level is > 30 mEq/L/24 h but the serum potassium level is low (3 mEq/L or less).

Definitive diagnosis rests on demonstration of an elevated urine or plasma aldosterone level or a

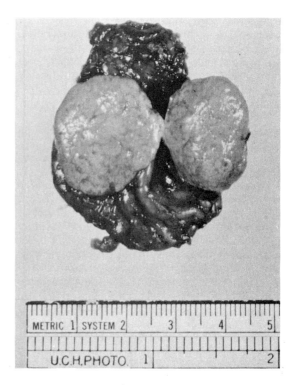

Figure 21–13. A typical canary yellow aldosteronoma associated with the syndrome of hypertension, hyperkalemia, and alkalosis. Note the relatively small size of this tumor compared to other types of adrenocortical neoplasms.

positive desoxycorticosterone acetate test (Table 21–2). Before aldosterone is measured, the patient should be loaded with salt (6 g/d) to avoid a decrease in plasma volume, which by itself raises the aldosterone level. In hyperaldosteronism, urinary aldosterone is more than 10 μg/d after suppression with desoxycorticosterone acetate or fludrocortisone.

C. Localization: Tomograms do not usually reveal the small adenoma ranging from 1–2 cm in diameter (Fig 21–13). CT scans may locate the tumor. ^{131}I-19-iodocholesterol scan (see Fig 21–8) is the noninvasive method of choice.

Differential Diagnosis

Secondary hyperaldosteronism may accompany renovascular hypertension. An abdominal bruit will suggest this condition initially. This too is associated with hypokalemic alkalosis. Differentiation requires estimation of blood volume and serum sodium. In primary aldosteronism, both tend to be elevated. In the secondary form, both may be low.

Essential hypertension does not cause changes in the electrolyte pattern. Definitive tests for hyperaldosteronism are negative.

The diagnosis of pheochromocytoma (see below) is based on catecholamine measurements, which in patients suffering from paroxysmal hypertension are not elevated during normotensive

Table 21–2. Desoxycorticosterone acetate test for primary aldosteronism.

Patient preparation
  (1) Withdraw all hypotensive drugs for 1 week.
  (2) Give 6+ g of salt for 3 days.
  (3) Give 100 mEq (7 g) of potassium chloride for 3 days.
Test procedure
  (1) Collect 24-hour urine sample for aldosterone determination.
  (2) Give 5 mg of desoxycorticosterone acetate (eg, Percorten Acetate) IM daily for 3 days or 1 mg fludrocortisone orally twice daily for 3 days.
  (3) On third day, repeat 24-hour urine test for aldosterone.
Results (aldosterone concentration in urine, μg/d)

	Normal	Primary Aldosteronism	Secondary Aldosteronism
Control day	9	18	25
Third day of suppression	3	17	9

intervals. Careful administration of glucagon, 1 mg intravenously, will cause a rise in both blood pressure and catecholamine levels. Aldosterone levels remain normal.

Cushing's syndrome is associated with hypertension, but physical examination and appropriate hormonal assays will establish the diagnosis.

Treatment

A. Aldosteronoma: If localization of the tumor has been established, only the affected adrenal need be removed. A flank incision with resection of the 11th or 12th rib will provide good exposure. Two-thirds of adenomas are in the left adrenal. They are practically never bilateral.

B. Bilateral Nodular Hyperplasia: Most authorities do not recommend resection of both adrenals, since the fall in blood pressure is only temporary and electrolyte imbalance may continue. Medical treatment is recommended.

C. Medical Treatment: If surgery must be postponed, if the hypertension is mild in an older person, or if bilateral hyperplasia is the cause, one may treat medically with spironolactone (Aldactone), 25–50 mg orally 4 times daily.

Prognosis

In rare cases, hypotension may persist for as long as 2 years after removal of the adenoma; this can be controlled by increased sodium intake. Following removal of an adenomatous adrenal, 60% of patients become normotensive and 40% show some lowering of hypertension. Bilateral nodular hyperplasia is not amenable to surgical treatment, and the results of medical treatment are only fair.

DISEASES OF THE ADRENAL MEDULLA

PHEOCHROMOCYTOMA

Pheochromocytoma, derived from the neural crest, is one of the surgically curable hypertensive syndromes. There is no sex predilection. Pheochromocytoma accounts for fewer than 1% of cases of hypertension, but it is readily diagnosed if the possibility is kept in mind. It usually occurs spontaneously but may result from a familial disease known as multiple endocrine neoplasia type 2, which is inherited as an autosomal dominant trait. In up to 5% of patients, pheochromocytoma occurs as part of a pluriglandular syndrome including medullary carcinoma of the thyroid, hyperparathyroidism (adenoma or hyperplasia), Cushing's syndrome with excess ACTH, and oral mucosal neuromas with neuroectodermal dysplasia, including neurofibromatosis. The tumor is bilateral or extra-adrenal in 5% of cases in adults and in an even greater percentage in children and is then most often familial.

Clinical Findings

A. Symptoms and Signs: Hypertension is both systolic and diastolic. The appearance of the retinal vessels on ophthalmoscopic examination is commensurate with the severity of the hypertension and the duration of the disease state. Hypertension may be either sustained and indistinguishable from ordinary blood pressure elevation, or paroxysmal, coming on for variable lengths of time and then subsiding to normal levels. Such attacks are usually precipitated by trigger mechanisms of various sorts, eg, emotional upsets or straining at stool.

Headache is a frequent complaint and is commensurate in severity with the degree of hypertension. Increased sweating without appropriate causes such as exertion or environmental heat resembles the phenomenon seen during menopause and may be accompanied by flushing or blanching. Tachycardia with palpitations occurs mainly as a consequence of epinephrine rather than norepinephrine excess. Postural hypotension is a frequent finding, partly as a result of diminished plasma volume and ganglionic blocking of normal pressor pathways by excess catecholamines.

Profound weakness may occur after an attack of hypertension. Weight loss is common, partly because of the anorexia that results from elevated blood glucose and fatty acid levels—the former caused by increased glycogenolysis and the latter by the increased lipolysis induced by elevated catecholamine levels.

Decreased gastrointestinal motility occurs, leading to nausea and vomiting, especially in children, and constipation. This effect is a direct pharmacologic consequence of excessive circulating catecholamines. Episodes of psychic instability verging on hysteria are frequent and are probably due to increased concentrations of catecholamines and other neurotransmitters in the brain, although circulating catecholamines, unlike some of their precursors, penetrate the blood-brain barrier to only a limited extent.

In the 5% of patients that have associated neuroectodermal disease, café au lait spots are found with smooth outlines ("coast of California") rather than the ragged ones ("coast of Maine") that occur only with the unrelated fibrous dysplasia of bone. Telangiectasia and, rarely, cerebellar involvement may coexist in neuroectodermal disease.

In a very few patients, the tumor is palpable. Even if it is not palpable, pressure over the site of the tumor may cause an exacerbation of hypertension. Thus, in a tumor embedded in the bladder, blood pressure rise occurs with micturition (Flanigan & others, 1980).

B. Laboratory Findings: The hematocrit is usually elevated, and the white cell count is high, with few lymphocytes. Serum proteins are elevated. The fasting plasma glucose level is often elevated and accompanied by a diabetic glucose tolerance curve.

Table 21–3. Catecholamines in urine and plasma.*

Urine
  Norepinephrine: 10–100 μg/24 h
  Epinephrine: Up to 20 μg/24 h
  Normetanephrine and metanephrine: < 1.5 mg/24 h
  Vanilmandelic acid (VMA): 2–9 mg/24 h
Plasma
  Norepinephrine: 100–200 pg/mL
  Epinephrine: 30–50 pg/mL

*The values listed represent the means of the normal ranges, which vary for each laboratory.

Urinary catecholamine levels must be measured. The patient must discontinue all medication except diuretics, digitalis, and barbiturates for at least 2 days. An exact 24-hour urine collection, in a bottle containing 15 mL of 6 N hydrochloric acid, is then obtained. The test must be performed within 48 hours. The normal limits are shown in Table 21–3.

In individual cases, epinephrine or norepinephrine (or both) may be elevated, but elevation of only epinephrine suggests that the tumor is in the adrenal medulla, in ectopic medullary tissue, or in the organ of Zuckerkandl, since the methylating enzyme necessary for transforming norepinephrine to epinephrine is present only in medullary tissue.

Urinary normetanephrine, metanephrine, and vanilmandelic acid (VMA) are breakdown products of epinephrine and norepinephrine. Whereas less than 5% of secreted catecholamines appear as such in the urine, over 50% appear as metabolites, such as metanephrine or normetanephrine, and these are usually independent of any medication taken by the patient. Before collection of urine for measurement of VMA, the patient must have no vanilla ice cream, chocolate, coffee, tea, or citrus fruits for at least 48 hours. The range of normal values is shown in Table 21–3.

If estimations of both urinary catecholamines and VMA are performed, the diagnostic accuracy is 98%. In patients with paroxysmal hypertension, the urine must be collected during an attack. A spot urine specimen obtained during a brief paroxysm is suitable for determination of catecholamines and VMA, which may be compared to the amount of simultaneously determined creatinine. Since the average urinary excretion of creatinine per 24 hours is 1.4 g, a finding of 0.2 g of creatinine in the aliquot means that the amount of catecholamines and VMA should be multiplied by 7 to obtain a rough estimate of the 24-hour excretion of these substances.

As a rule, a high ratio of VMA to catecholamines indicates a large tumor; a low ratio indicates a small one (Farndon & others, 1980).

Glucagon test. If pheochromocytoma as a cause of hypertension is suspected in a patient who may be in a period of remission (normotensive), give 1 mg of glucagon subcutaneously. If pheochro-

mocytoma is present, both blood pressure and catecholamine levels will rise markedly within 2 minutes. A hormonal assay can then be done. It is also advisable to determine plasma calcitonin, which will be elevated in cases of concurrent medullary carcinoma of the thyroid.

C. X-Ray Findings: Preoperative localization by x-ray can be attempted but is of limited importance, since up to 7% of the tumors are multiple, and 13% are extra-adrenal and require direct exploration. Since the tumors are often quite large (Fig 21–14), tomograms with or without excretory urograms will often reveal the tumor (Fig 21–15, left). CT scans may reveal more than one tumor (Laursen & Damgaard-Pedersen, 1980).

A retrograde arteriogram (Fig 21–15, right) or venogram will reveal small or multiple tumors. Determination of plasma catecholamine concentrations at different levels during catheterization of the vena cava is quite helpful as a means of localizing ectopic tumors (Modlin & others, 1979).

Differential Diagnosis

Thyrotoxicosis may be suggested because of the marked hypermetabolism, nervousness, and weight loss. However, normal thyroid indices, con-

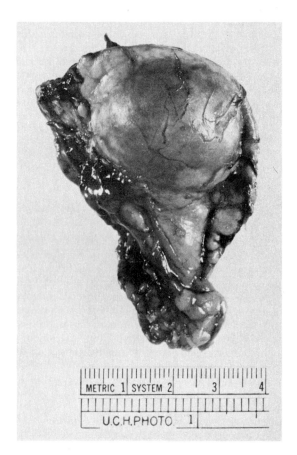

Figure 21–14. A typical large pheochromocytoma. Removal was followed by complete remission of hypertension.

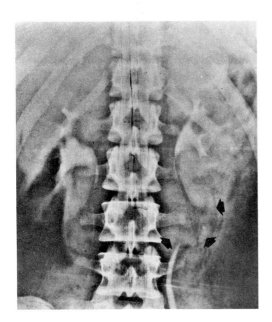
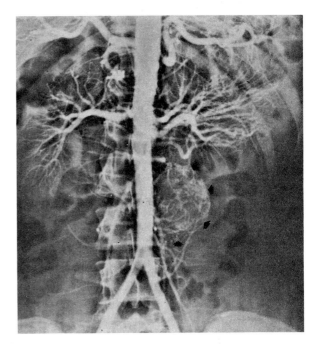

Figure 21–15. Extra-adrenal pheochromocytoma. *Left:* Excretory urogram showing normal kidneys but a soft tissue mass just below and medial to the left kidney. *Right:* Angiogram, same patient. Vascular mass below left renal arteries.

stipation rather than diarrhea, and a low rather than high blood lymphocyte count (as seen with pheochromocytoma) rule out thyrotoxicosis.

Diabetes mellitus must always be suspected because of the elevated fasting plasma glucose. With pheochromocytoma, epinephrine directly inhibits insulin secretion from the beta cells while transforming liver glycogen to glucose by stimulating the process of glycogenolysis. Only persistent hyperglycemia after removal of the pheochromocytoma shows whether permanent diabetes mellitus exists.

In many patients with pheochromocytoma, organic heart disease is suggested by findings of hypertension, cardiac murmurs, and ventricular hypertrophy. These features resolve in the majority of patients following correction of catecholamine excess; their persistence will establish a definite diagnosis of primary cardiac disease.

Treatment

The sooner hypertension can be cured, the better for the patient. Vascular accidents are common, and the longer the disease exists the more likely the hypertension is to become irreversible.

A. Preoperative Management: Hypovolemia has been noted in up to 80% of cases and may cause fatal postoperative vascular collapse. Blood and plasma volumes must be checked and normal volumes restored before surgery. Oral administration of an alpha-adrenergic blocking agent such as phenoxybenzamine (Dibenzylene), 40–200 mg/d in 2 divided doses, will control the blood pressure. If

this can be started at least 3 weeks before surgery, the hypovolemia can be corrected. For fine adjustment of blood pressure before and during induction of anesthesia, when the danger of development of hypertensive crisis is greatest, the alpha-adrenergic blocking agent phentolamine (Regitine), 5 mg in 200 mL of 5% dextrose in water, can be infused intravenously at a rate that will maintain the blood pressure at a nearly normal level.

B. Anesthetic Management: Thiopental (Pentothal) sodium and nitrous oxide combined are used with curare or other muscle relaxants as necessary for muscle relaxation, since they do not raise catecholamine secretion as some other agents do.

C. Operation: Since 10% of tumors (even more in children) are multiple and ectopic, a transperitoneal approach is recommended. An anterior transverse (subcostal) incision provides the best exposure. When an adrenal tumor is found, early ligation of the adrenal vein should be performed to avoid sudden blood pressure elevation from handling the tumor. Intravenous phentolamine during surgery will control blood pressure. After removal of the tumor, there is always a fall in systemic blood pressure of variable severity and duration. This can be minimized by preoperative restoration of blood volume (as discussed above). Hypotension should be treated by infusion of norepinephrine or related pressor agents. If hypotension still persists, hydrocortisone phosphate, 100 mg intravenously, may reestablish the pressure or response. Only when both adrenals are removed is there an absolute need for cortisol replacement.

D. Immediate Postoperative Care: Two to 3 days following surgery, a 24-hour urinary VMA level should be obtained. If it is normal, similar tests every 6 months need be done only in patients with a family history of pheochromocytoma. If the VMA value is still elevated immediately after surgery, another site of pheochromocytoma exists. Malignancies (and, therefore, functional metastases) are very rare.

E. Medical Treatment: Although often effective in decreasing catecholamine production, drugs such as metyrosine (Demser) that limit the production of catecholamines are not in general use because they do not prevent tumor growth and because numerous side-effects, including anxiety, sedation, diarrhea, lactation, and tremor, are reported. Antineoplastic drugs to inhibit the growth of metastases have been only moderately successful.

Prognosis

In general, the prognosis is good. With better understanding of the disease, surgical deaths are now rare. Blood pressure will fall to normal levels in about 70% of patients. In most of the remainder, blood pressure will remain elevated. In rare cases, the patient will become worse as a consequence of secondary vascular changes that have irreversibly activated various pressure systems. Although this persistent hypertension can be controlled with antihypertensive therapy, it is preferable to avoid the problem by early diagnosis and operation.

NEUROBLASTOMA

Neuroblastoma (Fig 21–16) is of neural crest origin and may therefore develop from any portion of the sympathetic chain. Most arise in the retroperitoneum, and 45% involve the adrenal gland. The latter offer the poorest prognosis. In childhood, neuroblastoma is the third most common neoplastic disease after leukemia and brain tumors. Most are encountered in the first 2½ years of life, but a few are seen as late as the sixth decade, when they seem to be less aggressive (Rowe, Oram, & Scott, 1979). Most patients have lymphocytes that are cytotoxic to neuroblastoma cells in tissue culture. Most members of the patient's family show the same lymphocytic reaction. It has been observed that the more lymphocytes found in the peripheral blood or the tumor, the better the prognosis. Abnormalities of muscle and heart and hemihypertrophy have been observed in association with neuroblastoma.

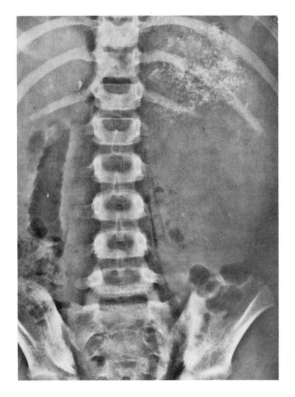

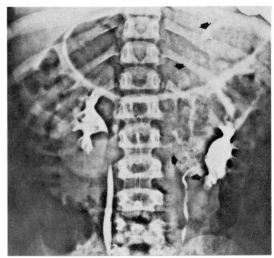

Figure 21–16. Neuroblastoma of adrenal gland. **Left:** Plain film, child age 7 years, showing large mass occupying left flank. Punctate calcification in upper portion that is typical of neuroblastoma. **Right:** Excretory urogram, child age 4 years, revealing lateral and downward displacement and rotation of left kidney by suprarenal mass. No caliceal deformity; calcific areas in mass are compatible with neuroblastoma.

Metastases spread through both the bloodstream and lymphatics. Common sites in children include the skull and long bones, regional lymph nodes, liver, and lungs. Local invasion is common. In infants, who enjoy the best prognosis, metastases are usually limited to the liver and subcutaneous fat.

Evans, D'Angio, & Randolph (1971) evolved the following staging of neuroblastoma:

Stage A: Tumors confined to the structure of origin.

Stage B: Tumors extending in continuity beyond the organ but not crossing the midline. Ipsilateral lymph nodes may be involved.

Stage C: Tumors extending in continuity beyond the midline. Regional lymph nodes may be involved.

Stage D: Remote disease involving skeletal organs, soft tissues, and distant lymph node groups.

Stage E: Stage A or B tumors locally but with distant metastases.

Clinical Findings

A. Symptoms: An abdominal mass is usually noted by parents, the physician, or the patient. About 70% of patients have metastases when first seen. Symptoms relating to metastases include fever, malaise, bone pain, failure to thrive, and constipation or diarrhea.

B. Signs: A flank mass is usually palpable and may even be visible; it often extends across the midline. The tumor is usually nodular and fixed, since it tends to be locally invasive. Evidence of metastases may be noted: ocular proptosis from metastases to the skull, enlarged nodular liver, or a mass in bone. Hypertension is often found.

C. Laboratory Findings: Anemia is common. Urinalysis and renal function are normal. Because 70% of neuroblastomas elaborate increased levels of norepinephrine and epinephrine, urinary vanilmandelic acid (VMA) and homovanillic acid (HVA) levels should be measured. Serial estimations of definitive treatment can be used as tumor markers. A return to normal levels is encouraging, while rising levels imply a residual tumor. Bone marrow aspiration may reveal tumor cells.

D. X-Ray Findings: Excretory urography usually reveals a large area of grayness in one of the upper abdominal quadrants. Intestinal gas is displaced by the mass. At least 50% of these tumors contain punctate calcific deposits. The ipsilateral kidney, which usually functions normally, is displaced by the suprarenal mass (Fig 21–16).

An inferior venacavogram may show occlusion from tumor invasion. Such a finding indicates the need for radiotherapy before surgical excision is attempted. Other necessary tests include a chest film, a complete bone survey, a total body bone scan (Howman-Giles, Gilday, & Ash, 1979), and a liver scan.

CT scans will not only delineate the tumor but may also yield information about invasion of adjacent tissues or organs.

Differential Diagnosis

Nephroblastoma (Wilms's tumor) is also a disease of childhood. Intravenous urograms show the caliceal distortion characteristic of an intrinsic renal tumor; no such distortion is shown in neuroblastoma, which merely displaces the kidney. Urinary catecholamines are normal with Wilms's tumor but are usually elevated in neuroblastoma. Urinary lactic dehydrogenase may be increased with Wilms's tumor but is normal with neuroblastoma. An aortogram will reveal the site of the lesion.

Hydronephrosis may also occur as a flank mass but is ordinarily neither hard nor nodular. Evidence of urinary infection is common. Hydronephrosis is often bilateral, in which case renal function is depressed. Excretory urograms will reveal the dilated pelvis and calices and the site of obstruction.

Polycystic renal disease usually presents with palpable masses in both flanks. Renal function is impaired, and urograms, renal scan, or angiography will establish the diagnosis.

Neonatal adrenal hemorrhage may be confused with neuroblastoma (Smith & Middleton, 1980). These infants have a palpable upper quadrant mass, are apt to be jaundiced, and have increased serum bilirubin and a low hematocrit. Excretory urograms show grayness in the area with displacement of bowel gas. The ipsilateral kidney is displaced downward. The mass is sonolucent on ultrasound (Mittelstaedt & others, 1979). Neuroblastomas cause the excretion of large amounts of catecholamines (eg, vanilmandelic acid).

Treatment

Surgical excision of a tumor should be followed by radiotherapy to the tumor bed. If the tumor is very large or is deemed unresectable, preoperative x-ray therapy should be given, followed by surgical excision. In disseminated disease, chemotherapy must be given. Useful drugs include cyclophosphamide (Cytoxan), vincristine (Oncovin), and dacarbazine. In the past, there has been little enthusiasm for chemotherapy, but Lopez, Kerakousis, & Rao (1980) treated 4 adults with chemotherapy following surgical excision of the tumor. Later study showed complete maturation of the metastases in 1 of them. Evans & others (1980) noted very good results in children who had widespread metastases (but not to bone).

Prognosis

About 90% of patients who die of the disease do so within 14 months following initiation of treatment. Infants have the best prognosis; their 2-year survival rate approaches 60%, and if the tumor is confined to the primary site with or without adjacent regional spread, the cure rate is about 80%. In children age 2 or older, less than 10% are cured. When the disease is disseminated, few cures are obtained.

In a few infants, spontaneous maturation of neuroblastoma to ganglioneuroma has been observed. It is thought by some that x-ray and chemotherapy can also accomplish this.

Serial estimation of urinary catecholamines following therapy will usually indicate the presence of residual tumor.

•   •   •

References

Cushing's Syndrome & Adrenocortical Tumors

Bailey RE: Periodic hormonogenesis—a new phenomenon: Periodicity in function of a hormone-producing tumor in man. *J Clin Endocrinol* 1971;**32**:317.

Baxter JD, Forsham PH: Tissue effects of glucocorticoids. *Am J Med* 1972;**53**:573.

Bennett AH & others: Surgical treatment of adrenocortical hyperplasia: 20 years' experience. *J Urol* 1973;**109**:321.

Birnholz JC: Ultrasound imaging of adrenal mass lesions. *Radiology* 1973;**109**:163.

Bledsoe T: Surgery and the adrenal cortex. *Surg Clin North Am* 1974;**54**:449.

Christy NP: Cushing's syndrome: The natural disease. Pages 359–395 in: *The Human Adrenal Cortex.* Christy NP (editor). Harper & Row, 1971.

Conn JW & others: Primary aldosteronism: Photoscanning of tumors after administration of [131]I-19-iodocholesterol. *Arch Intern Med* 1972;**129**:417.

Cushing H: The basophil adenomas of the pituitary body and their clinical manifestations (pituitary basophilism). *Bull Johns Hopkins Hosp* 1932;**50**:137.

Daughaday WH: Cushing's disease and basophilic microadenomas. (Editorial.) *N Engl J Med* 1978;**298**:793.

Dimopoulos C, Ikkos D: Localization of adrenal adenoma with [131]I-19-iodocholesterol. *Br J Urol* 1977;**49**:256.

Dunnick NR & others: Computed tomography in adrenal tumors. *AJR* 1979;**132**:43.

Eddy RL & others: Cushing's syndrome: A prospective study of diagnostic methods. *Am J Med* 1973;**55**:621.

Flint LD: Surgical exposures for adrenal endocrinopathies. *Surg Clin North Am* 1973;**53**:445.

Gabrilove JL, Nicolis GL, Sohval AR: The testes in Cushing's syndrome. *J Urol* 1974;**112**:95.

Ghandur-Mnaymneh L, Slim M, Muakassa K: Adrenal cyst: Pathogenesis and histologic identification with report of 6 cases. *J Urol* 1979;**122**:87.

Glenn F & others: Total adrenalectomy for Cushing's disease. *Ann Surg* 1972;**175**:948.

Herwig KR, Sonda LP III: Usefulness of adrenal venography and iodocholesterol scan in adrenal surgery. *J Urol* 1979;**122**:7.

Herwig KR & others: Localization of adrenal tumors by photoscanning. *J Urol* 1973;**109**:2.

Kearney GP & others: Functioning and nonfunctioning cysts of the adrenal cortex and medulla. *Am J Surg* 1977;**134**:363.

Lagerquist LG & others: Cushing's disease with cure by resection of a pituitary adenoma: Evidence against a primary hypothalamic defect. *Am J Med* 1974;**57**:826.

Liddle GW: The adrenal cortex. Pages 233–283 in: *Textbook of Endocrinology,* 5th ed. Williams RH (editor). Saunders, 1974.

Nelson DH & others: ACTH-producing pituitary tumors following adrenalectomy for Cushing's syndrome. *Ann Intern Med* 1960;**52**:560.

Schwartz DL, Gann DS, Haller JA Jr: Endocrine surgery in children. *Surg Clin North Am* 1974;**54**:363.

Tyrrell JB & others: Cushing's disease: Selective transsphenoidal resection of pituitary microadenomas. *N Engl J Med* 1978;**298**:753.

Wilson JM, Woodhead DM, Smith RB: Adrenal cysts: Diagnosis and management. *Urology* 1974;**4**:248.

Zaitoon MM, Mackie GG: Adrenal cortical tumors in children. *Urology* 1978;**12**:645.

Adrenogenital Syndromes

Biglieri EG, Herron MA, Brust N: 17-Hydroxylation deficiency in man. *J Clin Invest* 1966;**45**:1946.

Bongiovanni AM & others: Disorders of adrenal steroid biogenesis. *Recent Prog Horm Res* 1967;**23**:375.

Givens JR: Hirsutism and hyperandrogenism. *Adv Intern Med* 1976;**21**:221.

Gooding GA: Ultrasonic spectrum of adrenal masses. *Urology* 1979;**13**:211.

Hajjar RA, Hickey RC, Samaan NA: Adrenal cortical carcinoma: A study of 32 patients. *Cancer* 1975;**35**:549.

Hamilton HW: Congenital adrenal hyperplasia: Inborn errors of cortisol and aldosterone synthesis. *Clin Endocrinol Metabol* 1972;**1**:503.

Harrison JH, Mahoney E, Bennett AH: Tumors of the adrenal cortex. *Cancer* 1973;**32**:1227.

Hoffman DL, Mattox VR: Treatment of adrenocortical carcinoma with o,p'-DDD. *Med Clin North Am* 1972;**56**:999.

Liddle GW: The adrenal cortex. Pages 233–283 in: *Textbook of Endocrinology,* 5th ed. Williams RH (editor). Saunders, 1974.

Mitty HA, Nicolis GL, Gabrilove JL: Adrenal renography: Clinical-roentgenographic correlation in 80 patients. *Am J Roentgenol* 1973;**119**:564.

Parrott TS, Scheflan M, Hester TR: Reduction clitoroplasty and vaginal construction in a single operation. *Urology* 1980;**16**:367.

Shons AR, Gamble WG: Nonfunctioning carcinoma of the adrenal cortex. *Surg Gynecol Obstet* 1974;**138**:705.

Tang CM, Gray GF: Adrenocortical neoplasms: Prognosis and morphology. *Urology* 1975;**5**:691.

Zurbrügg RP: Congenital adrenal hyperplasia. Pages 476–500 in: *Endocrine and Genetic Diseases of Childhood and Adolescence,* 2nd ed. Gardner LI (editor). Saunders, 1975.

Hyperaldosteronism

Conn JW & others: Normokalemic primary aldosteronism. *JAMA* 1966;**195**:21.

Horton R, Finck E: Diagnosis and localization in primary

aldosteronism. *Ann Intern Med* 1972;**76**:885.

Hunt TK, Schambelan M, Biglieri EG: Selection of patients and operative approach in primary aldosteronism. *Ann Surg* 1975;**182**:353.

Liddle GW: The adrenal cortex. Pages 233–283 in: *Textbook of Endocrinology*, 5th ed. Williams RH (editor). Saunders, 1974.

Tarazi RC & others: Hemodynamic characteristics of primary aldosteronism. *N Engl J Med* 1973;**289**:1330.

Weinberger MH, Donohue JP: Aldosterone updated. *J Urol* 1973;**110**:1.

White EA & others: Use of computed tomography in diagnosing the cause of primary aldosteronism. *N Engl J Med* 1980;**303**:1503.

Pheochromocytomas & Related Tumors

Farndon JR & others: VMA excretion in patients with pheochromocytoma. *Ann Surg* 1980;**191**:259.

Flanigan RC & others: Malignant pheochromocytoma of urinary bladder. *Urology* 1980;**16**:386.

Freier DT, Tank ES, Harrison TS: Pediatric and adult pheochromocytomas: A biochemical and clinical comparison. *Arch Surg* 1973;**107**:252.

Funyu T & others: Familial pheochromocytoma: Case report and review of the literature. *J Urol* 1973;**110**:151.

Himathongkam T & others: Pheochromocytoma: Medical emergency management. *JAMA* 1974;**230**:1692.

Laursen K, Damgaard-Pedersen K: CT for pheochromocytoma diagnosis. *AJR* 1980;**134**:277.

Mahoney EM, Harrison JH: Malignant pheochromocytoma: Clinical course and treatment. *J Urol* 1977;**118**:225.

Melmon KL: Catecholamines and the adrenal medulla. Pages 283–322 in: *Textbook of Endocrinology*, 5th ed. Williams RH (editor). Saunders, 1974.

Modlin IM & others: Phaeochromocytoma in 72 patients: Clinical and diagnostic features, treatment and long term results. *Br J Surg* 1979;**66**:456.

Pont A: Multiple endocrine neoplasia syndromes. *West J Med* 1980;**59**:100.

Scott HW Jr & others: Pheochromocytoma: Present diagnosis and management. *Ann Surg* 1976;**183**:587.

Zelch JV, Meany TF, Belhobek GH: Radiologic approach to the patient with suspected pheochromocytoma. *Radiology* 1974;**111**:279.

Neuroblastoma

Bill AH: Immune aspects of neuroblastoma: Current information. *Am J Surg* 1971;**122**:142.

D'Angio GJ, Evans AE, Koop CE: Special pattern of widespread neuroblastoma with favorable prognosis. *Lancet* 1971;**1**:1046.

Evans AE, D'Angio GJ, Randolph J: A proposed staging for children with neuroblastoma. *Cancer* 1971;**27**:374.

Evans AE & others: A review of 17 IV-S neuroblastoma patients at the Children's Hospital of Philadelphia. *Cancer* 1980;**45**:833.

Gitlow SE & others: Diagnosis of neuroblastoma by qualitative and quantitative determination of catecholamine metabolites in urine. *Cancer* 1970;**25**:1377.

Harrison J & others: Results of combination chemotherapy, surgery, and radiotherapy in children with neuroblastoma. *Cancer* 1974;**34**:485.

Howman-Giles RB, Gilday DL, Ash JM: Radionuclide skeletal survey in neuroblastoma. *Radiology* 1979;**131**:497.

Liebner EJ: Serial catecholamines in the radiation management of children with neuroblastoma. *Cancer* 1973;**32**:623.

Lopez R, Karakousis C, Rao U: Treatment of adult neuroblastoma. *Cancer* 1980;**45**:840.

Mittelstaedt CA & others: The sonographic diagnosis of neonatal adrenal hemorrhage. *Radiology* 1979;**131**:453.

Rogers LE, Lyon GM Jr, Porter FS: Spot test for vanillylmandelic acid and other guaiacols in urine of patients with neuroblastoma. *Am J Clin Pathol* 1972;**58**:383.

Rowe PH, Oram JJ, Scott GW: Neuroblastoma in adults. *Postgrad Med J* 1979;**55**:579.

Smith JA Jr, Middleton RG: Neonatal adrenal hemorrhage. *J Urol* 1980;**122**:674.

Varkarakis MJ & others: Current status of prognostic criteria in neuroblastoma. *J Urol* 1973;**109**:94.

Wilson LMK, Draper GJ: Neuroblastoma, its natural history and prognosis: A study of 487 cases. *Br Med J* 1974;**3**:301.

22 | Disorders of the Kidneys

Donald R. Smith, MD

CONGENITAL ANOMALIES OF THE KIDNEYS

Congenital anomalies occur more frequently in the kidney than in any other organ. Some cause no difficulty, but many (eg, hypoplasia, polycystic kidneys) cause impairment of renal function. It has been noted that the child with a gross deformity of an external ear associated with ipsilateral maldevelopment of the facial bones is apt to have a congenital abnormality of the kidney (eg, ectopy, hypoplasia) on the same side as the visible deformity. Lateral displacement of the nipples has been observed in association with bilateral renal hypoplasia.

In association with congenital scoliosis and kyphosis, a significant incidence of renal agenesis, ectopy, malrotation, and duplication has been observed. Unilateral agenesis, hypoplasia, and dysplasia are often seen in association with supralevator imperforate anus. (See General References on p 430.)

AGENESIS

One kidney may be absent. This is probably because the ureteral bud (from the wolffian duct) failed to develop or, if it did develop, did not reach the metanephros (adult kidney). Without a drainage system, the metanephric mass undergoes atrophy. The ureter is usually absent on the side of the unformed kidney, although a blind duct may be found. (See Chapter 2.)

Renal agenesis causes no symptoms; it is usually found by accident on urography. It is not an easy diagnosis to establish even though the ureteral ridge is absent and no orifice is visualized, for the kidney could be present but be drained by a ureter whose opening is ectopic (into the urethra, seminal vesicle, or vagina). If definitive diagnosis seems essential, midstream angiography could be done. A suggestive clue is the presence of low ears.

There appears to be an increased incidence of infection, hydronephrosis, and stones in the contralateral organ. Other congenital anomalies associated with this defect include cardiac, vertebral column, and anal anomalies as well as those of the long bones, hands, and genitalia.

HYPOPLASIA

Hypoplasia implies a small kidney. The total renal mass may be divided in an unequal manner, in which case one kidney is small and the other correspondingly larger than normal. Some of these congenitally small kidneys prove, on pathologic examination, to be dysplastic. Qazi and others (1979) have observed unilateral or bilateral hypoplasia in infants suffering from the fetal alcohol syndrome.

Differentiation from acquired atrophy is difficult. Atrophic pyelonephritis usually reveals typical distortion of the calices. Vesicoureteral reflux in the infant may cause a dwarfed kidney even in the absence of infection. Stenosis of the renal artery leads to shrinkage of the kidney.

Cha, Kandzari, & Khoury (1972) noted that such kidneys have small renal arteries and branches and are associated with hypertension, which is relieved by nephrectomy. Selective renal venography is helpful in differentiating between a congenitally absent and a small, nonvisualized kidney.

SUPERNUMERARY KIDNEYS

The presence of a third kidney is very rare; the presence of 4 separate kidneys in one individual has only been reported once. This anomaly must not be confused with duplication (or triplication) of the pelvis in one kidney, which is not uncommon.

DYSPLASIA & MULTICYSTIC KIDNEY

Renal dysplasia presents protean manifestations. Multicystic kidney of the newborn is usually unilateral, nonhereditary, and characterized by an irregularly lobulated mass of cysts; the ureter is usually absent or atretic. It may develop because of faulty union of the nephron and the collecting system. At most, only a few embryonic glomeruli and tubules are observed. The only finding is the discovery of an irregular mass in the flank. Nothing is shown on urography, but in an occasional case, some radiopaque fluid may be noted (Warshawsky, Miller, & Kaplan, 1977). Bloom & Brosman (1978) have noted that if the cystic kidney is large, its mate is usually normal. When, however, the cystic organ is small, the contralateral kidney is apt to be abnormal. The cystic nature of the lesion may be revealed by sonography (Bearman, Hine, & Sanders, 1976). Friedberg, Mitnick, & Davis (1979) were able to establish the diagnosis by ultrasonography in utero. Cystoscopy usually fails to reveal the ipsilateral ureteral orifice. If the physician feels that the proper diagnosis has been made, no treatment is necessary (Bloom & Brosman, 1978). If in doubt about diagnosis then nephrectomy is considered the procedure of choice.

Dysplasia of the renal parenchyma is also seen in association with ureteral obstruction or reflux that was probably present early in pregnancy. It is relatively common as a segmental renal lesion involving the upper pole of a duplicated kidney whose ureter is obstructed by a congenital ureterocele. It may also be found in urinary tracts severely obstructed by posterior urethral valves; in this instance, the lesion may be bilateral.

Microscopically, the renal parenchyma is "disorganized." Tubular and glomerular cysts may be noted; these elements are fetal in type. Islands of metaplastic cartilage are often seen. The common denominator seems to be fetal obstruction (Fisher & Smith, 1975).

POLYCYSTIC KIDNEYS
(See Chapter 23.)

Polycystic kidney disease is hereditary and almost always bilateral (95% of cases). Lee, McLennan, & Kissane (1978) have discussed one case of unilateral polycystic disease, but it is not clear that their patient did not have multiple renal cysts or congenital multicystic kidney disease. The disease encountered in infancy is different from that seen in the adult, although Kaye & Lewy (1974) reported 4 cases from the literature of infants with the adult type. The former is an autosomal recessive disease and life expectancy is short, whereas that diagnosed in adulthood is autosomal dominant; symptoms ordinarily do not appear until after age 40. In association with both forms, cysts of the liver, spleen, and pancreas may be noted. The kidneys are larger than normal and are studded with cysts of various sizes.

Etiology & Pathogenesis
The evidence suggests that the cysts occur because of defects in the development of the collecting and uriniferous tubules and in the mechanism of their joining. Blind secretory tubules that are connected to functioning glomeruli become cystic. As these cysts enlarge, they compress adjacent parenchyma, destroy it by ischemia, and occlude normal tubules. The result is progressive functional impairment. It would appear that medullary sponge kidney is part of the spectrum but a milder form.

Pathology
Grossly, the kidneys are usually much enlarged. Their surfaces are studded with cysts of various sizes (Fig 22–1). On section, the cysts are found to be scattered throughout the parenchyma. Calcification is rare (Kutcher, Schneider, & Gordon, 1977). The fluid in the cyst is usually amber-colored but may be hemorrhagic.

Microscopically, the lining of the cysts consists of a single layer of cells. The renal parenchyma may show peritubular fibrosis and evidence of secondary infection. There appears to be a reduction in the number of glomeruli, some of which may be hyalinized. Renal arteriolar thickening is a prominent finding in the adult.

Clinical Findings
A. Symptoms: Pain over one or both kidneys may occur because of the drag on the vascular pedicles by the heavy kidneys, from obstruction or infection, or from hemorrhage into a cyst. Gross total hematuria is not uncommon and may be severe; the

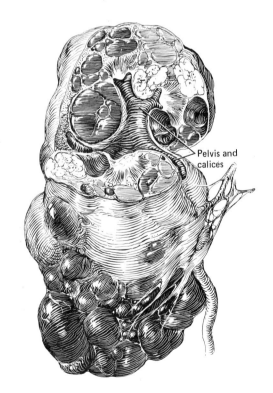

Pelvis and calices

Figure 22–1. Polycystic kidney. Multiple cysts deep in the parenchyma and on the surface. Note distortion of the calices by the cysts.

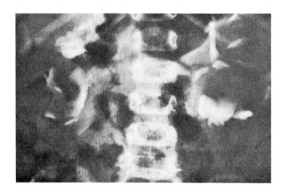

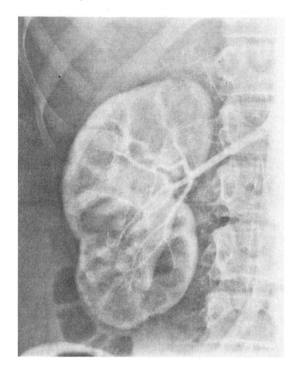

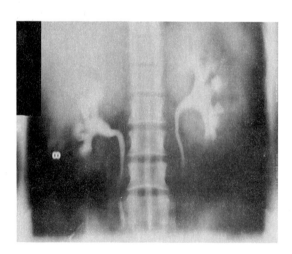

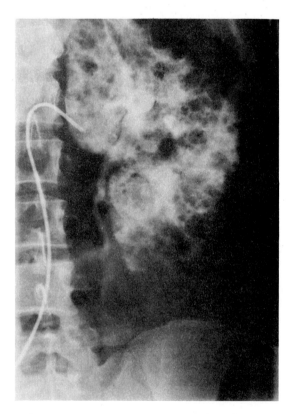

Figure 22–2. Polycystic kidneys. *Above left:* Excretory urogram in a child, showing elongation, broadening, and bending of the calices around cysts. Good renal function. *Above right:* Angiogram of right kidney, showing "negative" shadows of cysts. *Below left:* Angionephrotomogram showing kidneys of essentially normal size. All infundibula on left and infundibulum of right upper calix are widened, suggesting polycystic kidneys. *Below right:* Nephrogram phase of left selective angiogram (same patient) showing multiple small negative shadows representing the cysts.

cause for this is not clear. Colic may be present if blood clots or stones are passed. The patient may notice an abdominal mass (Segal, Spataro, & Barbaric, 1977).

Infection (chills, fever, renal pain) commonly complicates polycystic disease. Symptoms of vesical irritability may be the first complaint. When renal insufficiency ensues, headache, nausea and vomiting, weakness, and loss of weight occur.

B. Signs: One or both kidneys are usually palpable. They may feel nodular. If infected, they may be tender. Hypertension is found in 60–70% of these patients. Evidence of cardiac enlargement is then noted.

Fever may be present if pyelonephritis exists or if cysts have become infected. In the stage of uremia, anemia and loss of weight may be evident. Ophthalmoscopic examination may show changes typical of moderate or severe hypertension.

C. Laboratory Findings: Anemia may be noted, caused either by chronic loss of blood or, more commonly, by the hematopoietic depression accompanying uremia. Proteinuria and microscopic (if not gross) hematuria are the rule. Pus cells and bacteria are common.

Progressive loss of concentrating power occurs. The PSP and clearance tests will show varying degrees of renal impairment. About a third of patients with polycystic kidney disease are uremic when first seen.

D. X-Ray Findings: Both renal shadows are usually enlarged on a plain film of the abdomen, even as much as 5 times normal size. Kidneys more than 16 cm in length are suspect.

Excretory infusion urograms with tomography are helpful if, as is true in most cases, the PSP excretion is better than 30% in 1 hour, in which event excretion of the medium may be sufficient to delineate the caliceal system and thus establish the diagnosis. Tomography will reveal multiple lucencies representing cysts. On these or on retrograde urography the renal masses are usually enlarged, and the caliceal pattern is quite bizarre (spider deformity). The calices are broadened and flattened, enlarged, and often curved, as they tend to hug the periphery of adjacent cysts (Fig 22–2). Often the changes are only slight or may even be absent on one side, leading to the erroneous diagnosis of tumor of the other kidney.

If cysts are infected, perinephritis may obscure the renal and even the psoas shadows.

Angiography will reveal bending of small vessels around the cysts and the "negative" shadows (nonvascular) of the cysts (Fig 22–2).

Enlarged kidneys containing multiple cysts have a lobulated contour on computed tomography. The liver and spleen may contain cysts also (Sagel & others, 1977).

E. Isotope Studies: Photoscan (see Chapter 8) will reveal multiple "cold" avascular spots in large renal shadows.

F. Sonography: B scan sonography appears to be superior to both excretory urography and isotope scanning in diagnosis of the polycystic disorders (Lufkin & others, 1974).

G. Instrumental Examination: Cystoscopy may show evidence of cystitis, in which case the urine will contain abnormal elements. Bleeding from a ureteral orifice may be noted.

Ureteral catheterization and retrograde urograms are rarely indicated.

Differential Diagnosis

Bilateral hydronephrosis (on the basis of congenital or acquired ureteral obstruction) may present bilateral flank masses and signs of impairment of renal function, but urography and sonography will show changes quite different from those of the polycystic kidney.

Bilateral renal tumor is rare but may mimic polycystic kidney disease perfectly on urography. Differentiation of a unilateral tumor may be quite difficult if one of the polycystic kidneys shows little or no distortion on urography. However, tumors are usually localized to one portion of the kidney, whereas cysts are quite diffusely distributed. The total renal function should be normal with unilateral tumor but is usually depressed in the patient with polycystic kidney disease. Nephrotomograms or renal angiography may be needed at times, to differentiate between the 2 conditions (Fig 22–2). Photoscans or sonograms may also prove helpful in differentiation.

In **Lindau's disease** (angiomatous cerebellar cyst, angiomatosis of the retina, tumors or cysts of the pancreas), multiple bilateral cysts or adenocarcinomas of both kidneys may develop. Urograms or nephrotomograms may suggest polycystic kidney disease. The presence of other stigmas should make the diagnosis. Angiography, sonography, or scintophotography should be definitive (Lamiell, Stor, & Hsia, 1980).

Tuberous sclerosis (convulsive seizures, mental retardation, and adenoma sebaceum) is typified by hamartomatous tumors often involving the skin, brain, retinas, bones, liver, heart, and kidneys. (See Chapter 18.) The renal lesions are usually multiple and bilateral and microscopically are angiomyolipomas. Urograms obtained during the stage of uremia are apt to suggest polycystic disease; the presence of other stigmas and angiography or sonography should make the differentiation.

Simple cyst (see below) is usually unilateral and single; total renal function should be normal. Urograms usually show a single lesion (Fig 22–3), whereas polycystic kidney disease is bilateral and has multiple filling defects.

Complications

For reasons that are not clear, pyelonephritis is a common complication of polycystic kidney disease. It may be asymptomatic; pus cells in the

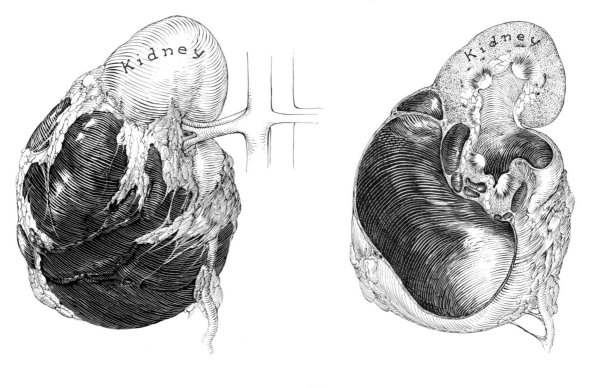

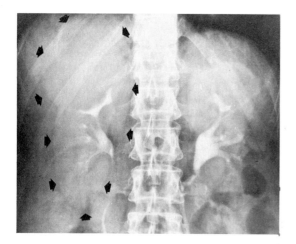

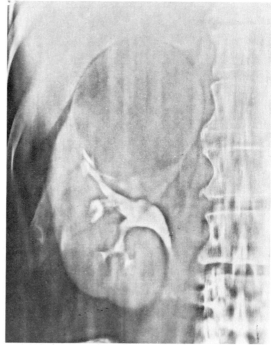

Figure 22–3. Simple cyst. *Above left:* Large cyst displacing lower pole laterally. *Above right:* Section of kidney showing one large and a few small cysts. *Below left:* Excretory urogram showing soft tissue mass in upper pole of right kidney. Elongation and distortion of upper calices by cyst. *Below right:* Infusion nephrotomogram showing large cyst in upper renal pole distorting upper calices and dislocating upper portion of kidney laterally.

urine may be few or absent. Stained smears or quantitative cultures make the diagnosis. A gallium-67 citrate scan will definitely reveal the sites of infection, including abscess (Waters, Hershman, & Klein, 1979).

Infection of cysts will be associated with pain and tenderness over the kidney and a febrile response. The differential diagnosis between infection of cysts and pyelonephritis may be difficult, but here again a gallium scan will prove helpful.

In rare instances gross hematuria may be so brisk and persistent as to endanger life.

Treatment

Except for unusual complications, the treatment is conservative and supportive.

A. General Measures: Place the patient on a low-protein diet (0.5–0.75 g/kg/d of protein) and force fluids to 3000 mL or more per day. Physical activity may be permitted within reason, but strenuous overexercise is contraindicated. When the patient is in the state of absolute renal insufficiency, treat as for uremia from any cause. Hypertension should be controlled. Hemodialysis may be indicated.

B. Surgery: There is no evidence that excision or decompression of cysts improves renal function (Milam, Magee, & Bunts, 1963). Should a large cyst be found to be compressing the upper ureter, causing obstruction and further embarrassing renal function, it should be resected or aspirated. When the degree of renal insufficiency becomes life-threatening, chronic dialysis or renal transplantation should be considered (Salvatierra, Kountz, & Belzer, 1973).

C. Treatment of Complications: Pyelonephritis must be rigorously treated to prevent further renal damage. Infection of cysts requires surgical drainage. If bleeding from one kidney is so severe as to threaten exsanguination, nephrectomy or embolization of the renal or preferably the segmental artery must be considered as a lifesaving measure.

Concomitant diseases (eg, tumor, obstructing stone) may require definitive surgical treatment.

Prognosis

When the disease affects children, it has a very poor prognosis. The large group presenting clinical signs and symptoms after age 35–40 years has a somewhat more favorable prognosis. Although there is wide variation, these patients usually do not live longer than 5 or 10 years after the diagnosis is made unless dialysis is made available or renal transplant is done.

SIMPLE (SOLITARY) CYST

Simple cyst (Figs 22–3 and 22–4) of the kidney is usually unilateral and single but may be multiple and multilocular and, more rarely, bilateral. It differs from polycystic kidneys both clinically and pathologically.

Etiology and Pathogenesis

Whether simple cyst is congenital or acquired is not clear. Its origin may be similar to that of polycystic kidneys, ie, the difference may be merely one of degree. On the other hand, simple cysts have been produced in animals by causing tubular obstruction and local ischemia, which suggests that the lesion can be acquired.

As a simple cyst grows it compresses and thereby may destroy renal parenchyma, but rarely is a significant amount of renal tissue destroyed so that function is impaired (Roth & Roberts, 1980). A solitary cyst may be placed in such a position as to compress the ureter, causing progressive hydronephrosis. Infection may then complicate the picture.

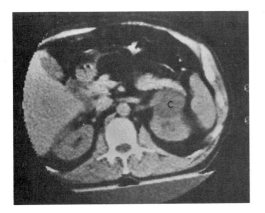 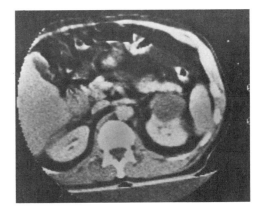

Figure 22–4. Left renal cyst. *Left:* CT scan shows a homogeneous low density mass (C) arising from anterior border of left kidney just posterior to tail of the pancreas. The CT attenuation value was similar to that of water, indicating a simple renal cyst. *Right:* After intravenous injection of contrast material, the mass did not increase in attenuation value, adding further confirmatory evidence of its benign cystic nature.

Pathology

Simple cysts usually involve the lower pole of the kidney. They average about 10 cm in diameter when producing symptoms, but a few are large enough to fill the entire flank. They usually contain a clear amber fluid. Their walls are quite thin, and the cysts are "blue-domed" in appearance. Calcification of the sac is occasionally seen. About 5% contain hemorrhagic fluid, and possibly one-half of these have papillary cancers on their walls.

Simple cysts are usually superficial but may be deeply situated. When a cyst is situated deep in the kidney, the cyst wall is adjacent to the epithelial lining of the pelvis or calices, from which it may be separated only with great difficulty. Cysts do not communicate with the renal pelvis (Fig 22–3). Microscopic examination of the cyst wall shows heavy fibrosis and hyalinization; areas of calcification may be seen. The adjacent renal tissue is compressed and fibrosed. A number of cases of simple cysts have been reported in children (Gordon & others, 1979; Bartholomew & others, 1980).

Clinical Findings

A. Symptoms: Pain in the flank or back, usually intermittent and dull, is not uncommon. Should bleeding suddenly distend the cyst wall, pain may come on abruptly and be severe. Gastrointestinal symptoms are frequently noted and may suggest peptic ulcer or gallbladder disease. The patient may discover a mass in the abdomen, although cysts of this size are unusual. If the cyst becomes infected, the patient usually complains of pain in the flank, malaise, and fever.

B. Signs: Physical examination is usually normal, although occasionally a mass in the region of the kidney may be palpated or percussed. Tenderness in the flank may be noted if the cyst becomes infected.

C. Laboratory Findings: Urinalysis is usually normal. Microscopic hematuria is rare. Renal function tests are normal unless the cysts are multiple and bilateral (rare). Even in the face of extensive destruction of one kidney, compensatory hypertrophy of the other kidney will maintain normal total function.

D. X-Ray Findings: An expansion of a portion of the kidney shadow or a mass superimposed upon it can usually be seen on a plain film of the abdomen (Fig 6–2, top left). The axis of the kidney may be abnormal because of rotation due to the weight or position of the cyst. Streaks of calcium can sometimes be seen in the border of the mass.

Excretory urograms establish the presumptive diagnosis of cyst. On the film taken 1–2 minutes after infusion of the radiopaque fluid, the vascularized parenchyma becomes white while the space-occupying cyst does not because it is avascular. The urographic series will show changes compatible with a mass. One or more calices or the pelvis will usually be indented or bent around the cyst and are often broadened and flattened, even obliterated (Figs 22–3 and 22–5). Oblique and lateral films may prove helpful. If a mass occupies the lower pole of the kidney, the upper part of the ureter may be displaced toward the spine. The kidney itself may be rotated. The psoas muscle may be seen through the radiolucent cyst fluid.

Should the routine urogram fail to significantly opacify the parenchyma, infusion nephrotomography should be done, thus increasing the contrast between vascular renal tissue and the cyst (Fig 22–3). Occasionally, a renal parenchymal tumor may be relatively avascular, thus being confused with cyst. In a few instances, carcinoma may grow on the cyst wall (Ambrose & others, 1977; Sufrin & others, 1975; Varma & others, 1974). Because of these phenomena, further steps in differential diagnosis should be performed.

E. Computed Tomography: CT scan appears to be the most accurate means of differentiating renal cyst and tumor (Fig 22–4) (Sagel & others, 1977). Cysts have an attenuation approximating that of water, whereas tumor density is similar to that of normal parenchyma (Fig 18–5). Parenchyma is made more dense with the intravenous injection of radiopaque fluid. A cyst remains unaffected. The wall of a cyst is sharply demarcated from the renal parenchyma; a tumor is not. The wall of a cyst is thin; that of a tumor is not. This test may well supplant cyst puncture in the differentiation of cyst and tumor in many cases.

F. Renal Sonography: Renal sonography is a noninvasive diagnostic technic that in a high percentage of cases differentiates between a cyst and a solid mass (Bartholomew & others, 1980). If this study is also compatible with cyst, a needle can be introduced into the cyst under fluoroscopic or ultrasonographic B scan control.

G. Isotope Scanning: A rectilinear scan will clearly delineate the mass but does not differentiate cyst from tumor. The technetium scan, made with the camera, will reveal that the mass is, indeed, avascular (see Chapter 8).

H. Percutaneous Cyst Aspiration With Cystography: If the above studies leave some doubt about the differentiation between cyst and tumor, this procedure should be done. (See Treatment, below, and p 87.)

Differential Diagnosis

Carcinoma of the kidney also occupies space but tends to lie more deeply in the organ and therefore causes more distortion of the calices. Hematuria is common with tumor, rare with cyst. If a solid tumor overlies the psoas muscle, the edge of the muscle is obliterated on the plain film; it can be seen through a cyst, however. Evidence of metastases (ie, loss of weight and strength, palpable supraclavicular nodes, chest film showing metastatic nodules), erythrocytosis, hypercalcemia, elevation of plasma or urinary CEA, and increased sedimen-

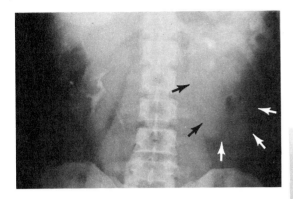

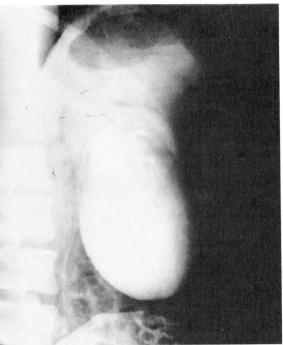

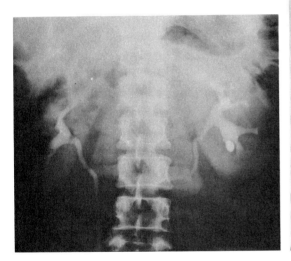

Figure 22–5. *Above left:* Excretory urogram showing large smooth mass in lower pole of left kidney with distortion of calices. *Right:* Cyst punctured and radiopaque fluid instilled. Cyst is smooth-walled. Iophendylate then instilled. *Lower left:* Excretory urogram 3 months later. Iophendylate occupies what is left of cyst in the lower medial calix. Urogram normal.

tation rate suggest cancer. It must be remembered, however, that the walls of a simple cyst may undergo cancerous degeneration. If the renal vein is occluded by cancer, the excretory urogram may be visualized only faintly or not at all. Sonography or CT scan should be almost definitive in differential diagnosis. Angiography (Fig 18–3) or nephrotomography (Fig 18–4) may reveal "pooling" of the medium in the highly vascularized tumor, whereas the density of a cyst is not affected (Fig 22–6). It is wise to assume that all space-occupying lesions of the kidneys are cancers until proved otherwise.

Polycystic kidney disease is almost always bilateral, as shown by urography (Fig 22–2). Diffuse caliceal and pelvic distortion is the rule. Simple cyst is usually solitary and unilateral. Polycystic kidney disease is usually accompanied by impaired renal function and hypertension. Simple cyst is not.

Renal carbuncle is a rare disease. A history of skin infection a few weeks before the onset of fever and local pain may be obtained. Urograms may show changes similar to cyst or tumor, but the renal outline as well as the edge of the psoas muscle may be obscured because of perinephritis. The kidney may be fixed, as demonstrated by comparing the position of the kidney in the supine and upright positions. Angiography will demonstrate an avascular lesion (Fig 12–8). A gallium-67 scan will demonstrate its inflammatory nature but might be similar if a simple cyst should become infected.

Hydronephrosis may present the same symptoms and signs as simple cyst, but the urograms are quite different. Cyst causes caliceal distortion; with hydronephrosis, dilatation of the calices and pelvis due to an obstruction is present. Acute or subacute hydronephrosis usually produces more local pain because of increased intrapelvic pressure and is more apt to be complicated by infection.

Extrarenal tumor (eg, adrenal, mixed retroperitoneal sarcoma) may displace a kidney, but rarely does it invade it and distort its calices.

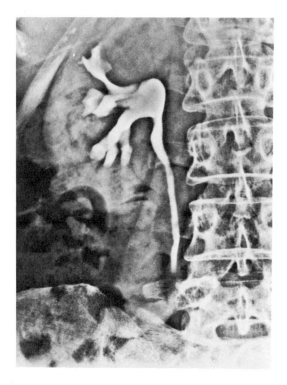 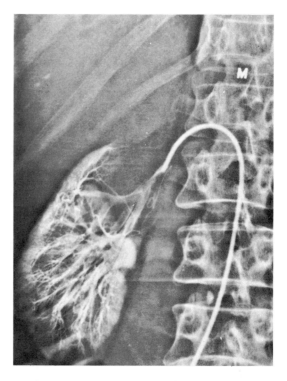

Figure 22–6. Diagnosis of simple renal cyst. **Left:** Excretory urogram showing lateral and inferior displacement and distortion of upper calix, right kidney. Differential diagnosis: cyst versus tumor. **Right:** Same patient. Selective femoral angiogram showing a completely avascular mass typical of cyst.

If an echinococcus cyst of the kidney does not communicate with the pelvis, it may be difficult to differentiate from solitary cyst, for no scoleces or hooklets will be present in the urine. The wall of a hydatid cyst often reveals calcification on x-ray examination (Fig 13–5). A skin sensitivity test (Casoni) for hydatid disease may prove helpful.

Complications (Rare)

Spontaneous infection in a simple cyst is rare, but when it occurs it is difficult to differentiate from carbuncle. Hemorrhage into the cyst sometimes occurs. If sudden, it causes severe pain. The bleeding may come from a complicating carcinoma arising on the wall of the cyst.

Hydronephrosis may develop if a cyst of the lower pole impinges upon the ureter. This in itself may cause pain from back pressure of urine in the pelvis. This obstruction may lead to renal infection.

Treatment

A. Specific Measures:

1. If excretory urography, nephrotomograms, sonograms, and CT scan do not lead to a definitive diagnosis, renal angiography might be necessary, but percutaneous needle aspiration of the cyst should probably be the next step. This may be done under either fluoroscopic or sonographic (see p 87) control (Hayt, Blatt, & Robinson, 1978; Gross,

1979). The recovery of clear fluid is an encouraging sign, but the fluid must be subjected to cytologic examination. Its fat content should be estimated. Increased levels are compatible with tumor. The cyst is then drained, and cyst fluid is replaced with a radiopaque fluid. Films are taken in various positions to prove that the cyst wall is smooth and that there are no excrescences that might represent tumor. Before the radiopaque fluid is removed, instill 3 mL of iophendylate (Pantopaque) into the cavity. This will decrease the chances for reaccumulation of fluid (Fig 22–5) (Wettlaufer & Modarelli, 1978). If simple aspiration alone is utilized, most cysts will refill (Raskin, Roen, & Viamonte, 1975).

Should the aspirate reveal blood, immediate nephrectomy should be considered, because the chances that the growth is cancerous are great.

2. If the diagnosis can be clearly established, one should consider leaving it alone, since it is rare for a cyst to harm the kidney.

3. Surgical exploration should be considered if the diagnosis is still in doubt. Ambrose & others (1977) prefer exploration in most cases diagnosed as cysts. Of the 55 cases they explored, 5 proved to be cancer (9%). Usually only the extrarenal portion of the cyst is excised. Should the kidney be badly damaged, nephrectomy may be indicated, but this is rare.

B. Treatment of Complications: If the cyst

should become infected, intensive antibiotic therapy should be instituted. If this proves unsuccessful, surgical excision of the extrarenal portion of the cyst wall and drainage will prove curative.

If, on exploration, the cyst appears to contain blood (and the other kidney is normal), immediate nephrectomy should be strongly urged without preliminary incision into the cyst, for this finding makes the presence of neoplasm likely. Drainage of the contents of a cancerous cyst, by either incision or needle, invites growth of carcinoma in the wound.

If hydronephrosis is present, excision of the obstructing cyst will relieve the ureteral obstruction (Hinman, 1978).

Pyelonephritis in the involved kidney should suggest urinary stasis secondary to impaired ureteral drainage. Removal of the cyst and consequent relief of urinary back pressure will make antimicrobial therapy more effective.

Prognosis

In masses compatible with cyst, aspiration and renal cystography afford a good prognosis. If the possibility of tumor cannot be ruled out, the kidney should be explored.

RENAL FUSION

About one out of 1000 individuals has some type of renal fusion, the most common being the horseshoe kidney. The fused renal mass almost always contains 2 excretory systems and therefore 2 ureters. The renal tissue may be divided equally between the 2 flanks, or the entire mass may be on one side. Even in the latter case, the 2 ureters open at their proper places in the bladder.

Etiology & Pathogenesis

It appears that this fusion of the 2 metanephroi occurs early in embryologic life, when the kidneys lie low in the pelvis. For this reason, they seldom ascend to the high position that normal kidneys assume. They may even remain in the true pelvis. Under these circumstances such a kidney may derive its blood supply from many vessels in the area (eg, aorta, iliacs).

In association with both ectopia and fusion, 78% of the patients will have extraurologic anomalies and 65% will exhibit other genitourinary defects (Kelalis, Malek, & Segura, 1973).

Pathology (Fig 22–7)

Because the renal masses fuse early, normal rotation cannot occur; therefore, each pelvis lies on the anterior surface of its organ. Thus, the ureter must ride over the isthmus of a horseshoe kidney or traverse the anterior surface of the fused kidney. Some degree of ureteral compression may arise

from this or from obstruction by one or more aberrant blood vessels. The incidence of hydronephrosis and, therefore, infection is high. Vesicoureteral reflux has frequently been noted in association with fusion.

In horseshoe kidney the isthmus usually joins the lower poles of each kidney; each renal mass lies lower than normal. The axes of these masses are vertical, whereas the axes of normal kidneys are oblique to the spine, since they lie along the edges of the psoas muscles.

On rare occasions the 2 nephric masses are fused into one mass containing 2 pelves and 2 ureters. The mass may lie in the midline to open into the bladder at the proper point (crossed renal ectopy with fusion).

Clinical Findings

A. Symptoms: Most patients with fused kidneys have no symptoms. Some, however, develop ureteral obstruction. Gastrointestinal symptoms (renodigestive reflex) mimicking peptic ulcer, cholelithiasis, or appendicitis may be noted. Infection is apt to occur if ureteral obstruction and hydronephrosis or calculus develop.

B. Signs: Physical examination is usually negative unless the abnormally placed renal mass can be felt. With horseshoe kidney it may be possible to palpate a mass over the lower lumbar spine (the isthmus). In the case of crossed ectopy, a mass may be felt in the flank or lower abdomen.

C. Laboratory Findings: Urinalysis is normal unless there is infection. Renal function is normal unless disease coexists in each of the fused renal masses.

D. X-Ray Findings: In the case of horseshoe kidney, the axes of the 2 kidneys, if visible on a plain film, are parallel to the spine. At times the isthmus can be identified. The plain film may also reveal a large soft tissue mass in one flank yet not show a renal shadow on the other side (Fig 22–8).

Excretory urograms establish the diagnosis if the renal parenchyma has maintained good function. The increased density of the kidney tissue may make its position or configuration more distinct. Urograms will also visualize the pelves and ureters.

1. With horseshoe kidney, the renal pelves lie on the anterior surfaces of their respective kidney masses, whereas the normal kidney has its pelvis lying mesial to it. The most valuable clue to the diagnosis of horseshoe kidney is the presence of calices in the region of the lower pole that point medially and overlie the psoas muscles or even reach the vertebrae (Figs 22–7 and 22–8).

2. Crossed renal ectopy with fusion shows 2 pelves and 2 ureters. One ureter must cross the midline in order to empty into the bladder at the proper point (Figs 22–7 and 22–8).

3. A cake or lump kidney may lie in the pelvis (fused pelvic kidney), but again its ureters and pelves will be shown (Figs 22–7 and 22–8).

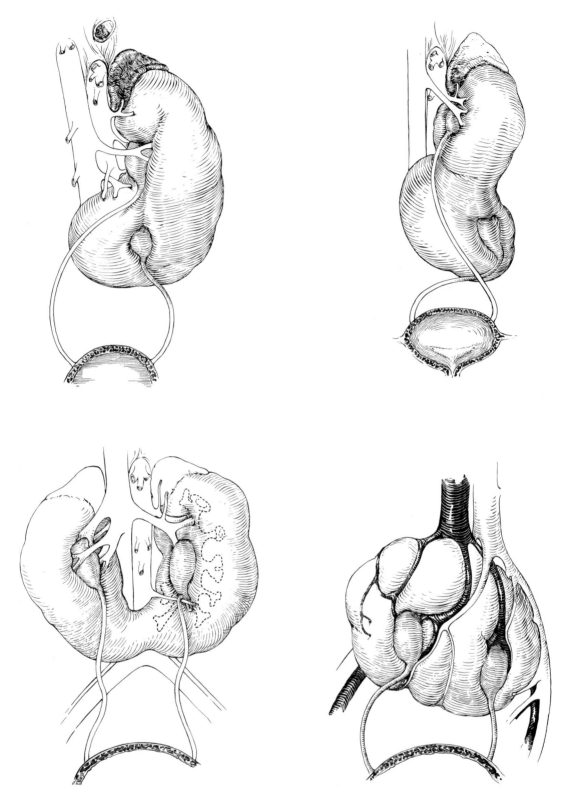

Figure 22–7. Renal fusion. *Above left:* Crossed renal ectopy with fusion. The renal mass lies in the left flank. The right ureter must cross over the midline. *Above right:* Example of "sigmoid" kidney. *Below left:* Horseshoe kidney. Pelves are anterior. Note aberrant artery obstructing left ureter and the low position of renal mass. *Below right:* Pelvic kidney. Pelves are placed anteriorly. Note aberrant blood supply.

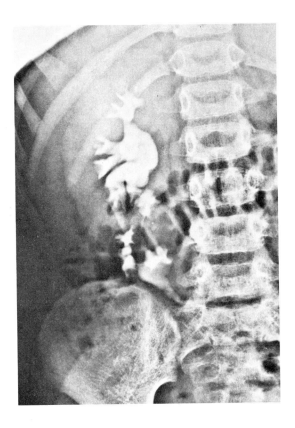
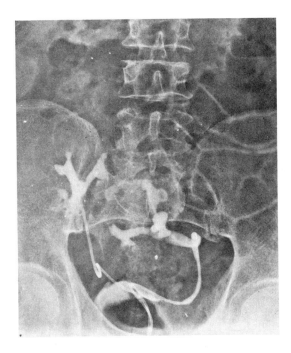
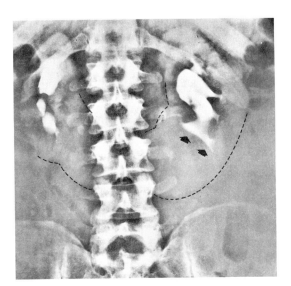
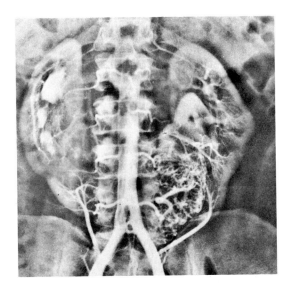

Figure 22–8. Renal fusion. *Above left:* Excretory urogram showing fused renal masses on the right side. Both kidneys are normal. Crossed renal ectopy. *Above right:* Retrograde urogram showing pelvic kidney. *Below left:* Excretory urogram showing horseshoe kidney with expansion of left side of isthmus and compression of lower left caliceal system. *Below right:* Angiogram on same patient. Hypervascular mass in left side of isthmus typical of adenocarcinoma.

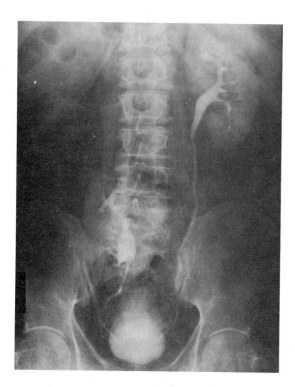

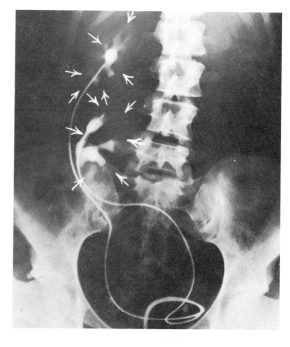

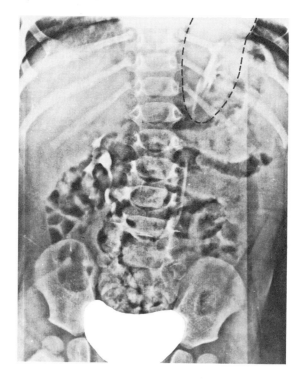

Figure 22–9. Renal ectopy. *Above left:* Excretory urogram showing congenital ectopy, right kidney. *Above right:* Retrograde urogram showing crossed renal ectopy. In this film the differentiation between fusion and nonfusion cannot be made. *Below:* Left kidney, ectopic in the chest.

Tomograms will clearly outline the renal mass but are seldom necessary for diagnosis.

With pelvic fused kidney or one lying in the flank, the plain film taken with ureteral catheters in place will give the first hint of the diagnosis. Retrograde urograms will show the position of the pelves and demonstrate changes compatible with infection or obstruction (Fig 22–9). Renal scanning will delineate the renal mass and its contour (see Chapter 8) as will sonography also.

Differential Diagnosis

Separate kidneys that fail to undergo the normal rotation may be confused with horseshoe kidney. They lie along the edges of the psoas muscles, whereas the poles of a horseshoe kidney lie parallel to the spine and their lower poles are placed on the psoas muscles. The calices in the region of the isthmus of a horseshoe kidney point medially and lie close to the spine.

The diagnosis of fused or lump kidney may be missed on excretory urograms if one of its ureters is markedly obstructed so that a portion of the kidney and its pelvis and ureter fail to visualize. Infusion urograms or retrograde urograms will demonstrate both excretory tracts in the renal mass.

Complications

Fused kidneys are prone to ureteral obstruction because of a high incidence of aberrant renal vessels and the necessity for one or both ureters to arch around or over the renal tissue. Hydronephrosis, stone, and infection therefore are common.

A large fused kidney occupying the concavity of the sacrum may cause dystocia.

Treatment

No treatment is necessary unless obstruction or infection is present. Drainage of a horseshoe kidney may be improved by dividing its isthmus. If one pole of a horseshoe is badly damaged, it may require surgical resection.

Prognosis

In most cases, the outlook is excellent. Should ureteral obstruction and infection occur, renal drainage must be improved by surgical means so that antimicrobial therapy will be effective.

ECTOPIC KIDNEY

Congenital ectopic kidney usually causes no symptoms unless complications such as ureteral obstruction or infection develop.

Simple Ectopy

Simple congenital ectopy is a low kidney on the proper side that failed to ascend normally. It may lie over the pelvic brim or in the pelvis. (Rarely, it may be found in the chest [Fig 22–9]). It takes its blood supply from adjacent vessels, and its ureter is short. It is prone to ureteral obstruction and infection, which may lead to pain or fever. At times such a kidney may be palpable, leading to an erroneous presumptive diagnosis (eg, cancer of the bowel, appendiceal abscess).

Excretory urograms (Fig 22–9) will reveal the true position. Hydronephrosis, if present, will be evident. There is no redundancy of the ureter, as is the case with nephroptosis or acquired ectopy (eg, displacement by large suprarenal tumor).

Obstruction and infection may complicate simple ectopy and should be treated by appropriate means.

Crossed Ectopy Without Fusion

In crossed ectopy without fusion, the kidney lies on the opposite side of the body but is not attached to its normally placed mate. Unless 2 distinct renal shadows can be seen, it may be difficult to differentiate this condition from crossed ectopy with fusion (Fig 22–7). Sonography or angiography would make the distinction.

ABNORMAL ROTATION

Normally, when the kidney ascends to the lumbar region the pelvis lies on its anterior surface. Later, the pelvis comes to lie mesially. Such rotation may fail to occur, although this seldom leads to renal disease. Urography demonstrates the abnormal position.

MEDULLARY SPONGE KIDNEY
(Cystic Dilatation of the Renal Collecting Tubules)

Medullary sponge kidney is a congenital autosomal recessive defect characterized by widening of the distal collecting tubules. It is usually bilateral, affecting all of the papillae, but it may be unilateral. At times, only one papilla is involved. Cystic dilatation of the tubules is often present also. Infection and calculi are occasionally seen as a result of urinary stasis in the tubules. Potter believes that medullary sponge kidney is related to polycystic renal disease. Its occasional association with hemihypertrophy of the body has been noted.

The only symptoms are those arising from infection and stone formation. The diagnosis is made on the basis of excretory urograms (Fig 22–10). The pelvis and calices are normal, but dilated (streaked) tubules are seen just lateral to them; many of the dilated tubules contain round masses of radiopaque material (the cystic dilatation). If stones are present, a plain film will reveal small, round calculi in the pyramidal regions just beyond the calices. Retrograde urograms often do not reveal the lesion

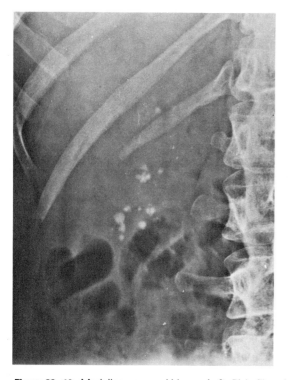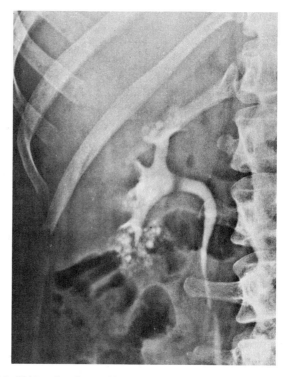

Figure 22–10. Medullary sponge kidneys. *Left:* Plain film of right kidney showing multiple small stones in its mid portion. *Right:* Excretory urogram showing relationship of calculi to calices. Typically, the calices are large; the stones are located in the dilated collecting tubules.

unless the mouths of the collecting ducts are widely dilated.

The differential diagnosis includes tuberculosis, healed papillary necrosis, and nephrocalcinosis. Tuberculosis is usually unilateral, and urography shows ulceration of calices; tubercle bacilli are found on bacteriologic study. Papillary necrosis may be complicated by calcification in the healed stage but may be distinguished by its typical caliceal deformity, the presence of infection, and, usually, impaired renal function (Figs 12–5 and 12–6). The tubular and parenchymal calcification seen in nephrocalcinosis is more diffuse than that seen with sponge kidney (Fig 15–5); the symptoms and signs of primary hyperparathyroidism or renal tubular acidosis may be found.

There is no treatment for medullary sponge kidney. Therapy is directed toward the complications (eg, pyelonephritis and renal calculi). Only a small percentage of people with sponge kidney develop complications. The overall prognosis is good. A few patients may pass small stones occasionally.

ABNORMALITIES OF RENAL VESSELS

As a rule, each kidney receives one renal artery from the aorta and has one vein passing to the vena cava. Aberrant veins and especially arteries are common. Three or 4 renal arteries may be depicted

on angiography. An aberrant artery passing to the lower pole of the kidney may compress and thereby obstruct the ureter, causing hydronephrosis. On urography, it may be difficult to differentiate between an obstructing vessel and intrinsic ureteral stenosis. The diagnosis can be made on angiography or at the operating table.

ACQUIRED LESIONS OF THE KIDNEYS

RENOALIMENTARY FISTULA

Over 100 instances of renoalimentary fistula have been reported. They usually involve the stomach, duodenum, or adjacent colon, although fistula formation with the esophagus, small bowel, appendix, and rectum has been reported.

The underlying cause is usually a pyonephrotic kidney that becomes adherent to a portion of the alimentary tract and then ruptures spontaneously, thus creating a fistula (Fig 22–11). A few cases following trauma have been reported. The patient is apt to suffer symptoms and signs of acute pyelonephritis. Urography may show radiopaque material escaping into the gastrointestinal tract. Gastrointestinal series may also reveal the connection with the

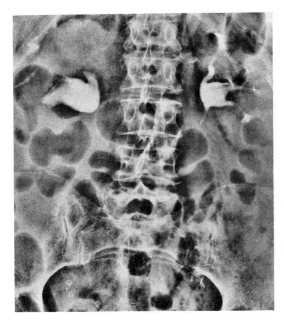
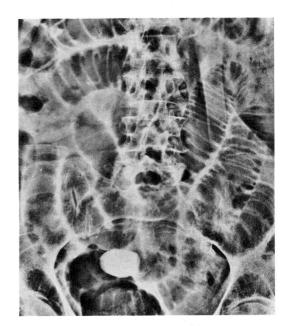

Figure 22–11. Nephroduodenal fistula and small bowel obstruction from renal staghorn calculus. *Left:* Excretory urogram showing nonfunction of right kidney; staghorn stone. *Right:* Patient presented with symptoms and signs of bowel obstruction 4 years later. Plain film showing dilated loops of small bowel down to a point just proximal to ileocecal valve. Obstruction due to stone extruded into duodenum. (Courtesy of CD King.)

kidney. The treatment is nephrectomy with closure of the opening into the gut.

ANEURYSM OF THE RENAL ARTERY

Aneurysm of the renal artery usually results from degenerative arterial disease that weakens the wall of the artery so that intravascular pressure may balloon it out. It is most commonly caused by arteriosclerosis or polyarteritis nodosa, but it may develop secondary to trauma or syphilis. Well over 300 cases have been reported. Congenital aneurysm has been recorded. Most represent an incidental finding on angiography (Hageman & others, 1978).

Aneurysmal dilatation has no deleterious effect upon the kidney unless the mass compresses the renal artery, in which case some renal ischemia and therefore atrophy is to be expected. A true aneurysm may rupture, producing a false aneurysm. This is especially likely to happen during pregnancy. The extravasated blood occupying the retroperitoneal space finally becomes encapsulated by a fibrous covering as organization occurs. An aneurysm may involve a small artery within the renal parenchyma. It may rupture into the renal pelvis or a calix.

Most aneurysms cause no symptoms unless they rupture, in which case there may be severe flank pain and even shock. If an aneurysm ruptures into the renal pelvis, marked hematuria occurs. The common cause of death is severe hemorrhage from rupture of the aneurysm. Hypertension is not usually present. A bruit should be sought over the costovertebral angle or over the renal artery anteriorly. If spontaneous or traumatic rupture has occurred, a mass may be palpated in the flank.

A plain film of the abdomen may show a ringlike calcification (Fig 22–12), either intra- or extrarenal. Urograms may be normal or reveal renal atrophy. Some impairment of renal function may be noted if compression or partial obstruction of the renal artery has developed. Aortography will delineate the aneurysm.

The differential diagnosis of rupture of an aneurysm and injury to the kidney is difficult unless a history or evidence of trauma is obtained. A hydronephrotic kidney may present a mass, but urography will clarify the issue.

Since the incidence of spontaneous rupture of noncalcified and large calcified aneurysms is significant, the presence of such a lesion is an indication for operation, particularly during pregnancy. The repair of extrarenal aneurysms may be considered, but complications (eg, thrombosis) are not uncommon. If an intrarenal aneurysm is situated in one pole, heminephrectomy may be feasible. If, however, it is in the center of the organ, nephrectomy will be required. Almgård & Fernström (1973) have reported therapeutic occlusion of an aneurysm by the intra-arterial injection of autologous muscle tissue. Those few patients with hypertension may become normotensive following definitive surgery.

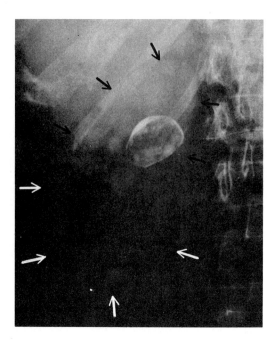 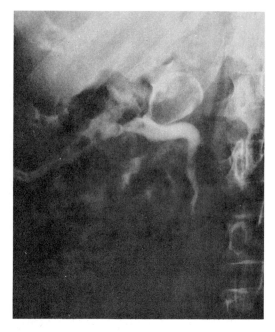

Figure 22–12. Intrarenal aneurysm of renal artery. *Left:* Plain film showing calcified structure over right renal shadow. *Right:* Excretory urogram relating calcific mass to pelvis and upper calix. (Courtesy of CD King.)

RENAL INFARCTS

Renal infarcts are caused by arterial occlusion. The major causes are subacute infective endocarditis, atrial or ventricular thrombi, arteriosclerosis, polyarteritis nodosa, and trauma. A thrombotic process in the abdominal aorta may gradually extend upward to occlude the renal artery. They may be unilateral or bilateral.

If smaller arteries or arterioles become obstructed, the tissue receiving blood from such a vessel will first become swollen and then undergo necrosis and fibrosis. Multiple infarcts are the rule. Should the main renal artery become occluded, the entire kidney will react in kind. The kidney may therefore become functionless and atrophic as it undergoes necrosis and fibrosis.

Partial renal infarction is usually a silent disease. Sudden and complete infarction may cause renal or chest pain and at times gross or microscopic hematuria. Proteinuria and leukocytosis are found. Tenderness over the flank may then be elicited. The kidney is not significantly enlarged by arterial occlusion. Serum glutamic-oxaloacetic transaminase and lactate dehydrogenase will be elevated for 1 or 2 days after the incident.

Excretory urograms may fail to visualize a portion of the kidney with partial infarction; with complete infarction, none of the radiopaque fluid is excreted. In this instance, retrograde urography will reveal no obstruction—and in fact, ureteropyelograms will be normal—but no urine will drain from the ureteral catheter, because the kidney has ceased to function. Even though complete loss of measurable function has occurred, renal circulation may be restored spontaneously in some instances.

Renal angiography makes the definitive diagnosis. A rectilinear scan may reveal no tubular function in a kidney of normal size. Lack of tracer activity may be noted in one pole if a segmental artery becomes occluded. A dynamic technetium scan will reveal no perfusion of the affected renal vasculature.

During the acute phase, infarction may mimic ureteral stone. With stone the excretory urogram may also show lack of renal function, but even so there is usually enough of the medium in the tubules so that a "nephrogram" is obtained (Fig 15–9). This will not occur with complete infarction. Evidence of a cardiac or vascular lesion is helpful in arriving at a proper diagnosis.

The complications are related to those arising from the primary cardiovascular disease, including emboli to other organs. In a few cases, hypertension may develop a few days or weeks after the infarction. It may later subside.

While emergency surgical intervention has been done, it has become clear that anticoagulation therapy is the treatment of choice. Renal function returns in most cases.

THROMBOSIS OF THE RENAL VEIN

Thrombosis of the renal vein is rare in the adult. It may develop secondary to various inflammatory lesions, including intrarenal or perirenal suppuration; from ascending thrombosis of the vena cava associated with phlebothrombosis; or from disseminated malignant disease. Thrombosis of the renal vein may occur as a complication of ileocolitis of infancy. The thrombosis may extend from the vena cava into the peripheral venules or may originate in the peripheral veins and propagate to the main renal vein. The severe passive congestion that develops causes the kidney to swell and become engorged. Degeneration of the nephrons ensues. There is usually flank pain, and symptoms and signs of sepsis are occasionally seen. Hematuria may be noted. A large, tender mass is often felt in the flank. The blood count may show changes compatible with sepsis. Thrombocytopenia may be noted. The urine contains albumin, red cells, and frequently pus cells and bacteria. In the acute stage, urograms show poor or absent secretion of the radiopaque material in a large kidney. Stretching and thinning of the caliceal infundibula may be noted. Clots in the pelvis may cause filling defects. Later the kidney may undergo atrophy. Urograms may then show notching of the upper ureter caused by dilated collateral veins. The typical picture of nephrotic syndrome develops in many of these patients. Renal biopsy reveals findings compatible with membranous glomerulonephritis.

B scan ultrasonography shows the thrombus in the vena cava in 50% of cases. The involved organ is enlarged (Fowler Jr & Paciulli, 1977). Renal angiography reveals stretching and bowing of small arterioles. In the nephrographic phase, the pyramids may become quite dense. Late films may show venous collaterals. Venacavography or, preferably, selective renal venography will demonstrate the thrombus in the renal vein (Fig 22–13) and, at times, in the vena cava. If washout from the vein gives poor filling, this may be enhanced by an injection of epinephrine into the renal artery.

The symptoms and signs may suggest acute renal infection or obstruction from a ureteral calculus. Acute pyelonephritis will cause the greatest difficulty in differential diagnosis, since the complaints and physical findings in the 2 diseases are similar. Excretory urography will prove helpful, for simple pyelonephritis will not appreciably depress renal function and there are no significant changes in the caliceal pattern. The presence of a stone in the ureter should be obvious; some degree of dilatation of the ureter and pelvis should then also be expected.

While thrombectomy and even nephrectomy have been recommended in the past, it has become increasingly clear that medical treatment is usually efficacious. In infants and children, it is essential to correct fluid and electrolyte problems, apply appropriate treatment if bacteriuria is found, and administer anticoagulants. Similar therapy is indicated for the adult. Renal function is usually fully recovered.

ARTERIOVENOUS FISTULA

Arteriovenous fistula may be congenital (25%) or acquired. A number of these fistulas have been reported following renal needle biopsy. A few have occurred following nephrectomy secondary to suture or ligature occlusion of the pedicle. These require surgical repair. A few have been recognized in association with adenocarcinoma of the kidney.

A thrill can often be palpated and a murmur heard both anteriorly and posteriorly. In cases with a wide communication, the systolic blood pressure is elevated and a widened pulse pressure is noted. Renal angiography or isotopic scan establishes the diagnosis. Arteriovenous fistula involving the renal artery and vein requires surgical repair or nephrectomy. Most, however, can be occluded by embolization, balloon or steel coil. Those that develop secondary to renal biopsy tend to heal spontaneously.

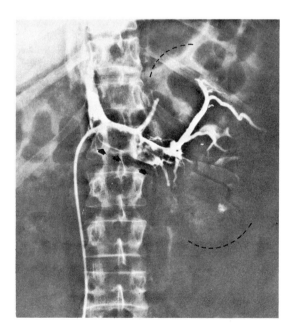

Figure 22–13. Thrombosis of renal vein. Selective left renal venogram showing almost complete occlusion of vein. Veins to lower pole failed to fill. Note large size of kidney.

ARTERIOVENOUS ANEURYSM

About 100 instances of this lesion have been reported (Fig 22–14). Most follow trauma. Hypertension is to be expected and is associated with high-output cardiac failure. A bruit is usually present.

Nephrectomy is usually indicated.

RENAL CORTICAL NECROSIS

Acute necrosis of the renal cortex is, with few exceptions, a complication of severe hemorrhage, often occurring secondary to premature separation of the placenta in the third trimester of pregnancy. The entire cortex of each kidney commonly exhibits coagulation necrosis. The cause is thought to be spasm of the glomerular afferent arteries and disseminated intravascular coagulation. Microscopically, the glomeruli and proximal convoluted tubules are necrotic. The medulla is intact. After a few weeks, peripheral cortical calcification may be noted. It may be seen on laminagrams.

The onset is usually characterized by sudden severe abdominal pain secondary to severe uterine hemorrhage. Oliguria develops promptly and leads to progressive uremia. (For a discussion of the differential diagnosis and treatment of oliguria, see Chapter 24.)

Blood loss must be promptly replaced. Hyperkalemia may require dialysis. The use of ganglionic blocking agents, eg, trimethaphan (Arfonad), may relieve the cortical ischemia.

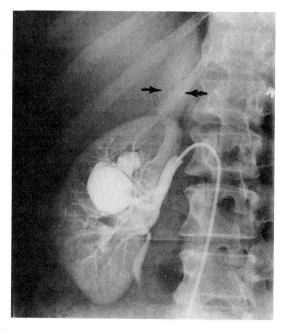

Figure 22–14. Arteriovenous aneurysm. Selective renal angiogram. Note aneurysm in center of kidney, with prompt filling of the vena cava (shown by arrows).

The prognosis depends upon the degree of renal damage. In many cases the renal lesion is irreversible. In most patients who recover, some degree of permanent renal damage is evident. Dialysis or renal transplantation may be necessary.

● ● ●

References

CONGENITAL ANOMALIES

General

Belman AB, King LR: Urinary tract abnormalities associated with imperforate anus. *J Urol* 1972;**108**:823.

Fleisher DS: Lateral displacement of the nipples, a sign of bilateral renal hypoplasia. *J Pediatr* 1966;**69**:806.

Taylor WC: Deformity of ears and kidneys. *Can Med Assoc J* 1965;**93**:107.

Vitko RJ, Cass AS, Winter RB: Anomalies of the genitourinary tract associated with congenital scoliosis and congenital kyphosis. *J Urol* 1972;**108**:655.

Agenesis

Athanasoulis CA, Brown B, Baum S: Selective renal venography in differentiation between congenitally absent and small contracted kidney. *Radiology* 1973;**108**:301.

Cain DR & others: Familial renal agenesis and total dysplasia. *Am J Dis Child* 1974;**128**:377.

Emanuel B & others: Congenital solitary kidney: A review of 74 cases. *J Urol* 1974;**111**:394.

Kohn G, Borns PF: The association of bilateral and unilateral renal aplasia in the same family. *J Pediatr* 1973;**83**:95.

Mauer SM, Dobrin RS, Vernier RL: Unilateral and bilateral renal agenesis in monoamniotic twins. *J Pediatr* 1974;**84**:236.

Hypoplasia

Cha EM, Kandzari S, Khoury GH: Congenital renal hypoplasia: Angiographic study. *Am J Roentgenol* 1972;**114**:710.

Kanasawa M & others: Dwarfed kidneys in children. *Am J Dis Child* 1965;**109**:130.

Dysplasia & Multicystic Kidney

Abt AB, Demers LM, Shochat SJ: Cystic nephroma: An ultrastructural and biochemical study. *J Urol* 1979;**122**:539.

Azimi F, Kodroff MB: Congenital renal dysplasia: Osathanondh-Potter type II polycystic kidneys. *Urology* 1976;**7**:550.

Baldauf MC, Schulz DM: Multilocular cyst of the kidney: Report of three cases and review of the literature. *Am J Clin Pathol* 1976;**65**:93.

Bearman SB, Hine PL, Sanders RC: Multicystic kidney: A sonographic pattern. *Radiology* 1976;**118**:685.

Bloom DA, Brosman S: The multicystic kidney. *J Urol* 1978;**120**:211.

De Klerk DP, Marshall FF, Jeffs RD: Multicystic dysplastic kidney. *J Urol* 1977;**118**:306.

Fisher C, Smith JF: Renal dysplasia in nephrectomy specimens from adolescents and adults. *J Clin Pathol* 1975;**28**:879.

Friedberg JE, Mitnick JS, Davis DA: Antipartum ultrasonic detection of multicystic kidney. *Radiology* 1979;**131**:198.

Gipson TG, Anderson EE, Bradford WD: Multicystic renal dysplasia. *Clin Pediatr (Phila)* 1976;**15**:896.

Hattery RR: Computed tomography of renal abnormalities. *Radiol Clin North Am* 1977;**15**:401.

Mackie GG, Stephens FD: Duplex kidneys: A correlation of renal dysplasia with position of the ureteral orifice. *J Urol* 1975;**114**:274.

Perrin EV & others: Renal duplication and dysplasia. *Urology* 1974;**4**:660.

Stecker JF Jr, Rose JG, Gillenwater JY: Dysplastic kidneys associated with vesicoureteral reflux. *J Urol* 1973;**110**:341.

Warshawsky AB, Miller KE, Kaplan GW: Urographic visualization of multicystic kidneys. *J Urol* 1977;**117**:94.

Polycystic Kidneys

Bernstein J: Heritable cystic disorders of the kidney: The mythology of polycystic disease. *Pediatr Clin North Am* 1971;**18**:435.

Hatfield PM, Pfister RC: Adult polycystic disease of the kidneys (Potter type 3). *JAMA* 1972;**222**:1527.

Kaye C, Lewy PR: Congenital appearance of adult-type (autosomal dominant) polycystic kidney disease. *J Pediatr* 1974;**85**:807.

Kendall AR, Pollack HM, Karafin L: Congenital cystic disease of kidney: Classification and manifestations. *Urology* 1974;**4**:635.

Kutcher R, Schneider M, Gordon DH: Calcification in polycystic disease. *Radiology* 1977;**122**:77.

Lamiell JM, Stor RA, Hsia YE: Von Hippel-Lindau disease simulating polycystic kidney disease. *Urology* 1980;**15**:287.

Lee JKT, McClennan BL, Kissane JM: Unilateral polycystic disease. *AJR* 1978;**130**:1165.

Levine E & others: Computed tomography in the diagnosis of renal carcinoma complicating Hippel-Lindau syndrome. *Radiology* 1979;**130**:703.

Lufkin EG & others: Polycystic kidney disease: Earlier diagnosis using ultrasound. *Urology* 1974;**4**:5.

Milam JH, Magee JH, Bunts RC: Evaluation of surgical decompression of polycystic kidneys by differential renal clearances. *J Urol* 1963;**90**:144.

Qazi Q & others: Renal anomalies in fetal alcohol syndrome. *Pediatrics* 1979;**63**:886.

Sagel SS & others: Computed tomography of the kidney. *Radiology* 1977;**124**:359.

Salvatierra O Jr, Kountz SL, Belzer FO: Polycystic renal disease treated by renal transplantation. *Surg Gynecol Obstet* 1973;**137**:431.

Segal AJ, Spataro RF, Barbaric ZL: Adult polycystic kidney disease: A review of 100 cases. *J Urol* 1977;**118**:711.

Thaysen JH & others: Involution of polycystic kidneys during active treatment of terminal uremia. *Acta Med Scand* 1975;**197**:257.

Wallack HI, Kandel G, Presman DC: Polycystic kidneys: Indications for surgical intervention. *Urology* 1974;**3**:552.

Waters WB, Hershman H, Klein L: Management of infected polycystic kidneys. *J Urol* 1979;**122**:383.

Wenzl JE, Lagos JC, Albers DD: Tuberous sclerosis presenting as polycystic kidneys and seizures in an infant. *J Pediatr* 1970;**77**:673.

Simple Cyst

Ambrose SS & others: Unsuspected renal tumors associated with renal cysts. *J Urol* 1977;**117**:704.

Bartholomew TH & others: The sonographic evaluation and management of simple renal cysts in children. *J Urol* 1980;**123**:732.

Branitz BH, Schlossberg IR, Freed SZ: Complications of renal cyst puncture. *Urology* 1976;**7**:578.

Evans AT, Coughlin JP: Urinary obstruction due to renal cysts. *J Urol* 1970;**103**:277.

Gordon RL & others: Simple serous cysts of the kidney in children. *Radiology* 1979;**131**:357.

Gross DM: Diagnostic renal cyst puncture and percutaneous nephrostomy. *Urol Clin North Am* 1979;**6**:409.

Harp GE, Goldstein AMB, Morrow JW: Bleeding solitary renal cysts. *Urology* 1974;**3**:649.

Harris RD, Goergen TG, Talner LB: The bloody cyst aspirate: A diagnostic dilemma. *J Urol* 1975;**114**:832.

Hattery RR: Computed tomography of renal abnormalities. *Radiol Clin North Am* 1977;**15**:401.

Hayt DB, Blatt CJ, Robinson SH: Renal cyst puncture: Utilization of pediatric guide wire technique and upright radiographic changes. *J Urol* 1978;**120**:530.

Hinman F Jr: Obstructive renal cysts. *J Urol* 1978;**119**:681.

Johanson K-E & others: Management of intrarenal peripelvic cysts. *Urology* 1974;**4**:514.

Lang EK & others: Assessment of avascular renal mass lesions: The use of nephrotomography, arteriography, cyst puncture, double contrast study and histochemical and histopathologic examination. *South Med J* 1972;**65**:1.

Mullin EM, Paulson DF: Renal cystic disease. *Urology* 1976;**8**:5.

Pollack HM, Goldberg BB, Bogash M: Changing concepts in the diagnosis and management of renal cysts. *J Urol* 1974;**111**:326.

Raskin MM & others: Percutaneous management of renal cysts: Results of a four-year study. *Radiology* 1975;**115**:551.

Roth JK Jr, Roberts JA: Benign renal cysts and renal function. *J Urol* 1980;**123**:625.

Sagel SS & others: Computed tomography of the kidney. *Radiology* 1977;**124**:359.

Stables DP, Jackson RS: Management of an infected simple renal cyst. *Br J Radiol* 1974;**47**:290.

Sufrin G & others: Hypernephroma arising in wall of simple renal cyst. *Urology* 1975;**6**:507.

Varma KR & others: Papillary carcinoma in wall of simple renal cyst. *Urology* 1974;**3**:762.

Wettlaufer JN, Modarelli RO: Triple contrast percutaneous nephrocystography and analysis of cyst aspirate. *Urology* 1978;**12**:373.

Zelch J & others: Complications of renal cyst exploration versus renal mass aspiration. *Urology* 1976;**7**:244.

Renal Fusion

Bietz DS, Merendino KA: Abdominal aneurysm and horseshoe kidney: A review. *Ann Surg* 1975;**181**:333.

Downs RA, Lane JW, Burns E: Solitary pelvic kidney: Its clinical implications. *Urology* 1973;**1**:51.

Friedland GW, de Vries P: Renal ectopia and fusion: Embryologic basis. *Urology* 1975;**5**:698.

Hendron WH, Donahoe PK, Pfister RC: Crossed renal ectopia in children. *Urology* 1976;**7**:135.

Kelalis PP, Malek RS, Segura JW: Observations on renal ectopia and fusion in children. *J Urol* 1973;**110**:588.

Kvarstein B, Mathisen W: Surgical treatment of horseshoe kidney: A follow-up study. *Scand J Urol Nephrol* 1974;**8**:10.

Pitts WR Jr, Muecke EC: Horseshoe kidneys: A 40-year experience. *J Urol* 1975;**113**:743.

Roy JB, Stevens RK: Polycystic horseshoe kidney. *Urology* 1975;**6**:222.

Ectopic Kidney

Hertz M & others: Crossed renal ectopia: Clinical and radiological findings in 22 cases. *Clin Radiol* 1977;**28**:339.

Hildreth TA, Cass AS: Crossed renal ectopia with familial occurrence. *Urology* 1978;**12**:59.

Malkin RB, Dodson AI Jr, Koontz WW Jr: Adenocarcinoma in a sigmoid kidney. *Urology* 1974;**4**:713.

Marshall FF, Freedman MT: Crossed renal ectopia. *J Urol* 1978;**119**:188.

Ramos AJ, Slovis TL, Reed JO: Intrathoracic kidney. *Urology* 1979;**13**:14.

Ward JN, Nathanson B, Draper JW: The pelvic kidney. *J Urol* 1965;**94**:36.

Medullary Sponge Kidney

Eisenberg RL, Pfister RC: Medullary sponge kidney associated with congenital hemihypertrophy (asymmetry): A case report and survey of the literature. *Am J Roentgenol* 1972;**116**:773.

Hayt DB & others: Direct magnification intravenous pyelography in re-evaluation of medullary sponge kidney. *Am J Roentgenol* 1973;**119**:701.

Potter EL, Osathanondh V: Medullary sponge kidney: Two cases in young infants. *J Pediatr* 1963;**62**:901.

Spence HM, Singleton R: What is sponge kidney disease and where does it fit in the spectrum of cystic disorders? *J Urol* 1972;**107**:176.

Swenson RS, Kempson RL, Friedland GW: Cystic disease of the renal medulla in the elderly. *JAMA* 1974;**228**:1404.

ACQUIRED LESIONS

Renoalimentary Fistulas

Bissada NK, Cole AT, Fried FA: Reno-alimentary fistula: An unusual urological problem. *J Urol* 1973;**110**:273.

Chowdhury SD, Higgins PM: An intrarenal foreign body. *Br J Urol* 1972;**44**:133.

Dunn M, Kirk D: Renogastric fistula: Case report and review of the literature. *J Urol* 1973;**109**:785.

Greene JE, Bucy JG, Wise L: Spontaneous pyeloduodenal and renocolic fistulas. *South Med J* 1975;**68**:641.

Newman JH, Jeans WD: Reno-colic fistula demonstrated by antegrade pyelography. *Br J Urol* 1972;**44**:692.

Schwartz DT & others: Pyeloduodenal fistula due to tuberculosis. *J Urol* 1970;**104**:373.

Aneurysm of the Renal Artery

Almgård LE, Fernström I: Embolic occlusion of an intrarenal aneurysm: A case report. *Br J Urol* 1973;**45**:485.

Altebarmakian VK & others: Renal artery aneurysm. *Urology* 1979;**13**:257.

Carron J & others: Renal artery aneurysm: Polyaneurysmal lesion of kidney. *Urology* 1975;**5**:1.

Cohen SG, Cashdan A, Berger R: Spontaneous rupture of a renal artery aneurysm during pregnancy. *Obstet Gynecol* 1972;**39**:897.

Hageman JH & others: Aneurysms of the renal artery: Problems of prognosis and surgical management. *Surgery* 1978;**84**:563.

Litvak AS, Lucas BA, McRoberts JW: Urologic manifestations of polyarteritis nodosa. *J Urol* 1976;**115**:572.

Poutasse EF: Renal artery aneurysms. *J Urol* 1975;**113**:443.

Soussou ID & others: Renal artery aneurysm: Long-term relief of renovascular hypertension by in situ operative correction. *Arch Surg* 1979;**114**:1410.

Renal Infarcts

Chehval MJ, Mehan DJ: Nonoperative management of renal artery embolus. *Urology* 1979;**14**:569.

Fay R & others: Renal artery thrombosis: A successful revascularization by autotransplantation. *J Urol* 1974;**111**:572.

Fergus JN, Jones NF, Thomas ML: Kidney function after arterial embolism. *Br Med J* 1969;**4**:587.

Frank PH & others: The cortical rim sign of renal infarction. *Br J Radiol* 1974;**47**:875.

Grablowsky OM & others: Renal artery thrombosis following blunt trauma: Report of four cases. *Surgery* 1970;**67**:895.

Lang EK, Mertz JHO, Nourse M: Renal arteriography in the assessment of renal infarction. *J Urol* 1968;**99**:506.

Lessman RK & others: Renal artery embolism: Clinical features and long-term follow-up of 17 cases. *Ann Intern Med* 1978;**89**:477.

Mounger EJ: Hypertension resulting from segmental renal artery infarction. *Urology* 1973;**1**:189.

Moyer JD & others: Conservative management of renal artery embolus. *J Urol* 1973;**109**:138.

Ranniger K, Abrams E, Borden TA: Pseudotumor resulting from a fresh renal infarct. *Radiology* 1969;**92**:343.

Schramek A & others: Survival following late renal embolectomy in a patient with a single functioning kidney. *J Urol* 1973;**109**:342.

Smith SP Jr & others: Occlusion of the artery to a solitary kidney: Restoration of renal function after prolonged anuria. *JAMA* 1974;**230**:1306.

Tse RL, Leberman PR: Acute renal artery occlusion—etiology, diagnosis and treatment: Report of a case with subsequent revascularization. *J Urol* 1972;**108**:32.

Thrombosis of the Renal Vein

Baum NH, Moriel E, Carlton CE Jr: Renal vein thrombosis. *J Urol* 1978;**119**:443.

Belman AB: Renal vein thrombosis in infancy and childhood: A contemporary survey. *Clin Pediatr (Phila)* 1976;**15**:1033.

Cade R & others: Chronic renal vein thrombosis. *Am J Med* 1977;**63**:387.

Clark RA, Wyatt GM, Colley DP: Renal vein thrombosis: An underdiagnosed complication of multiple renal abnormalities. *Radiology* 1979;**132**:43.

Fowler JE Jr, Paciulli J: Renal vein thrombosis: Diagnosis by B-scan ultrasonography. *J Urol* 1977;**118**:849.

Halvorsen JF, Moe PJ: Renal vein thrombosis in neonates: Report of three cases treated with nephrectomy. *Acta Paediatr Scand* 1975;**64**:373.

Kiruluta HG & others: The protean manifestations of renal vein thrombosis in the adult. *J Urol* 1976;**115**:634.

Llach F & others: On the incidence of renal vein thrombosis in the nephrotic syndrome. *Arch Intern Med* 1977;**137**:333.

Rosenberg ER & others: Ultrasonic diagnosis of renal vein thrombosis in neonates. *AJR* 1980;**134**:35.

Thompson IM, Schneider R, Lababidi Z: Thrombectomy for neonatal renal vein thrombosis. *J Urol* 1975;**113**:396.

Arteriovenous Fistula

Hart PL, Ingram DW, Peckham GB: Postnephrectomy arteriovenous fistula causing "stroke" and congestive heart failure. *Can Med Assoc J* 1973;**108**:1400.

Hawkins IF, Garin EH: Therapeutic renal embolization in children. *J Pediatr* 1979;**94**:415.

Kostiner AI, Burnett LL: Intrarenal arteriovenous fistula: Documented increase in size during an eight-year interval in one case and surgical treatment with renal salvage in another. *Radiology* 1973;**109**:531.

Lisbona R & others: Radionuclide detection of iatrogenic arteriovenous fistulas of the genitourinary system. *Radiology* 1980;**134**:201.

Mark LK: Arteriovenous malformations of kidney. *Urology* 1974;**4**:706.

Marshall FF & others: Treatment of traumatic renal arteriovenous fistulas by detachable silicone balloon embolization. *J Urol* 1979;**122**:237.

Tucci P, Doctor D, Diagonale A: Embolization of post-traumatic renal arteriovenous fistula. *Urology* 1979;**13**:192.

Wallace S & others: Intrarenal arteriovenous fistulas: Transcatheter steel coil occlusion. *J Urol* 1978;**120**:282.

Arteriovenous Aneurysm

Merritt BA, Middleton RG: Repair of a huge renal arteriovenous aneurysm with preservation of the kidney. *J Urol* 1972;**107**:521.

O'Donnel KF, Pais VM: Arteriovenous aneurysm of kidney after open renal biopsy. *Urology* 1976;**7**:305.

Renal Cortical Necrosis

Bloom R, Swenson RS, Coplon NS: Acute renal cortical necrosis: Variable course and changing prognosis. *Calif Med* (Oct) 1973;**119**:1.

Kleinknecht D & others: Diagnostic procedures and long-term prognosis in bilateral cortical necrosis. *Kidney Int* 1973;**4**:390.

Leonidas JC, Berdon WE, Gribetz D: Bilateral renal cortical necrosis in the newborn infant: Roentgenographic diagnosis. *J Pediatr* 1971;**79**:623.

Matlin RA, Gary NE: Acute cortical necrosis. *Am J Med* 1974;**56**:110.

Ramachandran S, Perera MVF: Survival in renal cortical necrosis due to snake bite. *Postgrad Med J* 1974;**50**:314.

23 | Diagnosis of Medical Renal Diseases

Marcus A. Krupp, MD

The medical renal diseases are those that involve principally the parenchyma of the kidneys. Many of the symptoms and signs of urinary tract disease are common to both medical and surgical diseases of the kidneys and other urologic organs. Hematuria, proteinuria, pyuria, oliguria, polyuria, pain, renal insufficiency with azotemia, acidosis, anemia, electrolyte abnormalities, hypertension, headache, and ocular involvement may occur in a wide variety of disorders affecting any portion of the parenchyma of the kidney, its blood vessels, or the excretory tract.

Every effort must be made to rule out nonsurgical disease of the urinary tract before resorting to diagnostic or therapeutic procedures that may prove to be unnecessary or dangerous.

A complete medical history and physical examination, a thorough examination of the urine, and blood chemistry examinations as indicated are essential initial steps in the work-up of any patient.

History

A. Family History: The family history may reveal disease of genetic origin, eg, tubular metabolic anomalies, polycystic kidneys, unusual types of nephritis, or vascular or coagulation defects that may be essential clues to the diagnosis.

B. Past History: The past history should cover infections, injuries, and exposure to toxic agents, anticoagulants, or drugs that may produce toxic or sensitivity reactions, including blood dyscrasias. A history of diabetes, hypertensive disease, and collagen disease may be obtained. The inquiry must also elicit symptoms of uremia, debilitation, and the vascular complications of chronic renal disease.

Physical Examination

One must look for such physical signs as pallor, edema, hypertension, retinopathy, and the stigmas of congenital disease (eg, enlarged kidneys with polycystic disease).

Urinalysis

Examination of the urine (see Chapter 5) is the essential part of the investigation.

A. Proteinuria: Proteinuria of any significant degree (2–4+) is suggestive of "medical" renal disease (parenchymal involvement). Proteinuria should be interpreted with consideration of the urine specific gravity, since a proteinuria of 1+ in a dilute urine may indicate a significantly great protein loss. Formed elements present in the urine usually establish the diagnosis. Only after careful examination of the patient and suitable urine specimens, as well as analysis of the chemical constituents of the blood, is urography or cystoscopy justified.

1. "Pathologic" proteinurias–Significant proteinuria is present in such disorders as glomerulonephritis, subacute or chronic nephritis, nephrotic syndrome, collagen disease, diabetic nephropathy, myeloma of the kidney, amyloid kidney, and polycystic kidney disease.

2. "Nonpathologic" proteinurias–When investigating causes, one must be careful not to overlook mild cases of glomerulonephritis or other parenchymal disease.

a. "Physiologic" proteinuria–Following vigorous exercise or protracted physical effort, protein, erythrocytes, casts, and tubule cells may appear transiently in urine samples. Repeat examination of the urine after a period of rest usually shows normal urine.

b. Orthostatic proteinuria–Some persons have proteinuria when they are up and about but not while recumbent. In any patient with proteinuria, the degree of proteinuria is usually more pronounced when the patient is upright, and especially when the patient is active. Absence of proteinuria when the patient is supine during the period of urine formation confirms the diagnosis of orthostatic proteinuria.

B. Red Cell Casts: Although red cells in the urine indicate extravasation of blood anywhere along the urinary tract, the occurrence of red cells in casts proves the renal origin of the bleeding. The erythrocytes forming typical red cell casts are from the glomeruli or the upper portions of the nephron.

C. Fatty Casts and Oval Fat Bodies: Tubule cells showing fatty changes occur in degenerative diseases of the kidney (nephrosis, glomerulonephritis, collagen disease, amyloidosis, and damage due to such toxins as mercury).

D. Other Findings: The presence of abnormal urinary chemical constituents may be the only indication of metabolic disorders involving the kidneys. These include diabetes mellitus, renal glycosuria, aminoacidurias (including cystinuria), oxaluria, gout, hyperparathyroidism, hemoglobinuria, and myoglobinuria.

Renal Biopsy

Renal biopsy is a valuable diagnostic procedure that also serves as a guide to rational treatment. The technic has become well established, frequently providing sufficient tissue for light and electron microscopy and for immunofluorescence examination. Absolute contraindications include anatomic presence of only one kidney; severe malfunction of one kidney even though function is adequate in the other; bleeding diathesis; the presence of hemangioma, tumor, or large cysts; abscess or infection; hydronephrosis; and an uncooperative patient. Relative contraindications are the presence of serious hypertension, uremia, severe arteriosclerosis, and unusual difficulty in doing a biopsy due to obesity, anasarca, or inability of the patient to lie flat.

Clinical indications for renal biopsy, in addition to the necessity for establishing a diagnosis, include the need to determine prognosis, to follow progression of a lesion and response to treatment, to confirm the presence of a generalized disease (collagen disorder, amyloidosis, sarcoidosis), and to follow rejection response in a transplanted kidney.

GLOMERULONEPHRITIS

Information obtained from experimentally induced glomerular disease in animals and from correlations with evidence derived by modern methods of examination of tissue obtained by biopsy and at necropsy have provided a new concept of glomerulonephritis.

The clinical manifestations of renal disease are apt to consist only of varying degrees of hematuria, excretion of characteristic formed elements in the urine, proteinuria, and renal insufficiency and its complications. Alterations in glomerular architecture as observed in tissue examined by light microscopy are also apt to be minimal and difficult to interpret. For these reasons, attempts to correlate clinical syndromes with histologic features of renal tissue have failed to provide a satisfactory basis for precise diagnosis, treatment, and prognosis.

More recently, however, immunologic technics for demonstrating a variety of antigens, antibodies, and complement fractions have led to new concepts of the origins and pathogenesis of glomerular disease. Electron microscopy has complemented the immunologic methods.

Briefly, then, glomerular disease resulting from immunologic reactions may be divided into 2 groups:

(1) Immune complex disease, in which soluble antigen-antibody complexes in the circulation are trapped in the glomeruli. The antigens are not derived from glomerular components; they may be

Table 23–1. Common patterns of abnormal urine composition in disease.*

Disease	Specific Gravity	Protein†	Red Cells†	Casts†	Microscopic (Casts and Cells) and Other Findings
Normal	1.003–1.030	0 to trace (up to 0.05 g)	0 to occ	0 to occ	Hyaline casts (urine must be acid and fresh or preserved).
Diseases with high fevers	Increased	Trace or +	0	0 to few	Hyaline casts, tubule cells.
Congestive heart failure	High; varies with renal function	1–2+	0 to +	+	Hyaline and granular casts.
Eclampsia	Increased	3–4+	0 to +	3–4+	Hyaline casts.
Diabetic coma	High	+	0	0 to +	Hyaline casts, glucose, ketone bodies.
Acute glomerulonephritis‡	Increased	2–4+	1–4+	2–4+	Blood, cellular, granular, hyaline casts; renal tubule epithelium.
Degenerative phase glomerulonephritis	Normal or increased	4+	1–2+	4+	Granular, waxy, hyaline, fatty casts; fatty tubule cells.
Terminal phase glomerulonephritis	Low, fixed	1–2+	Trace to +	1–3+	Granular, hyaline, fatty, broad casts.
Lipoid nephrosis	Very high	4+	0 to trace	4+	Hyaline, granular, fatty, waxy casts; fatty tubule cells.
Collagen diseases	Normal or decreased	1–4+	1–4+	1–4+	Blood, cellular, granular, hyaline, waxy, fatty, broad casts, fatty tubule cells.
Pyelonephritis	Normal or decreased	0 to +	0 to +	0 to +	Leukocyte and hyaline casts, pus cells, bacteria.
Benign hypertension (late)	Normal or low	0 to +	0 to trace	0 to +	Hyaline and granular casts.
Malignant hypertension	Low, fixed	1–2+	Trace to +	1–2+	Hyaline and granular casts.

*Modified from Krupp MA & others: *Physician's Handbook,* 19th ed. Lange, 1979.

†Scale of 0–4+.

‡May be anuric, or have low, fixed specific gravity.

exogenous (bacterial, viral, chemical) or endogenous (circulating native DNA, thyroglobulin). Factors in the pathogenic potential of the antigen include its origin, quantity, and route of entry and the host's duration of exposure to it. The immune response to the antigen depends on the severity of inflammation or infection and the host's capacity to respond (immunocompetency).

In the presence of antigen excess, antigen-antibody complexes form in the circulation and are trapped in the glomeruli as they are filtered through capillaries rendered permeable by the action of vasoactive amines. The antigen-antibody complexes bind components of complement, particularly C3. Activated complement provides chemoactive factors that attract leukocytes whose lysosomal enzymes incite the injury to the glomerulus.

On electron microscopy and with immunofluorescence methods, these complexes appear as lumpy deposits between the epithelial cells and the glomerular basement. IgG, IgM, occasionally IgA, β1C, and C3 are demonstrable.

(2) Anti-GBM (glomerular basement membrane) disease, in which antibodies are generated against the glomerular basement membrane of the kidney and often against lung basement membrane, which appears to be antigenically similar to GBM. The autoantibodies may be stimulated by autologous GBM altered in some way or combined with an exogenous agent. The reaction of antibody with GBM is accompanied by activation of complement, the attraction of leukocytes, and the release of lysosomal enzymes. The presence of thrombi in glomerular capillaries is often accompanied by leakage of fibrinogen and precipitation of fibrin in Bowman's space, with subsequent development of epithelial "crescents" in the space.

Immunofluorescence technics and electron microscopy show the anti-GBM complexes as linear deposits outlining the GBM. IgG and C3 are usually demonstrable.

The current classification of glomerulonephritis is based on the immunologic concepts described above. However, the discussions in the following pages will be organized according to traditional clinical categories.

I. Immunologic Mechanisms Likely
  A. Immune Complex Disease:
  Glomerulonephritis associated with infectious agents, including streptococci, staphylococci, pneumococci, infective endocarditis, secondary syphilis, malaria, viruses of hepatitis (HBAg) and measles
  Lupus erythematosus
  Glomerulonephritis associated with other systemic (?autoimmune) diseases such as polyarteritis nodosa, scleroderma, and idiopathic cryoglobulinemia

  Membranous glomerulonephritis, cause unknown
  Membranoproliferative glomerulonephritis, cause unknown
  Focal glomerulonephritis
  Rapidly progressive glomerulonephritis (some cases)
  B. Anti-GBM Disease:
  Goodpasture's syndrome
  Rapidly progressive glomerulonephritis (some cases)
II. Immunologic Mechanisms Not Clearly Demonstrated
  Lipoid nephrosis
  Focal glomerulonephritis (some cases)
  Chronic sclerosing glomerulonephritis
  Diabetic glomerulosclerosis
  Amyloidosis
  Hemolytic-uremic syndrome and thrombohemolytic thrombocytopenic purpura
  Wegener's granulomatosis
  Alport's syndrome
  Sickle cell disease

1. POSTSTREPTOCOCCAL GLOMERULONEPHRITIS

Essentials of Diagnosis

- History of preceding streptococcal infection.
- Malaise, headache, anorexia, low-grade fever.
- Mild generalized edema, mild hypertension, retinal hemorrhages.
- Gross hematuria; protein, red cell casts, granular and hyaline casts, white cells, and renal epithelial cells in urine.
- Elevated antistreptolysin O titer, variable nitrogen retention.

General Considerations

Glomerulonephritis is a disease affecting both kidneys. In most cases recovery from the acute stage is complete, but progressive involvement may destroy renal tissue, and renal insufficiency results. Acute glomerulonephritis is most common in children age 3–10 years, although 5% or more of initial attacks occur in adults over age 50. By far the most common cause is an antecedent infection of the pharynx and tonsils or of the skin with group A β-hemolytic streptococci, certain strains of which are nephritogenic. Nephritis occurs in 10–15% of children and young adults who have clinically evident infection with a nephritogenic strain. In children under age 6, pyoderma (impetigo) is the most common antecedent; in older children and young adults, pharyngitis is a common and skin infection a rare antecedent. Nephritogenic strains commonly encountered include, for the skin, M types 49 (Red Lake), 2, and provisional 55; for pharyngitis, types 12, 1, and 4. Rarely, nephritis may follow infections due to pneumococci, staphylococci, some bacilli and viruses, or *Plasmodium malariae* and exposure to some drugs. *Rhus* dermatitis and reactions to venom or chemical agents may be associated with renal disease clinically indistinguishable from glomerulonephritis.

The pathogenesis of the glomerular lesion has been further elucidated by the use of new immunologic technics (immunofluorescence) and electron microscopy. A likely sequel to infection by nephritogenic strains of β-hemolytic streptococci is injury to the mesangial cells in the intercapillary space. The glomerulus may then become more easily damaged by antigen-antibody complexes developing from the immune response to the streptococcal infection. β1C globulin of complement is deposited in association with IgG or alone in a granular pattern on the epithelial side of the basement membrane and occasionally in subendothelial sites as well.

Gross examination of the involved kidney shows only punctate hemorrhages throughout the cortex. Microscopically, the primary alteration is in the glomeruli, which show proliferation and swelling of the mesangial and endothelial cells of the capillary tuft. The proliferation of capsular epithelium produces a thickened crescent about the tuft, and in the space between the capsule and the tuft there are collections of leukocytes, red cells, and exudate. Edema of the interstitial tissue and cloudy swelling of the tubule epithelium are common. As the disease progresses, the kidneys may enlarge. The typical histologic findings in glomerulitis are enlarging crescents that become hyalinized and converted into scar tissue and obstruct the circulation through the glomerulus. Degenerative changes occur in the tubules, with fatty degeneration and necrosis and ultimate scarring of the nephron. Arteriolar thickening and obliteration become prominent.

Clinical Findings

A. Symptoms and Signs: Often the disease is very mild, and there may be no reason to suspect renal involvement unless the urine is examined. In severe cases, about 2 weeks following the acute streptococcal infection, the patient develops headache, malaise, mild fever, puffiness around the eyes and face, flank pain, and oliguria. Hematuria is usually noted as "bloody" or, if the urine is acid, as "brown" or "coffee-colored." Respiratory difficulty with shortness of breath may occur as a result of salt and water retention and circulatory congestion. There may be moderate tachycardia and moderate to marked elevation of blood pressure. Tenderness in the costovertebral angle is common.

B. Laboratory Findings: The diagnosis is confirmed by examination of the urine, which may be grossly bloody or coffee-colored (acid hematin) or may show only microscopic hematuria. In addition, the urine contains protein (1–3+) and casts.

Hyaline and granular casts are commonly found in large numbers, but the classic sign of glomerulitis, the erythrocyte cast (blood cast), may be found only occasionally in the urinary sediment. The erythrocyte cast resembles a blood clot formed in the lumen of a renal tubule; it is usually of small caliber, intensely orange or red, and under high power with proper lighting may show the mosaic pattern of the packed red cells held together by the clot of fibrin and plasma protein.

With the impairment of renal function (decrease in GFR and blood flow) and with oliguria, plasma or serum urea nitrogen and creatinine become elevated, the levels varying with the severity of the renal lesion. The sedimentation rate is rapid. A mild normochromic anemia may result from fluid retention and dilution. Infection of the throat with nephritogenic streptococci is frequently followed by increasing antistreptolysin O (ASO) titers in the serum, whereas high titers are usually not demonstrable following skin infections. Production of antibody against streptococcal deoxyribonuclease B (anti-DNase B) is more regularly observed following both throat and skin infections. Serum complement levels are usually low.

Confirmation of diagnosis is made by examination of the urine, although the history and clinical findings in typical cases leave little doubt. The finding of erythrocytes in a cast is proof that erythrocytes were present in the renal tubules and did not arise from elsewhere in the genitourinary tract.

Differential Diagnosis

Although erythrocyte casts are considered to be the hallmark of glomerulonephritis, they also occur along with other abnormal elements in any disease in which glomerular inflammation and tubule damage are present, eg, polyarteritis nodosa, disseminated lupus erythematosus, dermatomyositis, sarcoidosis, subacute infective endocarditis, "focal" nephritis, Goodpasture's syndrome, Henoch's purpura, or poisoning with chemicals toxic to the kidney.

Treatment

There is no specific treatment. Eradication of infection, prevention of overhydration and hypertension, and prompt treatment of complications such as hypertensive encephalopathy and heart failure require careful observation and management.

Prognosis

Most patients with the acute disease recover completely within 1–2 years; 5–20% show progressive renal damage. If oliguria, heart failure, or hypertensive encephalopathy is severe, death may occur during the acute attack. Even with severe acute disease, however, recovery is the rule, particularly in children.

2. CHRONIC GLOMERULONEPHRITIS

Progressive destruction of the kidney may continue for many years in a clinically latent or subacute form. The subacute form is similar to the latent form (see below) except that symptoms occur—malaise, mild fever, and sometimes flank pain and oliguria. Treatment is as for the acute attack. Exacerbations may appear from time to time, reflecting the stage of evolution of the disease.

3. LATENT GLOMERULONEPHRITIS

If acute glomerulonephritis does not heal within 1–2 years, the vascular and glomerular lesions continue to progress, and tubular changes occur. In the presence of smoldering, active nephritis, the patient is usually asymptomatic, and the evidence of disease consists only of the excretion of abnormal urinary elements.

The urinary excretion of protein, red cells, white cells, epithelial cells, and casts (including erythrocyte casts, granular casts, and hyaline and waxy casts) continues at levels above normal. As renal impairment progresses, signs of renal insufficiency appear (see below).

The differential diagnosis is the same as that given for acute glomerulonephritis. Recent studies of tissue obtained by renal biopsy in cases of recurrent or persistent hematuria indicate a high incidence of mesangial deposition of immune complexes made up of IgM or IgA (rarely IgG) and fractions of complement.

Prevention

Treat intercurrent infections promptly and vigorously as indicated. Avoid unnecessary vaccinations.

Prognosis

Worsening of the urinary findings may occur with infection, trauma, or fatigue. Exacerbations may resemble the acute attack and may be associated with intercurrent infection or trauma. Other exacerbations may be typical of the nephrotic syndrome (see below). Death in uremia is the usual outcome, but the course is variable, and the patient may live a reasonably normal life for 20–30 years.

4. IgA NEPHROPATHY
(Idiopathic Benign Hematuria; Primary Hematuria)

Primary hematuria (idiopathic benign and recurrent hematuria, Berger's disease) is now known to be an immune complex glomerulopathy in which deposition of IgA and occasionally IgG with C3 and fibrin-related antigens occurs in a granular pattern in the mesangium of the glomerulus.

Recurrent macroscopic and microscopic hematuria and mild proteinuria are usually the only manifestations of renal disease. Recent prospective studies have shown progression of the glomerular disease with destruction of glomeruli and loss of renal function, often with hypertension. Exacerbations have occurred with upper respiratory tract infections. Progression is usually slow, extending over decades.

Diagnosis is made by renal biopsy and demonstration of the mesangial immune complex deposits. Similar deposits may be seen in disseminated lupus erythematosus, eclampsia, Henoch-Schönlein purpura, membranous glomerulonephritis, acute postinfectious glomerulonephritis, and other rare causes of glomerulopathy. The urine sediment resembles that of any latent glomerulonephritis, with protein, red cells, and casts, including erythrocyte casts. The paucity of clinical manifestations and slow progress may be the determinative diagnostic features of the history.

No specific treatment is available for this indolent disease.

5. ANTI–GLOMERULAR BASEMENT MEMBRANE NEPHRITIS
(Goodpasture's Syndrome)

The patient usually gives a history of recent hemoptysis and often of malaise, anorexia, and headache. The clinical syndrome is that of a severe acute glomerulonephritis that may be accompanied by diffuse hemorrhagic inflammation of the lungs. The urine shows gross or microscopic hematuria, and laboratory findings of severely suppressed renal function are usually evident. Biopsy shows glomerular crescents, glomerular adhesions, and inflammatory infiltration interstitially. Electron microscopic examination shows an increase in basement membrane material and deposition of fibrin beneath the capillary endothelium. In some cases, circulating antibody against glomerular basement membrane can be identified. IgG, C3, and, often, other components of the classic complement pathway can be demonstrated as linear deposits on the basement membranes of the glomeruli and the lung. Anti-glomerular basement membrane antibody also reacts with lung basement membrane.

Only rare cases of survival have been documented. Adrenal corticosteroid therapy in combination with immunosuppressive therapy may be useful. Hemodialysis and nephrectomy with renal transplantation may offer the only hope for rescue. Transplantation should be delayed until circulating anti-glomerular basement antibodies have disappeared.

Occasionally, acute renal disease with a similar clinical and immunologic pattern may occur without associated lung disease. Termed **idiopathic rapidly progressive glomerulonephritis**, it characteristically progresses to severe renal insufficiency in a few weeks.

NEPHROTIC SYNDROME

Essentials of Diagnosis
- Massive edema.
- Proteinuria > 3.5 g/d.
- Hypoalbuminemia < 3 g/dL.
- Hyperlipidemia: Cholesterol > 300 mg/dL.
- Lipiduria: Free fat, oval fat bodies, fatty casts.

General Considerations
Because treatment and prognosis vary with the cause of nephrotic syndrome (nephrosis), renal biopsy and appropriate examination of an adequate tissue specimen are important. Light microscopy, electron microscopy, and immunofluorescence identification of immune mechanisms provide critical information for identification of most of the causes of nephrosis.

Glomerular diseases associated with nephrosis include the following:

A. Minimal Glomerular Lesions: Lipoid nephrosis accounts for about 20% of cases of nephrosis in adults. No abnormality is visible by examination of biopsy material with the light microscope. With the electron microscope, alterations of the glomerular basement membrane, with swelling and vacuolization and loss of organization of foot processes of the epithelial cells (foot process disease), are evident. There is no evidence of immune disease by immunofluorescence studies. The response to treatment with adrenocortical steroids is satisfactory. Renal function remains good.

B. Membranous Glomerulonephritis: (About 25–27% of cases.) Examination of biopsy material with the light microscope shows thickening of the glomerular capillary walls and some swelling of mesangial cells but no cellular proliferation. With the electron microscope, irregular lumpy deposits appear between the basement membrane and the epithelial cells, and new basement membrane material protrudes from the glomerular basement membrane as spikes or domes. Immunofluorescence studies show diffuse granular deposits of immunoglobulins (especially IgG) and complement (C3 component). As the membrane thickens, glomeruli become sclerosed and hyalinized.

This form of disease does not respond to any form of therapy. It usually progresses to renal failure in the course of a few to 10 years.

C. Membranoproliferative (Hypocomplementemic) Glomerulonephritis: (About 5% of cases.) Light microscopy shows thickening of glomerular capillaries, accompanied by mesangial proliferation and obliteration of glomeruli. With the electron microscope, subendothelial deposits and growth of mesangium into capillary walls are demonstrable. Immunofluorescence studies show the presence of the C3 component of complement and, rarely, the presence of immunoglobulins. There is no known treatment.

D. Proliferative Glomerulonephritis: (About 5% of cases.) This is considered to be a stage in the course of poststreptococcal nephritis.

E. Miscellaneous Diseases: A large number of metabolic, autoimmune, infectious, and neoplastic diseases and reactions to drugs and other toxic substances can produce glomerular disease. These include diabetic glomerulopathy, systemic lupus erythematosus, polyarteritis, Wegener's granulomatosis, amyloid disease, multiple myeloma, lymphomas, carcinomas, syphilis, reaction to toxins (bee venom, *Rhus* antigen), reaction to drugs (trimethadione, etc), and exposure to heavy metals.

Clinical Findings
A. Symptoms and Signs: Edema may appear insidiously and increase slowly; often it appears suddenly and accumulates rapidly. As fluid collects in the serous cavities, the abdomen becomes protuberant, and the patient may complain of anorexia and become short of breath. Symptoms other than those related to the mechanical effects of edema and serous sac fluid accumulation are not remarkable.

On physical examination, massive edema is apparent. Signs of hydrothorax and ascites are common. Pallor is often accentuated by the edema, and striae commonly appear in the stretched skin of the extremities. Hypertension, changes in the retina and retinal vessels, and cardiac and cerebral signs of hypertension may occur more often when collagen disease, diabetes mellitus, or renal insufficiency is present.

B. Laboratory Findings: The urine contains large amounts of protein, 4–10 g/24 h or more. The sediment contains casts, including the characteristic fatty and waxy varieties; renal tubule cells, some of which contain fatty droplets (oval fat bodies); and variable numbers of erythrocytes. A mild normochromic anemia is common, but anemia may be more severe if renal damage is great. Nitrogen retention varies with the severity of impairment of renal function. The plasma is often lipemic, and the blood cholesterol is usually greatly elevated. Plasma protein is greatly reduced. The albumin fraction may fall to less than 2 g or even below 1 g/dL. Some reduction of gamma globulin occurs in pure nephrosis, whereas in systemic lupus erythematosus the protein of the gamma fraction may be greatly elevated. Serum complement is usually low in active disease. The serum electrolyte concentrations are often normal, although serum sodium may be slightly low; total serum calcium may be low, in keeping with the degree of hypoalbuminemia and decrease in the protein-bound calcium moiety. During edema-forming periods, urinary sodium excretion is very low and urinary aldosterone excretion elevated. If renal insufficiency (see above) is present, the blood and urine findings are usually altered accordingly.

Renal biopsy is essential to confirm the diagnosis and to indicate prognosis.

Differential Diagnosis

The nephrotic syndrome (nephrosis) may be associated with a variety of renal diseases, including glomerulonephritis (membranous and proliferative), collagen diseases (disseminated lupus erythematosus, polyarteritis, etc), amyloid disease, thrombosis of the renal vein, diabetic nephropathy, myxedema, multiple myeloma, malaria, syphilis, reaction to toxins such as bee venom, *Rhus* antigen, or heavy metals, drugs such as trimethadione, and constrictive pericarditis. In small children, nephrosis may occur without clear evidence of any cause.

Treatment

An adequate diet with restricted sodium intake (0.5–1 g/d) and prompt treatment of intercurrent infection are the basis of therapy. Other measures may be added as required.

The corticosteroids have been shown to be of value in treating nephrotic syndrome in children and in adults when the underlying disease is the minimal glomerular lesion (lipoid nephrosis), systemic lupus erythematosus, proliferative glomerulonephritis, or idiosyncrasy to toxin or venom. These drugs are less often effective in the treatment of membranous disease and membranoproliferative lesions of the glomerulus. They are of little or no value in amyloidosis or renal vein thrombosis and are contraindicated in diabetic nephropathy.

Diuretics may be given but are often ineffective. The most useful are the thiazide derivatives, eg, hydrochlorothiazide, 50–100 mg every 12 hours; other thiazides, chlorthalidone, and other diuretics may be employed in comparable effective dose levels. Spironolactone may be helpful when employed concurrently with thiazides. Salt-free albumin, dextran, and other oncotic agents are of little help, and their effects are transient.

Immunosuppressive drugs (aklylating agents, cyclophosphamide, mercaptopurine, azathioprine, etc) are under trial in the treatment of nephrotic syndrome. Combination therapy with corticosteroids is similar to that employed in reversing rejection of homotransplants in humans. Encouraging early results have been reported in children and adults with proliferative or membranous lesions and with systemic lupus erythematosus. Those with minimal lesions refractory to corticosteroid therapy did no better when immunosuppressive agents were added. Improvement was noted in the glomerular changes and renal function in many patients responding well to treatment. It is not known what percentage of patients can be expected to benefit from these drugs.

Both the corticosteroids and the cytotoxic agents are commonly associated with serious side-effects. At present, this form of therapy should be employed only by those experienced in treating nephrotic syndrome in patients who have proved refractory to well-established treatment regimens.

For renal vein thrombosis, treatment with heparin and long-term use of coumarin drugs is directed against progress of thrombus formation.

Prognosis

The course and prognosis depend upon the basic disease responsible for nephrotic syndrome. In about 50% of cases of childhood nephrosis, the disease appears to run a rather benign course when properly treated and to leave insignificant sequelae. Of the others, most go inexorably into the terminal state with renal insufficiency. Adults with nephrosis fare less well, particularly when the fundamental disease is glomerulonephritis, systemic lupus erythematosus, amyloidosis, renal vein thrombosis, or diabetic nephropathy. In those with minimal lesions, remissions, either spontaneous or following corticosteroid therapy, are common. Treatment is more often unsuccessful or only ameliorative when other glomerular lesions are present. Hypertension and nitrogen retention are serious signs.

RENAL INVOLVEMENT IN COLLAGEN DISEASES

The collagen diseases often produce symptoms and signs of renal disease indistinguishable from acute or chronic glomerulonephritis, nephrosis, renal vein thrombosis, and renal infarction. Although it may not be accurate to classify all of these disorders as collagen diseases, acute disseminated lupus erythematosus, polyarteritis nodosa, scleroderma, dermatomyositis, Wegener's granulomatosis, and thrombotic thrombocytopenic purpura have been implicated in producing a syndrome resembling glomerulonephritis. In about one-third to one-half of cases, the urine sediment is diagnostic, containing red blood cells and red blood cell casts; renal tubule cells, including some filled with fat droplets; and waxy and granular broad casts. The presence of these formed elements is indicative of active glomerular and tubular disease with extensive focal destruction of nephrons. The symptoms and signs of the primary disease and a variety of new tests of autoimmune disease help to differentiate the form of collagen disease present. When collagen disease involves the kidneys, complete recovery from the disease is not likely to occur, although steroid and immunosuppressive drugs (alone or in combination) may be effective for long-term amelioration.

DISEASES OF THE RENAL TUBULES & INTERSTITIUM

1. INTERSTITIAL NEPHRITIS

Acute interstitial disease may be due to systemic infections such as syphilis and sensitivity to drugs, including antibiotics (penicillins, colistin, sulfonamides), phenindione, and phenytoin. Recovery may be complete.

Chronic interstitial nephritis is characterized by focal or diffuse interstitial fibrosis accompanied by infiltration with inflammatory cells ultimately associated with extensive atrophy of renal tubules. It represents a nonspecific reaction to a variety of causes: analgesic abuse, lead and cadmium toxicity, nephrocalcinosis, urate nephropathy, radiation nephritis, sarcoidosis, Balkan nephritis, and some instances of obstructive uropathy. There are a few cases in which antitubule basement membrane antibodies have been identified.

2. ANALGESIC NEPHROPATHY

Renal papillary necrosis has usually been associated with fulminating urinary tract infection in the presence of diabetes mellitus. Since 1953, however, increasing numbers of cases have been associated with long-term ingestion of nonsteroidal analgesic and anti-inflammatory drugs. The typical patient is a middle-aged woman with chronic and recurrent headaches or a patient with chronic arthritis who habitually consumes large amounts of the drugs. Phenacetin was implicated initially, but even with elimination of phenacetin from the mixtures, the incidence of analgesic nephropathy has not decreased. The ensuing damage to the kidneys usually is detected late, after renal insufficiency has developed.

The kidney lesion is pathologically nonspecific, consisting of peritubular and perivascular inflammation with degenerative changes of the tubule cells (chronic interstitial nephritis). There are no glomerular changes. Renal papillary necrosis extending into the medulla may involve many papillae.

Hematuria is a common presenting complaint. Renal colic occurs when necrotic renal papillae slough away. Polyuria may be prominent. Signs of acidosis (hyperpnea), dehydration, and pallor of anemia are common. Infection is a frequent complication. The history of excessive use of analgesics may be concealed by the patient.

The urine usually is remarkable only for the presence of blood and small amounts of protein. Hemolytic anemia is usually evident. Elevated blood urea nitrogen and creatinine and the electrolyte changes characteristic of renal failure are typically present.

Urograms show typical cavities and ring shadows of areas of destruction of papillae.

Treatment consists of withholding analgesics containing phenacetin and aspirin. Renal failure and infection are treated as outlined elsewhere in this chapter.

3. URIC ACID NEPHROPATHY

Crystals of urate produce an interstitial inflammatory reaction. Urate may precipitate out in acid urine in the calices to form uric acid stones. Patients with myeloproliferative disease under treatment may develop hyperuricemia and are subject to occlusion of the upper urinary tract by uric acid crystals. Alkalinization of the urine and a liberal fluid intake will help prevent crystal formation. Allopurinol is a useful drug to prevent hyperuricemia and hyperuricosuria.

4. OBSTRUCTIVE UROPATHY

Interstitial nephritis due to obstruction may not be associated with infection. Tubular conservation of salt and water is impaired. Following relief of obstruction, diuresis may be massive and may require vigorous but judicious replacement of water and electrolyte.

5. MYELOMATOSIS

Features of myelomatosis that contribute to renal disease include proteinuria (including filtrable Bence Jones protein and κ and λ chains) with precipitation in the tubules leading to accumulation of abnormal proteins in the tubule cells, hypercalcemia, and occasionally an increase in viscosity of the blood associated with macroglobulinemia. A Fanconi-like syndrome may develop.

Plugging of tubules, giant cell reaction around tubules, tubular atrophy, and, occasionally, the accumulation of amyloid are evident on examination of renal tissue.

Renal failure may occur acutely or may develop slowly. Hemodialysis may rescue the patient during efforts to control the myeloma with chemical agents.

HEREDITARY RENAL DISEASES

The importance of inheritance and the familial incidence of disease warrants inclusion of the classification of hereditary renal diseases suggested by Perkoff (see reference below). Although relatively uncommon in the population at large, hereditary renal disease must be recognized to permit early diagnosis and treatment in other family members and to prepare the way for genetic counseling.

1. HEREDITARY CHRONIC NEPHRITIS

Evidence of the disease usually appears in childhood, with episodes of hematuria often following an upper respiratory infection. Renal insufficiency commonly develops in males but only rarely in females. Survival beyond age 40 is rare.

In many families, deafness and abnormalities of the eyes accompany the renal disease. Another form of the disease is accompanied by polyneuropathy. Infection of the urinary tract is a common complication.

The anatomic features in some cases resemble proliferative glomerulonephritis; in others, there is thickening of the glomerular basement membrane or podocyte proliferation and thickening of Bowman's capsule. In a few cases there are fat-filled cells (foam cells) in the interstitial tissue or in the glomeruli.

Laboratory findings are commensurate with existing renal function.

Treatment is symptomatic.

2. CYSTIC DISEASES OF THE KIDNEY

Congenital structural anomalies of the kidney must always be considered in any patient with hypertension, pyelonephritis, or renal insufficiency. The manifestations of structural renal abnormalities are related to the superimposed disease, but management and prognosis are modified by the structural anomaly.

Polycystic Kidneys

Polycystic kidney disease is familial and often involves not only the kidney but the liver and pancreas as well.

The formation of cysts in the cortex of the kidney is thought to result from failure of union of the collecting tubules and convoluted tubules of some nephrons. New cysts do not form, but those present enlarge and, by exerting pressure, cause destruction of ajacent tissue. Cysts may be found in the liver and pancreas. The incidence of cerebral vessel aneurysms is higher than normal.

Cases of polycystic disease are discovered during the investigation of hypertension, by diagnostic study in patients presenting with pyelonephritis or hematuria, or by investigation of families of patients with polycystic disease. At times, flank pain due to hemorrhage into a cyst will call attention to a kidney disorder. Otherwise the symptoms and signs are those commonly seen in hypertension or renal insufficiency. On physical examination the enlarged, irregular kidneys are easily palpable.

The urine may contain leukocytes and red cells. With bleeding into the cysts there may also be bleeding into the urinary tract. The blood chemical findings reflect the degree of renal insufficiency. Examination by echography or x-ray shows the en-larged kidneys, and urography demonstrates the classic elongated calices and renal pelves stretched over the surface of the cysts.

No specific therapy is available, and surgical interference is contraindicated unless ureteral obstruction is produced by an adjacent cyst. Hypertension, infection, and uremia are treated in the conventional manner.

Because persons with polycystic kidneys may live in reasonable comfort with slowly advancing uremia, it is difficult to determine when renal transplantation is in order. Hemodialysis can extend the life of the patient, but recurrent bleeding and continuous pain indicate the need for a transplant.

Although the disease may become symptomatic in childhood or in early adult life, it usually is discovered in the fourth or fifth decade. Unless fatal complications of hypertension or urinary tract infection are present, uremia develops very slowly, and patients live longer than with other causes of renal insufficiency.

Cystic Disease of the Renal Medulla

Two syndromes have been recognized with increasing frequency as their diagnostic features have become better known.

Medullary cystic disease is a familial disease that may become symptomatic during adolescence. Anemia is usually the initial manifestation, but azotemia, acidosis, and hyperphosphatemia soon become evident. Hypertension may develop. The urine is not remarkable, although there is often an inability to produce a concentrated urine. Many small cysts are scattered through the renal medulla. Renal transplantation is indicated by the usual criteria for the operation.

Sponge kidney is asymptomatic and is discovered by the characteristic appearance of the urogram. Enlargement of the papillae and calices and small cavities within the pyramids are demonstrated by the contrast media in the excretory urogram. Many small calculi often occupy the cysts, and infection may be troublesome. Life expectancy is not affected, and only symptomatic therapy for ureteral impaction of a stone or for infection is required.

3. ANOMALIES OF THE PROXIMAL TUBULE

Defects of Amino Acid Reabsorption

A. Congenital Cystinuria: Increased excretion of cystine results in the formation of cystine calculi in the urinary tract. Ornithine, arginine, and lysine are also excreted in abnormally large quantities. There is also a defect in absorption of these amino acids in the jejunum. Nonopaque stones should be examined chemically to provide a specific diagnosis.

Maintain a high urine volume by giving a large

fluid intake. Maintain the urine pH above 7.0 by giving sodium bicarbonate and sodium citrate plus acetazolamide at bedtime to ensure an alkaline night urine. In refractory cases, a low-methionine (cystine precursor) diet may be necessary. Penicillamine has proved useful in some cases.

B. Aminoaciduria: Many amino acids may be poorly absorbed, resulting in unusual losses. Failure to thrive and the presence of other tubular deficits suggest the diagnosis.

There is no treatment.

C. Hepatolenticular Degeneration: In this congenital familial disease, aminoaciduria is associated with cirrhosis of the liver and neurologic manifestations. Hepatomegaly, evidence of impaired liver function, spasticity, athetosis, emotional disturbances, and Kayser-Fleischer rings around the cornea constitute a unique syndrome. There is a decrease in synthesis of ceruloplasmin, with a deficit of plasma ceruloplasmin and an increase in free copper that may be etiologically specific.

Give penicillamine to chelate and remove excess copper. Edathamil (EDTA) may also be used to remove copper.

Multiple Defects of Tubular Function (De Toni-Fanconi-Debré Syndrome)

Aminoaciduria, phosphaturia, glycosuria, and a variable degree of renal tubular acidosis characterize this syndrome. Osteomalacia is a prominent clinical feature; other clinical and laboratory manifestations are associated with specific tubular defects described separately above.

The proximal segment of the renal tubule is replaced by a thin tubular structure constituting the "swan neck" deformity. The proximal segment also is shortened to less than half the normal length.

Treatment consists of replacing cation deficits (especially potassium), correcting acidosis with bicarbonate or citrate, replacing phosphate loss with isotonic neutral phosphate (mono- and disodium salts) solution, and a liberal calcium intake. Vitamin D is usually useful, but the dose used must be controlled by monitoring serum calcium and phosphate.

Defects of Phosphorus & Calcium Absorption

A. Vitamin D-Resistant Rickets: Excessive loss of phosphorus and calcium results in rickets or osteomalacia that responds poorly to vitamin D therapy. Treatment consists of giving large doses of vitamin D and calcium supplementation of the diet.

B. Pseudohypoparathyroidism: As a result of excessive reabsorption of phosphorus, hyperphosphatemia and hypocalcemia occur. Symptoms include muscle cramps, fatigue, weakness, tetany, and mental retardation. The signs are those of hypocalcemia; in addition, the patients are short, round-faced, and characteristically have short fourth and fifth metacarpal and metatarsal bones.

The serum phosphorus is high, serum calcium low, and serum alkaline phosphatase normal. There is no response to parathyroid hormone.

Vitamin D therapy and calcium supplementation may prevent tetany.

Defects of Glucose Absorption (Renal Glycosuria)

This results from an abnormally low ability to reabsorb glucose, so that glycosuria is present when blood glucose levels are normal. Ketosis is not present. The glucose tolerance response is usually normal. In some instances, renal glycosuria may precede the onset of true diabetes mellitus.

There is no treatment for renal glycosuria.

Defects of Glucose & Phosphate Absorption (Glycosuric Rickets)

The symptoms and signs are those of rickets or osteomalacia, with weakness, pain, or discomfort of the legs and spine, and tetany. The bones become deformed, with bowing of the weight-bearing long bones, kyphoscoliosis, and, in children, signs of rickets. X-ray shows markedly decreased density of the bone, with pseudofracture lines and other deformities. Nephrocalcinosis may occur with excessive phosphaturia, and renal insufficiency may follow. Urinary calcium and phosphorus are increased and glycosuria is present. Serum glucose is normal, serum calcium is normal or low, serum phosphorus is low, and serum alkaline phosphatase is elevated.

Treatment consists of giving large doses of vitamin D and calcium supplementation of the diet.

Defects of Bicarbonate Reabsorption

Proximal renal tubular acidosis (RTA, type II) is due to a deficiency in the production of H^+ in the proximal tubule, with resultant loss of bicarbonate in the urine and decreased bicarbonate concentration in extracellular fluid. Accompanying the limitation of H^+ secretion are increased K^+ secretion into the urine and retrieval of Cl^- instead of HCO_3^-. The acidosis is therefore associated with hypokalemia and hyperchloremia. Transport of glucose, amino acids, phosphate, and urate may be deficient as well and may result in Fanconi's syndrome.

4. ANOMALIES OF THE DISTAL TUBULE

Defects of Hydrogen Ion Secretion & Bicarbonate Reabsorption (Classic Renal Tubular Acidosis, Type I)

Failure to secrete hydrogen ion and to form ammonium ion results in loss of "fixed base": sodium, potassium, and calcium. There is also a high rate of excretion of phosphate. Vomiting, poor growth, and symptoms and signs of chronic metabolic acidosis are accompanied by weakness due to potassium deficit and the bone discomfort due to osteomalacia. Nephrocalcinosis, with calcification in the medullary portions of the kidney, occurs in about half of cases. The urine is alkaline and contains larger than normal quantities of sodium, potassium, calcium, and phosphate. The blood chemical findings are those of metabolic acidosis (low HCO_3^- or CO_2) with hyperchloremia, low serum calcium and phosphorus, low serum potassium, and, occasionally, low serum sodium.

Treatment consists of replacing deficits and increasing the intake of sodium, potassium, calcium, and phosphorus. Sodium and potassium should be given as bicarbonate or citrate. Additional vitamin D may be required.

Excess Potassium Secretion (Potassium "Wastage" Syndrome)

Excessive renal secretion or loss of potassium may occur in 4 situations: (1) chronic renal insufficiency with diminished H^+ secretion; (2) renal tubular acidosis and the De Toni-Fanconi syndrome, with cation loss resulting from diminished H^+ and NH_4^+ secretion; (3) hyperaldosteronism and hyperadrenocorticism; and (4) tubular secretion of potassium, the cause of which is as yet unknown. Hypokalemia indicates that the deficit is severe. Muscle weakness, metabolic alkalosis, and polyuria with dilute urine are signs attributable to hypokalemia.

Treatment consists of correcting the primary disease and giving supplementary potassium.

Defects of Water Absorption (Renal Diabetes Insipidus)

Nephrogenic diabetes insipidus occurs more frequently in males. Unresponsiveness to antidiuretic hormone is the key to differentiation from pituitary diabetes insipidus.

In addition to congenital refractoriness to antidiuretic hormone, obstructive uropathy, lithium, methoxyflurane, and demeclocycline may also render the tubule refractory.

Symptoms are related to an inability to reabsorb water, with resultant polyuria and polydipsia. The urine volume approaches 12 L/d, and osmolality and specific gravity are low. Mental retardation, atonic bladder, and hydronephrosis occur frequently.

Treatment consists primarily of an adequate water intake. Chlorothiazide may ameliorate the diabetes; the mechanism of action is unknown, but the drug may act by increasing isosmotic reabsorption in the proximal segment of the tubule.

5. UNSPECIFIED RENAL TUBULAR ABNORMALITIES

In **idiopathic hypercalciuria**, decreased reabsorption of calcium predisposes to the formation of renal calculi. Serum calcium and phosphorus are normal. Urine calcium excretion is high; urine phosphorus excretion is low.

See treatment of urinary stones containing calcium.

● ● ●

References

General

Black DAK (editor): *Renal Disease,* 4th ed. Lippincott, 1978.

Brenner BM, Rector FC Jr: *The Kidney.* Saunders, 1981.

Heptinstall RH: *Pathology of the Kidney,* 2nd ed. Little, Brown, 1974.

Krupp MA: Genitourinary tract. Chapter 15 in: *Current Medical Diagnosis & Treatment 1981.* Krupp MA, Chatton MJ (editors). Lange, 1981.

Lindheimer MD & others: The kidney in pregnancy. *N Engl J Med* 1970;**283**:1095.

Schrier RW (editor): *Renal and Electrolyte Disorders,* 2nd ed. Little, Brown, 1980.

Symposium on diseases of the kidney. *Med Clin North Am* 1971;**55**:1. [Entire issue.]

Symposium on glomerulonephritis. *Bull NY Acad Med* 1970;**46**:747. [Entire issue.]

Urinalysis

Brody LH & others: Urinalysis and the urinary sediment. *Med Clin North Am* 1971;**55**:243.

Haber MH: *Urine Casts: Their Microscopy and Clinical Significance.* American Society of Clinical Pathologists, 1975.

Sternheimer R: A supravital cytodiagnostic stain for urinary sediments. *JAMA* 1975;**231**:826.

Glomerulonephritis

Baldwin DS: Poststreptococcal glomerulonephritis: A progressive disease? *Am J Med* 1977;**62**:1.

Carpenter CB: Immunologic aspects of renal disease. *Annu Rev Med* 1970;**21**:1.

Clarkson AR & others: IgA nephropathy: A syndrome of uniform morphology, diverse clinical features, and uncertain prognosis. *Clin Nephrol* 1977;**8**:459.

Dixon FJ: The pathogenesis of glomerulonephritis. *Am J Med* 1968;**44**:493.

Gutman RA & others: The immune complex glomerulonephritis of subacute bacterial endocarditis. *Medicine* 1972;**51**:1.

Lehman DH: Drug-induced nephritis. *Drug Ther Bull* (April) 1976;**6**:182.

Lewis EJ: Rapidly progressive glomerulonephritis. *The Kidney* (Jan) 1973;**6**:1.

Mahieu P & others: Detection of humoral and cell mediated immunity to kidney basement membrane in human renal disease. *Am J Med* 1972;**53**:185.

Merrill JP: Glomerulonephritis. (3 parts.) *N Engl J Med* 1974;**290**:257, 313, 374.

Morel-Maroger L, Leathem A, Richet G: Glomerular abnormalities in nonsystemic diseases. *Am J Med* 1972;**53**:170.

Van de Putte LBA & others: Recurrent or persistent hematuria. *N Engl J Med* 1974;**290**:1165.

Wilson CB: Immunological mechanisms of glomerulonephritis. *Calif Med* (Jan) 1972;**116**:47.

Nephrotic Syndrome

Hayslett JP & others: Clinicopathological correlation in the nephrotic syndrome due to primary renal disease. *Medicine* 1973;**52**:93.

Hopper J Jr & others: Lipoid nephrosis in 31 adult patients: Renal biopsy study by light, electron and fluorescence microscopy with experience in treatment. *Medicine* 1970;**49**:321.

Kaplan BS & others: Glomerular injury in patients with neoplasia. *Annu Rev Med* 1976;**27**:117.

Llach F & others: Renal vein thrombosis and nephrotic syndrome. *Ann Intern Med* 1975;**83**:8.

Skinner MD, Schwartz RS: Immunosuppressive therapy. (2 parts.) *N Engl J Med* 1972;**287**:221, 281.

Steinberg AD & others: Cytotoxic drugs in treatment of nonmalignant diseases. *Ann Intern Med* 1972;**76**:619.

Trew PA & others: Renal vein thrombosis in membranous glomerulonephropathy: Incidence and association. *Medicine* 1978;**57**:69.

Interstitial Nephritis

Graber ML & others: Idiopathic acute interstitial nephritis. *West J Med* 1978;**129**:72.

Kincaid-Smith P: Analgesic abuse and the kidney. *Kidney Int* 1980;**17**:250.

Lehman DH: Using drugs for compromised patient: Drug-induced nephritis. *Drug Ther* (April) 1976;**6**:31.

Ooi BS: Acute interstitial nephritis: A clinical and pathological study based on renal biopsies. *Am J Med* 1975;**59**:614.

Cystic Disease

Gardner KD Jr (editor): *Cystic Diseases of the Kidney.* Wiley, 1976.

Hatfield PM, Pfister RC: Adult polycystic disease of the kidneys (Potter type 3). *JAMA* 1972;**222**:1527.

Wahlqvist L: Cystic disorders of kidney: Review of pathogenesis and classification. *J Urol* 1967;**97**:1.

Tubule Disorders

Courey WR, Pfister RC: The radiographic findings in renal tubular acidosis. *Radiology* 1972;**105**:497.

Frimpter GW: Aminoacidurias due to inherited disorders of metabolism. (2 parts.) *N Engl J Med* 1974;**289**:835, 895.

Gennari FJ, Cohen JJ: Renal tubular acidosis. *Annu Rev Med* 1978;**29**:521.

Lee DBN & others: The adult Fanconi syndrome. *Medicine* 1972;**51**:107.

Perkoff GT: Hereditary renal diseases. (2 parts.) *N Engl J Med* 1967;**277**:79, 129.

Rector FC, Cogan MC: The renal acidoses. *Hosp Pract* (April) 1980;**15**:99.

Stanbury JB, Wyngaarden JB, Fredrickson DS (editors): *The Metabolic Basis of Inherited Disease,* 4th ed. McGraw-Hill, 1978.

24 | Oliguria; Acute Renal Failure

William J.C. Amend, Jr., MD, & Flavio G. Vincenti, MD

Oliguria literally means "too little" urine volume in response to the body's excretory needs. Oliguria is present when the daily urine volume is not sufficient to remove the endogenous solute loads that are the end products of metabolism. No precise figure for 24-hour urine volume can be used in defining oliguria, since urine volumes normally vary with fluid intake and the concentrating ability of the kidney. If the kidney can concentrate urine in a normal fashion to a specific gravity of 1.035, oliguria is present at urine volumes under 400 mL/d. On the other hand, if the kidney concentration is impaired and the patient can achieve a specific gravity of only 1.010, oliguria is present at urine volumes under 1000–1500 mL/d.

Acute renal failure is a condition in which the glomerular filtration rate is abruptly reduced, causing a sudden retention of endogenous metabolites (urea, potassium, phosphate, sulfate, creatinine) that are normally cleared by the kidneys. Low urine volumes (under 400 mL/d) are usually present. However, if renal concentrating mechanisms are impaired (see above), the daily urine volume may be normal or even high ("high-output" or "nonoliguric" renal failure). Rarely, there is no urine output at all (anuria) in acute renal failure.

The causes of acute renal failure are listed in Table 24–1. Prompt differentiation of one cause of acute renal failure from the other categories is important in determining appropriate therapy. Prerenal renal failure is reversible if treated promptly, whereas a delay in therapy may allow progression into a fixed, nonspecific form of intrinsic renal failure (eg, acute tubular necrosis). The other causes are classified on the basis of their involvement with vascular lesions, intrarenal disorders, or postrenal disorders.

PRERENAL RENAL FAILURE

The term prerenal denotes inadequate renal perfusion because of inadequate or ineffective intravascular volume. The most common cause of this form of acute renal failure is dehydration due to renal or extrarenal fluid losses from diarrhea, vomiting, excessive use of diuretics, etc. Less common

Table 24–1. Etiology of acute renal failure.

I. Prerenal renal failure:
1. Dehydration.
2. Vascular collapse due to sepsis, antihypertensive drug therapy.
3. Reduced cardiac output.
II. Vascular:
1. Atheroembolism.
2. Dissecting arterial aneurysms.
3. Malignant hypertension.
III. Parenchymal (intrarenal):
1. Specific:
a. Glomerulonephritis.
b. Interstitial nephritis.
c. Toxin, dye-induced.
2. Nonspecific:
a. Acute tubular necrosis.
b. Acute cortical necrosis.
IV. Postrenal:
1. Calculus in patients with solitary kidney.
2. Bilateral ureteral obstruction.
3. Outlet obstruction.
4. Leak, posttraumatic.

causes are septic shock and excessive use of antihypertensive drugs, which cause relative or absolute depletion of intravascular fluid volume. Heart failure with reduced cardiac output can also reduce effective renal blood flow. Careful clinical assessment may identify the primary condition responsible for prerenal renal failure.

Clinical Findings

A. Symptoms and Signs: Except for rare cases with associated cardiac or "pump" failure, patients usually complain of thirst or of dizziness in the upright posture (orthostatic dizziness). There may be a history of overt fluid loss. Sudden weight loss usually reflects the degree of dehydration.

Physical examination frequently reveals poor skin turgor, collapsed neck veins, dry mucous membranes and axillas, and, most importantly, orthostatic or postural changes in blood pressure and pulse.

B. Laboratory Findings:

1. Urine—The urine volume is usually low. Ac-

Table 24—2. Acute renal failure versus prerenal azotemia.

	Acute Renal Failure	Prerenal Azotemia
Urine osmolality (mOsm/L)	< 350	> 500
Urine/plasma urea	< 10	> 20
Urine/plasma creatinine	< 20	> 40
Urine Na (mEq/L)	> 40	< 20
Renal failure index = $\dfrac{U_{Na}}{U/P_{Cr}}$	> 1	< 1
*$F_{E\,Na}$ = $\dfrac{U/P_{Na}}{U/P_{Cr}}$ × 100	> 1	< 1

*Excreted fraction of filtered sodium. See Espinel CH: *JAMA* 1976;**236**:579; and Miller TR & others: *Ann Intern Med* 1978; **89**:47.

curate assessment may require bladder catheterization followed by hourly output measurements (which will also rule out lower urinary tract obstruction; see below). High urine specific gravity (> 1.025) and urine osmolality (> 600 mOsm/kg) also are noted in this form of acute renal failure. Routine urinalysis is generally not helpful.

2. Urine and blood chemistries–The blood urea nitrogen/creatinine ratio, normally 10:1, is usually increased with prerenal renal failure. Other findings are set forth in Table 24–2. These assessments should not be done if mannitol or other diuretics have been given prior to the measurements, since these agents affect the delivery and tubular handling of urea, sodium, and creatinine.

3. Central venous pressure–A low central venous pressure indicates hypovolemia, which may be due to blood loss or dehydration. If severe cardiac failure is the principal cause of prerenal renal failure (it is rarely the sole cause), a reduced cardiac output and high central venous pressure will be apparent.

4. Fluid challenge–An increase in urine output in response to a carefully administered fluid challenge is both diagnostic and therapeutic in prerenal renal failure. Rapid intravenous administration of 300–500 mL of physiologic saline or of 125 mL of 20% mannitol (25 g/125 mL) is the usual initial treatment. Urine output is measured over the subsequent 1–3 hours. A urine volume of more than 50 mL/h is considered a favorable response that warrants continued intravenous infusion with physiologic solutions to restore plasma volume and correct dehydration. If the urine volume does not increase, results of the blood and urine chemistry tests should be carefully reviewed, the patient's fluid status should be reassessed, and a repeat physical examination should be done to determine if an additional fluid challenge (with or without furosemide) might be worthwhile.

Treatment

In states of dehydration, rapid correction of measured and estimated fluid losses is necessary to treat oliguria of prerenal origin. Inadequate fluid management may cause further renal hemodynamic deterioration and eventual renal tubular degeneration (fixed acute tubular necrosis; see below). If oliguria persists in a well hydrated patient, vasopressor drugs are indicated in an effort to correct the hypotension associated with sepsis or cardiogenic shock. Pressor agents that restore systemic blood pressure while maintaining renal blood flow and renal function (eg, dopamine, 1–5 μg/kg/min) are most useful. Discontinuance of antihypertensive medications or diuretics can, by itself, cure the apparent acute renal failure resulting from prerenal causes.

VASCULAR RENAL FAILURE

Common causes of acute renal failure due to vascular disease include atheroembolic disease, dissecting arterial aneurysms, and malignant hypertension. Atheroembolic disease is rare before age 60 and in patients who have not undergone vascular procedures or angiographic studies. Dissecting arterial aneurysms and malignant hypertension are usually clinically evident. Acute renal venous thrombosis, unless it affects both kidneys, has no deleterious effect on renal clearance function.

Rapid assessment of the arterial blood supply to the kidney requires arteriography. The cause of malignant hypertension may be identified on physical examination (scleroderma, etc). Primary management of the vascular process is necessary to affect any renal failure.

INTRARENAL DISEASE STATES; INTRARENAL ACUTE RENAL FAILURE

Diseases in this category can be divided into specific and nonspecific parenchymal processes.

1. SPECIFIC INTRARENAL DISEASE STATES

The most common causes of intrarenal acute renal failure are acute or rapidly progressive glomerulonephritis, acute interstitial nephritis, and toxic nephropathies.

Clinical Findings

A. Symptoms and Signs: Usually there are some salient historical data such as sore throat or upper respiratory infection, use of antibiotics, or intravenous use of drugs (often illicit types). Bilateral back pain, at times severe, is occasionally noted. Gross hematuria may be present. It is unusual for pyelonephritis to present as acute renal failure unless there is (1) associated sepsis or dehydration, (2) obstruction, or (3) involvement of a solitary kidney. Systemic diseases in which acute renal failure occurs include Henoch-Schönlein purpura, thrombotic thrombocytopenic purpura, systemic lupus erythematosus, and scleroderma.

B. Laboratory Findings:

1. Urine–Urinalysis discloses many red and white cells and multiple types of cellular and granular casts ("telescopic urine"). In allergic interstitial nephritis, eosinophils may be noted. The urine sodium concentration may range from 10 to 40 mEq/L.

2. Serum–Components of serum complement are often diminished during deposition of immune complexes. In a few laboratories, circulating immune complexes can be identified. Other tests may disclose systemic diseases such as lupus erythematosus and thrombotic thrombocytopenic purpura.

3. Renal biopsy–Biopsy examination will show characteristic changes of acute interstitial nephritis or glomerulonephritis. There may be extensive crescents involving Bowman's space.

C. X-Ray Findings: Poor visualization on intravenous urography or radionuclide renal scans is characteristic.

Treatment

Therapy is directed toward eradication of infection, removal of antigen, elimination of toxic materials and drugs, suppression of autoimmune mechanisms, removal of autoimmune antibodies, or a reduction in effector-inflammatory responses. Immunotherapy may involve drugs, anticoagulants, or the temporary use of plasmapheresis.

2. NONSPECIFIC INTRARENAL STATES

These include acute tubular necrosis and acute cortical necrosis. The latter presents with anuria and associated intrarenal intravascular coagulation and has a generally poorer prognosis than acute tubular necrosis.

Acute tubular necrosis was initially described by Lücke in World War II in patients suffering crush injuries and shock. Degenerative changes of the more distal tubules (lower nephron nephrosis) were believed to be due to ischemia. When dialysis became available, most of these patients recovered—sometimes completely—provided that intrarenal intravascular coagulation and cortical necrosis had not occurred.

Elderly patients are more prone to develop this form of oliguric acute renal failure following hypotensive episodes. It appears that exposure to certain drugs (eg, prostaglandin inhibitors such as nonsteroidal anti-inflammatory agents) may predispose patients to a greater risk of acute tubular necrosis. Although the classic picture of lower nephron nephrosis may not develop, a similar nonspecific acute renal failure is noted in some cases of mercury (especially mercuric chloride) poisoning and following exposure to radiocontrast agents in patients with diabetes mellitus or myeloma.

Clinical Findings

A. Symptoms and Signs: Usually the clinical picture is that of the associated clinical state. Dehydration and shock may be present concurrently but fail to improve following administration of intravenous fluids as with prerenal renal failure (see above). There may be only signs of excessive fluid retention in post-radiocontrast cases of acute renal failure. Symptoms of uremia per se (ie, altered mentation or gastrointestinal symptoms) are unusual in acute renal failure (in contrast to patients with chronic renal failure).

B. Laboratory Findings: (See also Table 24–2.)

1. Urine–Although the specific gravity may be high immediately after the acute event, it usually becomes low or fixed in the 1.005–1.015 range. Urine osmolality is also low (< 450 mOsm/kg and U/P osmolal ratio < 1.5:1). Urinalysis often discloses tubular cells and granular casts; the urine may be muddy brown. If the test for occult blood is positive, one must be concerned about the presence of myoglobin as well as hemoglobin. Tests for differentiating myoglobin pigment are available.

2. Central venous pressure is usually normal to slightly elevated.

3. Fluid challenges–There is no increase in urine volume following administration of intravenous mannitol or physiologic saline. Occasionally following the use of furosemide, a low urine output will be converted to a high fixed urine output (low-output renal failure to high-output renal failure), but there is no change in the rates of increases in blood urea nitrogen or creatinine.

Treatment

If there is no response to the initial fluid or mannitol challenge, the volume of administered fluid must be sharply curtailed and the amount given related to the measured urine volume. An early assessment of the rate of rise of serum creatinine and blood urea nitrogen and of the concentrations of electrolytes is necessary to provide criteria for possible use of dialysis therapy. There is some evidence that early use of hyperalimentation might be beneficial in both reducing the need for dialysis and for reducing morbidity and mortality rates. With appropriate regulation of the volume of fluid administered, use of solutions of glucose and essential amino acids to provide 30–35 kcal/kg may correct or reduce the severity of the catabolic state accompanying acute tubular necrosis.

Serum or plasma potassium must be closely monitored and serial ECGs done to ensure early recognition of hyperkalemia. This condition can be treated with (1) intravenous sodium bicarbonate administration; (2) Kayexalate, 25–50 g (with sorbitol), orally or by enema; (3) intravenous glucose and insulin; and (4) intravenous calcium preparations to prevent cardiac irritability. Peritoneal dialysis or hemodialysis should be used as necessary to avoid or correct uremia, hypokalemia, or fluid overload.

Prognosis

Most cases are reversible within 7–14 days. Residual renal damage may be noted, particularly in elderly patients.

POSTRENAL ACUTE RENAL FAILURE

The conditions listed in Table 24–1 involve primarily urologic diagnostic and therapeutic interventions. Following lower abdominal surgery, urethral or ureteral obstruction should be considered. The causes of bilateral ureteral obstruction are (1) peritoneal or retroperitoneal neoplastic involvement, with masses or nodes; (2) retroperitoneal fibrosis; (3) calculous disease; or (4) postsurgical or traumatic interruption. With a solitary kidney, ureteral stones can produce total urinary tract obstruction and acute renal failure. Urethral or bladder neck obstruction is a frequent cause of renal failure, especially in elderly men. Posttraumatic urethral tears are discussed in Chapter 16.

Clinical Findings

A. Symptoms and Signs: Renal pain and renal tenderness may often be present. If there has been an operative ureteral injury with associated urine extravasation, urine may leak through a wound. Edema from overhydration may be noted. Ileus is often present along with associated abdominal distention and vomiting.

B. Laboratory Findings: Urinalysis is usually not helpful. A large volume of urine obtained by catheterization may be both diagnostic and therapeutic for lower tract obstruction.

C. X-Ray Findings: Poor visualization is the usual finding on intravenous urography. Radionuclide renal scans may show a urine leak or, in cases of obstruction, retention of the isotope in the renal pelvis. Ultrasound examination will often reveal a dilated upper collecting system with deformities characteristic of hydronephrosis.

D. Instrumental Examination: Cystoscopy and retrograde ureteral catheterization will demonstrate ureteral obstruction.

Treatment

For further discussion of ureteral injuries, see Chapter 16.

● ● ●

References

Abel RM & others: Improved survival from acute renal failure after treatment with intravenous essential L-amino acids and glucose: Results of a prospective, double-blind study. *N Engl J Med* 1973;**288**:695.

Cohn HE, Capelli JP: The diagnosis and management of oliguria in the postoperative period. *Surg Clin North Am* 1967;**47**:1187.

Davis BB Jr, Knox FG: Current concepts of the regulation of urinary sodium excretion: A review. *Am J Med Sci* 1970;**259**:373.

Espinel CH: The $F_{E_{Na}}$ test: Use in the differential diagnosis of acute renal failure. *JAMA* 1976;**236**:579.

Figueroa JE: Acute renal failure: Its unusual causes and manifestations. *Med Clin North Am* 1967;**51**:995.

Hall JW & others: Immediate and long-term prognosis in acute renal failure. *Ann Intern Med* 1970;**73**:515.

Harrington JT, Cohen JJ: Acute oliguria. *N Engl J Med* 1975;**292**:89.

Jones LW, Weil MH: Water, creatinine and sodium excretion following circulatory shock with renal failure. *Am J Med* 1971;**51**:314.

Levinsky NG: Pathophysiology of acute renal failure. *N Engl J Med* 1977;**296**:1453.

Lewers DJ & others: Long-term follow up of renal function and histology after acute tubular necrosis. *Ann Intern Med* 1970;**73**:523.

Lyon RP: Nonobstructive oliguria: Differential diagnosis. *Calif Med* 1963;**99**:83.

McMurray SD & others: Prevailing patterns and predictor values in patients with acute tubular necrosis. *Arch Intern Med* 1978;**138**:950.

Merrill JP: Acute renal failure. *JAMA* 1970;**211**:289.

Swartz RD & others: Renal failure following major angiography. *Am J Med* 1978;**65**:31.

Thurau K, Boylan JW: Acute renal success: The unexpected logic of oliguria in acute renal failure. *Am J Med* 1976;**61**:308.

Vertel RM, Knochel JP: Nonoliguric acute renal failure. *JAMA* 1967;**200**:598.

25 | Chronic Renal Failure & Dialysis

William J.C. Amend, Jr., MD, & Flavio G. Vincenti, MD

In renal failure, the clearance of endogenous solutes from the kidney is reduced, and the concentrations of these solutes in the body become elevated. The most common solutes measured as indicators of renal failure are blood urea nitrogen and serum creatinine. However, marked elevation of blood urea nitrogen can be due to nonrenal causes such as prerenal azotemia, gastrointestinal hemorrhage, or high protein intake. If the serum creatinine has remained constant or risen to a new steady state, creatinine clearance can be measured as an indicator of the glomerular filtration rate (GFR).

Renal failure may be classified as acute or chronic depending on the rapidity of onset and the subsequent course of azotemia. An analysis of the acute or chronic development of renal failure is important in understanding physiologic adaptations, disease mechanisms, and ultimate therapy. In individual cases, it is often difficult to establish the duration of renal failure. Historic clues such as preceding hypertension or radiologic findings such as small, shrunken kidneys favor a more chronic process. Certain forms of acute renal failure tend to progress to irreversible chronic renal failure.

For a discussion of acute renal failure, see Chapter 24.

The general incidence of chronic renal failure in the USA, defined as "people who can benefit from hemodialysis or renal transplantation," is 50 per million population per year. The medical acceptance criteria are strict. All age groups are affected. The severity and the rapidity of development of uremia are hard to predict. Rapidly expanding use of dialysis and transplantation is worldwide. Forty-eight thousand patients are currently being treated with either dialysis or transplantation, and it is estimated that 56,000 patients will be treated each year by 1982.

Historical Background

There are various causes of progressive renal dysfunction leading to end stage or terminal renal failure. Bright in the 1800s described several cases that presented with edema, hematuria, and proteinuria, ending in death. Early chemical analyses of patients' sera drew attention to retained nonpro-tein nitrogen (NPN) compounds, and an association was made between this and the clinical findings of uremia. Although the pathologic state of uremia was well described in the intervening years, it remained for technics of chronic dialysis and renal transplantation to solve the therapeutic problems.

Etiology

A variety of disorders are associated with end stage renal disease. Either a primary renal process (eg, glomerulonephritis, pyelonephritis, congenital hypoplasia) or a secondary one (eg, a kidney affected by a systemic process such as diabetes mellitus or lupus erythematosus) may be at fault. Minor physiologic alterations secondary to dehydration, infection, or hypertension often "tip the scale" and put a borderline patient into uncompensated clinical uremia.

Clinical Findings

A. Symptoms and Signs: Symptoms such as pruritus, generalized malaise, lassitude, forgetfulness, loss of libido, nausea, and altered behavior patterns are subtle complaints in this chronic disorder. There is often a strong family history of renal disease. Growth failure is a primary complaint in preadolescent patients. Symptoms of a multisystem disorder (eg, arthritis in lupus erythematosus) may be present coincidentally. Most patients with renal failure have elevated blood pressure secondary to volume overload and overhydration. Occasionally, hyperreninemic conditions may be present. However, the blood pressure may be normal or low if patients are on a very low sodium diet or have marked salt-losing tendencies (eg, medullary cystic disease). The pulse and respiratory rates are rapid as manifestations of anemia and metabolic acidosis. Clinical findings of uremic fetor, pericarditis, neurologic findings of asterixis, reduced mentation, and peripheral neuropathy are often present. Terry's nails—pallor of the proximal nail beds—can sometimes distinguish chronic from acute renal failure. Palpable kidneys suggest polycystic disease. Ophthalmoscopic examination may show hypertensive or diabetic retinopathy. Alterations involving the cornea have been associated with metabolic disease (eg, Fabry's disease).

B. Laboratory Findings:

1. Urine composition—Urine volumes vary depending on the severity and type of renal disease. Quantitatively, normal amounts of water and salt losses in urine can be associated with polycystic and interstitial forms of disease. Usually, however, urine volumes are quite low when the GFR falls below 5% of normal. Daily salt losses become more fixed, and a state of sodium retention occurs soon after. If the patient has had proteinuria in the nephrotic range preceding the uremic stage, this degree of proteinuria will be absent due to reduced GFR.

2. Blood studies—Anemia is the rule, but the hematocrit may be normal in polycystic disease. Platelet dysfunction or thrombasthenia is characterized by abnormal bleeding times. Platelet counts and prothrombin content are normal.

Elevated serum creatinine, blood urea nitrogen, and nonprotein nitrogen are the hallmarks of this disorder. Metabolic acidosis is usual, but normokalemia will be present unless the patient has minimal residual renal function (GFR less than 5 mL/min), is dehydrated, or has an excessive potassium intake or catabolism rate (due to infection, gastrointestinal bleeding, etc). Progressive reduction of body buffer stores and an inability to excrete titratable acids lead to progressive acidosis characterized by reduced serum bicarbonate and compensatory respiratory hyperventilation. In the presence of this acidemia, serum potassium levels may be elevated and reflect intra- to extracellular shifts of potassium. Serum phosphate is elevated, and serum calcium is reduced secondary to multiple factors. Uremic patients have a reduced appetite and, consequently, reduced calcium ingestion. There is diminished vitamin D activity because of reduced conversion of vitamin D_2 to active vitamin D_3 in the kidney. Phosphate retention (due to reduced phosphate clearance) is noted. These alterations may lead to uremic osteodystrophy with elements of both osteomalacia and secondary hyperparathyroidism. Uric acid levels are elevated secondary to reduced renal tubular clearances. It is unusual, however, for these elevated uric acid levels to be clinically important (ie, gouty attacks or renal urate depositions). Creatinine and urea clearances are markedly reduced.

C. X-Ray Findings: Infusion nephrotomograms are required if the serum creatinine is 3 mg/dL or more. They will usually reveal small kidneys, congenital hypoplasia, polycystic disease, or some other structural disorder. Bone x-rays may show retarded growth, osteomalacia (renal rickets), or secondary hyperparathyroidism. Soft tissue calcification may be present.

D. Other Examinations: Renal sonograms are helpful in determining renal size and cortical thickness and in localizing tissue for percutaneous renal biopsy. Renal biopsies, however, may not reveal much except end stage scarring and glomerulosclerosis. There may be pronounced vascular changes consisting of thickening of the media, fragmentation of elastic fibers, and intimal proliferation, which may be secondary to uremic hypertension or may be due to arteriolar nephrosclerosis. Percutaneous or open biopsies of end stage shrunken kidneys are associated with a high morbidity rate, particularly bleeding. However, if kidney size is still normal, a renal biopsy may be diagnostic. Appropriate examination by light microscopy, immunofluorescence, and electron microscopy is also indicated.

Treatment

Management should be conservative until it becomes impossible for patients to continue their customary life-styles. This conservative management includes dietary protein and potassium restriction as well as close sodium balance in the diet so that patients do not retain sodium or become sodium depleted. Use of bicarbonate can be helpful when mild to moderate acidemia occurs. Transfusions may be helpful, but fresh blood should be used to avoid excessive release of potassium. Prevention of possible uremic osteodystrophy requires close attention to calcium and phosphorus balance through phosphate-retaining antacids and administration of calcium or vitamin D. Extreme care must be paid to this management, however, since a Ca × P product of greater than 65 mg/dL can cause metastatic calcifications, and a product of less than 25 mg/dL may encourage osteomalacia.

A. Chronic Peritoneal Dialysis: Chronic peritoneal dialysis is used electively or when circumstances (ie, no available vascular access) prohibit chronic hemodialysis. Improved soft catheters (Tenckhoff) have allowed for repetitive use. In comparison to hemodialysis, small molecules (such as creatinine and urea) are cleared less effectively than larger molecules (vitamin B_{12}), but excellent treatment can be accomplished. Either intermittent thrice-weekly treatment (IPPD) or chronic ambulatory peritoneal dialysis (CAPD) is possible. With the latter, the patient performs 3–5 daily exchanges with 1–2 L of dialysate each exchange. Bacterial contamination and peritonitis are becoming less common with improvements in technology.

B. Chronic Hemodialysis: Chronic hemodialysis using semipermeable dialysis membranes is now widely used. Access to the vascular system is by means of Scribner shunts, arteriovenous fistulas, and grafts. The actual dialyzers may be of a parallel plate, coil, or hollow fiber type. Clearance of body solutes and excessive body fluids can be easily accomplished by using dialysate fluids of known chemical composition.

Treatment is intermittent—usually 3–5 hours 3 times weekly. It may be given in a kidney center, in a satellite unit, or in the home. Very ill patients or those who for any reason cannot be trained in the use of the equipment with an assistant require treatment in a dialysis center. Home dialysis is optimal because it provides greater scheduling flexibility and is generally more comfortable and convenient for the patient, but only 30% of a dialysis population meets the medical and training requirements for this type of therapy.

More widespread use of dialytic technics has permitted a more normal degree of patient mobility. Treatment on vacations and business trips can be provided by prior arrangement.

Common problems with either type of chronic dialysis include infection, bone symptoms, technical accidents, persistent anemia, and psychologic disorders. The morbidity associated with atherosclerosis often occurs with long-term treatment. Bilateral nephrectomy should be avoided, because it increases the transfusion requirements of dialysis patients as well as the attendant morbidity and mortality risk from the procedure. Nephrectomy in dialysis patients should be performed in cases of refractory hypertension, reflux, and polycystic disease with recurrent bleeding and pain.

Yearly costs range from an average of $10,000 for patients who receive dialysis at home to as much as $25,000–$30,000 for patients treated at dialysis centers, but much of this is absorbed under HR-1 (Medicare) legislation. The mortality rates are 8–10% per year once maintenance dialysis therapy is instituted. Despite these medical, psychologic, social, and financial difficulties, most patients lead productive lives while receiving dialysis treatments.

C. Renal Transplantation:* After immunosuppression technics and genetic matching were developed, renal homotransplantation became an acceptable alternative to maintenance hemodialysis. The great advantage of transplantation is reestablishment of nearly normal constant body physiology and chemistry without intermittent dialysis. Diet can be more normal. The disadvantages include bone marrow suppression, susceptibility to infection, cushingoid body habitus, and the psychologic uncertainty of the homograft's future. Most of the disadvantages of transplantation are related to the medicines (azathioprine and corticosteroids) that are given to counteract the rejection. Later problems with transplantation include recurrent disease in the transplanted kidney. Genitourinary infection appears to be of minor importance if structural urologic complications (eg, leak) do not occur.

Nephrology centers, with close cooperation between medical and surgical staff, attempt to use these treatment alternatives of dialysis and transplantation in an integrated fashion.

*For a more detailed review, see Chapter 26.

• • •

References

Anderson CF & others: Nutritional therapy for adults with renal disease. *JAMA* 1973;**223**:68.

Bell PRF, Calman KC: *Surgical Aspects of Hemodialysis.* Churchill Livingstone, 1974.

Bricker NS: Adaptations in chronic uremia: Pathophysiologic "trade-offs." *Hosp Pract* (July) 1974;**9**:119.

Friedman E & others: Pragmatic realities in uremia therapy. *N Engl J Med* 1978;**298**:368.

Hampers CL, Schupak E: *Long-Term Hemodialysis,* 2nd ed. Grune & Stratton, 1973.

Lazarus JM: Complications in hemodialysis: An overview. *Kidney Int* 1980;**18**:783.

Lindner A & others: Accelerated atherosclerosis in prolonged maintenance hemodialysis. *N Engl J Med* 1974;**290**:697.

Merrill JP, Hampers CL: Uremia. (2 parts.) *N Engl J Med* 1970;**282**:953, 1014.

Nsouli KA & others: Bacteremic infection in hemodialysis. *Arch Intern Med* 1979;**139**:1255.

Popovich RP & others: Continuous ambulatory peritoneal dialysis. *Ann Intern Med* 1978;**88**:449.

Proceedings of a conference on adequacy of dialysis: Eighth Scientific Conference of the Artificial Kidney-Chronic Uremia Program. *Kidney Int* 1975;7 (**Suppl 2**):S1–S265. [Entire issue.]

Rubin J & others: Peritonitis during continuous ambulatory peritoneal dialysis. *Ann Intern Med* 1980;**92**:7.

Snydman DR, Bryan JA, Hanson B: Hemodialysis-associated hepatitis in the United States–1972. *J Infect Dis* 1975;**132**:109.

Strange PD, Sumner AT: Predicting treatment costs and life expectancy in end stage renal disease. *N Engl J Med* 1978;**298**:372.

Renal Transplantation | 26

Oscar Salvatierra, Jr., MD, & Nicholas J. Feduska, MD

Renal transplantation is an effective therapeutic modality for patients with end stage renal disease. Approximately 1700 renal transplants have been performed at the University of California, San Francisco (UCSF), and many of the conclusions in this chapter are based on that experience. Although the immunologic problems of rejection remain unchanged, technical complications and patient mortality rates have been significantly reduced by detailed attention to cadaver organ recovery, preservation, surgical technics, and elimination of prolonged corticosteroid therapy in high doses. Graft survival has been significantly improved by use of the mixed lymphocyte culture (MLC) in selecting living related donors and, recently, by use of pretransplant, donor-specific blood transfusions when the related donor and recipient are poorly matched.

Selection & Preparation of Recipients

The principal indication for renal transplantation is end stage renal failure. According to the Thirteenth Report of the Human Renal Transplant Registry, the following are the most common diseases treated by renal transplantation: chronic glomerulonephritis (54%); chronic pyelonephritis (12%); polycystic kidney disease (5%); and malignant nephrosclerosis (6%). Other diseases, including hereditary nephritis, account for 23% of cases.

A. Exclusions: Patients with active infections, as well as those whose end stage renal failure is due to primary oxalosis, are generally not accepted for transplantation. Patients with systemic diseases such as juvenile diabetes mellitus and lupus erythematosus, however, are acceptable.

B. Preliminary Nephrectomy: Approximately 90% of all patients now receive transplants with their own kidneys left in situ. The indications for preliminary nephrectomy are as follows:

1. Severe hypertension uncontrolled by medications or dialysis.

2. Anatomic abnormalities of the urinary tract with or without infection, eg, hydronephrosis or ureteral reflux. In patients with reflux or ureteral abnormalities, nephroureterectomy should be performed with removal of the ureter to the ureterovesical junction.

3. Some cases of polycystic renal disease. If the patient has pyelonephritis or a history of hematuria requiring blood transfusions, preparation by nephrectomy is an absolute prerequisite to transplantation. If the history is negative, transplantation without nephrectomy is preferred and has proved to be safe. The size of the polycystic kidneys is not an indication for preliminary nephrectomy in our experience.

C. Splenectomy: Some transplant centers perform splenectomy before transplantation, but there is still no clear evidence that it modifies the immunologic reaction. In addition, there is evidence that patients (particularly children) who have undergone splenectomy are predisposed to pneumococcal and other infections.

Donor Selection

The kidney to be transplanted can be obtained from either a living related donor or a cadaver donor.

A. Related Donor: Living related donors currently accepted are usually siblings or parents, but in some cases, more distant relatives may be accepted if histocompatibility testing shows a high probability of graft survival. Histocompatibility is determined as follows: (1) by determination of human leukocyte antigens (HLA) to establish the inheritance pattern in a family group; (2) by mixed lymphocyte culture (MLC) to measure the stimulation between donor and recipient lymphocytes incubated in the test tube by their uptake of tritiated thymidine; and (3) by donor-recipient (B lymphocyte) typing, which is done by serologic testing. The best donor-recipient combinations are siblings who share all HLA antigens (HLA-identical) and are nonstimulating in the mixed lymphocyte culture. The prognosis for long-term graft survival in this case is over 95%.

B. Poorly Matched Related Donor: In 1978, a new method of transplantation was begun at the University of California, San Francisco, in which poorly matched relatives were allowed to serve as donors. Such donors were formerly not accepted, because graft survival in such cases was no better than could be achieved with cadaver transplants. The new method involves donor-recipient pairs who are poorly matched by MLC testing. Three donor-specific blood transfusions (DSTs) are administered to the recipient according to a uniform protocol, and serial immunologic monitoring for T-warm and B-warm cytotoxic antibodies (directed against T and B lymphocytes) is performed during and following the transfusion period. The transplant is performed no earlier than 4 weeks after the third transfusion and only if the recipient does not become sensitized to the donor. Sixty-two patients treated in this manner have received transplants from their poorly matched donor. Sensitization appears to occur in about 25% of first-transplant candidates and in about 75% of second-transplant candidates. Fifty-nine of the 62 transplants are presently functioning, and only one of the 3 transplant losses was for immunologic reasons. Graft survival with this new method is 98% and 95% at 1 and 2 years, respectively. Donor-specific blood transfusions have also led to good results for poorly matched transplants in patients with juvenile-onset diabetes mellitus. For our group of patients, graft survival is 93% and 84% at 1 and 3 years. In addition, patients who do show evidence of sensitization following DSTs do not appear to have difficulty in receiving cadaver transplants.

C. Cadaver Donor: If a suitable living related donor is not available, patients with end stage renal disease must depend upon cadaver organs for transplantation.

1. Unacceptable cadaver donors–Cadaver kidneys are unacceptable in the following circumstances:

a. Kidneys from newborns and those over age 55. Early thrombosis and poor function is the fate of most newborn kidneys. Data from the Renal Transplant Registry show that kidneys from donors over age 55 do not give results that are comparable to those achieved with kidneys from younger donors. Kidneys from children age 10 months and older have provided an excellent source of grafts, as renal hypertrophy occurs rapidly after transplantation.

b. History of generalized or intra-abdominal sepsis.

c. Preexisting disease that imposes a risk of renal involvement, such as hypertension, diabetes, and lupus erythematosus.

d. History of malignant neoplastic disease, except in the case of some types of brain tumors, because of the risk of transplanting tumor cells with the renal graft.

2. Donor-recipient matching–

a. No correlation between the quality of the HLA match at the conventional A and B loci and cadaver graft survival has been observed with more than 1000 cadaver transplants at UCSF. We have also shown that sensitive cross-matching is especially important for recipients with preformed cytotoxic antibodies. Cross-matching is the incubation of recipient serum with donor lymphocytes. At UCSF, there has been no evidence of impaired

graft survival in recipients with high levels of preformed cytotoxic antibodies.

b. Currently, efforts are being made to define new determinants on the major histocompatibility complex, located on chromosome 6. Perhaps the most important recent innovation in tissue typing has been the development of donor-recipient typing.

c. It is now evident that blood transfusions prior to transplantation enhance graft survival. Transfusions were formerly withheld from patients on dialysis, but the poorer graft survival in those who had not received transfusions has led to a more favorable assessment of the possible beneficial effects of transfusions.

Although no correlation between conventional HLA typing and graft survival could be shown in our cadaver series, we did find an excellent correlation between the results of the MLC and subsequent graft survival. However, the 5-day incubation period required for the MLC prevents use of this test for cadaver kidney screening.

Organ Preservation

Preservation of the cadaver kidney prior to transplantation can be accomplished in 2 ways: by simple hypothermic storage or by pulsatile perfusion.

A. Hypothermic Storage: In simple hypothermic storage, the kidneys are removed from the cadaver donor and then are rapidly cooled, usually by a combination of a flush-out solution and external cooling to reduce the core temperature. The kidneys are stored in a simple container immersed in another container packed with crushed ice. The disadvantages of this method are that preservation is not consistently reliable after 24 hours have passed, especially if warm ischemia has occurred at the time of organ recovery, and that it provides no clues to the viability or physiologic quality of the kidney.

B. Pulsatile Perfusion: The perfusate for continuous pulsatile perfusion can be either cryoprecipitated plasma or a modified albumin solution. The 2 major advantages of continuous pulsatile perfusion are that no kidneys need be discarded because of the time limitations of the storage method and that a sudden influx of several cadaver organs to a single transplant center can be satisfactorily transplanted by a small team. The average storage time at UCSF in over 750 cadaver transplants has been 31 hours, and some kidneys have been transplanted after storage periods of up to 3 days. Continuous perfusion also allows viability testing to be performed after donor nephrectomy and prior to transplantation. Viability testing is essential if donors are accepted who have been in prolonged shock or have abnormal renal function prior to death. The 3 criteria for organ viability are fully reliable if perfusion preservation is started immediately after donor nephrectomy. These criteria are a warm ischemia time of less than 1 hour, adequate perfusion characteristics, and a donor serum creatinine that is less than twice normal at the time of nephrectomy. These criteria are insufficient if the kidney has also been subjected to a period of simple cold storage prior to perfusion preservation.

When perfusion preservation was started immediately after donor nephrectomy, the postoperative dialysis rate following transplantation was 24%, and an average of only 2 or 3 dialysis treatments was required for each patient.

The Human Renal Transplant Registry has shown that the use of perfusion or cold storage has no influence on long-term survival of cadaver grafts.

Donor Nephrectomy

Strict adherence to technical detail during donor nephrectomy is of the utmost importance.

A. Technic of Donor Nephrectomy: Donor nephrectomy in both cadaver and living related donors must be performed so that the blood supply to the ureter from the renal vessels is preserved. Although the blood supply of the ureter in situ has multiple origins, the ureter of the transplanted kidney receives its blood supply only from renal vessel branches that course in hilar and upper periureteral fat. Thus, no dissection should be performed in the area of the renal pelvis or the hilus of the kidney. As the ureteral blood supply courses in the adventitia, the ureter must also be meticulously removed with adequate surrounding tissue. For maximum assurance of preservation of the ureteral blood supply, hilar and periureteral fatty tissue is removed en bloc with the kidney and ureter.

B. Management of Multiple Vessels: If multiple vessels are found in a cadaver kidney, the kidney is removed en bloc with the aorta, so that it can be perfused through the aorta. Subsequently, the kidney can be transplanted with a Carrel patch of aorta including the multiple vessels. If the vessels are in close proximity to each other, a single Carrel patch will suffice, but if the vessels are some distance apart, 2 Carrel patches are preferable. Since all living related donors have preoperative arteriograms, the presence of multiple arteries is determined prior to transplantation. Most donors have a single artery to at least one of their kidneys. Sometimes, a related donor kidney with multiple arteries must be used but without a Carrel patch, because removal of a portion of the donor aorta would involve increased donor risk.

C. Treatment of Living Related Donor: Anesthesia is not started in the donor until intravenous hydration has resulted in excellent diuresis. If anesthesia is induced prior to diuresis, the ADH effect will make it difficult to obtain diuresis after induction of anesthesia. In donor nephrectomy, it is also important to avoid traction on the pedicle and to feel the kidney frequently during manipulation in order to be certain that the kidney is well perfused. It is stimulation of the nerve supply to the kidney

during dissection that produces vasospasm and causes the kidney to become soft, with no urine output. If the kidney becomes soft, dissection should be discontinued until the kidney has again become firm. Mannitol is given in divided doses during dissection of the renal pedicle. It is imperative that the kidney be firm and that urine be spurting from the ureter prior to division of the renal vessels. By using this approach to donor nephrectomy, postoperative dialysis is rarely necessary in related transplants.

D. Treatment of the Cadaver Donor: The potential cadaver donor is often hypovolemic and receiving vasopressors, so that rapid infusion of intravenous fluids is initially necessary to readjust the contracted blood volume. Subsequently, alpha-adrenergic blocking agents such as phenoxybenzamine (Dibenzyline) and phentolamine (Regitine) are given to prevent renal vasospasm. These agents are especially important when kidneys are removed after cardiac arrest. Once renal vasospasm is established, it will persist during preservation, resulting in inadequate tissue perfusion and organ damage.

Technic of Renal Transplantation

The surgical technic of renal transplantation involves vascular anastomoses and establishment of urinary tract continuity. Specific considerations may be outlined as follows:

In adults, the kidney is placed through an oblique lower abdominal incision and the iliac and hypogastric arteries are mobilized. The iliac veins are similarly mobilized so that an end-to-side renal vein-to-iliac vein anastomosis can be performed. An end-to-end renal artery–to–hypogastric artery anastomosis is usually accomplished unless the hypogastric artery is unsuitable because of arteriosclerotic changes, in which case the renal artery is transplanted end-to-side to the common iliac artery. (See Fig 26–1.)

When multiple arteries are present in cadaver donors, the kidneys are transplanted with anastomosis of a Carrel patch of aorta to the common iliac artery.

In small children, a midline abdominal incision is used and the cecum and ascending colon are mobilized, exposing the aorta and vena cava. An end-to-side anastomosis of the renal vessels to the vena cava and aorta is then easily accomplished, following which the kidney is placed retroperitoneally by repositioning the previously mobilized right colon.

When small pediatric cadaver kidneys are used, donor nephrectomy is carried out en bloc with the aorta and vena cava. The kidneys are then stored by hypothermic pulsatile perfusion through the aorta. Subsequently, pediatric kidneys are transplanted as single units, with each donor providing kidneys for 2 recipients. Arterial anastomosis is performed by using a Carrel patch of donor aorta and, whenever possible, a Carrel patch of the vena

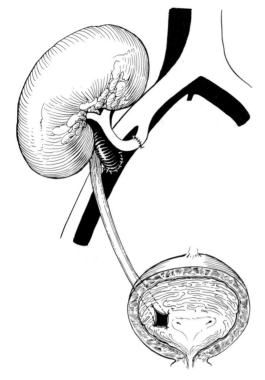

Figure 26–1. Renal transplantation (anastomoses to hypogastric artery, iliac vein, and bladder).

cava is used for the venous anastomosis. If a Carrel patch of vena cava is not used, interrupted sutures for the venous anastomosis are used instead. Arterial and venous anastomoses are usually carried out on the iliac vessels, and the aorta and vena cava are utilized only in very small children.

Establishment of urinary tract continuity can be performed by pyeloureterostomy, ureteroureterostomy, or ureteroneocystostomy. Ureteroneocystostomy by a modified Politano-Leadbetter technic is used at UCSF. The primary ureteral leak rate with this method has been less than 1%.

Immediate Posttransplant Care

Postoperative management does not differ essentially from that of other surgical patients except that emphasis is placed upon the following areas:

Foley catheter drainage is maintained for 1 week, because of the impaired wound healing associated with immunosuppressive therapy. This method has essentially eliminated urinary leakage from the bladder. If bacteriuria develops, it is detected by appropriate urinary cultures and specifically treated.

Intravenous fluids are given immediately after the operation at a rate to maintain a good diuresis. The urinary output in the immediate posttransplant patient may be abundant, and this volume must be considered in determining the rate of administration of replacement fluids.

Renal scintiphotography is useful in the immediate posttransplant period as a base line for future comparative studies and to evaluate the patency of vascular and ureteral anastomoses. Good isotope uptake in the renal cortex indicates adequate perfusion, while normal drainage of urine confirms patency of the ureteral anastomosis. Renal scintiphotography with excretion of 131 I-orthoiodohippurate is the principal method used to evaluate the graft and to complement clinical impressions and chemical determinations.

The differential diagnosis of renal failure following transplantation can be extremely difficult in 2 situations: (1) when urinary output suddenly decreases shortly after transplantation, and (2) with the diagnosis of rejection superimposed upon acute tubular necrosis. Our experience with more than 6000 scintiphotographic studies in renal transplant patients has shown these studies to be of great value in the evaluation of the structure, function, and viability of the transplanted kidney. The study causes no discomfort or harm to the patient. Furthermore, good renal visualization is possible in patients with oliguria or anuria.

Rejection

Hyperacute rejection is mediated by humoral antibodies. It occurs in patients who have preexisting circulating cytotoxic antibodies that react with the donor kidney. The classic picture of hyperacute rejection is seen when, after release of the vascular clamps following vascular anastomoses, the kidney appears normal but very rapidly turns into a bluish-black, nonviable organ. The only treatment is immediate nephrectomy. Subliminal sensitization can also occur in which irreversible renal failure and graft nonviability take several days to become completely established. This is called accelerated rejection.

Acute rejection generally presents during the first several months following transplantation. This type of rejection is usually characterized by fever, oliguria, weight gain, tenderness and enlargement of the graft, hypertension, and chemical evidence of renal functional impairment. Treatment is by increased corticosteroid dosage, and in most cases the process is reversible.

Chronic rejection is a late cause of renal deterioration. Chronic rejection is most often diagnosed by evidence of slowly decreasing renal function in association with proteinuria and hypertension. This type of rejection is resistant to standard methods of corticosteroid rejection treatment, and graft loss will eventually occur, though at times not for several years after the inception of impaired renal function.

Immunosuppressive Therapy

The principal immunosuppressive drugs are prednisone used in combination with either azathioprine (Imuran)—an antimetabolite—or cyclophosphamide (Cytoxan)—an alkylating agent. The latter is used instead of azathioprine in patients with past or present hepatic dysfunction, and also when allopurinol (Zyloprim) is used concurrently. In general, the basic prednisone dosage at the time of transplantation is 120 mg daily in adults, with appropriate lower dosages in children. Dosage is then rapidly reduced to maintenance levels. During an acute rejection episode, prednisone is increased to 2–3 mg/kg daily, followed by a rapidly progressive decrease to maintenance dosages. By 2 years after transplantation, all patients are on a maximum prednisone dosage of 10 mg/d.

Since 1972, emphasis at our transplant center has been on patient survival rather than graft survival. This has been accomplished by abolishing prolonged high-dose immunosuppressive therapy for graft rejection. Full prednisone pulse therapy is limited to only 2 rejection episodes. Although graft rejection is now treated less vigorously, our results show that graft survival has not been jeopardized by emphasizing patient survival.

Complications

A. Urologic: The urologic complication rate, including bladder leaks, ureteral obstruction, and ureteral urinary leaks, is less than 1% in our center.

B. Vascular: Renal artery stenosis has occurred in 15 of our patients, an incidence of less than 1%. Stenosis has been of 2 types: (1) that limited to the suture line and secondary to reaction to the suture material, and (2) generalized stenosis of the main renal artery to its bifurcation due to extensive periadventitial cicatricial formation, ·probably a part of the generalized reaction to the graft. All 15 cases of renal artery stenosis were successfully corrected surgically.

C. Infection: The primary wound infection rate is 0.7%. Topical use of antibiotics, strict adherence to careful surgical technic, and omission of wound drainage are mainly responsible for this low incidence.

D. Complications Secondary to Immunosuppressive Therapy: These complications, such as infection and sepsis, can be kept to a minimum by emphasizing low-dose immunosuppressive therapy.

Results

A. Patient Survival: After a policy of low-dose immunosuppressive therapy was adopted in 1972, the cumulative patient mortality rate has been reduced to 2% at 1 year and 3% at 2 years for related transplants and 9% and 12% for cadaver transplants.

B. Graft Survival:

a. Survival of primary cadaver grafts at 2 and 5 years is 50% and 40%. Second cadaver grafts are equally successful. If an individual lacks a suitable living related donor and must rely on cadaver transplantation, the use of both primary and secondary grafting can potentially provide good long-term renal function.

b. Related grafts prospectively selected by low-stimulating MLCs provide the following 2-year survival rate: 96% for HLA-identical recipients and 91% for non–HLA identical recipients.

c. Related grafts performed according to the DST protocol show survival rates of 98% and 95% at 1 and 2 years.

● ● ●

References

Advisory Committee to the Renal Transplant Registry: The 13th Report of the Human Renal Transplant Registry. *Transplant Proc* 1977;**9**:9.

Cochrum K, Salvatierra O, Belzer FO: The correlation between MLC stimulation and graft survival in living related and cadaver kidney transplants. *Ann Surg* 1974;**180**:617.

Feduska NJ & others: An alternative to cadaver kidney transplants for patients with insulin-dependent diabetes mellitus. *Transplantation* [In press.]

Feduska NJ & others: Cadaver kidney transplantation provided from one center within a large geographical region. *Trans Am Soc Artif Intern Organs* 1978;**24**:270.

Feduska NJ & others: Comparative study of albumin solution and cryoprecipitated plasma for renal preservation: A preliminary report. *Transplant Proc* 1979;**11**:472.

Feduska NJ & others: Do blood transfusions enhance the possibility of a compatible transplant? *Transplantation* 1979;**27**:35.

Feduska NJ & others: Graft survival with high levels of cytotoxic antibodies. *Transplant Proc* 1981;**13**:73.

Feduska NJ & others: A ten year experience with cadaver kidney preservation using cryoprecipitated plasma. *Am J Surg* 1978;**135**:356.

Hamburger J & others: *Renal Transplantation.* Williams & Wilkins, 1972.

Najarian JS, Simmons RL: *Transplantation.* Lea & Febiger, 1972.

Salvatierra O, Kountz SL, Belzer FO: Prevention of ureteral fistula after renal transplantation. *J Urol* 1974;**112**:445.

Salvatierra O & others: The advantages of 131 I-orthoiodohippurate scintiphotography in the management of patients after renal transplantation. *Ann Surg* 1974;**180**:336.

Salvatierra O & others: Deliberate donor-specific blood transfusions prior to living related renal transplantation. *Ann Surg* 1980;**192**:543.

Salvatierra O & others: End-stage polycystic kidney disease: Management by renal transplantation and selective use of preliminary nephrectomy. *J Urol* 1976;**115**:5.

Salvatierra O & others: HLA typing and primary cadaver graft survival. *Transplant Proc* 1977;**9**:495.

Salvatierra O & others: The impact of 1000 renal transplants at one center. *Ann Surg* 1977;**186**:424.

Salvatierra O & others: Improved patient survival in renal transplantation. *Surgery* 1976;**79**:166.

Salvatierra O & others: Incidence, characteristics and outcome of recipients sensitized after donor-specific blood transfusions. *Transplantation* [In press.]

Salvatierra O & others: The influence of presensitization on graft survival rate. *Surgery* 1977;**81**:146.

Salvatierra O & others: Procurement of cadaver kidneys. *Urol Clin North Am* 1976;**3**:457.

Salvatierra O & others: 1500 renal transplants at one center: The evolution of a strategy for optimum success. *Am J Surg* [In press.]

Salvatierra O & others: Urological complications of renal transplantation can be prevented or controlled. *J Urol* 1977;**117**:421.

Starzl TE: *Experience in Renal Transplantation.* Saunders, 1964.

Terasaki PI & others: Microdroplet testing for HLA-A_1-B_1-C_1 and -D antigens. *Am J Clin Pathol* 1978;**69**:103.

Disorders of the Ureters | 27

Donald R. Smith, MD

CONGENITAL ANOMALIES OF THE URETER

Congenital ureteral anomalies are common. Since most of them cause urinary obstruction or stasis, hydronephrosis with secondary renal infection is a common sequel.

INCOMPLETE URETER

The ureter may be entirely absent or may extend from the bladder only part way to the renal area. Either the ureteral bud fails to develop from the urogenital segment during embryologic development, or it is arrested in its development before it reaches the kidney. It is demonstrated by retrograde urography. Absence of the kidney or multicystic renal disease is to be expected.

DUPLICATION OF THE URETER

Complete or incomplete duplication of the ureter is one of the most common congenital ureteral anomalies. The family pattern of inheritance suggests an autosomal dominant gene of incomplete penetrance. The incomplete (Y) type (Fig 27–1) is more common than 2 complete ureters on one side (Figs 27–1, 27–3). The condition may be bilateral. Duplication presupposes 2 renal pelves in the renal mass. Most cases occur in females. An instance of 5 ureters on one side has been reported.

These abnormalities usually cause no difficulty; in the Y type, however, obstruction may occur at the point where the 2 ureters join. One segment may become dilated because of retrograde flow (reflux) from one ureter into the other.

In complete duplication, the ureter from the upper pole opens at a point closest to the bladder neck. It follows that the ureter to the major lower pole has a relatively short intravesical ureteral segment. Thus, vesicoureteral reflux to the lower portion of the kidney may be seen (Fig 11–5) (Kaplan, Nasrallah, & King, 1978). Most ureteroceles in children involve the ureter that drains the upper

portion of the duplicated kidney. The ureter to the upper renal pole may open ectopically into the vulva, urethra, or seminal vesicle (Fig 27–1). Such ureters are always obstructed to some degree (Figs 27–1, 27–6).

Duplication of the ureter is clinically significant only when obstruction or reflux is present, in which case dilatation and tortuosity of the ureter and hydronephrosis are found (Fig 27–1).

The symptoms and signs are those of persistent or recurrent infection. Urologic investigation (urograms) will reveal the congenital abnormality. If complete hydronephrotic atrophy of one renal pole has occurred, excretory urograms may show only one normal pelvis and ureter (Fig 27–4). The clue to duplication will be the observation that the visualized pelvis and calices fail to drain a relatively large area of the renal shadow. The visualized ureter may be displaced laterally by its dilated obstructed mate.

If the anomaly causes obstruction or reflux, surgical repair should be attempted if at all practicable. It may be necessary to resect the hydronephrotic pole of the kidney with its ureter. Nephrectomy may be indicated if renal damage is severe. At times it may be feasible to construct a side-to-side anastomosis of an obstructed ureter to its normal mate (Amar, 1978).

URETEROCELE

A ureterocele is a ballooning of the submucosal ureter into the bladder, secondary probably to congenital stenosis of the epithelial lining at the vesical end of the ureter; thus the urine cannot easily escape into the bladder. The pressure produced by ureteral peristalsis pushes the periureteral vesical mucosa into the bladder, causing a cystic protrusion. This urine-filled cyst is covered by vesical mucosa on the outside and lined by ureteral mucosa internally (Fig 27–2). Its complications, basically caused by the obstruction, are hydroureter, hydronephrosis, and upper tract infection. Stones may develop in the cyst. If large enough, ureterocele may cause bladder neck obstruction (ectopic ureterocele) and may even prolapse

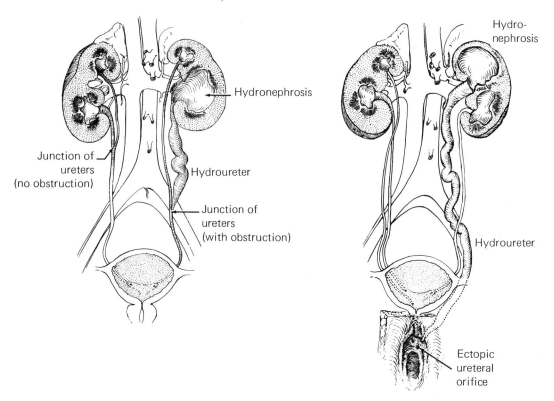

Figure 27–1. Duplication of ureters. *Left:* Incomplete Y type with hydroureteronephrosis on left. *Right:* Complete duplication with obstruction to one ureter with ectopic orifice on left. The ureter with the ectopic opening always drains the upper pole of the kidney.

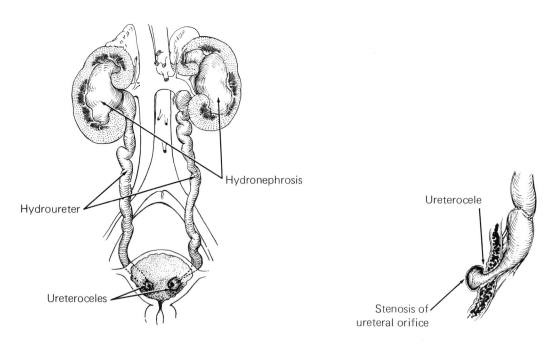

Figure 27–2. Ureterocele. *Left:* Obstructing ureteroceles (adult type) with hydroureteronephrosis. *Right:* Sagittal section through ureterocele and ureter to show pathologic changes. Resection of this ureterocele will be followed by vesicoureteral reflux.

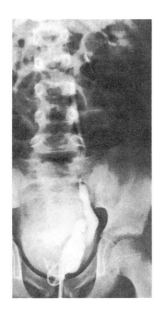

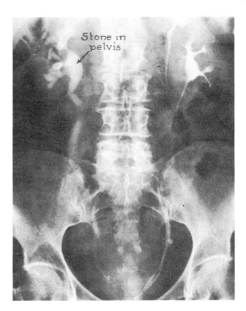

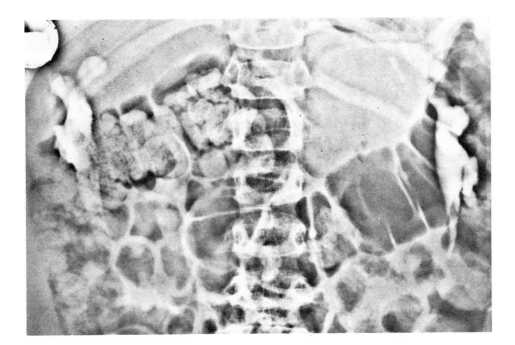

Figure 27–3. Duplication of ureters. *Above left:* Ureteral catheters passed through opening in region of verumontanum. Injection of radiopaque fluid reveals duplicated ureter to upper renal pole joining seminal vesicle (ectopic ureteral ostium). Second ureter not shown. *Above right:* Excretory urogram showing complete duplication of left ureters and renal pelves, which are otherwise normal. Staghorn calculus in right kidney; dilatation of upper ureter suggests possibility of presence of stone in lower portion of right ureter. *Below:* Excretory urogram showing marked displacement of visualized renal masses by giant functionless hydronephroses of upper renal segments. Ureters to upper poles opened into prostatic urethra.

through the female urethra (Klauber & Crawford, 1980).

Ureterocele is most commonly encountered in little girls and usually involves the ureter that drains the upper pole of a duplicated kidney (Figs 11–5 and 27–4). The obstructed portion is often dysplastic. Ureteroceles in adults tend to be bilateral and are smaller and less obstructive than those in children.

The history and physical signs are compatible with ureteral obstruction or urinary tract infection. A history of an obstructed urinary stream, even incontinence, may be elicited if the ureterocele impinges on the bladder neck. Pyuria and bacteriuria may be present. Total renal function is normal unless both kidneys are affected. Excretory urograms may show cystic dilatation of the lower end of the ureter (Fig 27–4, left) or a round space-occupying lesion in a cystogram. Some changes from back pressure above this point are to be expected (eg, hydroureter, hydronephrosis, changes due to infection). A cystogram may reveal reflux into the lower renal pole (Bauer & Retik, 1978).

Catheterization of the pinpoint ureteral opening may be impossible, but it is helpful in establishing the presence of infection in the kidney. If poor renal function has precluded adequate secretion of opaque material given intravenously, retrograde urography should be attempted.

The small, mildly obstructive ureterocele can usually be destroyed transurethrally. In children it may be necessary to open the bladder suprapubically so that the cyst can be resected. This may be followed, however, by vesicoureteral reflux because the obstruction has caused wide dilatation of the ureteral hiatus, thus shortening the intravesical ureter (Fig 11–5). At times, the obstructing ureterocele may so dilate the intramural ureter that reflux up the noninvolved ureter may occur. Excision of the cystic structure combined with simultaneous vesicoureteroplasty should, therefore, probably be done (Hendren & Mitchell, 1979; Kroovand & Perlmutter, 1979; Brock & Kaplan, 1978). Removal of this obstruction will usually cause the pathologic changes of the ureter and kidney to regress. Secondary infection can then more readily be controlled or cured. If the affected portion of a duplicated kidney is destroyed, heminephrectomy and complete ureterectomy are indicated.

POSTCAVAL URETER

The rare postcaval or retrocaval ureter is one that (from above downward) passes medially and behind the vena cava, turns forward along the great vein's left wall, and then passes laterally on the anterior surface of the vena cava and resumes its

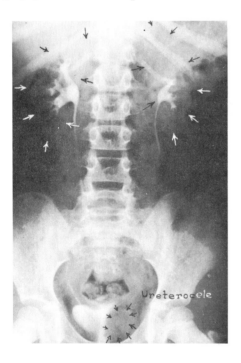
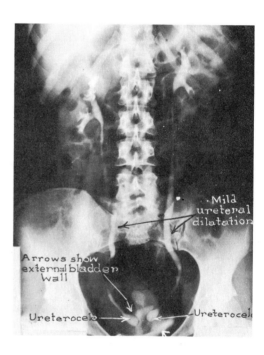

Figure 27–4. Ureterocele. *Left:* Excretory urogram in a girl 8 years old, showing a space-occupying lesion on the left side of the bladder caused by ureterocele. Absence of a caliceal system in the upper portion of the left kidney implies duplication of the ureters and pelves and nonfunction (advanced hydronephrosis) of the upper pole; its dilated ureter drains into the obstructing ureterocele and displaces the visualized ureter laterally just below the kidney. *Right:* Excretory urogram in an adult female, showing "cobra head" deformity of the distal ends of both ureters; bilateral ureteroceles causing minimal obstruction; pressure on bladder from uterus. No treatment is indicated.

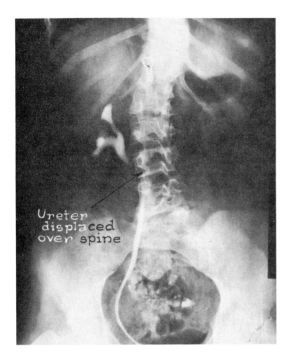 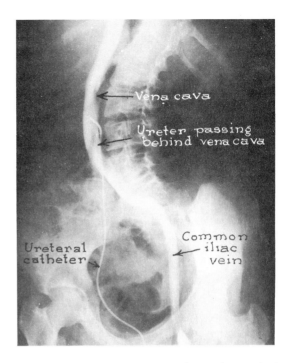

Figure 27–5. Postcaval ureter. **Left:** Retrograde ureteropyelogram showing upper ureter displaced onto the vertebral bodies, suggesting postcaval ureter. Note the congenital deformity of the spine. **Right:** Femoral venacavogram (right oblique view) showing ureter in retrocaval position.

normal course to the bladder. It actually "hooks" around the cava. This anomalous position is due to an abnormal development of the vena cava.

The significance of postcaval ureter lies in the ureteral obstruction that is usually caused by the cava. This leads to hydronephrosis and, at times, infection. A catheter passed up such a ureter will take a course, in its mid portion, overlying the spine. Excretory urograms will show deviation of the mid ureter over the spine. A retrograde ureterogram will show this defect graphically. A simultaneous venacavogram will relate the vena cava to the ureter (Fig 27–5) (Carrion & others, 1979).

Division of the ureter where it courses around the cava, with end-to-end anastomosis in the normal position, relieves the obstruction. It has also been recommended that the vena cava be divided, the ureter replaced in its normal position, and the vena cava then repaired. Nephrectomy may be necessary if secondary renal damage is advanced.

RETROILIAC URETER

A few cases of retroiliac ureter have been reported. They, too, are obstructed. On urography the ureter is deviated and compressed at the pelvic brim. The hydronephrosis is treated by division of the ureter with reanastomosis anterior to the vessels.

ECTOPIC URETERAL ORIFICE

In rare instances the ureter opens at a point other than the lateral horn of the interureteric ridge. If it drains distal to the external sphincter (this is seen only in the female), a constant dripping (incontinence) of urine is noted. Ectopy results from an abnormality of embryologic development (see Chapter 2). The wolffian duct arises from the cloaca and acts as the drainage tube for the pronephros (primitive kidney) and the mesonephros. From this duct, at a point near the cloaca (which divides to form the rectum and lower urinary tract), the ureteral bud develops, then extends to and joins the metanephros. This junction forms the permanent kidney. As development progresses, the ureteral opening in the wolffian duct gradually moves caudally until the wolffian and ureteral ducts have separate openings in the urethrovesical area. Normally in the male, the wolffian ducts form the vasa deferentia and seminal vesicles. Their cranial ends drain the spermatogenic tubules of the testes. In the female, the superior portion atrophies and the caudal portion becomes Gartner's duct.

If abnormalities of development occur, the ureter may enter the urinary tract at a position below the normal point. In the male, its orifice may be found in the posterior urethra; in the female, just outside the bladder neck.

If the ureteral orifice does not disengage itself from the proximal end of the wolffian duct, it is

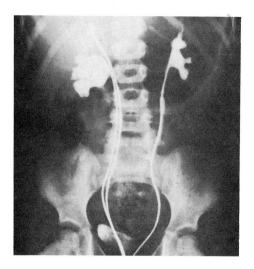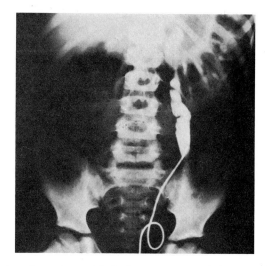

Figure 27–6. Ectopic ureter. (Girl, age 6, complained of partial urinary incontinence.) **Left:** Cystoscopy revealed 2 ureteral orifices on right, one on left; these were catheterized and urograms made. **Right:** Same patient. Ectopic ureteral orifice near urethral meatus catheterized. Retrograde urogram demonstrates second left hydronephrotic renal pelvis. Resection of upper pole and ureter cured incontinence.

obvious that in the male the ureter will drain into the seminal tract (eg, seminal vesicle, vas deferens). In the female it will drain into the remnants of Gartner's duct, and urine will empty into the vagina, cervix, uterus, or most commonly, the vaginal vestibule (Figs 27–1 and 27–6). Drainage into the rectum is rare. Most ectopic orifices are seen in the female.

Most ureters with ectopic openings are one of a pair to a single kidney, and the ectopic ureter almost always drains the rudimentary upper renal pole. Since ureters that open in abnormal positions are usually obstructed at their terminations, hydroureter and hydronephrosis develop. Secondary infection is common. Those ureters opening in the proximal urethra usually reveal vesicoureteral reflux on cystography.

In the male, since all ectopic orifices are proximal to the external sphincter, no incontinence ensues. In the female, vaginal or vestibular ureters are devoid of sphincteric control, and a constant drainage of urine occurs in spite of normal voiding.

Symptoms therefore depend upon the site of the opening. If proximal to the external sphincter, there may be flank pain, fever, and vesical irritability. If the opening is distal to the external sphincter, "incontinence" is the complaint. Symptoms of renal infection and pain may also be experienced. In the female, careful inspection of the vestibule or anterior vaginal wall may reveal an orifice from which urine or purulent material may drain. Renal tenderness or enlargement may be present. Epididymitis is a common complication when the ureter drains into the seminal vesicle.

The urine may be infected. Excretory urograms will usually show duplication of the renal pelves, with hydronephrosis of the upper pole, whose ureter may be markedly dilated and tortuous. Distally it may be traced beyond the trigonal area. If renal destruction is severe, no opaque medium may be excreted. Absence of calices in the upper portion of the renal shadow and lateral displacement of the upper portion of the visualized ureter will suggest the diagnosis.

Cystoscopy may reveal the orifice in the urethra. If catheterization can be performed (it may be possible if a vaginal or vestibular orifice is identified), urine can be obtained for study and urograms made (Fig 27–6).

It may be feasible to resect the lowermost portion of the ureter and to implant the distal end of the ureter into the bladder. However, resection of the superior renal pole and its ureter is usually indicated because of the degree of parenchymal damage.

STRICTURE OF THE URETER
(See also Chapter 10.)

Evidence of obstruction at the ureteropelvic or ureterovesical junction has heretofore been interpreted as stricture. It is now clear that most cases of the latter type really represent changes secondary to ureterovesical reflux (Fig 27–7). Some ureteropelvic obstructions also develop as a complication of reflux. Most resolve when ureterovesicoplasty has been done. A few may require surgical correction. A similar picture develops secondary to hypertrophy of the trigone that arises in association with distal obstruction, eg, posterior urethral valves. Creevy has observed what he calls achalasia of the lower ureteral segment that produces a functional obstruction. Tanagho, Smith, & Guthrie

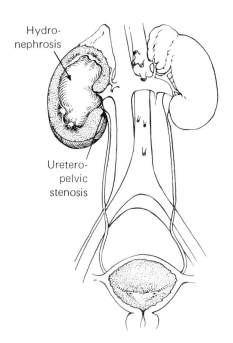
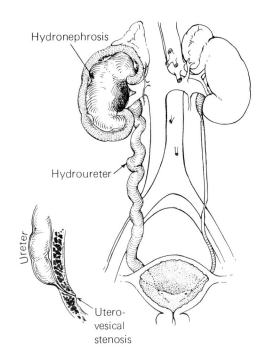

Figure 27–7. Congenital ureteral obstruction. *Left:* Right ureteropelvic stenosis with hydronephrosis. *Right:* Ureterovesical obstruction with hydroureteronephrosis. The common causes are (1) reflux, (2) hypertrophy of the ureterotrigonal complex secondary to distal obstruction, and (3) hypertrophy of the circular musculature of the juxtavesical ureter (Tanagho).

(1970) find that this obstruction is caused by congenital hypertrophy of the circular smooth musculature of the juxtavesical ureter. A few cases of ureteral-obstructing valves (Maizels & Stephens, 1980) and aberrant vessels have been recorded. Kirks and Currarino (1978) have noted transverse defects in the proximal ureter representing nonobstructing mucosal folds of no clinical importance.

Symptoms are often absent, for many of these strictures are so mild that sudden renal capsular distention does not take place even though the kidney is completely destroyed by hydronephrotic atrophy. Some patients, however, may have costovertebral angle pain from the obstruction; others may have only reflex gastrointestinal complaints; and some have both. Ureteral stricture on the right side not uncommonly simulates appendicitis. Symptoms of infection may be elicited. It should be remembered, however, that chronic pyelonephritis may cause no symptoms.

Physical examination may reveal nothing unless the hydronephrotic kidney is large and tense and can be felt or percussed. Tenderness may be present with complicating pyelonephritis. Urinalysis may provide evidence of urinary infection. Renal function will be normal unless there is bilateral renal disease.

A plain film of the abdomen may reveal an enlarged renal shadow. Excretory urograms will demonstrate dilatation of the excretory tract above the site of constant narrowing (Fig 27–8); one must

not be confused by "pseudostrictures," which represent normal systolic ureteral contraction. Advanced renal damage may cause lack of excretion of the radiopaque medium. A voiding cystourethrogram may reveal ureterovesical reflux.

Retrograde passage of a ureteral catheter may be arrested by a severe stricture. It may, however, pass through the site of obstruction, only to be stopped by the acute ureteral angulations proximal to the stricture. On the other hand, an area of functional obstruction may accept a large catheter easily although stasis persists. Retrograde ureteropyelograms will furnish a graphic picture of the obstruction and the changes secondary to it.

Little significance should be attached to the ease of passage of various sizes of catheters in the diagnosis of stricture. Unjustified diagnoses of stricture have also been made by passing a catheter with a fusiform bulge at its tip up the ureter. On withdrawal, a "hang" or sudden resistance to withdrawal is sometimes mistaken for evidence of stricture. It should be pointed out that it is the nature of the ureter to go into spasm even on being touched lightly during surgery. The diagnosis of true stricture is made on urographic study, preferably the "nontraumatic" intravenous type. The point of narrowing should show in every film, and dilatation above this point should be demonstrated.

Repair of the stricture is usually indicated if the kidney retains some degree of function. Severe renal damage is treated by nephrectomy. Should

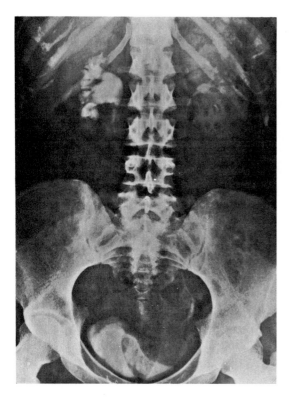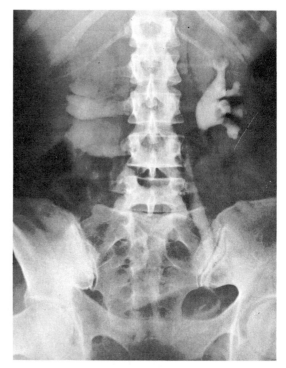

Figure 27–8. Ureteral obstruction. *Left:* Right ureteropelvic stenosis with mild hydronephrosis due to aberrant blood vessel. Pressure defect of left side of bladder from uterus. *Right:* Excretory urogram taken 2 weeks after Wertheim operation, showing bilateral ureteral obstruction and advanced hydronephrosis on right.

the changes be secondary to vesicoureteral reflux or muscular hypertrophy of the juxtavesical ureter, repair of this junction may be indicated.

ACQUIRED DISEASES OF THE URETER

ACQUIRED URETERAL STRICTURE

Most ureteral strictures are congenital, but some are acquired. The most common causes of acquired stenosis are the following:

(1) Injury to the ureters during extensive pelvic surgery or from intensive radiotherapy (Fig 27–8).

(2) Renal or ureteral injury secondary to external trauma, with perirenal and periureteral hematoma that leaves periureteral scar tissue following absorption.

(3) Compression of the ureters by lymph nodes involved by cancer (metastases, lymphomas) (Fig 18–17).

(4) Contracture due to infection, and ischemia caused by prolonged impaction of a ureteral stone.

(5) Ureteral stenosis due to uterine prolapse.

(6) Tuberculous or bilharzial infection (pyeloureteritis) may cause fibrosis of the ureter, which may lead in turn to contracture or functional obstruction (Fig 13–2).

(7) Retroperitoneal fibrosis.

(8) Aneurysm of the aorta or iliac artery or following aortofemoral bypass grafts (Peters & Cowie, 1978).

(9) Ureteropelvic or ureterovesical obstruction secondary to vesicoureteral reflux (see Chapter 11).

(10) Occlusion of the ureterovesical junction by cancer of the bladder, cervix, or prostate (Fig 18–16) (Richie, Withers, & Ehrlich, 1979).

(11) Obstruction of the ureterovesical junction caused by hypertrophy of the trigone secondary to benign prostatic hyperplasia or posterior urethral valves.

(12) Compression of the lower ureters secondary to severe constipation in women and children.

(13) Endometriosis involving the ureter (Moore, 1979).

(14) Compression of the ureter by the right ovarian vein (rare).

(15) Retroperitoneal scarring with ureteral obstruction secondary to granulomatous bowel (Crohn's) disease (Siminovitch & Fazio, 1980).

(16) Associated with uterine prolapse.

The effects upon the kidney and the clinical findings, complications, and treatment of acquired ureteral stricture are the same as those described under congenital stricture and urinary obstruction and stasis.

RETROPERITONEAL FASCIITIS
(Chronic Retroperitoneal Fibroplasia, Retroperitoneal Fibrosis)

One or both ureters may be compressed by a chronic inflammatory process that involves the retroperitoneal tissues over the lower lumbar vertebrae. Patients treated for migraine with methysergide (Sansert), an ergot derivative, may also develop retroperitoneal fibrosis. Analgesic abuse has been suspected (Lewis & others, 1975). Sclerosing Hodgkin's disease and other malignancies have occasionally been found to cause this reaction. Phils & others (1973) have observed the development of retroperitoneal fasciitis in 3 siblings with sickle cell trait. Recently, lysergic acid diethylamide (LSD; an ergot alkaloid) has been reported as a cause of retroperitoneal fibrosis (Stecker & others, 1974). Willscher, Mozden, & Olsson (1978) reported an instance caused by *Actinomyces israelii*. A few cases have been reported in children (Chan, Johnson, & McLoughlen, 1979; Wacksman, Weinerth, & Kredich, 1978). Brock & Soloway (1980) have observed an increasing incidence of retroperitoneal fibrosis associated with aortic aneurysm.

The symptoms, which are nonspecific, include renal pain, low back pain, weight loss, anorexia, and the syndrome of uremia. Claudication of the legs may be noted, and ischemia may cause impotence. The only pathognomonic sign is the presence of a palpable firm mass over the sacral promontory.

Infection of the urinary tract is not usually present. Renal function tests are normal unless both ureters are obstructed; anemia may be found during the stage of uremia.

The diagnosis can be made if excretory urograms reveal medial deviation of the ureters involved in the fibrous plaque in the lumbar area (Fig 27–9). It should be pointed out, however, that such ureteral deviation is occasionally seen in normal persons. Dilatation of the ureters and renal pelves may occur proximal to the point of obstruction. When uremia has supervened, retrograde urograms may be needed to delineate the excretory tracts. Sanders & others (1977) diagnosed this disease by sonography, which revealed a smooth-

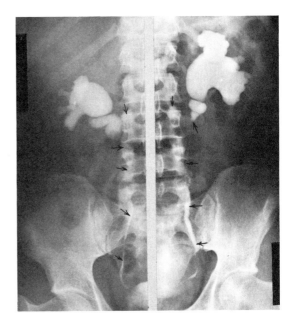

Figure 27–9. Retroperitoneal fasciitis. Right and left kidneys of same patient as shown by excretory urography. Note medial deviation of the upper portions of the ureters (see arrows) with marked obstruction. (Courtesy of JA Hutch.)

bordered, relatively echo-free mass anterior to the promontory of the sacrum.

If radiographic changes are moderate and the patient is not uremic, corticosteroid therapy should be instituted; rather dramatic response in a matter of a few weeks has been reported (Moody & Vaughan Jr, 1979). Begin with 30–60 mg of prednisone per day. If serial urograms show lessening hydronephrosis, the dosage can be gradually decreased to a maintenance dose of 5–15 mg/d. If the degree of obstruction is severe, the ureters should be freed from the fibrous plaque, which should be subjected to multiple biopsies, and either transplanted intraperitoneally or displaced lateral to the psoas muscles so that they do not again become involved (Lepor & Walsh, 1979). Since there is a tendency for the disease to progress, prophylactic corticosteroid therapy should be instituted.

If the patient has been on methysergide, withdrawal of the drug is often followed by spontaneous regression of the obstruction.

Unless the cause is malignancy, the prognosis is fair to good. Autotransplantation has been accomplished in a few patients after failure of ureterolysis.

• • •

References

Incomplete Ureter

Rao KG: Blind-ending bifid ureter. *Urology* 1975;
6:81.

Duplication of the Ureter

Amar AD: Ipsilateral ureteroureterostomy for single ureteral disease in patients with ureteral duplication: A
review of 8 years of experience with 16 patients. *J Urol*
1978;**119**:472.

Kaplan WE, Nasrallah P, King LR: Reflux in complete
duplication in children. *J Urol* 1978;**120**:220.

Mascatello VJ & others: Ultrasonic evaluation of the
obstructed duplex kidney. *AJR* 1977;**129**:113.

Perkins PJ, Kroovand RL, Evans AT: Ureteral triplication.
Radiology 1973;**108**:533.

Peterson C Jr, Silbiger ML: Five ureters: A case report. *J
Urol* 1968;**100**:160.

Whitaker J, Danks DM: A study of the inheritance of
duplication of the kidneys and ureters. *J Urol*
1966;**95**:176.

Ureterocele

Amar AD: Congenital hydronephrosis of lower segment in
duplex kidney. *Urology* 1976;7:480.

Barrett DM, Malek RS, Kelalis PP: Problems and solutions
in surgical treatment of 100 consecutive ureteral dupli-
cations in children. *J Urol* 1975;**114**:126.

Bauer SB, Retik AB: The non-obstructive ectopic
ureterocele. *J Urol* 1978;**119**:804.

Brock WA, Kaplan GW: Ectopic ureteroceles in children.
J Urol 1978;**119**:800.

Hendren WH, Mitchell ME: Surgical correction of
ureteroceles. *J Urol* 1979;**121**:590.

Klauber GT, Crawford DB: Prolapse of ectopic ureterocele
and bladder trigone. *Urology* 1980;**15**:164.

Kroovand RL, Perlmutter AD: A one-stage surgical
approach to ectopic ureterocele. *J Urol* 1979;**122**:
367.

Mitty HA, Schapira HE: Ureterocele and pseudouretero-
cele: Cobra versus cancer. *J Urol* 1977;**117**:557.

Nash AG, Knight M: Ureterocele calculi. *Br J Urol*
1973;**45**:404.

Snyder HM, Johnston JH: Orthotopic ureteroceles in children. *J Urol* 1978;**119**:543.

Soderdahl DW, Shiraki IW, Schamber DT: Bilateral ureteral quadruplication. *J Urol* 1976;**116**:255.

Tanagho EA: Embryologic basis for lower ureteral anomalies: A hypothesis. *Urology* 1976;7:451.

Postcaval Ureter

Carrion H & others: Retrocaval ureter: Report of 8
cases and the surgical management. *J Urol* 1979;**121**:
514.

Kenawi MM, Williams DI: Circumcaval ureter: A report of
four cases in children with a review of the literature and
a new classification. *Br J Urol* 1976;**48**:183.

Morganstern SL, Seery WH, Cole AT: Periureteric vena
cava. *Urology* 1977;9:664.

Retroiliac Ureter

Hanna MK: Bilateral retroiliac-artery ureters. *Br J Urol*
1972;**44**:339.

Hock E, Purkayastha A, Jay BD: Retroiliac ureter: A case
report. *J Urol* 1972;**107**:37.

Ectopic Ureteral Orifice

Brannan W, Henry HH Jr: Ureteral ectopia: Report of 39
cases. *J Urol* 1973;**109**:192.

Gordon HL, Kessler R: Ectopic ureter entering the seminal vesicle associated with renal dysplasia. *J Urol*
1972;**108**:389.

Mogg RA: The single ectopic ureter. *Br J Urol* 1974;**46**:3.

Persky L, Noseworthy J: Adult ureteral ectopia. *J Urol*
1976;**116**:156.

Stricture of the Ureter

Albertson KW, Tainter LB: Valves of the ureter. *Radiology*
1972;**103**:91.

Allen TD: Congenital ureteral strictures. *J Urol*
1970;**104**:196.

Javadpour N, Solomon T, Bush IM: Obstruction of the
lower ureter by aberrant vessels in children. *J Urol*
1972;**108**:340.

Tanagho EA, Smith DR, Guthrie TH: Pathophysiology of
functional ureteral obstruction. *J Urol* 1970;**104**:73.

Acquired Ureteral Stricture

Bagby RJ & others: Genitourinary complications of granulomatous bowel disease. *Am J Roentgenol* 1973;**117**:
297.

Bissada NK, Redman JF: Ureteral complications in diverticulitis of the colon. *J Urol* 1974;**112**:454.

Bosch A, Frias Z, de Valda GC: Prognostic significance of
ureteral obstruction in carcinoma of the cervix uteri.
Acta Radiol [*Ther*] *(Stockh)* 1973;**12**:47.

Chapman RH: Ureteric obstruction due to uterine prolapse. *Br J Urol* 1975;**47**:531.

Geller SA, Lin C-S: Ureteral obstruction from metastatic
breast carcinoma. *Arch Pathol* 1975;**99**:476.

Glassberg KI: Dilated ureter: Classification and approach.
Urology 1977;9:1.

Heal MR: Primary obstructive megaloureter in adults. *Br J
Urol* 1973;**45**:490.

Kirks DR, Currarino G, Weinberg AG: Transverse folds in
the proximal ureter: A normal variant in infants. *AJR*
1978;**130**:463.

Lang EK & others: Complications in the urinary tract
related to treatment of carcinoma of the cervix. *South
Med J* 1973;**66**:228.

Maizels M, Stephens FD: Valves of the ureter as a cause of
primary obstruction of the ureter: Anatomic, embryologic and clinical aspects. *J Urol* 1980;**123**:742.

Moore JG: Urinary tract endometriosis: Enigmas in diagnosis and management. *Am J Obstet Gynecol*
1979;**134**:162.

Peck DR, Bhatt GM, Lowman RM: Traction displacement
of the ureter: A sign of aortic aneurysm. *J Urol*
1973;**109**:983.

Peters JL, Cowie AG: Ureteric involvement with abdominal aortic aneurysm. *Br J Urol* 1978;**50**:313.

Peterson LJ, McAninch JW, Weinerth JL: Ureteral
obstruction of solitary kidneys by iliac artery aneurysms.
Urology 1977;9:17.

Petrone AF, Dudzinski PJ, Maniatis W: Ureteral obstruction secondary to aortic femoral bypass. *Ann Surg*
1974;**179**:192.

Pollack HM, Popky GL, Blumberg ML: Hernias of the
ureter: An anatomic-roentgenographic study. *Radiology* 1975;**117**:275.

Richie JP, Withers G, Ehrlich RM: Ureteral obstruction secondary to metastatic tumors. *Surg Gynecol Obstet* 1979;**148**:355.

Riddle PR, Shawdon HH, Clay B: Procidentia and ureteric obstruction. *Br J Urol* 1975;**47**:387.

Safran R, Sklenicka R, Kay H: Iliac artery aneurysm: A common cause of ureteral obstruction. *J Urol* 1975;**113**:605.

Schapira HE, Mitty HA: Right ovarian vein septic thrombophlebitis causing ureteral obstruction. *J Urol* 1974;**112**:451.

Siminovitch JMP, Fazio VW: Ureteral obstruction secondary to Crohn's disease: A need for ureterolysis? *Am J Surg* 1980;**139**:95.

Whitaker RH, Johnston JH: A simple classification of wide ureters. *Br J Urol* 1975;**47**:781.

Williams G, Peet TND: Bilateral ureteral obstruction due to malignant lymphoma. *Urology* 1976;**7**:649.

Retroperitoneal Fasciitis

Bree RL & others: Medial deviation of the ureters secondary to psoas muscle hypertrophy. *Radiology* 1976;**118**:691.

Brock J, Soloway MS: Retroperitoneal fibrosis and aortic aneurysm. *Urology* 1980;**15**:14.

Chan SL, Johnson HW, McLoughlin MG: Idiopathic retroperitoneal fibrosis in children. *J Urol* 1979;**122**:103.

Lepor H, Walsh PC: Idiopathic retroperitoneal fibrosis. *J Urol* 1979;**122**:1.

Lewis CT & others: Analgesic abuse, ureteric obstruction, and retroperitoneal fibrosis. *Br Med J* 1975;**2**:76.

Linke CA, May AG: Autotransplantation in retroperitoneal fibrosis. *J Urol* 1972;**107**:196.

Moody TE, Vaughan ED Jr: Steroids in the treatment of retroperitoneal fibrosis. *J Urol* 1979;**121**:109.

Nitz GL & others: Retroperitoneal malignancy masquerading as benign retroperitoneal fibrosis. *J Urol* 1970;**103**:46.

Phils JA & others: Retroperitoneal fibrosis in three siblings with sickle cell trait. *Can Med Assoc J* 1973;**108**:1025.

Sanders RC & others: Sonography in the diagnosis of retroperitoneal fibrosis. *J Urol* 1977;**118**:944.

Snow N & others: Peripheral ischemia due to retroperitoneal fibrosis. *Am J Surg* 1977;**133**:640.

Stecker JF Jr & others: Retroperitoneal fibrosis and ergot derivatives. *J Urol* 1974;**112**:30.

Thomas MH, Chisholm GD: Retroperitoneal fibrosis associated with malignant disease. *Br J Cancer* 1973;**28**:453.

Usher SM, Brendler H, Ciavarra VA: Retroperitoneal fibrosis secondary to metastatic neoplasm. *Urology* 1977;**9**:191.

Wacksman J, Weinerth JL, Kredich D: Retroperitoneal fibrosis in children. *Urology* 1978;**12**:438.

Willscher MK, Mozden PJ, Olsson CA: Retroperitoneal fibrosis with ureteral obstruction secondary to Actinomyces israeli. *Urology* 1978;**12**:569.

Disorders of the Bladder, Prostate, & Seminal Vesicles

Donald R. Smith, MD

CONGENITAL ANOMALIES OF THE BLADDER*

EXSTROPHY

Exstrophy of the bladder is a complete ventral defect of the urogenital sinus and the overlying skeletal system (see Chapter 2). Other congenital anomalies are frequently associated with it. The lower central abdomen is occupied by the inner surface of the posterior wall of the bladder, whose mucosal edges are fused with the skin. Urine spurts onto the abdominal wall from the ureteral orifices.

The rami of the pubic bones are widely separated. The pelvic ring thus lacks rigidity, the femurs are rotated externally, and the child "waddles like a duck." Since the rectus muscles insert on the rami, they are widely separated from each other inferiorly. A hernia, made up of the exstrophic bladder and surrounding skin, is therefore present. Epispadias almost always accompanies it.

Many exstrophic bladders reveal fibrosis, derangement of the muscularis mucosae, and chronic infection (Rudin, Tannenbaum, & Lattimer, 1972). These changes tend to defeat efforts to form a bladder of proper capacity. About 60 instances of adenocarcinoma developing in such bladders have been reported.

Renal infection is common, and hydronephrosis caused by ureterovesical obstruction is often found on urography. These films also reveal the separation of the pubic bones.

Many attempts have been made to free the bladder from surrounding skin, close it primarily, and repair sphincteric mechanisms in the hope of achieving bladder continence and thus avoiding progressive upper urinary tract damage. Lattimer & others (1978), persistent pioneers in this field, have followed their 17 reconstructed patients for as long as 20 years. They report that the quality of life of these patients has been good. Ansell (1979) has performed neonatal reconstruction in 28 patients in an attempt to protect the bladder from later del-

*Congenital vesicorectal fistulas are discussed with urethrorectal fistulas.

eterious changes. Half of his patients in the series did well, and most were continent. DeMaria & others (1980) found renal function to be normal in all of their 22 patients. Toguri & others (1978) report that their 21 patients were continent at the end of 1 year.

Boyce (1972) and Gregoir & Schulman (1978) perform vesicorectal anastomosis after closure of the bladder; proximal colostomy is necessary with this procedure.

Most urologists, however, divert the urine (using an isolated loop of sigmoid or ileum or by ureterosigmoidostomy) after it has been established that the anal sphincter is competent.

The last stage is to remove the bladder and repair the external genitalia.

PERSISTENT URACHUS

Embryologically, the allantois connects the urogenital sinus with the umbilicus. Normally the allantois is obliterated and is represented by a fibrous cord (urachus) extending from the dome of the bladder to the navel (see Chapter 2).

Incomplete obliteration sometimes occurs. If obliteration is complete except at the superior end, a draining umbilical sinus may be noted. If it becomes infected, the drainage will be purulent. If the inferior end remains open it will communicate with the bladder, but this does not usually produce symptoms. Rarely, the entire tract remains patent, in which case urine drains constantly from the umbilicus. This is apt to become obvious within a few days of birth. If only the ends of the urachus seal off, a cyst of that body may form and may become quite large, presenting a low midline mass (Fig 28–1). If the cyst should become infected, signs of general and local sepsis will develop.

Adenocarcinoma may occur in a urachal cyst, particularly at its vesical extremity, and will tend to invade the tissues beneath the anterior abdominal wall. It may be seen cystoscopically. Stones may develop in a cyst of the urachus. These can be identified on a plain x-ray film.

Treatment consists of excision of the urachus, which lies on the peritoneal surface. If adenocarci-

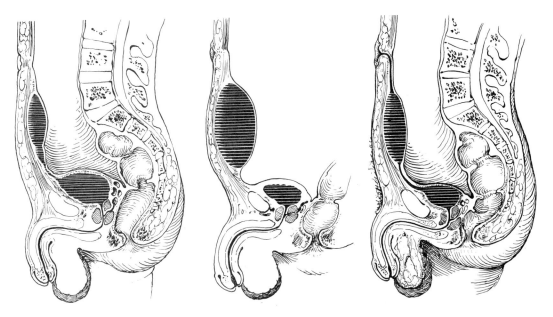

Figure 28–1. Types of persistent urachus. *Left:* Communicating urachus continuous with the bladder. This is a "pseudodiverticulum" and usually causes no symptoms. *Center:* Urachal cyst; usually causes no symptoms or signs unless it becomes larger or infected. *Right:* Patent urachus. There is constant drainage of urine from the umbilicus.

noma is present, radical resection is required.

Unless other serious congenital anomalies are present, the prognosis is good. The complication of adenocarcinoma offers a poor prognosis.

CONTRACTURE OF THE BLADDER NECK

There is considerable debate about the incidence of congenital narrowing of the bladder neck. Some feel that its presence is a common cause of vesicoureteral reflux, vesical diverticula, a bladder of large capacity, and the syndrome of irritable bladder associated with enuresis. A few observers consider this contracture a rare phenomenon and believe that the diagnosis is purely presumptive. The diagnosis is based upon endoscopic observation, which is an unreliable method. Voiding cystourethrography has been used to depict such narrowing, but interpretation of the films varies from urologist to urologist and radiologist to radiologist.

Nunn (1965) studied the intravesical and urethral pressures during voiding in cases with the signs mentioned above. He found no evidence of bladder neck obstruction. The 2 recorded pressures were essentially equal. It appears that the bladder neck would have to be extremely stenotic to truly obstruct urine flow. It is becoming increasingly clear that in little girls, the obstructive lesion is spasm of the periurethral striated muscle which develops secondary to distal urethral stenosis (see Chapter 30).

Empirical treatment is often employed, consisting of suprapubic bladder neck revision or transurethral resection. Making the bladder neck incompetent in the male child may later cause retrograde ejaculation and, therefore, infertility. Revision of the bladder neck in the female may cause urinary incontinence. The diagnosis must therefore be made with caution.

ACQUIRED DISEASES OF THE BLADDER

INTERSTITIAL CYSTITIS
(Hunner's Ulcer, Submucous Fibrosis)

Interstitial cystitis is primarily a disease of middle-aged women. It is characterized by fibrosis of the vesical wall, with consequent loss of bladder capacity. Frequency is the principal symptom.

Pathogenesis & Pathology

Infection does not appear to be the cause of fibrosis of the bladder wall, for the urine is usually normal. It has been postulated that the fibrosis is due to obstruction of the vesical lymphatics secondary to pelvic surgery or infection, but many of these patients fail to give such a history. It may be secondary to thrombophlebitis complicating acute infections of the bladder or pelvic organs, or may be the result of prolonged intrinsic arteriolar spasm secondary to psychogenic impulses.

Recently, however, evidence has been adduced which suggests that interstitial cystitis is an autoimmune collagen disease. Oravisto, Alfthan, & Jokinen (1970) studied 54 women afflicted with this disease. Antinuclear antibodies were found in 85%. A significant number had allergy of the reagin type or hypersensitivity to drugs. Jacobo, Stamler, & Culp (1974) and Gordon & others (1973) have confirmed these findings. An allergic cause would explain the favorable responses to corticosteroids.

The primary change is fibrosis in the deeper layers of the bladder. The capacity of the organ is decreased, sometimes markedly. The mucosa is thinned, especially where mobility is greatest as the bladder fills and empties (ie, over the dome), and small ulcers or cracks in the mucous membrane may be seen in this area. In the most severe cases, the normal mechanism of the ureterovesical junctions is destroyed, leading to vesicoureteral reflux. Hydroureteronephrosis and pyelonephritis may then ensue.

Microscopically, the mucosa may be thinned or even denuded. The capillaries of the tunica propria are often engorged, and signs of inflammation are apparent. The muscle is replaced by varying amounts of fibrous tissue, which is often quite avascular. The lymphatics may be engorged. Increased mast cells and lymphocytic infiltration are seen (Jacobo, Stamler, & Culp, 1974).

Clinical Findings

Interstitial cystitis should be considered when a middle-aged woman with clear urine complains of severe frequency and nocturia and suprapubic pain on vesical distention.

A. Symptoms: There is a long history of slowly progressive frequency and nocturia, both of which may be severe. The history does not suggest infection (burning on urination, cloudy urine). Suprapubic pain is usually marked when the bladder is full. Pain may also be experienced in the urethra or perineum. It is relieved on voiding. Gross hematuria is occasionally noted, usually when urination has had to be postponed (ie, following vesical overdistention). The patient is tense and anxious. Whether this is secondary to the prolonged and severe symptoms or is the primary cause of the vesical changes is not clear (see Chapter 36). A history of allergy may be obtained.

B. Signs: Physical examination is usually normal. Some tenderness in the suprapubic area may be noted. There may be some tenderness in the region of the bladder when it is palpated through the vagina.

C. Laboratory Findings: If the patient has had no previous treatment (eg, instrumentation), the urine is almost always free of infection. Microscopic hematuria may be noted. Renal function (as measured by the PSP test) is normal except in the occasional patient in whom vesical fibrosis has led to vesicoureteral reflux or obstruction.

D. X-Ray Findings: Excretory urograms are usually normal unless reflux has occurred, in which case hydronephrosis is found. The accompanying cystogram will reveal a bladder of small capacity; reflux into a dilated upper tract may be noted on cystography.

E. Instrumental Examination: Cystoscopy is usually diagnostic. As the bladder fills, increasing suprapubic pain is experienced. The vesical capacity may be as low as 60 mL. In a patient not previously treated (by fulguration or hydraulic overdistention), the bladder lining may look fairly normal. But if a second distention is done (Messing & Stamey, 1978), punctate hemorrhagic areas may appear over the most distensible portion of the wall. With further distention, an arcuate split in the mucosa will occur and bleeding from it may be profuse.

Lapides (1975) believes this disease is common in young women whose only complaint is frequency due to a small bladder capacity. In these cases he finds no vesical lesion, however.

Differential Diagnosis

Tuberculosis of the bladder may cause true ulceration but is most apt to involve the region of the ureteral orifice which drains the tuberculous kidney. Typical tubercles may be identified, pyuria is present, and tubercle bacilli can usually be found. Furthermore, urograms will often show the typical lesion of renal tuberculosis.

Nonspecific vesical infection seldom causes ulceration. Pus and bacteria will be found in the urine. Antimicrobial treatment will be effective.

Utz & Zinke (1974) have observed that 20% of their male patients who had been diagnosed as having interstitial cystitis actually had carcinoma. They stress the need for cytologic study and transurethral biopsy.

Complications

Gradual ureteral stenosis or reflux and its sequelae (eg, hydronephrosis) may develop.

Treatment

A. Specific Measures: There appears to be no definitive treatment for interstitial cystitis. The therapy usually employed frequently affords partial relief but may be completely ineffective.

Hydraulic overdistention, with or without anesthesia, sometimes gradually improves the bladder capacity. Vesical lavage with increasing strengths of silver nitrate (1:5000–1:100) may have the same effect. Superficial (transcystoscopic) electrocoagulation of the split mucosa is commonly practiced and may afford temporary relief of pain. Greenberg & others (1974) believe that transurethral resection of the lesion affords better results than fulguration.

Stewart & Shirley (1976) report good symptomatic relief following the instillation of 5 mL of 50% dimethyl sulfoxide (DMSO) into the bladder every 2 weeks. It is left in for 15 minutes.

Messing & Stamey (1978) claim their best results were obtained with vesical irrigations of 0.4% oxychlorosene sodium (Clorpactin WCS-90). At 10 cm of water pressure, the bladder is repeatedly filled to capacity until 1 L has been used. This must be done under anesthesia. Cystography should be done before instituting this therapy. The presence of vesicoureteral reflux has caused ureteral fibrosis (Messing & Freiha, 1979).

Cortisone acetate, 100 mg, or prednisone (Meticorten), 10–20 mg/d, in divided doses orally for 21 days, followed by decreasing amounts for an additional 21 days, has also been found effective (Badenoch, 1971). Transcystoscopic injection of the lesions with prednisone has its proponents.

Antihistamines (eg, pyribenzamine, 50 mg 4 times a day) may also afford some relief. Heparin sodium (long-acting), 20,000 units/d intravenously, also blocks the action of histamine, and its use in the treatment of Hunner's ulcer is encouraging.

Freiha, Faysal, & Stamey (1980) performed cystolysis in 5 patients who did not respond to oxychlorosene; 5 were improved. If the bladder becomes fibrotic and the capacity small, ceco- or ileocystoplasty can be done, thereby augmenting vesical capacity (Dounis, Abel, & Gow, 1980; Shirley & Mirelman, 1978). The majority are cured or greatly improved; those who are not may require urinary diversion.

B. General Measures: General or vesical sedatives may be prescribed but seldom afford relief. If urinary infection is found (usually following instrumentation), it should be treated by appropriate antibiotics. If senile urethritis is discovered, diethylstilbestrol vaginal suppositories may prove helpful.

C. Treatment of Complications: If progressive hydronephrosis develops secondary to ureteral stenosis, little will be gained by ureteral dilatations. Diversion of the urinary stream (eg, ureteroileocutaneous anastomosis) may therefore be necessary.

Prognosis

Most patients respond to vesical irrigations with oxychlorosene. Those that do not may require operation.

EXTERNAL VESICAL HERNIATION

The bladder of a young girl may protrude through a patulous urethra and present itself externally. Treatment requires gentle pressure upon the mass, with the patient in the Trendelenburg position. After reduction, a small urethral catheter should be left in the bladder for a few days. If herniation recurs, the bladder and urethra should be sutured to the linea alba.

INTERNAL VESICAL HERNIATION

One side of the bladder may become involved in an inguinal hernia (in men) or a femoral hernia (in women) (Fig 28–2). Such a mass may recede on urination. It is most often found as a previously unsuspected complication during the surgical correction of a hernia (Bell & Witherington, 1980). Weitzenfeld & others (1980) have reported a case in which the right kidney and ureter as well as the left ureter were in scrotal inguinal hernias.

URINARY STRESS INCONTINENCE

Stress incontinence, the loss of urine with physical strain (eg, coughing, sneezing), is a common complaint of older women. Although it usually occurs as an aftermath of childbirth, it has been observed in girls and nulliparous women also.

Normal urethral resistance is about 100 cm of water; this is the sum of the smooth muscle urethral sphincter (50 cm of water) and the striated midurethral sphincter (50 cm of water). Normally, with strain or cough, intraperitoneal pressure rises sharply but the resistance in the mid urethra rises also, thus maintaining the relatively high urethra-to-detrusor pressure ratio. In patients with stress incontinence, the basic lesion is loss of normal midurethral resistance caused by a severe sagging of the vesical base and urethra caused by poor support of these structures. The sphincter muscles are usually normal, but with the descent of the urethra and bladder they cannot work efficiently. Normally, the length of the urethra is 4 cm. Urethral pressure studies show that the proximal half of the urethra reveals little closure pressure. Thus, the functional length of their urethras is about 2 cm (Tanagho, 1979). In addition, the area of the posterior urethra and bladder neck has fallen out of the true pelvis, so that the strain that suddenly increases intravesical pressure is associated with decreased resistance in the proximal and mid urethra, thereby leading to incontinence.

Susset & others (1976) and Gershon & Diakno (1978) have also published definitive studies on the urodynamics of this affliction.

Clinical Findings

Patients complain of loss of urine only with straining in the upright position. They remain dry while in bed. Some degree of urethrocele is usually noted. Of some diagnostic value is the demonstration that support to the bladder neck will cause the patient to be continent with cough or strain. This test must be performed with the patient standing. The region of the bladder neck is lifted well up under the pubic symphysis with 2 fingers or 2 clamps. (If clamps are used, infiltration with a local anesthetic is required.) False position tests, however, are sometimes elicited.

An important test in establishing the diagnosis of true stress incontinence is the lateral cystogram taken both with and without straining. A beaded chain or catheter should be placed in the bladder to delineate the urethrovesical junction (Fig 28–2). In the normal female, the base of the bladder lies about 2 cm above a line drawn from the inferior margin of the pubis to the sacrococcygeal joint (the SCIPP line). With straining, the vesical base should descend no more than 1.5 cm. With true stress incontinence, the static lateral cystogram may reveal some sagging of the bladder, and this is markedly accentuated on the film taken when the patient strains to void (Noll & Hutch, 1969; Susset & others, 1976).

Differential Diagnosis

Careful history taking will usually differentiate between stress and urgency incontinence. The latter implies the presence of either local inflammatory disease or nervous tension. The following diseases must be differentiated from the lesion causing stress incontinence if good surgical results are to be obtained: ectopic ureteral orifice, neurogenic bladder, senile urethritis, urethral diverticulum, and local lesions of the urethra and bladder (eg, cystitis, urethritis). The history, physical examination, urinalysis, and PSP test as well as cystoscopy, excretory urography, lateral cystography, and cystometry should make the differentiation. If urodynamic study can be done, the diagnosis becomes highly accurate.

Treatment

If hypoestrogenism of the vagina and urethra is discovered, give estrogens locally or by mouth (see Chapter 30). If the degree of incontinence is mild, Stewart, Banowsky, & Montague (1976) recommend Ornade Spansules, a sustained release preparation containing phenylpropanolamine 50 mg, chlorpheniramine 8 mg, and isopropamide iodide 2.5 mg, 1 capsule daily. This treatment appears to be worth trying before surgery is recommended.

Although a vaginal approach designed to afford support to the bladder neck is most commonly employed, it appears that retropubic urethrovesical suspension (Marshall-Marchetti operation) affords a better result (Tanagho, 1976). Stamey, Schaeffer, & Condy (1975) employ a similar procedure done through the endoscope with good results. Cobb & Ragde (1978) also report good results with this technic.

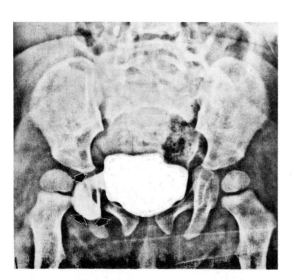

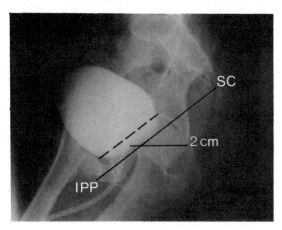

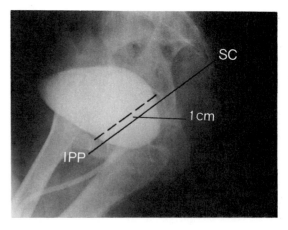

Figure 28–2. Internal vesical hernia; lateral cystograms in stress incontinence. *Above left:* Female, 6 months old. Cystogram of excretory urogram showing tongue of bladder in right femoral hernia (see arrows). In the 2 films shown below, the dashed line shows the normal position of the base of the normal bladder. Line SCIPP is a reference line drawn from the sacrococcygeal (SC) joint to the inferior point of the pubic bone (IPP). *Below left:* Resting cystogram in stress incontinence. The bladder base lies 2 cm below the normal position. *Right:* Cystogram taken with straining in a patient with stress incontinence. The base of the bladder descends about 4 cm, revealing poor support of the urethrovesical junction. (Courtesy of John A Hutch.)

Prognosis

If the proper diagnosis has been made, the cure rate approaches 85%. Unfortunately, after a year or so, stress incontinence recurs in a few cases. Reoperation may therefore be necessary.

URINARY INCONTINENCE

Partial or complete urinary incontinence may develop after prostatectomy, particularly the transurethral type. Intrinsic damage to the smooth muscle urethral sphincter is implied. Though it is common to incriminate damage to or resection of the external voluntary sphincter, this is very rare. Such a patient can stop the voiding stream by contracture of the latter sphincter, but prolonged control is impossible because of fatigue of striated muscle. Only the smooth muscle with its constant tone can afford continence.

Scott, Bradley, & Timm (1974) and Scott (1978) have described an ingenious method for affording urinary control. The entire silicone prosthesis is buried in the patient. It consists of a reservoir of fluid in a plastic bag placed deep to the abdominal wall near the bladder and a collar of plastic material which can encircle either the bladder neck or the perineal urethra. The former is used in the female, the latter in the male. One plastic bulb is placed in one scrotal (or labial) sac and another is implanted in the other sac. These are connected by tubing in such a way that pumping one scrotal (or labial) bulb forces fluid into the collar, thus closing off the urethra; pressure on the other allows the fluid to return to the reservoir. This device has been successful in affording control in most instances. A newer model requires only one scrotal (or labial) bulb that can both pump fluid into the collar and cause it to return to the reservoir (Scott: personal communication, 1978). Rosen (1978) has designed a similar mechanism that is very effective (Small, 1980).

Numerous operations for cure of total incontinence have been devised.

Kaufman has devised a number of procedures that apply pressure to the perineal urethra just distal to the prostate. These include apposition or transposition of the ischiocavernosus muscles and implantation of a plastic prosthesis. His most recent device (Kaufman & Raz, 1979) consists of a plastic container embedded in the perineum over the bulbous urethra. Silicon gel is instilled into the container until the desired occlusive pressure is reached. If leakage still occurs in the postoperative period, more silicon can be instilled percutaneously. Of his 184 patients, 33% achieved perfect control and 28% had some stress incontinence. Politano (1978) injects Polytef (Teflon) into the perineal periurethral tissues to afford suitable compression.

Some of the mild cases may respond to ephedrine. Diokno & Taub (1975) prescribed up to 200 mg/d in 4 divided doses with good response. Children were also benefited by the elixir, which contains 11 mg/5 mL.

Tanagho & Smith (1972) have designed a procedure based upon sound anatomic principles that has been quite successful in restoring urinary continence. A strip of the heavy layer of the middle circular layer of the detrusor muscle, anteriorly, is formed into a tube, thus affording sphincteric action. This is anastomosed to the bladder neck or prostatic urethra. Preliminary results are encouraging. Williams & Snyder (1976) have successfully utilized this procedure in children.

ENURESIS

Enuresis originally meant "incontinence of urine," but usage has caused the term to be restricted to bedwetting after age 3 years. Most children have achieved normal bladder control by that time, girls earlier than boys. At age 6 years, 10% have enuresis. Even at age 14, 5% still wet the bed (Simonds, 1977). It is difficult to be sure, but it seems that more than 50% of cases are caused by delayed maturation of the nervous system or an intrinsic myoneurogenic bladder dysfunction; 30% are of psychic origin; and 20% are secondary to more obvious organic disease. Most children with functional enuresis gain spontaneous nocturnal control by age 10 years.

Psychodynamics

Training in bladder control should begin after the age of 1½ years; attempts made before this are usually fruitless and may be harmful. If the parents fail in this teaching, the child may not develop cerebral inhibitory control over the infantile uninhibited bladder until much later in childhood. If the parents are emotionally unstable, their anxieties may be transmitted to the child, who may express tension through enuresis.

The birth of a sibling may cause loss of the child's paramount position in the family. The child may then regress to an infancy pattern in order to recapture the parents' affection. An acute illness may be accompanied or followed by recurrence of incomplete nocturnal control. Physiologic or psychologic stress (fear and anxiety) may reestablish an uninhibited bladder.

Possibly 40% of enuretic children have electroencephalograms that are borderline or compatible with epilepsy or delayed maturation of the central nervous system.

Clinical Findings

A. Symptoms: A child may wet the bed occasionally or regularly. Careful questioning of the parents or observation by the physician reveals that the patient voids a free stream of normal caliber. This tends to rule out obstruction of the lower tract as a cause of the enuresis. Children with daytime incontinence are apt to have more than psychogenic enuresis. Many void frequently and are found to have a diminished vesical capacity, though under anesthesia capacity is normal. This is probably a reflection of delayed maturation.

There is no burning, although frequency and urgency are common. The urine is clear.

Observation of the parents often reveals that they are anxious and tense, traits that can only be aggravated by the child's bedwetting.

B. Signs: General physical and urologic examinations are normal.

C. Laboratory Findings: In the emotional and delayed maturation group, all tests, including urinalysis, are normal. An electroencephalogram may be abnormal, however.

D. X-Ray Findings: Excretory urograms show no abnormality. The accompanying cystogram reveals no trabeculation; a film of the bladder taken immediately after voiding shows no residual urine.

E. Instrumental Examination: A catheter of suitable size passes readily to the bladder, thereby ruling out stricture. If the catheter is passed after urination, no residual urine is found. Urethrocystoscopy is normal. Cystometric studies are usually normal, but a curve typical of the "uninhibited" (hyperirritable) neuropathic bladder (Fig 19–5) is often obtained. Unless infection or some more obvious organic disease is discovered, instrumentation, x-ray, and urodynamic studies are not necessary.

Differential Diagnosis

A. Obstruction: Lower tract obstruction (eg, posterior urethral valves, meatal stenosis) causes a urinary stream of decreased caliber. Painful, frequent urination during the day and night, pyuria, and fever (eg, pyelonephritis) are often present, and the bladder may be distended. Urinalysis usually reveals evidence of infection. Anemia and impairment of renal function may be demonstrated.

Excretory urograms may show dilatation of the bladder and the upper urinary tract. Incomplete vesical emptying may be seen on the postvoiding film. Cystography may demonstrate distal urethral stenosis or reflux. Urethrocystoscopy reveals the organic cause.

Severe obstruction from severe spasm of the entire pelvic floor musculature on a psychosomatic basis can cause damage to the bladder and kidneys; infection is the rule.

B. Infection: Chronic urinary tract infection not due to obstruction usually produces frequency both day and night and pain on urination, although such infections may occur without symptoms of vesical irritability. Recurrent fever with exacerbations is common.

General examination may be normal. Anemia may be noted. Urinalysis will show pus cells or bacteria, or both. Renal function may be deficient.

Excretory urograms may be essentially normal, although changes compatible with healed pyelonephritis are often seen. Cystoscopy will show the changes caused by infection. Urine specimens obtained by ureteral catheter may reveal renal infection. Cystography may show vesicoureteral reflux.

C. Neurogenic Disease: Children suffering from sacral cord or root abnormality (eg, myelodysplasia) may have incomplete urinary control both day and night. Since they ordinarily have significant amounts of residual urine, infection is usually found on urinalysis. The passage of a catheter, or the postvoiding film taken in conjunction with excretory urograms, will demonstrate the presence of residual urine. A plain film of the abdomen may reveal spina bifida.

The cystometrogram is usually typical of a flaccid neurogenic bladder. Cystoscopy demonstrates an atonic bladder with moderate trabeculation and evidence of infection.

D. Distal Urethral Stenosis: This congenital anomaly is the cause of enuresis in many young girls, even in the absence of cystitis. Urethral calibration will establish this diagnosis.

Complications

The complications of functional enuresis are psychic, not organic. These children are particularly disturbed when they begin to attend school. Even more pressure is brought to bear by their parents; these children find it impossible to stay overnight at the homes of their playmates. Unhealthy introversion may be their lot. Enuresis may be prolonged because of undue emphasis on dryness or as a result of punitive or shaming measures.

Late Sequelae

Occasionally an adult is seen who, under stress, develops nocturnal frequency without comparable diurnal frequency. Thorough urologic investigation proves to be negative. Many of these people will give histories of enuresis of long duration in childhood. It is suggested that their cerebrovesical pathways again break down under undue emotional tension; nocturnal frequency may be the adult expression of enuresis.

Treatment

Treatment should be considered if enuresis persists after age 3 years.

A. General Measures: Fluids should be limited after supper. The bladder should be completely emptied at bedtime, and the child should be completely awakened a little before the usual time of bedwetting and allowed to void.

Drug therapy has its proponents.

1. Imipramine has been reported to cure 50–70% of patients and is probably the drug of choice. Start with 25 mg before dinner. Increase the dose as needed to 50 mg. Twenty-five mg usually suffice (Kass, Diokno, & Montealegre, 1979).

2. Parasympatholytic drugs such as atropine or belladonna, by decreasing the tone of the detrusor, may at times be of value. Methantheline bromide, 25–75 mg at bedtime, is more potent.

3. Sympathomimetic drugs, eg, dextroamphetamine sulfate, 5–10 mg at bedtime, may cause enough wakefulness so that the child perceives the urge to void.

4. Phenytoin has been found to control some of those children whose electroencephalograms are abnormal.

5. The use of mechanical devices such as metal-covered pads that when wet cause an alarm to ring may be of benefit in cases of delayed maturation by setting up a conditioned reflex (Close, 1980).

6. Urologic treatments (eg, urethral dilatation, urethral instillations of silver nitrate), though often recommended, should be condemned in the absence of demonstrable local disease. They are physically and psychically traumatic and can only cause further apprehension and fear in an already disturbed child.

B. Psychotherapy: Analytic evaluation and treatment may be indicated for some of the children and their parents. Responsibility for correction of the patient's feelings of insecurity rests with the parents, who must be cautioned not to punish the child or in any way contribute further to existing feelings of guilt and insecurity. The handling of the parents may prove difficult, in which case psychiatric referral may be necessary.

Prognosis

Retraining the enuretic child and, above all, reeducating the parents is difficult and time-consuming. Psychiatric referral for the parents and, at times, for the child may be necessary. Most patients conquer their enuresis by age 10 years. A few, however, do not, and they may later develop vesical irritability of the psychogenic type in response to acute or chronic tension or anxiety.

FOREIGN BODIES INTRODUCED INTO THE BLADDER & URETHRA

Numerous objects have been found in the urethra and bladder of both men and women. Some of them find their way into the urethra in the course of inquisitive self-exploration. Others are introduced (in the male) as contraceptive devices in the hope that plugging the urethra will block the drainage of the ejaculate.

The presence of a foreign body causes cystitis. Hematuria is not uncommon. Embarrassment may cause the victim to delay medical consultation. A plain x-ray of the bladder area will disclose metal objects. Nonopaque objects sometimes become coated with calcium. Cystoscopy will visualize them all.

Cystoscopic or suprapubic removal of the foreign body is indicated. If not removed, the foreign body will lead to infection of the bladder. If the infecting organisms are urea-splitting, the alkaline urine (which causes increased insolubility of calcium salts) contributes to rapid formation of stone upon the foreign object (Fig 15–10).

VESICAL MANIFESTATIONS OF ALLERGY

So many mucous membranes are affected by allergens that the possibility of allergic manifestations involving the bladder must be considered. Hypersensitivity is occasionally suggested in cases of recurrent symptoms of acute "cystitis" in the absence of urinary infection or other demonstrable abnormality. During the attack, general erythema of the vesical mucosa may be seen and some edema of the ureteral orifices noted.

A careful history may reveal that these attacks follow the ingestion of a certain food not ordinarily eaten (eg, fresh lobster). Sensitivity to spermicidal creams is occasionally observed. If vesical allergy is suspected, it may be aborted by the subcutaneous injection of 0.5–1 mL of 1:1000 epinephrine. Control may also be afforded by the use of one of the antihistamines. Skin testing has not generally proved helpful in determining the source of allergy.

DIVERTICULUM

Most vesical diverticula are acquired and are secondary to either obstruction distal to the vesical neck or the upper motor neuron type of neurogenic bladder. Increased intravesical pressure causes vesical mucosa to insinuate itself between hypertrophied muscle bundles, so that a mucosal extravesical sac develops. Often, this sac lies just superior to the ureter and causes vesicoureteral reflux (Hutch saccule; see Chapter 11). The diverticulum is devoid of muscle and therefore has no expulsive power; residual urine is the rule, and infection is perpetuated. If the diverticulum has a narrow opening that interferes with its emptying, transurethral resection of its neck will improve drainage (Vitale & Woodside, 1979). Reece & others (1974) suggest the use of a fiberoptic bronchoscope passed through a panendoscope sheath to inspect the wall of the diverticulum because carcinoma occasionally develops on its wall. At the time of open prostatectomy, resection of the diverticulum should be considered.

VESICAL FISTULAS

Vesical fistulas are common. The bladder may communicate with the skin, intestinal tract, or

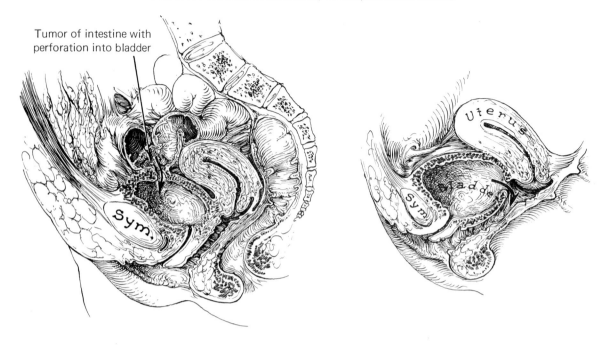

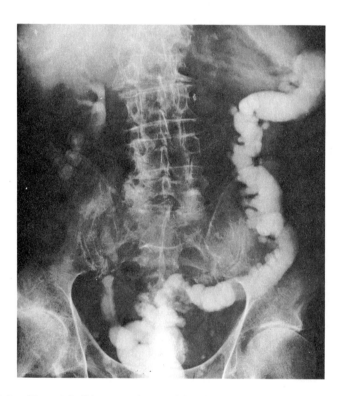

Figure 28–3. Vesical fistulas. *Above left:* Primary carcinoma of the sigmoid, with perforation through bladder wall. *Above right:* Injury to base of bladder following delivery by forceps. *Below:* Cystogram showing radiopaque fluid entering sigmoid containing multiple diverticula; right ureteral reflux, gallbladder calculi.

gynecologic organs. The primary disease is usually not urologic. The causes are as follows: (1) Primary intestinal disease—diverticulitis, 50–60%; cancer of the colon, 20–25%; and Crohn's disease, 10%. (2) Primary gynecologic disease—pressure necrosis during difficult labor; advanced cancer of the cervix. (3) Treatment for gynecologic disease following hysterectomy, low cesarean section, or radiotherapy for tumor. (4) Trauma.

Malignant tumors of the small or large bowel, uterus, or cervix may invade and perforate the bladder. Inflammations of adjacent organs may also erode through the vesical wall. Severe injuries involving the bladder may lead to perivesical abscess formation, and these abscesses may rupture through the skin of the perineum or abdomen. The bladder may be inadvertently injured during gynecologic or intestinal surgery; cystotomy for stone or prostatectomy may lead to a persistent cutaneous fistula.

Clinical Findings

A. Vesicointestinal Fistula: Symptoms arising from a vesicointestinal fistula include vesical irritability, the passage of feces and gas through the urethra, and usually a change in bowel habits (eg, obstipation, abdominal distention, diarrhea) caused by the primary intestinal disease. Signs of bowel obstruction may be elicited; abdominal tenderness may be found if the cause is inflammatory. The urine is always infected.

A barium enema, upper gastrointestinal series, or sigmoidoscopic examination may demonstrate the communication. Following a barium enema, centrifuged urine should be placed on an x-ray cassette and an exposure made. The presence of radiopaque barium will establish the diagnosis of vesicocolonic fistula. Cystograms may reveal gas in the bladder or reflux of the opaque material into the bowel (Fig 28–3). Cystoscopic examination, the most useful diagnostic procedure, will show a severe localized inflammatory reaction from which bowel contents may exude. Catheterization of the fistulous tract may be feasible; the instillation of radiopaque fluid will often establish the diagnosis (Carson, Malek, & Remine, 1978).

B. Vesicovaginal Fistula: This relatively common fistula is secondary to obstetric, surgical, or radiation injury or to invasive cancer of the cervix. The constant leakage of urine is most distressing to the patient. Pelvic examination usually reveals the fistulous opening, which can also be visualized with the cystoscope. It may be possible to pass a ureteral catheter through the fistula into the vagina. Vaginography often successfully shows ureterovaginal, vesicovaginal, and rectovaginal fistulas. A 30-mL Foley catheter is inserted into the vagina and the balloon is distended. A radiopaque solution is then instilled and appropriate x-rays are taken. Biopsy of the edges of the fistula may show carcinoma. Persky, Forsythe, & Herman (1980) describe this

lesion in 6 children; all occurred as a complication of surgery, 3 following transurethral resection of the bladder neck.

C. Vesicoadnexal Fistula: This rare fistula can be diagnosed by vaginal examination and by seeing the fistulous opening through the cystoscope.

Differential Diagnosis

It is necessary to differentiate ureterovaginal from vesicovaginal fistula.

Give pyridium by mouth to color the urine orange. One hour later, insert 3 cotton pledgets into the vagina and then instill methylene blue solution into the bladder. Then have the patient walk around. If the proximal cotton ball is wet and stained orange, the fistula is ureterovaginal. If the deep cotton pledget contains blue fluid, the diagnosis is vesicovaginal fistula. If only the distal pledget is blue, the patient probably has urinary incontinence (Raghavaiah, 1974).

Treatment

A. Vesicointestinal Fistula: If the lesion is in the rectosigmoid, treatment consists of proximal colostomy. When the inflammatory reaction has subsided, resection of the involved bowel may be done with closure of the opening in the bladder. Later the colostomy can be closed. Some authors recommend that the entire procedure be performed in one stage, thus avoiding the need for preliminary colostomy. Small bowel or appendiceal vesical fistulas require bowel or appendiceal resection and closure of the vesical defect.

B. Vesicovaginal Fistula: Tiny fistulous openings may seal following the introduction into the fistula of an electrode. As the electrode is withdrawn, the fistula is coagulated with the electrosurgical unit to destroy the epithelium of the tract. An indwelling catheter should be left in place for 2 weeks or more. Aycinena (1977) reports good results in such cases by inserting a metal screw through the vaginal stoma. It is moved up and down to act as a curet. The vaginal mucosa is then closed and an indwelling catheter placed for 3 weeks.

Larger fistulas secondary to obstetric or surgical injuries respond readily to surgical repair, which may be done either through the vagina or transvesically. Persky, Herman & Guerrier (1979) advise immediate repair rather than waiting for 3–6 months as counseled by most surgeons. Fistulas that develop following radiation therapy for cancer of the cervix are much more difficult to close because of the avascularity of the tissues (Patil, Waterhouse, & Laungani, 1980). Surgical closure of fistulas which arise from direct invasion of the bladder by cervical carcinoma is impossible; diversion of the urinary stream above the level of the bladder (eg, ureterosigmoidostomy) is therefore necessary.

C. Vesicoadnexal Fistula: These fistulas are cured by removal of the involved gynecologic organs, with closure of the opening in the bladder.

Prognosis

The surgical repair of fistulas caused by benign disease or operative trauma is highly successful. Postirradiation necrosis offers a more guarded prognosis. Fistulas secondary to invading cancers present difficult problems.

PERIVESICAL LIPOMATOSIS

The cause of this lesion is not known. The disorder seems to affect principally black males in the 20–40 year age group. There are no pathognomonic symptoms. There may be some dysuria or mild urinary obstructive symptoms. Examination may demonstrate a distended or enlarged pear-shaped bladder. Excretory urograms and cystography may show dilatation of both upper tracts and an upward displacement and lateral compression of the bladder. In the perivesical area, x-ray reveals areas of radiolucency compatible with fatty tissue. A barium x-ray may show extrinsic pressure on the rectosigmoid. Angiography shows no evidence of neoplastic vessels.

CT scan in association with the above findings establishes the diagnosis by clearly demonstrating the fatty nature of the perivesical tissue (Levine, Farber, & Lee, 1978; Susmano & Dolin, 1979). Church & Kazam (1979) found sonography equally helpful.

On surgical exploration, lipomatous tissue is found surrounding the bladder and rectosigmoid. Though it is tempting to proceed with its resection, there are no cleavage planes. Such dissections have usually failed to relieve the ureteral obstruction. Sacks & Dresnick (1975) report that a low-calorie diet led to relief of ureteral obstruction in one case. Dilatation recurred when the patient again gained weight.

Ballesteros (1977) feels that surgical excision is feasible and reported excellent results in one such case. Crane & Smith (1977) found, after a 5-year follow-up, that hydronephrosis progressed in most. Many finally required urinary diversion.

RADIATION CYSTITIS

Many women receiving radiation treatment for carcinoma of the cervix develop some degree of vesical irritability. These symptoms may develop months after cessation of treatment. The urine may or may not be sterile. Vesical capacity is usually appreciably reduced. Cystoscopy will reveal a pale mucous membrane with multiple areas of telangiectatic blood vessels. Vesical ulceration may be noted, and vesicovaginal fistulas may develop. If symptoms are severe and prolonged, diversion of urine from the bladder may be necessary.

NONINFECTIOUS HEMORRHAGIC CYSTITIS

Some patients, following radiotherapy for carcinoma of the cervix or bladder, are prone to intermittent, often serious vesical hemorrhage. The same is true of those given cyclophosphamide.

In the case of the latter, the drug must be stopped. To control bleeding, cystoscopic fulguration can be tried, though it usually fails. The instillation of 3.9% formalin (prepared by diluting the standard 39% solution 10 times) is more efficacious. Clamp the catheter for 30 minutes and then lavage the bladder with 10% alcohol. A second or third instillation may be necessary on subsequent days. Holstein & others (1973) recommend the transurethral placement of a large balloon in the bladder. The balloon is filled to a pressure level equal to the systolic blood pressure and left in place for 6 hours. McGuire & others (1974) consider this the procedure of choice.

Pyeritz & others (1978) were unable to stop the hemorrhage with formalin or $AgNO_3$, but a continuous intravenous infusion of vasopressin caused it to cease. Giulani & others (1979) report success by selective transcatheter embolization of the internal iliac arteries.

EMPYEMA OF THE BLADDER

If supravesical diversion of the urine is performed without cystectomy, severe infection of the bladder may develop because of lack of washout. In the male, cystostomy or cutaneous vesicostomy may be necessary. In the female, the formation of a vesicovaginal fistula will permit drainage (Spence & Allen, 1971). Occasionally, cystectomy may be necessary.

CONGENITAL ANOMALIES OF THE PROSTATE & SEMINAL VESICLES

Congenital anomalies of the prostate are rare. Cysts of the prostate and the seminal vesicles have been reported. Enlargements of the prostatic utricle are often found in association with penoscrotal or perineal hypospadias. They are usually small, lying in the midline posterior to the prostate and emptying through the verumontanum. These cysts represent embryologic remnants of the distal end of the müllerian ducts (see Chapter 2). Rarely, they become large enough to be easily palpable rectally or even abdominally. Through local pressure, they may cause symptoms of obstruction of the bladder neck.

BLOODY EJACULATION

Hemospermia is a not uncommon complaint of middle-aged men. It is the wife that usually recognizes the symptom. It is thought by some to be caused by hyperplasia of the mucosa of the seminal vesicles. For this reason, the use of diethylstilbestrol, 5 mg/d for 1 week, has been suggested. In the author's hands, it has worked well. Tolley & Castro (1975) stated that thorough urologic investigation of men without other symptoms never reveals a pathologic lesion. The cause is therefore not clear. Stein, Prioleau, & Catalona (1980) have observed this symptom caused by adenomatous polyps in 3 men and in another with a prostatic intraductal carcinoma.

● ● ●

References

Exstrophy

Ansell JS: Surgical treatment of exstrophy of the bladder with emphasis on neonatal primary closure: Personal experience with 28 consecutive cases treated at the University of Washington hospitals from 1962 to 1977: Techniques and results. *J Urol* 1979;**121**:650.

Boyce WH: A new concept concerning treatment of exstrophy of the bladder: 20 years later. *J Urol* 1972;**107**:476.

DeMaria JE & others: Renal function in continent patients after surgical closure of bladder exstrophy. *J Urol* 1980;**124**:85.

Gregoir W, Schulman CC: Exstrophy of the bladder: Treatment by trigonosigmoidostomy: Long-term results. *Br J Urol* 1978;**50**:90.

Jeffs RD: Exstrophy and cloacal exstrophy. *Urol Clin North Am* 1978;**5**:127.

Johnston JH: The genital aspects of exstrophy. *J Urol* 1975;**113**:701.

Kandzari SJ & others: Exstrophy of urinary bladder complicated by adenocarcinoma. *Urology* 1974;**3**:496.

Lattimer JK & others: Long-term followup after exstrophy closure: Late improvement and good quality of life. *J Urol* 1978;**119**:664.

Rudin L, Tannenbaum M, Lattimer JK: Histologic analysis of the exstrophied bladder after anatomical closure. *J Urol* 1972;**108**:802.

Spence HM, Hoffman WW, Pate VA: Exstrophy of the bladder. 1. Long-term results in a series of 37 cases treated by ureterosigmoidostomy. *J Urol* 1975;**114**:133.

Stanton SL: Gynecologic complications of epispadias and bladder exstrophy. *Am J Obstet Gynecol* 1974;**119**:749.

Toguri AG & others: Continence in cases of bladder exstrophy. *J Urol* 1978;**119**:538.

Weed JC, McKee DM: Vulvoplasty in cases of exstrophy of the bladder. *Obstet Gynecol* 1974;**43**:512.

Persistent Urachus

Bauer SB, Retik AB: Urachal anomalies and related umbilical disorders. *Urol Clin North Am* 1978;**5**:195.

Blichert-Toft M, Koch F, Nielsen OV: Anatomic variants of the urachus related to clinical appearance and surgical treatment of urachal lesions. *Surg Gynecol Obstet* 1973;**137**:51.

Morin ME & others: Urachal cyst in the adult: Ultrasound diagnosis. *AJR* 1979;**132**:831.

Walden TB, Karafin L, Kendall AR: Urachal diverticulum in a 3-year-old boy. *J Urol* 1979;**122**:554.

Contracture of the Bladder Neck

Grieve J: Bladder neck stenosis in children: Is it important? *Br J Urol* 1967;**39**:13.

Kaplan GW, King LR: An evaluation of Y-V vesicourethroplasty in children. *Surg Gynecol Obstet* 1970;**130**:1059.

Leadbetter GW Jr: Urinary tract infection and obstruction in children. *Clin Pediatr (Phila)* 1966;**5**:377.

Moir JC: Vesicovaginal fistulae caused by wedge-resection of the bladder neck. *Br J Surg* 1966;**53**:102.

Nunn IN: Bladder neck obstruction in children. *J Urol* 1965;**93**:693.

Ochsner MG, Burns E, Henry HH Jr: Incidence of retrograde ejaculation following bladder neck revision in the child. *J Urol* 1970;**104**:596.

Shopfner CE: Roentgenologic evaluation of bladder neck obstruction. *Am J Roentgenol* 1967;**100**:162.

Smith DR: Critique on the concept of vesical neck obstruction in children. *JAMA* 1969;**207**:1686.

Interstitial Cystitis

Badenoch AW: Chronic interstitial cystitis. *Br J Urol* 1971;**43**:718.

Bell ED, Witherington R: Bladder hernias. *Urology* 1980;**15**:127.

Dounis A, Abel BJ, Gow JG: Cecocystoplasty for bladder augmentation. *J Urol* 1980;**123**:164.

Freiha FS, Faysal MH, Stamey TA: The surgical treatment of intractable interstitial cystitis. *J Urol* 1980;**123**:632.

Gordon HL & others: Immunologic aspects of interstitial cystitis. *J Urol* 1973;**109**:228.

Greenberg E & others: Transurethral resection of Hunner's ulcer. *J Urol* 1974;**111**:764.

Jacobo EJ, Stamler FW, Culp DA: Interstitial cystitis followed by total cystectomy. *Urology* 1974;**3**:481.

Jokinen EJ, Oravisto KJ, Alfthan OS: The effect of cystectomy on antitissue antibodies in interstitial cystitis. *Clin Exp Immunol* 1973;**15**:457.

Lapides J: Observations on interstitial cystitis. *Urology* 1975;**5**:610.

Messing EM, Freiha FS: Complication of clorpactin WCS90 therapy for interstitial cystitis. *Urology* 1979;**13**:389.

Messing EM, Stamey TA: Interstitial cystitis: Early diagnosis, pathology and treatment. *Urology* 1978;**12**:381.

Oravisto KJ, Alfthan OS, Jokinen EJ: Interstitial cystitis: Clinical and immunological findings. *Scand J Urol Nephrol* 1970;**4**:37.

Rosin RD & others: Interstitial cystitis. *Br J Urol* 1979;**51**:524.

Shirley SW, Mirelman S: Experiences with colocystoplasties, cecocystoplasties and ileocystoplasties in urologic surgery. *J Urol* 1978;**120**:165.

Stewart BH, Shirley SW: Further experience with intravesical dimethyl sulfoxide in the treatment of interstitial cystitis. *J Urol* 1976;**116**:36.

Utz DC, Zinke H: The masquerade of bladder cancer as interstitial cystitis. *J Urol* 1974;**111**:160.

Weitzenfeld MB & others: Scrotal kidney and ureter: An unusual hernia. *J Urol* 1980;**123**:437.

Worth PHL, Turner-Warwick R: The treatment of interstitial cystitis by cystolysis with observations on cystoplasty. *Br J Urol* 1973;**45**:65.

External Vesical Herniation

Ray B & others: Massive inguinoscrotal bladder herniation. *J Urol* 1977;**118**:330.

Redman JF & others: The treatment of massive scrotal herniation of the bladder. *J Urol* 1973;**110**:59.

Internal Vesical Herniation

Liebeskind AL, Elkin M, Goldman SH: Herniation of the bladder. *Radiology* 1973;**106**:257.

McCarthy MP: Obturator hernia of urinary bladder. *Urology* 1976;**7**:312.

Urinary Stress Incontinence

Beck RP & others: Recurrent urinary stress incontinence treated by the fascia lata sling procedure. *Am J Obstet Gynecol* 1974;**120**:613.

Biggers RD, Soderdahl DW: Per os pubis (POP) urethropexy. *Urology* 1980;**16**:36.

Cobb OE, Ragde H: Simplified correction of female stress incontinence. *J Urol* 1978;**120**:418.

Gershon CR, Diokno AC: Urodynamic evaluation of female stress urinary incontinence. *J Urol* 1978;**119**:787.

McGuire EJ, Lytton B: Pubovaginal sling procedure for stress incontinence. *J Urol* 1978;**119**:82.

McGuire EJ & others: Stress urinary incontinence. *Obstet Gynecol* 1976;**47**:255.

Noll LE, Hutch JA: The SCIPP line: An aid in interpreting the voiding lateral cystourethrogram. *Obstet Gynecol* 1969;**33**:680.

Stamey TA, Schaeffer AJ, Condy M: Clinical and roentgenographic evaluation of endoscopic suspension of the vesical neck for urinary incontinence. *Surg Gynecol Obstet* 1975;**14**:355.

Stewart BH, Banowsky HW, Montague DK: Stress incontinence: Conservative therapy with sympathomimetic drugs. *J Urol* 1976;**115**:558.

Susset JG & others: Urodynamic assessment of stress incontinence and its therapeutic implications. *Surg Gynecol Obstet* 1976;**142**:343.

Tanagho EA: Colpocystourethropexy: The way we do it. *J Urol* 1976;**116**:751.

Tanagho EA: Simplified cystography in stress urinary incontinence. *Br J Urol* 1974;**46**:295.

Tanagho EA: Urodynamics of female urinary incontinence with emphasis on stress incontinence. *J Urol* 1979;**122**:200.

Urinary Incontinence

Cook WA & others: Techniques and results of urodynamic evaluation of children. *J Urol* 1977;**117**:346.

Diokno AC, Taub M: Ephedrine in treatment of urinary incontinence. *Urology* 1975;**5**:624.

Furlow WL: Postprostatectomy urinary incontinence: Etiology, prevention, and selection of surgical treatment. *Urol Clin North Am* 1978;**5**:347.

Kaufman JJ, Raz S: Urethral compression procedure for the treatment of male urinary incontinence. *J Urol* 1979;**121**:605.

McGuire EJ, Woodside JR: Suprapubic suspension of Kaufman urinary incontinence prosthesis. *Urology* 1980;**15**:256.

Merrill DC: Failure to control postprostatectomy urinary incontinence by urethral compression. *Urology* 1977;**9**:36.

Pagani JJ & others: Radiographic evaluation of an artificial urinary sphincter. *Radiology* 1980;**134**:311.

Politano VA: Periurethral teflon injection for urinary incontinence. *Urol Clin North Am* 1978;**5**:415.

Raezer DM & others: A clinical experience with the Scott genitourinary sphincter in the management of urinary incontinence in the pediatric age group. *J Urol* 1980;**123**:546.

Raney AM: Reconstruction of bladder neck and prostatic urethra: Clinical experience with bladder-flap. *Urology* 1974;**3**:324.

Raz S: Diagnosis of urinary incontinence in the male. *Urol Clin North Am* 1978;**5**:305.

Raz S: Pathophysiology of male incontinence. *Urol Clin North Am* 1978;**5**:295.

Rosen M: The Rosen inflatable incontinence prosthesis. *Urol Clin North Am* 1978;**5**:405.

Scott FB: The artificial sphincter in the management of incontinence in the male. *Urol Clin North Am* 1978;**5**:375.

Scott FB, Bradley WE, Timm GW: Treatment of urinary incontinence by implantable prosthetic urinary sphincter. *J Urol* 1974;**112**:75.

Small MP: The Rosen incontinence procedure: A new artificial urinary sphincter for the management of urinary incontinence. *J Urol* 1980;**123**:507.

Tanagho EA, Smith DR: Clinical evaluation of a surgical technique for the correction of complete urinary incontinence. *J Urol* 1972;**107**:402.

Williams DI, Snyder H: Anterior detrusor tube repair for urinary incontinence in children. *Br J Urol* 1976;**48**:671.

Enuresis

Andersen OO, Petersen KE: Enuresis: An attempt at classification of genesis. *Acta Paediatr Scand* 1974;**63**:512.

Arnold ST, Ginsburg A: Enuresis: Incidence and pertinence of genitourinary disease in healthy enuretic children. *Urology* 1973;**2**:437.

Bradley WE, Anderson JT: Techniques for analysis of micturition reflex disturbances in childhood. *Pediatrics* 1977;**59**:546.

Butcher C, Donnai D: Vaginal reflux and enuresis. *Br J Radiol* 1972;**45**:501.

Buttarazzi PJ: Oxybutynin chloride (Ditropan) in enuresis. *J Urol* 1977;**118**:46.

Campbell EW, Young JD Jr: Enuresis and its relationship to electroencephalographic disturbances. *J Urol* 1966;**96**:947.

Close GC: Nocturnal enuresis and the buzzer alarm: Role of the general practitioner. *Br Med J* 1980;**281**:483.

Forsythe WI, Redmond A: Enuresis and spontaneous cure

rate: Study of 1129 enuretics. *Arch Dis Child* 1974;**49**:259.

Fraser MS: Nocturnal enuresis. *Practitioner* 1972;**208**:203.

Gibbon NO & others: Transection of the bladder for adult enuresis and allied conditions. *Br J Urol* 1973;**45**:306.

Kass EJ, Diokno AC, Montealegre A: Enuresis: Principles of management and results of treatment. *J Urol* 1979;**121**:794.

Kolvin I: Enuresis in childhood. *Practitioner* 1975;**214**:33.

Linderholm BE: The cystometric findings in enuresis. *J Urol* 1966;**96**:718.

Marshall S, Marshall HH, Lyon RP: Enuresis: An analysis of various therapeutic approaches. *Pediatrics* 1973;**52**:813.

Martin GI: Imipramine pamoate in the treatment of childhood enuresis. *Am J Dis Child* 1971;**122**:42.

Murphy S & others: Adolescent enuresis: A multiple contingency hypothesis. *JAMA* 1971;**218**:1189.

Oppel WC, Harper PA, Rider RV: Social, psychological, and neurological factors associated with nocturnal enuresis. *Pediatrics* 1968;**42**:627.

Simonds JF: Enuresis: A brief survey of current thinking with respect to pathogenesis and management. *Clin Pediatr (Phila)* 1977;**16**:79.

Foreign Bodies Introduced into the Bladder & Urethra

Najafi E, Maynard JF: Foreign body in lower urinary tract. *Urology* 1975;**5**:117.

Prasad S & others: Foreign bodies in urinary bladder. *Urology* 1973;**2**:258.

Vesical Manifestations of Allergy

Pastinszky I: The allergic diseases of the male genitourinary tract with special reference to allergic urethritis and cystitis. *Urol Int* 1960;**9**:288.

Rubin L, Pincus MB: Eosinophilic cystitis: The relationship of allergy in the urinary tract to eosinophilic cystitis and the pathophysiology of eosinophilia. *J Urol* 1974;**112**:457.

Diverticulum

Barrett DM, Malek RS, Kelalis PP: Observations on vesical diverticulum in childhood. *J Urol* 1976;**116**:234.

Bauer SB, Retik AB: Bladder diverticula in infants and children. *Urology* 1974;**3**:712.

Goldman HJ: A rapid safe technique for removal of a large vesical diverticulum. *J Urol* 1971;**106**:379.

Ostroff EB, Alperstein JB, Young JD Jr: Neoplasm in vesical diverticula: Report of 4 patients, including a 21-year-old. *J Urol* 1973;**110**:65.

Peterson LJ, Paulson DF, Glenn JF: The histopathology of vesical diverticula. *J Urol* 1973;**110**:62.

Reece RW & others: Evaluation of bladder diverticulum using fiberoptic bronchoscope. *Urology* 1974;**3**:790.

Vitale PJ, Woodside JR: Management of bladder diverticula by transurethral resection: Re-evaluation of an old technique. *J Urol* 1979;**122**:744.

Vesical Fistulas

Aycinena JF: Small vesicovaginal fistula. *Urology* 1977;**9**:543.

Birkhoff JD, Wechsler M, Romas NA: Urinary fistulas: Vaginal repair using labial fat pad. *J Urol* 1977;**117**:595.

Carson CC, Malek RS, Remine WH: Urologic aspects of vesicoenteric fistulas. *J Urol* 1978;**119**:744.

Farringer JL Jr & others: Vesicolic fistula. *South Med J* 1974;**67**:1043.

Goodwin WE, Scardino PT: Vesicovaginal and ureterovaginal fistulas: A summary of 25 years of experience. *J Urol* 1980;**123**:370.

Gross M, Peng B: Appendico-vesical fistula. *J Urol* 1969;**102**:697.

Hutch JA, Noll LE: Prevention of vesicovaginal fistulas. *Obstet Gynecol* 1970;**35**:924.

Krompier A & others: Vesicocolonic fistulas in diverticulitis. *J Urol* 1976;**115**:664.

Landes RR: Simple transvesical repair of vesicovaginal fistula. *J Urol* 1979;**122**:604.

Patil U, Waterhouse K, Laungani G: Management of 18 difficult vesicovaginal and urethrovaginal fistulas with modified Ingelman-Sundberg and Martius operations. *J Urol* 1980;**123**:653.

Persky L, Forsythe WE, Herman G: Vesicovaginal fistulas in childhood. *Urology* 1980;**15**:36.

Persky L, Herman G, Guerrier K: Nondelay in vesicovaginal fistula repair. *Urology* 1979;**13**:273.

Raghavaiah NV: Double-dye test to diagnose various types of vaginal fistulas. *J Urol* 1974;**112**:811.

Shatila AH, Ackerman NB: Diagnosis and management of colovesical fistulas. *Surg Gynecol Obstet* 1976;**143**:71.

Shield DE & others: Urologic complications of inflammatory bowel disease. *J Urol* 1976;**115**:701.

Wolfson JS: Vaginography for demonstration of ureterovaginal, vesicovaginal and rectovaginal fistulas, with case reports. *Radiology* 1964;**83**:438.

Perivesical Lipomatosis

Ambos MA & others: The pear-shaped bladder. *Radiology* 1977;**122**:85.

Ballesteros JJ: Surgical treatment of perivesical lipomatosis. *J Urol* 1977;**118**:329.

Church PA, Kazam E: Computed tomography and ultrasound in diagnosis of pelvic lipomatosis. *Urology* 1979;**14**:631.

Crane DB, Smith MJV: Pelvic lipomatosis: Five-year follow-up. *J Urol* 1977;**118**:547.

Levine E, Farber B, Lee KR: Computed tomography in diagnosis of pelvic lipomatosis. *Urology* 1978;**12**:606.

Radinsky S, Cabal E, Shields J: Pelvic lipomatosis. *Urology* 1976;**7**:108.

Sacks SA, Dresnick EJ: Pelvic lipomatosis: Effect of diet. *Urology* 1975;**6**:609.

Susmano DE, Dolin EH: Computed tomography in diagnosis of pelvic lipomatosis. *Urology* 1979;**13**:215.

Radiation Cystitis

Mallik MKB: Study of radiation necrosis of the urinary bladder following treatment of carcinoma of the cervix. *Am J Obstet Gynecol* 1962;**83**:393.

Noninfectious Hemorrhagic Cystitis

Bennett AH: Cyclophosphamide and hemorrhagic cystitis. *J Urol* 1974;**111**:603.

Giulani L & others: Gelatin foam and isobutyl-2-cyanoacrylate in the treatment of life-threatening bladder haemorrhage by selective transcatheter embolisation of the internal iliac arteries. *Br J Urol* 1979;**51**:125.

Holstein P & others: Intravesical hydrostatic pressure treatment: New method for control of bleeding from bladder mucosa. *J Urol* 1973;**109**:234.

McGuire EJ & others: Hemorrhagic radiation cystitis: Treatment. *Urology* 1974;**3**:204.

Marshall FF, Klinefelter HF: Late hemorrhagic cystitis following low-dose cyclophosphamide therapy. *Urology* 1979;**14**:573.

Pyeritz RE & others: An approach to the control of massive hemorrhage in cyclophosphamide-induced cystitis by intravenous vasopressin: A case report. *J Urol* 1978;**120**:253.

Scott MP Jr, Marshall S, Lyon RP: Bladder rupture following formalin therapy for hemorrhage secondary to cyclophosphamide therapy. *Urology* 1974;**3**:364.

Spiro LH & others: Formalin treatment for massive bladder hemorrhage. *Urology* 1973;**2**:669.

Yalla SV & others: Cystitis glandularis with perivesical lipomatosis: Frequent association of two unusual proliferative conditions. *Urology* 1975;**5**:383.

Empyema of the Bladder

Dretler SP: The occurrence of empyema cystitis: Management of the bladder to be defunctionalized. *J Urol* 1972;**108**:82.

Spence HM, Allen TD: Vaginal vesicostomy for empyema of the defunctionalized bladder. *J Urol* 1971;**106**:862.

Congenital Anomalies of the Prostate & Seminal Vesicles

Donohue RE, Greenslade NF: Seminal vesical cyst and ipsilateral renal agenesis. *Urology* 1973;**2**:66.

Feldman RA, Weiss RM: Urinary retention secondary to Müllerian duct cyst in a child. *J Urol* 1972;**108**:647.

Rieser C, Griffin TL: Cysts of the prostate. *J Urol* 1964;**91**:282.

Warren MM, Greene LF: Calculus in the prostatic utricle. *J Urol* 1972;**107**:82.

Bloody Ejaculation

Ross JC: Haemospermia. *Practitioner* 1969;**203**:59.

Stein AJ, Prioleau PG, Catalona WJ: Adenomatous polyps of the prostatic urethra: A cause of hematospermia. *J Urol* 1980;**124**:298.

Tolley DA, Castro JE: Hemospermia. *Urology* 1975;**6**:331.

CONGENITAL ANOMALIES OF THE PENIS & MALE URETHRA

Congenital absence of the penis (apenia) is rare. The urethra opens on the perineum or just inside the rectum. These patients must be assigned a female role. Castration should be done and a vaginoplasty performed later. Estrogen treatment should start at puberty.

Megalopenis may be seen in boys suffering from interstitial cell tumor or hyperplasia or tumor of the adrenal cortex.

Micropenis is often seen in male intersex individuals who have other feminizing traits (eg, hypospadias) and sometimes in otherwise normal-appearing boys with palpable normal-size scrotal testes. In these cases, penile growth is usually obtained by the local application of 0.2% testosterone propionate in a water-miscible ointment base twice daily, or 5% topical testosterone cream once a day (Jacobs, Kaplan, & Gittes, 1975). These authors noted that this therapy caused a significant increase in serum testosterone, so its beneficial effect was not local. Kogan & Williams (1977) are concerned about the boy with micropenis who has no palpable testes. In this type of patient, they recommend a buccal smear and 17-ketosteroid determination. In order to determine the existence or absence of testicular tissue, they administer hCG to see if the 17-ketosteroid level is affected. If it is not, testicular tissue is probably absent, so they would consider sex reversal procedures. (See also Jones, Park, & Rock, 1978.)

Hinman (1972) reports that surgical release of the corpora allows a significant gain in length. He points out (Hinman, 1980) that boys with endocrinopathy (eg, low FSH) may respond to hormonal therapy, whereas those with anomalous micropenis will not. Klugo & Cerney (1978) recommend a combination of hCG and 10% topical testosterone cream for boys with hypogonadotropic hypogonadism.

Duplication of the urethra is occasionally seen. The structures may be complete or incomplete (Naparstek & others, 1980). Wirtshafter & others (1980) report a case with 3 complete urethras. Resection of all but one complete urethra is recommended.

URETHRAL STRICTURE

Congenital urethral stricture occasionally occurs in male infants. The 2 most common sites are in the region of the corona (fossa navicularis) and in the membranous urethra. Severe strictures cause back pressure from obstruction, which is followed by dilatation of the urethra, hypertrophy of the vesical musculature, and functional ureterovesical obstruction or reflux, both leading to hydronephrosis. Symptoms may be those of obstruction (eg, urinary stream of small caliber, hyperdistended bladder) or secondary infection (eg, fever, dysuria).

Excretory urograms may show the changes caused by obstruction (vesical trabeculation, hydronephrosis). The postvoiding film may reveal residual urine. A urethrogram (Figs 6–10 and 29–1) will delineate the degree and length of the stricture.

Every child with the symptoms mentioned above should be examined cystoscopically. The passage of the instrument will be arrested by the stricture. Urethral dilatations with sounds or filiforms and followers will keep the stricture open, but the prognosis depends upon the degree of damage suffered by the upper urinary tract. Surgical repair of the stricture is usually necessary. Congenital diaphragmatic strictures respond well to overdilatation or internal urethrotomy (Fig 29–1).

POSTERIOR OR PROSTATIC URETHRAL VALVES

Posterior (prostatic) urethral valves or diaphragms are folds of mucous membrane on the floor of the prostatic urethra (Fig 29–2). Uehling (1980) recognizes 3 clinical presentations: (1) mild obstructive symptoms, hematuria, normal excretory urograms; (2) moderate obstruction, abnormal urograms; and (3) severe obstruction with uremia. Severe obstruction is usually associated with renal dysplasia, dilatation of the prostatic urethra, hypertrophy of the detrusor (trabeculation), vesical diverticula, and hypertrophy of the trigonal muscles. Trigonal hypertrophy tends to cause functional obstruction of the intravesical ureter and hydroureteronephrosis. In the advanced stage, vesicoureteral reflux may occur, but less than half of

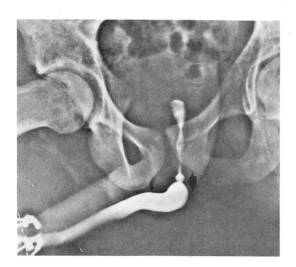

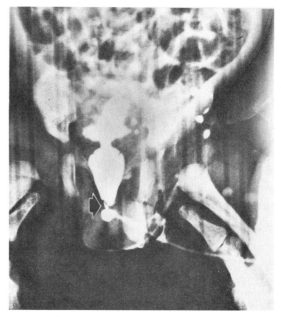

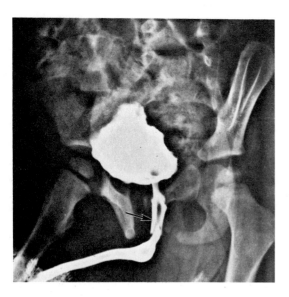

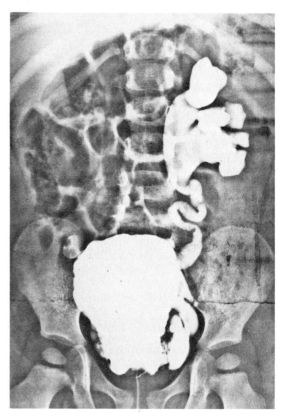

Figure 29–1. *Above left:* Retrograde urethrogram showing congenital diaphragmatic stricture. *Above right:* Posterior urethral valves revealed on voiding cystourethrography. Arrow points to area of severe stenosis at distal end of prostatic urethra. *Below left:* Posterior urethral valves. Patient would not void with cystography. Retrograde urethrogram showing valves (see arrow). *Below right:* Cystogram, same patient. Free vesicoureteral reflux and vesical trabeculation with diverticula.

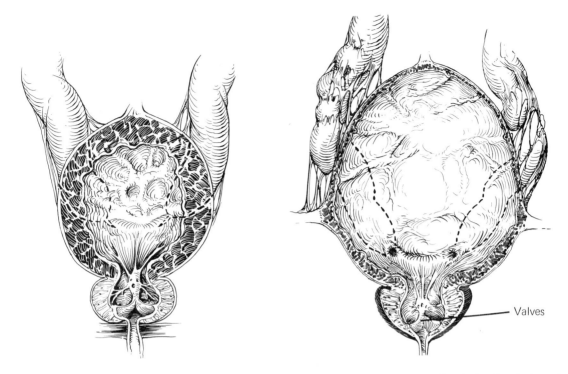

Figure 29–2. Posterior urethral valves. *Left:* Dilatation of the prostatic urethra, hypertrophy of vesical wall and trigone in stage of compensation; bilateral hydroureters secondary to trigonal hypertrophy. *Right:* Attenuation of bladder musculature in stage of decompensation; advanced ureteral dilatation and tortuosity, usually secondary to vesicoureteral reflux.

these boys exhibit reflux. Infection under these circumstances is almost inevitable, but it is apt to occur late because of the normally sterile proximal urethra. A number of cases of intraperitoneal rupture of the kidney with urinary ascites have been reported in newborns with prostatic valves. In a few, ascites is severe enough to cause respiratory difficulty. Paracentesis may be necessary to save life (Kellett, Turner, & Levkoff, 1973). Tank, Carey, & Seifert (1980) recommend percutaneous or surgical nephrostomy if ascites persists. In milder cases, relief of the prostatic obstruction will cause the urinary extravasation to subside.

Clinical Findings

A. Symptoms: Difficulty in initiating urination and a very weak urinary stream are the principal symptoms. A distended bladder may be noted by the parents. Infection causes frequency, enuresis, and burning on urination. High fever suggests renal infection, but infection can be present without febrile response or vesical symptoms.

In the later stages, after renal insufficiency has developed, the child may suffer from anorexia, loss of weight, and anemia and fails to thrive.

B. Signs: A distended bladder may be seen, felt, or percussed. More commonly, however, a hard mass is felt deep in the pelvis. This represents the severely hypertrophied bladder. A poor urinary stream may be observed. Often, however, examina-

tion may reveal nothing more than evidence of chronic illness.

C. Laboratory Findings: Anemia due to chronic infection or uremia may be noted. The urine is often infected. Impairment of renal function may be discovered by noting loss of concentrating power of the kidneys or elevation of the blood urea nitrogen and serum creatinine.

A diaper PSP test (see Chapter 5) should be performed on all infants suspected of having urinary tract obstruction. Excretion of less than 30% of the dye in 3 hours requires explanation. Little dye will be recovered when valves are present because of the combination of impaired renal function and transport of urine.

D. X-Ray Findings: Excretory urograms may demonstrate hydroureters and hydronephroses as well as irregularity in the outline of the bladder (trabeculation) or diverticula. The postvoiding film will reveal considerable retention of urine. Voiding cystourethrograms may reveal wide dilatation of the prostatic urethra and the negative shadows representing the valves (Fig 29–1). This procedure is the definitive diagnostic step. The cystograms may demonstrate reflux of the radiopaque material into the ureters and kidneys. The resulting urograms usually preclude the need for ureteral catheterization and retrograde urograms. If the child cannot be induced to void, retrograde urethrography may show the valves (Fig 29–1).

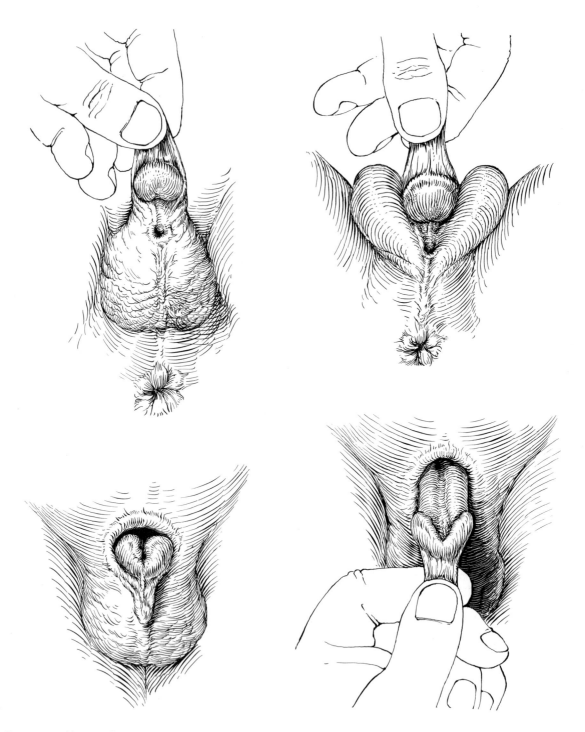

Figure 29–3. Hypospadias and epispadias. *Above left:* Hypospadias, penoscrotal type. Redundant dorsal foreskin that is deficient ventrally; ventral chordee. *Above right:* Hypospadias, midscrotal type. Chordee more marked. Penis often small. *Below left:* Epispadias. Redundant ventral foreskin that is absent dorsally; severe dorsal chordee. *Below right:* Traction on foreskin reveals dorsal defect.

E. Instrumental Examination: A catheter can usually be passed without difficulty, thereby ruling out stricture. These valves are only obstructive from within outward. Cystoscopy and panendoscopy show trabeculation of the bladder wall, occasionally diverticula, and hypertrophy of the trigone. The mucosal diaphragms may be visualized on the floor of the prostatic urethra, although they may be torn during instrumentation and therefore may be missed.

Treatment

Treatment consists of destruction of the valves. The simplest method is to pass very large sounds (up to 30F) through a perineal urethrotomy, thus tearing the valves. Transurethral resection has its advocates. If the changes proximal to the valves are not severe, destruction of the valves is all that is necessary. Johnston & Kulatilake (1971) found that the majority of their cases fell into this category.

Almost half of the boys will show vesicoureteral reflux, but in one-third, reflux will cease after relief of the primary obstruction. Johnston (1979) found that bilateral reflux had a worse prognosis than the unilateral type. He also observed that continuing reflux usually results in a functionless kidney on that side, whereas useful function can be achieved if reflux is corrected. Because of hypertrophy of the trigone, functional obstruction of the ureterovesical junctions may develop. After treatment of the valves, the hypertrophy of the trigone subsides with lessening of the abnormal pull on the intramural ureters; secondary hydroureteronephrosis may subside.

In the most severe cases of hydronephrosis, removal of the primary obstruction may not be sufficient because of ureteral atony or obstruction; therefore, loop cutaneous ureterostomies may have to be done to preserve renal function (Pinto, Markland, & Fraley, 1978). This will lead to resolution of ureteral dilatation and hydronephrosis. When optimum repair is obtained, reconstruction of the urinary tract can usually be accomplished. Otherwise, permanent drainage (eg, via cutaneous ureterostomy) may be all that can be offered.

The period of urinary diversion should be as short as possible. Tanagho (1974) has observed that, after prolonged proximal diversion, permanent vesical contracture occurs in some patients.

Following destruction of the posterior urethral valves, about one-third of patients will have normal urinary control, another third will suffer stress incontinence, and the remainder will have poor control (Whitaker, Keeton, & Williams, 1972). Johnston & Kulatilake (1971) have observed that control is apt to improve appreciably at puberty.

Complicating urosepsis should be treated by whatever drug is indicated by culture and sensitivity tests. In many cases infection cannot be eradicated even after definitive surgical repair; suppressive therapy should then be applied.

Prognosis

The prognosis depends upon the degree of destruction of the upper urinary tract. Too often, the diagnosis is not made until renal damage has become severe. Some of these children continue to lose function from incurable renal infection even after the obstruction has been relieved.

Early diagnosis requires that the pediatrician or a nurse in the newborn nursery make it a point to observe the size and force of the urinary stream in all male infants before they leave the hospital.

ANTERIOR URETHRAL VALVES

A few instances of anterior urethral valves in boys have been reported. Patients may suffer from enuresis or leakage of urine and an impaired urinary stream. A voiding cystourethrogram or a retrograde urethrogram will reveal the valve. Panendoscopy will visualize the lesion, which can be destroyed by fulguration or fragmentation by the passage of sounds (Golimbu & others, 1978; Firlit, Firlit, & King, 1978).

URETHRORECTAL & VESICORECTAL FISTULAS

Urethrorectal and, more rarely, vesicorectal fistulas are sometimes seen. They are almost always associated with imperforate anus occurring when the urorectal fold that divides the rectum from the urogenital sinus fails to develop completely. This permits a communication between the rectum and the urethra (in the region of the verumontanum) or bladder. (See Chapter 2.)

An infant with such a fistula passes fecal material and gas through the urethra. The anus may develop normally (open externally), in which case urine may be passed through the rectum.

Cystoscopy and panendoscopy usually visualize the fistulous opening. Barium given by mouth will reach the blind rectal pouch, and appropriate radiograms will measure the distance between the end of the rectum and the perineum. The imperforate anus must be opened immediately and the fistula closed, or, if the rectum lies quite high, temporary sigmoid colostomy must be performed. Definitive surgery, with repair of the urethral fistula, can be undertaken later.

HYPOSPADIAS

Hypospadias in the male is evidence of feminization. The hypospadiac penis presents ventral curvature (chordee) distal to the urethral meatus. The meatus opens on the ventral side of the penis proximal to the tip of the glans penis; it may present as far back as the perineum. When the orifice is in the scrotal or perineal area, the scrotum is bifid, thereby assuming the appearance of labia majora. The foreskin is deficient on the ventrum (Fig 29–3). In extreme degrees of hypospadias, the penis may be unusually small, simulating a hypertrophied clitoris. Aarskog (1979) has noted that the incidence of this anomaly is increasing. He suspects that in some instances, ingestion of progestins or contraceptive pills by the mother may be the cause. Bauer, Bull, & Retik (1979) feel that the condition is hereditary, since 14% of boys with hypospadias have a brother similarly afflicted and 9% of their fathers have hypospadias. Other anomalies are apt to be observed. Shima & others (1979) noted undescended testes, enlarged utricle, prepenile scrotum, and hypoplastic testes. The more severe the degree of hypospadias, the more anomalies are found.

The penoscrotal and perineal types (Fig 29–3) are usually associated with enlargement of the prostatic utricle, which represents a remnant of the fused ends of the müllerian ducts (Devine & others, 1980). At times a rudimentary or even complete vaginal tract and uterus are present. For this reason, chromatin (genetic) sex should be established by a buccal smear. Dwoskin & Kuhn (1974) have found that half of these patients have a hernia, and of these, 50% are bilateral. This was demonstrated by instilling radiopaque fluid into the peritoneal cavity; then, with the patient prone, 3–4 x-rays were taken during the next 45 minutes. There is no deficiency of the sphincters, so incontinence does not occur.

Routine excretory urograms are apt to reveal that 5–10% of these boys have minor congenital anomalies of the kidney. Rarely do these require surgical intervention, however.

Adequate surgical correction demands, above all, straightening of the shaft so that normal intercourse is possible. This must be followed by formation of a urethra that extends to or near the tip of the glans so that semen can be deposited deep in the vagina. For psychologic reasons, it is best that this corrective surgery be completed before school age.

CHORDEE WITHOUT HYPOSPADIAS

Congenital ventral chordee without hypospadias is occasionally seen. It appears to be caused by a short urethra that acts as a bow-string, particularly with erection. Such a lesion interferes with intercourse. If the penis has adequate length, the dorsal surface can be shortened by (1) excising elliptical portions of the tunica albuginea on the dorsum of the penis on either side of the midline (Redman, 1978), or (2) by making transverse cuts in a similar position and then closing them longitudinally, thus shortening the dorsum (Udall, 1980).

Devine & Horton (1973) have found that in most cases, fibrous tissue will be found in associa-

tion with the urethra and corpus spongiosum. Resection of this tissue leads to a straight penis.

EPISPADIAS

Epispadias is considerably less common than hypospadias, but it is more disabling. It is quite rare in females. The urethra opens on the dorsum of the penis at some point proximal to the glans. The most common site is at the abdominopenile junction. Dorsal curvature (chordee) is also present (Fig 29–3). More serious, however, is the fact that this dorsal defect usually extends proximally, so that a defect of the urinary sphincters is present. This causes urinary incontinence. The pubic bones are separated as in exstrophy of the bladder. It should be noted that epispadias is nothing more than a relatively mild degree of exstrophy.

Treatment requires correction of urinary incontinence and of the inability to copulate. Repair of the urinary sphincters has not been too successful, but Tanagho & Smith (1972) have obtained complete continence by interposing a tubed flap of anterior bladder wall between the bladder and the prostatic urethra. Plastic repair of the penis requires reduction of the chordee followed by urethroplasty, which advances the urinary orifice to the distal end of the shaft (Duckett, 1978; Hendren, 1979). If urinary continence cannot be achieved, some type of urinary diversion may have to be provided (eg, ureteroileal conduit).

ACQUIRED DISEASES OF THE PENIS & MALE URETHRA

PRIAPISM

Priapism is a rather rare affliction. It consists of a prolonged erection, unassociated with sexual stimulation, which is usually painful. The blood in the corpora cavernosa becomes sludgelike rather than clotted. Unlike an erection caused by psychic stimuli, the corpus spongiosum is not involved; the glans remains soft. This erection may last for days. About 25% of cases are associated with leukemia, metastatic carcinoma, local trauma, or sickle cell disease, but as a rule the mechanism is not clear. Priapism is occasionally seen following injuries to the spinal cord.

Fitzpatrick (1973) has shown obstruction of the deep dorsal vein on corpora cavernosograms as the basic cause of the erection.

If spontaneous subsidence of priapism does not occur within a few hours, the following regimen should be instituted: ice-water enemas should first be ordered; temporary (even permanent) subsidence of the erection may occur. Evacuation of the sludged blood of the corpora by needle and syringe should next be tried. The corpora should then be thoroughly irrigated with an anticoagulant, followed by bandage compression. Unless the erection subsides promptly, either spontaneously or in response to treatment, the septa of the corpora cavernosa undergo fibrosis. This results in impotence—inability to gain an erection.

Using arteriography, Evans & Young (1973) demonstrated occlusion of the internal pudendal arteries at the level of the urogenital diaphragm. This appears to be an obvious cause of the impotence.

In patients with sickle cell anemia, Seeler (1973) suggests giving a massive transfusion of packed red cells to double the hematocrit. Cessation of pain and subsidence of the erection occurred in 24 hours. Kinney & others (1975) and Baron & Leiter (1978) agree that in these cases exchange transfusions were indicated. They found that at times a vascular shunt was necessary. Shreibman, Gee, & Grabstald (1974) lowered the peripheral blood count in patients with chronic granulocytic leukemia by administering either cytarabine or hydroxyurea, with good results.

If conservative treatment fails, prompt operation is mandatory. Either saphenous vein-corpus cavernosum or bilateral corpora cavernosa-spongiosum shunt (Guerriera, 1978) should be considered. Once the erection subsides, normal blood flow may return, in which case the shunts close spontaneously. Permanent inability to gain an erection often persists, however.

Because the ultimate sexual result has been poor, other methods of therapy have recently been advocated. In a patient with priapism following perineal trauma, pelvic angiography revealed dilatation of both internal pudendal arteries, with one artery occluded by autologous clot. Removal of the clot did not cause loss of potency. The result was excellent (Wear, Crummy, & Munson, 1977). Douglas (1976) and Gates & Middleton (1980) placed a cannula into the corpora and connected it to an arm vein. The corpora were decompressed by means of a pump. The patients treated in this manner maintained potency. A recent technic described by Winter (1978) seems to have merit. He formed a fistula between the glans penis and the corpora cavernosa by means of a Travenol biopsy needle. This appears to be the quickest and simplest method of shunting.

PLASTIC INDURATION OF THE PENIS
(Peyronie's Disease)

Fibrosis of the covering sheaths of the corpora cavernosa occurs without known cause, usually in men over age 45 years. This fibrotic area will not permit lengthening of the involved surface (dorsum) with erection, so that the penis bends toward the involved area (chordee). In the early stages, erection is accompanied by pain. The degree of curvature may finally preclude coitus. Apparently the process begins as vasculitis in the connective tissue beneath the tunica albuginea of the penis and then extends to adjacent structures. This leads to fibrosis and at times calcification or even ossification.

Palpation of the shaft reveals a well-demarcated, raised plaque of fibrosis that is usually in the midline of the dorsum near the base of the organ, although it may be placed more laterally or distally. X-ray may reveal areas of calcification within the indurated area.

Treatment is unsatisfactory. Low-dosage x-ray therapy has some value. Recently there has been some enthusiasm for operation. Poutasse (1972) exposes the center of the plaque and chips away the scar tissue for a distance of 2–3 cm down to cavernous tissue. This maneuver allows separation of the remaining plaque. Wild, Devine, & Horton (1979) excise the plaque and replace it with a dermal graft taken from the abdomen. Hall & Turner (1977) and Hicks & others (1978) have experienced good results with this technic. Such procedures should be considered if intercourse is difficult or impossible.

Bruskewitz & Raz (1980) incise the plaque and then place Small-Carrion prostheses in the corpora cavernosa. These keep the penis straight and correct the impaired erection that is often noticed distal to the plaque. Pryor & Fitzpatrick (1979) make longitudinal incisions in the tunica albuginea of the ventral side of the penis on either side of the corpus spongiosum. The incisions are closed transversely, thus foreshortening the ventrum and correcting the chordee.

PHIMOSIS

Phimosis is a disease in which it is impossible to retract the foreskin over the glans. It may be a complication of circumcision when too much skin is left behind. It is usually secondary to infection beneath a redundant foreskin. Poor hygiene frequently contributes to the infection. Such a reaction causes tissue injury, and healing is by fibrosis. The preputial opening thereby becomes contracted, so that the foreskin cannot be retracted. This further facilitates the infectious process, usually by mixed organisms, including anaerobes, vibrios, and spirochetes. Such chronic irritation of many years' standing may be the cause of squamous epithelioma. Stones may form in the preputial sac.

The patient may complain only of inability to retract the foreskin, but more commonly he is disturbed by symptoms and signs of infection (eg, redness and swelling of the foreskin, purulent discharge, and local pain).

Treatment consists of measures to control the infection (hot soaks, antibiotics). A dorsal slit of the foreskin is necessary if infection is marked. Circumcision should be performed when the inflammatory reaction has subsided.

PARAPHIMOSIS

Paraphimosis is a condition in which the foreskin, once retracted behind the glans, cannot be replaced in its normal position. This is due to chronic inflammation under the redundant foreskin, which leads to contracture of the preputial skin ring.

This tight ring of skin, caught behind the glans, causes venous occlusion that leads to edema of the glans and further disproportion between the size of the glans and the caliber of the preputial opening. If neglected, arterial occlusion may supervene and gangrene of the glans may develop.

Paraphimosis can usually be treated by squeezing the glans firmly for at least 5 minutes, thus reducing its size. The glans is then pushed proximally as the prepuce is moved distally. If manual reduction fails, incision of the constricting tissue is indicated. Once the inflammation and edema have subsided, circumcision should be performed.

CIRCUMCISION

In most countries, routine circumcision is practiced at birth. Unfortunately, in unskilled hands, the use of various mechanical devices has at times caused removal of too much penile skin or even resection of a portion or all of the glans. It seems that the most common cause of urethral meatal stenosis is excoriation of the denuded meatus following circumcision.

Circumcision does prevent phimosis, paraphimosis, and balanoposthitis in adolescence and adult life. The diabetic suffers a high incidence of the latter. Circumcision is indicated in this instance. It is rare for the male circumcised at birth to develop penile cancer, which carries a mortality rate of 33%. For these reasons, routine neonatal circumcision seems indicated.

URETHRAL STRICTURE

Today, acquired urethral stricture is a rare complication of severe gonococcal urethritis but a common sequela of urethral injury, particularly that caused by injury to the membranous urethra secondary to fracture of the pelvis (see Chapter 16). It sometimes follows endoscopy. In all cases the urethra heals by the proliferation of fibroblasts, producing contraction.

Pathogenesis & Pathology

A severe degree of stenosis causes changes typical of obstruction. These include (1) dilatation of the urethra proximal to the stricture, (2) ectasia of the prostatic ducts, (3) compensatory changes in the bladder musculature, and (4) hydroureteronephrosis secondary to hypertrophy of the ureterotrigonal complex or vesicoureteral reflux. Because of stasis, infection occurs that may cause periurethral abscess, urethrocutaneous fistulas, prostatitis, cystitis, and pyelonephritis. If the organisms split urea, vesical or renal calculi may form. Urethral stricture, then, may cause severe damage to the urinary tract.

Clinical Findings

A. Symptoms: The most common symptom is gradual diminution of the force and caliber of the urinary stream. Sudden urinary retention may occur if an infection at the site of stricture is exacerbated. A history of urethral injury or severe untreated gonorrhea can usually be obtained. Symptoms of cystitis may be noted. There may be fever secondary to prostatitis or pyelonephritis.

B. Signs: Periurethral induration may be found at the site of the stricture. A tender mass may be present if periurethral abscess has developed. Perineal urinary fistulas may be noted. A visible or palpable bladder may be found if urinary retention has supervened. Prostatic massage and culture of the secretions may reveal evidence of prostatitis.

C. Laboratory Findings: If infection is present, the white blood count may be elevated and pus and bacteria will be found in the urine. PSP excretion may be diminished if there is renal damage or residual urine.

D. X-Ray Findings: A urethrogram and voiding cystourethrogram will reveal the site and degree of the stricture. Fistulas may be demonstrated (Fig 29–4). After urethral dilatation, a cystogram may show a thickened, trabeculated bladder and, possibly, ureteral reflux. Excretory urograms may reveal urinary calculi or changes compatible with healed pyelonephritis.

E. Instrumental Examination: A catheter or sound of average size (22F) will be arrested at the site of stricture. Panendoscopy may visualize it. Cystoscopy (done after urethral dilatation) will show hypertrophy of the vesical muscle and, often, inflammation.

Differential Diagnosis

Prostatic or bladder neck obstruction may cause similar symptoms but does not impede passage of a urethral catheter. An enlarged (or cancerous) gland is usually found on rectal examination.

Carcinoma of the urethra can mimic urethral stricture, but panendoscopy and biopsy of the visualized tumor will establish the proper diagnosis.

Complications

Prostatitis, cystitis, and pyelonephritis are common complications. Periurethral abscess may

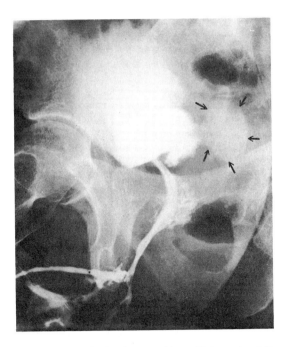

Figure 29–4. Urethral stricture with multiple perineal fistulas. Voiding cystourethrogram showing stricture of perineal urethra, multiple fistulas, dilated prostatic ducts, and vesical diverticulum outlined by arrows.

develop at the stricture site and may resolve or rupture through the skin, causing a urethrocutaneous fistula. Urinary stones may form secondary to stasis and infection.

Treatment

A. Specific Measures:

1. Dilatation–After local urethral or general anesthesia has been achieved and the urethra distended with water-soluble lubricant, a 22F sound should be gently passed (Fig 9–4). If this is arrested, a 20F sound should be tried. Smaller sounds should not be used, for their tips may perforate the friable urethra at the site of the stricture.

Next, passage of a filiform should be attempted (Figs 9–5 and 9–6). If one passes to the bladder, an appropriate follower can be screwed onto its end. If the smallest follower will not penetrate the stricture, the filiform should be taped in place; the patient will be able to void around it. This maneuver will allow subsidence of the inflammatory reaction, so that after a day or so dilatation will be possible. If a filiform cannot be passed and the patient is in urinary retention, suprapubic cystostomy must be done.

Once an instrument has been passed through the stricture, 2 methods for urethral dilatation are available:

a. The stricture should be dilated to 18–20F. A 14–16F catheter should then be passed into the bladder and left indwelling. After 48 hours, the next

size can usually be easily passed; this procedure can be repeated every 2 days until a 24–26F catheter has been placed. This method is relatively painless.

b. Sounds of increasing sizes should be passed to the point of urethral tolerance. This procedure can then be repeated, using larger sounds at weekly intervals until a 24–26F sound can be passed. This method achieves results more quickly but is more painful.

Dilatation of a urethral stricture is palliative treatment. Sounds should be passed at increasing intervals (eg, 2 weeks, 1 month, 3 months, 6 months). Periodic sounding must be done indefinitely.

2. Surgery–

a. Endoscopic internal urethrotomy–Optical urethrotomy is currently in vogue, although "blind" internal urethrotomy has been performed for many years. The urethrotome is passed and the stricture visualized. The stricture is then cut through dorsally. A catheter is left in place for 1–4 days. The results are quite satisfactory in 70–80% of patients (Smith, Dunn, & Dounis, 1979; Sacknoff & Kerr, 1980; Walther, Parsons, & Schmidt, 1980).

b. Surgical reconstruction–If the above methods fail, open surgical methods must be resorted to. If there is a short stricture in the perineal or pendulous urethra, it should be excised and an end-to-end anastomosis done (Azoury & Freiha, 1976). Long strictures of the pendulous urethra are best handled by splitting the stricture and suturing the edges of the open urethra to adjacent skin. A Denis-Browne type of repair can then be accomplished.

Strictures involving the membranous urethra present the most difficult problem. The perineal or transpubic operations described by Turner-Warwick (1977), Badenoch (Tilak, Dhayagude, & Joshi, 1976), Pierce (1979), and Waterhouse, Laungani, & Patil (1980) are satisfactory. Devine, Wendelken, & Devine Jr (1979) excise the stricture and replace it with a tube made of full-thickness skin or incise the stricture and enlarge the diameter with a patch graft. Betts, Texter, & Crane (1978) and Oswalt, Lloyd, & Bueschen (1979) also claim excellent results utilizing this technic.

B. Treatment of Complications: Infection of the kidneys or bladder requires antimicrobial therapy, particularly at the time of urethral dilatation (which may exacerbate preexisting infection). Periurethral abscess may resolve with medical treatment. If it does not, surgical drainage will be necessary. Urethrocutaneous fistulas may close spontaneously once the stricture is dilated. If they do not, surgical correction must be done.

Prognosis

Most urethral strictures can be kept open by periodic dilatations; a few will require surgical treatment. Their deleterious effects on renal function must always be kept in mind.

URETHRAL WARTS
(Condylomata Acuminata)
(See also Chapter 32.)

Men with cutaneous condylomas may complain of bloody spotting from the urethra or a wart just inside the meatus. Diagnosis can be made by panendoscopy or urethrography (Pollack & others, 1978). Treatment by transurethral fulguration is adequate if only a few warts are present; if a great many must be so treated, extensive electrocoagulation could lead to stricture formation.

Rosenberg & al-Askari (1973) recommend intraurethral instillation of thiotepa once a week for 7–10 weeks. Sixty milligrams of the drug are dissolved in 5 mL of water and mixed with 10 mL of a mixture of water and water-soluble lubricant. The drug should be retained for 30 minutes by clamping the glans. Before each instillation, a white blood cell and platelet count must be done to be sure absorption has not caused an adverse hematopoietic effect.

Bissada, Redman, & Sulieman (1974) had similar success with the use of fluorouracil. They instilled 5 mL of a 5% solution for 20 minutes twice a week for 5 weeks. The drug was retained for 20 minutes. If a few lesions persist, they recommend its use once a week for another 6–8 weeks. Weimar & others (1978) observed that the use of fluorouracil liquid or cream led to irritation of the scrotum from leakage. They made up suppositories of this drug, inserting them twice a day for 7–10 days, with good results.

Gigax & Robison (1971) recommend the instillation of 0.5% colchicine, which was successful in eradicating the warts in 4 cases. The author, however, knows of 2 cases in which urethral absorption of the drug endangered life. Fuselier & others (1980) destroyed meatal condylomas with the CO_2 laser and recommend this technic when other methods fail. They noted no side-effects.

Occasionally, giant condylomas (Buschke-Loewenstein tumors) may be seen that involve the glans penis and often the urethra. They are often confused with fungating carcinoma. Biopsy is diagnostic. Surgical extirpation is the treatment of choice.

FISTULA

Fistulas between the urethra and penile skin usually follow an exacerbation of infection just proximal to a stricture. A fistula may develop secondary to a carcinoma of the urethra or to a foreign body that has been inserted into the channel (eg, bobby pin). Periurethritis and abscess formation may then develop. Spontaneous drainage may occur. Urethroscopy (panendoscopy) and urethrography will reveal the site and cause of the fistulous opening. Biopsy may be indicated. When all evidence of inflammation has disappeared, surgical closure can be performed.

STENOSIS OF THE EXTERNAL URINARY MEATUS

Mild stenosis of the external meatus is fairly common and should be sought in newborn males. It may be congenital or acquired after circumcision (Belman & others, 1978). Damage to the proximal urinary tract is exceedingly rare. Stenosis is often seen in hypospadias, but it is usually more apparent than real. Passage of a forceful urinary stream is evidence against a harmful lesion. In a few cases, bloody spotting may occur, which usually implies meatal stenosis with a small ulcer just proximal to it. Meatotomy is indicated.

THROMBOPHLEBITIS OF THE SUPERFICIAL PENILE VEINS

Not infrequently, thrombophlebitis of the circumferential veins just proximal to the corona develops. The patient notes a firm ridge of tender tissue and redness of the overlying skin. Examination reveals thrombosis of the vein; this may also involve the longitudinal superficial dorsal vein. No treatment is required. Recanalization takes place in a few months.

• • •

References

CONGENITAL ANOMALIES

Penis & Male Urethra

Farah R, Reno G: Congenital absence of the penis. *J Urol* 1972;**107**:154.

Hinman F Jr: Microphallus: Characteristics and choice of treatment from a study of 20 cases. *J Urol* 1972;**107**:499.

Hinman F Jr: Microphallus: Distinction between anomalous and endocrine types. *J Urol* 1980;**123**:412.

Jacobs SC, Kaplan GW, Gittes RF: Topical testosterone therapy for penile growth. *Urology* 1975;**6**:708.

Johnston WG Jr, Yeatman GW, Weigel JW: Congenital absence of the penis. *J Urol* 1977;**117**:508.

Jones HW Jr, Park IJ, Rock JA: Technique of surgical sex reassignment for micropenis and allied conditions. *Am J Obstet Gynecol* 1978;**132**:870.

Klugo RC, Cerny JC: Response of micropenis to topical testosterone and gonadotropin. *J Urol* 1978;**119**:667.

Kogan SJ, Williams DI: The micropenis syndrome: Clinical observations and expectations for growth. *J Urol* 1977;**118**:311.

Naparstek S & others: Complete duplication of male urethra in children. *Urology* 1980;**16**:391.

Wirtshafter A & others: Complete trifurcation of the urethra. *J Urol* 1980;**123**:431.

Stenosis of the External Urinary Meatus

Allen JS, Summers JL: Meatal stenosis in children. *J Urol* 1974;**112**:526.

Belman AB & others: Urethral meatal stenosis in males. *Pediatrics* 1978;**61**:778.

Urethral Stricture

Cobb BG, Wolf JA Jr, Ansell JS: Congenital stricture of the proximal urethral bulb. *J Urol* 1968;**99**:629.

Leadbetter GW Jr: The etiology, symptoms, and treatment of urethral strictures in male children. *Pediatrics* 1963;**31**:80.

Redman JF, Fraiser LP: Apparent congenital anterior urethral strictures in brothers. *J Urol* 1979;**122**:707.

Posterior or Prostatic Urethral Valves

Friedland GW & others: Posterior urethral valves. *Clin Radiol* 1977;**27**:367.

Johnston JH: Vesicoureteric reflux with urethral valves. *Br J Urol* 1979;**51**:100.

Johnston JH, Kulatilake AE: The sequelae of posterior urethral valves. *Br J Urol* 1971;**43**:743.

Kellett JW, Turner WR Jr, Levkoff AH: Paracentesis in the management of neonatal ascites. *Urology* 1973;**2**:672.

Pinto MH, Markland C, Fraley EE: Posterior urethral valves managed by cutaneous ureterostomy with subsequent ureteral reconstruction. *J Urol* 1978;**119**:696.

Rabinowitz R & others: Upper tract management when posterior urethral valve ablation is insufficient. *J Urol* 1979;**122**:370.

Schoenberg HW, Miyai K, Gregory JG: Posterior urethral valves. *Urology* 1976;**7**:611.

Scott TW: Urinary ascites secondary to posterior urethral valves. *J Urol* 1976;**116**:87.

Tanagho EA: Congenitally obstructed bladder: Fate after prolonged defunctionalization. *J Urol* 1974;**111**:102.

Tank ES, Carey TC, Seifert AL: Management of neonatal urinary ascites. *Urology* 1980;**16**:270.

Uehling DT: Posterior urethral valves: Functional classification. *Urology* 1980;**15**:27.

Whitaker RH: The ureter in posterior urethral valves. *Br J Urol* 1973;**45**:395.

Whitaker RH, Keeton JE, Williams DI: Posterior urethral valves: A study of urinary control after operation. *J Urol* 1972;**108**:167.

Anterior Urethral Valves

Firlit RS, Firlit CF, King LR: Obstructing anterior urethral valves in children. *J Urol* 1978;**119**:819.

Golimbu M & others: Anterior urethral valves. *Urology* 1978;**12**:343.

Urethrorectal & Vesicorectal Fistulas

Wesolowski S, Bulinski W: Vesico-intestinal fistulae and recto-urethral fistulae. *Br J Urol* 1973;**45**:34.

Hypospadias

Aarskog D: Current concepts in cancer: Maternal progestins as a possible cause of hypospadias. *N Engl J Med* 1979;**300**:75.

Allen TD, Spence HM: The surgical treatment of coronal hypospadias and related problems. *J Urol* 1968;**100**:504.

Bailen J, Howerton LW: Decreased fistula formation with modified Denis Browne hypospadias repair. *J Urol* 1980;**123**:754.

Bauer SB, Bull MJ, Retik AB: Hypospadias: A familial study. *J Urol* 1979;**121**:474.

Devine CJ Jr, Franz JP, Horton CE: Evaluation and treatment of patients with failed hypospadias repair. *J Urol* 1978;**119**:223.

Devine CJ Jr, Horton CE: Hypospadias repair. *J Urol* 1977;**118**:188.

Devine CJ Jr & others: Utricular configuration in hypospadias and intersex. *J Urol* 1980;**123**:407.

Dwoskin JY, Kuhn JP: Herniograms and hypospadias. *Urology* 1974;**3**:458.

Gearhart JP, Witherington R: The Denis-Browne hypospadias repair revisited. *J Urol* 1979;**122**:66.

Genetics of hypospadias. *Br Med J* 1972;**4**:189.

Golimbu M, al-Askari S, Morales P: One-stage hypospadias repair. *Urology* 1977;**9**:672.

Kelalis PP, Benson RC Jr, Culp OS: Complications of single and multistage operations for hypospadias: A comparative review. *J Urol* 1977;**118**:657.

Lutzker LG, Kogan SJ, Levitt SB: Is routine intravenous urography indicated in patients with hypospadias? *Pediatrics* 1977;**59**:630.

McArdle R, Lebowitz R: Uncomplicated hypospadias and anomalies of the upper urinary tract: Need for screening? *Urology* 1975;**59**:630.

Sadlowski RW, Belman AB, King LR: Further experience with one-stage hypospadias repair. *J Urol* 1974;**112**:677.

Shima H & others: Developmental anomalies associated with hypospadias. *J Urol* 1979;**122**:619.

Smith DR: Repair of hypospadias in the preschool child: A report of 150 cases. *J Urol* 1967;**97**:723.

Wettlaufer JN: Cutaneous chordee: Fact or fancy? *Urology* 1974;**4**:293.

Wray RC, Ribaudo JM, Weeks PM: The Byars hypospadias

repair: A review of 253 consecutive patients. *Plast Reconstr Surg* 1976;**58**:329.

Chordee Without Hypospadias

Devine CJ Jr, Horton CE: Chordee without hypospadias. *J Urol* 1973;**110**:264.

Devine CJ Jr, Horton CE: Use of dermal graft to correct chordee. *J Urol* 1975;**113**:56.

Kaplan GW, Lamm DL: Embryogenesis of chordee. *J Urol* 1975;**114**:769.

Perlmutter AD, Vatz AD: Meatal advancement for distal hypospadias without chordee. *J Urol* 1975;**113**:850.

Redman JF: Extended application of Nesbit ellipses in the correction of childhood penile curvature. *J Urol* 1978;**119**:122.

Udall DA: Correction of 3 types of congenital curvature of the penis, including the first reported case of dorsal curvature. *J Urol* 1980;**124**:50.

Epispadias

Ambrose SS, O'Brien DP III: Surgical embryology of the exstrophy-epispadias complex. *Surg Clin North Am* 1974;**54**:1379.

Dey DL, Cohen D: The surgery of female epispadias. *Surgery* 1971;**69**:542.

Duckett JW Jr: Epispadias. *Urol Clin North Am* 1978;**5**:107.

Hendren WH: Penile lengthening after previous repair of epispadias. *J Urol* 1979;**121**:527.

Tanagho EA, Smith DR: Clinical evaluation of a surgical technique for the correction of complete urinary incontinence. *J Urol* 1972;**107**:402.

ACQUIRED DISEASES

Priapism

Baron M, Leiter E: The management of priapism in sickle cell anemia. *J Urol* 1978;**119**:610.

Carter RG, Thomas CE, Tomsky GC: Cavernospongiosum shunts in treatment of priapism. *Urology* 1976;**7**:292.

Douglas LL: Extracorporeal circulatory management of priapism. *Urology* 1976;**7**:198.

Evans IL, Young AE: Internal pudendal arteriography after priapism. *Br J Surg* 1973;**60**:329.

Fitzpatrick TJ: Spongiograms and cavernosograms: A study of their value in priapism. *J Urol* 1973;**109**:843.

Gates CL Jr, Middleton RG: Extracorporeal corpusvenous shunting for priapism. *J Urol* 1980;**123**:595.

Goulding FJ: Modification of cavernoglandular shunt for priapism. *Urology* 1980;**15**:64.

Guerriero WG: Corpus cavernosum-corpus spongiosum shunts. *Surg Gynecol Obstet* 1978;**146**:792.

Kinney TR & others: Priapism in association with sickle hemoglobinopathies in children. *J Pediatr* 1975;**86**:241.

Persky L, Kursh E: Post-traumatic priapism. *J Urol* 1977;**118**:397.

Resnick MI & others: Priapism in boys: Management with cavernosaphenous shunt. *Urology* 1975;**5**:492.

Schreibman SM, Gee TS, Grabstald H: Management of priapism in patients with chronic granulocytic leukemia. *J Urol* 1974;**111**:786.

Seeler RA: Intensive transfusion therapy for priapism in boys with sickle cell anemia. *J Urol* 1973;**110**:360.

Wear JB Jr, Crummy AB, Munson BO: A new approach to the treatment of priapism. *J Urol* 1977;**117**:252.

Winter CC: Priapism cured by creation of fistulas between glans penis and corpora cavernosa. *J Urol* 1978;**119**:227.

Plastic Induration of the Penis

Bruskewitz R, Raz S: Surgical considerations in treatment of Peyronie disease. *Urology* 1980;**15**:134.

Byström J & others: Induratio penis plastica (Peyronie's disease). *Scand J Plast Reconstr Surg* 1973;**7**:137.

Chesney J: Peyronie's disease. *Br J Urol* 1976;**48**:209.

Devine CJ Jr, Horton CE: Surgical treatment of Peyronie's disease with a dermal graft. *J Urol* 1974;**111**:44.

Hall WT, Turner RW: Experience with Devine-Horton dermal patch graft for Peyronie's disease. *Urology* 1977;**9**:407.

Helvie WW, Ochsner SF: Radiation therapy in Peyronie's disease. *South Med J* 1972;**65**:1192.

Hicks CC & others: Experience with the Horton-Devine dermal graft in the treatment of Peyronie's disease. *J Urol* 1978;**119**:504.

Oosterlinck W, Renders G: Treatment of Peyronie's disease with procarbazine. *Br J Urol* 1976;**48**:219.

Poutasse EF: Peyronie's disease. *J Urol* 1972;**107**:419.

Pryor JP, Fitzpatrick JM: New approach to correction of penile deformity in Peyronie's disease. *J Urol* 1979;**122**:622.

Raz S, deKernion JB, Kaufman JJ: Surgical treatment of Peyronie's disease: A new approach. *J Urol* 1977;**117**:598.

Wild RM, Devine CJ Jr, Horton CE: Dermal graft repair of Peyronie's disease: Survey of 50 patients. *J Urol* 1979;**121**:47.

Phimosis

Redman AJ, Scribner LJ, Bissada NK: Postcircumcision of phimosis and its management. *Clin Pediatr (Phila)* 1975;**14**:407.

Paraphimosis

Oster J: Further fate of the foreskin: Incidence of preputial adhesions, phimosis, and smegma among Danish boys. *Arch Dis Child* 1968;**43**:200.

Skoglund RW Jr, Chapman WH: Reduction of paraphimosis. *J Urol* 1970;**104**:137.

Circumcision

Dagher R, Selzer ML, Lapides J: Carcinoma of the penis and the anti-circumcision parade. *J Urol* 1973;**110**:79.

Murdock MI, Selikowitz SM: Diabetes-related need for circumcision. *Urology* 1974;**4**:60.

Trier WC, Drach GW: Concealed penis: Another complication of circumcision. *Am J Dis Child* 1973;**125**:276.

Urethral Stricture

Azoury BS, Freiha FS: Excision of urethral stricture and end to end anastomosis. *Urology* 1976;**8**:138.

Betts JM, Texter JH Jr, Crane DB: Single stage urethroplasty as treatment for stricture disease. *J Urol* 1978;**120**:412.

Blandy JP & others: Urethroplasty in context. *Br J Urol* 1976;**48**:697.

Devine PC, Wendelken JR, Devine CJ Jr: Free full thickness skin graft urethroplasty: Current technique. *J Urol* 1979;**121**:282.

Khan AU, Furlow WL: Transpubic urethroplasty. *J Urol* 1976;**116**:447.

Madduri S, Kamat MH, Seebode J: Urethral stricture treated with soft catheter dilatation: Reappraisal of an old technique. *Urology* 1974;4:504.

Malek RS, O'Dea MJ, Kelalis PP: Management of ruptured posterior urethra in childhood. *J Urol* 1977;117:105.

Oswalt GC Jr, Lloyd LK, Bueschen AJ: Full thickness skin graft urethroplasty for anterior urethral strictures. *Urology* 1979;13:45.

Pierce JM Jr: Posterior urethral stricture repair. *J Urol* 1979;121:739.

Sacknoff EJ, Kerr WS Jr: Direct vision cold knife urethrotomy. *J Urol* 1980;123:492.

Schwarz RD & others: The assessment of sphincteric activity in patients following trans-sphincteric urethral reconstruction. *Br J Urol* 1976;48:643.

Smith PJB, Dunn M, Dounis A: The early results of treatment of stricture of the male urethra using the Sachse optical urethrotome. *Br J Urol* 1979;51:224.

Strong DW, Hodges CV: Transpubic urethroplasty for membranous urethral strictures. *Urology* 1977;9:27.

Tilak GH, Dhayagude HC, Joshi SS: Badenoch's pull-through operation for urethral stricture. *Br J Urol* 1976;48:83.

Turner-Warwick R: Complex traumatic posterior urethral strictures. *J Urol* 1977;118:564.

Walther PC, Parsons CL, Schmidt JD: Direct vision internal urethrotomy in the management of urethral strictures. *J Urol* 1980;123:497.

Waterhouse K, Laungani G, Patil U: The surgical repair of membranous urethral strictures: Experience with 105 consecutive cases. *J Urol* 1980;123:500.

Urethral Warts

Bissada NK, Redman JF, Sulieman JS: Condyloma-acuminatum of the male urethra: Successful management with 5-fluorouracil. *Urology* 1974;3:499.

Bruns TNC & others: Buschke-Lowenstein giant condylomas: Pitfalls in management. *Urology* 1975;5:773.

Dretler SP, Klein LA: The eradication of intraurethral condyloma acuminatum with 5 percent 5-fluorouracil cream. *J Urol* 1975;113:195.

Fuselier HA Jr & others: Treatment of condylomata acuminata with carbon dioxide laser. *Urology* 1980;15:265.

Gigax JH, Robison JR: The successful treatment of intraurethral condyloma acuminatum with colchicine. *J Urol* 1971;105:809.

Pollack HM & others: Urethrographic manifestations of venereal warts (condyloma acuminata). *Radiology* 1978;126:643.

Rosenberg JW, al-Askari S: Management of intraurethral condyloma acuminatum. *J Urol* 1973;110:686.

Weimar GW & others: 5-Fluorouracil urethral suppositories for the eradication of condyloma acuminata. *J Urol* 1978;120:174.

Fistula

Blandy JP, Singh M: Fistulae involving the adult male urethra. *Br J Urol* 1972;44:632.

Thrombophlebitis of the Superficial Penile Veins

Harrow BR, Sloane JA: Thrombophlebitis of superficial penile and scrotal veins. *J Urol* 1963;89:841.

30 | Disorders of the Female Urethra

Emil A. Tanagho, MD

CONGENITAL ANOMALIES OF THE FEMALE URETHRA

DISTAL URETHRAL STENOSIS IN INFANCY & CHILDHOOD
(Spasm of the External Urinary Sphincter)

There has been considerable confusion about the site of lower tract obstruction in little girls who suffer from enuresis, a slow and interrupted urinary stream, recurrent cystitis, and pyelonephritis and who, on thorough examination, often exhibit vesicoureteral reflux. Treatment has largely been directed to the bladder neck on rather empirical grounds. Most of these children, however, have congenital distal urethral stenosis with secondary spasm of the striated external sphincter rather than bladder neck contracture.

At birth, calibration of the urethra with bougies à boule reveals no evidence of a distal ring of urethral stenosis (Fisher & others, 1969). Within a few months, however, such a ring develops as a normal anatomic structure. After puberty, the ring disappears. The inference is that the absence of estrogens leads to the development of this lesion. Lyon & Tanagho (1965) found that the ring calibrates at 14F at age 2 and at 16F between the ages of 4 and 10. Even though from the hydrodynamic standpoint such a stenotic area should not be obstructive, almost all observers agree that destruction of the ring does relieve symptoms in these children and that it results in cure or correction of persistent infection or vesical dysfunction in 80% of cases. Lyon and Tanagho thought it possible that the basic cause of these urinary difficulties might be reflex spasm of the periurethral striated sphincter and noted that voiding cystourethrograms supported that view (Fig 30–1).

Tanagho & others (1971) measured pressures in the bladder and in the proximal and mid urethra simultaneously in symptomatic girls and found resting pressures in the midurethral segment as high as 200 cm of water (normal, 100 cm of water). Attempts at voiding caused intravesical pressures as high as 225 cm of water (normal, 30–40 cm of water) to develop. Under curare, the urethral closing pressures dropped to normal (40–50 cm of water), proving that these obstructing pressures were caused by spasm of the striated sphincter muscle. If the distal urethral ring was treated and symptoms abated, repeat pressure studies showed normal midurethral and intravesical voiding pressures. If, on the other hand, symptoms persisted, pressures were found to remain at extremely high levels.

It seems clear, therefore, that the major cause of urinary problems in little girls is spasm of the external sphincter and not vesical neck stenosis (Smith, 1969).

In addition to recurrent urinary tract infections, these patients have hesitancy in initiating micturition and a slow, hesitant, or interrupted urinary stream. Enuresis and involuntary loss of urine during the day are common complaints. Abdominal straining may be required. Small amounts of residual urine are found, thus impairing the vesical defense mechanism (Hinman, 1966). A voiding cystourethrogram may reveal an open bladder neck and ballooning of the proximal urethra secondary to the spastic external sphincter (Fig 30–1).

The voiding cystourethrogram may reveal evidence of the distal ring, but typical findings are not always seen, particularly if the flow rate is slow. Definitive diagnosis is made by bougienage.

The simplest and least harmful treatment is overdilatation with sounds up to 32–36F or with the Kollmann dilator (Lyon & Tanagho, 1965; Lyon & Marshall, 1971; Hendry, Stanton, & Williams, 1973). With either method, the ring "cracks" anteriorly, with some bleeding. Recurrence is rare. Internal urethrotomy has its proponents (Immergut & Gilbert, 1973; Hradec & others, 1973), but Kaplan, Sammons, & King (1973) achieved poor results with urethrotomy, since incising the urethra along its entire length does not cut the internal sphincter, whose abnormal tone is the cause of the obstruction, whereas "cracking" the ring by overdilatation accomplishes this purpose.

Walker & Richard (1973) have little to say about this syndrome, and their bibliography does not include the work of writers who have reported success in its management. Eighty percent of children can be helped to overcome enuresis and achieve a normal free voiding pattern, along with

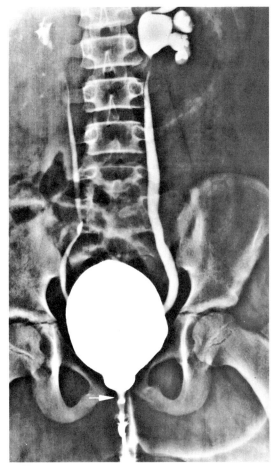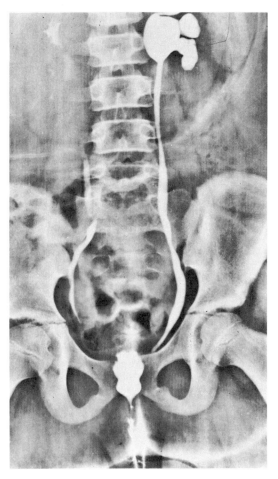

Figure 30–1. Distal urethral stenosis with reflux spasm of voluntary urethral sphincter. *Left:* Voiding cystourethrogram showing bilateral vesicoureteral reflux, a wide-open vesical neck, and severe spasm of the striated urethral sphincter in the midportion of the urethra (see arrow) secondary to distal urethral stenosis. *Right:* Postvoiding film. Bladder empty, vesical neck open, but dilated urethra contains radiopaque fluid proximal to the stenotic zone. Urethral bacteria thus can flow back into the bladder. (Courtesy of AD Amar.)

cure of recurrent cystitis or persistent bacteriuria (Lyon & Marshall, 1971). Correction of reflux is possible only in the case of "borderline" valves that tend to give way in the presence of increased voiding pressure and infection.

Since the ring normally disappears at puberty, it is commonly said that spontaneous cure can be awaited. Even though this is true, the ring should be broken if symptoms have been severe enough to bring the child to the attention of a urologist.

LABIAL FUSION
(Synechia Vulvae)

Some children with recurring urinary infection are found to have fusion of the labia minora, which is apt to obstruct the flow of urine so that it tends to pool in the vagina. Local application of estrogen cream twice daily for 2–4 weeks usually causes

spontaneous separation (Capraro & Greenberg, 1972). Forceful separation or dissection has its advocates (Podolsky, 1973; Christensen & Øster, 1971).

ACQUIRED DISEASES OF THE FEMALE URETHRA

ACUTE URETHRITIS

Acute urethritis frequently occurs with gonorrheal infection in women. Urinary symptoms are often present at the onset of the disease. Cultures and smears establish the diagnosis. Prompt cure can be achieved with antibiotic drugs.

The detergents in bubble bath or certain spermicidal jellies may cause vaginitis and urethritis. Symptoms of vesical irritability may occur.

CHRONIC URETHRITIS

Chronic urethritis is one of the most common urologic problems of females. The distal urethra normally harbors pathogens, and the risk of infection may be increased by wearing contaminated diapers, by insertion of an indwelling catheter, by spread from cervical or vaginal infections, or by intercourse with an infected partner. Urethral inflammation may also occur from the trauma of intercourse or childbirth, particularly if urethral stenosis, either congenital or following childbirth, is present.

Clinical Findings

The urethral mucosa is reddened and quite sensitive, often stenotic. Granular areas are often seen, and polypoid masses may be noted just distal to the bladder neck.

A. Symptoms: The symptoms resemble those of cystitis, although the urine may be clear. Complaints include burning on urination, frequency, and nocturia. Discomfort in the urethra may be felt, particularly when walking.

B. Signs: Examination may disclose redness of the meatus, hypersensitivity of the meatus and of the urethra on vaginal palpation, and evidence of cervicitis or vaginitis. There is no urethral discharge.

C. Laboratory Findings: Collection of the initial and midstream urine in separate containers reveals pus in the first glass and none in the second (Marshall, Lyon, & Schieble, 1970). *Ureaplasma urealyticum* (formerly called T-strain *Mycoplasma*) is often identifiable in the first glass. These findings are similar to those of nongonococcal (chlamydial) urethritis in the male. Clinically, the presence of white blood cells in the absence of bacteria on a routine stain or culture suggests nongonococcal urethritis.

In other instances, various bacteria may be found on culture (eg, *Streptococcus faecalis, Escherichia coli*) in both the urethral washings and in a specimen taken from the introitus. Bruce & others (1973) recommend the regular local application of an antiseptic (eg, hexachlorophene, chlorhexidine cream) to the introitus in order to prevent bacteria from the perineum-vagina-vulva from reinfecting the urethra.

D. Instrumental Examination: A catheter, bougie à boule, or sound may meet resistance because of urethral stenosis. Panendoscopy reveals redness and a granular appearance of the mucosa. Inflammatory polyps may be seen in the proximal portion of the urethra. Cystoscopy may show increased injection of the trigone (trigonitis), which often accompanies urethritis.

Differential Diagnosis

Differentiation from cystitis depends upon bacteriologic study of the urine; panendoscopy demonstrates the urethral lesion. Both diseases may be present.

Psychologic disorders may cause symptoms identical to those of chronic urethritis. A history of short bouts of frequency without nocturia is suggestive of functional illness. The neurotic makeup of the patient is usually obvious (Zufall, 1963).

Treatment & Prognosis

Gradual urethral dilatations (up to 36F in the adult) are indicated for urethral stenosis; this allows for some inevitable contracture. Immergut & Gilbert (1973) prefer internal urethrotomy. *Ureaplasma urealyticum* is fairly sensitive to tetracycline or erythromycin. Chlamydial urethritis usually responds to sulfonamides or tetracyclines.

SENILE URETHRITIS

After physiologic (or surgical) menopause, hypoestrogenism occurs and retrogressive (senile) changes take place in the vaginal epithelium, so that it becomes rather dry and pale. Similar changes develop in the lower urinary tract, which arises from the same embryologic tissues as the female generative organs. Some eversion of the mucosa about the urethral orifice, from foreshortening of the vaginal canal, is usually seen. This is commonly misdiagnosed as caruncle.

Clinical Findings

A. Symptoms: Many postmenopausal women have symptoms of vesical irritability (burning, frequency, urgency) and stress incontinence. They may complain of vaginal and vulval itching and some discharge.

B. Signs: The vaginal epithelium is dry and pale. The mucosa at the urethral orifice is often reddened and hypersensitive; eversion of its posterior lip from foreshortening of the urethrovaginal wall is commonly seen.

C. Laboratory Findings: The urine is usually free of organisms. The diagnosis can be made by the following procedure: A dry smear of vaginal epithelial cells is stained with Lugol's solution. The slide is then washed with water and immediately examined microscopically while wet. In hypoestrogenism, the cells take up the iodine poorly and are therefore yellow. When the mucosa is normal, these cells stain deep brown because of their glycogen content. The diagnosis may also be confirmed by the Papanicolaou technic.

D. Instrumental Examination: Panendoscopy usually demonstrates a reddened and granular urethral mucosa. Some urethral stenosis may be noted.

Differential Diagnosis

Senile urethritis is often mistaken for urethral caruncle. Eversion of the posterior lip of the urinary meatus is evident in both conditions; however, a hypersensitive vascular tumor is not present in senile urethritis.

Before operations to relieve stress incontinence are performed, estrogenic (or androgenic) therapy should be tried.

Treatment

Senile urethritis responds well to diethylstilbestrol vaginal suppositories, 0.1 mg nightly for 3 weeks. Estrogen creams applied locally are also effective. Estrogen urethral suppositories have been recommended, but they offer no advantages and are difficult to insert. After 3 weeks of treatment, the drug is withheld for 1 week and the course is then repeated. Three or more courses are occasionally indicated, depending upon the symptoms and the appearance of the vaginal smear stained as outlined above.

If vaginal irritation or bleeding upon discontinuing estrogen suppositories is a problem, methyltestosterone buccal tablets can be used as vaginal suppositories. Insert one 5-mg tablet vaginally daily for 5–8 weeks. Diethylstilbestrol, 0.1 mg/d by mouth, is also effective.

Prognosis

Senile urethritis usually responds promptly to estrogen or androgen therapy.

URETHRAL CARUNCLE

Urethral caruncle is a benign, red, raspberrylike, friable vascular tumor involving the posterior lip of the external urinary meatus. It is rare before the menopause. Microscopically, it consists of connective tissue containing many inflammatory cells and blood vessels and is covered by an epithelial layer.

Clinical Findings

Symptoms include pain on urination, pain with intercourse, and bloody spotting from even mild trauma. A sessile or pedunculated red, friable, tender mass is seen at the posterior lip of the meatus.

Differential Diagnosis

Carcinoma of the urethra may involve the urethral meatus. Palpation reveals definite induration. Biopsy will establish the true diagnosis.

Senile urethritis is often associated with a polypoid reaction of the urinary meatus and in fact is the most common cause of masses in this region. The diagnosis can be made by verifying the patient's hypoestrogenic status and by demonstrating a favorable response to estrogen replacement therapy. Biopsy should be done if doubt exists.

Thrombosis of the urethral vein presents as a bluish, swollen, tender lesion involving the posterior lip of the urinary meatus. It has the appearance of a thrombosed hemorrhoid. It subsides without treatment.

Treatment

Local excision is indicated only if symptoms are troublesome.

Prognosis

True caruncle is usually cured by excision, but in a few instances it does recur.

THROMBOSIS OF THE URETHRAL VEIN

Spontaneous thrombosis of the urethral vein on the floor of the distal urethra occurs in older women, who complain of a sudden onset of local pain followed shortly thereafter by the appearance of a mass at the urethral orifice. Examination reveals a purple mass protruding from the posterior lip of the urethra; early, it is quite tender. The abrupt onset tends to rule out caruncle or cancer. If there is doubt about the true nature of the lesion, biopsy should be done.

No treatment is usually required, since the process gradually resolves. Evacuation of the clot has been recommended.

PROLAPSE OF THE URETHRA

Prolapse of the female urethra is not common. It usually occurs only in children or in paraplegics suffering from a lower motor neuron lesion. The protruding urethral mucosa presents as an angry red mass that may become gangrenous if it is not reduced promptly. A protruding mass in a little girl must be differentiated from prolapse of a ureterocele.

After reduction, cystoscopy should be done to rule out ureterocele. Recurrences are rare following reduction; the accompanying inflammation probably "fixes" the tissue in place as healing progresses. If the prolapsed urethra cannot be reduced or if it recurs, an indwelling catheter should be inserted, traction placed upon it, and a heavy piece of suture material tightly tied over the tissue and catheter just proximal to the mass. The tissue later sloughs off. Using this same technic, the tissue can be resected, preferably with an electrosurgical cautery.

URETHROVAGINAL FISTULA

Urethrovaginal fistulas may follow local injury secondary to fracture of the pelvis or obstetric or surgical injury (see Chapter 16). A common cause is accidental trauma to the urethra or its blood supply in the course of surgical repair of a cystocele. Vaginal urethroplasty is indicated.

URETHRAL DIVERTICULUM

Diverticulation of the urethral wall is not common. Diverticula are at times multiple. Most cases are probably secondary to obstetric urethral trauma or severe urethral infection. A few cases of carcinoma in such diverticula have been reported. This disease is usually associated with recurrent attacks of cystitis. Purulent urethral discharge is sometimes noted as the infected diverticulum empties. Dyspareunia sometimes results. On occasion the diverticulum may be large enough to be discovered by the patient.

The diagnosis is usually made on feeling a rounded cystic mass in the anterior wall of the vagina that leaks pus from the urethral orifice when pressure is applied. Endoscopy may reveal the urethral opening. The postvoiding film of an excretory urographic series may demonstrate the lesion (Houser & von Eschenbach, 1974). It may be possible to introduce a small catheter through which radiopaque fluid can be instilled. Appropriate x-ray films are then exposed (Fig 30–2). The plain film may show a stone in the diverticulum. If these methods fail, the following procedures can be used:

(1) Empty the diverticulum manually. Catheterize, and instill 5 mL of indigo carmine and 60 mL of contrast medium into the bladder. Remove the catheter and have the patient begin to void. Occlude the meatus with a finger. This maneuver usually causes filling of the diverticulum with the test solution. Take appropriate x-rays and do panendoscopy, looking for leakage of blue dye from the mouth of the diverticulum (Borski & Stutzman, 1965).

(2) Insert a Davis-TeLinde catheter. This looks like a Foley catheter but is surrounded by a second movable balloon. Pass the catheter to the bladder and inflate the proximal balloon. While exerting tension on the catheter, slide the second balloon against the urinary meatus and inflate it. In the catheter, between the balloons, is a hole through which injected radiopaque fluid will escape, thus filling the urethra and diverticulum. X-rays are then exposed.

Treatment consists of removal of the sac through an incision in the anterior vaginal wall, care being taken not to injure the urethral sphincteric musculature. Incision is carried down to the diverticular mucosa, and the plane of cleavage is then followed all around to the neck of the diverticulum. The diverticular sac is completely excised, and the defect in the urethra must be repaired. Ellik (1957) recommends opening the diverticulum and stuffing it with Oxycel, then closing the diverticulum. The inflammatory reaction that results destroys the cyst. An indwelling urethral catheter (or suprapubic cystostomy) should be left in place for 10 days following treatment.

The outcome is usually good unless the diverticulum is so situated that its excision injures the external urinary sphincter mechanism. In a few cases, urethrovaginal fistula may develop. If the fistula does not close with prolonged catheter drainage, surgical repair will be necessary.

URETHRAL STRICTURE

True organic stricture of the adult female urethra is not common. (Functional urethral obstruction is more common.) It may be congenital or acquired. The trauma of intercourse and especially of childbirth may lead to periurethral fibrosis with contracture, or the stricture may be caused by the

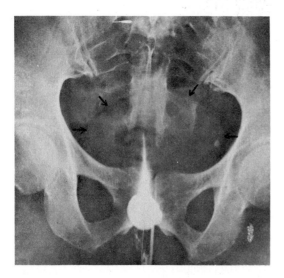 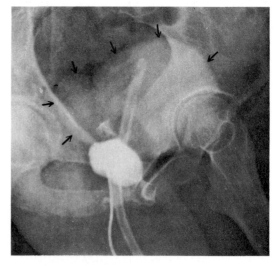

Figure 30–2. Urethral diverticulum containing stone. *Left:* Plain film showing stone. Arrows outline bladder. *Right:* Diverticulum filled with radiopaque fluid instilled through ureteral catheter. Bladder outlined by arrows.

surgeon during vaginal repair. It may develop secondary to acute or chronic urethritis.

Persistent hesitancy in initiating urination and a slow urinary stream are the principal symptoms of stricture. Burning, frequency, nocturia, and urethral pain may occur from secondary urethritis or cystitis. If secondary infection of the bladder is present, pus and bacteria will be found in the urine. A fairly large catheter (22F) may pass to the bladder only with difficulty. Panendoscopy may demonstrate the point of narrowness and disclose evidence of urethritis. Cystoscopy often reveals trabeculation (hypertrophy) of the bladder wall.

Chronic cystitis may cause similar symptoms, but urinalysis will reveal evidence of infection. Cancer of the urethra causes progressive narrowing of the urethra, but induration and infiltration of the urethra will be found on vaginal examination.

Panendoscopy with biopsy establishes the diagnosis. Vesical tumor involving the bladder neck will cause hesitancy and impairment of the urinary stream. Cystoscopy is definitive. Chronic urethritis commonly accompanies urethral stenosis; either may be primary. Recurrent or chronic cystitis is often secondary to stenosis.

Treatment consists of gradual urethral dilatation (up to 36F) at weekly intervals. Slight overstretching is necessary, since some contracture will occur after therapy is discontinued. Measures to combat urethritis and cystitis must also be employed. Internal urethrotomy also has its proponents.

With proper overdilatation of the urethra and specific therapy of the urethritis that is usually present, the prognosis is good.

● ● ●

References

Distal Urethral Stenosis

Farrar DJ, Green NA, Ashken MH: An evaluation of Otis urethrotomy in female patients with recurrent urinary tract infections: A review after 6 years. *Br J Urol* 1980;**52:**68.

Firlit CF: Urethral anomalies. *Urol Clin North Am* 1978;**5:**31.

Fisher RE & others: Urethral calibration in newborn girls. *J Urol* 1969;**102:**67.

Hendry WF, Stanton SL, Williams DI: Recurrent urinary infections in girls: Effects of urethral dilatation. *Br J Urol* 1973;**45:**72.

Hinman F Jr: Mechanisms for the entry of bacteria and the establishment of urinary infection in female children. *J Urol* 1966;**96:**546.

Hojsgaard A: The urethral pressure profile in female patients with meatal stenosis. *Scand J Urol Nephrol* 1976;**10:**97.

Hradec E & others: Significance of urethral obstruction in girls. *Urol Int* 1973;**28:**440.

Immergut MA, Gilbert EC: Internal urethrotomy in recurring urinary infections in girls. *J Urol* 1973;**109:**126.

Kaplan GW, Sammons TA, King LR: A blind comparison of dilatation, urethrotomy and medication alone in the treatment of urinary tract infection in girls. *J Urol* 1973;**109:**917.

Kilner TP, Peet EW: *Urethra and Bladder: Congenital Malformations.* Butterworth, 1953.

Lyon RP, Marshall S: Urinary tract infections and difficult urination in girls: Long-term follow-up. *J Urol* 1971;**105:**314.

Lyon RP, Tanagho EA: Distal urethral stenosis in little girls. *J Urol* 1965;**93:**379.

Obrink A, Bunne G, Hedlund PO: Cultures from different parts of the urethra in female urethral syndrome. *Urol Int* 1979;**34:**70.

Smith DR: Critique on the concept of vesical neck obstruction in children. *JAMA* 1969;**207:**1686.

Tanagho EA, Lyon RP: Urethral dilatation versus internal urethrotomy. *J Urol* 1971;**105:**242.

Tanagho EA, Meyers FH, Smith DR: Urethral resistance: Its components and implications. 1. Smooth muscle component. 2. Striated muscle component. *Invest Urol* 1969;**7:**136, 195.

Tanagho EA & others: Spastic external sphincter and urinary tract infection in girls. *Br J Urol* 1971;**43:**69.

Uehling DT: The normal caliber of the adult female urethra. *J Urol* 1978;**120:**176.

Van Gool J, Tanagho EA: External sphincter activity and recurrent urinary tract infection in girls. *Urology* 1977;**10:**348.

Vermillion CD, Halverstadt DB, Leadbetter GW Jr: Internal urethrotomy and recurrent urinary tract infection in female children. 2. Long-term results in the management of infection. *J Urol* 1971;**106:**154.

Walker D, Richard GA: A critical evaluation of urethral obstruction in female children. *Pediatrics* 1973;**51:**272.

Labial Fusion

Aribarg A: Topical oestrogen therapy for labial adhesions in children. *Br J Obstet Gynaecol* 1975;**82:**424.

Capraro VJ, Greenberg H: Adhesions of the labia minora: A study of 50 patients. *Obstet Gynecol* 1972;**39:**65.

Christensen EH, Oster J: Adhesions of labia minora (synechia vulvae) in childhood. *Acta Paediatr Scand* 1971;**60:**709.

Podolsky ML: Labial fusion: A cause of recurrent urinary tract infections. *Clin Pediatr (Phila)* 1973;**12:**345.

Acute Urethritis

Bass HN: "Bubble bath" as an irritant to the urinary tract of children. *Clin Pediatr (Phila)* 1968;**7:**174.

Marshall S: The effect of bubble bath on the urinary tract. *J Urol* 1965;**93:**112.

Chronic Urethritis

Bruce AW & others: Recurrent urethritis in women. *Can Med Assoc J* 1973;**108:**973.

Immergut MA, Gilbert EC: The clinical response of women to intestinal urethrotomy. *J Urol* 1973;**109:**90.

Marshall S, Lyon RP, Schieble J: Nonspecific urethritis in females. *Calif Med* (June) 1970;**112**:9.

Moore T, Hira NR, Stirland RM: Differential urethro-vesical urinary cell-count. *Lancet* 1965;**1**:626.

Zimskind PD, Mannes HA: Approach to bladder neck and urethral obstruction in women. *Surg Clin North Am* 1973;**53**:571.

Zufall R: Treatment of the urethral syndrome in women. *JAMA* 1963;**184**:894.

Senile Urethritis

Quinlivan LG: The treatment of senile vaginitis with low doses of synthetic estrogens. *Am J Obstet Gynecol* 1965;**92**:172.

Smith P: Age changes in the female urethra. *Br J Urol* 1972;**44**:667.

Caruncle

Marshall FC, Uson AC, Melicow MM: Neoplasms and caruncles of the female urethra. *Surg Gynecol Obstet* 1960;**110**:723.

Thrombosis of the Urethral Veins

Falk HC: Treatment of urethral vein thrombosis. *Obstet Gynecol* 1964;**23**:85.

Harrow BR: The thrombosed urethral hemorrhoid: 3 case reports. *J Urol* 1967;**98**:482.

Prolapse

Capraro VJ, Bayonet-Rivera NP, Magoss I: Vulvar tumor in children due to prolapse of urethral mucosa. *Am J Obstet Gynecol* 1970;**108**:572.

Devine PC, Kessel HC: Surgical correction of urethral prolapse. *J Urol* 1980;**123**:856.

Klaus H, Stein RT: Urethral prolapse in young girls. *Pediatrics* 1973;**52**:645.

Potter BM: Urethral prolapse in girls. *Radiology* 1971;**98**:287.

Smith HW Jr, Campbell EW Jr: Benign periurethral masses in women. *J Urol* 1976;**116**:451.

Turner RW: Urethral prolapse in female children. *Urology* 1973;**2**:530.

Urethrovaginal Fistula

Gray L: Urethrovaginal fistulas. *Am J Obstet Gynecol* 1968;**101**:28.

Hendren WH: Construction of female urethra from vaginal wall and perineal flap. *J Urol* 1980;**123**:657.

Tehan TJ, Nardi JA, Baker R: Complications associated with surgical repair of urethrovaginal fistula. *Urology* 1980;**15**:31.

Diverticulum

Benjamin J & others: Urethral diverticulum in adult female: Clinical aspects, operative procedure, and pathology. *Urology* 1974;**3**:1.

Borski AA, Stutzman RE: Diverticulum of female urethra: A simplified diagnostic aid. *J Urol* 1965;**93**:60.

Bracken RB & others: Primary carcinoma of the female urethra. *J Urol* 1976;**116**:188.

Dretler SP, Vermillion CD, McCullough DL: The roentgenographic diagnosis of female urethral diverticula. *J Urol* 1972;**107**:72.

Elik M: Diverticulum of the female urethra: A new method of ablation. *J Urol* 1957;**77**:243.

Glassman TA, Weinerth JL, Glenn JF: Neonatal female urethral diverticulum. *Urology* 1975;**5**:249.

Golimbu M, al-Askari S: High pressure voiding urethrography. *Urology* 1974;**3**:717.

Houser LM II, von Eschenbach AC: Diverticula of female urethra: Diagnostic importance of postvoiding film. *Urology* 1974;**3**:453.

Lapides J: Transurethral treatment of urethral diverticula in women. *J Urol* 1979;**121**:736.

Marshall S, Hirsch K: Carcinoma within urethral diverticula. *Urology* 1977;**10**:161.

Palagiri A: Urethral diverticulum with endometriosis. *Urology* 1978;**11**:271.

Presman D, Rolnick D, Zumerchek J: Calculus formation within a diverticulum of the female urethra. *J Urol* 1964;**91**:376.

Roberts TW, Melicow MM: Pathology and natural history of urethral tumors in females: Review of 65 cases. *Urology* 1977;**10**:583.

Sholem SL, Wechsler M, Roberts M: Management of the urethral diverticulum in women: A modified operative approach. *J Urol* 1974;**112**:485.

Spence HM, Duckett JW Jr: Diverticulum of the female urethra: Clinical aspects and presentation of a simple operative technique for cure. *J Urol* 1970;**104**:432.

Torres SA, Quattlebaum RB: Carcinoma in a urethral diverticulum. *South Med J* 1972;**65**:1374.

Stricture

Essenhigh DM, Ardran GM, Cope V: A study of the bladder outlet in lower urinary tract infections in women. *Br J Urol* 1968;**40**:268.

Immergut MA, Gilbert EC: The clinical response of women to internal urethrotomy. *J Urol* 1973;**109**:90.

Surgical Repair

Hajj SN, Evans MI: Diverticula of the female urethra. *Am J Obstet Gynecol* 1980;**136**:335.

Symmonds RE, Hill LM: Loss of the urethra: A report on 50 patients. *Am J Obstet Gynecol* 1978;**130**:130.

Disorders of the Testis, Scrotum, & Spermatic Cord | 31

Donald R. Smith, MD

DISORDERS OF THE SCROTUM

Hypoplasia of the scrotum accompanies cryptorchidism. Bifid scrotum is present with midscrotal or perineal hypospadias and in certain cases of intersexuality. In both instances the 2 scrotal sacs simulate labia majora.

Idiopathic edema of the scrotum is occasionally seen in children. It may involve one or both sacs and also the penis, the perineum, or the inguinal region. The exact cause is not known; it may represent an allergic response or angioneurotic edema (Evans & Snyder, 1977). Antihistamines may be of value, though the condition does resolve spontaneously.

Conn (1971) has observed scrotal edema caused by development of a fistula between the peritoneum and the subcutaneous tissue following paracentesis for cirrhosis of the liver. In women, the edema involves the labia. Futter (1980) observed 3 instances of scrotal emphysema (1) following treatment of rectal polyp, (2) following an open renal biopsy, and (3) in traumatic pneumothorax. It must be remembered, however, that torsion of the spermatic cord may affect the scrotal skin in a similar manner.

In association with healed meconium peritonitis, masses may develop in the scrotum (or in the inguinal area) (Heydenrych & Marcus, 1976). Examination at birth may lead to the diagnosis of hydrocele, but a month later the scrotal masses will have become firm. A plain film of the abdomen will reveal calcification in both the masses and the abdomen. This will differentiate the masses from teratoma.

CONGENITAL ANOMALIES OF THE TESTIS

ANOMALIES OF NUMBER

Absence of one or both testes is very rare. Brothers, Weber, & Ball (1978) stress the need for a careful search for the absent organ. They cite 13 cases of testicular tumor in intra-abdominal cryptorchidism, most of which were seminomas.

Pelander, Luna, & Lilly (1978), in a review of the literature, report 53 instances of polyorchidism. A spermatocele or tumor of the spermatic cord is often mistaken for a third gonad.

HYPOGONADISM

Males suffering from either congenital or prepuberal primary testicular eunuchoidism or pituitary hypogonadism (congenital or secondary to a brain lesion) are tall and have disproportionately long extremities because of delay in fusion of the epiphyses. The testes are small, and there is lack of development of secondary sexual characteristics associated with some deficiency in libido and potency. These men are sterile. A somewhat feminine fat distribution may be noted, and there are wrinkles about the eyes. The primary gonadal defect is often associated with color blindness and mental retardation.

X-ray studies of the bones reveal delay in closure of the epiphyses. The differential diagnosis of these 2 disorders often depends upon determination of FSH and 17-ketosteroid (or serum testosterone) excretion in the urine. The pituitary type will excrete no FSH; the androgen level is very low. The gonadal eunuch excretes high levels of FSH (above 80 mouse units/24 h) but only moderately decreased amounts of urinary 17-ketosteroids or serum testosterone. The pituitary eunuchoid male may have an enlarged sella turcica or visual field defects secondary to tumor.

Both conditions are treated with long-acting esters of testosterone, 200 mg/mo intravenously, or a comparable preparation by mouth daily.

Stearns & others (1974) have studied declining testicular function due to age. They found that serum testosterone levels remained normal to age 70 years. After age 40, however, a slight but steady increase in serum LH and FSH was observed.

For a discussion of Klinefelter's syndrome, see Chapter 33.

ECTOPY & CRYPTORCHIDISM

In ectopy the testis has strayed from the path of normal descent; in cryptorchidism it is arrested in the normal path of descent. Ectopy may be due to an abnormal connection of the distal end of the gubernaculum testis that leads the gonad to an abnormal position. The ectopic sites are as follows (Fig 31–1):

(1) Superficial inguinal (most common site): After passing through the external inguinal ring, the testis proceeds superolaterally to a position superficial to the aponeurosis of the external oblique muscle.

(2) Perineal (rare): The testis is found just in front of the anus and to one side of the midline (Middleton, Beamon, & Gillenwater, 1976).

(3) Femoral or crural (rare): The testis is found in Scarpa's triangle superficial to the femoral vessels. The cord passes under the inguinal ligament.

(4) Penile (rare): The testis is placed under the skin at the root of the dorsum of the penis (Concodora, Evans, & Smith, 1976).

(5) Transverse or paradoxic descent (rare): Both testes descend the same inguinal canal. Fujita (1980) has collected some 85 examples from the literature.

(6) Pelvic (rare): The testis is found in the true pelvis (discovered only by surgical exploration).

Cryptorchidism is a condition in which a testicle is arrested at some point in its normal descent anywhere between the renal and scrotal areas. Unilateral arrest is more common than bilateral. At the time of birth (9-month gestation), the incidence of maldescent is 3.4%; half of these descend in the first month of life. The incidence in the adult is 0.7–0.8%. In the premature infant, it is 30%. A few cryptorchid testes may descend at puberty.

Dewald, Kelalis, & Gordon (1977) did chromosomal studies in cases of cryptorchidism. No abnormality was observed.

Etiology

The cause of maldescent is not clear. The following possibilities must be considered.

A. Abnormality of the Gubernaculum Testis: Differential growth of the embryo appears to cause descent of the gonad from its lumbar origin. Descent is guided by the gubernaculum, a cordlike structure that extends from the lower pole of the testis to the scrotum. In the embryo, of course, it is very short. Absence or abnormality of this structure may be a cause of maldescent (Shafik, 1977).

B. Intrinsic Testicular Defect: Maldescent may be caused by a congenital gonadal (dysgenetic) defect that makes the testicle insensitive to gonadotropins. This theory is the best explanation for unilateral cryptorchidism. It would also explain why many patients with bilateral cryptorchidism are sterile, even when given definitive therapy at the optimum age.

C. Deficient Gonadotropic Hormonal Stimulation: Lack of adequate maternal gonadotropins may be a cause of incomplete descent. This seems to be the obvious explanation for bilateral cryptorchidism in the premature infant, since the elaboration of maternal gonadotropins remains at a low level until the last 2 weeks of gestation. It is difficult, however, to apply this theory to unilateral cryptorchidism.

Rajfer & Walsh (1977) have shown that testicular descent is an androgen-mediated event that is regulated by pituitary gonadotropin. This process leads to high levels of dihydrotestosterone. They point out that the testis must also have free access to the scrotum for normal descent.

Pathogenesis & Pathology

Moore has clearly shown the efficacy of the

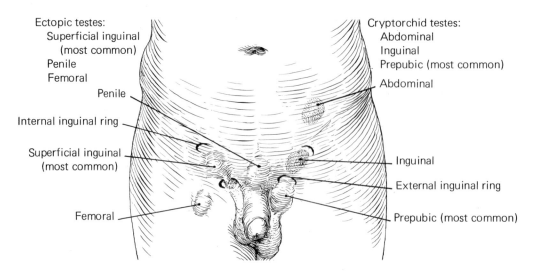

Figure 31–1. Undescended testes. Position of testes in various types of ectopy and cryptorchidism.

scrotum as a temperature regulator for the testes, which are kept about 1 C (1.8 F) cooler than body temperature. The spermatogenic cells are sensitive to body temperature. Cooper has demonstrated microscopic changes in the retained organ in boys at age 2. Robinson and also Engle and co-workers have reported diminished size of spermatogenic tubules and fewer spermatogonia in undescended testes in boys as young as age 6 years.

After age 6 years, changes become more obvious. The diameter of the tubules is smaller than normal. The number of spermatogonia decreases, and fibrosis between the tubules becomes marked. The cryptorchid testis after puberty may be fairly normal in size, but it is markedly deficient in spermatogenic components; infertility is the rule.

It must be remembered that about 10% of these testes are congenitally defective (primary hypogonadism, hypogonadism secondary to hypopituitarism). These gonads will show subnormal spermatogenic activity in spite of treatment.

Fortunately, the Leydig cells are not affected by body temperature and are therefore usually found in normal numbers in the cryptorchid organ. An endocrinologic cause of impotence is rare in this group.

In a study employing the latest analytical methods, Dewald, Kelalis, & Gordon (1977) could find no chromosomal abnormalities in biopsies of undescended testes. Maldescent and carcinomatous degeneration cannot be attributed to defects in chromosomes in the undescended organ.

Marshall & Shermeta (1979) point out that epididymal abnormalities are commonly found in these testes. The anomalies include agenesis, atresia, and elongated epididymides poorly connected to the gonad.

Clinical Findings

A. Symptoms: The cardinal symptom of ectopy or cryptorchidism is the absence of one or both testes from the scrotum. The patient may complain of pain from trauma to the testis, which may be situated in a vulnerable position (eg, over the pubic bone). The adult patient with bilateral cryptorchidism may present with a complaint of infertility.

B. Signs: In true maldescent, the scrotum on the affected side is atrophic. The testis either is not palpable (lying within or even proximal to the inguinal canal) or can be felt external to the inguinal ring. It cannot be manipulated into the scrotum. A common position for such a testis is in the region of the inguinal canal. A testis felt in this area would have to be a superficial inguinal ectopic testis (lying subcutaneously), for it would be impossible to palpate a small testis through the heavy external oblique aponeurosis. Inguinal hernia may be present on the affected side.

C. Laboratory Findings: Studies of the urinary 17-ketosteroids, gonadotropins, and serum testosterone may help in tracing the cause of cryptorchidism. In primary hypogonadism, the urinary gonadotropins (FSH) are markedly elevated, whereas the androgens are moderately reduced. In primary hypopituitarism, the androgens and pituitary gonadotropins are definitely depressed. In "primary" cryptorchidism, the androgens and pituitary gonadotropins are often moderately diminished.

If neither testis can be demonstrated, Shapiro & Bodai (1978) suggest using herniography, venography, and arteriography. If these are unrevealing, they suggest using the human chorionic gonadotropin test. This is done by establishing a baseline serum testosterone level and then giving hCG, 2000 units daily for 4 days. On the fifth day, the serum testosterone estimation should be repeated. If testes are present, this hormone will be elevated as much as 10 times.

D. X-Ray Findings: Freeny, Cummings, & Simmons (1978), and Weiss, Glickman, & Lytton (1979) use selective gonadal venography via the percutaneous femoral vein for localization of the nonpalpable testis. The testis is identified by visualization of its pampiniform plexus. Proof of agenesis makes operation unnecessary.

E. Computed Tomography: Using CT scan, Lee & others (1980) demonstrated 3 lower abdominal and 5 inguinal testes in the 8 patients they studied.

F. Ultrasonography: Madrazo & others (1979) used sonography to locate the undescended organ. The inguinal testis was easily identified, but the more deeply placed testis was not.

Differential Diagnosis

Physiologic cryptorchidism (retractile or migratory testis) is a common phenomenon requiring no treatment. Because of the small mass of the prepuberal testis and the strength of the cremaster muscle, which inserts upon the spermatic cord, the testes are apt to be involuntarily retracted out of the scrotum in cold weather or with excitement or physical activity. The diagnosis is made by noting that the scrotum on the suspected side is normally developed and that the "inguinal" testis can be pushed into and to the bottom of the scrotum. It may be necessary to place the child in a warm tub to afford maximum muscular relaxation, in which case the testis is found in the normal position. Such a testis descends at puberty and has been found to be normal (Puri & Nixon, 1977).

Complications

Associated inguinal hernia is found in 25% of patients with maldescent. At surgery, 95% of cases have a patent processus vaginalis. For diagnosis, Dwoskin & Kuhn (1973) recommend that radiopaque fluid be injected intraperitoneally. With the patient prone, a hernia sac will fill and be visible on serial films.

Torsion of the spermatic cord is occasionally seen as a complication of cryptorchidism. Phillips & Holmes (1972) believe it is most commonly seen in spastic neurologic disease, which must be differentiated from strangulated hernia, appendicitis, and diverticulitis (Riegler, 1972).

Most authorities agree that malignancy in a misplaced testis is significantly more common than in the normally descended organ. This further substantiates the theory that many of these testes are dysgenetic. Martin (1979) collected 220 instances of cancer in undescended testes. It is rare before age 10. Because of this evidence, he suggests that the undescended testis in a patient 10 years of age or older should be removed rather than treated by orchidopexy. Hinman (1979) recommends orchidectomy for the unilateral abdominal testis, because it is less likely to be fertile, more prone to malignancy, and more difficult to place in the scrotum.

Treatment

Since definite histologic change can be demonstrated in the cryptorchid testis by age 6 years, placement of the testis in the scrotum should be accomplished by age 5. Scorer (1967) recommends surgical correction at about age 1 year. He found that 83% of patients had an associated inguinal hernia. A successful operation will not ensure fertility if the testis is congenitally defective.

A. Hormone Therapy: Chorionic gonadotropin should be administered in doses of 5000 IU intramuscularly daily for 3–5 days, depending upon the size of the child. Methyltestosterone, 5 mg/d, may be given by mouth for 1 month if the child refuses to accept the injections. Illig & others (1977) treated 84 young boys with synthetic luteinizing hormone intranasally. The dosage was 1.2 mg/d in 6 divided doses for 4 weeks. No side-effects were observed. They found this therapy to be as effective as injection of chorionic gonadotropic hormone. The degree of success depended upon the position of the testis; impalpable testes failed to respond.

If physiologic cryptorchidism has been ruled out, hormone therapy will cause descent in about a month in 10–20% of cases, with more success in bilateral than unilateral cryptorchidism. Some of these cases may have been physiologic retractile testes that were misdiagnosed despite frequent examination. Descent with hormone therapy will save the child an operation and the surgeon embarrassment, although, if this treatment is successful, the testis would probably have descended spontaneously at puberty.

B. Surgical Treatment: If hormone therapy fails, or if inguinal hernia can be demonstrated, orchiopexy (and hernioplasty) should be done immediately. The testis must be placed at the bottom of the scrotum, without tension; the blood supply to the organ must be meticulously preserved. Dissection of the inguinal area sometimes reveals that the vascular pedicle is too short to allow placement of the testis in the bottom of the scrotum. If so, the organ should be placed as low as possible, and 2 years later, the testicle should be advanced to the scrotum. In 62 cases, Zer, Wolloch, & Dintsman (1975) found that 17% of patients with atrophy of the testis required orchiectomy. In the past, a few authors have recommended division of the spermatic artery if the vascular pedicle was too short. They claimed that viability of the testis was preserved. Datta & others (1977) divided this artery at the internal ring, taking care to preserve collateral arteries to the vas deferens, cremaster muscle, and scrotum. They observed radionuclide evidence of normal vascular perfusion of the testicle. This is probably the procedure of choice for the short cord. Gibbons, Cromie, & Duckett Jr (1979) also recommend this procedure. However, Jones & Bagley (1979) used an extraperitoneal approach to place the testis in the scrotum in 85 of 86 subjects. Microsurgery has been used to place the abdominal testis in the scrotum by anastomosing the artery and vein of the testis to the inferior epigastric artery and vein (Martin & Salibian, 1980; Romas, Janecka, & Krisiloff, 1978). If the testis is not discovered or is very atrophic and is therefore removed, a prosthesis can be placed in the scrotum (Lattimer & others, 1973).

Prognosis

Success of treatment is measured by fertility. The man with one untreated cryptorchid testis produces fewer sperms than the man with normally descended testes (Lipshultz & others, 1976). Untreated bilateral cryptorchidism almost always causes infertility, but with treatment at the optimal age, 60% of these males will be fertile.

CONGENITAL ANOMALIES OF THE EPIDIDYMIS

Congenital absence of the epididymis is rare. At times the epididymis may be anterior rather than posterior to the testis. Fusion of the epididymis and testis may not occur.

DISORDERS OF THE SPERMATIC CORD*

SPERMATOCELE

A spermatocele is a painless cystic mass containing sperm. It lies just above and posterior to the

*The only congenital anomaly that affects the spermatic cord is absence of the vas deferens. If the vas is absent on both sides, infertility results.

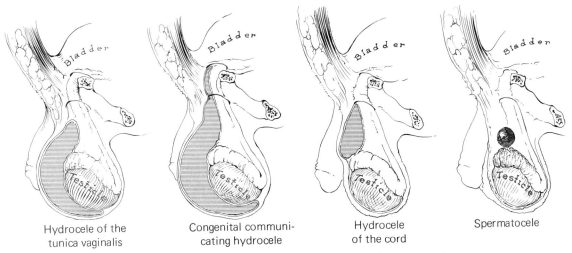

Hydrocele of the
tunica vaginalis

Congenital communi-
cating hydrocele

Hydrocele
of the cord

Spermatocele

Figure 31–2. Hydrocele of the tunica vaginalis and cord; spermatocele.

testis but is separate from it (Fig 31–2). Most spermatoceles are less than 1 cm in diameter, although they are occasionally quite large and may be mistaken for hydroceles. They may be firm, simulating solid tumor. The cause is not entirely clear, although they probably arise from the tubules that connect the rete testis to the head of the epididymides (vasa efferentia) or from cystic structures on the upper pole of the testis or epididymis.

Since they are relatively small, spermatoceles are usually discovered by the physician during routine examination of the genitalia; at times they may be large enough to come to the attention of the patient. Examination reveals a freely movable transilluminating cystic mass lying above the testicle. Microscopic examination of aspirated contents reveals sperms, usually dead. Grossly, the fluid is thin, white, and cloudy.

Spermatocele is differentiated from hydrocele of the tunica vaginalis in that the latter covers the entire anterior surface of the testicle. Aspiration of hydrocele recovers yellow but clear fluid. A tumor of the coverings of the spermatic cord (eg, mesothelioma, fibroma) may feel like a tense spermatocele. It does not, however, contain fluid and will not transilluminate.

Spermatocele requires no therapy unless it is large enough to annoy the patient, in which case it should be excised.

VARICOCELE*

Varicocele is common in young men and consists of dilatation of the pampiniform plexus above the testis, with the left side most commonly affected. These veins drain into the internal spermatic vein in the region of the internal inguinal

*See also p 551.

ring. The internal spermatic vein passes lateral to the vas deferens at the internal inguinal ring and, on the left side, drains into the renal vein. On the right it empties into the vena cava.

Incompetent valves are more common in the left internal spermatic vein. This condition, combined with the effect of gravity, may lead to poor drainage of the pampiniform plexus, the veins of which gradually undergo dilatation and elongation. The area may be painful, particularly in sexually continent men. Sexual activity (including masturbation) may relieve symptoms.

The sudden development of a varicocele in an older man is sometimes a late sign of renal tumor when tumor cells have invaded the renal vein, thereby occluding the spermatic vein.

Examination of a man with varicocele when he is upright reveals a mass of dilated, tortuous veins lying posterior to and above the testis. It may extend up to the external inguinal ring and is often tender. The degree of dilatation can be increased by the Valsalva maneuver. In the recumbent position, venous distention abates. Testicular atrophy from impaired circulation may be present.

No treatment is required unless the varicocele is thought to contribute to infertility or is painful or so large as to disturb the patient. A scrotal support will often relieve discomfort; otherwise, ligation of the internal spermatic vein at the internal inguinal ring is indicated. Results from this operation are uniformly excellent.

HYDROCELE

A hydrocele consists of a collection of fluid within the tunica or processus vaginalis. Although it may occur within the spermatic cord, it is most often seen surrounding the testis. A number of cases of hydrocele of the canal of Nuck have been reported. A hydrocele may develop rapidly secondary to local injury, radiotherapy (Streit & others, 1978), acute nonspecific or tuberculous epididymitis, or orchitis. It may complicate testicular neoplasm. Chronic hydrocele is more common. Its cause is usually unknown, and it usually afflicts men past age 40 years. Fluid collects about the testis, and the mass grows gradually (Fig 31–2). It may be soft and cystic or quite tense. The fluid is clear and yellow.

Hydrocele of the tunica vaginalis is common in the newborn, probably due to late closure of the processus vaginalis, which is continuous with the peritoneum. Most of these fluid collections subside spontaneously during the first few weeks of life.

Clinical Findings

Young boys with hydrocele commonly have a history of a cystic mass that is small and soft in the morning but larger and more tense at night. This indicates that a small communication exists in the processus vaginalis between the peritoneal cavity and the tunica vaginalis (Fig 31–2). Hernia or communicating hydrocele is therefore the proper diagnosis. Hydrocele is painless unless it is accompanied by acute epididymal infection. The patient may, however, complain of its bulk or weight.

The diagnosis is made by finding a rounded cystic intrascrotal mass that is not tender unless underlying inflammatory disease is present. The mass transilluminates. If the hydrocele is enclosed within the spermatic cord, a cystic fusiform swelling is noted in the groin or in the upper scrotum.

A tense hydrocele must be differentiated from tumor of the testis, which does not transilluminate. However, if hydrocele develops in a young man without apparent cause, it should be aspirated so that careful palpation of the testicle and epididymis can be done in order to rule out cancer or tuberculosis.

Complications include compression of the blood supply of the testicle, which leads to atrophy; hemorrhage into the hydrocele sac following trauma or aspiration (hematocele); or, rarely, infection complicating aspiration.

Treatment

Unless complications are present, active therapy is not required. The indications for treatment are a very tense hydrocele that might embarrass circulation to the testicle or a large, bulky mass that is cosmetically unsightly and perhaps uncomfortable for the patient.

A hydrocele present during the first few months of life is often cured by a single aspiration. Periodic aspiration is usually the treatment of choice in chronic hydrocele. Most chronic hydroceles refill slowly over a period of 6–20 weeks, at which time aspiration can be repeated. If the sac refills rapidly or if the patient requests definitive therapy, the parietal tunica vaginalis should be re-

sected. Lord has described a simple operation wherein the hydrocele sac, after being opened, is merely stitched together to collapse the wall (Haas & others, 1978). The results of both procedures are good, though in a few cases the hydrocele recurs. Secondary infection may require incision and drainage. Hematocele should be treated by resection of the hydrocele sac.

TORSION OF THE SPERMATIC CORD

Torsion of the spermatic cord (torsion of the testicle) is an uncommon affliction that is almost completely limited to prepuberal males. It has been observed in the newborn (Kay, Strong, & Tank, 1980). It causes strangulation of the blood supply to the testis. Unless treatment is given within 3 or 4 hours, testicular atrophy may occur.

The cryptorchid testis is prone to undergo torsion (Mowad & Konvolinka, 1978). In about half of patients, this disorder occurs during sleep. In most instances, congenital abnormality of the tunica vaginalis or spermatic cord is present. Torsion seems to be most often due to a voluminous tunica vaginalis that inserts well up on the cord. This allows the testis to rotate within the tunica. The initiating factor seems to be spasm of the cremaster muscle, which inserts obliquely on the cord. The contraction of this muscle causes the patient's left testis to rotate counterclockwise and his right testis clockwise (as the physician observes the patient from the foot of the bed). With vascular occlusion there is edema of the testis and the cord up to the point of occlusion. This leads to gangrene of the testis and epididymis.

Clinical Findings

Diagnosis is suggested when a young boy suddenly develops severe pain in one testicle, followed by swelling of the organ, reddening of the scrotal skin, lower abdominal pain, and nausea and vomiting. However, torsion of the cord may be accompanied only by moderate scrotal swelling and little or no pain (Lyon, 1961).

Examination usually reveals a swollen, tender organ that is retracted upward as a result of shortening of the cord by volvulus. Corriere (1972) observed that the testis is apt to lie in the horizontal position. Greaney (1975) noted that testes that are apt to undergo torsion lie horizontally with the patient standing. He recognized this abnormality in a number of boys who had, in the past, suffered from transient testicular pain representing torsion with spontaneous detorsion. Pain may be increased by lifting the testicle up over the symphysis. (The pain from epididymitis, rare in children, is usually alleviated by this maneuver.) Within a few hours after onset, moderate fever and leukocytosis may develop.

The diagnosis may be made in the early stages

if the epididymis can be felt in an abnormal position (eg, anterior). After a few hours, however, the entire gonad becomes so swollen that the epididymis cannot be distinguished from the testis by palpation. Torsion can be differentiated from epididymitis by using the Doppler stethoscope in conjunction with ultrasound. The testis made ischemic by torsion will not echo sound; the hypervascularity of epididymitis will increase sound (Smith & King, 1979). This is a quick and simple method. Differentiation can also be done by a rectilinear scan following intravenous injection of ^{99m}Tc (Boedecker, Sty, & Jona, 1979). The Doppler stethoscope can be used in conjunction with ultrasound for a simple and quicker diagnosis. There is no sound echoing from an ischemic testis; sound is increased with the hypervascularity of epididymitis (Smith & King, 1979).

Differential Diagnosis

The differential diagnosis includes acute epididymitis, acute mumps orchitis, and trauma. Epididymitis is rare before puberty and is often accompanied by pyuria. Mumps orchitis, also rare before puberty, is usually accompanied by parotitis. Without a history or findings of injury, traumatic orchitis may be misdiagnosed as torsion of the cord.

Epididymitis is unusual before age 25. Differential diagnosis from torsion may be difficult if epididymitis is not complicated by pyuria, for fever is associated with both conditions. In case of doubt, the testis should be exposed.

Treatment

If the patient is seen within a few hours of onset, manual detorsion may be attempted (King & others, 1974). Torsion causes the left testis to rotate counterclockwise and the right one clockwise; therefore, one may twist a testis in the opposite direction. The right testis should be "unscrewed" and the left one "screwed up" (Editorial, *Br Med J*, 1972). This maneuver is facilitated by infiltration of the spermatic cord, near the external inguinal ring, with 10–20 mL of 1% procaine hydrochloride. Even if this is successful, surgical fixation of both testes should be done within the next few days. If manual detorsion fails, immediate surgical detorsion must be performed, although after 4–6 hours infarction usually will have occurred in those testes subjected to a 720-degree twist of the cord. Whether the testis appears to be viable or not, it should be sutured down to preclude subsequent torsion. Even though the seminiferous tubules may become necrotic, the more hardy interstitial cells may remain viable. Excision of the parietal tunica vaginalis will cause agglutination of the testicle to the scrotal wall. Since the opposite testicle usually is affected by the same abnormal attachments, prophylactic fixation of that organ is imperative.

Prognosis

Unfortunately, the diagnosis is usually made and treatment instituted too late, and atrophy is to be expected in most instances. Wright (1977) has observed that detorsion within 12 hours of onset affords a good result; that recovery is possible if treatment is given 12–24 hours later; and that preservation is doubtful after 24 hours. If detorsion is delayed beyond 48 hours, orchiectomy is advised.

•   •   •

TORSION OF THE APPENDICES OF THE TESTIS AND EPIDIDYMIS

On the upper poles of both the testis and epididymis there are small vestigial appendages that may be sessile or pedunculated (Fig 1–7). The latter type may spontaneously undergo torsion, which leads to an inflammatory reaction followed by ischemic necrosis and absorption.

This phenomenon usually affects boys up to age 16 years, though Altaffer & Steele (1980) were able to find reports of 350 instances of torsion in adults. Sudden onset of testicular pain is noted. Shortly after onset, a small tender lump may be felt at the upper pole of the testis or epididymis; this sign is pathognomonic, particularly if the lump appears to be blue when the skin is held tight over the mass (Dresner, 1973; Puri & Boyd, 1976).

At later examination, the entire testicle is swollen and tender. The differential diagnosis is then between torsion of these appendages and of the spermatic cord. Immediate surgical exploration is indicated, for time is a critical factor in the treatment of torsion of the cord. If an appendix is twisted, it should be excised.

•   •   •

References

SCROTUM

Futter NG: Scrotal emphysema. *Urology* 1980;**15**:360.

Heydenrych JJ, Marcus PB: Meconium granulomas of the tunica vaginalis. *J Urol* 1976;**115**:596.

Kaplan GW: Acute idiopathic scrotal edema. *J Pediatr Surg* 1977;**12**:647.

TESTIS

Anomalies of Number

Brothers LR III, Weber CH Jr, Ball TP Jr: Anorchism versus cryptorchidism: The importance of a diligent search for intra-abdominal testes. *J Urol* 1978;**119**:707.

Goldberg LM, Skaist LB, Morrow JW: Congenital absence of the testes: Anorchism and monorchism. *J Urol* 1974;**111**:840.

Lazarus BA, Tessler AN: Polyorchidism with normal spermatogenesis. *Urology* 1974;**3**:615.

Pelander WM, Luna G, Lilly JR: Polyorchidism: Case report and literature review. *J Urol* 1978;**119**:705.

Reckler JM, Rose LI, Harrison JH: Bilateral anorchism. *J Urol* 1975;**113**:869.

Hypogonadism

Bryson MF, Reichlin S: Neuroendocrine regulation of sexual function and growth. *Pediatr Clin North Am* 1966;**13**:423.

Federman DD: The assessment of organ function–the testis. *N Engl J Med* 1971;**285**:901.

Stearns EL & others: Declining testicular function with age. *Am J Med* 1974;**57**:761.

Wilson JD: Recent studies on the mechanism of action of testosterone. *N Engl J Med* 1972;**287**:1284.

Ectopy & Cryptorchidism

Concodora JA, Evans RA, Smith MJV: Ectopic penile testis. *Urology* 1976;**8**:263.

Datta NS & others: Division of spermatic vessels in orchiopexy: Radionuclide evidence of preservation of testicular circulation. *J Urol* 1977;**118**:447.

Dewald GW, Kelalis PP, Gordon H: Chromosomal studies in cryptorchidism. *J Urol* 1977;**117**:110.

Dwoskin JY, Kuhn JP: Herniagrams in undescended testes and hydroceles. *J Urol* 1973;**109**:520.

Freeny PC, Cummings KB, Simmons JR: Selective testicular venography for localization of nonpalpable testis. *Urology* 1978;**12**:617.

Fujita J: Transverse testicular ectopia. *Urology* 1980;**16**:400.

Gibbons MD, Cromie WJ, Duckett JW Jr: Management of the abdominal undescended testicle. *J Urol* 1979;**122**:76.

Hinman F Jr: Unilateral abdominal cryptorchidism. *J Urol* 1979;**122**:71.

Illig R & others: Treatment of cryptorchidism by intranasal synthetic luteinising-hormone releasing hormone. *Lancet* 1977;**2**:518.

Jones PF, Bagley FH: An abdominal extraperitoneal approach for the difficult orchidopexy. *Br J Surg* 1979;**66**:14.

Lattimer JK & others: A natural-feeling testicular prosthesis. *J Urol* 1973;**110**:81.

Lee JKT & others: Utility of computed tomography in the localization of the undescended testis. *Radiology* 1980;**135**:121.

Lipshultz LI & others: Testicular function after orchiopexy for unilaterally undescended testis. *N Engl J Med* 1976;**295**:15.

Madrazo BL & others: Ultrasonographic demonstration of undescended testes. *Radiology* 1979;**133**:181.

Marshall FF, Shermeta DW: Epididymal abnormalities associated with undescended testis. *J Urol* 1979;**121**:341.

Martin DC: Germinal cell tumors of the testis after orchiopexy. *J Urol* 1979;**121**:422.

Martin DC, Salibian AH: Orchiopexy using microvascular surgical technique. *J Urol* 1980;**123**:435.

Miller HC: Transseptal orchiopexy for cryptorchism. *J Urol* 1967;**98**:503.

Puri P, Nixon HH: Bilateral retractile testes: Subsequent effects on fertility. *J Pediatr Surg* 1977;**12**:563.

Rajfer J, Walsh PC: Hormonal regulation of testicular descent: Experimental and clinical observations. *J Urol* 1977;**118**:985.

Riegler HC: Torsion of intra-abdominal testis: An unusual problem in diagnosis of the acute surgical abdomen. *Surg Clin North Am* 1972;**52**:371.

Romas NA, Janecka I, Krisiloff M: Role of microsurgery in orchiopexy. *Urology* 1978;**12**:670.

Scorer CG: Early operation for the undescended testis. *Br J Surg* 1967;**54**:694.

Shapiro SR, Bodai BI: Current concepts of the undescended testis. *Surg Gynecol Obstet* 1978;**147**:617.

Weiss RM, Glickman MG, Lytton B: Clinical implications of gonadal venography in the management of the nonpalpable undescended testis. *J Urol* 1979;**121**:745.

SPERMATIC CORD

Spermatocele

Clarke BG, Bamford SB, Gherardi GJ: Spermatocele: Pathologic and surgical anatomy. *Arch Surg* 1963;**86**:351.

Lord PH: A bloodless operation for spermatocele or cyst of the epididymis. *Br J Surg* 1970;**57**:641.

Schoenberg HW, Murphy JJ: The differential diagnosis of intrascrotal masses. *GP* (March) 1962;**25**:82.

Varicocele

Ahlberg NE & others: Phlebography in varicocele scroti. *Acta Radiol [Diagn] (Stockh)* 1966;**4**:517.

Clarke BG: Incidence of varicocele in normal men and among men of different age groups. *JAMA* 1966;**198**:1121.

Kiska EF, Cowart GT: Treatment of varicocele by high ligation. *J Urol* 1960;**83**:713.

Shafik A, Khalil AM, Saleh M: The fasciomuscular tube of the spermatic cord: A study of its surgical anatomy and relation to varicocele: A new concept for the pathogenesis of varicocele. *Br J Urol* 1972;**44**:147.

Hydrocele

Ariyan S: Hydrocele of the canal of Nuck. *J Urol* 1973;**110**:172.

Haas JA & others: Operative treatment of hydrocele: Another look at Lord's procedure. *Urology* 1978;**12**:578.

Parekh BP, Reinboth G, Mishra OP: Abdominoscrotal hydrocele. *Br J Surg* 1975;**62**:629.

Streit CC & others: Hydrocele formation from sandwich irradiation therapy for testicular tumor. *Urology* 1978;**12**:222.

Wilkinson JL: An operation for large scrotal hydrocele. *Br J Surg* 1973;**60**:450.

Torsion of the Spermatic Cord

Abu-Sleiman R, Ho JE, Gregory JG: Scrotal scanning: Present value and limits of interpretation. *Urology* 1979;**13**:326.

Boedecker RA, Sty JR, Jona JZ: Testicular scanning as a diagnostic aid in evaluating scrotal pain. *J Pediatr* 1979;**94**:760.

Corriere JN Jr: Horizontal lie of the testicle: A diagnostic sign of torsion of the testicle. *J Urol* 1972;**107**:616.

Greaney MG: Torsion of the testis—A review of 22 cases: Improved diagnosis and earlier correction. *Br J Surg* 1975;**62**:57.

Kay R, Strong DW, Tank ES: Bilateral spermatic cord torsion in the neonate. *J Urol* 1980;**123**:293.

Lyon RP: Torsion of the testicle in childhood: A painless emergency requiring contralateral orchiopexy. *JAMA* 1961;**178**:702.

Mowad JJ, Konvolinka CW: Torsion of undescended testis. *Urology* 1978;**12**:567.

Schneider RE, Laycob LM, Griffin WT: Testicular torsion in utero. *Am J Obstet Gynecol* 1973;**117**:1126.

Smith SP, King LR: Torsion of the testis: Techniques of assessment. *Urol Clin North Am* 1979;**6**:429.

Torsion of the testicle again. (Editorial.) *Br Med J* 1972;**4**:505.

Williams JD, Hodgson NB: Another look at torsion of testis. *Urology* 1979;**14**:36.

Wright JE: Torsion of the testis. *Br J Surg* 1977;**64**:274.

Appendices of the Testis & Epididymis

Altaffer LF III, Steele SM Jr: Torsion of testicular appendages in men. *J Urol* 1980;**124**:56.

Dresner ML: Torsed appendage diagnosis and management: Blue dot sign. *Urology* 1973;**1**:63.

Puri P, Boyd E: Torsion of the appendix testis: A survey of 22 cases. *Clin Pediatr (Phila)* 1976;**15**:949.

Williamson RCN: Torsion of the testis and allied conditions. *Br J Surg* 1976;**63**:465.

32 | Skin Diseases of the External Genitalia*

Rees B. Rees, Jr., MD, MS

Almost any skin condition, including psoriasis, seborrheic dermatitis, lichen planus, eczema, etc, can affect the region of the external genitalia and perineum. The patient should be questioned and examined for other possible areas of involvement. In any case of itching or infected dermatitis in this area, it is important to rule out diabetes and pediculosis or scabies.

Associated vaginal and other urologic conditions should be corrected. Self-treatment and over-treatment may alter and complicate genital lesions. Emotional factors associated with repeated scratching and rubbing tend to prolong and complicate genital conditions.

Many individuals with involvement in this area have a fear of venereal disease; if there is no question of this, the fear should be dispelled.

ECZEMATOID DERMATITIS

Eczematoid dermatitis is a broad descriptive term which denotes changes such as redness, vesiculation, scaling, weeping, lichenification (accentuation and thickening of skin markings), and excoriation. This type of eruption may become secondarily infected through scratching. Included in this group are such conditions as contact dermatitis, localized neurodermatitis, pruritus vulvae and scroti, atopic dermatitis, and intertriginous dermatitis. These conditions usually overlap in producing an eczematoid dermatitis, and treatment must take this into consideration.

Contact Dermatitis

Contact dermatitis includes changes produced by both primary irritants and true allergic sensitizers. Possible causes are cosmetics, feminine deodorant sprays, douches, contraceptives, soaps, local medications ("overtreatment dermatitis"), wearing apparel, plants (poison oak and ivy), etc.

Treatment must include removal of the suspected agent, if possible. Cool wet dressings consti-

*Venereal disease is discussed in Chapter 14; tumors in Chapter 18.

tute excellent treatment, and corticosteroid creams may be used topically if infection is not present. The fluorinated corticosteroid creams such as fluocinolone, triamcinolone, betamethasone, and fluocinonide are more likely to produce atrophic striae in the groin than is 1% hydrocortisone.

Circumscribed Neurodermatitis (Lichen Simplex Chronicus)

These thickened lesions are of great importance in the persistence of any vulval or scrotal skin condition regardless of the original cause. Rubbing and scratching can prolong any eruption indefinitely, and it is usually this problem that causes the patient to seek medical care. This may be done almost subconsciously. A continuing itch-scratch cycle is established which must be broken before healing can occur.

Treatment is as for contact dermatitis (above) plus counseling about the dangers of persistent trauma.

Itching of Vulva & Scrotum

These are merely nonspecific terms used to classify some cases of marked pruritus of these areas with little or no skin changes. Treatment is as for contact dermatitis (above). Refractory cases call for biopsy, direct microscopic examination for fungi in skin scales or exudate (using 15% sodium or potassium hydroxide for clearing), examination for parasites (including *Trichomonas*), and a careful search of the rest of the body for evidence of skin disease.

Atopic Dermatitis

This lesion presents as dry lichenified dermatitis on the penis and scrotum, in the groins, and on the vulva. Similar changes are usually present also on the face and neck and in the antecubital and popliteal spaces. Generalized dryness is present. There is usually a personal or family history of asthma or hay fever.

Hydrocortisone cream, 1%, should be rubbed in thinly twice daily.

Triamcinolone acetonide suspension, 20–40 mg given deeply intragluteally at monthly or less frequent intervals, may give dramatic relief in this and other eczematous disorders. It may disturb the menstrual cycle in women. Observe the precautions that apply to all internal corticosteroids.

Intertrigo

Intertrigo (sodden, macerated dermatitis) is due to chafing and friction of contiguous surfaces. It occurs in the groins, inframammary areas, skin folds, etc, usually in obese individuals, and is more common during hot, humid weather. Treatment must be directed toward drying the area and reducing chafing. Hydrocortisone, 1%, and iodochlorhydroxyquin, 3% in hydrophilic ointment base, may be rubbed into the areas twice daily, then dusted over with ZeaSorb Powder.*

COMMON SUPERFICIAL INFECTIONS OF THE EXTERNAL GENITALIA

Pyodermas

Staphylococci are present in most of the infections discussed below, but streptococci may be found in as many as 40% of cases. A smear stained with Giemsa's stain will usually show many cocci within the polymorphonuclear leukocytes. Systemic antibiotic treatment is mandatory, even though it will not prevent the development of nephritis caused by nephritogenic strains of streptococci in the individual. It will prevent other complications and is essential from an epidemiologic viewpoint. Pediculosis and scabies should be ruled out.

Sodium cloxacillin is the drug of choice, since it is not destroyed by penicillinase. If the patient is allergic to penicillin, the drug of second choice is erythromycin. A polymyxin-bacitracin ointment such as Polysporin may be used topically.

Pyodermas frequently complicate some other primary condition, such as pediculosis and scabies.

A. Folliculitis and Furunculosis: Infection of a hair follicle is usually acute but may be chronic and recurrent. Sharply pointed, extremely tender and hot swellings with central pustulation may be found.

B. Impetigo: Impetiginous involvement is more superficial and is characterized by "stuck-on crusts" and weeping. The mons pubis may be the sole site of involvement, but other areas are usually involved also.

C. Infectious Eczematoid Dermatitis: This is an acute reddened, weeping, spreading eruption. It is often associated with a draining process such as a furuncle or abscess.

D. Hidradenitis Suppurativa: This is a deep chronic inflammatory infection of the apocrine sweat glands, characterized by cystic involvement and interconnecting sinus tracts. It usually involves

---

*Parachlorometaxylenol 0.5%, microporous cellulose 45%, and aluminum dihydroxy allantoinate 0.2%.

the axillas and groins and may be an accompaniment of severe cystic acne. In addition to giving antibiotics, it may be necessary to unroof ("saucerize") or actually excise the lesions, with or without grafting.

Fungal Infections

Heat, moisture, and darkness favor these infections. They are frequently aggravated by overtreatment.

A. Tinea Cruris: Tinea cruris is characterized by marginated, slightly elevated, scaling patches on the inner thighs and in the groins. There may be an active vesicular border. Pruritus may be intense. Direct microscopic examination of skin scrapings in 15% potassium or sodium hydroxide solution will reveal hyphae or spores. The differential diagnosis includes seborrheic dermatitis, psoriasis, intertrigo, and localized neurodermatitis. Tinea cruris usually responds to treatment with 3% precipitated sulfur and 1% salicylic acid in an emulsion base applied twice daily. Miconazole, 2% cream or lotion, or clotrimazole, 1% cream or lotion, and haloprogin, 1% cream, applied twice daily, are good alternatives. If they are irritating, 1% hydrocortisone cream may be used concomitantly. Griseofulvin (micronized), 500 mg orally, may be given daily after supper.

B. Anogenital Candidiasis: Infection with *Candida albicans* is characterized by erythematous, weeping, circumscribed lesions with peripheral epidermal undermining and satellite vesiculopustules. "Ping-pong" infections between sexual partners may occur. Pregnancy, diabetes, obesity, and hyperhidrosis are predisposing factors. Broad-spectrum antibiotic therapy or estrogen therapy may be followed by an overgrowth of candidal organisms. The skin involvement may be secondary to vaginal involvement. Lesions occur under the prepuce. High-power microscopic examination of skin scrapings in 15% potassium or sodium hydroxide solution shows clusters of tiny spores and fine mycelial filaments. Nystatin appears to be effective in most instances. It is available as dusting powder, cream, vaginal inserts, and oral tablets. Miconazole, 2% cream or lotion, clotrimazole, 1% cream or lotion, and 1% haloprogin cream, applied twice daily, are good alternatives to nystatin.

Virus Infections

A. Warts: Warts are common in the vulval region, under the prepuce, and on the shaft of the penis. If present on the mucous or mucocutaneous surfaces, they are called condylomata acuminata. They are usually moist and macerated. They frequently respond to topical treatment with podophyllum resin, 25% in compound tincture of benzoin applied sparingly once weekly. Severe discomfort may follow application of podophyllum. Fulguration may be necessary if podophyllum is not successful. Liquid nitrogen can be used with a cotton-tipped applicator. Each lesion may be frozen for 10–30 seconds.

B. Herpes Simplex (Cold Sore, Fever Blister): Genital herpes is usually due to recurrent herpesvirus type 2 and is characterized by grouped vesiculopustular lesions. There may be secondary adenopathy. This can be a painful recurrent condition and has been implicated in the genesis of cervical carcinoma. Rarely, a primary herpes simplex infection is seen, with severe vulvovaginitis and systemic manifestations. Lesions may be painted weekly with fresh Castellani's paint or 1% aqueous gentian violet, after which they are dabbed thoroughly dry with cotton.

A wet styptic pencil (aluminum sulfate) may be rubbed into the lesions frequently. A simple dusting powder such as BFI (bismuth formic iodide) may be useful.

OTHER INFLAMMATORY DISORDERS

Drug Eruptions

Drug eruptions may involve the genitals. A fixed drug eruption, due usually to phenolphthalein, broad-spectrum antibiotics, or barbiturates, may cause a perfectly round, bright-red to purplish macular lesion which comes and goes with each reexposure to the drug. Other drug eruptions usually have manifestations elsewhere as well as on the circumscribed area.

Urticaria & Angioneurotic Edema

These lesions ("hives" and "giant hives") may present on the vulva or male genitalia as a sole sign, at least initially. They may be confused with acute contact dermatitis, which can have an urticarial component. There may be a history of ingestion of an urticariogenic food such as shellfish, pork and pork products, strawberries, or yeast-containing foods. Penicillin is the most common drug cause. Treatment consists of removal of the cause, if known, plus soothing baths with oatmeal (Aveeno baths), and hydroxyzine, 25 mg 2–4 times daily, or cyproheptadine, 4 mg 2–4 times daily.

Erythema Multiforme

Erythema multiforme may present as an acute inflammatory erosive process on the genitalia, although signs are usually present elsewhere, eg, the lips, tongue, and mouth, possibly with conjunctivitis. Erythema multiforme and its more severe variant, Stevens-Johnson disease, may be idiopathic or may be caused by drug reaction, herpes simplex, or other infection. Finding a typical "target" herpes iris or "bull's-eye" lesion may make the diagnosis. Severe forms must be managed symptomatically with supportive treatment and hospitalization. Systemic corticosteroids may be necessary (unless contraindicated), and broad-spectrum antibiotics may be helpful as well.

"Jock Itch"

"Jock Itch" is a common term usually intended to denote tinea cruris, but any of the following may give rise to irritated and pruritic dermatitis in anogenital folds: tinea cruris and candidiasis (see above); intertrigo, due to maceration from heat moisture, darkness, friction, and chafing; seborrheic dermatitis and psoriasis inversus (look for stigmas of these conditions elsewhere on the body); and lichen simplex chronicus. Management of any type of "jock itch," in addition to measures described under tinea cruris and candidiasis, include airing the affected parts, painting them from time to time with Castellani's paint (caution), use of a highly absorbent powder such as Zeasorb (made of ground-up corncobs), and the application morning and night of a very thin layer of cream containing 3% iodochlorhydroxyquin (Vioform) and 1% hydrocortisone. In tropical climates, successful treatment has been bed rest with the patient nude, covered by a cradle with a sheet over it and an electric fan playing on the affected parts. Associated tinea pedis must be treated also.

PAPULOSQUAMOUS ERUPTIONS

Psoriasis

Psoriasis may involve flexural surfaces (inverse psoriasis) such as the groin and the perianal, internatal cleft, and intermammary areas. It tends to be bright red and moist, and usually free of scales. Itching may be intense. Occasionally the only involvement may be in the anogenital area. A solitary plaque may present on the penis, leading to confusion with Bowen's disease or some other more serious disorder. The diagnosis usually can be made by inspection and by noting other areas of involvement such as in the scalp and on the elbows and knees. Pitting of the nails, when present, is almost pathognomonic of psoriasis. Treatment is with 0.1% anthralin ointment rubbed in sparingly morning and night for intertriginous lesions. Hydrocortisone cream, 1%, may be used concomitantly.

Seborrheic Dermatitis

Seborrheic dermatitis may appear as scurfy, scaly, erythematous patches and is easily confused with candidiasis, intertrigo, and psoriasis. Typical areas of involvement are usually present elsewhere, eg, the scalp, brows, creases of the cheeks and chin, in and around the ears, on the presternum, and in the axillas. Corticosteroid creams are very useful. Twice daily application of sulfur (3%) and salicylic acid (1%) in an emulsion base is also effective. Highly potent corticosteroid creams should not be used on the face for prolonged periods because of the appearance of temporary atrophy and "steroid rosacea" in susceptible individuals.

Lichen Planus

Lichen planus may appear on the glans penis or on the labia and introitus. The lesions are small polygonal violet-hued papules about 2–3 cm in diameter which have milky striations over their shiny surfaces. They may become clustered together to form plaques. Itching is usually a problem. There may be generalized involvement or typical lesions in the buccal mucosa that look like spilled milk.

Corticosteroid creams may be helpful in relieving the pruritus. The disease usually disappears after a course of several months.

LICHEN SCLEROSUS ET ATROPHICUS

This is a distinct entity characterized by flat-topped white papules which coalesce to form white patches without infiltration. The surface shows comedonelike plugs or dells. The end stages may resemble very thin parchment or tissue paper. It occurs most frequently in patches on the upper back, chest, and breasts, mostly in women. It almost inevitably involves the anogenital regions, where painful fissures may develop and severe itching may be a distressing symptom. On the penis this condition occurs as balanitis xerotica obliterans, which may lead to urethral stenosis and atrophy with telangiectasia about the meatus and on the glans, with some shrinkage of the prepuce. There is a direct relationship between these conditions and carcinoma, although this is quite rare and should not call for prophylactic surgery of these genital lesions. Anogenital lichen sclerosus et atrophicus may be misdiagnosed as kraurosis vulvae with or without leukoplakia. At present, kraurosis is regarded as a descriptive term for the manifestation in a number of diseases.

Lichen sclerosus et atrophicus may involute spontaneously, especially in young girls.

Vitamin A ointment may be tried. For severe itching, one may use intralesional corticosteroids such as triamcinolone (Kenalog) suspension injected into the skin with the Dermajet apparatus or by syringe. Topical corticosteroids may give relief.

Circumcision for balanitis xerotica obliterans that is lichen sclerosus is not particularly helpful.

In the author's hands, vitamin E acetate (D-α-tocopheryl acetate), 1600 IU daily by mouth, has been associated with involution of these lesions.

Testosterone, 1–2% in a creamy vehicle, is said to cause some lesions to involute in the female.

● ● ●

References

General

Domonkos AN, Arnold HL Jr, Odom RB: *Andrews' Diseases of the Skin: Clinical Dermatology,* 7th ed. Saunders, 1981.

Fitzpatrick TB & others: *Dermatology in General Medicine.* McGraw-Hill, 1980.

Moschella SL, Pillsbury DM, Hurley JF Jr: *Dermatology.* Saunders, 1975.

Noojin RO: *Practitioner's Guide to Dermatology.* Medical Examination Publishing Co., 1977.

Rook A, Wilkinson DS, Ebling FJ: *Textbook of Dermatology.* Blackwell, 1979.

Contact Dermatitis

Fisher AA: *Contact Dermatitis.* Lea & Febiger, 1973.

Circumscribed Neurodermatitis

Runne U, Orfanos C: Cutaneous neural proliferation in highly pruritic lesions of chronic prurigo. *Arch Dermatol* 1977;**113**:787.

Atopic Dermatitis

Hanifin J, Lobitz WC Jr: Newer concepts of atopic dermatitis. *Arch Dermatol* 1977;**113**:663.

Pyodermas

Noble WC, Somerville DA: *Microbiology of Human Skin.* Saunders, 1974.

Fungal Infections

De Villez RL, Lewis CW: Candidiasis seminar. *Cutis* 1977;**19**:69.

Smith EB: New topical agents for dermatophytosis. *Cutis* 1976;**17**:54.

Virus Infections

Rees RB: How I treat warts. *Med Times* (March) 1980;**108**:31.

Conant MA: Cutaneous virology: Recent advances relating to dermatology. *Cutis* 1975;**15**:339.

Drug Eruptions

Arndt KA, Jick H: Rates of cutaneous reactions to drugs: A report from the Boston Collaborative Drug Surveillance Program. *JAMA* 1976;**235**:918.

Urticaria

Monroe EW, Jones HE: Urticaria. *Arch Dermatol* 1977;**113**:80.

Erythema Multiforme

Orfanos CE, Schaumberg-Lever G, Lever WF: Dermal and epidermal types of erythema multiforme. *Arch Dermatol* 1974;**109**:682.

"Jock Itch"

Rees RB: Tinea cruris (jock itch). Page 65 in: *Current Medical Diagnosis & Treatment,* 20th ed. Krupp MA, Chatton MJ (editors). Lange, 1981.

Psoriasis

Farber EM, Cox AJ (editors): *Psoriasis: Proceedings of the Second International Symposium.* Yorke Medical Books, 1977.

Seborrheic Dermatitis

Rees RB: Seborrheic dermatitis. Page 575 in: *Current Therapy 1975.* Conn HF (editor). Saunders, 1975.

Lichen Planus

Michel B, Sy EK: Tissue-fixed immunoglobulins in lichen planus. In: *Immunopathology of the Skin.* Beutner EH & others (editors). Dowden, Hutchinson, & Ross, 1973.

Lichen Sclerosus et Atrophicus

Ridley CM: *The Vulva.* Saunders, 1975.

Abnormalities of Sexual Differentiation | 33

Felix A. Conte, MD, & Melvin M. Grumbach, MD

Advances in cytogenetics, experimental embryology, steroid biochemistry, and methods of evaluation of the interaction between the hypothalamus, pituitary, and gonads have helped to clarify problems of sexual differentiation. Such anomalies may occur at any stage of intrauterine maturation and can lead to gross ambisexual development or to subtle abnormalities that do not become manifest until sexual maturity is achieved.

Figs 33–1 to 33–4, 33–7 to 33–10, and 33–14 and Tables 33–2, 33–4, and 33–5 are reproduced, with permission, from Grumbach MM, Van Wyk JJ: Disorders of sex differentiation. Chap 8, pp 423–501, in: *Textbook of Endocrinology*, 5th ed. Williams RH (editor). Saunders, 1974.

NORMAL SEX DIFFERENTIATION

Chromosomal Sex

The normal human diploid cell contains 22 autosomal pairs of chromosomes and 2 sex chromosomes (two X or one X and one Y). Arranged serially and numbered according to size and centromeric position, they are known as a karyotype. Recent advances in the technics of staining chromosomes (Fig 33–1) permit positive identification of each chromosome by its unique "banding" pattern. Bands can be produced with the fluorescent dye quinacrine (Q bands), in the region of the centromere (C bands), and with Giemsa's stain (G bands). Fluorescent banding (Fig 33–2) is particularly useful because the Y chromosome stains so brightly that it can be identified easily in both interphase and metaphase cells. The standard nomenclature for describing the human karyotype is shown in Table 33–1.

Studies in patients with abnormalities of sexual differentiation indicate that the sex chromosomes—the X and Y chromosomes—carry genes that influence sexual differentiation by causing the bipotential gonad to develop either as a testis or as an ovary. Two normally functioning X chromosomes, in the absence of a Y chromosome and the genes for testicular organogenesis, lead to the formation of an ovary.

Careful examination of the karyotype in humans reveals a marked discrepancy in size between the X and Y chromosomes. There is evidence that gene dosage compensation is achieved in all persons with 2 or more X chromosomes in their genetic

constitution by inactivation of all X chromosomes except one. This phenomenon, the so-called Lyon hypothesis, is thought to be a random process that occurs in each cell in the late blastocyst stage of embryonic development. The result of this process is formation of a sex chromatin body (Barr body) in the interphase cells of persons having 2 or more X chromosomes (Fig 33–3). In buccal mucosal smears

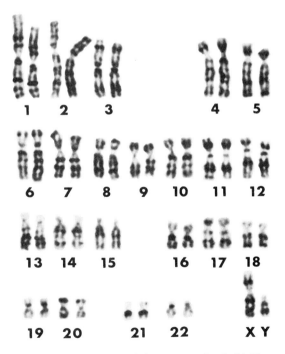

Figure 33–1. A normal 46,XY karyotype stained with Giemsa's stain to produce G bands. Note that each chromosome has a specific banding pattern.

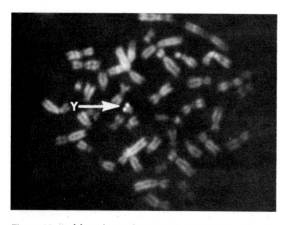
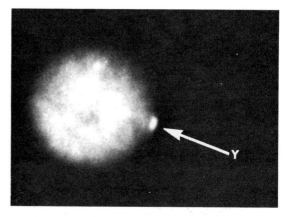

Figure 33–2. Metaphase chromosomes stained with quinacrine and examined through a fluorescence microscope. Note the bright fluorescence of the distal arms of the Y chromosome, which can also be seen in interphase cells ("Y body" at right).

Table 33–1. Nomenclature for describing the human karyotype pertinent to designating sex chromosome abnormalities.

Paris Conference	Description	Former Nomenclature
46,XX	Normal female karyotype	XX
46,XY	Normal male karyotype	XY
47,XXY	Karyotype with 47 chromosomes including an extra X chromosome	XXY
45,X	Monosomy X	XO
45,X/46,XY	Mosaic karyotype composed of 45,X and 46,XY cell lines	XO/XY
p	Short arm	p
q	Long arm	q
46,X, del (X) (:p21 qter)	Deletion of the short arm of the X distal to band Xp21	Xp–
46,X, del (X) (pter q21:)	Deletion of the long arm of the X distal to band Xq21	Xq–
46,X,i (Xq)	Isochromosome of the long arm of X	Xqi
46,X,i (Xp)	Isochromosome of the short arm of X	Xpi
46,X,r (X)	Ring X chromosome	Xr
46,X,del (Y) (pter → q11:), t(7;Y) (7pter 7q36::Yq11 → Yqter)	Translocation of the distal fluorescent portion of the Y chromosome to the long arm of chromosome 7.	46,XYt (Yq–7q+)

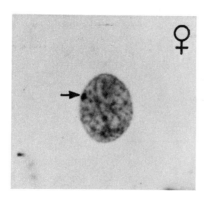

Figure 33–3. X chromatin body in the nucleus of a buccal mucosal cell from a normal female.

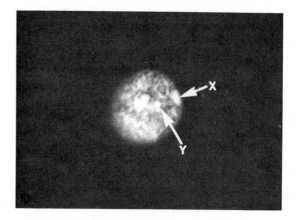

Figure 33–4. An interphase nucleus stained with quinacrine and examined by fluorescence microscopy. This cell reveals a "Y body" and an X chromatin body. The patient has a 47,XXY karyotype.

Table 33–2. Sex chromosome complement correlated with X chromatin and Y bodies in somatic interphase nuclei.*

Sex Chromosomes	Maximum Number in Diploid Somatic Nuclei	
	X Bodies	Y Bodies
45,XO	0	0
46,XX	1	0
46,XY	0	1
47,XXX	2	0
47,XXY	1	1
47,XYY	0	2
48,XXXX	3	0
48,XXXY	2	1
48,XXYY	1	2
49,XXXXX	4	0
49,XXXXY	3	1
49,XXXYY	2	2

*The maximum number of X chromatin bodies in diploid somatic nuclei is one less than the number of Xs, whereas the maximum number of Y fluorescent bodies is equivalent to the number of Ys in the chromosome constitution.

of 46,XX females, a sex chromatin body is evident in 20–30% of the nuclei examined, whereas in normal 46,XY males, a comparable sex chromatin body is absent. In patients with more than two X chromosomes, the maximum number of sex chromatin bodies in any diploid nucleus is one less than the total number of X chromosomes. By utilizing sex chromatin and Y fluorescent staining (Fig 33–4), one can determine indirectly the sex chromosome complement (Table 33–2).

H-Y Antigen

In 1955, Eichwald and Silmser showed that among inbred strains of mice, most male-to-female skin grafts were rejected, whereas male-to-male and female-to-female grafts survived. This phenomenon was attributed to a specific Y-linked histocompatibility locus, the H-Y antigen.

Utilizing a sperm cytotoxicity test to test for this antigen, Wachtel and his co-workers expanded the study of H-Y antigen from inbred mice to rats, guinea pigs, rabbits, and humans. They demonstrated the invariable association of H-Y antigen with the heterogametic sex (usually the male) in a wide range of vertebrates. In mammals, H-Y antigen is expressed in the heterogametic male but not usually in the homogametic XX female.

Wachtel and Ohno and their associates noted the striking conservation throughout evolution of this ubiquitous minor cross-reacting plasma membrane histocompatibility antigen, its appearance early in embryonic development (in the 8-cell male mouse embryo), and its association with heterogametic sex. These observations led them to suggest that this phylogenetically conserved antigen is the factor responsible for inducing testicular organogenesis of the bipotential fetal gonads. They examined their hypothesis by testing patients with testicular tissue who had XX karyotypes, eg, XX

males and XX true hermaphrodites. Despite the absence of a Y chromosome in these patients, H-Y antigen was detected in all patients tested. In addition, the gonad of the bovine freemartin (the intersex XX twin of a male fetus) is positive for H-Y antigen. Further evidence indicates that even in the absence of a discrete Y chromosome, or karyotypic evidence of a Y-to-X chromosome, or Y-to-autosome translocation or insertion, the presence of testicular tissue is invariably associated with a positive test for H-Y antigen. The chromosome sites of the structural and regulatory genes for the expression of H-Y antigen are uncertain. Evidence suggests that there are sites in the pericentromeric region of the Y chromosome, on the short arm of the X chromosome, and possibly on autosomes that affect the synthesis and action of H-Y antigen.

According to Ohno, biologically active H-Y antigen is a protein composed of hydrophobic peptide units with a molecular weight of 16,000–18,000 which are linked by intersubunit disulfide bonds. The only gonadal cell known to disseminate H-Y antigen is the primitive Sertoli cell. H-Y antigen has been detected on all cell membranes from normal XY males except those of immature germ cells. Apparently, cells have 2 receptors for H-Y antigen. Ohno has proposed that one receptor is nonspecific and ubiquitous and represents the stable cell membrane anchorage sites for H-Y antigen on all male cells; this anchorage site is conceived as an association of "major histocompatibility complex" cell surface antigens (HLA) with β_2-microglobulin. The second receptor is found only on gonadal cells, both male and female, and binds free H-Y antigen with a greater affinity than the nonspecific anchorage sites.

A hypothesis for the organogenesis of the indifferent embryonic gonad as testis can be summarized as follows: The pericentromeric region of the Y chromosome contains a locus (or loci) that either codes for H-Y antigen or regulates its expression. H-Y antigen is disseminated by cells in the gonadal blastema, binds to gonad-specific H-Y receptors, and induces differentiation of the primitive gonad as a testis by the seventh week of gestation (Fig 33–5). In the absence of H-Y antigen and in the

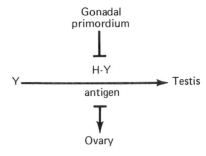

Figure 33–5. Interaction of H-Y antigen, germ cells, and somatic elements of the primordial gonad in testicular differentiation.

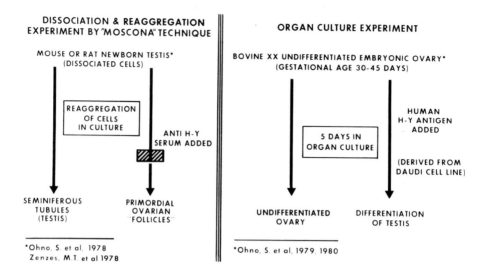

Figure 33–6. Diagrammatic scheme summarizing experimental evidence supporting H-Y antigen as the inducer of the testis in gonadal organogenesis. (Reproduced, with permission, from Grumbach MM, Conte FA: *Textbook of Endocrinology,* 6th ed. Williams RH [editor]. Saunders, 1981.)

presence of 2 structurally normal X chromosomes, an ovary will develop. Indirect evidence suggests the presence of a specific ovarian organizing antigen.

All of the evidence discussed previously in support of the testis-organizing function of H-Y antigen is indirect and circumstantial. However, recent experimental data provide more direct evidence for this hypothesis. In a series of experiments, Ohno and Zenzius and their co-workers have reported cell dissociation and reaggregation experiments on newborn rat and mouse gonads (Fig 33–6). Using the Moscona technic, a suspension of single cells from newborn mouse or rat testes was obtained. The free cell suspension was exposed to excess anti-H-Y serum and incubated in rotation culture. The H-Y antibody-treated dissociated testicular cells reaggregated to form ovarian "primordial-like follicles," whereas untreated testicular cells reorganized as "seminiferous tubule-like structures." In a converse group of experiments, free cell suspensions of rat newborn or bovine fetal ovarian cells exposed to H-Y antigen reorganized to form "seminiferous tubule-like" structures. In a further experiment (Fig 33–6), Ohno and his co-workers purified H-Y antigen from culture media of a "Daudi" human male Burkitt lymphoma cell line, which lacks the putative β_2-microglobulin H-Y anchorage site. Bovine fetal XX indifferent gonads exhibited testicular organization in the presence of purified H-Y antigen. Thus, these experiments directly demonstrate the capacity of H-Y antigen to induce differentiation of the indifferent fetal gonad into a testis.

Recently, several groups have reported the detection of H-Y antigen in unexplained circumstances, ie, patients with XO karyotypes and Turner's syndrome and female-to-male transsexual patients. Questions of the specificity, reproducibility, and quantification of these technically difficult serologic assays for H-Y antigen must be addressed before one can interpret these discrepancies between a putative immunoreactive H-Y antigen and gonadal and chromosomal sex.

TESTICULAR & OVARIAN DIFFERENTIATION

Until the 12-mm stage (approximately 42 days of gestation), the embryonic gonads of males and females are indistinguishable. By 42 days, 300–1300 primordial germ cells have seeded the undifferentiated gonad. These large cells later become oogonia and spermatogonia, and lack of these cells is incompatible with further gonadal differentiation. Under the influence of the genes that code for the H-Y antigen, the gonad will begin testicular differentiation by 43–50 days of gestation. Leydig cells are apparent by about 60 days, and differentiation of male external genitalia occurs by 65–77 days of gestation.

In the gonad destined to be an ovary, the lack of differentiation persists. At 77–84 days, long after differentiation of the testis in the male fetus, a significant number of germ cells enter meiotic prophase to characterize the transition of oogonia into oocytes, which marks the onset of ovarian differentiation from the undifferentiated gonads (Fig 33–7).

Differentiation of Genital Ducts (Fig 33–8)

By the seventh week of intrauterine life, the fetus is equipped with the primordia of both male

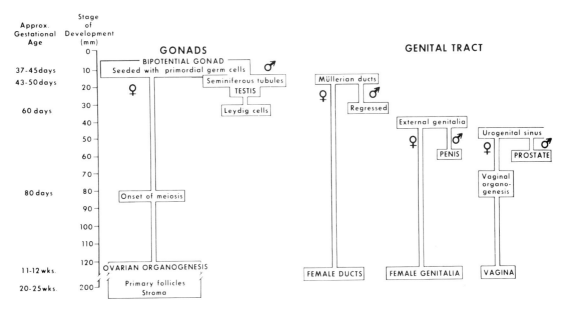

Figure 33–7. Schematic sequence of sexual differentiation in the human fetus. Note that testicular differentiation precedes all other forms of differentiation.

and female genital ducts. The müllerian ducts, if allowed to persist, form the uterine tubes, the uterus, the cervix, and the upper third of the vagina. The wolffian ducts, on the other hand, have the potential for differentiating into the epididymis, vas deferens, seminal vesicles, and ejaculatory ducts of the male. In the presence of a functional testis, the müllerian ducts involute under the influence of "müllerian duct inhibitory factor," a nonsteroid macromolecule secreted by Sertoli cells. This substance acts "locally" to cause müllerian duct repression ipsilaterally. The differentiation of the wolffian duct is stimulated by testosterone secretion from the testis. In the presence of an ovary or in the absence of a functional fetal testis, müllerian duct differentiation occurs, and the wolffian ducts involute.

Differentiation of External Genitalia (Fig 33–9)

Up to the eighth week of fetal life, the external genitalia of both sexes are identical and have the capacity to differentiate into the genitalia of either sex. Female sex differentiation will occur in the presence of an ovary or streak gonads or if no gonad is present (Fig 33–10). Differentiation of the external genitalia along male lines depends on the action of testosterone and particularly dihydrotestosterone, the 5α-reduced metabolite of testosterone. In the male fetus, testosterone is secreted by the Leydig cells, first under the influence of chorionic gonadotropin and thereafter by stimulation from fetal pituitary LH and FSH. Masculinization of the external genitalia and urogenital sinus of the fetus results from the action of dihydrotestosterone, which is converted from testosterone in the target

cells by the enzyme 5α-reductase. Dihydrotestosterone is bound to a cytosol receptor (binding protein) in the target cell. It is then translocated to the nucleus of the cell, where chromatin binding occurs, which initiates DNA-directed, RNA-mediated transcription and results in androgen-induced differentiation and growth of the cell. The gene that codes for the cytosol androgen-binding protein is located on the X chromosome. Thus, an X-linked gene controls the androgen response of all somatic cell types by specifying the cytosol androgen receptor protein.

As in the case of the genital ducts, there is an inherent tendency for the external genitalia and urogenital sinus to develop along female lines. Differentiation of the external genitalia along male lines requires androgenic stimulation early in fetal life. The testosterone metabolite dihydrotestosterone and its specific cytosol receptor must be present to effect masculinization. Dihydrotestosterone stimulates growth of the genital tubercle, fusion of the urethral folds, and descent of the labioscrotal swellings to form the penis and scrotum. Androgens also inhibit descent and growth of the vesicovaginal septum and differentiation of the vagina. There is a critical period for action of the androgen. After about the 12th week of gestation, fusion of the labioscrotal folds will not occur even under intense androgen stimulation, although phallic growth can be induced. Impairment in the synthesis or secretion of fetal testosterone or in its conversion to dihydrotestosterone, deficient or defective androgen receptor activity, or defective production and local action of müllerian duct inhibitory factor leads to incomplete mas-

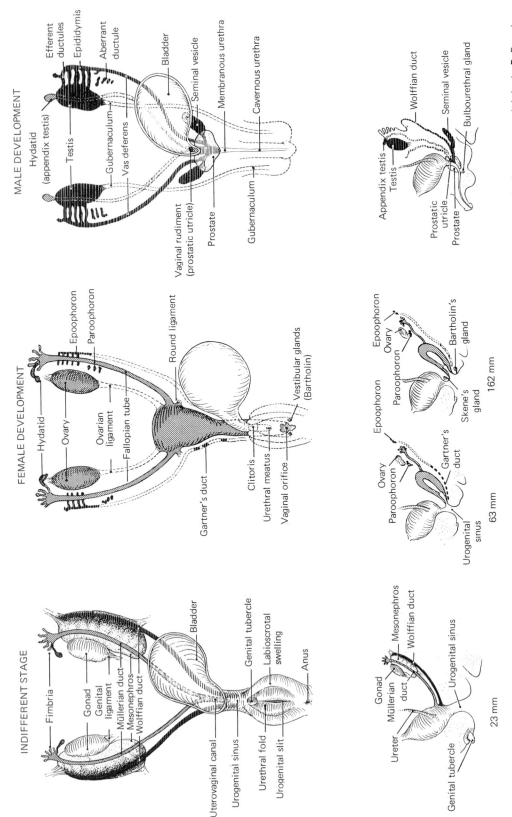

Figure 33–8. Embryonic differentiation of male and female genital ducts from wolffian and müllerian primordia. *A*: Indifferent stage showing large mesonephric body. *B*: Female ducts. Remnants of the mesonephros and wolffian ducts are now termed the epoophoron, paroophoron, and Gartner's duct. *C*: Male ducts before descent into scrotum. The only müllerian remnant is the testicular appendix. The prostatic utricle (vagina masculina) is derived from the urogenital sinus. (Redrawn from Corning and Wilkins.)

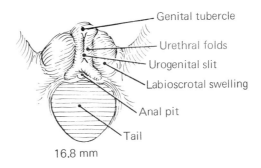

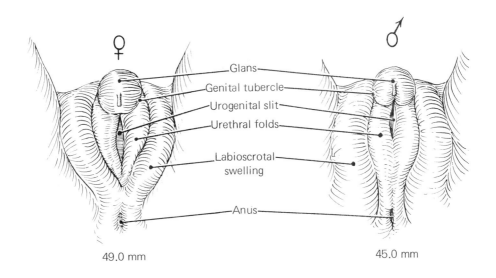

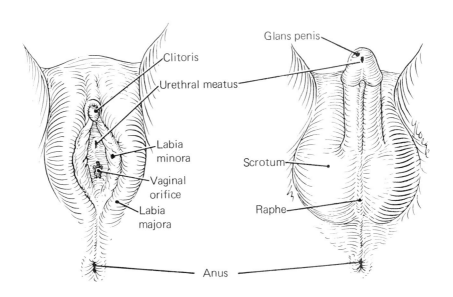

Figure 33–9. Differentiation of male and female external genitalia from bipotential primordia.

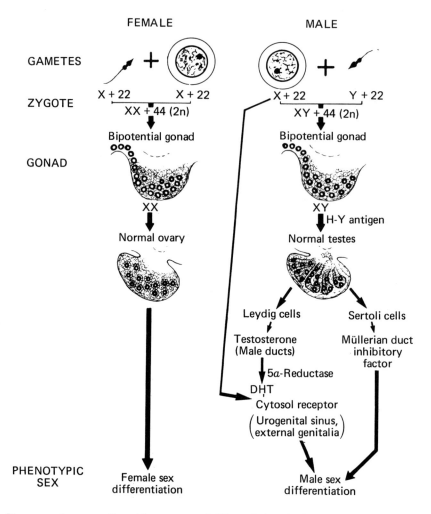

Figure 33–10. Diagrammatic summation of human sexual differentiation. DHT = dihydrotestosterone. (Modified, with permission, from Grumbach MM, Van Wyk WW: *Textbook of Endocrinology,* 5th ed. Williams RH [editor]. Saunders, 1974.)

culinization of the male fetus (Fig 33–10). Exposure of the female fetus to abnormal amounts of androgens from either endogenous or exogenous sources, especially before the 12th week of gestation, can result in virilization of the external genitalia.

PSYCHOSEXUAL DIFFERENTIATION

Gender role is a psychosocial term used to denote a person's sexual designation as well as identification of self in relationship to other members of the same or opposite sex. Studies in humans indicate that gender role is not coded for by the sex chromosomes, the gonads, or the sex steroids. Rather, it has been suggested that gender role is imprinted by words, attitudes, clothes, and comparison of one's body with that of others. In the absence of ambiguous attitudes on the part of the parent and child, Money postulated that gender role—ie, sexual identity—was established by

18–30 months of age. He postulated that once gender identity is fixed, even the paradoxic development of secondary sexual characteristics of the opposite sex may not shake this conviction of sexual identity. Recently, Imperato-McGinley and her co-workers have challenged the concept of "fixed gender identity" on the basis of their studies of a group of pseudohermaphrodites with 5α-reductase deficiency, primarily from a genetic isolate in the Dominican Republic. These patients, presumably raised unambiguously as girls, became virilized at puberty and changed their gender identity. Although these studies demonstrate that gender identity may not be irrevocably "fixed" and thus may be more "plastic" than previously believed, they should not be applied to assignment of sex in patients with abnormalities of sex differentiation, since in our cultural setting, the weight of evidence strongly supports environmental factors as the principal determinant of gender identity.

ABNORMAL SEX DIFFERENTIATION

Classification of Errors in Sex Differentiation
(Table 33–3)

Disorders of sexual differentiation are the result of abnormalities in the complex processes of sexual differentiation, which originate in genetic information on the X and Y chromosomes as well as on the autosomes. A true hermaphrodite is defined as a person who possesses both ovarian and testicular tissue. A male pseudohermaphrodite is one whose gonads are exclusively testes but whose genital ducts or external genitalia, or both, exhibit incomplete masculinization. A female pseudohermaphrodite is a person whose gonadal tissue is exclusively ovarian but whose genital development exhibits an ambiguous or male appearance.

SEMINIFEROUS TUBULE DYSGENESIS: CHROMATIN-POSITIVE KLINEFELTER'S SYNDROME & ITS VARIANTS

Klinefelter's syndrome is one of the most common forms of primary hypogonadism and infertility in males. These patients usually have an XXY sex chromosome constitution and an X chromatin-positive buccal smear, although patients with a variety of sex chromosome constitutions, including mosaicism, have been described. Virtually all of these variants have in common the presence of at least two X chromosomes and a Y chromosome, except for the rare group in which only an XX sex chromosome complement is found.

Surveys of the prevalence of XXY fetuses by karyotype analysis of unselected newborn infants indicate an incidence of one per 1000 newborn

Table 33–3. Classification of anomalous sexual development.

Disorders of Gonadal Differentiation
- A. Seminiferous tubular dysgenesis (Klinefelter's syndrome).
- B. Syndrome of gonadal dysgenesis and its variants (Turner's syndrome).
- C. Complete and incomplete forms of XX and XY gonadal dysgenesis.
- D. True hermaphroditism.

Female Pseudohermaphroditism
- A. Congenital virilizing adrenal hyperplasia.
- B. Androgens and synthetic progestins transferred from maternal circulation.
- C. Malformations of intestine and urinary tract (nonadrenal female pseudohermaphroditism).
- D. Other teratologic factors.

Male Pseudohermaphroditism
- A. Testicular unresponsiveness to hCG and LH.
- B. Inborn errors of testosterone biosynthesis:
    - 1. Enzyme defects affecting synthesis of both corticosteroids and testosterone (variants of congenital adrenal hyperplasia).
        - a. Cholesterol desmolase complex deficiency (congenital lipoid adrenal hyperplasia).
        - b. 3β-Hydroxysteroid dehydrogenase deficiency.
        - c. 17α-Hydroxylase deficiency.
    - 2. Enzyme defects primarily affecting testosterone biosynthesis by the testes.
        - a. 17,20-Desmolase (lyase) deficiency.
        - b. 17β-Hydroxysteroid oxidoreductase deficiency.
- C. Defects in androgen-dependent target tissues:
    - 1. End organ insensitivity to androgenic hormones (androgen receptor and postreceptor defects):
        - a. Complete syndrome of androgen insensitivity and its variants (testicular feminization and its variant forms).
        - b. Incomplete syndrome of androgen insensitivity and its variants (Reifenstein's syndrome).
        - c. Androgen insensitivity in infertile men.
    - 2. Defects in testosterone metabolism by peripheral tissues: 5α-Reductase deficiency—Male pseudohermaphroditism with normal virilization at puberty (familial perineal hypospadias with ambiguous development of urogenital sinus and male puberty; pseudovaginal perineoscrotal hypospadias).
- D. Dysgenetic male pseudohermaphroditism:
    - 1. X chromatin-negative variants of the syndrome of gonadal dysgenesis (eg, XO/XY,XYp–).
    - 2. Incomplete form of XY gonadal dysgenesis.
    - 3. Associated with degenerative renal disease.
    - 4. "Vanishing testes" (embryonic testicular regression; XY agonadism → XY gonadal agenesis → rudimentary testes → anorchia).
- E. Defects in synthesis, secretion, or response to müllerian duct inhibitory factor: Female genital ducts in otherwise normal men—"uteri herniae inguinale"; persistent müllerian duct syndrome.
- F. Maternal ingestion of estrogens and progestins.

Unclassified Forms of Abnormal Sexual Development
- A. In males:
    - 1. Hypospadias.
    - 2. Ambiguous external genitalia in XY males with multiple congenital anomalies.
- B. In females: Absence or anomalous development of the vagina, uterus, and uterine tubes (Rokitansky-Küstner syndrome).

males. The invariable clinical features of Klinefelter's syndrome in adults are a male phenotype; small, firm testes less than 3 cm in length; and azoospermia. Prepubertally, the disorder is characterized by disproportionately long legs, small testes, and personality and behavioral disorders with or without mental retardation. Gynecomastia and other signs of androgen deficiency such as diminished facial and body hair, a small phallus, poor muscular development, and a eunuchoidal body habitus occur postpubertally in affected patients. Adult males with an XXY karyotype tend to be taller than average, mainly because of the disproportionate length of their legs. They also have an increased incidence of mild diabetes mellitus, varicose veins, chronic pulmonary disease, and carcinoma of the breast. Sexual precocity due to an hCG-secreting polyembryoma has recently been described in six XXY males.

The testicular lesion appears to be progressive and gonadotropin-dependent. It is characterized in the adult by extensive seminiferous tubular hyalinization and fibrosis, absent or severely deficient spermatogenesis, and pseudoadenomatous clumping of the Leydig cells. Although hyalinization of the tubules is usually extensive, it varies considerably from patient to patient and even between testes in the same patient. Spermatogenesis is rarely found, and patients who have been reported to be fertile have been XY/XXY mosaics.

Advanced maternal age and meiotic nondisjunction have been found to play a role in the genesis of the XXY karyotype. Pedigree studies indicate that both X chromosomes are of maternal origin in 67% of XXY patients.

The diagnosis of Klinefelter's syndrome is suggested by the classic phenotype and hormonal changes. It is confirmed by the finding of an X chromatin–positive buccal smear and demonstration of an XXY karyotype in blood, skin, or gonads. Serum and urinary gonadotropin levels, especially FSH, are elevated, whereas plasma testosterone levels can be low or normal. Testicular biopsy reveals the classic findings of hyalinization of the seminiferous tubules, severe deficiency of spermatogonia, and pseudoadenomatous clumping of Leydig cells.

Treatment of patients with Klinefelter's syndrome is directed toward androgen replacement, if necessary. Testosterone enanthate in oil, 200 mg intramuscularly every 2 weeks, is recommended as an adult replacement dose. Gynecomastia is not amenable to hormone therapy and should be corrected by reduction mammoplasty if it is severe or psychologically disturbing to the patient.

Variants of Chromatin-Positive Seminiferous Tubule Dysgenesis

A. XY/XXY Mosaicism: This is the second most common chromosome complement associated with the Klinefelter phenotype. Mosaicism with any XY cell line may modify the clinical syndrome and result in less severe gynecomastia, as well as a lesser degree of testicular pathology. Some of these patients are fertile. Mean testosterone levels tend to be higher in XY/XXY mosaics than in XXY patients. In order to rule out XY/XXY mosaicism, cultures for karyotype analysis should be obtained from 2 or more tissues, and a sufficient number of cells (50 or more) should be examined from each tissue. Therapy depends on the severity of the clinical and gonadal aberrations associated with the XXY cell line.

B. XXYY: These patients comprise 3% of chromatin-positive males. In addition to exhibiting the usual characteristics of Klinefelter's syndrome, they tend to be tall, and almost all reported patients have been mentally retarded. Therapy with testosterone is similar to that in patients with XXY Klinefelter's syndrome.

C. XXYY and XXXYY: All of these patients have had significant mental retardation; developmental anomalies (short neck, epicanthal folds, radioulnar synostosis, and clinodactyly) are present in half of patients.

D. XXXXY: These patients are more severely affected than those with a lesser number of X chromosomes. In addition to severe mental retardation, they exhibit radioulnar synostosis, hypoplastic external genitalia, and cryptorchid testes. Other anomalies such as congenital heart disease, cleft palate, strabismus, and microcephaly may be present. The facies is characteristic, with prognathism, hypertelorism, and myopia.

E. XX Males: Over 100 phenotypic males with a 46,XX karyotype have been described since 1964. In general, they have a male phenotype, male psychosocial gender identity, and testes with histologic features similar to those observed in patients with an XXY karyotype. At least 10% of patients have had hypospadias or ambiguous external genitalia. XX males have normal body proportions and a mean final height that is shorter than patients with an XXY karyotype or normal males but taller than normal females. As in XXY males, testosterone levels are low or low normal, gonadotropins are elevated, and spermatogenesis is impaired. Gynecomastia is present in approximately one-third of the patients.

The presence of testes and male sexual differentiation in 46,XX individuals has been a perplexing problem. However, the paradox has been clarified by the discovery that XX males are H-Y antigen–positive.

Three theories have been advanced to explain this rare example of sex reversal: (1) the presence of hidden sex chromosome mosaicism in an XX male with an undetected cell line containing a Y chromosome; (2) interchange or translocation between a Y and an X chromosome or an autosome that results in relocation of masculinizing genes from the Y chromosome onto an X chromosome or an autosome; and (3) a mutant autosomal gene that leads to the differentiation of testes in an XX embryo, as in the "Saanen" goat and the sex-reversed mouse. There is evidence to support each of these possibilities in the pathogenesis of this abnormality, and all would lead to an XX individual who is H-Y antigen–positive. The presence of XX males and true hermaphrodites in the same family in mammals suggests that these conditions are linked.

SYNDROME OF GONADAL DYSGENESIS: TURNER'S SYNDROME & ITS VARIANTS

Turner's Syndrome: XO Gonadal Dysgenesis

One in 10,000 newborn females has an XO sex chromosome constitution. The cardinal features of XO gonadal dysgenesis are a variety of somatic anomalies, sexual infantilism at puberty secondary to gonadal dysgenesis, and short stature. Patients with an XO karyotype can be recognized in infancy usually because of lymphedema of the extremities and loose skin folds over the nape of the neck. In later life, the typical patient is often recognizable by her distinctive facies, in which micrognathia, epicanthal folds, prominent low-set ears, a fishlike mouth, and ptosis are present to varying degrees. The chest is shieldlike and the neck short, broad, and webbed (40%). Additional anomalies associated with Turner's syndrome include coarctation of the aorta (10%), hypertension, renal abnormalities (50%), pigmented nevi, cubitus valgus, a tendency to keloid formation, puffiness of the dorsum of the hands, short fourth metacarpals, and recurrent otitis media. Routine intravenous urography is indicated for all patients to rule out a surgically correctable renal abnormality. The internal ducts and external genitalia of these patients are female.

Short stature is an invariable feature of the syndrome of gonadal dysgenesis. Mean final height in XO patients is 142 cm, with a range of 133–153 cm. Current data suggest that the short stature found in patients with the syndrome of gonadal dysgenesis is not due to a deficiency of growth hormone, somatomedin, sex steroids, or thyroid hormone. No significant increase in final height has been documented in these patients after therapy with growth hormone, anabolic steroids, and estrogens.

Gonadal dysgenesis is another feature of patients with an XO sex chromosome constitution. The gonads are typically streaklike and usually contain only a fibrous stroma arranged in whorls. Longitudinal studies of both basal and LRF-evoked gonadotropin secretion in patients with gonadal dysgenesis indicate a lack of feedback inhibition of the hypothalamic-pituitary axis by the dysgenetic gonads in affected infants and children (Fig 33–11). Thus, plasma and urinary gonadotropins, particularly FSH, are elevated, especially in early infancy and after 10 years of age. Since ovarian function is impaired, puberty does not usually ensue spontaneously; thus, sexual infantilism is a hallmark of this syndrome.

A variety of disorders are associated with this syndrome, including obesity, diabetes mellitus, Hashimoto's thyroiditis, rheumatoid arthritis, and inflammatory bowel disease.

Phenotypic females with the following features should have a buccal smear for sex chromatin or a karyotype analysis: (1) short stature (> 2.5 SD below the mean value per age); (2) somatic anomalies associated with the syndrome of gonadal dysgenesis; and (3) delayed adolescence and increased concentration of plasma gonadotropins. In normal XX females, 20–30% of the nuclei are sex chromatin-positive. Although sex chromatin is useful, karyotype analysis should be performed for definitive diagnosis.

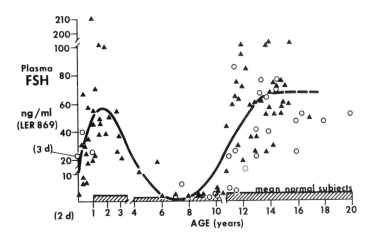

Figure 33–11. Diphasic variation in basal levels of plasma FSH (ng/mL-LER 869) in patients with an XO karyotype (Δ) and patients with structural abnormalities of the X chromosome, and mosaics (O). Note that mean basal levels of plasma FSH in patients with gonadal dysgenesis are in the castrate range before 4 years and after 10 years of age. (Reproduced, with permission, from Grumbach MM, Conte FA, Kaplan SL: *J Clin Endocrinol Metab* 1975;**40**;670.)

Therapy is directed toward the institution of estrogen therapy in order to produce secondary sexual characteristics and menarche at an age commensurate with normal peers. We routinely initiate therapy at age 12–13 years with either 0.3 mg (or less) of conjugated estrogens, or ethinyl estradiol, 5 μg by mouth for the first 21 days of the calendar month. Thereafter, the dose of estrogen is gradually increased over the next 2–3 years to 0.6–1.25 mg of conjugated estrogens daily or 10–20 μg of ethinyl estradiol daily. The patient is maintained on the minimum dose of estrogen necessary to maintain secondary sexual characteristics and menses. Medroxyprogesterone acetate, 5 mg daily, is given on the 12th–21st days of the cycle to ensure physiologic menses and to perhaps reduce the risk of endometrial carcinoma from sustained estrogen stimulation.

X Chromatin-Positive Variants of the Syndrome of Gonadal Dysgenesis

Patients with structural abnormalities of the X chromosome (deletions and additions) and mosaicism with XX cell lines may manifest the somatic as well as the gonadal features of the syndrome of gonadal dysgenesis (Table 33–4). Evidence suggests that genes on both the long and short arms of the X chromosome control gonadal differentiation, whereas genes on the short arms of the X prevent the short stature and somatic anomalies that are seen in XO patients. In general, mosaicism with an XX cell line in association with an XO cell line will modify the phenotype toward normal and can even result in normal gonadal function.

X Chromatin-Negative Variants of the Syndrome of Gonadal Dysgenesis

These patients usually have mosaicism with an XO- and a Y-bearing cell line—XO/XY, XO/XYY, XO/XY/XYY—or perhaps a structurally abnormal Y chromosome. They range from phenotypic females with the features of Turner's syndrome through patients with ambiguous genitalia to (rarely) completely virilized males with a few stigmas of Turner's syndrome. The gonadal differentiation varies from bilateral streaks to bilateral dysgenetic testes, along with asymmetric development, ie, a streak on one side and a dysgenetic testicle (or, rarely, a nearly normal testis) on the other side, sometimes called "mixed gonadal dysgenesis." The development of the external genitalia as well as the internal ducts correlates well with the degree of testicular differentiation and, presumably, the capacity of the fetal testes to secrete müllerian duct inhibitory factor and testosterone.

The risk of development of gonadal tumors is greatly increased in patients with XO/XY mosaicism, and prophylactic removal of streak gonads or dysgenetic undescended testes in this syndrome is indicated. Breast development at or after the age of puberty in these patients is associated with a gonadal neoplasm, usually a gonadoblastoma. Pelvic sonography as well as CT scan may be useful in screening for neoplasms in these patients. Gonadoblastomas are calcified, so that they may be visible even on a plain film of the abdomen.

The diagnosis of XO/XY mosaicism can be established by the demonstration of both XO and XY cells in blood, skin, or gonadal tissue. The decision as to the sex of rearing of the child should be based on the age at diagnosis and the potential for normal function of the external genitalia. In patients assigned a female gender role, the gonads should be removed and the external genitalia repaired. Estrogen therapy should be initiated at the age of puberty, as in patients with an XO karyotype (see above). In affected infants who are assigned a male gender role, all gonadal tissue except that which appears histologically normal and is in the scrotum should be removed. Removal of the müllerian structures and repair of hypospadias are also indicated. At puberty, depending on the functional integrity of the retained gonad, androgen replacement therapy may be indicated in doses similar to those for patients with XY gonadal dysgenesis (see p 531).

Table 33–4. Relationship of structural abnormalities of the X and Y to clinical manifestations of the syndrome of gonadal dysgenesis.*

Type of Sex Chromosome Abnormality	Karyotypes	Phenotype	Sexual Infantilism	Shortness of Stature	Somatic Anomalies of Turner's Syndrome
Loss of an X or Y	XO	Female	+	+	+
†Deletion of short arm of an X	XXqi	Female	+ (occ. ±)	+	+
	XXp−	Female	+, ±, or −	+ (−)	+ (−)
†Deletion of long arm of an X	XXpi	Female	+	−	− or (±)
	XXq−	Female	+	− (+)	− or (±)
Deletion of ends of both arms of an X	XXr	Female	− or +	+	+ or (±)
Loss of short arm of Y	XYp−	Ambiguous	+	+	+

*Modified and reproduced, with permission, from Williams RH (editor): *Textbook of Endocrinology,* 5th ed. Saunders, 1974.
†In Xp− and Xq−, the extent and site of the deleted segment is variable.
Xqi = isochromosome for long arm of an X; Xp− = deletion of short arm of an X; Xpi = isochromosome for short arm of an X; Xq− = deletion of long arm of an X; Xr = ring chromosome derived from an X; Yp− = deletion of short arm of the Y chromosome.

COMPLETE & INCOMPLETE FORMS OF XX & XY GONADAL DYSGENESIS

The terms XX and XY gonadal dysgenesis have been applied to XX or XY patients who have bilateral streak gonads, a female phenotype, and no stigmas of Turner's syndrome. After puberty, they exhibit sexual infantilism, castrate levels of plasma and urinary gonadotropins, normal or tall stature, and eunuchoid proportions.

XX Gonadal Dysgenesis

Familial and sporadic cases of XX gonadal dysgenesis have been reported. Pedigree analysis of familial cases is consistent with autosomal recessive inheritance. In 3 families, XX gonadal dysgenesis was associated with deafness of the sensorineural type. In several affected groups of siblings, a spectrum of clinical findings occurred, eg, varying degrees of ovarian function, including breast development and menses followed by secondary amenorrhea. The diagnosis of XX gonadal dysgenesis should be suspected in phenotypic females with sexual infantilism and normal müllerian structures who lack the somatic stigmas of the syndrome of gonadal dysgenesis (Turner's syndrome). Karyotype analysis reveals only 46,XX cells. As in Turner's syndrome, gonadotropins are elevated, estrogens are low, and treatment consists of cyclic estrogen replacement.

Sporadic cases of XX gonadal dysgenesis may represent a heterogeneous group of patients from a pathogenetic point of view. XX gonadal dysgenesis should be distinguished from ovarian failure due to infections such as mumps, antibodies to gonadotropin receptors, biologically inactive FSH, and gonadotropin-insensitive ovaries as well as errors in estrogen biosynthesis.

XY Gonadal Dysgenesis

XY gonadal dysgenesis occurs both sporadically and in familial aggregates. Patients with this syndrome have female external genitalia, normal or tall stature, bilateral streak gonads, müllerian development, sexual infantilism, eunuchoid habitus, and a 46,XY karyotype. Clitoromegaly is common, and in familial cases a continuum of involvement ranging from the complete syndrome to ambiguity of the external genitalia has been described. The phenotypic difference between the complete form of XY gonadal dysgenesis and the variant form is due to the degree of differentiation of the testicular tissue and its functional capacity to produce testosterone and müllerian duct inhibitory factor.

Analysis of familial cases suggests that XY gonadal dysgenesis is transmitted as an X-linked recessive or sex-limited autosomal dominant trait. Both H-Y antigen–positive and H-Y antigen–negative forms of this syndrome have been described and reflect the genetic heterogeneity of this syndrome. XY gonadal dysgenesis may result from a mutant gene that affects the expression of H-Y antigen (H-Y negative); from a defect in the gonad-specific H-Y antigen receptor (H-Y positive); or possibly from the production of a serologically reactive but abnormal H-Y antigen that lacks affinity for H-Y antigen receptors on gonadal cells (H-Y antigen–positive). Sporadic cases may represent teratologic defects in gonadal morphogenesis.

Therapy for patients with XY gonadal dysgenesis who have female external genitalia involves prophylactic gonadectomy and estrogen substitution at puberty. In the variant form of XY gonadal dysgenesis, assignment of a male gender role is possible. It depends upon the degree of ambiguity of the genitalia and the potential for normal function in the future. Prophylactic gonadectomy should be performed, since fertility is unlikely and there is an increased risk of malignant gonadal transformation in these patients. Prosthetic testes should be implanted at the time of gonadectomy, and androgen substitution therapy is instituted at the age of puberty. Testosterone enanthate in oil is utilized, beginning with 50 mg intramuscularly monthly and gradually increasing the dose over 3–4 years to a full replacement dose of 200 mg intramuscularly every 2 weeks.

TRUE HERMAPHRODITISM

True hermaphrodites have both ovarian and testicular tissue present in either the same or opposite gonads. Differentiation of the internal and external genitalia is highly variable. The external genitalia may simulate those of a male or female, but most often they are ambiguous. Cryptorchidism and hypospadias are common. In all cases, a uterus is present. The differentiation of the genital ducts usually follows that of the ipsilateral gonad. The ovotestis is the most common gonad found in true hermaphrodites, followed by the ovary and, least commonly, the testis. At puberty, breast development is usual in the untreated patients and menses occurs in over 50% of cases. Whereas the ovary or the ovarian portion of an ovotestis may function normally, the testis or testicular portion of an ovotestis is almost always dysgenetic.

Sixty percent of true hermaphrodites have a 46,XX karyotype, 20% have 46,XY and about 20% have mosaicism or XX/XY chimerism. True hermaphroditism may result from (1) sex chromosome mosaicism or chimerism, (2) Y-to-autosome or Y-to-X chromosome translocation or interchange, and (3) an autosomal mutant gene. There is evidence to support each of these possibilities in the pathogenesis of this clinically and anatomically heterogeneous syndrome, and all could lead to the serologic expression of H-Y antigen.

The diagnosis of true hermaphroditism should be considered in all patients with ambiguous genitalia. The finding of an XX/XY karyotype or a bilobed gonad compatible with an ovotestis in the inguinal region or labioscrotal folds suggests the diagnosis. If all other forms of male and female pseudohermaphroditism have been excluded, laparotomy and histologic confirmation of both ovarian and testicular tissue establishes the diagnosis. The management of true hermaphroditism is contingent upon the age at diagnosis and a careful assessment of the functional capacity of the gonads and the internal and external genitalia.

Gonadal Neoplasms in Dysgenetic Gonads

While gonadal tumors are rare in patients with Klinefelter's syndrome and XO gonadal dysgenesis, the prevalence of gonadal neoplasms is greatly increased in patients with certain types of dysgenetic gonads. Dysgerminomas, seminomas, teratomas, and gonadoblastomas are found most frequently. The frequency is increased (1) in XO/XY mosaicism and in patients with a structurally abnormal Y chromosome and (2) in XY gonadal dysgenesis, either with a female phenotype or with ambiguous genitalia. Prophylactic gonadectomy is advised in these 2 categories as well as in individuals with gonadal dysgenesis who manifest signs of virilization, regardless of karyotype.

The gonad should be preserved in patients who are being raised as males only if it is a relatively normal testicle that can be relocated in the scrotum. The fact that a gonad is palpable in the scrotum does not preclude malignant degeneration and spread, since seminomas tend to metastasize at an early stage before a local mass is obvious.

FEMALE PSEUDOHERMAPHRODITISM

These individuals have normal ovaries and müllerian derivatives associated with ambiguous external genitalia. In the absence of testes, a female fetus will be masculinized if subjected to increased circulating levels of androgens derived from an extragonadal source. The degree of masculinization depends upon the stage of differentiation at the time of exposure (Fig 33–12). After 12 weeks of gestation, androgens will produce only clitoral hypertrophy. Rarely, ambiguous genitalia that superficially resemble those produced by androgens are the result of teratogenic malformations.

Congenital Adrenal Hyperplasia (Fig 33–13)

There are 6 major types of adrenal hyperplasia, all transmitted as autosomal recessive disorders. The common denominator of all 6 types is a defect in the synthesis of cortisol that results in an increase in ACTH and in adrenal hyperplasia. Both males and females can be affected, but males are rarely diagnosed at birth unless they have ambiguous genitalia or are salt losers and manifest adrenal crises. Types I–III are defects confined to the adrenal gland that produce virilization. Types IV–VI have in common blocks in cortisol and sex steroid synthesis, in both the adrenals and the gonads. The latter 3 types produce primarily incomplete masculinization in the male and little or no virilization in the female (Table 33–5). Consequently, these will be discussed primarily as forms of male pseudohermaphroditism.

A. Type I–C$_{21}$ Hydroxylase Deficiency Primarily Affecting C$_{21}$ Hydroxylation in the Zona Fasciculata (Simple Virilization): This is the most common type of congenital adrenal hyperplasia, with a prevalence of 1:5000 to 1:15,000 live births in Caucasians. Recent data indicate that the locus for the gene which codes for 21-hydroxylation is on the short arm of chromosome No. 6 in close proximity to the locus for the histocompatibility gene HLA-B. Thus, the gene for 21-hydroxylase deficiency is closely linked to the HLA gene complex. In addition, certain specific HLA subtypes are found to be statistically increased in patients with 21-hydroxylase deficiency.

A defect in 21-hyroxylase activity in the zona

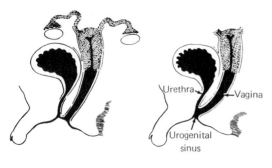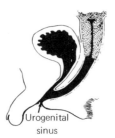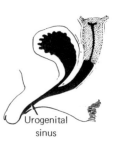

Figure 33–12. Female pseudohermaphroditism induced by prenatal exposure to androgens. Exposure after the 12th fetal week leads only to clitoral hypertrophy (diagram on left). Exposure at progressively earlier stages of differentiation (depicted from left to right in drawings) leads to retention of the urogenital sinus and labioscrotal fusion. If exposure occurs sufficiently early, the labia will fuse to form a penile urethra. (Reproduced, with permission, from Grumbach MM, Ducharme J: *Fertil Steril* 1960;11:757.)

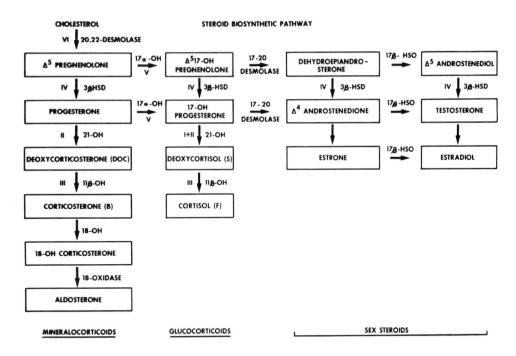

Figure 33–13. A diagrammatic representation of the steroid biosynthetic pathways in the adrenal and gonads. I to VI correspond to enzymes whose deficiency results in congenital adrenal hyperplasia. OH = hydroxylase, 3β-HSD = 3β-hydroxysteroid dehydrogenase, and 17β-HSO = 17β-hydroxysteroid oxidoreductase. (Reproduced, with permission, from Conte FA, Grumbach MM: Pathogenesis, classification, diagnosis, and treatment of anomalies of sex. Chapter 106, in: *Endocrinology.* DeGroot L [editor]. Grune & Stratton, 1979.)

fasciculata of the adrenal cortex results in impaired cortisol synthesis, increased ACTH levels, and increased adrenal androgen and androgen precursor production. Prior to 12 weeks of gestation, high fetal androgen levels lead to a varying degree of labioscrotal fusion and clitoral enlargement in the female fetus; exposure to androgen after 12 weeks induces clitoromegaly alone. In the male fetus, no structural abnormalities in the external genitalia are evident at birth, but the phallus may be enlarged. These patients produce sufficient amounts of aldos-

terone to prevent the signs and symptoms of mineralocorticoid deficiency.

B. Type II–C_{21} Hydroxylase Deficiency Affecting C_{21} Hydroxylation in the Zona Fasciculata and Glomerulosa (Virilization With Salt Wasting): The salt-losing variant of 21-hydroxylase deficiency involves a more severe deficit of 21-hydroxylase in the zona fasciculata and zona glomerulosa of the adrenal cortex, which leads to impaired secretion of both cortisol (fasciculata) and aldosterone (glomerulosa). This results in electrolyte and fluid

Table 33–5. Clinical manifestations of the various types of congenital adrenal hyperplasia.

Enzymatic Defect	Cholesterol Desmolase System (Cholesterol 20α-Hydroxylase)		3β-Hydroxysteroid Dehydrogenase		17α-Hydroxylase		11β-Hydroxylase		21α-Hydroxylase	
Type	VI		IV		V		III		II and I	
Chromosomal	XX	XY	XX	XY	XX	XY	XX	XY	XX	XY
External genitalia	Female	Female	Female (clitoromegaly)	Ambiguous	Female	Female or ambiguous	Ambiguous	Male	Ambiguous	Male
Postnatal virilization	— (Sexual infantilism at puberty)		±	Mild to moderate	— (Sexual infantilism at puberty)		+		+	
Addisonian crises	+		+		—		—		+ in 40% (type II)	
Hypertension	—		—		+		+		—	

losses after the fifth day of life which are manifested as hyponatremia, hyperkalemia, acidosis, dehydration, and vascular collapse. Masculinization of the external genitalia of affected females tends to be more severe than that found in patients with simple 21-hydroxylase deficiency. Recently, the heterogeneity of 21-hydroxylase deficiency has been demonstrated by the finding that classic adrenal hyperplasia, acquired (late-onset) adrenal hyperplasia, and "cryptic" adrenal hyperplasia are all HLA-linked and thus represent forms of 21-hydroxylase deficiency with a wide range of clinical and biochemical severity.

The diagnosis of 21-hydroxylase deficiency should always be considered (1) in patients with ambiguous genitalia who have an XX karyotype and are thus female pseudohermaphrodites; (2) in apparent cryptorchid males; (3) in any infant who presents with shock, hypoglycemia, and serologic findings compatible with adrenal insufficiency; and (4) in males and females with signs of virilization prior to puberty. In the past, the diagnosis of 21-hydroxylase deficiency was based on the finding of elevated levels of 17-ketosteroids and pregnanetriol in the urine. Although still valid and useful, urinary steroid determinations have been replaced by the measurement of plasma 17-hydroxyprogesterone. The concentration of plasma 17-hydroxyprogesterone is normally elevated in umbilical cord blood but rapidly decreases into the range of 100–200 ng/dL by 24 hours after delivery. In patients affected with 21-hydroxylase deficiency, the 17-hydroxyprogesterone values usually range from 3000 to 40,000 ng/dL, depending on the age of the patient and the severity of 21-hydroxylase deficiency. Patients with mild 21-hydroxylase deficiency, ie, late-onset and cryptic forms, may have borderline basal 17-hydroxyprogesterone values, but they can be distinguished from heterozygotes on the basis of an augmented 17-hydroxyprogesterone response to the administration of ACTH. Salt losers can be ascertained clinically, usually by chemical evidence of hyponatremia and hyperkalemia on a regular or low-salt diet. In these patients, aldosterone levels in both plasma and urine are low in relation to the serum electrolyte pattern, while plasma renin activity is elevated.

C. Type III–C_{11} Hydroxylase Deficiency (Virilization With Hypertension): A defect in hydroxylation at C_{11} leads to the hypersecretion of 11-deoxycorticosterone and 11-deoxycortisol in addition to adrenal androgens. Patients with this form of adrenal hyperplasia exhibit virilization secondary to increased androgen production and hypertension caused by increased 11-deoxycorticosterone secretion. Recent data suggest that the defect in 11β-hydroxylation may be primarily in the zona fasciculata. The 11β-hydroxylase gene is not linked to the HLA complex. As in other forms of congenital adrenal hyperplasia, mild forms of 11β-hydroxylase deficiency may not become manifest until adolescence or early adulthood.

The diagnosis of 11β-hydroxylase deficiency can be confirmed by demonstration of elevated plasma levels of 11-deoxycortisol and 11-deoxycorticosterone and increased excretion of their metabolites in urine (mainly tetrahydro 11-deoxycortisol).

D. Type IV–3β-Hydroxysteroid Dehydrogenase Deficiency (Male or Female Pseudohermaphroditism and Adrenal Insufficiency): See p 535.

E. Type V–17α-Hydroxylase Deficiency (Male Pseudohermaphroditism, Sexual Infantilism, Hypertension, and Hypokalemic Alkalosis): See p 536.

F. Type VI–Cholesterol Desmolase Complex Deficiency (Congenital Lipoid Adrenal Hyperplasia, Male Pseudohermaphroditism, Sexual Infantilism, and Adrenal Insufficiency): See p 535.

Treatment

Treatment of patients with adrenal hyperplasia may be divided into acute and chronic phases. In acute adrenal crises, a deficiency of both cortisol and aldosterone results in hypoglycemia, hyponatremia, hyperkalemia, hypovolemia, and shock. An infusion of 5% glucose in isotonic saline should be started immediately. In the first hour, if the patient is in shock, 20 mL/kg of saline may be given; thereafter, fluid and electrolyte replacement is calculated on the basis of deficits and standard maintenance requirements. Hydrocortisone sodium succinate, 50 mg/m², should be given as a bolus and another 50–100 mg/m² added to the infusion fluid over the first 24 hours of therapy. If profound hyponatremia and hyperkalemia are present, deoxycorticosterone acetate, 1–3 mg, may be given every 12–24 hours intramuscularly. The amount of deoxycorticosterone acetate and the concentration and amount of saline solution must be adjusted according to the results of frequent electrolyte determinations, assessment of the state of hydration, and blood pressure measurements. Excess deoxycorticosterone acetate and salt can result in hypokalemia, hypertension, congestive heart failure, and hypertensive encephalopathy, whereas too little salt and deoxycorticosterone acetate will fail to correct the electrolyte imbalance.

Once the patient is stabilized and a definitive diagnosis with appropriate steroid studies has been made, the patient should receive maintenance doses of glucocorticoids to permit normal growth, development, and bone maturation (approximately 18 mg/m²/d of hydrocortisone by mouth in 3 divided doses). Salt losers need treatment with mineralocorticoids and added dietary salt. The dose of mineralocorticoid should be adjusted to maintain plasma renin activity in the normal range.

Patients with ambiguous external genitalia must have plastic repair of the external genitalia before age 1 year. Clitoral recession or clitoroplasty rather than clitoridectomy is preferred. Of major importance to the family with an affected child is the assurance that their child will grow and develop into a normal functional adult. In patients with the most common form of adrenal hyperplasia—21-hydroxylase deficiency—fertility in males and feminization, menstruation, and fertility in females can be expected with adequate treatment. Long-term psychologic guidance and support for the patient and family by the physician is essential.

Aberrant adrenal rests are common in males with adrenal hyperplasia and may be mistaken for either adult testicular maturation or testicular neoplasms. These adrenal rests are often bilateral and are made up of cells that appear indistinguishable from Leydig cells histologically except for the fact that they lack Reinke crystalloids.

MATERNAL ANDROGENS & PROGESTINS

Masculinization of the external genitalia of female infants can occur following ingestion by the mother of testosterone or synthetic progestational agents during the first trimester of pregnancy. After the 12th week of gestation, exposure results in clitoromegaly only. Norethindrone, ethisterone, norethynodrel, and medroxyprogesterone acetate have also been implicated in masculinization. In rare instances, masculinization of a female fetus may be secondary to an ovarian or adrenal tumor, adrenal hyperplasia, or luteoma of pregnancy.

The diagnosis of female pseudohermaphroditism arising from transplacental passage of androgenic steroids is based on exclusion of other forms of female pseudohermaphroditism and a history of drug exposure. Surgical correction of the genitalia, if needed, is the only therapy necessary.

MALE PSEUDOHERMAPHRODITISM

Male pseudohermaphrodites have gonads that are testes, but the genital ducts or external genitalia are not completely masculinized. Male pseudohermaphroditism can result from deficient testosterone secretion as a consequence of (1) failure of testicular differentiation, (2) failure of secretion of testosterone or müllerian duct inhibitory factor, (3) failure of target tissue response to testosterone or dihydrotestosterone, and (4) failure of conversion of testosterone to dihydrotestosterone.

Testicular Unresponsiveness to hCG & LH

Male sexual differentiation is dependent upon the production of testosterone by fetal Leydig cells. Data indicate that Leydig cell testosterone secretion is under the influence of placental hCG and, thereafter, fetal pituitary LH during gestation. Absence, hypoplasia, or unresponsiveness of Leydig cells to hCG-LH would result in deficient testos-

terone production and, consequently, male pseudohermaphroditism. The extent of the genital ambiguity is a function of the degree of testosterone deficiency. A small number of patients with absent, hypoplastic, or unresponsive Leydig cells (attributed to a lack of receptor activity for hCG-LH) have been reported, as well as an animal model—the "vet" rat.

The finding of normal male sexual differentiation in XY males together with anencephaly, apituitarism, and congenital hypothalamic hypopituitarism suggests that male sex differentiation can occur independently of the secretion of fetal pituitary gonadotropins.

Inborn Errors of Testosterone Biosynthesis

Fig 33–14 demonstrates the major pathways in testosterone biosynthesis in the gonads; each step is associated with an inherited defect that results in testosterone deficiency and, consequently, male pseudohermaphroditism. Steps 1, 2, and 3 are enzymatic deficiencies that occur in both the adrenals and gonads and result in defective synthesis of both corticosteroids and testosterone. Thus, they represent forms of congenital adrenal hyperplasia.

(1) 20,22-Desmolase deficiency, cholesterol desmolase complex defect, type VI adrenal hyperplasia, congenital lipoid adrenal hyperplasia (male pseudohermaphroditism, sexual infantilism, and adrenal insufficiency): This is a very early defect in the synthesis of all steroids and results in severe adrenal and gonadal insufficiency. On intravenous urography, large lipid-laden adrenals may be visualized that displace the kidneys downward. Death in early infancy from adrenal insufficiency is not uncommon. Affected males have female-appearing external genitalia. The diagnosis is confirmed by the lack of or low levels of all steroids in plasma and urine.

(2) 3β-Hydroxysteroid dehydrogenase deficiency, type IV congenital adrenal hyperplasia (male or female pseudohermaphroditism and adrenal insufficiency): 3β-Hydroxysteroid dehydrogenase deficiency is an early defect in steroid synthesis that results in inability of the adrenals and gonads to convert 3β-hydroxy-Δ^5 steroids to 3-keto-Δ^4 steroids. This defect in its complete form results in a deficiency of aldosterone, cortisol, testosterone, and estradiol. Mild forms of this defect may not be manifested clinically until adolescence. Males with this defect are incompletely masculinized, and females have mild clitoromegaly. Salt loss and adrenal crises usually occur in early infancy in affected patients.

The diagnosis of 3α-hydroxysteroid dehydrogenase deficiency is based on finding elevated concentrations of dehydroepiandrosterone and its sulfate as well as other 3β-hydroxy-Δ^5 steroids in the plasma and urine of patients with a consistent clinical picture. Suppression of the increased plasma and urinary 3β-hydroxy-Δ^5 steroids by the adminis-

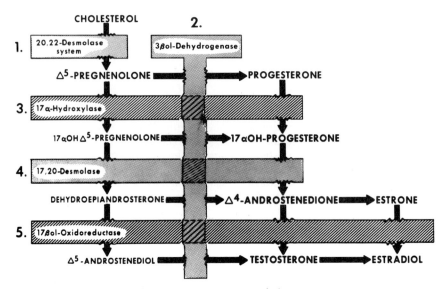

Figure 33–14. Enzymatic defects in the biosynthetic pathway for testosterone. All 5 of the enzymatic defects cause male pseudohermaphroditism in affected males. Although all of the blocks affect gonadal steroidogenesis, those at steps 1, 2, and 3 are associated with major abnormalities in the biosynthesis of glucocorticoids and mineralocorticoids in the adrenal.

tration of dexamethasone distinguishes 3β-hydroxysteroid dehydrogenase deficiency from a virilizing adrenal tumor.

(3) 17α-Hydroxylase deficiency, type V congenital adrenal hyperplasia (male pseudohermaphroditism, sexual infantilism, hypertension, and hypokalemic alkalosis): A defect in 17α-hydroxylation in the zona fasciculata of the adrenal and in the gonads results in impaired synthesis of 17α-hydroxyprogesterone and 17α-hydroxypregnenolone and, consequently, cortisol and sex steroids. The secretion of large amounts of corticosterone and deoxycorticosterone leads to hypertension, hypokalemia, and alkalosis. Increased 11-deoxycorticosterone secretion with resultant hypertension produces suppression of renin and aldosterone secretion.

The clinical manifestations result from the adrenal and gonadal defect. XX females have normal development of internal ducts and external genitalia but manifest sexual infantilism with elevated gonadotropins at puberty. In males, impaired testosterone synthesis by the fetal testes results in female or ambiguous genitalia.

The diagnosis of 17α-hydroxylase deficiency should be suspected in XY males with ambiguous genitalia or phenotypic females with sexual infantilism, who also manifest hypertension associated with hypokalemic alkalosis. Elevated levels of progesterone, Δ5-pregnenolone, deoxycorticosterone, and corticosterone in plasma and increased excretion of their urinary metabolites establishes the diagnosis. Plasma renin activity is markedly diminished in these patients.

The following errors affect testosterone and estrogen biosynthesis in the gonads only:

(4) 17,20-Desmolase (lyase) deficiency: This is a rare defect in testosterone synthesis that affects the conversion of the C_{21} steroids 17α-hydroxyprogesterone and 17α-hydroxy-Δ5 pregnenolone to the C_{19} steroids androstenedione and dehydroepiandrosterone. Patients described with 17,20-desmolase deficiency have been male pseudohermaphrodites with female or ambiguous genitalia and inguinal or intra-abdominal testes. Müllerian derivatives are absent, presumably as a result of the secretion of müllerian duct inhibitory factor. At puberty, incomplete virilization without gynecomastia may occur.

Patients with 17,20-desmolase deficiency have low circulating levels of testosterone, androstenedione, dehydroepiandrosterone, and estradiol. The diagnosis can be confirmed by demonstration of an increased ratio of 17α-hydroxy C_{21} deoxysteroids to C_{19} steroids (testosterone, dehydroepiandrosterone, Δ5-androstenediol, and androstenedione) after hCG or ACTH stimulation.

(5) 17β-Hydroxysteroid oxidoreductase deficiency: The last step in testosterone and estradiol biosynthesis by the gonads involves the reduction of androstenedione to testosterone and estrone to estradiol. At birth, males with a deficiency of the enzyme 17β-hydroxysteroid oxidoreductase have female or mildly ambiguous external genitalia resulting from testosterone deficiency during male differentiation. They have male duct development, absent müllerian structures with a blind vaginal pouch, and inguinal or intra-abdominal testes. At puberty, progressive virilization with clitoral hypertrophy occurs, often associated with the concurrent development of gynecomastia. Plasma gonadotropins are elevated, as are androstenedione and estrone levels, while testosterone and estradiol concentrations are low.

17β-Hydroxysteroid oxidoreductase deficiency should be included in the differential diagnosis of (1) male pseudohermaphrodites with absent müllerian derivatives who have no abnormality in glucocorticoid or mineralocorticoid synthesis and (2) male pseudohermaphrodites who virilize at puberty, especially if gynecomastia is present. The diagnosis of 17β-hydroxysteroid oxidoreductase deficiency can be confirmed by the demonstration of inappropriately high plasma levels of estrone and androstenedione and decreased ratios of plasma testosterone to androstenedione and estradiol to estrone before or after hCG stimulation.

Management of the patients, as with other forms of male pseudohermaphroditism, depends on the age at diagnosis and the degree of ambiguity of the external genitalia. In the patient assigned a male gender identity, plastic repair of the genitalia and replacement testosterone therapy at puberty will be necessary. In patients reared as females (the usual case), the appropriate treatment is castration, followed by estrogen replacement therapy at puberty.

Defects in Androgen-Dependent Target Tissues

The complex mechanism of action of steroid hormones at the cellular level has recently been clarified (Fig 33–15). Free testosterone enters the target cells and undergoes 5α reduction to dihydrotestosterone, which in turn is bound to a receptor protein; the receptor protein complex is translocated into the nucleus of the target cell. In the nucleus, the receptor-dihydrotestosterone complex binds to chromatin and initiates transcription. mRNA is synthesized, modified, and exported to the cytoplasm of the cell, where ribosomes translate

mRNA into new proteins that have an androgenic effect on the cell. A lack of androgen effect at the end-organ and male pseudohermaphroditism may result from abnormalities in 5α-reductase activity, dihydrotestosterone receptor activity, translocation of the steroid-receptor complex, nuclear binding, transcription, exportation, or translation.

End-Organ Insensitivity to Androgenic Hormones (Androgen Receptor & Postreceptor Effects)

A. Complete Syndrome of Androgen Insensitivity and Its Variants (Testicular Feminization): The complete syndrome of androgen insensitivity (testicular feminization) is characterized by a 46,XY karyotype, bilateral testes, female-appearing external genitalia, a blind vaginal pouch, and absent müllerian derivatives. At puberty, female secondary sexual characteristics develop, but menarche does not ensue. Pubic and axillary hair are usually sparse and in one-third of patients totally absent. Some patients have a variant form of this syndrome and exhibit slight clitoral enlargement. At puberty, these patients may exhibit mild virilization in addition to the development of breasts and a female habitus.

Androgen insensitivity during embryogenesis prevents masculinization of the external genitalia and differentiation of the wolffian ducts. Secretion of müllerian duct inhibitory factor by the fetal Sertoli cells leads to regression of the müllerian ducts. Thus, affected patients are born with female external genitalia and a blind vaginal pouch. At puberty, androgen insensitivity results in augmented LH secretion with subsequent increases in testosterone and estradiol. Estradiol arises from conversion of testosterone and androstenedione as well as from direct secretion by the testes. Androgen insensitivity coupled with increased estradiol secretion re-

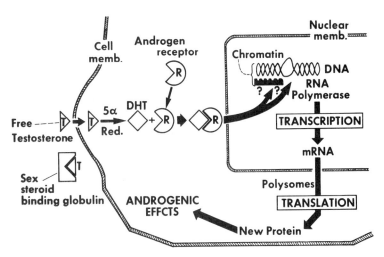

Figure 33–15. A simplified diagrammatic representation of the mechanism of action of testosterone at the target organ. 5α-Red. = 5α-reductase. DHT = dihydrotestosterone. (Reproduced, with permission, from Conte FA, Grumbach MM: Pathogenesis, classification, diagnosis, and treatment of anomalies of sex. Chapter 106, in: *Endocrinology.* DeGroot L [editor]. Grune & Stratton, 1979.)

sults in the development of female secondary sexual characteristics at puberty.

Data in rodents as well as mammals indicate that androgen insensitivity is modulated, at least in part, by abnormalities in androgen receptor activity in androgen-sensitive tissues. Studies utilizing fibroblasts cultured from genital skin indicate that patients with complete androgen insensitivity are genetically heterogeneous. Patients have been described who have (1) an undetectable or low amount of androgen receptor activity, (2) an unstable (thermolabile) androgen receptor, and (3) a normal amount of androgen receptor activity (a presumed postreceptor defect). Inheritance in all forms appears to be X-linked.

The diagnosis of complete androgen insensitivity can be suspected from the clinical features. Prepubertally, testislike masses in the inguinal canal or labia in a phenotypic female suggest the diagnosis. Postpubertally, the patients present with primary amenorrhea, normal breast development, and absent or sparse sexual hair. Characteristically, the concentrations of LH and testosterone are markedly elevated. This latter finding is an important hormonal feature of androgen insensitivity. The family history, phenotype, endocrine evaluation, androgen receptor studies, and, if necessary, the metabolic response to testosterone will help confirm the diagnosis.

Therapy of patients with complete androgen insensitivity involves affirmation and reinforcement of their female gender identity. Castration, either prior to or after puberty, is indicated because of the increased risk of gonadal neoplasms with age.

B. Incomplete Syndrome of Androgen Insensitivity and Its Variants (Reifenstein's Syndrome): Patients with incomplete androgen insensitivity manifest a wide spectrum of phenotypes as far as masculinization is concerned. The external genitalia at birth can range from ambiguous, with a blind vaginal pouch, to hypoplastic male genitalia. Müllerian duct derivatives are absent and wolffian duct derivatives present, but they are usually hypoplastic. At puberty, virilization is poor; pubic and axillary hair as well as gynecomastia are usually present. The testes remain small and exhibit azoospermia as a consequence of germinal cell arrest.

As in the case of patients with complete androgen insensitivity, there are high levels of plasma LH, testosterone, and estradiol. However, the degree of feminization in these patients despite elevated estradiol is less than that found in the complete syndrome of androgen insensitivity.

Androgen receptor studies in these patients have revealed (1) a partial deficiency of androgen receptor activity and (2) normal androgen receptor activity (a presumed postreceptor defect). As in the complete syndrome of androgen insensitivity, inheritance appears to be X-linked.

Androgen Insensitivity in Infertile Men

Partial androgen insensitivity with a partial deficiency of androgen receptor activity has been described in a group of infertile men who have a normal male phenotype but may exhibit gynecomastia. Like other patients with androgen insensitivity, they have increased plasma levels of testosterone and LH. Inheritance appears to be X-linked.

Defects in Testosterone Metabolism by Peripheral Tissues; 5α-Reductase Deficiency (Male Pseudohermaphroditism With Masculinization at Puberty, Pseudovaginal Perineoscrotal Hypospadias)

The defective conversion of testosterone to dihydrotestosterone produces a unique form of male pseudohermaphroditism (Fig 33–16). At birth, ambiguous external genitalia are manifested by a small hypospadiac phallus bound down in chordee, a bifid scrotum, and a urogenital sinus that opens onto the perineum. A blind vaginal pouch is present. The testes are either inguinal or labial. The müllerian structures are absent, and the wolffian structures are well-differentiated. At puberty, affected males virilize; the voice deepens, muscle mass increases, and the phallus enlarges. The bifid scrotum becomes rugate and pigmented. The testes enlarge and descend into the labioscrotal folds, and spermatogenesis ensues. Gynecomastia is notably absent in these patients. Of note also is the absence of acne, temporal hair recession, and hirsutism. A remarkable feature of this form of male pseudohermaphroditism has been the reported change

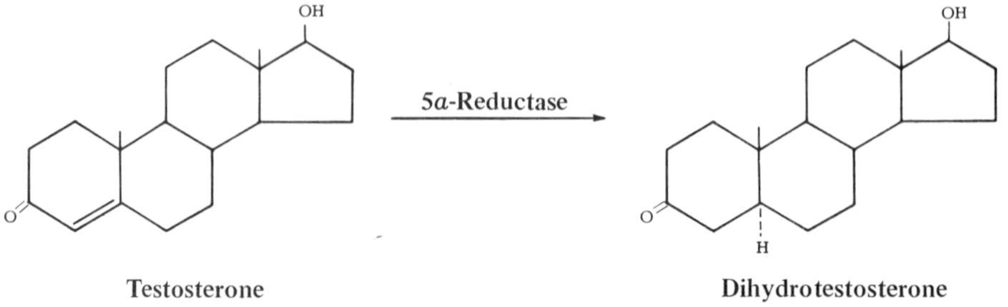

Figure 33–16. Metabolism of testosterone.

in gender identity from female to male at puberty, primarily in affected individuals living in rural communities in the Dominican Republic.

After the onset of puberty, patients with 5α-reductase deficiency have normal to elevated testosterone levels and elevated plasma concentrations of LH. As expected, plasma dihydrotestosterone is low and the testosterone/dihydrotestosterone ratio is abnormally high. Apparently, lack of 5α reduction of testosterone to dihydrotestosterone in utero during the critical phases of male sex differentiation results in incomplete masculinization of the external genitalia, while testosterone-dependent wolffian structures are normally developed. The marked virilization that occurs at puberty in these patients is in sharp contrast to that which occurs in utero and is as yet not well explained. Since the androgen receptor binds both dihydrotestosterone and testosterone (but with a lower affinity), the sustained high levels of circulating testosterone attained at puberty may be a factor in the virilization achieved. In addition, the enzyme defect is incomplete, and at puberty the plasma concentration of dihydrotestosterone, while low, is detectable. Also, the hormonal development is markedly different at puberty in that large quantities of competitive steroids (estrogens and progestins) are not present as they are in utero. In particular, high concentrations of progesterone may have a marked effect on 5α-reductase activity in utero, whereas at puberty progesterone levels are quite low in males. 5α-Reductase deficiency is inherited as an autosomal recessive, and the enzymatic defect exhibits genetic heterogeneity.

5α-Reductase deficiency should be suspected in male pseudohermaphrodites with a blind vaginal pouch. The diagnosis can be confirmed by demonstration of an abnormally high testosterone/dihydrotestosterone ratio, either under basal conditions or after hCG stimulation. Other confirmatory studies include an increased $5\beta/5\alpha$ ratio of urinary 11-deoxy C_{19} steroid metabolites of testosterone, a decreased level of 5α-reductase activity in genital skin in vitro, and a decreased conversion of infused testosterone to dihydrotestosterone in vivo.

The early diagnosis of this condition is particularly critical. Affected males can be assigned a male gender identity, treated with dihydrotestosterone, and have appropriate plastic repair of their external genitalia. In patients who are diagnosed after infancy, in whom gender identity is unequivocally female, we feel that prophylactic orchidectomy and estrogen substitution therapy is still the treatment of choice until further experience with this biochemical entity and sex reversal in our culture is available.

Dysgenetic Male Pseudohermaphroditism (Ambiguous Genitalia Due to Dysgenetic Gonads)

Defective gonadogenesis results in ambiguous development of the genital ducts, urogenital sinus, and external genitalia. Patients with XO/XY mosaicism, structural abnormalities of the Y chromosome, and forms of XY gonadal dysgenesis manifest defective gonadogenesis and thus defective virilization. These disorders are classified under disorders of gonadal differentiation but also are included as a subgroup of male pseudohermaphroditism.

A. Ambiguous Genitalia Associated With Degenerative Renal Disease: Several cases are recorded of male pseudohermaphroditism associated with degenerative renal disease and hypertension as well as with Wilms's tumor. In this syndrome, both the kidneys and the testes are dysgenetic and a predisposition for renal neoplasms exists.

B. Vanishing Testes Syndrome (Embryonic Testicular Regression Syndrome; XY Agonadism; Rudimentary Testes Syndrome; Congenital Anorchia): Cessation of testicular function during the critical phases of male sex differentiation can lead to varying clinical syndromes depending on when testicular function ceases. At one end of the clinical spectrum of these heterogeneous conditions are the XY patients in whom testicular functional deficiency occurred prior to 8 weeks of gestation, which results in female differentiation of the internal and external genitalia. At the other end of the spectrum are the patients with "anorchia" or "vanishing testes." These patients have perfectly normal male differentiation of their internal and external structures, but gonadal tissue is absent. The diagnosis of anorchia should be considered in all cryptorchid males. Administration of hCG, 1000–2000 units intramuscularly every 3 days for 5 doses, is a useful test of Leydig cell function. In the presence of normal Leydig cell function, there will be a rise in plasma testosterone from concentrations of less than 20 ng/dL to over 200 ng/dL in prepubertal males. In infants under 4 years of age and children over 10 years of age, plasma FSH levels are a sensitive index of gonadal integrity. The gonadotropin response to a 100-μg bolus injection of luteinizing hormone–releasing factor (LRF) can also be utilized to diagnose the absence of gonadal feedback on the hypothalamus and pituitary. In agonadal children, LRF will elicit a rise in LH and FSH that is greater than that achieved in prepubertal children with normal gonadal function. Patients with elevated gonadotropins and no testosterone response to hCG are usually found to lack recognizable gonadal tissue at laparotomy.

Defects in the Synthesis, Structure, or Response to Müllerian Duct Inhibitory Factor

A small number of patients have been described in whom normal male development of the external genitalia has occurred but in whom the müllerian ducts persist. The retention of müllerian structures can be ascribed to failure of the Sertoli cells to synthesize müllerian duct inhibitory factor or to a defect in the response of the duct to that factor. This condition appears to be transmitted as an autosomal recessive trait. Therapy involves removal of the müllerian structures.

UNCLASSIFIED FORMS OF ABNORMAL SEXUAL DEVELOPMENT IN MALES

Hypospadias

Hypospadias occurs as an isolated finding in one in 700 newborn males. Although on an embryologic basis, deficient virilization of the external genitalia implies subnormal Leydig cell function in utero or end-organ resistance, in most patients there is little reason to suspect either mechanism. Thus, nonendocrine factors that affect differentiation of the primordia may be found in a variety of genetic syndromes. Aarskog prospectively studied 100 patients with hypospadias and found one patient to be a genetic female with congenital adrenal hyperplasia, 5 with sex chromosome abnormalities, and one with the incomplete form of XY gonadal dysgenesis. Nine patients were from pregnancies in which the mother had taken progestational compounds during the first trimester. Thus, a pathogenetic mechanism was found in 15% of these patients.

Microphallus

Microphallus can result from a heterogeneous group of disorders. There are data in mammals to indicate that testosterone synthesis by the fetal Leydig cell during the critical period of male differentiation (8–12 weeks) may be autonomous or under the influence of placental hCG. After midgestation fetal pituitary LH as well as placental hCG seems to modulate fetal testosterone synthesis by the Leydig cell and, consequently, growth of the phallus. Growth hormone also appears to play a role in growth of the phallus. Thus, males with congenital hypopituitarism as well as isolated gonadotropin deficiency can present with normal male differentiation and microphallus at birth (phallus less than 2 cm in length) along with hypoglycemia. After appropriate evaluation of anterior pituitary function (ie, growth hormone, ACTH, cortisol, TSH, and gonadotropins) and stabilization of the patient with hormone replacement, if necessary, a trial of testosterone therapy should be administered to all patients with microphallus before definitive gender assignment is made. Patients with fetal testosterone deficiency as a cause of their microphallus respond to 25–50 mg of testosterone enanthate intramuscularly monthly for 3 months with a mean increase of 2 cm in phallic length (Fig 33–17). If a trial of testosterone therapy does not result in a reasonable increase in phallic size, castration and assignment of a female gender is then a prudent course to follow in the management of patients with microphallus.

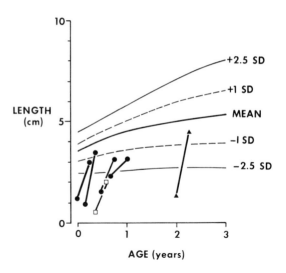

Figure 33–17. The response in phallic length to a 3-month course of testosterone in 6 patients with microphallus under 2 years of age. Each patient was given 25 mg of testosterone enanthate in oil intramuscularly monthly for 3 months. Δ, □ indicate 2 patients who subsequently underwent a second course of testosterone therapy. (Reproduced, with permission, from Burstein S, Grumbach MM, Kaplan SL: Early determination of androgen-responsiveness is important in the management of microphallus. *Lancet* 1979;2:983.)

UNCLASSIFIED FORMS OF ABNORMAL SEXUAL DEVELOPMENT IN FEMALES

Congenital absence of the vagina occurs in one in 5000 female births. It can be associated with müllerian derivatives that vary from normal to absent. Ovarian function is usually normal. Therapy involves plastic repair of the vagina, if indicated.

MANAGEMENT OF PATIENTS WITH INTERSEX PROBLEMS

Choice of Sex

The goal of the physician in the management of patients with ambiguous genitalia is to establish a diagnosis and to assign a sex for rearing that is most compatible with a well-adjusted life and sexual adequacy. Once the sex for rearing is assigned, the gender role is reinforced by the use of appropriate surgical, hormonal, or psychologic measures. Except in female pseudohermaphrodites, ambiguities of the genitalia are caused by lesions that almost always make the patient infertile. In recommending male sex assignment, the adequacy of the size of the phallus should be the most important consideration.

History: family history, pregnancy (hormones), "crises," virilization inspection
Palpation of inguinal region and labioscrotal folds and rectal examination
X chromatin pattern; karyotype analysis
Urinary 17-ketosteroids and pregnanetriol; plasma 17-hydroxyprogesterone
Serum electrolytes and urocytogram
Provisional diagnosis

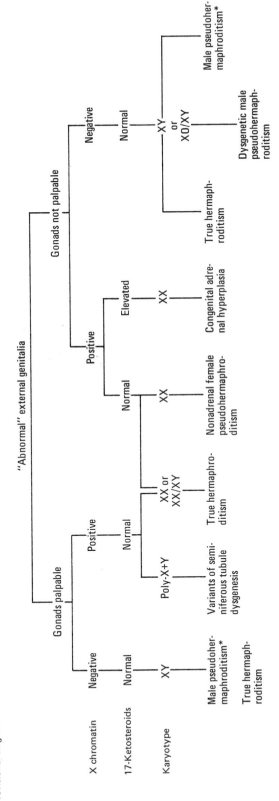

"Vaginogram" (urogenital sinus): selected cases
Endoscopy, laparotomy, gonadal biopsy: restricted to suspected male pseudohermaphrodites,
true hermaphrodites, and selected instances of nonadrenal female pseudohermaphroditism

*Excretion of 17-ketosteroids is increased in male pseudohermaphrodites who have congenital adrenal hyperplasia due to a defect in 3β-hydroxysteroid dehydrogenase.

Figure 33–18. Steps in the diagnosis of intersexuality in infancy and childhood. (Modified, with permission, from Grumbach MM: In: *Pediatrics*, 13th ed. Holt LE Jr, McIntosh R, Barnett HL [editors]. Appleton-Century-Crofts, 1962.)

Differential Diagnosis

The steps in the diagnosis of intersexuality are delineated in Fig 33–18.

Reassignment of Sex

Reassignment of sex in infancy and childhood is always a difficult psychosocial problem for the patient, the parents, and the physicians involved. While easier in infancy than after 2 years of age, it should always be undertaken with much deliberation and with provision for long-term medical and psychiatric supervision and counseling.

Reconstructive Surgery

It is desirable to initiate plastic repair of the external genitalia prior to 6–12 months of age. In children raised as females, the clitoris should be salvaged, if possible, by clitoroplasty or clitoral recession. Reconstruction of a vagina, if necessary, can be deferred until adolescence.

Removal of the gonads in children with the variant forms of gonadal dysgenesis should be performed at the time of initial repair of the external genitalia, because gonadoblastomas, seminomas, and dysgerminomas have been reported to occur during the first decade.

In a patient with testicular feminization, the gonads may be left in situ (provided they are not situated in the labia majora) to provide estrogen until late adolescence. The patient may then undergo prophylactic castration, having had her female identity reinforced by normal feminization at puberty.

In patients with incomplete testicular feminization reared as females or in patients with errors of testosterone biosynthesis in whom some degree of masculinization occurs at puberty, gonadectomy should be performed prior to puberty.

Hormonal Substitution Therapy

Cyclic estrogen and progestin treatment is used in individuals reared as females in whom a uterus is present (see p 530). In males, virilization is achieved by the administration of repository testosterone (see p 531).

Psychologic Management

Sex is not a single biologic entity but the summation of many morphogenetic, functional, and psychologic potentialities. There must never be any doubt in the mind of the parent or child as to the child's true sex. Chromosomal and gonadal sex are secondary matters; the sex of rearing is paramount. With proper surgical reconstruction and hormone substitution, the individual whose psychosexual gender is discordant with chromosomal gender need not have any psychologic catastrophes as long as the sex of rearing is accepted with conviction by the family and others during the critical early years. Anatomic abnormalities, it must be stressed, do not predispose to homosexual tendencies. These individuals should reach adulthood as well-adjusted men or women capable of normal sexual interaction, albeit usually not of procreation.

•   •   •

References

Conte FA, Grumbach MM: Pathogenesis, classification, diagnosis, and treatment of anomalies of sex. Chapter 106, in: *Endocrinology.* DeGroot L (editor). Grune & Stratton, 1979.

Griffen JE, Wilson JD: The syndrome of androgen resistance. *N Engl J Med* 1980;**302**:198.

Grumbach MM, Conte FA: Disorders of sex differentiation. In: *Textbook of Endocrinology,* 6th ed. Williams RH (editor). Saunders, 1981.

Hamerton JL: *Human Cytogenetics.* Vols 1 and 2. Academic Press, 1971.

Imperato-McGinley JL & others: Androgens and the evolution of male-gender identity among male pseudohermaphrodites with 5α-reductase deficiency. *N Engl J Med* 1979;**300**:1233.

Lee PA & others (editors): *Congenital Adrenal Hyperplasia.* University Park Press, 1977.

McKusick VA: *Mendelian Inheritance in Man,* 5th ed. Johns Hopkins Univ Press, 1978.

Money J, Ehrhardt AA: *Man and Woman, Boy and Girl: The Differentiation and Dimorphism of Gender Identity from Conception to Maturity.* Johns Hopkins Univ Press, 1972.

New MI & others: An update of congenital adrenal hyperplasia. *Recent Prog Horm Res.* [In press, 1981.]

Ohno S: *Major Sex Determining Genes.* Springer-Verlag, 1979.

Peters H, McNulty KP: *The Ovary.* Univ of California Press, 1980.

Peterson RE & others: Male pseudohermaphrodism due to steroid 5α-reductase deficiency. *Am J Med* 1977;**62**:170.

Rosenfield RL, Lucky AW, Allen TD: The diagnosis and management of intersex. *Curr Probl in Pediatr* 1980;**10**:7. [Entire issue.]

Simpson JL: *Disorders of Sexual Differentiation, Etiology and Clinical Delineation.* Academic Press, 1976.

Simpson JL, Photopulos G: The relationship of neoplasia to disorders of abnormal sexual differentiation. *Birth Defects* 1976;**12**(Suppl 1):15.

Vallet HL, Porter IH (editors): *Symposium on Genetic Mechanisms of Sexual Development.* Academic Press, 1979.

Van Niekerk WA: *True Hermaphrodism.* Harper & Row, 1974.

Wachtel SS, Ohno S: The immunogenetics of sexual development. *Prog Med Genet* 1979;**3**:109.

Wilson JD, MacDonald PC: Male pseudohermaphroditism due to androgen resistance: Testicular feminization and related syndromes. In: *Metabolic Basis of Inherited Disease,* 4th ed. Stanbury JB (editor). McGraw-Hill, 1978.

Renovascular Hypertension | 34

Donald R. Smith, MD

Urologic renal disease is a not uncommon cause of hypertension. However, most cases of high blood pressure (ie, essential hypertension) are of unknown cause. Coarctation of the aorta, polycystic kidneys, glomerulonephritis, and polyarteritis nodosa are often accompanied by hypertension.

Etiology

Many years have passed since Goldblatt demonstrated in experimental animals that protracted renal ischemia could produce hypertension. In dogs, unilateral renal ischemia can cause transient hypertension, or it can cause no change at all if the other kidney is not removed or rendered ischemic. In humans, however, there is unequivocal evidence that unilateral renal ischemia causes hypertension that can be cured by nephrectomy or reconstruction of the renal artery.

Pathogenesis

It is now clear that in the ischemic kidney, there is decreased blood flow through the afferent glomerular arteries, which causes an increased number of secretory granules in the juxtaglomerular bodies that elaborate renin. Renin reacts with an alpha$_2$ globulin to produce angiotensin I, a somewhat inert substance. When acted upon by a converting enzyme, it is changed to angiotensin II, a potent vasoconstrictor that also acts on the adrenal cortex to increase aldosterone secretion. Thus, hypertension is established.

In severe hypertension caused by stenosis of the renal artery, renin has been recovered in increased amounts from the renal vein of the ischemic organ, and evidence of hyperaldosteronism (hypokalemic alkalosis) has been observed. However, in milder cases, such increased humoral activity may not be found. The recent observation that saralasin, a competitive inhibitor of angiotensin II, caused lowering of blood pressure in patients with renal ischemia gave rise to speculation that this response might serve as a definitive test for renal ischemia. However, the test has given false-negative results in about 7–10% of cases—ie, some patients whose hypertension was cured by vascular reconstruction did not respond to saralasin. False-positive results have been reported also in patients with essential hypertension who have increased renin secretion and therefore respond positively to saralasin. Despite these errors, the test is an important screening procedure in patients with suspected renovascular hypertension (Vaughan, 1979). It is discussed further below.

Pathology

The common causes of stenosis of the renal artery are arteriosclerotic plaques, fibromuscular hyperplasia of the media (which usually affects relatively young females and children) (Rushton, 1980), neurofibromatosis (most often seen in children), and embolism or thrombosis. Stenosis in a renal artery may protect a kidney from the deleterious effects of hypertension while the other kidney remains hypertensive. Thus, the ischemic kidney may ultimately be the better of the two; it should be preserved unless considerable atrophy has occurred.

At autopsy, there does not appear to be a high correlation between stenosis of the renal artery and the presence of hypertension. A lesion producing at least a 70% reduction in luminal diameter appears to be necessary in order to reduce renal plasma flow to the point where clinically significant ischemia is produced. Therefore, the significance of a stenosis shown on aortography can only be determined by measurement of renal vein renin levels, by observation of a drop in blood pressure after saralasin, and, in selected cases, by split renal function studies.

The changes observed in the pyelonephritic kidney have already been described (Chapter 12). From the standpoint of the genesis of hypertension, the most striking lesion is the marked thickening of the arteriolar walls. Pfau & Rosenmann (1978) believe that pyelonephritis is a rare cause of hypertension, but Poutasse & others (1978) and Savage & others (1978) have reported on a number of children with the disorder who had increased levels of renin from the involved kidney and were cured by nephrectomy.

Other urologic renal lesions causing hypertension include ureteral and ureteropelvic junction obstruction with hydronephrosis (Pak, Kawamura, & Yoshida, 1980), renal cyst, radiation nephritis, severe perinephritis following trauma (Page kid-

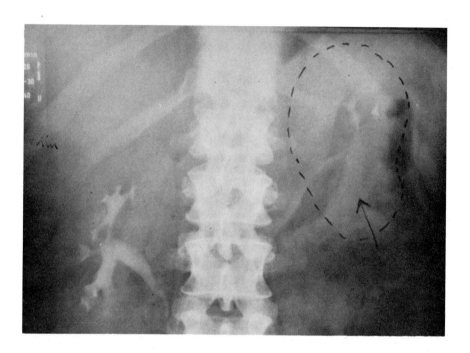

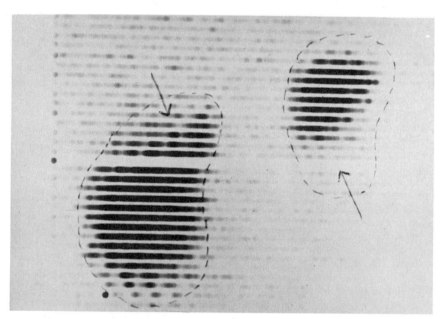

Figure 34–1. Renovascular hypertension. *Above:* Excretory urogram shows contraction of lower half of left kidney and failure of visualization of lower pole calices. Right urogram normal. *Below:* Rectilinear scan, same patient, demonstrating ischemia of lower half of left kidney. Small area of upper pole of right kidney also ischemic. Renal angiogram showed stenosis of artery to lower pole of left kidney.

ney), aneurysm of the renal artery, renal hypoplasia, ligation of a segmental branch of a renal artery, and tuberculosis. Preoperatively, elevated renin concentrations have been demonstrated in such cases. Hypertension is common with Wilms's tumor and is occasionally observed in patients with renal adenocarcinoma. Nephrectomy is apt to lead to normotension.

Clinical Findings

The clinical features of renal diseases that may cause hypertension have already been discussed (see chronic pyelonephritis, thrombosis of the renal artery, aneurysm of the renal artery, hydronephrosis, renal tumors, and renal tuberculosis).

A. Symptoms: Hypertension from renal ischemia should be suspected (1) if there is a recent onset of hypertension in the absence of a family history of hypertension, particularly if the patient is under age 25 or over age 50 years; (2) if the patient has had severe flank or abdominal pain or trauma (suggesting embolism or thrombosis of a renal artery or an organized perirenal hematoma), with or without hematuria; (3) if there is abrupt worsening of preexisting hypertension, especially in an older person; or (4) in the presence of severe hypertension at any age.

B. Signs: In addition to a relatively sustained diastolic hypertension, changes typical of malignant hypertension may be found in the retinas. A systolic bruit should be sought anteriorly and posteriorly over the renal areas. A renal mass may be felt (eg, tumor). The presence of an aortic aneurysm or vascular insufficiency of the extremities is suggestive.

C. Laboratory Findings: Bacteria and pus cells in the urine may indicate chronic pyelonephritis. In the malignant phase of hypertension, proteinuria, casts, and red cells will be seen. Unless malignant hypertension, polycystic disease, bilateral atrophic pyelonephritis, or bilateral renal artery stenosis is present, total renal function (as measured by PSP test and creatinine clearance) is usually normal. Hypokalemic alkalosis suggestive of aldosteronism may be found. Lactic acid dehydrogenase may be elevated in the presence of bilateral chronic pyelonephritis or malignant hypertension.

D. X-Ray Findings: Excretory urography is a useful screening test for the presence of renal ischemia (Figs 34–1 and 34–2). It suggests the presumptive diagnosis in 60–70% of cases. The bowel should be well prepared. Since delay in appearance of the radiopaque medium is an important sign, exposures should be made immediately and at 2, 3, 4, and 5 minutes after rapid injection. The following findings are suggestive of renal ischemia: (1) a kidney at least 1 cm shorter than its mate (normally, the right kidney is 0.5 cm shorter than the left); (2) lack of function of one kidney (with normal pyelocaliceal architecture as shown by retrograde urography); (3) delayed appearance of visualization on the early films; (4) the occurrence, at times, of hyperconcentration of the radiopaque medium due to marked overreabsorption of water (a phenomenon that may be accentuated by making urograms with the patient hydrated); (5) narrow, delicate renal calices, renal pelvis, and ureter because of diminution in the volume of urine excreted; (6) partial

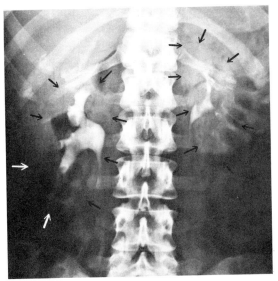 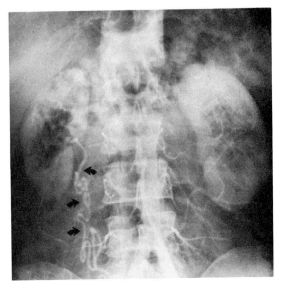

Figure 34–2. Hypertension caused by stenosis of left renal artery. *Left:* Ten-minute excretory urogram showing small left kidney with delayed and impaired excretion of radiopaque fluid. Because of diminution of urine volume, calices and pelvis are smaller than in the contralateral kidney. *Right:* Angiogram in patient with complete occlusion of right main renal artery. Marked secondary periureteral collateral circulation allows persistence of some renal function.

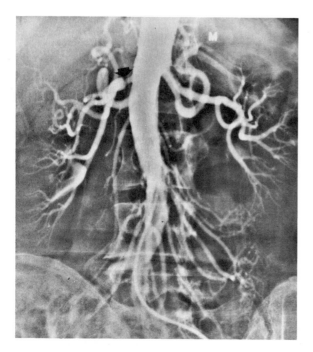 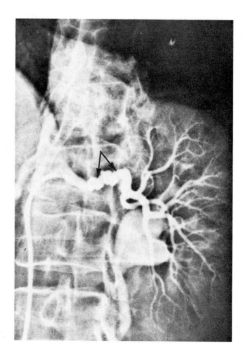

Figure 34–3. *Left:* Renal angiogram, "midstream" type, showing significant arteriosclerotic plaque at takeoff of right renal artery (see arrow). *Right:* Selective angiogram of left kidney, right posterior oblique position. Fibromuscular hyperplasia of renal artery.

atrophy (contraction) of one pole; (7) normal, but small, caliceal pattern in a small kidney; and (8) scalloping or notching of the upper ureter caused by secondary arterial collaterals.

The urographic changes of chronic pyelonephritis, hydronephrosis, tumor, and polycystic kidneys should be obvious.

Renal angiography (including selective angiography) will demonstrate stenosis of the renal artery caused by an atheromatous plaque (usually proximal), fibromuscular hyperplasia (usually distal), and neurofibromatosis (proximal) (Fig 34–3). Oblique views are helpful. When stenosis is severe, secondary periureteral collateral circulation may be seen (Fig 34–2).

E. Renal Isotope Studies:

1. The ^{131}I-hippurate isotope renogram—This has proved to be a fairly good screening test for renovascular hypertension. Because of the over-reabsorption of water by the tubules in the ischemic kidney, transport of the isotope to the pelvis is slow, and its escape down the ureter is slowed. Furthermore, diminished renal blood flow decreases the amount of the iodide that reaches the kidney. Hence, the vascular spike from such a kidney is lower than that of its mate; its secretory phase is prolonged. Instead of the counts beginning to drop 3–5 minutes after injection, they tend to persist because of lack of "washout" (Fig 8–5). Stamey (1976) believes that if the intravenous urograms are equivocal, a renogram should be performed. Unfor-

tunately, the pyelonephritic kidney is apt to show a similar reaction.

2. The ^{203}Hg-chlormerodrin rectilinear scan—This measures renal tubular function and renal blood flow. It depicts the size and shape of the kidney. Thus, it may reveal polar atrophy (Fig 34–1), but it does not differentiate chronic pyelonephritis or renal infarct from ischemia.

3. Anger camera scan—(Fig 8–4.) The ^{131}I-hippurate photos will show slow uptake of the isotope in the ischemic kidney. Because of the over-reabsorption of water, there is slow transport of the iodide to the pelvis. Therefore, by 8–10 minutes there is apt to be hyperconcentration of the isotope in the parenchyma as compared to the normal kidney. At 15 minutes, the normal kidney may have cleared the isotope, but it still lingers in the renal pelvis of the ischemic kidney. An isotope renogram can be constructed from the counts that are recorded.

The ^{99m}Tc scan will reflect diminution of blood supply to the ischemic kidney. These tests are less helpful if the disease is bilateral.

F. Estimation of Venous Renin Levels: In renovascular hypertension, the peripheral venous renin may be normal or elevated. The level of elevation depends on the sodium balance. In order to accentuate the difference between these plasma renin concentrations, salt intake should be limited for a few days before the test. Furosemide should be administered the evening before. It is most convenient to perform renal vein catheterization at the time of angiography; renin concentrations from each vein can then be measured. If the difference in levels is 1.5:1 or more, surgery is likely to be curative or beneficial. If the ratio is 2:1 or more, an excellent surgical result can be obtained. If the ratio is less than 1.5:1, only one-third of patients will respond. Unfortunately, some false-positives and false-negatives are seen. A number of patients with equal renin levels also respond to reconstructive surgery or nephrectomy.

G. Angiotensin II Blockade (Saralasin Test): Saralasin blocks the conversion of angiotensin I to angiotensin II. In hypertension associated with elevated renal vein levels of renin, the administration of 10 mg/kg/min of saralasin causes an appreciable drop in blood pressure in 20–30 minutes. Patients with normal or low peripheral renin do not respond. Unfortunately, some patients with essential hypertension also have elevated renin secretion and therefore respond positively to saralasin.

Buda & others (1978) found a high correlation between elevated renin levels and response to saralasin. Poutasse & others (1980) report a 19% rate of false-negative saralasin tests in patients who later responded to surgery. They recommend using additional tests. Gillespie & others (1980) found the saralasin test to be particularly valuable in hypertensive children.

H. Relative Renal Function Tests: These tests have now been largely replaced by renal vein renin measurements and the saralasin test. Renal function tests should be considered if the newer tests are equivocal and the index of suspicion is high. In the presence of heart failure or shock (diminished renal blood flow), normal kidneys modify their function and respond in the following manner: urine volume, urine sodium, chloride, and blood urea nitrogen concentrations, total PSP excretion (test of renal blood flow), and urinary pH are reduced; and responses to clearance tests, such as creatinine, iodopyracet (Diodrast), and PAH, are lowered. In addition, there is increased osmolality and increased concentration of creatinine, nitrogen, and potassium in the urine.

The ischemic kidney reacts in a similar manner. Its basic functional characteristic is marked reabsorption of water by the renal tubules; to an even greater extent, salt (both sodium and chloride) is absorbed. On the other hand, potassium and creatinine—though excreted in amounts smaller than those excreted by the normal kidney—are poorly reabsorbed, leading to an increase in their concentrations per unit volume.

In the presence of renal ischemia, urea—as opposed to creatinine—is significantly reabsorbed, because of the slow flow of urine through the tubules. Thus, the urea nitrogen:creatinine ratio in the urine will be low. There is also a decrease in total PSP excretion but an increase in PSP concentration per milliliter of urine (because of overreab-

Table 34–1. Interpretation of Stamey test.

Lesion	Urine Volume	PAH Concentration
Stenosis of main artery, unilateral	↓ 67% or more	↑ 100% or more
Stenosis of main artery, bilateral	↓ 40% or more	↑ 36% or more
Stenosis of segmental artery, unilateral. Also essential hypertension, glomerulonephritis, chronic pyelonephritis (rare).	↓ 50% or more	↑ 16% or more

sorption of water) and an increase in osmolality of at least 15%.

The **sodium chloride-urea-ADH-PAH test (Stamey test)** is based upon the demonstration of abnormal reabsorption of water by the ischemic kidney; it is designed to exaggerate the evidence of this phenomenon. A normal saline infusion containing 8% urea and PAH is given after the placement of 8F plastic catheters in the mid ureters. (Stamey prefers to leave these catheters in place for 12–24 hours. This appears to lessen the incidence of postinstrumental ureteral obstruction.) Three collections of urine from each kidney at 10-minute intervals are analyzed for volume and PAH concentration. The latter is significantly increased by the kidney affected by renovascular disease. (The reader is referred to Stamey's monograph [1963] for a detailed description of the test technic.)

The ischemic kidney is revealed by its diminished urine volume and its increased concentration of PAH as compared to its mate (Table 34–1).

Summary of Plan of Study

If the history and physical examination are compatible with a presumptive diagnosis of renovascular hypertension, further studies are indicated. The following approach seems rational.

(1) Excretory urogram reveals suggestive abnormalities in more than half of patients.

(2) Radioactive renogram is simple and noninvasive though not definitive; it may correlate with other tests.

(3) The saralasin test is an office procedure. A significant drop in blood pressure suggests hyperreninism, though this reaction may also occur in some cases of essential hypertension. If the test is positive, even with determination of equal renal vein renin levels on both sides, or if it is negative but the index of suspicion is high, the next step is—

(4) Peripheral and separate renal vein renin determinations done in conjunction with—

(5) Angiography to find significant renal artery stenosis. The probable response to surgery cannot be estimated from these films alone.

(6) Split renal function studies should be considered if the diagnosis is still doubtful.

In an appendix to Poutasse's report (1980), Kaufman lists the percentages of false-negative responses: 39% with peripheral renin estimations; 27% with divided renal vein renin estimations; 30% with rapid sequence urograms; and 7% with the saralasin test.

Differential Diagnosis

Essential hypertension usually develops between ages 25 and 50 in a person with a family history of hypertension. Intravenous urograms, excretory urograms, and renograms are usually normal. Patients with essential hypertension may have elevated peripheral renin levels and therefore may respond positively to saralasin. Angiography will probably reveal normal renal vasculature.

Coarctation of the aorta is characterized by relatively low blood pressure in the legs, a bruit over the vascular lesion, and evidence of collateral circulation.

Pheochromocytoma may be considered, especially if hypertension occurs in paroxysms associated with sweating and palpitation. The glucagon test is usually positive (see Chapter 21). Urinary vanilmandelic acid or serum or urinary catecholamines are elevated during hypertensive seizures. Excretory urograms may reveal displacement of a kidney by the tumor. Angiography will reveal the tumor. The saralasin test is negative.

Secondary aldosteronism may accompany renovascular hypertension. In both primary and secondary aldosteronism, hypokalemic alkalosis is present; it responds to the administration of spironolactone (Aldactone). Differentiation requires estimation of blood volume, serum sodium, and peripheral venous renin. In primary aldosteronism, blood volume and sodium tend to be elevated, whereas peripheral venous renin is low. In secondary aldosteronism, blood volume and sodium are apt to be low with peripheral renin normal or elevated.

Cushing's disease usually causes hypertension. Physical examination and hormonal assays establish the diagnosis.

The rare renal juxtaglomerular cell tumors elaborate increased amounts of renin (Warshaw & others, 1979). Findings consistent with hyperaldosteronism are present. The saralasin test is usually positive, and the renal vein renin on the tumor side is elevated. Angiography reveals normal renal arteries but may show neovascularity in the tumor.

Treatment

Since some risk is involved in arterial repair, medical antihypertensive treatment should be tried. If hypertension cannot be adequately controlled, however, angioplasty should be done.

A. Percutaneous Transluminal Dilatation of the Stenotic Renal Artery (Transluminal Angioplasty): Renal angiographers have recently developed a technic for dilating the stenotic renal artery with a balloon. Preliminary reports are encouraging (Martin, Diamond, & Casarella, 1980). In most cases, postdilatation angiograms show improved diameter of the renal artery, and renal vein renin levels return to normal. This technic is comparable in effectiveness to surgical angioplasty, which has a mortality rate of 5–6%. In a few cases, restenosis requires a second dilatation (Millan, Mast, & Madias, 1979). Restenosis can also be treated surgically (Katzen & others, 1979). Both fibromuscular and arteriosclerotic lesions have been treated successfully (Kuhlmann & others, 1980). In some cases, the severity and length of stenosis or the tortuosity of the vessel may impede passage of the dilator, and surgery will be required. The efficacy of balloon dilatation is not yet regarded as established.

B. Surgical Renal Artery Reconstruction: Nephrectomy is indicated in hypertension associated with serious unilateral renal lesions. The kidney should be removed only if its function is markedly impaired (eg, due to atrophic pyelonephritis, stenosis of the renal artery with marked atrophy, or advanced hydronephrosis) or in order to save life (eg, in cancer of the kidney). In the high-risk patient with a short life expectancy, nephrectomy should be considered, for it offers much lower mortality and morbidity rates than renal artery reconstruction. Recently, there have been a number of reports of successful revascularization where the renal artery was totally occluded (Scheft & others, 1980; Libertino & others, 1980). If severe perinephritis (Page kidney) is diagnosed, the kidney must be completely removed surgically. Hypertension is usually relieved (Conrad & others, 1976).

Endarterectomy, homograft, sleeve resection of the involved arterial segment, or arterial shunt or graft is indicated in unilateral renal artery stenosis when the involved kidney reveals fairly good function. This is potentially the better kidney, since it has been protected from the adverse effects of hypertension. Postoperatively, a "reversal" of the Howard test occurs; the repaired kidney excretes more PSP, water, and salt than its mate.

Bilateral stenosis of the renal arteries, found in 50% of cases, should be treated in a similar manner, though Gittes & McLaughlin (1974) found that with repair of the most serious lesion only, hypertension was controlled in 85% of cases.

Fibromuscular hyperplasia may involve intrarenal portions of the arteries, so that it may be necessary to remove the kidney and reconstruct it "on the bench." Autotransplantation should then be accomplished (Lawson, 1980).

Reuter & others (1976) recommend embolic occlusion of segmental renal artery stenosis by catheter rather than surgical intervention.

Prognosis

Surgery is indicated if either the intravenous

urogram or the isotope renogram suggests renal ischemia, if the renin level of the renal vein on the suspected side is significantly increased, if the saralasin test is positive, and if the selective angiogram reveals renal artery stenosis. If preliminary screening tests are suggestive and the angiogram reveals renal artery stenosis but renal vein renin measurements on both sides are essentially equal, a positive saralasin test should indicate the need for surgery. If, at operation, there is a pressure gradient of at least 50 mm Hg between the aorta and a point distal to the renal artery lesion, successful arterial repair or nephrectomy will cure renal hypertension in about 40% of cases and lead to significant improvement in another 40%. If angioplasty fails, nephrectomy is usually necessary.

The best results are obtained in patients with fibromuscular hyperplasia (90% improvement). Only 60% of those with atherosclerosis will respond. In unilateral lesions, nephrectomy offers the lowest mortality rate and the best response. Children respond particularly well (Pinkerton, Crouch, & Sharma, 1979; Pechan & others, 1979; Chung & Salvian, 1979).

• • •

References

Baer L & others: Detection of renovascular hypertension with angiotensin II blockade. *Ann Intern Med* 1977;**86**:257.

Biglieri EG: Evaluation of renal vascular hypertension and primary hyperaldosteronism. *Calif Med* (Dec) 1971;**115**:40.

Buda JA & others: Evaluation of surgical response in renovascular hypertension using angiotensin II blockade. *Surgery* 1978;**84**:664.

Chassin MRG, Sullivan JM: Pharmacologic management of renovascular hypertension. *JAMA* 1974;**227**:421.

Chung WB, Salvian AJ: Surgical treatment of renovascular hypertension. *Am J Surg* 1979;**138**:143.

Conrad MR & others: Sonography of the Page kidney. *J Urol* 1976;**116**:293.

Dean RH & others: Bilateral renal artery stenosis and renovascular hypertension. *Surgery* 1977;**81**:53.

Dillon MJ, Shah V, Barratt TM: Renal vein renin measurements in children with hypertension. *Br Med J* 1978;**2**:168.

Erikson U & others: On the use of renal angiography and intravenous urography in the investigation of renovascular hypertension. *Acta Med Scand* 1975;**198**:39.

Freed TA, Tavel FR: Diagnosis and surgical treatment of Page kidney: Selected aspects. *Urology* 1976;**7**:330.

Gillespie L & others: Use of saralasin to detect renovascular hypertension in childhood. *Urology* 1980;**16**:453.

Gittes RF, McLaughlin AP III: Unilateral operation for bilateral renovascular disease. *J Urol* 1974;**111**:292.

Hoard TD, O'Brien DP III: Simple renal cyst and high renin hypertension cured by cyst decompression. *J Urol* 1976;**115**:326.

Johnston JH, Mix LW: The Ask-Upmark kidney: A form of ascending pyelonephritis? *Br J Urol* 1976;**48**:393.

Katzen BT & others: Percutaneous transluminal angioplasty for treatment of renovascular hypertension. *Radiology* 1979;**131**:53.

Kaufman JJ: Renovascular hypertension: The UCLA experience. *J Urol* 1979;**121**:139.

Knochel JP, White MG: The role of aldosterone in renal physiology. *Arch Intern Med* 1973;**131**:876.

Korobkin M, Perloff DL, Palubinskas AJ: Renal arteriography in the evaluation of unexplained hypertension in children and adolescents. *J Pediatr* 1976;**88**:388.

Kuhlmann U & others: Renovascular hypertension: Treatment by percutaneous transluminal dilatation. *Ann Intern Med* 1980;**92**:1.

Lawson RK: Extracorporeal renal surgery. *J Urol* 1980;**123**:301.

Libertino JA & others: Renal artery revascularization: Restoration of renal function. *JAMA* 1980;**244**:1340.

Marks LS, Poutasse EF: Hypertension from renal tuberculosis: Operative cure predicted by renal vein renin. *J Urol* 1973;**109**:149.

Marks LS & others: Detection of renovascular hypertension: Saralasin test versus renin determinations. *J Urol* 1976;**116**:406.

Martin EC, Diamond NG, Casarella WJ: Percutaneous transluminar angioplasty in non-atherosclerotic disease. *Radiology* 1980;**135**:27.

Mena E & others: Neurofibromatosis and renovascular hypertension in children. *Am J Roentgenol* 1973;**118**:39.

Millan VG, Mast WE, Madias NE: Nonsurgical treatment of severe hypertension due to renal-artery intimal fibroplasia by percutaneous transluminal angioplasty. *N Engl J Med* 1979;**300**:1371.

More IAR, Jackson AM, MacSween RNM: Renin-secreting tumor associated with hypertension. *Cancer* 1974;**34**:2093.

Nemoy NJ, Fichman MP, Sellers A: Unilateral ureteral obstruction: A cause of reversible high renin content hypertension. *JAMA* 1973;**225**:512.

Novick AC, Straffon RA, Stewart BH: Surgical management of branch renal artery disease: In situ versus extracorporeal methods of repair. *J Urol* 1980;**123**:311.

Novick AC & others: Surgical treatment of renovascular hypertension in the pediatric patient. *J Urol* 1978;**119**:794.

Pak K, Kawamura J, Yoshida O: Hypertension with elevated renal vein renin secondary to unilateral hydronephrosis. *Urology* 1980;**16**:499.

Paster SB, Adams DF, Abrams HL: Errors in renal vein renin collections. *Am J Roentgenol* 1974;**122**:804.

Peart WS: Renin-angiotensin system. *N Engl J Med* 1975;**292**:302.

Pechan BW & others: Endarterectomy and patchgraft angioplasty in treatment of atherosclerotic renovascular hypertension. *Urology* 1979;**14**:487.

Pfau A, Rosenmann E: Unilateral chronic pyelonephritis and hypertension: Coincidental or causal relationship? *Am J Med* 1978;**65**:499.

Pinkerton JA, Crough TT, Sharma JN: Surgical treatment of renovascular hypertension. *Am J Surg* 1979;**138**:759.

Poutasse EF & others: Malignant hypertension in children

secondary to chronic pyelonephritis: Laboratory and radiologic indications for partial or total nephrectomy. *J Urol* 1978;**119**:264.

Poutasse EF & others: Saralasin test as a diagnostic and prognostic aid in renovascular hypertensive patients subjected to renal operation. *J Urol* 1980;**123**:306.

Rose HJ, Pruitt AW: Hypertension, hyperreninemia and a solitary renal cyst in an adolescent. *Am J Med* 1976;**71**:579.

Rushton AR: The genetics of fibromuscular dysplasia. *Arch Intern Med* 1980;**140**:233.

Savage JM & others: Renin and blood-pressure in children with renal scarring and vesicoureteric reflux. *Lancet* 1978;**2**:441.

Scheft P & others: Renal revascularization in patients with total occlusion of the renal artery. *J Urol* 1980;**124**:184.

Schiff M Jr, McGuire EJ, Baskin AM: Hypertension and unilateral hydronephrosis. *Urology* 1975;**5**:178.

Shapiro AP & others: Hypertension in radiation nephritis. *Arch Intern Med* 1977;**137**:848.

Silver D, Clements JB: Renovascular hypertension from renal artery compression by congenital bands. *Ann Surg* 1976;**183**:161.

Stamey TA: *Renovascular Hypertension.* Williams & Wilkins, 1963.

Stamey TA: Unilateral renal disease causing hypertension. *JAMA* 1976;**235**:2340.

Stanley JC, Fry WJ: Surgical treatment of renovascular hypertension. *Arch Surg* 1977;**112**:1291.

Stanley P & others: Renovascular hypertension in children and adolescents. *Radiology* 1978;**129**:123.

Stecker JF Jr, Read BP, Poutasse EF: Pediatric hypertension as a delayed sequela of reflux-induced chronic pyelonephritis. *J Urol* 1977;**118**:644.

Sufrin G: The Page kidney: A correctable form of arterial hypertension. *J Urol* 1975;**113**:450.

Vaughan ED Jr: Laboratory tests in the evaluation of renal hypertension. *Urol Clin North Am* 1979;**6**:485.

Vaughan TJ & others: Renal artery aneurysms and hypertension. *Radiology* 1971;**99**:287.

Warshaw BL & others: Hypertension secondary to a renin-producing juxtaglomerular cell tumor. *J Pediatr* 1979;**94**:247.

Urologic Aspects of Andrology | 35

Donald R. Smith, MD

INFERTILITY

A couple can be judged infertile if conception does not occur after 12 months of adequate cohabitation. About 10% of marriages are barren; spermatogenic deficiencies in the male are responsible in at least 30% of these.

From the clinical standpoint, male fertility is judged through study of the sperms, including number, the percentage of motile sperms, and their viability and morphology. If sperms are absent from the ejaculate, testicular biopsy is indicated to differentiate between intrinsic deficiency of the germ cells (common) and obstruction of the conduction system (rare).

Pathogenesis

The common causes of male infertility are as follows:

A. Deficiencies in Maturation of Germ Cells: At least 85% of infertile men have intrinsic spermatogenic defects. The germ cells of the seminiferous tubules may be congenitally imperfect (aplastic), or incomplete maturation (spermatogenic arrest) may be observed secondary to hypogonadism or hypopituitarism.

Orchitis due to mumps or trauma and exposure to x-ray radiation frequently exert a deleterious effect upon spermatogenesis. In the cryptorchid testis, the temperature of the body causes injury to the germ cells.

B. Obstruction of the Conduction System: Bilateral epididymitis may cause occlusion of the ducts. Absence of connection between the vas deferens and the epididymis may be congenital or acquired (eg, vasoligation) (Rubin, 1975).

C. Hyperadrenalism: Hyperadrenalism causes an increase in volume of the ejaculate, diminished sperm count and motility, and an increased percentage of abnormal forms, with evidence of desquamation. Plasma testosterone is elevated. A similar picture is seen in association with varicocele.

D. Hypopituitarism: Hypopituitarism leads to lack of normal maturation of spermatogenic cells (germinal aplasia). Urine levels of FSH are low.

E. Hypogonadism: In testicular failure (eg, Klinefelter's syndrome), degeneration of the seminiferous tubules is seen. Urinary FSH is elevated. Serum testosterone or urinary 17-ketosteroid values are normal or only slightly subnormal, since Leydig cells are numerous.

F. Sperm Antibodies: It would appear that 3 immune mechanisms are involved in some cases of infertility: (1) autoimmunization in men, (2) circulatory antibodies against sperms in women, and (3) tissue antibodies against semen in women.

In men, autoimmune antibodies cause sperm agglutination and may immobilize sperms. In women, penetrating sperms may be immobilized; the cervical mucus may become impenetrable. In the investigation of infertile couples, about 7% of men and 13% of women will show antisperm antibodies (Haas, Cines, & Schreiber, 1980). Wall & others (1975) performed immunologic studies in infertile men. They found testicular germinal cell antibodies in 14%, sperm antibodies in 21%, and positive macrophage inhibitory factor tests in 33%. These factors were positive in only 5% of the controls.

G. Tight Clothing: The use of shorts or supporters that hold the testes close to the body leads to increase in testicular temperature deleterious to spermatogenesis.

H. Varicocele: The presence of varicocele causes (1) an increase in the percentage of immature forms, (2) a decrease in sperm count, and (3) a decrease in the percentage of motile sperms (seminal stress pattern). The cause is not known. It has been shown that it is not due to increased scrotal heat from the pooled blood. It has been postulated that adrenal corticosteroids might move in a retrograde manner down the spermatic vein to the testes. This theory has little support. Caldamone, Al-Juburi, & Cockett (1980) studied varicoceles in dogs and found that blood from the varicocele had increased levels of serotonin. Some men with varicocele also have increased serotonin. The authors postulate that serotonin may inhibit spermatogenesis and androgen synthesis.

I. Males of Mothers Exposed to Diethylstilbestrol: Bibbo & others (1977) studied the spermatology of 163 such men. Volumes were less than 1.5 mL and sperm counts were half of normal but still in the fertile range. Poor quality semen was found in 28%.

J. Dysplastic Testes: On exploration and biopsy of the testes of men with azoospermia, Lingårdh & others (1975) found a few examples of dysplasia.

K. Cryptorchidism: Lipshultz (1976) observed that the cryptorchid testis, treated or not, is subfertile. Such a testis is always smaller than normal; FSH is often elevated.

L. Habitual Abortion: Byrd, Askew, & McDonough (1977) studied the cytogenic characteristics of 55 couples with recurrent fetal wastage. About 6% were found to have a balanced chromosomal translocation. Though this was more often found in women, they recommended karyotype studies for these couples. Joël (1966) observed that highly abnormal semen is associated with 6% of habitual abortions.

Testicular Histology & Pathology

(Amelar & Dubin, 1975; Wong & others, 1978.)

A. Normal Development: Up to the age of 4 or 5 years, the testes are in a relatively quiescent state. The spermatogenic tubules are small. Adjacent to the basement membrane, a number of ovoid or round cells are seen. Few spermatogonia are present. The interstitial tissue contains a few clumps of Leydig cells.

Between ages 5 and 10 years, the germinal tubules become more tortuous and their lumens increase in diameter. More spermatogonia are present. The interstitial tissues show a decrease in the number of fibroblasts.

At puberty, probably stimulated by increasing amounts of pituitary gonadotropins (FSH, LH), active spermatogenesis begins and mature spermatozoa make their appearance. Hyperplasia of the interstitial (Leydig) cells develops (Fig 1–7).

B. Abnormal Development: The pathologic changes found in the infertile testis have been carefully studied by gonadal biopsy. Many degrees of damage may be noted.

1. Germinal aplasia–The seminiferous tubules show a complete or almost complete lack of germ cells. Normal numbers of Sertoli cells are present, however. The cause of this change may be either congenital or secondary to lack of follicle-stimulating hormone (FSH) from the pituitary gland. If pituitary function is normal, increased amounts of FSH may be found in the urine (Klinefelter's syndrome).

2. Spermatogenic arrest–The tubule and its cells are normal in appearance, but maturation fails to reach the adult stage.

3. Peritubular fibrosis–Normally, the basement membrane of the tubule is quite thin. For some unknown reason, progressive peritubular fibrosis may occur. In all probability, this impairs

cellular nutrition, and the sperm cells gradually disappear. At this stage, FSH excretion in the urine is increased.

4. Incomplete spermatogenesis–Some tubules may be quite normal, whereas others show lack of complete maturation. Both mature and immature sperms may be found in the tubular lumens. Men suffering from this defect have lowered sperm counts and an increase in the number of abnormal forms.

C. Spermatology: Clinically, there are 3 important criteria for normal semen (Sobrero & Rehan, 1975; MacLeod & Wang, 1979).

1. Number–Most authorities state that "normal" semen contains at least 40 million sperms per milliliter in 2 mL of fluid. One researcher has found that 25% of fertile men have counts below 50 million/mL. He considers that true oligospermia consists of less than 20 million/mL, but he observes that, with excellent motility, conception may occur when the sperm count is as low as 10 million/mL.

2. Percentage of motile sperms and degree of motility–In most fertile men, at least 60% of the sperms are actively motile when the specimen is fresh. The fewer the motile forms, the greater the impairment of fertility. The degree of motility is also quite significant. The more sluggish the sperms, the greater the degree of infertility.

Generally speaking, the greater the percentage of motile forms, the more vigorous their motility.

3. Morphology–A differential count of normal and abnormal sperms yields considerable information. At least 60–70% of the sperms in most fertile men are normal (Fig 35–1).

Clinical Findings

A. History: The chief complaint of the patient is the inability to cause conception. Other information of importance includes childhood and adult illnesses (eg, mumps orchitis, cryptorchidism, tuberculosis); operations, especially those that might cause injury to the testes or their ducts (eg, repair of inguinal hernia, orchiopexy); trauma to the external genitalia; genital infections, particularly epididymitis; pregnancy in present or previous partner; frequency of intercourse; and exposure to toxins (eg, x-rays).

Evidence of retrograde ejaculation or lack of emission should be sought. This is common in diabetics, those undergoing repair of aortic aneurysms or radical retroperitoneal lymph node dissection (eg, testis tumor), and following any type of prostatectomy.

Certain drugs have a deleterious effect upon spermatogenesis. These include antitumor chemotherapeutic agents and nitrofurantoin. Vaginal lubricants are often spermatocidal.

The patient should be questioned about the use of shorts that support the scrotum, thus increasing testicular temperature.

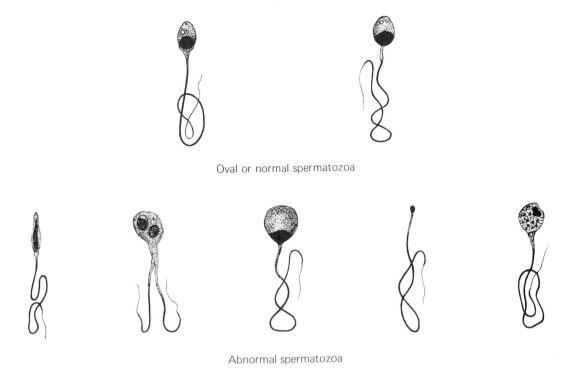

Oval or normal spermatozoa

Abnormal spermatozoa

Figure 35–1. Normal and abnormal spermatozoa. (Redrawn and reproduced, with permission, from Hotchkiss: *Fertility in Men.* Lippincott, 1944.)

B. Signs: A complete physical examination should never be neglected. Evidence of endocrinologic abnormality should be sought, including weight, height, body build, amount and distribution of hair, and gynecomastia. The degree of development of the penis should be noted and the scrotal contents carefully examined. (The testes of infertile men are usually normal in size and consistency.) Unilateral or bilateral changes may be noted. The small, flabby testes or the hard, pea-sized testes of Klinefelter's syndrome are usually azoospermic. Other testicular abnormalities may include cryptorchidism and thickening of the epididymides (old epididymitis). The vas deferens should be carefully felt, for it may be absent or may fail to join the epididymis. Varicocele should be sought, since this lesion offers the best hope for successful treatment.

Rectal examination should include prostatic massage, although the significance of prostatitis in infertility is not clear. Fjällbrant (1970) believes that there is an increased incidence of sperm antibodies in some men who harbor this infection.

C. Laboratory Findings: Proteinuria or pyuria may be clues to chronic renal disease, which may depress spermatogenesis. Tests for nitrogen retention should be ordered.

1. Examination of the semen–This is the most important step in the investigation of suspected infertility.

a. Method of collection–The ejaculate should be obtained after at least 4 days of abstinence from

intercourse. It is best produced by masturbation in the physician's office. This ensures that the entire specimen is collected in a clean, dry glass. Condoms must not be used, for the sperms are quickly killed on contact with them. The specimen must be examined within 2 hours of its collection. Normally, the semen is quite gelatinous and ropy. Within a few minutes, at room temperature, the fluid becomes thin and homogeneous. Failure to liquefy is abnormal.

b. Sperm count–The technic is simple, requiring only a Neubauer blood cell counting chamber and a white cell pipette. Semen is drawn up to the 0.5 mark, and the rest of the chamber is filled with a saturated solution of sodium bicarbonate containing 1% phenol, which immobilizes the sperms. This mixture is then flooded over the counting chamber and covered with a coverslip. The number of sperms in the 5 blocks (80 small squares) is determined. To this number are added 6 zeros. This equals the number of sperms per milliliter.

Most fertile men have at least 40 million sperms per milliliter. The absence of sperms means a severe defect of the seminiferous tubules or obstruction of the conducting system. The finding of a few dead sperms rules out obstruction.

Oligospermia is almost always due to disease of the germ cells. The lower the count, the poorer the prognosis.

c. Percentage of motile sperms and degree of motility–Semen is placed on a slide and covered with a coverslip sealed with petroleum jelly. An estimate should be made of the percentage of motile forms, the degree of motility, and the duration of life of the sperms. The average normal is 65%.

d. Morphology–(Fig 35–1.) Morphology may be judged by counting the normal and abnormal forms in a smear stained as follows:

(1) Dry a thin smear of semen in air.
(2) Flood with 10% formalin for 1 minute.
(3) Wash.
(4) Stain with Meyer's hematoxylin for 1½ minutes.
(5) Wash in lukewarm water.

Normal forms are found in 75%.

2. Testicular biopsy–Biopsy is usually indicated only if azoospermia is present. Perhaps 40% of men showing defects on sperm examination will have serious irreversible lesions of the seminiferous tubules. Study of the seminiferous tubules will permit differentiation between severe intrinsic gonadal disease and blockage of the conducting system. In the latter case, spermatogenesis is normal. There is, however, evidence that sperm counts are apt to be temporarily depressed after biopsy.

3. Buccal smear–A buccal smear should undergo nuclear chromatin analysis. If chromatin sex is positive (female), the diagnosis of Klinefelter's syndrome should be entertained. These patients are irreversibly sterile.

4. FSH test–Pituitary gonadotropins (FSH) in the urine should be measured. An increase means primary gonadal deficiency, though this may be noted in men with unilateral cryptorchidism, treated or not; if FSH is decreased, hypopituitarism is present.

5. Other tests–Estimation of plasma testosterone levels should be obtained. If this cannot be done, urinary 17-ketosteroids should be measured. These levels are depressed in chronic heavy marihuana users (Kolodny & others, 1974). They are elevated with hyperadrenocorticism. Segal & others (1979) found hyperprolactinemia in 4% of infertile men who also had hypogonadism, impotence, and galactorrhea. This condition can be caused by pituitary adenoma, hypothalamic dysfunction, or drug use, or it may be idiopathic. The spermogram shows low volume, normal or low count, and normal or diminished motility.

D. X-Ray Findings: If blockage of the vasa is suspected, vasoseminal vesiculography may be indicated (Hébert, Bouchard, & Charron, 1971). A No. 23 needle pointing to the epididymis is introduced into the lumen of the vas. Two or 3 mL of radiopaque fluid are injected and films exposed. The needle is then pointed toward the prostate and the procedure is repeated.

E. Immunologic Survey: If both the man and the woman are found to have normal fertility or if the man's sperms show agglutination or are immobile, both should be tested for the presence of sperm antibodies.

Treatment

The results of treatment of infertility in the male are unsatisfactory except when a varicocele is found. Morphologic changes in the various components of the seminiferous tubules are largely irreversible.

A. Abnormalities Based on Spermatology:

1. Idiopathic oligospermia–

a. Cortisone acetate–Stewart & Montie (1973) prescribed 2.5 mg of this drug 4 times daily.

b. Clomiphene citrate–Jones & others (1980) and Paulson (1979) report good results with this drug. They both recommend 2.5 mg/d. Jones suggests 3 weeks of treatment followed by 1 week with no drug; Paulson prefers 25 days with treatment and 5 days without. The regimen should be continued for 6–12 months. The number of sperms increased in most patients and pregnancy was produced by 40%. However, Charny (1979) did not see much improvement with clomiphene.

c. Arginine–Schachter, Goldman, & Zuckerman (1973) found that 1 g of arginine per day improved sperm count and motility in 65% of their patients, but Pryor & others (1978) recognized no improvement in their 64 patients. No pregnancies ensued.

d. Mesterolone–Schellin & Beek (1972) and Hendry & others (1973) recommend this hormone, 75–100 mg/d for 1 year. They noted improvement in semen quality in more than 50% of their patients.

2. Asthenospermia (low motility)–Stewart & Montie (1973) observed a good response to hCG, 10,000 units given intramuscularly twice a week for 3 months. Chehval & Meehan (1979) treated 64 men with 50,000 units of hCG in 10 divided doses. Improvement was noted in 69% and pregnancy ensued with 36%.

3. Low volume of ejaculate (less than 1 mL)–Amelar & Dubin (1973) have observed improvement after administering hCG, 2000–4000 units intramuscularly twice a week for 8 weeks. They suggest coitus interruptus in those with normal spermatology but with abnormally high volumes. The first portion of such ejaculate contains an increased concentration of sperms (Eliasson & Lindholmer, 1972).

B. Abnormal Endocrinologic Tests:

1. If the plasma testosterone or urinary 17-ketosteroid levels are low, androgen therapy should be prescribed (Hendry & others, 1973). If the androgen levels are increased (hyperadrenalism), corticosteroid should be given to suppress adrenal activity.

2. If urinary FSH is low (hypopituitarism), give hCG, 2000–4000 units intramuscularly twice a week (Amelar & Dubin, 1973). An increased level of FSH reflects severe seminiferous tubular defects.

If hyperprolactinemia is present, the primary cause should be treated. Segal & others (1979) found that bromocriptine corrected the semen abnormality in all of their 7 patients.

C. Retrograde Ejaculation or Lack of Emission: Immediately after ejaculation, the urine should be examined for the presence of sperms. Such urine should be centrifuged and the sperms instilled into the cervix. Abrahams & others (1975) were able to correct this defect, which had been caused by a YV-plasty of the bladder neck. They reversed the operation, thus tightening the neck. If the urine contains no sperms and an operation has been performed that might have damaged the thoracolumbar sympathetic nerves, prescribe ephedrine, 50–75 mg, one-half hour before coitus. This may cause ejaculation, and the ejaculate may contain sperms. Stockamp, Schreiter, & Altwein (1974) noted some effect following the administration of 60 mg of phenylephrine intravenously. Cunningham (1978) found oronade to be superior to ephedrine in correcting this problem.

D. General Measures: Sexual technic should be discussed. The couple should be apprised of the "fertile" period in the menstrual cycle. Intercourse should be avoided for 3 or 4 days before this time in order that the man can then deliver the best quantity and quality of semen. This is particularly important if the sperm count is deficient. Psychic factors should be sought.

If nonliquefaction of the semen is observed, Wilson & Bunge (1975) recommend that the woman insert a cocoa butter suppository containing 5 mg of alpha amylase powder into the vagina immediately after intercourse performed during the time of ovulation. They observed the phenomenon of nonliquefaction in 12% of infertile couples. Dougherty, Cockett, & Urry (1978) have confirmed the efficacy of this treatment.

The general health of the patient should be improved by regulating his diet and eradicating infections, particularly of the prostate gland. A reducing diet should be utilized if the man is overweight. Alcoholic excesses should be curbed.

Vitamin B complex should be prescribed to ensure the normal inactivation of estrogens by the liver.

If the man wears a supporter or shorts that hold the scrotal contents close to the body, he should be instructed not to do so.

If treatment fails to improve the number, form, and motility of the sperms, and if conception does not occur, a cap containing the inadequate semen can be placed over the cervix. This may improve the chances for conception (Ulstein, 1973).

White & Glass (1976) recommend cervical instillation of the semen, if it is fairly normal, in instances where the cervical mucus is too thick for penetration or when the sperms become immobilized in the vagina.

It has been recommended that large doses of testosterone (50 mg intramuscularly 3 times a week) should be administered to men whose sperms are markedly inadequate in quality and quantity (Lamensdorf, Compere, & Begley, 1975). This should be continued until complete azoospermia is observed. This may take as long as 4–5 months. After cessation of treatment, a "rebound" phenomenon may occur and the semen may show improvement over its pretreatment level in 30% of patients. Five percent may be made worse, however.

If the temperature of the testis is increased for a few months by hot soaks or by an insulated athletic supporter, the sperm count is significantly decreased. Cessation of this treatment may result in a rebound of spermatogenic activity and a consequent increase in the sperm count that may culminate in pregnancy.

E. Surgical Measures: The surgical procedures available for the correction of specific abnormalities are as follows:

1. Vasovasostomy–Silber, Galle, & Friend (1977); Belker (1980); and Willscher & Novicki (1980), using microsurgical technics, obtained 90% satisfactory results as measured by spermatology. They observed a pregnancy rate of 50%. Though a few patients may develop sperm antibodies after this procedure, all tests are negative within 3 months (Bullock, Gilmore, & Wilson, 1977).

2. Epididymovasostomy–If azoospermia is present but the testicular biopsy shows normal spermatogenesis and there is evidence of epididymal occlusion, epididymovasostomy should be considered. It may make conception possible in 10–20% of otherwise sterile matings (Silber, 1978).

3. Treatment of varicocele–Ligation of the spermatic vein at the internal inguinal ring as a cure for varicocele improves motility, quality, and numbers of sperms. Pregnancy results in 40–50% of couples (Lome & Ross, 1977; Dubin & Amelar, 1975; Greenberg, Lipshultz, & Wein, 1978).

4. Orchiopexy–Orchiopexy for undescended testes is of no value in the treatment of infertility after puberty.

F. Miscellaneous Factors in Therapy:

1. Noxious drugs should be stopped unless they appear to be lifesaving (Stewart [1973], Timmermans [1974]).

2. Friberg & Gnarpe (1973) examined 54 infertile couples where the women harbored *Ureaplasma urealyticum* (T-mycoplasmas). They prescribed doxycycline, 100 mg/d from days 7 to 16 following the beginning of the last menstrual cycle, for 3 months. If the organism was still present, the dose of doxycycline was increased to 200 mg/d for 10 days. The partner was also treated for 10 days, and *U urealyticum* was abolished in all. Pregnancy then occurred in 25%. De Louvois & others (1974) and Matthews & others (1975) were, however, unable to corroborate these claims.

3. Schoenfeld, Amelar, & Dubin (1975) observed that the addition of caffeine to the ejaculate led to improved motility. Instillation of this fluid into the vagina or into the uterus might prove helpful when the major problem is impaired motility.

A. Incisions

B. Sheath of right vas opened

C. Right vas cut

D. Fulguration

E. Mucosa of lumen destroyed

F. Sheath closed over proximal vas

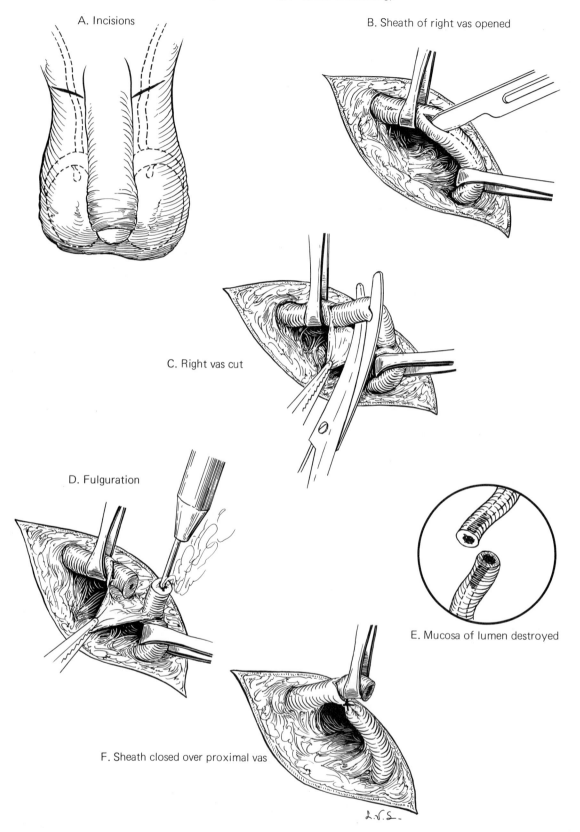

Figure 35–2. Steps in vasectomy. (Modified from a drawing by S Taft. Reproduced, with permission, from Schmidt S: Vasectomy should not fail. *Contemp Surg* [May] 1974;**4**:13.)

4. If the woman is found to have sperm antibodies, her partner should use a condom for 1 year. This allows subsidence of the antibody titer. Ansbacher, Keung-Yeung, & Behrman (1973) found that pregnancy then occurred in 50% of cases. If the man has antisperm antibodies, he should receive methylprednisolone, 32 mg orally 3 times a day for 10 days beginning on day 21 of the menstrual cycle, followed by gradually decreased doses for the next 3 days (Haas, Cines, & Schreiber, 1980). Shulman, Harlin, & Davis (1978) prefer 96 mg/d for 1 week.

Prognosis

The poorer the quality of the semen, the poorer the outlook for success in treatment. When the count is under 1 million/mL, there is little room for optimism. Azoospermia, unless caused by obstruction of the tubules of the epididymis, cannot be treated successfully.

VASECTOMY

During the past few years, there has been a striking increase in the utilization of vasectomy to prevent conception. Many women have had adverse reactions to the "pill"; others have suffered complications from the intrauterine device. Men are beginning to accept the fact that they must share the responsibility for population control. The usual indication for the operation, therefore, is the desire to be made sterile. The medical indications are (1) routine vasectomy performed at the time of prostatectomy to prevent postoperative epididymitis, and (2) prevention of recurrent epididymitis.

Some men have deep-seated resistance to undergoing vasectomy. They may feel that the operation will cause them to become impotent out of some primitive feeling that if a man cannot cause conception he is not really a man. Thorough discussion of these matters before the operation is essential, for if a man expects to become impotent he will become so (Cass, 1979; Brown & Magarick, 1979).

Preoperative Discussion With the Patient

The man must realize that 2 types of cells are harbored in the testes: seminiferous tubules and Leydig cells. Interrupting the vas stops sperm migration to the urethra. The Leydig cells are unaffected, for their androgens are picked up by blood vessels that continue to nourish them. Thus, androgen levels remain normal and the cells viable. Many men find intercourse even more satisfactory than before because the fear of conception has been removed (Nash & Rich, 1972).

The man must be told that he will suffer some discomfort during the operation from instillation of the local anesthetic. Minor discomfort for a few days postoperatively can be controlled with simple analgesics. Occasionally, an incision may open prematurely and drain for a few days. The patient must be warned that a small amount of bleeding may occur on the day of surgery. Some ecchymosis of the scrotal skin is to be expected. Significant bleeding (hematoscrotum) is rare but may require immediate operation.

The patient must realize that viable sperms are still harbored in the ampulla of the vas and that he cannot have intercourse for a time without continuing contraceptive practices. The ejaculate must be examined and shown to be free of sperms before the doctor can verify that the patient is infertile. This takes at least 12 ejaculations and often more (Marshall & Lyon, 1972).

In the discussion of vas repair it should be made clear that, although anatomically a high success rate can be expected, the formation of sperm antibodies as a complication of vasoligation has been reported. Should they persist, even with successful reanastomosis, pregnancy might not occur. Recently, however, it has been found that this rise in titer is transient and is gone within 3 months (Bullock, Gilmore, & Wilson, 1977; Jenkins & others, 1979).

Should the patient feel that he might desire a child later and if vasovasostomy is unacceptable, he may wish to deposit his semen in a frozen semen bank. There is a gradual loss of motility—approaching 50%—during the first 36 months; little change occurs thereafter (Smith & Steinberger, 1973). Friberg & Gemzell (1973) report 26 pregnancies out of 187 specimens after storing. Witherington, Black, & Karow (1977) state that high-quality sperms are preserved, whereas the less adequate sperms die. This leads to improvement in the semen. Amelar & Dubin (1979) found the quality of frozen semen poor after 3 years.

Technic of Vasectomy (Schmidt, 1974)
(Fig 35–2)

The spermatic cord is isolated so that the skin over it is taut. The vas is manipulated so it is just under the skin, which is infiltrated with a local anesthetic. The needle is then advanced to infiltrate the perivasal tissues.

A 10-mm transverse incision should be made over the vas (Fig 35–2A). The tissues around the vas are separated and the vas is grasped with 2 Allis clamps (Fig 35–2B). The fascia covering the vas should be incised for a distance of 15 mm and the vas freed from it. The vas can then be divided (Fig 35–2C). Though occlusion by ligature is commonly practiced, there is a risk that the tissue distal to the tie may slough, allowing recanalization. Schmidt experienced no failures if he merely inserted the needle electrode of the electrosurgical machine into the lumen of each vasal end and delivered a mild coagulation current as he withdrew the electrode to destroy the mucous membrane (Fig 35–2D). It had been recommended that sterile water be instilled into the proximal ends of the vasa at the time of vasoligation in order to decrease the time ordinarily needed for complete absence of sperms in the ejaculate. Berthelson (1976) found this to be of no value. Albert, Mininberg, & Davis (1975) were able to cause immediate sterility by injecting either 3 mL of nitrofurantoin sodium (20 mg/mL) or nitrofurazone (1 mg/mL) into the vasa. Urquhart-Hay (1975) had similar success using 2.5 mL of a 1:1000 solution of euflavine. Mumford and Davis (1979) found no chemical irrigant that was immediately 100% successful.

The proximal end of the vas is placed back in its fascial sheath, which is closed with plain catgut (Fig 35–2E). This burial technic further prevents recanalization. After hemostasis is achieved, the skin is closed with chromic catgut.

Hormonal Changes Following Vasectomy

Whitby, Gordon, & Blair (1979), Skegg & others (1976), and Rosenberg & others (1974) have found that the levels of serum testosterone and urinary FSH and LH were unchanged following the operation.

Complications of Vasectomy & Their Treatment

Sperm granuloma, due to extravasation of sperms, presents as a mass felt in the region of the vasectomy. The patient may complain of local pain, and the mass is found to be tender. At times, such a lesion is asymptomatic. The incidence has been estimated at 5–18% (Kwart & Coffey, 1973), most cases occurring when ligation of the vasa has been done. Electrocoagulation markedly reduces the incidence of this complication. Excision may be necessary to produce comfort.

Sperm granuloma may develop in the epididymis from rupture of the tubules due to high pressure distal to the vasectomy site. This will cause occlusion of the epididymal ducts, making later successful vasovasostomy impossible.

Congestive epididymitis is occasionally seen. The patient complains of testicular discomfort, and the organ is found to be enlarged and tender. It usually subsides with time.

Recanalization has an incidence of about 0.6% (Klapproth & Young, 1973). This can be reduced by using the surgical technic described above. Rarely, failure may be attributed to a mistake in properly identifying the vas (Leader & others, 1974); reoperation is indicated.

The development of both immobilizing and agglutinating sperm antibodies may occur as a result of extravasation of sperms, but their persistence seems short-lived.

Profuse bleeding into the scrotum is rare. Because of the distensibility of the scrotal wall, it has no hemostatic effect. Drainage is at times necessary.

Though the wound may open prematurely and drain for a few days, frank infection is rare. It may necessitate surgical drainage.

Prognosis

If the patient is well prepared psychologically by the physician and if the operation is properly performed, the success rate should approach 100%. Zufall (1980) found that over a period of 10 years, 200 vasectomy patients had no negative effects or sexual problems.

Bremner & deKretser (1976) have discussed possible medical means of causing sterility in men, including both hypothalamic-pituitary and direct testicular suppression, inhibition of epididymal function, and immunologic technics. Brueschke & others (1975) have developed various types of occlusive devices for the vas deferens, but, following their removal, stenosis of the duct developed.

SEXUAL DYSFUNCTION
Ira D. Sharlip, MD, FACS

Knowledge of male reproductive physiology and pathology is expanding rapidly. Changes in social attitudes have encouraged this trend. Sexuality is now more widely accepted as an important and integral part of overall physical and emotional well-being. More accurate diagnosis and effective therapy are now available for organic male sexual dysfunction because of (1) identification of vasculogenic impotence due to arteriosclerosis of the internal pudendal and penile arteries; (2) the discovery, by new diagnostic technics, that the incidence of organic impotence is much higher than was previously suspected; and (3) the development of highly effective surgical treatment for impotence.

Anatomy & Physiology of the Normal Male Sexual Response

There are 4 parts to the male sexual response: erection, emission, ejaculation, and orgasm. Each part has a separate neurologic mechanism. It is possible—and common—to find impairment of any one or combination of the 4 while the others remain intact.

A. Erection: The ability to have an erection depends on intact neural and vascular function in the presence of an adequate hormonal and psychologic milieu. Erection is predominantly a parasympathetic function, although increasing histochemical and neuropharmacologic evidence shows a sympathetic role as well. Blood flow and pressure are increased within the corpora cavernosa during erection. The mechanism of the increase in vascularity is currently a matter of controversy. A series of coussinets or polsters in the penile arteries and veins may act to shunt blood toward or away from the cavernous tissue, altering the state of penile tumescence. Recently, however, it has been suggested that the penile polsters are degenerative structures that have no function in the mechanism of erection. Erection and detumescence may be due to the alternating contraction of smooth muscle and endothelium. The role of the venous system in erection is also unclear. Recent studies indicate that outflow regulation probably does play an important role in the mechanism of erection. The mechanism of detumescence has not yet been clarified; current theories include the simple termination of parasympathetic stimulation, increase in sympathetic tone causing inflow vasoconstriction, or an active mechanism involving the pudendal nerves.

With erotic stimuli, psychogenic erections occur via cerebral stimulation of sympathetic centers at T12–L2 and parasympathetic centers at S2–4. When the lower center is inactivated by spinal cord injury or disease, psychogenic erections continue to occur through the alternate sympathetic pathway that communicates from the thoracolumbar cord to the penis via the superior and inferior hypogastric plexuses. Conversely, elimination of the sympathetic pathway—eg, by surgical sympathectomy—usually does not cause impotence as long as the parasympathetic pathway is intact. Reflex erections occurring through the local reflex arc at S2–4 may also be activated by tactile stimuli of the genitalia. This explains how approximately 95% of patients with upper spinal cord injuries continue to have reflex erections (Comarr, 1971).

B. Emission: Emission is a manifestation of sympathetic activity. Usually, following initiation of erection, sensory nerve impulses from the glans penis reach the sacral cord and ascend to the sympathetic nuclei at T12–L2. Sympathetic discharge causes secretions from the prostate, seminal vesicles, vas deferens, and cauda epididymis to enter the prostatic urethra.

C. Ejaculation: Ejaculation occurs by somatic nervous system stimulation of the pudendal nerves. Distention of the prostatic urethra by emission stimulates a reflex via S2–4, resulting in efferent activity of the pudendal nerve. Spasmodic contractions of the urogenital diaphragm and the bulbocavernosus and ischiocavernosus muscles occur, forcing jets of semen down the urethra.

D. Orgasm: Orgasm is a psychic integration of these various events. It is a unique, intense, and exquisite sensation, usually associated with ejaculation. However, in certain pathologic states, orgasm may occur in the absence of erection, emission, or ejaculation.

Causes of Sexual Dysfunction

The causes of sexual dysfunction can be grouped into several broad categories.

A. Psychogenic Causes: In the early 1950s, 90% of cases of impotence were thought to be psychogenic. That figure had no valid statistical basis but nonetheless has been carried forward in the medical literature to the present time. Recent advances in diagnostic technics have identified or-ganic disease, especially of vasculogenic origin, in many patients formerly thought to have psychogenic or idiopathic impotence.

A new approach to psychotherapy for sexual dysfunction was developed in the 1960s (Masters & Johnson, 1976), using technics of behavioral modification in a 2-week course of treatment. This therapy produced up to 80% improvement for some problems, although other therapists have not been able to reproduce this success rate.

Certain symptoms are pathognomonic of psychogenic sexual dysfunction. These include normal and sustained erection in foreplay lost at the moment of intromission; normal erection with some sexual partners but failure with others; normal erection with masturbation but failure with partners; sudden onset of total impotence in a man under 40; and alternating periods of normal function and total impotence. Organic disease, especially vasculogenic disorders, may be present even though morning, nocturnal, or partial erections occur, since vasculogenic, pharmacologic, diabetic, endocrine, and neurogenic impotence often have waxing and waning periods of erectile function.

B. Vasculogenic Causes:

1. Arteriogenic disease–Studies identifying the existence of arteriosclerotic disease of the penile arterial tree and theories about its relationship to impotence were presented starting in 1973. This clinical entity may account for many of the cases of impotence that failed to respond to psychotherapy or were of unknown cause. Arteriosclerotic lesions identified include intimal proliferation, medial fibrosis, calcification, and narrowing of the lumen, leading to thrombotic obliteration of these vessels. These changes are related to both aging and diabetes.

New diagnostic technics such as penile sphygmomanometry, analysis of the penile arterial pulse waves, penile plethysmography, and penile arteriograms indicate that small arterial occlusive disease in the internal pudendal and penile arteries is a common cause of impotence, although accurate statistics are not yet available.

Arterial insufficiency of the penis may occur in one or more areas. Aortoiliac occlusive disease was the first identified (LeRiche, 1923). The incidence of impotence associated with atheromatous aortoiliac disease and other forms of atheromatous peripheral vascular disease is 50–70%. Obstruction may also occur at the hypogastric artery, internal pudendal artery, and dorsal or central penile arteries. Data in the literature and the opinions of andrologic surgeons in Western countries, where there is a high incidence of all forms of arteriosclerotic disease, indicate that stenosis of the pudendal and penile arteries may be the most common cause of penile vascular insufficiency.

2. Venogenic abnormalities–Ebbehoj & Wagner (1979) have shown that both primary and secondary impotence may be caused by excessive venous drainage of the corpus cavernosum. Fistulas between the corpus cavernosum and glans penis and, in one case, a venous malformation of the tunica albuginea were surgically closed, resulting in complete and normal erections.

3. Arteriovenous fistula–Zorgniotti & others (1979) identified an arteriovenous fistula of the pudendal vessels by arteriography in a 20-year-old man with primary partial impotence.

C. Pharmacologic Causes: Many commonly used drugs have undesirable effects on sexual function. The most common of these are the antihypertensive agents. The incidence of erectile impotence with some antihypertensive drugs was as follows: spironolactone, 5%; rauwolfia agents, 1%; guanethidine, 31%; methyldopa, 1.3–83%; clonidine, 0–24%; and propranolol, 4.7–15%. Thiazides, hydralazine, phazocin and phenoxybenzamine have not been associated with erectile dysfunction and are among the drugs of choice for use with hypertensive patients.

Anticholinergic drugs have also been associated with impotence, as have phenothiazines, antihistamines, and tricyclic antidepressants, all of which have significant anticholinergic action. These agents affect central nervous system function, but the mechanism by which they cause impotence has not been determined. Estrogens and antiandrogens produce impotence by altering hormonal status.

Many psychotropic agents have been associated with impotence. Alcohol has been found to depress central nervous system function, to elevate plasma estrogen by causing hepatic dysfunction (Adlercreutz, 1974), and to decrease effective circulating testosterone levels by directly causing testicular dysfunction (Gordon & others, 1976). Barbiturates, sedatives, and tranquilizers also cause central nervous system depression and have been associated with impotence. Marijuana, which can cause reversible depression of serum testosterone (Kolodny & others, 1974), has been said both to inhibit erections and intensify orgasm. Heroin is also known to reduce serum testosterone. Impaired libido and impotence have been reported by chronic users of heroin and amphetamines.

D. Diabetes: Impotence is reported in up to 59% of diabetic men (Ellenberg, 1971) and is unrelated to the duration, severity, or adequacy of control of diabetes. It is rarely the presenting manifestation (Rubin & Babbott, 1958). The pathogenesis may be neurogenic (Ellenberg, 1971; Faerman & others, 1974) or vasculogenic (Abelson, 1975; Ruzbarsky & Michal, 1977; Sharlip [*West J Med*], 1981). Recent studies indicate that vasculogenic factors are more common than neurogenic ones in diabetic impotence (Jevtich & others, 1980).

E. Surgery: Certain surgical procedures cause impotence. Following aortoiliac surgery, 10–34% of male patients will become impotent (May & others, 1969; Weinstein & Machleder, 1975), and 30–60% will suffer ejaculatory disturbance. The lat-

ter is caused by surgical injury to the sympathetic nervous system, whereas erectile impotence is either neurogenic or vasculogenic. Several forms of radical pelvic surgery for cancer result in sexual dysfunction, especially abdominoperineal resection for rectal carcinoma, radical prostatectomy (either perineal or retropubic), and radical cystectomy.

Surgery for benign prostatic hypertrophy is only infrequently complicated by impotence. Erectile impotence has recently been reported in 5–7% of transurethral prostatectomies, 7–13% of suprapubic prostatectomies, and 29% of perineal prostatectomies (Hargreave & Stephenson, 1977; Finkle & Prian, 1966).

Transurethral external sphincterotomy performed at the 3 and 9 o'clock positions is complicated by impotence in widely varying percentages, but generally in one-third of cases. This is presumably due to damage to the adjacent penile arteries during sphincterotomy. The same procedure performed at the 12 o'clock position results in impotence in 2.8% of cases (Carrion & others, 1979).

Certain neurosurgical procedures such as bilateral pudendal neurectomy or complicated spinal cord surgery may interfere with the neurophysiology or psychology of erection, producing impotence.

Interference with sympathetic innervation to the pelvic organs is responsible for ejaculatory disturbances. About 30–60% of aortoiliac surgical procedures result in a dry ejaculate. Kedia & others (1975) found total absence of ejaculation in 35 of 36 patients who had undergone retroperitoneal lymphadenectomy for a testis tumor. Whitelaw & Smithwick (1951) found that sympathectomy for peripheral vascular disease may produce loss of ejaculation.

F. Neurogenic Causes: Intact neurologic innervation to the penis is necessary for erection and ejaculation. Thus, encephalopathy, myelopathy, or peripheral neuropathy that interferes with the cerebral, spinal cord, or peripheral structures necessary for erection may cause sexual dysfunction. Prominent among these are spinal cord injuries, tabes dorsalis, multiple sclerosis, myelodysplasia, spinal cord injury or tumor, and various causes of peripheral neuropathy, including diabetes. Comarr (1971) found that about 95% of patients with upper motor neuron injury retained reflexogenic erections. When the injury involved the lower motor neuron, only 26% of patients with complete lesions retained erections; these occurred through the psychogenic pathway. Of those retaining erection, 70–80% were capable of intercourse. Patients with complete upper motor neuron lesions lost emission and orgasm, but patients with lower motor neuron lesions retained emission and orgasm in 17% of complete and 60% of incomplete lesions.

G. Renal Failure: Impotence occurs frequently with renal failure. The reported incidence in patients stabilized on hemodialysis is 36–87%.

The reported incidence following renal transplantation is 22–54% (Brannen & others, 1980). The pathogenesis of impotence in renal failure is multifactorial (Sherman, 1975; Brannen & others, 1980) and may include accelerated arteriosclerosis, antihypertensive agents, uremic neuropathy, low testosterone due to Leydig cell dysfunction, low serum zinc levels, and psychologic factors. Restoration of erections has followed zinc replacement therapy in some dialysis patients (Antoniou & others, 1977).

H. Endocrinopathy: Endocrinopathy accounts for only about 10% of organic impotence. Most cases have pituitary dysfunction. The second most common endocrinopathy is testicular dysfunction.

Hyperprolactinemia is being diagnosed more frequently as a cause of impotence, infertility, and galactorrhea. The serum testosterone level is usually normal or slightly diminished, and the serum FSH and LH levels are usually normal. Treatment for low testosterone without treatment for hyperprolactinemia does not improve erectile dysfunction.

Feminizing tumors and estrogen therapy cause impotence by elimination of the normal androgenic stimulus. Pituitary conditions such as acromegaly cause impotence probably through alteration of the normal pituitary-testis axis. Hyper- and hypothyroid states have also been associated with impotence.

I. Trauma: Penile fractures and injuries may result in damage to the erectile tissue, with subsequent partial or total impotence. The mechanism of impotence in these cases may be neurogenic, but penile arteriography has shown that injury to the internal pudendal vessels produces vasculogenic impotence as well (Sharlip, [in press], 1981). Normal ejaculation is almost always regained after surgical correction of the urethral stricture that frequently follows posterior urethral trauma.

J. Local Penile Diseases: Peyronie's disease usually does not prevent erection, although the erectile curvature it produces may make erection painful and intromission impossible. About half of patients experience impotence after priapism (Winter, 1979); impotence occurs because of fibrosis of the trabeculae of the corpora cavernosa (Hinman, 1960). Local penile tumors may involve the corpora cavernosa and prevent erection.

K. Chronic Disease States: Sexual dysfunction may complicate many chronic systemic illnesses. The pathogenesis is poorly defined. Psychogenic factors, especially decreased libido, are the most obvious, but organic factors are also present.

Chronic prostatitis and prostatic hypertrophy have been unfairly blamed for impotence. There is currently no documented causal relationship between chronic prostate disease and erectile impotence. Acute prostatitis may be a temporary cause of erectile dysfunction due to local pain and decreased libido.

Diagnosis

A. Sexual History: Information should be obtained concerning libido, erection, ejaculation, orgasm, the patient's sexual background, previous sexual experience, sexual expectations, marriage, and methods of adjusting to the state of dysfunction.

B. Medical History: The review of systems and past medical history should focus on the causes of erectile dysfunction discussed in the previous section.

C. Physical Examination: A thorough physical examination will often give clues to organic causes of impotence. Examination of the vascular, neurologic, endocrine, and genitourinary systems is especially important. Specific tests of S2–4 function should include perianal sensation, rectal sphincter tone, and bulbocavernosus reflex.

D. Laboratory Diagnosis: Basic laboratory studies should include complete blood count, urinalysis, examination of expressed prostatic secretions, measurement of blood sugar and serum creatinine, and the VDRL test. Initial endocrine screening should include measurement of serum testosterone and serum prolactin. Serum FSH and LH may be measured if either the testosterone or prolactin level is abnormal.

E. Advanced Diagnostic Technics: Several recently developed diagnostic technics are being widely used to determine the causes of impotence.

1. Nocturnal penile tumescence monitoring (NPTM)–Nocturnal erections occur in healthy males of all ages. Eighty to ninety percent of the nocturnal episodes occur with rapid eye movement (REM) phases of sleep. Four or 5 erectile episodes per night, each lasting 20–40 minutes, are normal for most adult men.

The NPT monitoring device consists of a pair of ring-shaped strain gauges that are placed about the penile shaft, one at the base and one at the tip behind the glans. These are connected to a portable recorder. A ring of postage stamps to test for the occurrence of nocturnal erections is a cheap equivalent. The "stamp test" can be used as a screening test to determine which patients might require more sophisticated sleep studies.

NPT monitoring is valuable in distinguishing psychogenic from organic impotence. Patients with psychogenic impotence are thought to be unable to suppress nocturnal erections and will therefore show normal patterns on the monitor. Organic impotence is revealed by abnormal patterns of nocturnal erections (Fig 35–3).

2. Penile blood pressure and pulse measurements–Penile blood pressure and blood flow can be measured with a Doppler probe, which will detect sounds in the penile arteries. The penile systolic pressures can be compared to brachial systolic pressures. Standards of normal and abnormal are not yet firmly established. Many clinicians differentiate normal from abnormal pressure using a penile to brachial systolic ratio of 0.75. By compar-

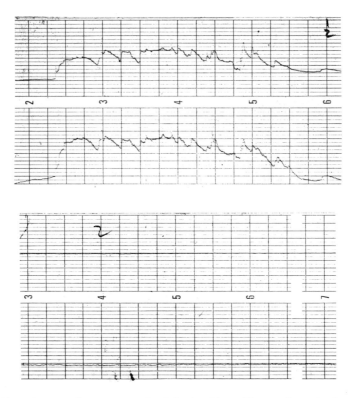

Figure 35–3. *Above:* Normal nocturnal tumescent episode lasting 1 hour. Three to five episodes per night lasting 20–40 minutes each are indicative of psychogenic impotence. *Below:* Abnormal NPT study in a totally impotent diabetic male with severe neuropathy and flaccid bladder. The study was perfectly flat for 3 consecutive nights, which indicates organic impotence.

ing the acceleration phase of the radial and penile pulses, Velcek has developed a penile flow index that adds a quantitative measure to analysis.

The significance of penile blood pressure and pulse wave forms in identifying vasculogenic impotence remains to be clearly defined. However, Velcek & others (1980) and Jevtich (1980) have reported an excellent correlation between Doppler studies of the penile arteries and penile arteriography in clinical impotence.

3. Penile arteriography–Penile arteriograms will conclusively establish diagnosis of vasculogenic impotence. The patient must be in the oblique position. Interpretation of the arteriograms requires experience. Abnormalities such as arterial stenosis or complete obstruction, congenital dysplasia or hypoplasia, collateralization and hyperplasia, or anomalous anatomy of the arteries and their branches can be demonstrated (Fig 35–4).

4. Bulbocavernosus reflex latency (BCRL) time–The bulbocavernosus reflex is a somatic reflex closely related to the erectile reflex, and measurement of its latency time provides an objective assessment of the integrity of the S2–4 reflex arc. A surface-stimulating electrode is applied to the distal penile skin, and response to the stimulus is obtained from a sensing needle electrode inserted into the bulbocavernosus muscle. The normal range of latency time is 27–42 ms (Krane & Siroky, 1980). BCRL time testing is a new technic that may provide a means of identifying otherwise obscure neurogenic causes of impotence.

5. Corpus cavernosography–Cavernosograms will occasionally demonstrate an area of unsuspected Peyronie's disease or other anatomic abnormality of the corpus cavernosum.

Treatment of Organic Sexual Dysfunction

A. Medical Treatment of Ejaculatory Dysfunction: Treatment of dry ejaculation with sympathomimetic agents such as ephedrine, 25–50 mg orally one-half hour before intercourse, has had some success.

Premature ejaculation can be treated by training the patient to control ejaculatory demand. Semans (1956) described a technic of repetitive stimulation to just short of ejaculation, alternating with rest periods. This gradually builds tolerance for a high degree of sexual excitement without ejaculation. Masters & Johnson emphasized the squeeze technic, whereby, as ejaculation approaches, the sexual partner squeezes the glans firmly for 3 or 4 seconds, inhibiting ejaculation and reducing erection.

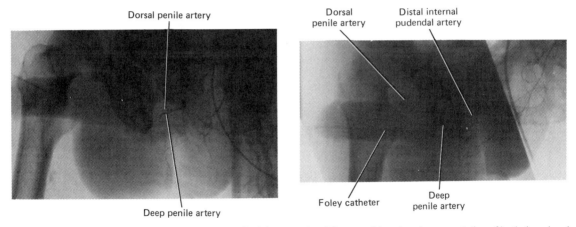

Figure 35–4. *Left:* Abnormal left penile arteriogram in right posterior oblique position showing amputation of both dorsal and deep penile arteries (arrows). Later films did not show any arterial visualization beyond these points. *Right:* Normal left penile arteriogram in right posterior oblique position. Penis points to patient's right thigh with glans penis at left margin of figure. Dorsal and deep penile arteries appear normal. A Foley catheter in the urethra and the distal internal pudendal artery are indicated.

B. Medical Treatment of Erectile Impotence: In general, medical therapy for erectile dysfunction is of limited usefulness. However, some patients are helped by the following types of medical management. Drugs that affect sexual function should be discontinued, according to clinical indications. Any basic endocrine abnormality should be treated. This may require removal of a pituitary tumor; normalization of hormone levels by intramuscular injections of long-acting testosterone or, occasionally, oral testosterone; or treatment of hyperprolactinemia. In the latter, removal of a pituitary tumor, if present, should be the first step in treatment. Rare forms of neurogenic impotence are reversible, particularly those related to vitamin deficiency, pernicious anemia, and chemotoxic neuropathies. Uremic impotence may be improved by oral zinc replacement (Antoniou, 1977) or by intramuscular testosterone if Leydig cell dysfunction complicates uremia.

C. Surgical Treatment of Erectile Impotence: Effective surgical treatment for impotence became available in the 1970s and is one of the major recent developments in the field of sexual dysfunction.

1. Semirigid penile prosthesis–The Small-Carrion prosthesis was the first of the currently successful prostheses. A pair of silicone rods is placed within the corpora cavernosa through a perineal, penoscrotal, or dorsal penile incision, imparting permanent semirigidity to the penis. The overall surgical and functional success rate is 90–97%. Partner acceptance is excellent when proper preoperative counseling of patient and partner is carried out.

To solve the problem of positioning of the semirigid penis and to allow for better concealment, a silicone prosthesis with a soft area at the penoscrotal junction has been developed; this hinged prosthesis allows the penis to assume a normal de-pendent position when the patient is standing, though it maintains sufficient rigidity for vaginal penetration.

The Jonas malleable penile prosthesis is also a paired silicone prosthesis, but it has a silver wire center rod that permits the penis to be directed and stabilized in different positions.

2. Inflatable penile prosthesis–The inflatable penile prosthesis consists of a pair of cylinders, a reservoir of radiopaque fluid, a pump to transfer the fluid, and tubing connecting these parts. The inflatable cylinders are placed within the corpora cavernosa, the pump is placed within the scrotum, and the reservoir is placed behind the abdominal wall. All components are placed through the same incision. To achieve an erection, the pump in the scrotum is digitally compressed 10–15 times, transferring fluid from the reservoir to the cylinders. Detumescence is achieved by pressing a release valve on the side of the pump, allowing the fluid to flow back into the reservoir. One-third of patients have undergone second or third surgical procedures to correct mechanical malfunction, which has been much reduced by recent design changes.

3. Corpus cavernosum revascularization–The newest surgical treatment of impotence is corpus cavernosum revascularization. Interest in revascularization procedures to correct penile arterial insufficiency escalated following the identification of arteriogenic impotence and initial reports of surgical treatment by Michal & others (1974, 1977). These procedures should be performed only for vasculogenic impotence.

Vasculogenic disease in the penile arteries has been treated by microsurgical anastomosis of the inferior epigastric artery directly to the corpus cavernosum or by vein interposition from the inferior epigastric artery or femoral artery to the corpus cavernosum. This procedure was developed to pus cavernosum. Success rates have been variable, ranging from nil (LeVeen & Diaz, 1980) to 77% (Ginestie, 1980), with an average range of functional success of 30–40% (Zorgniotti & others, 1980; Casey, 1979; Sharlip [*West J Med*], 1981). Long-term patency has been the main problem with this

technic. To solve this and to place the neovascular flow under normal neurophysiologic regulation, the latest technic of revascularization is a vein graft from the femoral artery directly to the dorsal or central penile arteries. Initial reports using microsurgical technics are encouraging.

• • •

References

Infertility

Abrahams JI & others: The surgical correction of retrograde ejaculation. *J Urol* 1975;**114**:888.

Amelar RD, Dubin L: Basic and practical aspects of the etiology and management of male infertility. *Urol Dig* (May) 1975;**14**:19.

Amelar RD, Dubin L: Male infertility: Current diagnosis and treatment. *Urology* 1973;**1**:1.

Amelar RD, Dubin L, Walsh PC: *Male Infertility.* Saunders, 1977.

Ansbacher R, Keung-Yeung K, Behrman SJ: Clinical significance of sperm antibodies in infertile couples. *Fertil Steril* 1973;**24**:305.

Belker AM: Microsurgical two-layer vasovasostomy. *Urology* 1980;**16**:376.

Bibbo M & others: Male and female offspring of DES-exposed mothers. *Obstet Gynecol* 1977;**49**:1.

Bullock JY, Gilmore LL, Wilson JD: Autoantibodies following vasectomy. *J Urol* 1977;**118**:604.

Byrd JR, Askew DE, McDonough PG: Cytogenic findings in fifty-five couples with recurrent fetal wastage. *Fertil Steril* 1977;**28**:246.

Caldamone AA, Al-Juburi A, Cockett ATK: Varicocele: Elevated serotonin and infertility. *J Urol* 1980;**123**:683.

Charny CW: Clomiphene therapy in male infertility: A negative report. *Fertil Steril* 1979;**32**:551.

Chehval MJ, Mehan DJ: Chorionic gonadotropins in the treatment of the subfertile male. *Fertil Steril* 1979;**31**:666.

Comhaire F, Monteyne R, Kunnen M: The value of scrotal thermography as compared with selective retrograde venography of the internal spermatic vein for the diagnosis of "subclinical" varicocele. *Fertil Steril* 1976;**27**:694.

Cunningham GR: Medical treatment of the subfertile male. *Urol Clin North Am* 1978;**5**:537.

De Louvois J & others: Frequency of mycoplasma in fertile and infertile couples. *Lancet* 1974;**1**:1073.

Dougherty KA, Cockett AT, Urry RL: Effect of amylase on sperm motility and viability. *J Urol* 1978;**120**:425.

Dubin L, Amelar RD: Varicocele. *Urol Clin North Am* 1978;**5**:563.

Dubin L, Amelar RD: Varicocelectomy in male infertility: 504 cases. *J Urol* 1977;**113**:640.

Eliasson R, Lindholmer C: Distribution and properties of spermatozoa in different fractions of split ejaculates. *Fertil Steril* 1972;**23**:252.

Fjällbrant B: Localization of human male antibodies on spermatozoa. *Am J Obstet Gynecol* 1970;**108**:550.

Friberg J, Gnarpe H: Mycoplasma and human reproduction failure. *Am J Obstet Gynecol* 1973;**116**:23.

Greenberg SH, Lipshultz LI, Wein AJ: Experience with

425 subfertile male patients. *J Urol* 1978;**119**:507.

Haas GG Jr, Cines DB, Schreiber AD: Immunologic infertility: Identification of patients with antisperm antibody. *N Engl J Med* 1980;**303**:722.

Hafez ESE, Thibault CG: International symposium on the biology of spermatozoa: Transport, survival, and fertilizing ability. *Fertil Steril* 1974;**25**:825.

Hébert G, Bouchard R, Charron J: Vasoseminal vesiculography. *Am J Roentgenol* 1971;**113**:735.

Hendry WF & others: Investigation and treatment of the subfertile male. *Br J Urol* 1973;**45**:684.

Joël CA: Male factor in habitual abortion. *Fertil Steril* 1966;**17**:374.

Jones TM & others: Parameters of response to clomiphene citrate in oligospermic men. *J Urol* 1980;**124**:53.

Kolodny RC & others: Depression of plasma testosterone levels after chronic intensive marihuana use. *N Engl J Med* 1974;**290**:872.

Lamensdorf H, Compere D, Begley G: Testosterone rebound therapy in the treatment of male infertility. *Fertil Steril* 1975;**26**:469.

Lingårdh G & others: Dysplasia of the testis and epididymis. *Scand J Urol Nephrol* 1975;**9**:1.

Lipshultz LI: Cryptorchidism in the subfertile male. *Fertil Steril* 1976;**27**:609.

Lome LG, Ross L: Varicocelectomy and infertility. *Urology* 1977;**9**:416.

McFadden MR, Mehan DJ: Testicular biopsies in 101 cases of varicocele. *J Urol* 1978;**119**:372.

MacLeod J, Wang Y: Male fertility potential in terms of semen quality: A review of the past, a study of the present. *Fertil Steril* 1979;**31**:103.

Matthews CD & others: The frequency of genital mycoplasma infection in human fertility. *Fertil Steril* 1975;**26**:988.

Mumford DM: Immunology and male infertility. *Urol Clin North Am* 1978;**5**:463.

Paulson DF: Cortisone acetate versus clomiphene citrate in pre-germinal idiopathic oligospermia. *J Urol* 1979;**121**:432.

Pedersen H: The human spermatozoon. *Dan Med Bull* 1974;**21** (**Suppl 1**):1.

Pryor JP & others: Controlled clinical trial of arginine for infertile men with oligozoospermia. *Br J Urol* 1978;**50**:47.

Rubin S-O: Congenital absence of the vas deferens: An analysis of fourteen personal cases. *Scand J Urol Nephrol* 1975;**9**:94.

Schachter A, Goldman JA, Zukerman Z: Treatment of oligospermia with the amino acid arginine. *J Urol* 1973;**110**:311.

Schellen TM, Beek JM: The influence of high doses of

mesterolone on the spermiogram. *Fertil Steril* 1972;23:712.

Schellen TM, Beek JM: The use of clomiphene treatment for male sterility. *Fertil Steril* 1974;25:407.

Schoenfeld C, Amelar RD, Dubin L: Stimulation of ejaculated human spermatozoa by caffeine. *Fertil Steril* 1975;26:158.

Sciarra JJ, Markland C, Speidel JJ: *Control of Male Fertility.* Harper & Row, 1975.

Segal S & others: Male hyperprolactinemia: Effects on fertility. *Fertil Steril* 1979;32:556.

Shulman S, Harlin B, Davis P: New method of treatment of immune infertility. *Urology* 1978;12:582.

Silber SJ: Microscopic vasoepididymostomy: Specific microanastomosis to the epididymal tubule. *Fertil Steril* 1978;30:565.

Silber SJ, Galle J, Friend D: Microscopic vasovasostomy and spermatogenesis. *J Urol* 1977;117:299.

Snyder PJ: Endocrine evaluation of the infertile male. *Urol Clin North Am* 1978;5:451.

Sobrero AJ, Rehan NE: The semen of fertile men. 2. The semen characteristics of 100 fertile men. *Fertil Steril* 1975;26:1048.

Stewart BH: Drugs as cause and cure in male infertility. *Drug Ther* (April) 1973;3:34.

Stewart BH, Montie JE: Male infertility: An optimistic report. *J Urol* 1973;110:216.

Stockamp K, Schreiter F, Altwein JE: α-Adrenergic drugs in retrograde ejaculation. *Fertil Steril* 1974;25:817.

Timmermans L: Influence of antibiotics on spermatogenesis. *J Urol* 1974;112:348.

Ulstein M: Fertility of husbands at homologous insemination. *Acta Obstet Gynecol Scand* 1973;52:5.

Walker HE: Psychiatric aspects of infertility. *Urol Clin North Am* 1978;5:481.

Wall JR & others: Immunologic studies of male infertility. *Fertil Steril* 1975;26:1035.

White RD, Paulson DF: Obstruction of the male reproductive tract. *J Urol* 1977;118:266.

White RM, Glass RH: Intrauterine insemination with husband's semen. *Obstet Gynecol* 1976;47:119.

Willscher MK, Novicki DE: Simplified technique for microscopic vasovastostomy. *Urology* 1980;15:147.

Wilson VB, Bunge RG: Infertility and semen nonliquefaction. *J Urol* 1975;113:509.

Wong TW & others: Pathological aspects of the infertile testis. *Urol Clin North Am* 1978;5:503.

Zorgniotti AW: Testis temperature, infertility, and the varicocele paradox. *Urology* 1980;16:7.

Vasectomy

Albert PS, Mininberg DT, Davis JE: The nitrofurans as sperm immobilizing agents: Their tissue toxicity and their clinical application. *Br J Urol* 1975;47:459.

Amelar RD, Dubin L: Frozen semen: A poor form of fertility insurance. *Urology* 1979;14:53.

Berthelson JG: Preoperative irrigation of the vas deferens during vasectomy. *Scand J Urol Nephrol* 1976;10:100.

Bremner WJ, deKretser DM: The prospects for new, reversible male contraceptives. *N Engl J Med* 1976;295:1111.

Brown RA, Magarick RH: Psychological effects of vasectomy in voluntarily childless men. *Urology* 1979;14:55.

Brueschke EE & others: Development of a reversible vas deferens occlusive device. 4. Rigid prosthetic devices.

5. Flexible prosthetic devices. *Fertil Steril* 1975;26:29, 40.

Bullock JY, Gilmore LL, Wilson JD: Autoantibodies following vasectomy. *J Urol* 1977;118:604.

Cass AS: Unsatisfactory psychosocial results of vasectomy resulting in modification of preoperative counseling. *Urology* 1979;14:588.

Esho JO, Ireland GW, Cass AS: Vasectomy: Comparison of ligation and fulguration methods. *Urology* 1974;3:337.

Friberg J, Gemzell C: Inseminations of human sperm after freezing in liquid nitrogen vapors with glycerol or glycerol-egg-yolk-citrate as protection media. *Am J Obstet Gynecol* 1973;116:330.

Jenkins IL & others: Consequences of vasectomy: An immunological and histological study related to subsequent fertility. *Br J Urol* 1979;51:406.

Klapproth HJ, Young IS: Vasectomy, vas ligation and vas occlusion. *Urology* 1973;1:292.

Kwart AM, Coffey DS: Sperm granulomas: An adverse effect of vasectomy. *J Urol* 1973;110:416.

Leader AJ & others: Complications of 2711 vasectomies. *J Urol* 1974;111:365.

Marshall S, Lyon RP: Variability of sperm disappearance from the ejaculate after vasectomy. *J Urol* 1972;107:815.

Moss WM: Sutureless vasectomy, an improved technique: 1300 cases performed without failure. *Fertil Steril* 1976;27:1040.

Mumford SD, Davis JE: Flushing of distal vas during vasectomy: Current status and review of literature. *Urology* 1979;14:433.

Nash JL, Rich JD: The sexual aftereffects of vasectomy. *Fertil Steril* 1972;23:715.

Rosenberg E & others: Serum levels of follicle stimulating and luteinizing hormones before and after vasectomy in men. *J Urol* 1974;111:626.

Schmidt SS: Vasectomy should not fail. *Contemp Surg* (May) 1974;4:13.

Schmidt SS & others: Vas cautery: Battery powered instrument for vasectomy. *Urology* 1974;3:604.

Skegg DCG & others: Hormonal assessment before and after vasectomy. *Br Med J* 1976;1:621.

Smith KD, Steinberger E: Survival of spermatozoa in a human sperm bank. *JAMA* 1973;223:774.

Urquhart-Hay D: Immediate sterility after vasectomy. *NZ Med J* 1975;81:11.

Whitby RM, Gordon RD, Blair BR: The endocrine effects of vasectomy: A prospective five-year study. *Fertil Steril* 1979;31:518.

Witherington R, Black JB, Karow AM Jr: Semen cryopreservation: An update. *J Urol* 1977;118:510.

Zufall R: Vasectomy: Five to ten-year follow-up of 200 cases. *Urology* 1980;15:278.

Impotence

Abelson D: Diagnostic value of the penile pulses and blood pressure: A Doppler study of impotence in diabetics. *J Urol* 1975;113:636.

Adlecreutz H: Hepatic metabolism of estrogens in health and disease. *N Engl J Med* 1974;290:1081.

Antoniou LD & others: Reversal of uremic impotence by zinc. *Lancet* 1977;2:895.

Barry JM: Clinical experience with hinged silicone penile implants for impotence. *J Urol* 1980;123:178.

Barry JM & others: Nocturnal penile tumescence monitoring with stamps. *Urology* 1980;15:171.

Benson GS, McConnell J, Lipshultz LI: Penile "polsters":

Normal functional structures or arteriosclerotic changes? *J Urol* 1981. [In press.]

Blaivas JG & others: Comprehensive laboratory evaluation of impotent men. *J Urol* 1980;**124**:201.

Bors E, Comarr AE: *Neurological Urology.* University Park Press, 1971.

Bossart MI, Spjut HJ, Scott FB: Ultrastructural analysis of human penile corpus cavernosum. *Urology* 1980;**15**:448.

Brannen GE & others: Impotence after kidney transplantation. *Urology* 1980;**15**:138.

Brooks ME & others: Treatment of retrograde ejaculation with imipramine. *Urology* 1980;**15**:353.

Carrion H & others: External sphincterotomy at the 12 o'clock position. *J Urol* 1979;**121**:462.

Carter JN & others: Prolactin secreting tumors and hypogonadism in 22 men. *N Engl J Med* 1978;**299**:847.

Casey WC: Revascularization of corpus cavernosum for erectile failure. *Urology* 1979;**14**:135.

Cohen MS & others: Morphology of the corpus cavernosum arterial bed in impotence. Chapter 13 in: *Vasculogenic Impotence.* Zorgniotti AW, Rossi G (editors). Thomas, 1980.

Comarr AE: Sexual concepts in traumatic cord and cauda equina lesions. *J Urol* 1971;**106**:375.

Conti G: L'erection du penis humaine et ses hases morphologico-vasculaires. *Acta Anat* 1952;**5**:217.

Cruz JFJ, Solano BE: Impotence secondary to postpuberal hypogonadism. *Eur Urol* 1979;**5**:168.

Ebbehoj J, Wagner G: Insufficient penile erections due to abnormal drainage of cavernous bodies. *Urology* 1979;**13**:507.

Ellenberg M: Impotence in diabetes: The neurologic factor. *Ann Intern Med* 1971;**75**:213.

Engel G & others: Penile blood pressure in the evaluation of erectile impotence. *Fertil Steril* 1978;**30**:687.

Faerman I & others: Impotence and diabetes: Histological studies of the autonomic nervous fibers of the corpora cavernosa in impotent diabetic males. *Diabetes* 1974;**23**:971.

Finkle A, Prian D: Sexual potency in elderly men before and after prostatectomy. *JAMA* 1966;**196**:125.

Finkle JE, Finkle ES, Finkle A: Encouraging preservation of sexual function post prostatectomy. *Urology* 1975;**6**:697.

Finney RP & others: Finney hinged penile implant: Experience with 100 cases. *J Urol* 1980;**124**:205.

Fisher C & others: Evaluation of nocturnal penile tumescence in the differential diagnosis of sexual impotence. *Arch Gen Psychiatry* 1979;**36**:431.

Forsberg L & others: Impotence, smoking and beta-blocking drugs. *Fertil Steril* 1979;**31**:589.

Franks S & others: Hyperprolactinaemia and impotence. *Clin Endocrinol (Oxf)* 1978;**8**:277.

Frantz AG: Prolactin. *N Engl J Med* 1978;**298**:201.

Furlow WL: Inflatable penile prosthesis: Mayo Clinic experience with 175 patients. *Urology* 1979;**13**:166.

Gerstenberger DL & others: Inflatable penile prosthesis: Follow-up study of patient-partner satisfaction. *Urology* 1979;**14**:583.

Ginestie J: Results of revascularization of the corpus cavernosum. Chapter 26 in: *Vasculogenic Impotence.* Zorgniotti AW, Rossi G (editors). Thomas, 1980.

Ginestie J, Romieu A: *Radiologic Exploration of Impotence.* Martinus Nijhoff, 1978.

Ginestie J, Romieu A: Traitement des impuissances d'or-

igine vasculaire: La revascularisation des corps caverneux. *J Urol Nephrol* 1976;**82**:853.

Gordon G & others: Effect of alcohol (ethanol) administration on sex-hormone metabolism in normal men. *N Engl J Med* 1976;**295**:793.

Gottesman JE & others: The Small-Carrion prosthesis for male impotency. *J Urol* 1977;**117**:289.

Hargreave TB, Stephenson TP: Potency and prostatectomy. *Br J Urol* 1977;**49**:683.

Hinman F: Priapism: Reasons for failure of therapy. *J Urol* 1960;**83**:240.

Houttuin E, Gregory JE: Hemodynamic studies of penile erection in dogs. Chapter 5 in: *Vasculogenic Impotence.* Zorgniotti AW, Rossi G (editors). Thomas, 1980.

Jevtich MJ: Importance of penile arterial pulse sound examination in impotence. *J Urol* 1980;**124**:820.

Jevtich MJ & others: Erectile failure in diabetes. Paper presented at Second International Conference on Vasculogenic Impotence, Monaco, 1980.

Jewett JS: The results of radical perineal prostatectomy. *JAMA* 1969;**210**:324.

Kaplan HS: *The New Sex Therapy.* Brunner/Mazel, 1974.

Karacan I & others: The ontogeny of nocturnal penile tumescence. *Waking & Sleeping* 1976;**1**:27.

Karacan I & others: Sleep related penile tumescence as a function of age. *Am J Psychol* 1975;**132**:9.

Kedia RK & others: Sexual function following high retroperitoneal lymphadenectomy. *J Urol* 1975;**114**:237.

Kelly ME, Needle MA: Imipramine for aspermia after lymphadenectomy. *Urology* 1979;**13**:414.

Kirby RW & others: Hyperprolactinemia: A review of recent clinical advances. *Arch Intern Med* 1979;**139**:1415.

Kolodny RC & others: Depression of plasma testosterone levels after chronic intensive marijuana use. *N Engl J Med* 1974;**290**:872.

Kramer SA & others: Complications of Small-Carrion penile prosthesis. *Urology* 1979;**13**:49.

Krane RJ, Siroky MB: Studies in sacral-evoked potentials. *J Urol* 1980;**124**:872.

Leiblum SR, Plevin LA: *Principles and Practice of Sex Therapy.* Guilford Press, 1980.

LeRiche R: Des obliterations arterielles hautes (obliterations de la termination de l'aorte) comme cause d'insuffisance circulatoire des membres inferieures. *Bull Soc Chirurgie Inter Paris* 1923;**49**:1404.

LeVeen HH, Diaz C: Treatment by corpus cavernosum revascularization. Chapter 25 in: *Vasculogenic Impotence.* Zorgniotti AW, Rossi G (editors). Thomas, 1980.

Madorsky ML & others: Postprostatectomy impotence. *J Urol* 1976;**115**:401.

Malloy TR & others: Further experiences with the inflatable penile prosthesis. *J Urol* 1979;**122**:478.

Masters WH, Johnson VE: Principles of the new sex therapy. *Am J Psychol* 1976;**133**:548.

May AG & others: Changes in sexual function following operation. *Surgery* 1969;**65**:41.

Michal V, Pospichal J: Phalloarteriography in the diagnosis of erectile impotence. *World J Surg* 1978;**2**:239.

Michal V & others: Aortoiliac occlusive disease. Chapter 24 in: *Vasculogenic Impotence.* Zorgniotti AW, Rossi G (editors). Thomas, 1980.

Michal V & others: Arterial epigastric-cavernous anastomosis for treatment of sexual impotence. *World J Surg* 1977;**1**:515.

Michal V & others: Femoropudendal bypass in treatment of sexual impotence. *J Cardiovasc Surg* 1974;**15**:356.

Montague DR & others: Diagnostic evaluation, classification, and treatment of men with sexual dysfunction. *Urology* 1979;**14**:545.

Morgan RJ, Pryor JP: Investigation of organic impotence. *Br J Urol* 1980;**52**:571.

Newman HF, Tchertkoff V: Penile vascular cushions and erection. *Invest Urol* 1980;**18**:43.

Nowinski J: *Becoming Satisfied: A Man's Guide to Sexual Fulfillment.* Prentice-Hall, 1980.

Papadopoulos C: Cardiovascular drugs and sexuality. *Arch Intern Med* 1980;**140**:1341.

Reichgott MJ: Problems of sexual function in patients with hypertension. *Cardiovasc Med* 1979;**4**:149.

Rubin A, Babbott D: Impotence and diabetes mellitus. *JAMA* 1958;**168**:498.

Ruzbarsky V, Michal V: Morphologic changes in the arterial bed of the penis with aging. *Invest Urol* 1977;**15**:194.

Scott FB & others: Erectile impotence treated with an implantable, inflatable prosthesis. *JAMA* 1979;**241**:2609.

Semans JH: Premature ejaculation: A new approach. *South Med J* 1956;**49**:353.

Semans JH, Langworthy OR: Observations on neurophysiology of sexual function in the male cat. *J Urol* 1938;**40**:836.

Sharlip ID: Penile arteriography in impotence due to pelvic trauma. *J Urol* 1981. [In press.]

Sharlip ID: Penile revascularization in the treatment of impotence. *West J Med* 1981;**134**:206.

Sherman FP: Impotence in patients with chronic renal failure on dialysis: Its frequency and etiology. *Fertil Steril* 1975;**26**:221.

Shrom SH & others: Clinical profile of experience with 130 consecutive cases of impotent men. *Urology* 1979;**13**:511.

Siroky MB, Krane RJ: Physiology of sexual function. Chapter 3 in: *Clinical Neuro-Urology.* Krane RJ, Siroky MB (editors). Little, Brown, 1979.

Small MP: Small-Carrion penile prosthesis: A report on 160 cases and review of the literature. *J Urol* 1978;**119**:365.

Sparks RF & others: Impotence is not always psychogenic. *JAMA* 1980;**243**:750.

Velcek D & others: Penile flow index utilizing a Doppler pulse wave analysis to identify penile vascular insufficiency. *J Urol* 1980;**123**:669.

Wagner G, Uhrenholdt A: Blood flow measurement by the clearance method in the human corpus cavernosum in the flaccid and erect status. Chapter 6 in: *Vasculogenic Impotence.* Zorgniotti AW, Rossi G (editors). Thomas, 1980.

Wasserman MD & others: The differential diagnosis of impotence. *JAMA* 1980;**243**:2038.

Weinstein M, Machleder H: Sexual function after aorto-iliac surgery. *Ann Surg* 1975;**181**:787.

Weinstein M, Roberts M: Sexual potency following surgery for rectal carcinoma. *Ann Surg* 1977;**185**:295.

Whitelaw GP, Smithwick RA: Some secondary effects of sympathectomy. *N Engl J Med* 1951;**245**:121.

Winter CC: Priapism treated by modification of creation of fistulas between glans penis and corpora cavernosa. *J Urol* 1979;**121**:743.

Zilbergeld B: *Male Sexuality.* Little, Brown, 1978.

Zohar J & others: Factors influencing sexual activity after prostatectomy: A prospective study. *J Urol* 1976;**116**:332.

Zorgniotti AW & others: Diagnosis and therapy of vasculogenic impotence. *J Urol* 1980;**123**:674.

Zorgniotti AW & others: Impotence caused by pudendal arteriovenous fistula. *Urology* 1979;**14**:161.

36 | Effects of the Psyche on Renal & Vesical Function

Donald R. Smith, MD

PSYCHOSOMATIC URINARY FREQUENCY & RETENTION

Psychologic disturbances are not infrequently reflected in dysfunction of the bladder and kidneys. The literature on this subject is scanty, despite the fact that functional disturbances of the gastrointestinal tract, cardiovascular and respiratory systems, and skin are well documented. These organ systems are affected by various hormones and by autonomic nerve impulses that affect the tone of smooth muscle. Since the bladder is also innervated by the parasympathetics and is composed of smooth muscle, the development of vesical spasm or atony could be expected under conditions of stress. Kidney function is influenced by changes in renal blood flow and by various hormones, including antidiuretic hormone (ADH), aldosterone, and epinephrine.

Hormonal and autonomic influences on urinary tract function have been documented and are summarized in the discussions of specific entities below.

EFFECTS ON VESICAL FUNCTION

Mosso and Pellacani in 1881 were the first investigators to perform cystometry in both dogs and humans. They found that psychic stimuli had a profound effect on vesical tone and function. Stimuli such as loud noises, the sound of running water, strong emotional reactions, or intense intellectual work caused vesical contractions.

Straub, Ripley, & Wolf (1949) studied, by cystometry, a group of neurotic patients who complained of vesical dysfunction. Small elevations of pressure occurred with cough or straining. When the patient was tranquil, the pressure remained low. If, however, the interviewer touched upon sensitive subjects (eg, relations with the husband, conditions of employment), intravesical pressure would immediately rise to 40–70 cm of water. When the conversation returned to more prosaic subjects, intravesical pressure returned to normal. Often, even though the patient complained of the frequent voiding of small amounts of urine, at the end of the interview the volume of fluid in the bladder, augmented by urine secretion, was apt to be 700 mL, yet the patient complained of no feeling of fullness.

In patients who had gone into acute urinary retention without apparent previous urinary difficulty, cystometrograms showed vesical atony. After acute psychotherapy and resumption of voiding, the test results reverted to normal.

Frequency was the most common complaint in this group and was associated with feelings of tension, anxiety, and resentment. Urinary retention was associated with feelings of hysteria and of being overwhelmed.

Acute vesical irritability is a common response to stress. A student may suffer from urinary frequency before final examinations. A female dog may wet the floor when the family returns from vacation.

EFFECTS ON RENAL FUNCTION

Blomstrand & Löfgren (1956) demonstrated the effects of fear or rage on renal blood flow. Catheters were passed to the level of the renal arteries of cats. In the controls, the injection of India ink caused diffuse staining of the renal cortex and, to a lesser extent, the medulla. Seventeen cats were subjected to the trauma of a barking dog and were then injected with India ink. The renal cortices were blanched. The authors believed that this phenomenon was caused by liberation of epinephrine. They noted that Homer Smith had recorded altered diuretic reactions that he thought were secondary to psychogenic renal vasoconstriction. They cited the work of Bycow and Alexjew-Berkman, who had dogs drink water while a bell rang. Once the conditioned reflex had been established, merely ringing the bell led to diuresis.

Levi (1965) studied the urinary excretion of epinephrine and norepinephrine in various psychologic states. Women were shown films that contained some exciting episodes. Catecholamine excretion was low during tranquil intervals on the screen, but during exciting or anxiety-provoking scenes, the level of urinary catecholamines rose significantly. When feelings of fear or anxiety were induced in a group of students, isotope renograms showed increased secretion of catecholamines (DeMaria & others, 1963).

Verney (1958) and Wakim (1967) showed that emotional tension causes increased secretion of ADH. Tranquility led to diuresis. Schottstaedt, Grace, & Wolff (1956) studied the excretion of water and electrolytes in a group of neurotic people. They found that when patients were subjected to stress, diuresis or antidiuresis occurred. When the patient was alert and tense (eg, occupied by intellectual work), urinary excretion fell 20%. Return to tranquility was followed by diuresis. If the patient became angry, a 300% increase in urine excretion was immediately observed, but if the patient was listless and depressed, 30% less urine was passed. A return to a normal emotional state was accompanied by diuresis.

Barnes & Schottstaedt (1960) noted that patients with congestive heart failure retained more water and salt than is customary with this disease if they suffered from excitement, anger, or apprehension.

Gerbner, Altman, & Mészáros (1959) hypnotized a group of patients and had them drink water. Eventually, drinking from an empty glass was a sufficient stimulus for diuresis.

It is clear from these reports that psychic stimuli influence vesical function—both of the detrusor and of the sphincters—and renal function, where changes in the secretion of catecholamines and ADH occur.

Jules Janet (1890) published a monograph on the effects of the psyche on vesical observations. Montassut, Chertok, & Aboulker (1951) and Chertok, Aboulker, & Cahen (1953) have written excellent studies.

PSYCHOGENIC SPASTIC BLADDER REACTION

Clinical Findings

Most of these patients are women; a few cases occur in children. It appears that during childhood, each person develops a preference for venting emotional responses through one organ or another; later in life, tension or anxiety continues to be expressed through that organ. Men are more apt to develop peptic ulcer.

A. Symptoms: An anxious patient complains of periodic frequency, mostly in the morning. It may be noticed for a few days and then subside spontaneously. Comparable nocturia is absent. In a period of dysfunction, urgency to the point of incontinence may occur (Jeffcoate & Francis, 1966; Frewen, 1972). The patient may complain of "burning," but careful questioning reveals that this sensation is not related to urination. It is probably secondary to spasm of the external urinary sphincter.

Frequency is initiated or increased following emotional upsets (eg, "scenes" with husband or children) and after sexual intercourse, which is, almost without exception, unsatisfactory. The common denominator seems to be unrelieved pelvic congestion precipitated by sexual frustration. A history of prolonged enuresis is often obtained.

Careful questioning reveals that the tense woman develops a functionally small-capacity bladder, so that she voids small amounts. After sleeping all night, however, she voids a normal volume on arising. This change in vesical capacity from hour to hour is an important clue to the psychosomatic spastic bladder.

Many of these women complain of obstructive voiding, but questioning will reveal that though some voidings are slow and hesitant, others are quite free. This rules out organic obstruction and defines a periodic spasm of the striated external urinary sphincter due to tension (Raz & Smith, 1976).

It is wise, when psychosomatic bladder reaction is suspected, to ask what the patient believes to be the cause. A surprising number will volunteer the information that they relate their attacks to acute emotional upsets, sometimes even before they are questioned.

B. Signs: A woman suffering from this syndrome tends to be aggressive and seemingly confident, yet is tense and anxious. A man with the same problem is usually meek and mild, with a poor sense of masculinity. The anal sphincter in women may be hypertonic. On vaginal examination, the urethra, the base of the bladder, and the cervix may be unduly sensitive, but no lesion is found.

C. Laboratory Findings: Urinalysis is normal. Renal function is intact.

D. Instrumental Examination: Cystoscopy may be unduly painful, indicating a low pain threshold. The trigone and urethra may be hyperemic, so that a diagnosis of "urethrotrigonitis" may be made. These changes are secondary to pelvic congestion resulting from the incomplete sexual act. The bladder wall may be trabeculated secondary to spasm of the external urinary sphincter; this must not be regarded as evidence of organic obstruction (eg, vesical neck stenosis). There is no residual urine. Findings with cystometry may be compatible with uninhibited neurogenic bladder, yet often, with relaxation, the capacity is found to be normal.

E. Recording of Intake and Output: Have the patient record, over a period of a few days, the time and volume of fluid intake and the time and volume of each voiding. During an attack, each urine volume in the morning may be 60–100 mL, whereas during the rest of the day and at night the volumes are normal (350–400 mL). This phenomenon is not present with organic disease.

Differential Diagnosis

Psychogenic diuresis (see below) also causes

periodic morning frequency, but the volumes of each voiding are normal.

In true cystitis, both acute and chronic, the urine will contain bacteria. Frequency is consistent both day and night.

Nonspecific urethritis causes symptoms similar to those of bacterial cystitis. Symptoms are not periodic, nor do they occur only in the morning.

Senile urethritis may cause some vesical irritability or even stress incontinence, but symptoms are persistent. Senile vaginitis is observed, and the vaginal epithelial cells fail to stain with iodine.

Multiple sclerosis often causes aberrations in vesical function typified by urgency, frequency, and nocturia. These symptoms, however, are not periodic as are those caused by psychic stimuli.

Complications

Some cases of interstitial cystitis may actually be the end stage of the psychogenic bladder (Bowers, Schwartz, & Leon, 1958), though there is evidence that this disease may be due to an autoimmune collagen reaction (see p 471).

Treatment

It is helpful to explain to patients how "nerves" can play tricks on vesical function. They often fear that they have cancer or some other serious disease. If patients understand the mechanism of symptoms, they will often accept symptoms with equanimity. Since their troubles are secondary to significant psychosexual problems, they are best referred to a psychiatrist.

Anticholinergics during attacks may give some relief.

Erroneous organic diagnoses are apt to lead to various empirical treatments, including urethral dilatations and even transurethral resection of the bladder neck. Such procedures are not only harmful but may further convince patients that they have a serious disease.

Ramsden & others (1976), however, felt that some relief could be provided by overdistention of the bladder under epidural anesthesia. Fluid was introduced into the bladder until the intravesical pressure equaled the systolic blood pressure plus 15 cm of water. This was retained for 4–30 minutes. About 25% of patients required a second treatment. Cure or significant relief was claimed in 80% of patients.

Kaplan, Firlit, & Schoenberg (1980) performed urodynamic studies in women suffering from "urethral syndrome." These studies revealed spasm of the external urinary sphincter that responded to prolonged diazepam therapy given for 2–6 months. Symptoms were relieved, and urodynamic studies showed return to normal function. Zufall (1978), however, noted little success with any form of therapy, including drug regimens.

Prognosis

This type of urinary frequency is difficult to relieve permanently by medical means. Considerable relief is usually achieved with psychotherapy.

EFFECTS OF THE PSYCHE ON VESICAL FUNCTION IN GIRLS

Little girls may suffer from the acute spastic bladder reaction, which is manifested by bouts of frequency and urgency. Enuresis is common in this group; even pantswetting may occur. Constipation is often noted. Voiding at times may seem obstructed, yet at other times it is free (Malmquist, 1971; Galdston & Perlmutter, 1973). There are usually obvious behavioral problems that are reflected in the parents' attitudes.

Urinalysis is usually negative, although in the little girl who suffers from periodic spasm of the external sphincter, bacteria in the proximal urethra may be washed back into the bladder by the resulting turbulent flow (see Distal Urethral Stenosis in Chapter 30). Excretory urograms are usually normal, and the postvoiding film usually reveals no significant residual urine. Urethrocystoscopy findings are usually normal, though at times some vesical trabeculation secondary to sphincter spasm may be seen. Urodynamic studies in children with this disorder have been reported by Firlit, Smey, & King (1978) and by Allen & Bright (1978). Both teams of investigators found combinations of spastic external sphincter and atonic bladder.

Bacterial cystitis is differentiated from this disorder because it usually is associated with urgency, frequency, nocturia, and burning on urination. Bacteriuria is found. There may be attacks of febrile pyelonephritis if vesicoureteral reflux is present.

No significant complications—except cystitis—are seen.

Raz (1978) and Smey, Firlit, & King (1978) report good responses to drug therapy. For hyperactivity of the external sphincter, they recommend diazepam, 1.5 mg 2–4 times daily, or phenoxybenzamine, 5–10 mg daily; for uninhibited bladder, propantheline bromide, 15–30 mg 4 times daily. Another useful regimen is to give Enuretrol (a combination of ephedrine 7.5 mg and atropine 1.5 mg as chewable tablets), 1–2 tablets twice daily, plus imipramine, 75–150 mg twice daily. Psychiatric treatment of the child and in some cases psychologic counseling for the parents may be necessary in addition to other measures. Even with no treatment, however, vesical irritability may subside at puberty, perhaps recurring only in response to stressful situations in the teen years or adult life.

EFFECTS OF THE PSYCHE ON VESICAL FUNCTION IN BOYS

Two important papers dealing with this subject have been published (Hinman & Baumann, 1973; Baumann & Hinman, 1974). These authors found that certain personality problems could lead to incoordination of function of the vesical detrusor and its sphincters. All of their patients suffered from enuresis, pantswetting, urinary tract infection, and constipation with soiling. Secondary changes in the morphology of the urinary tract ranged from mild to severe.

Neurologic examination was normal in all patients. No evidence of organic lower tract obstruction was revealed on endoscopy or voiding cystourography, though vesical trabeculation and residual urine were found. The majority (73 boys) had normal upper tracts without renal infection. Fourteen patients, however, had significant upper tract damage (hydroureteronephrosis) caused by ureterovesical obstruction, though a few did have vesicoureteral reflux (Fig 36–1 left).

The psychologic outlook of these patients was significant. Their self-concept was one of personal failure, and they were shy, timid, depressed, and anxious. The authors concluded that the constipation, enuresis, residual urine, and urinary infection were secondary to spasm of the entire pelvic floor, including the external urinary sphincter, which caused functional urethral obstruction. Allen (1977) corroborated these observations.

In more advanced cases, severe hypertrophy of the trigone led to functional ureteral obstruction caused by an increased pull on the ureterovesical junctions.

Treatment was as follows: (1) Antibiotic drugs were given for infection. (2) Anticholinergic medication was prescribed. The most beneficial was imipramine, 25 mg 4 times daily. (3) Constipation was treated with cleansing enemas followed by a stool softener at bedtime. (4) The parents were instructed to praise all successes but never to punish for wetting. A positive approach was emphasized, including giving rewards for dryness.

Physicians must also take a positive approach in suggesting to the patient ways in which urinary function can be improved. The boy should be en-

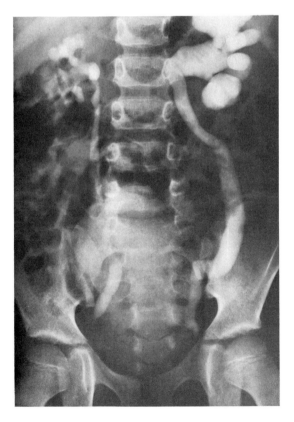 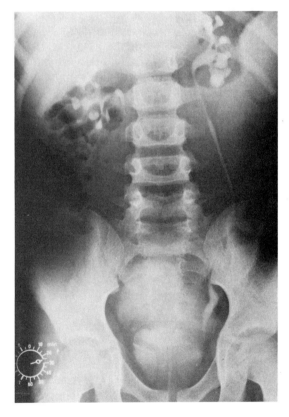

Figure 36–1. Pretreatment x-ray studies. *Left:* Excretory urogram showing dilated bladder reaching top of L5. Right ureter dilated throughout its length. Advanced hydroureteronephrosis, left. Voiding cystogram showed left vesicoureteral reflux. *Right:* Excretory urogram 1 year following institution of therapy. Right ureter now normal, left hydroureteronephrosis almost completely resolved. Cystogram negative. (Reproduced, with permission, from Hinman F, Baumann FW: Vesical and ureteral damage from voiding dysfunction in boys without neurologic or obstructive disease. *J Urol* 1972;**64**:116.)

couraged to try hard to please himself (not the doctor or the parents). Positive suggestive therapy can be enhanced by hypnosis.

In patients with lower tract findings only, 85% were relieved of all symptoms and infection. In the 14 boys with upper tract damage, all complaints were resolved, infection was eradicated, and moderate to marked improvement of the upper urinary tracts was demonstrated (Fig 36–1 right).

These authors warn against operation for this condition, since the cause is functional and not organic (Hinman & Baumann, 1976).

PSYCHOGENIC URINARY RETENTION

This phenomenon is much less common than acute spastic bladder reaction. Most patients are women, though the author has observed psychogenic urinary retention in homosexuals following acute psychosexual stress. Godec (1979) has also observed this phenomenon; he postulates that anal dilatation causes reflex inhibition of detrusor action. Women who suffer from sudden urinary retention express feelings of being overwhelmed (eg, by the threat of rape) and exhibit severe depressive reactions.

Typically, the patient has been voiding in a perfectly normal manner when, suddenly, acute urinary retention occurs. It is difficult to think of any organic disease that would cause this symptom in an otherwise healthy person. The patient may give a history of periodic difficulty with urination, suggesting external sphincter spasm.

The patient appears depressed. Some acute psychologic trauma has precipitated the attack. Abdominal examination will usually reveal a distended bladder. Neurologic examination is normal. Urinalysis and renal function tests are normal.

A catheter passes to the bladder with ease. A cystometrogram may reveal changes compatible with an atonic bladder. Cystoscopy may show some trabeculation secondary to prolonged intermittent sphincter spasm. The urethra is normal.

An acute neurologic deficit (eg, stroke, trauma) may cause urinary retention, but neurologic signs are usually obvious. Postoperative urinary retention usually responds to one or more catheterizations.

Bacterial cystitis may occur as a complication of periodic catheterization or the use of an indwelling catheter.

Intermittent catheterization is mandatory until normal vesical function returns. Prophylactic antimicrobial therapy should be considered.

Psychosomatic urinary retention usually responds well to acute psychotherapy, but on-going analysis is required to solve the patient's basic difficulties. In the author's experience, most patients respond (Montague & Jones, 1979).

Cholinergic drugs (eg, bethanechol chloride) may be tried, but in the author's experience, little is gained. Allen (1972), suspecting severe spasm of the external urinary sphincter in 6 patients, observed spontaneous voiding after bilateral block of the pudendal nerves.

A diagnosis of organic disease (eg, urethral or vesical neck stenosis) will lead to useless empirical therapy that will further convince the patient that a serious local lesion exists. Such therapy should be condemned.

PSYCHOSOMATIC ANTIDIURESIS–DIURESIS

Most patients suffering from periodic diuresis are women. They may be seemingly competent but also tense and anxious, or they may be subdued and repressed.

Clinical Findings

A. Symptoms: These patients complain of periodic frequency, mostly in the morning; there is usually no nocturia. A few, however, describe significant periodic nocturia without day frequency. Questioning reveals that, during the attacks of frequency, each voiding is of normal volume—in contrast to acute spastic bladder reaction. Such a history suggests diuresis.

The patient should be asked about significant changes in body weight. There is usually a history of weight gain of 2–5 kg over a period of 2–4 days. After the inevitable diuresis, weight returns to normal. As weight increases, signs of edema appears (rings tightening on fingers, ankle swelling, puffy facies). These changes subside following diuresis. This type of history is pathognomonic of the syndrome.

The attack usually follows an acute emotional experience (eg, an argument with the husband, an incomplete sexual act, trouble with the children at school). It resolves when tension or anxiety subsides.

With anger or rage, immediate diuresis may occur without the usual antecedent antidiuresis.

B. Signs: Examination reveals little unless the patient is in an antidiuretic stage, in which case evidence of fluid retention may be noted.

C. Laboratory Findings: Noncontributory.

D. Instrumental Findings: Urethrocystoscopy does not seem necessary, and in any case the findings are normal.

E. Recording of Intake and Output: Have the patient record the time and volume of fluid taken and voided as well as the body weight both morning and night for a few days. The typical record shows a gradual increase in body weight and relative oliguria. When diuresis occurs, the patient will void frequent but normal volumes of urine over a period of 3–4 hours in the morning; weight is normal by evening.

Differential Diagnosis

Patients suffering from acute spastic bladder reaction have frequency in the morning, but each voiding is of small volume.

Organic diseases of the bladder tend to cause frequency both day and night. The symptoms, which are not periodic, include a contracted bladder, significant residual urine, or bladder infection.

Complications

The only complications are those resulting from misdiagnosis and the use of organic therapy (eg, transurethral resection of the bladder neck).

Treatment

Most patients are helped by an explanation of the cause of diuresis. Some relief may be obtained by limiting salt intake. When body weight begins to increase, administration of a diuretic may prevent an attack. Psychotherapy, however, should be encouraged, for these patients have significant psychosexual problems.

Prognosis

The treatment outlined above tends to ease or abolish the attacks. Even if attacks recur, these patients are better able to live with the problem if they understand the mechanism. Women often understand better than men the relationship between emotions and bodily functions.

COMPULSIVE POLYDIPSIA

Frequency of urination can also be caused by drinking large volumes of fluid, a habit that may not be consciously recognized by the patient. Some tense, nervous people develop a dry mouth that they attribute to thirst, and this may lead to excessive fluid intake.

The patient complains of frequency day and night. Questioning reveals that each voiding is of good volume. There is no burning or other symptoms. The patient may deny polydipsia. Most revealing on urinalysis is a consistently low specific gravity, approaching 1.000. Infection is absent.

Excretory urograms are usually normal, though some hydroureteronephrosis may be noted (as in diabetes insipidus) because more urine is excreted than the ureterovesical junctions can pass (Shapiro & others, 1978).

Instruct the patient to record times and volumes of fluid intake and the times and volumes of voiding. The typical intake is 6–8 L of fluid and frequent voidings of 350–450 mL. This establishes the diagnosis.

A patient may have difficulty in reducing fluid intake to normal even after learning the physiologic cause of the disorder. Chapdelaine & Lanthier (1963) have described 2 such patients who eventually were unable to concentrate urine. Psychotherapy may be needed to bring about cure.

• • •

References

General

Chertok L & others: Urethral syndrome in the female ("irritable bladder"): The expression of fantasies about the urogenital area. *Psychosom Med* 1977;**39:**1.

Smith DR, Auerback A: Functional diseases. Pages 1–57 in: *Encyclopedia of Urology.* Vol 12. Springer, 1960.

Turner RD, Bors E: Some interesting observations in neurological urology. *Urol Int* 1963;**16:**30.

Effects of Psyche on Vesical Function

Allen JD: Psychogenic urinary retention. *South Med J* 1972;**65:**302.

Kaplan WE, Firlit CF, Schoenberg HW: The female urethral syndrome: External sphincter spasm as etiology. *J Urol* 1980;**124:**48.

Straub LR, Ripley HS, Wolf S: Disturbances of bladder function associated with emotional states. *JAMA* 1949;**141:**1139.

Zufall R: Ineffectiveness of treatment of urethral syndrome in women. *Urology* 1978;**12:**337.

Zufall R: Treatment of the urethral syndrome in women. *JAMA* 1963;**184:**894.

Effects of Psyche on Renal Function

Barnes R, Schottstaedt WW: The relation of emotional state to renal excretion of water and electrolytes in patients with congestive heart failure. *Am J Med* 1960;**29:**217.

Blomstrand R, Löfgren F: Influence of emotional stress on the renal circulation. *Psychosom Med* 1956;**18:**420.

Chertok L, Aboulker P, Cahen M: Perspectives psychosomatiques en urologie. *Evol Psychiatr* 1953;**3:**457.

DeMaria WJA & others: Renal conditioning. *Psychosom Med* 1963;**25:**538.

Dykman RA & others: Inhibition of urine flow as a component of the conditioned defense reaction. *Psychosom Med* 1962;**24:**177.

Gerbner M, Altman K, Mészáros I: The mechanism of the increase in diuresis induced by hypnotic suggestion. *J Psychosom Res* 1959;**3:**282.

Jammes JL, Tigchelaar PV, Rosenberger PB: Habituation and urinary retention. *JAMA* 1975;**232:**1264.

Janet J: *Les Troubles Psychopathiques de la Miction: Essai de Psycho-physiologie Normale et Pathologique.* Librairie Lefrançais (Paris), 1890.

Levi L: The urinary output of adrenalin and noradrenalin during pleasant and unpleasant emotional states: A preliminary report. *Psychosom Med* 1965;**27:**80.

Montassut ML, Chertok L, Aboulker P: De quelques investigations psychiatriques en urologie. *Sem Hop Paris* 1951;**27:**3002.

Ramsden PD & others: Distension therapy for the unstable

bladder: Later results including an assessment of repeat distensions. *Br J Urol* 1976;**48**:623.

Raz S, Smith RB: External sphincter spasticity syndrome in female patients. *J Urol* 1976;**115**:443.

Schottstaedt WW, Grace WJ, Wolff HG: Life situations, behavior, attitudes, emotions and renal excretion of fluid and electrolytes. (5 parts.) *J Psychosom Res* 1956;**1**:75, 147, 203, 287, 292.

Verney EB: Some aspects of water and electrolyte excretion. *Surg Gynecol Obstet* 1958;**106**:441.

Wakim KG: Reassessment of the source, mode and locus of action of antidiuretic hormone. *Am J Med* 1967;**42**:394.

Psychogenic Spastic Bladder Reaction

Bowers JE, Schwartz BE, Leon MJ: Masochism and interstitial cystitis: Report of a case. *Psychosom Med* 1958;**20**:296.

Frewen WK: Urgency incontinence: Review of 100 cases. *J Obstet Gynaecol Br Commonw* 1972;**79**:77.

Jeffcoate TNA, Francis WJA: Urgency incontinence in the female. *Am J Obstet Gynecol* 1966;**94**:604.

Effects of Psyche on Vesical Function in Girls

Allen TD, Bright TC III: Urodynamic patterns in children with dysfunctional voiding problems. *J Urol* 1978;**119**:247.

Firlit CF, Smey P, King LR: Micturition urodynamic flow studies in children. *J Urol* 1978;**119**:250.

Galdston R, Perlmutter AD: The urinary manifestations of anxiety in child. *Pediatrics* 1973;**52**:818.

Malmquist CP: Hysteria in childhood. *Postgrad Med* (Aug) 1971;**50**:112.

Raz S: Pharmacological treatment of lower urinary tract dysfunction. *Urol Clin North Am* 1978;**5**:323.

Smey P, Firlit CF, King LR: Voiding pattern abnormalities in normal children: Results of pharmacologic manipulation. *J Urol* 1978;**120**:574.

Effects of Psyche on Vesical Function in Boys

Allen TD: The non-neurogenic neurogenic bladder. *J Urol* 1977;**117**:232.

Baumann FW, Hinman F: Treatment of incontinent boys with non-obstructive disease. *J Urol* 1974;**111**:114.

Hinman F: Urinary tract damage in children who wet. *Pediatrics* 1974;**54**:143.

Hinman F, Baumann FW: Vesical and ureteral damage from voiding dysfunction in boys without neurologic or obstructive disease. *J Urol* 1973;**109**:727.

Hinman F Jr, Baumann FW: Complications of vesicoureteral operations from incoordination of micturition. *J Urol* 1976;**116**:638.

Psychogenic Urinary Retention

Allen JD: Psychogenic urinary retention. *South Med J* 1972;**65**:302.

Godec CJ: Acute urinary retention in young homosexuals. *Urology* 1979;**14**:581.

Khan AU: Psychogenic urinary retention in a boy. *J Urol* 1971;**106**:432.

Larson JW & others: Psychogenic urinary retention in women. *JAMA* 1963;**184**:697.

Montague DK, Jones LR: Psychogenic urinary retention. *Urology* 1979;**13**:30.

Wahl CM, Golden JS: Psychogenic urinary retention. *Psychosom Med* 1973;**25**:543.

Compulsive Polydipsia

Chapdelaine A, Lanthier A: Compulsive polydipsia with defective renal concentrating powers. *Can Med Assoc J* 1963;**88**:1184.

Linshaw MA, Hipp T, Gruskin A: Infantile psychogenic water drinking. *J Pediatr* 1974;**85**:520.

Shapiro SR & others: Diabetes insipidus and hydronephrosis. *J Urol* 1978;**119**:715.

Stevko RM, Balsley M, Segar WE: Primary polydipsia: Compulsive water drinking. *J Pediatr* 1968;**73**:845.

Appendix:
Normal Laboratory Values

Marcus A. Krupp, MD

HEMATOLOGY
(Blood [B], Plasma [P])

Bleeding time: 1–7 minutes (Ivy).

Cellular measurements of red cells: Average diameter = 7.3 μm (5.5–8.8 μm).
Mean corpuscular volume (MCV): Men, 80–94 fL; women, 81–99 fL (by Coulter counter).
Mean corpuscular hemoglobin (MCH): 27–32 pg.
Mean corpuscular hemoglobin concentration (MCHC): 32–36 g/dL red blood cells (0.32–0.36%).
Color, saturation, and volume indices: 1 (0.9–1.1).

Clot retraction: Begins in 1–3 hours; complete in 24 hours.

Coagulation time (Lee-White): At 37 C, 6–12 minutes; at room temperature, 10–18 minutes.

Fragility of red cells: Begins at 0.45–0.38% NaCl; complete at 0.36–0.3% NaCl.

Hematocrit (PCV): Men, 40–52%; women, 37–47%.

Hemoglobin: [B] Men, 14–18 g/dL (2.09–2.79 mmol/L); women, 12–16 g/dL (1.86–2.48 mmol/L). (Serum hemoglobin: 2–3 mg/dL.)

Platelets: 150–400 thousand/μL (0.15–0.4 $\times$ 10^{12}/L).

Prothrombin: [P] 75–125%.

Red blood count (RBC): Men, 4.5–6.2 million/μL (4.5–6.2 $\times$ 10^{12}/L); women, 4–5.5 million/μL (4–5.5 $\times$ 10^{12}/L).

Reticulocytes: 0.2–2% of red cells.

Sedimentation rate: Less than 20 mm/h (Westergren); 0–10 mm/h (Wintrobe).

White blood count (WBC) and differential: 5–10 thousand/μL (5–10 $\times$ 10^9/L).

Myelocytes	0 %
Juvenile neutrophils	0 %
Band neutrophils	0–5 %
Segmented neutrophils	40–60%
Lymphocytes	20–40%
Eosinophils	1–3 %
Basophils	0–1 %
Monocytes	4–8 %

BLOOD (B), PLASMA (P), OR SERUM (S) CHEMICAL CONSTITUENTS

Below are listed the specimen used, the source—blood [B], plasma [P], or serum [S]—the fasting state, and the normal values. Values vary with the procedure employed.

Acetone and acetoacetate: [S] 0.3–2 mg/dL (3–20 mg/L).

Aldolase: [S] 3–8 units/mL (Sibley-Lehninger). Men, < 33 units; women, < 19 units (Warburg and Christian).

α-Amino acid nitrogen: [S, fasting] 3–5.5 mg/dL (2.2–3.9 mmol/L).

Ammonia*: [B] 80–110 μg/dL (47–65 μmol/L) (diffusion method).

Amylase: [S] 80–180 units/dL (Somogyi) (0.8–3.2 IU/L).

α_1-Antitrypsin: [S] 210–500 mg/dL.

Ascorbic acid: [P] 0.4–1.5 mg/dL (22.7–85.3 μmol/L).

Base, total serum: [S] 145–160 mEq/L (145–160 mmol/L).

*Do not use anticoagulant containing ammonium oxalate.

Bicarbonate: [S] 24–28 mEq/L (24–28 mmol/L).

Bilirubin: [S] Total, 0.2–1.2 mg/dL (3.4–20.4 μmol/L). Direct, 0.1–0.4 mg/dL (1.7–6.8 μmol/L).

Calcium: [S] 8.5–10.5 mg/dL; 4.2–5.2 mEq/L (2.1–2.6 mmol/L) (varies with protein concentration).

Calcium, ionized: [S] 4.25–5.25 mg/dL; 2.1–2.6 mEq/L (1.05–1.3 mmol/L).

β-Carotene: [S, fasting] 50–300 μg/dL (0.9–5.58 μmol/L).

Ceruloplasmin: [S] 25–43 mg/dL (250–430 mg/L).

Chloride: [S] 96–106 mEq/L (96–106 mmol/L).

Cholesterol: [S] 150–280 mg/dL (3.9–7.28 mmol/L). (See Lipid Fractions.)

Cholesteryl esters: [S] 65–75% of total cholesterol.

CO_2 content: [S or P] 24–29 mEq/L (24–29 mmol/L).

Complement: [S] C3 (β_1C), 100–190 mg/dL; C4 (β_{1E}), 20–60 mg/dL.

Copper: [S or P] 100–200 μg/dL (16–31 μmol/L).

Cortisol: [P] 8:00 AM, 5–20 μg/dL; 8:00 PM, < 10 μg/dL (138–552 nmol/L).

Creatine kinase: [S] 10–50 IU/L at 30 C. Varies with method.

Creatinine: [S] 0.7–1.5 mg/dL (62–132 μmol/L).

Epinephrine: [P] < 0.1 μg/L.

Ferritin: [S] Women, 20–120 ng/mL; men, 30–300 ng/mL.

Folic acid: [S] 4–25 ng/mL; (9.1–57 nmol/L) [RBC] > 140 ng/mL (> 318 nmol/L).

Glucose: [S, fasting] 65–110 mg/dL (3.6–6.1 mmol/L).

Iron: [S] 50–175 μg/dL (9–31.3 μmol/L).

Iron-binding capacity, total: [S] 250–410 μg/dL (44.7–73.4 μmol/L). Percent saturation: 20–55%.

Lactate: [B, special handling] Venous: 4–16 mg/dL (0.44–1.8 mmol/L).

Lactate dehydrogenase (SLDH): [S] 55–140 IU/L at 30 C; SMA, 100–225 IU/L at 37 C; SMAC, 60–200 IU/L at 37 C.

Lipase: [S] 0.2–1.5 units/mL of 0.1 N NaOH.

Lipid fractions: [P, S] Desirable levels: HDL cholesterol, > 40 mg/dL; LDL cholesterol, < 180 mg/dL; VLDL cholesterol, < 40 mg/dL. (To convert to mmol/L, multiply by 0.026.)

Lipids, total: [S] 450–1000 mg/dL (4.5–10 g/L).

Magnesium: [P] 1.8–3 mg/dL (0.75–1.25 mmol/L).

Nonprotein nitrogen (NPN)*: [S] 15–35 mg/dL (10.7–25 mmol/L).

Norepinephrine: [P] < 0.5 μg/L.

Osmolality: [S] 275–295 mOsm/kg water.

Oxygen:
  Capacity: [B] 16–24 vol% (varies with hemoglobin concentration).
  Arterial content: [B] 15–23 vol% (varies with hemoglobin concentration).
  Arterial % saturation: 94–100% of capacity.
  Arterial P_{O_2} (Pa_{O_2}): 80–100 mm Hg (10.67–13.33 kPa) (sea level). (Varies with age.)

Pa_{CO_2}: [B, arterial] 35–45 mm Hg (4.67–6 kPa).

pH (reaction): [B, arterial] 7.35–7.45 (H^+ 44.7–45.5 nmol/L).

Phosphatase, acid: [S] 1–5 units (King-Armstrong), 0.1–0.63 units (Bessey-Lowry).

Phosphatase, alkaline: [S] 5–13 units (King-Armstrong); Adults, 0.8–2.3 (Bessey-Lowry); SMA, 30–85 IU/L at 37 C; SMAC, 30–115 IU/L at 37 C.

Phospholipid: [S] 145–200 mg/dL (1.45–2 g/L).

Phosphorus, inorganic: [S, fasting] 3–4.5 mg/dL (1–1.5 mmol/L).

Potassium: [S or P] 3.5–5 mEq/L (3.5–5 mmol/L).

Protein:
  Total: [S] 6–8 g/dL (60–80 g/L).
  Albumin: [S] 3.5–5.5 g/dL (35–55 g/L).
  Globulin: [S] 2–3.6 g/dL (20–36 g/L).
  Fibrinogen: [P] 0.2–0.6 g/dL (2–6 g/L).

Prothrombin clotting time: [P] By control.

---

*Do not use anticoagulant containing ammonium oxalate.

Pyruvate: [B] 0.6–1 mg/dL (70–114 μmol/L).

Serotonin: [B] 0.05–0.2 μg/mL.

Sodium: [S] 136–145 mEq/L (136–145 mmol/L).

Specific gravity:
   [B] 1.056 (varies with hemoglobin and protein concentration).
   [S] 1.0254–1.0288 (varies with protein concentration).

Sulfate: [P or S] as sulfur. 0.5–1.5 mg/dL (156–468 μmol/L).

Transaminases: [S]
   Glutamic-oxaloacetic (SGOT), 6–25 IU/L at 30 C; SMA, 10–40 IU/L at 37 C; SMAC, 0–41 IU/L at 37 C.
   Glutamic-pyruvic (SGPT), 3–26 IU/L at 30 C; SMAC, 0–45 IU/L at 37 C.

Transferrin: [S] 200–400 mg/dL (23–45 μmol/L).

Triglycerides: [S] < 165 mg/dL (5.4 mEq/L or 1.9 mmol/L). (See Lipid Fractions.)

Urea nitrogen*: [S] 8–25 mg/dL (2.9–8.9 mmol/L).

Uric Acid: [S] Men, 3–9 mg/dL (0.18–0.53 mmol/L); women, 2.5–7.5 mg/dL (0.15–0.45 mmol/L).

Vitamin A: [S] 15–60 μg/dL (0.53–2.1 μmol/L).

Vitamin B$_{12}$: [S] > 200 pg/mL (> 148 pmol/L).

Vitamin D: [S]. Cholecalciferol (D$_3$): 25-Hydroxycholecalciferol, 10–80 ng/mL; 1,25-dihydroxycholecalciferol, 21–45 pg/mL.

Volume, blood (Evans blue dye method): Adults, 2990–6980 mL. Women, 46.3–85.5 mL/kg; men, 66.2–97.7 mL/kg.

Zinc: [S] 50–150 μg/dL (7.65–22.95 μmol/L).

HORMONES, SERUM [S] OR PLASMA [P]

Pituitary:
   Growth (HGH): [S] Adults, 1–10 ng/mL (by RIA).
   Thyroid-stimulating (TSH): [S] < 10 μU/mL.
   Follicle-stimulating hormone (FSH): [S] Prepuberal, 2–12 mIU/mL; men, 1–15 mIU/mL; women, 1–30 mIU/mL; castrate or postmenopausal, 30–200 mIU/mL (by RIA).

   Luteinizing hormone (LH): [S] Prepuberal, 2–12 mIU/mL; men, 1–15 mIU/mL; women, < 30 mIU/mL; castrate or postmenopausal, > 30 mIU/mL.
   Corticotropin (ACTH): [P] 8–10 AM: up to 100 pg/mL.
   Prolactin: [S] 0–20 ng/mL.
   Somatomedin C: [P] 0.4–2 U/mL.

Adrenal:
   Aldosterone: [P] Supine, normal salt intake, 2–9 ng/dL; increased when upright.
   Cortisol: [S] 8:00 AM, 7–18 μg/dL; 5:00 PM, 2–9 μg/dL.
   Dopamine: [P] < 135 pg/mL.
   Epinephrine: [P] < 80 pg/mL.
   Norepinephrine: [P] < 400 pg/mL.
   See also Miscellaneous Normal Values.

Thyroid:
   Thyroxine, free (FT$_4$): [S] 0.8–2.4 ng/dL.
   Thyroxine, total (TT$_4$): [S] 4–11 μg/dL T$_4$ (by CPB); 5–14 μg/dL (by RIA).
   Thyroxine-binding globulin: [S] 2–4.8 mg/dL.
   Triiodothyronine: [S] 80–220 ng/dL.
   Reverse triiodothyronine: [S] Adult 30–80 ng/dL.
   Triiodothyronine uptake (RT$_3$U): [S] 25–36%; as TBG assessment (RT$_3$U ratio), 0.85–1.15.
   Calcitonin: [S] < 400 pg/mL.

Parathyroid: Parathyroid hormone levels vary with method and antibody. Correlate with serum calcium.

Islets:
   Insulin: [S] 4–25 μU/mL (0.17–1.04 μg/L).

Stomach:
   Gastrin: [S, special handling] Up to 100 pg/mL. Elevated, > 200 pg/mL.
   Pepsinogen I: [S] 25–100 ng/mL.

Kidney:
   Renin activity: [P, special handling] Supine, normal sodium intake, 1–3 ng/mL/h; standing or while on low-sodium diet or diuretics, 3–6 ng/mL/h.

Gonad:
   Testosterone: [S] Prepuberal, < 100 ng/dL; men, 300–1000 ng/dL; women, 20–80 ng/dL; luteal phase, up to 120 ng/dL.
   Estradiol (E$_2$), RIA: [S, special handling] Men, 12–34 pg/mL; women, menstrual cycle 1–10 days, 24–68 pg/mL; 11–20 days, 50–186 pg/mL; 21–30 days, 73–149 pg/mL.
   Progesterone, RIA: [S] Follicular phase, 20–150 ng/dL; luteal phase, 300–2400 ng/dL; pregnancy, > 2400 ng/dL; men, < 100 ng/dL.

*Do not use anticoagulant containing ammonium oxalate.

Placenta:
Estriol (E_3), RIA: [S] Men and nonpregnant women, < 0.2 μg/dL.

Chorionic gonadotropin: [S] Normal men and nonpregnant women, none detected.

NORMAL CEREBROSPINAL FLUID VALUES

Appearance: Clear and colorless.

Chlorides (as NaCl): 120–130 mEq/L (120–130 mmol/L).

IgG: 2–6 mg/dL (0.02–0.06 g/L).

Glucose: 50–85 mg/dL (2.8–4.7 mmol/L). (Draw serum glucose at same time.)

Cells: Adults, 0–5 mononuclears/μL. Infants, 0–20 mononuclears/μL.

Pressure (reclining): Newborn, 30–80 mm water. Children, 50–100 mm water. Adults, 70–200 mm water (avg = 125).

Proteins, total: 20–45 mg/dL (200–450 mg/L) in lumbar cerebrospinal fluid.

Specific gravity: 1.003–1.008.

RENAL FUNCTION TESTS

p-**Aminohippurate (PAH) clearance (RPF):** Men, 560–830 mL/min; women, 490–700 mL/min.

Creatinine clearance, endogenous (GFR): Approximates inulin clearance (see below).

Filtration fraction (FF): Men, 17–21%; women, 17–23%. (FF = GFR/RPF.)

Inulin clearance (GFR): Men, 110–150 mL/min; women, 105–132 mL/min (corrected to 1.73 m^2 surface area).

Maximal glucose reabsorptive capacity (Tm$_G$): Men, 300–450 mg/min; women, 250–350 mg/min.

Maximal PAH excretory capacity (Tm$_{PAH}$): 80–90 mg/min.

Specific gravity of urine: 1.003–1.030.

Urine osmolality: On normal diet and fluid intake, range 500–850 mOsm/kg water. Achievable range for normal kidney, dilution 40–80 mOsm; concentration (dehydration) up to 1400 mOsm/kg water (at least 3–4 times plasma osmolality).

MISCELLANEOUS NORMAL VALUES
(Urine [U], Serum [S])

Addis urine sediment count: Maximum values per 24 hours are as follows:

Red cells, 1 million
White and epithelial cells, 2 million
Casts, 100 thousand
Protein, 30 mg

Aldosterone: [U] 2–26 μg/24 h (5.5–72 nmol); varies with sodium and potassium intake.

Catecholamines: [U] Total < 100 μg/24 h. < 10 μg epinephrine (< 55 nmol); < 100 μg norepinephrine/24 h (< 591 nmol); varies with method.

Cortisol, free: [U] 20–100 μg/24 h (0.55–2.76 μmol).

Fecal fat: Less than 30% dry weight.

11,17-Hydroxycorticoids: [U] Men, 4–12 mg/24 h; women, 4–8 mg/24 h. Varies with method used.

Insulin tolerance: (0.1 unit insulin/kg IV.) [S] Glucose level decreases to half of fasting level in 20–30 minutes; returns to fasting level in 90–120 minutes.

17-Ketosteroids: [U] Under 8 years, 0–2 mg/24 h; adolescents, 2–20 mg/24 h. Men, 10–20 mg/24 h; women, 5–15 mg/24 h. Varies with method used.

Lead: [U] < 0.12 mg/24 h (< 0.57 μmol).

Metanephrine: [U] < 1.3 mg/24 h (< 6.6 μmol) or < 2.2 μg/mg creatinine. Varies with method.

Porphyrins: [U]
Delta-aminolevulinic acid: Adult, 1.5–7.5 mg/24 h (11.4–57.2 μmol).
Coproporphyrin: < 230 μg/24 h (< 345 nmol).
Uroporphyrin: < 50 μg/24 h (< 60 nmol).
Porphobilinogen: < 2 mg/24 h (< 8.8 μmol).

Urobilinogen, fecal: 40–280 mg/24 h (68–474 μmol).

Urobilinogen: [U] 0–2.5 mg/24 h (< 4.23 μmol).

Vanilmandelic acid (VMA): [U] Up to 7 mg/24 h (< 35 μmol).

Index